Breastfeeding

A GUIDE FOR THE MEDICAL PROFESSION

Madonna and Child, School of Bruges, Flemish, 15th century colored drawing. *(Reproduced with permission from Memorial Art Gallery of the University of Rochester.)*

Breastfeeding

A GUIDE FOR THE MEDICAL PROFESSION

Ruth A. Lawrence, MD

Professor of Pediatrics, Obstetrics and Gynecology
University of Rochester School of Medicine and Dentistry
Department of Pediatrics
Rochester, New York

Robert M. Lawrence, MD

Assistant Professor of Pediatrics and Microbiology
New York University School of Medicine
Bellevue Hospital Medical Center
New York, New York

Fifth Edition

with 170 illustrations

 Mosby

St. Louis Baltimore Boston Carlsbad Chicago Minneapolis New York Philadelphia Portland
London Milan Sydney Tokyo Toronto

Mosby
Dedicated to Publishing Excellence

A Times Mirror Company

Publisher: Susie H. Baxter
Editor: Elizabeth M. Fathman
Senior Developmental Editor: Ellen Baker Geisel
Project Manager: Carol Sullivan Weis
Senior Production Editor: Karen M. Rehwinkel
Designer: Jen Marmarinos
Manufacturing Supervisor: Karen Boehme
Cover Art: Rosemary Disney

Fifth Edition

Composition/lithography by Graphic World, Inc.
Printing/binding by R. R. Donnelley & Sons Company

Mosby, Inc.
11830 Westline Industrial Drive
St. Louis, Missouri 63146

Library of Congress Cataloging-in-Publication Data

Lawrence, Ruth A.,
    Breastfeeding : a guide for the medical profession / Ruth A.
Lawrence, Robert M. Lawrence. — 5th ed.
        p.   cm.
    Includes bibliographical references and index.
    ISBN 0-8151-2615-8
    1. Breastfeeding—Physiological aspects.   2. Lactation.
3. Breast milk—Physiological effect.   4. Infants—Nutrition.
    I. Lawrence, Robert M. (Robert Michael).   II. Title.
    [DNLM: 1. Breastfeeding.   WS 125 L422b 1999]
    RJ216.L358   1999
    613.2′69—dc21
    DNLM/DLC   98-42918
    for Library of Congress   CIP

98 99 00 01 02 / 9 8 7 6 5 4 3 2 1

Affectionately dedicated to
Rob, Barbara, Timothy, Kathleen,
David, Mary Alice, Joan, John, *and* **Stephen**
for their love and patient understanding
and to **Bob**
for his boundless faith, trust, and inspiration.

ℱoreword

The 5 years since the publication of the last edition of this excellent book have been a time of incredible advances in understanding several previously unknown physiologic and behavioral processes directly linked or associated with breast-feeding and beautifully described in this new volume.

These findings change our view of the mother-infant relationship and signal an urgent need to completely review present perinatal care procedures. These new research results include the observation that when the infant suckles from the breast there is a large outpouring of 19 different gastrointestinal hormones in both the mother and infant, including cholecystokinin, gastrin, and insulin. Several of these hormones stimulate the growth of the baby's and mother's intestinal villi, thus increasing the surface area for the absorption of additional calories with each feeding. The stimuli for these changes are touching the nipple of the mother or the inside of the infant's mouth. The stimuli in both infant and mother result in the release of oxytocin in the periventricular area of the brain, which leads to production of these hormones via the vagus nerve. These pathways were essential for survival thousands of years ago when periods of famine were common, before the development of modern agriculture and the storage of grain.

The discovery of the additional significance of the mother's breast and chest to the infant comes from the studies of Swedish workers who have shown that the normal infant, when dried, placed on the mother's chest, and covered with a light blanket, will warm or maintain body temperature as well as an infant warmed with elaborate, high-tech heating devices. The same researchers found that when infants are skin-to-skin with their mothers for the first 90 minutes after birth, they hardly cry at all compared with infants who are dried, wrapped in a towel, and placed in a bassinet. In addition, the researchers demonstrated that if a newborn is left quietly on the mother's abdomen after birth he will, after about 30 minutes, crawl gradually up to her breast, find the nipple, self-attach, and start to suckle on his own.

It would appear that each of these features—the crawling ability of the infant, the absence of crying when skin-to-skin with the mother, and the warming capabilities of the mother's chest—evolved genetically more than 400,000 years ago to help preserve the infant's life.

New research findings related to the 1991 Baby Friendly Hospital Initiative (BFHI) of WHO and UNICEF provided insight into an additional basic process. After the introduction of the BFHI, which emphasized mother-infant contact with an opportunity for suckling in the first 30 minutes after birth and mother-infant rooming-in throughout the hospital stay, there has been a significant drop in neonatal abandonment reported in maternity hospitals in Thailand, Costa Rica, the Philippines, and St. Petersburg, Russia.

A key to understanding this behavior is the observation that if the lips of the infant touch the mother's nipple in the first half hour of life, the mother will decide to keep the infant in her room 100 minutes longer on the second and third day of hospitalization than another mother whose infant does not touch her nipple in the first 30 minutes. It appears that the remarkable changes in maternal behavior that occur with just the touch of the infant's lips on the mother's nipple (i.e., the decrease in abandonment of young infants who have early contact and are rooming-in with the mother [two elements of the BFHI]) are probably related to increased brain oxytocin levels shortly after birth. These changes, in conjunction with known sensory, physiologic, immunologic, and behavioral mechanisms, all help attract the mother and infant to each other and start the attachment of the mother to the infant and the infant to the mother. As we pointed out in the fourth edition, a strong, affectionate bond is most likely to develop successfully with breastfeeding, in which close contact and interaction occur repeatedly when the infant wishes and at a pace that fits the needs and wishes of the mother and the infant, resulting in gratification for both. Thus breastfeeding plays a central role in the development of a strong mother-infant attachment when begun with contact immediately after birth, which in turn has been shown to be a simple maneuver to significantly increase the success of breastfeeding. All of these exciting findings provide further evidence why breastfeeding has been so crucial in the past and now again deserves our strong support.

In addition, these past few years have been associated with fundamental biochemical findings, including the importance of docosahexaenoic acid (DOCA) in optimal brain development. All in all, the many new observations described in this fifth edition place milk and the process of breastfeeding in a key position in the development of many critical functions in human infants and their mothers. We salute the author for her special skill in bringing together these many unique and original observations in this new and most valuable book.

SUGGESTED READINGS

1. Christensson K et al: Separation distress call in the human neonate in the absence of maternal body contact. In *Care of the newborn infant: satisfying the need for comfort and energy conservation,* thesis of Kyllike Christensson (Stockholm, Karolinska Institute, 1994).
2. Christensson K et al: Temperature, metabolic adaptation and crying in healthy newborn cared for skin-to-skin or in a cot, *ACTA Paediatrica Scandinavica* 81:488, 1992.
3. Uvnäs-Moberg K: The gastrointestinal tract in growth and reproduction, *Sci Am* 261(1):78, 1989.
4. Widström AM et al: Gastric suction in healthy newborn infants: effects on circulation and developing feeding behavior, *ACTA Paediatrica Scandinavica* 76:566, 1987.
5. Widström AM et al: Short-term effects of early suckling and touch of the nipple on maternal behavior, *Early Hum Dev* 21:153, 1990.

JOHN H. KENNELL
MARSHALL J. KLAUS

$\mathscr{P}$reface to the fifth edition

It was more than 2 decades ago that work began on the first edition of this text. Much has changed in the field of human lactation and in the world at large. The trickle of scientific work on the subject has swollen to a river overflowing its banks. The Lactation Study Center has over 20,000 documents on file reporting peer-reviewed scientific studies and reports, and there are thousands more unfiled recounting individual experience and anecdotal reports of events. The field has moved from a dogma of rules about breastfeeding that demanded rigid scheduling and specific managements through a brief period in which thoughtful contemplation and recognition of the variability of the human condition were recommended. Well-trained, skilled clinicians recognized the value of flexibility and individualizing care. Once again, however, ritual and protocol are being enforced. The Baby Friendly approach, whose very being was spawned to set us free from rigid dictums, is requiring protocols and policies. Mothers tell us they cannot breastfeed because there are too many rules. Medicine, itself in the era of managed care, has come forth with care guidelines for one disease or circumstance after another. Will breastfeeding be next?

In 1994, the Academy of Breastfeeding Medicine was founded for the promotion and support of breastfeeding. It is designed to provide physicians all over the world and from every discipline a forum for scientific learning and discussion about breastfeeding and human lactation. Its members form a nucleus of medical professionals dedicated to the advancement of breastfeeding. The American Academy of Pediatrics proclaimed with renewed energy in December 1997 that mothers should breastfeed for six months exclusively, then continue breastfeeding while introducing weaning foods through the first year and then for as long thereafter as desired by mother and infant. The health care provider can promote these goals most effectively when armed with information.

It is the intent of this volume to provide the basic tools of knowledge and experience that will enable the clinician to provide the thoughtful counseling and guidance to the breastfeeding family that is most applicable to that breastfeeding dyad and its circumstances, problems, and lifestyle. No protocol should ever replace thinking, however.

As the field became more complex, it was clear that one of the most difficult issues centers around infection in the mother or in the infant and sometimes in both. Thus Robert Michael Lawrence, MD, Assistant Professor of Pediatrics and Microbiology at New York University School of Medicine and Bellevue Hospital, has joined in the work of producing this volume to bring the most accurate information in these areas to these pages. He has also assisted in the editing of many other topics. Linda R. Friedman, PhD, has worked tirelessly on the drug database and has thoroughly revamped Appendix D, Drugs in Human Milk. Dr. James Woods, Professor of Obstetrics and Gynecology, provided wise counsel on contraceptive issues. The thousands of queries to the Lactation

Study Center have served as a basis for new topics and new clinical discussions.

The fifth edition was assembled with the help of many. Anita Matthews continues to provide the artwork with her scientifically accurate and artistically sensitive drawings. Carole Sydelnik prepared the typed manuscripts from hand-written, re-edited drafts with great skill and precision. Andrew McCooey has been an invaluable information stalker and library sleuth. The undergraduate students at the Center—Allison, Amy, Chris, Doug, Jimmy, and Sheila—have been loyal filers, copiers, and errand runners. A special thanks to medical editor Ellen Baker Geisel at Mosby for her generous support and attention to the details.

RUTH A. LAWRENCE

$\mathscr{P}$reface to the first edition

This book was written in an effort to provide the medical profession with an easily accessible reference for the clinical management of the mother-infant nursing couple. After many decades of championing formula for the newborn and infant, the medical profession has recognized that human milk is preferable for the human infant. The world literature reflects scientists' work on breastfeeding in the fields of nutrition, biochemistry, immunology, psychology, anthropology, and sociology. These researchers have demonstrated what most mothers have long believed: human milk is specifically designed for human infants.

Although reports in dozens of journals have contributed information valuable in the clinical management of lactation, it has remained difficult for the practitioner to gain access to it when an emergency arises. There are other topics, such as the pharmacokinetics of human milk, on which more knowledge and data are needed. This book is intended to provide the information that is available as well as identify areas of deficient information. The first part of this book is basic data on the anatomical, physiological, biochemical, nutritional, immunological, and psychological aspects of human lactation. The remainder centers on the problems of clinical management and, I hope, maximizes scientific data and minimizes anecdotal information. The goal is to provide practical information for managing individual mothers and their infants. It is also hoped that a balance has been struck between basic science, on which rational management should rest, and advice gar-

nered by experience. Through use of the bibliographies, interested readers may seek out the original works for details and supporting data.

I recognized some years ago that specific data were accumulating rapidly but remained in scattered, sometimes inaccessible, references. The increasing requests for consultation about breastfeeding sparked the idea for a more formal publication to replace the information sheets and brochures that I had been putting together. My interest in breastfeeding started during internship and residency at Yale–New Haven Hospital where Dr. Edith Jackson, Dr. Grover Powers, and Dr. Milton Senn expressed genuine concern for the declining rate of breastfeeding. Dr. Jackson provided excellent training in the art of breastfeeding for families and professionals in the rooming-in project in New Haven.

This book does not speak to world issues or the political issues of nutrition, since they have been eloquently discussed by Derrick and E.P. Patrice Jelliffe in their many works.

Throughout this book, because a nursing mother is a female, the personal pronoun *she* has been used. In referring to the infant, the choice between *he* or *she* has been made, using the male pronoun only to enhance clarity between reference to mother or child. The physician has been referred to as *he*, although I am thoroughly cognizant of the inordinate injustice perpetrated by this historical usage.

I should like to acknowledge the help and support of the many colleagues who encouraged me to investigate this subject and the hosts of nursing mothers who helped me learn what I am sharing here.

Extensive library research was done by Nancy Hess and Cathy Goodfellow, who worked as professional volunteers. Editing and tracking specific data were done by Timothy Lawrence, whom I also wish to thank. No writing is accomplished without diligent preparation of the manuscript. Loretta H. Anderson prepared many of the rough drafts. Carleen Wilenius was invaluable for her many skills with manuscripts, not the least of which were final preparation and typing of many of the lengthy charts and bibliographies. I also wish to thank Rosemary E. Disney, who designed the cover art.

RUTH A. LAWRENCE

Contents

APPENDIXES

Breastfeeding

A GUIDE FOR THE MEDICAL PROFESSION

$\mathcal{B}$reastfeeding in modern medicine

There is a reason behind everything in nature.
ARISTOTLE

Until recently, breastfeeding has been a subject considered too imprecise and nonspecific to justify consideration by scientists and clinicians confronted with questions of infant nutrition. Decades have been spent in the laboratory deciphering the nutritional requirements of the growing neonate. A considerably greater investment in time, talent, and money has been put toward the development of an ideal substitute for human milk. On the other hand, artificial feeding has been described as the world's largest experiment without controls.[90] In veterinary medicine, a careful study of the science of lactation in other species, especially bovine, has been made because of the commercial significance of a productive herd.

Advances in technology have allowed the gathering of much data about human milk, which unarguably is for human infants.

Some of the world's finest scientists have turned their attention to human lactation. Time and talent are providing a wealth of resource information about a remarkable fluid—human milk. Past dogmas are being reviewed in the light of new data, and previous data are being reworked with newer methods and technology. An interface is developing for the exchange of scientific information worldwide around issues of human lactation, breastfeeding, and human milk. The more detail that is deciphered about the specific macro and micro nutrients in human milk, the clearer it becomes that human milk is precisely engineered for the human infant.[46] The clinician should not have to justify the recommendation for breastfeeding; instead, the pediatrician should have to justify the replacement with a cow's milk substitute. Harnessing the continuing stream of scientific information into a clinically applicable resource has been encumbered by the need to identify reproducible, peer-reviewed scientific information and to cull the uncontrolled, poorly designed studies and reports appearing in print as a result of the widening interest in the clinical field of lactation.

The *Healthy People 2000* goals, first published in 1978 and restated in 1989, are that the nation will "increase to at least 75 percent the proportion of mothers who exclusively or partially breastfeed their babies in the early postpartum period and to at least 50 percent the proportion

TABLE 1-1   National health promotion and disease prevention objectives

14.9 Increase to at least 75 percent the proportion of mothers who exclusively or partially breastfeed their babies in the early postpartum period and to at least 50 percent the proportion who continue breastfeeding until their babies are 5 to 6 months old. (Baseline: 54 percent at discharge from birth site and 21 percent at 5 to 6 months in 1988)

Mothers breastfeeding their babies (special population targets)	1988 baseline	2000 target
During early postpartum period		
14.9a Low-income mothers	32%	75%
14.9b Black mothers	25%	75%
14.9c Hispanic mothers	51%	75%
14.9d American Indian/Alaskan Native mothers	47%	75%
At age 5-6 months		
14.9a Low-income mothers	9%	50%
14.9b Black mothers	8%	50%
14.9c Hispanic mothers	16%	50%
14.9d American Indian/Alaskan Native mothers	28%	50%

Healthy People 2000 is a statement of national opportunities. Although the Federal Government facilitated its development, it is not intended as a statement of Federal standards or requirements. It is the product of a national effort, involving 22 expert working groups, a consortium that has grown to include almost 300 national organizations and all the state health departments, and the Institute of Medicine of the National Academy of Sciences, which helped the U.S. Public Health Service to manage the consortium, convene regional and national hearings, and receive testimony from more than 750 individuals and organizations. After extensive public review and comment, involving more than 10,000 people, the objectives were revised and refined to produce this report. (From DHHS Pub No (PHS) 91-50213, US Government Printing Office, Washington, DC, 1990.

who continue breastfeeding until their babies are 5 to 6 months old."*

The report further states that special populations should be targeted (Table 1-1) because breastfeeding is the optimal way of nurturing infants while simultaneously benefiting the lactating mother. Former Surgeon General of the United States, C. Everett Koop, MD, ScD, agreed, noting: "We must identify and reduce the barriers which keep women from beginning or continuing to breastfeed their infants."[67]

In 1984 the surgeon general convened a workshop to address these barriers and devise a plan to reach the breastfeeding goals.[67] One barrier identified was the lack of training and

education of health care professionals in human milk and the physiology of lactation. A second workshop was convened[68] to bring together representatives of the professional organizations—American Academy of Pediatrics, American Academy of Family Practice, American College of Nurse Midwives, American College of Obstetrics and Gynecology, American Dietetic Association, National Association of Pediatric Nurse Practitioners, Nurses' Association of American College of Obstetrics and Gynecology—charged with the education and accreditation of their respective members. Through individual action of their boards of trustees, the organizations endorsed a statement supporting breastfeeding and human lactation. They also devised a plan of ensuring appropriate education for their members and the inclusion of the material in the certifying examination for their respective specialties (see Appendix M for model curriculum).

*Healthy People 2000: National Health Promotion and Disease Prevention Objectives, DHHS Pub No (PHS) 91-50213, US Department of Health and Human Services, Public Health Service, Washington, DC, 1990, US Government Printing Office.

Another targeted need for the nation was public education about the subject.[92] Education to put breastfeeding in the mainstream and to classify it as normal behavior has to start with preschoolers and continue through the educational system. Courses in biology, nutrition, health, and human sexuality should all include the breast and its functions.

New York State has taken a leadership position with respect to education of its youth. In 1994 a curriculum from kindergarten through twelfth grade was jointly developed by the Department of Education and the Department of Health* and reviewed by teachers and school districts. The curriculum is not a separate course but provides recommendations about how to include age-appropriate information on breastfeeding and human lactation throughout the school years. The senior high school materials are more detailed and designed to be included in the subject matter regarding reproduction and family life.

The media should include breastfeeding, not always bottle feeding, in reference to young infants. Dolls should not come with bottles. Public policy should facilitate breastfeeding and provide space to breastfeed in public buildings and at the workplace. Of interest were the results of a national survey conducted by professional poll takers for the surgeon general's office to explore ideas and feelings about breastfeeding.[68] The pollsters obtained a statistically representative sample of all age groups from youth to old age, both genders, married and unmarried, and all socioeconomic and ethnic groups. The majority in all age groups knew breastfeeding was best for infants and would want their child breastfed (75%). Very few people were embarrassed by breastfeeding or thought it should not be done in public.

This commitment to policy for breastfeeding has been part of the Code for Infant Feeding of the World Health Organization (WHO Code) to protect developing countries from being inundated with formula products, which discourage breastfeeding where infant survival depends on being nourished at the breast.[90]

Although the major countries of the world endorsed the WHO Code in 1981, the United States did not. Finally on May 9, 1994, signaling a tremendous policy shift, President Clinton made the WHO's International Code of Marketing of Breast-milk Substitutes worldwide policy by joining with the other member nations at the World Health Assembly in Geneva. Despite many efforts by the United States, Italy, and Ireland, to add weakening amendments the Swaziland delegation speaking for the African nations voted to strengthen the resolution even more, and all amendments were dropped. One by one all of the countries, including the United States, agreed to Resolution 47.5, and it was ratified.[8]

The battle to control formula distribution worldwide has not been won. The pandemic of acquired immunodeficiency syndrome (AIDS) has provided a new reason to provide formula to developing countries to stop the spread of human immunodeficiency virus (HIV) to infants from their HIV-positive mothers. This requires serious consideration of the risk/benefit ratio for breastfeeding.

In 1987 the Nutrition Taskforce of the Better Health Commission of Australia[14] set as targets for the year 2000 that 90% of mothers would be breastfeeding on discharge from the hospital and that 80% of babies would still be breastfed at 3 months of age. The rate of breastfeeding in Australia in a survey in 1984-1985 was 80% of mothers exclusively breastfeeding on leaving the hospital.[5] The rate at 3 months was 50%. These rates had been accomplished without public health intervention. The efforts now target high-risk groups with low rates. They have worksite-based programs that encompass prenatal care, pregnancy-related nutrition and drug education, and preparation for infant feeding during pregnancy.

In 1991 the rate in Australia was reported as 92% for initiating breastfeeding and 50% for those still breastfeeding at 6 months. The rate of initiating breastfeeding in 1996 was 80%, and 50% were still breastfeeding at 6 months.

---

*New York State Health Dept.: Breastfeeding—first step to good health: a breastfeeding education activity package for grades K-12, Albany, NY, 1995, NYS Health Research Inc.

BOX 1-1   Key elements for promotion of breastfeeding in the continuum of maternal and infant health care

1. Primary-care settings for women of childbearing age should have:
   - a supportive milieu for lactation
   - educational opportunities (including availability of literature, personal counseling, and information about community resources) for learning about lactation and its advantages
   - ready response to requests for further information
   - continuity allowing for the exposure to and development over time of a positive attitude regarding lactation on the part of the recipient of care

2. Prenatal-care settings should have:
   - a specific assessment at the first prenatal visit of the physical capability and emotional predisposition to lactation. This assessment should include the potential role of the father of the child as well as other significant family members. An educational program about the advantages of and ways of preparing for lactation should continue throughout the pregnancy.
   - resource personnel—such as nutritionists/dietitians, social workers, public health nurses, La Leche League members, childbirth education groups—for assistance in preparing for lactation
   - availability and utilization of culturally suitable patient-education materials
   - an established mechanism for a predelivery visit to the newborn care provider to ensure initiation and maintenance of lactation
   - a means of communicating to the in-hospital team the infant-feeding plans developed during the prenatal course

3. In-hospital settings should have:
   - a policy to determine the patient's infant-feeding plan on admission or during labor
   - a family-centered orientation to childbirth, including the minimum use of intrapartum medications and anesthesia
   - a medical and nursing staff informed about and supportive of ways to facilitate the initiation and continuation of breastfeeding (including early mother-infant contact and ready access by the mother to her baby throughout the hospital stay)
   - the availability of individualized counseling and education by a specially trained breastfeeding coordinator to facilitate lactation for those planning to breastfeed and to counsel those who have not yet decided about their method of infant feeding
   - ongoing inservice education about lactation and ways to support it. This program should be conducted by the breastfeeding coordinator for all relevant hospital staff.
   - proper space and equipment for breastfeeding in the postpartum and neonatal units. Attention should be given to the particular needs of women breastfeeding babies with special problems.
   - the elimination of hospital practices/policies that have the effect of inhibiting the lactation process (e.g., rules separating mother and baby)
   - the elimination of standing orders that inhibit lactation (e.g., lactation suppressants, fixed feeding schedules, maternal medications)
   - discharge planning that includes referral to community agencies to aid in the continuing support of the lactating mother. This referral is especially important for patients discharged early.
   - a policy to limit the distribution of packages of free formula at discharge to only those mothers who are not lactating
   - the development of policies to support lactation throughout the hospital units (e.g., medicine, surgery, pediatrics, emergency room)
   - the provision of continued lactation support for those infants who must remain in the hospital after the mother's discharge

From *Report of the Surgeon General's Workshop on Breastfeeding and Human Lactation.* Presented by US Department of Health and Human Services, June 1984, DHHS Pub No HRS-D-MC 84-2.

BOX 1-1   Key elements for promotion of breastfeeding in the continuum of maternal and infant health care—cont'd

4. Postpartum ambulatory settings should have:
   - a capacity for telephone assistance to mothers experiencing problems with breastfeeding
   - a policy for telephone follow-up 1-3 days after discharge
   - a plan for an early follow-up visit (within first week after discharge)
   - the availability of lactation counseling as a means of preventing or solving lactation problems
   - access to lay support resources for the mother
   - the presence of a supportive attitude by all staff
   - a policy to encourage bringing the infant to postpartum appointments
   - the availability of public-community-health nurse referral for those having problems with lactation
   - a mechanism for the smooth transition to pediatric care of the infant, including good communication between obstetric and pediatric care providers

The Queensland Anti-Discrimination Act, which took effect on June 30, 1992, prohibits discrimination on the grounds of gender, marital status, breastfeeding, lawful sexual activity, age, disability, religion, political belief, or trade-union activity. Under this act, breastfeeding mothers cannot be asked to leave restaurants, cinemas, or other public places. Nursing mothers have fed their infants in places such as pubs, parks, and banks. Any transgressions can be reported to the Anti-Discrimination Tribunal, whose decisions are legally binding.

A similar law has been enacted in Florida to encourage breastfeeding and "authorize" it in public (March 1993). The law provides that breastfeeding a baby does not violate prohibitions against unnatural and lascivious acts; exposure of sexual organs; or lewd, lascivious, or indecent conduct in the presence of a child. Nor is breastfeeding an obscenity, harmful to minors, or unlawful nudity or sexual conduct (Appendix L contains the text of the law). Illinois, Indiana, Michigan, New York, Nevada, North Carolina, Texas, Utah, and Virginia also have enacted legislation, with additional states starting the process one by one.

In general, the two types of interventions to promote breastfeeding are supply and demand.[4] Supply interventions in relation to breastfeeding increase the availability of breast milk while decreasing the availability of substitutes. Making hospital routines more conducive to breastfeeding is a supply intervention and involves early contact, early breastfeeding, rooming-in, or time available at work to breastfeed. Restricting the casual use of milk substitutes in the hospital or in Women, Infants, and Children (WIC) clinics is also a supply intervention. Demand interventions, on the other hand, affect the mother's motivation and attitude about infant feeding. Demand interventions tend to be educational, utilizing facts, such as breast is best; motivations, such as breastfeeding is a great mothering opportunity; or risk messages, such as using substitutes is a health risk.[4]

Box 1-1 provides a summary of interventions presented at the surgeon general's workshop.[67]

Although these recommendations have been promoted since 1984, many hospitals and health care facilities have not achieved them.[90] As a result, UNICEF and the WHO initiated the Baby Friendly Hospital Initiative, which has been implemented in developing countries with considerable success. Box 1-2 lists the 10 steps to becoming a designated Baby Friendly Hospital. A joint WHO/UNICEF statement, *Protecting, Promoting and Supporting Breastfeeding,* describes suggested actions for maternity services. Promotion in the United States has been facilitated by the Healthy Mothers/Healthy Babies Coalition.

In 1996, Evergreen Hospital in Kirkland, Wash., was the first Baby Friendly Hospital so designated in the United States. This initiative has been

BOX 1-2   Toward becoming a Baby Friendly Hospital: 10 steps to successful breastfeeding

Every facility providing maternity services and care for newborn infants should:

1. Have a written breastfeeding policy that is routinely communicated to all health care staff.
2. Train all health care staff in skills necessary to implement this policy.
3. Inform all pregnant women about the benefits and management of breastfeeding.
4. Help mothers initiate breastfeeding within a half hour of birth.
5. Show mothers how to breastfeed and how to maintain lactation even if they should be separated from their infants.
6. Give newborn infants no food or drink other than breast milk, unless *medically* indicated.
7. Practice rooming-in—allow mothers and infants to remain together—24 hours a day.
8. Encourage breastfeeding on demand.
9. Give no artificial teats or pacifiers (also called *dummies* or *soothers*) to breast-feeding infants.
10. Foster the establishment of breastfeeding support groups and refer mothers to them on discharge from the hospital or clinic.

From WHO/UNICEF: *Protecting, promoting and supporting breastfeeding: the special role of maternity services,* a joint WHO/UNICEF statement, Geneva, 1989, World Health Organization.

reorganized and reestablished through *Healthy Children 2000* as a not-for-profit organization called *Baby Friendly, USA.* Ten more hospitals were certified in the first 6 months of 1997, and the program is expanding. For certification, the hospital must provide evidence that it has met the 10 criteria (Box 1-2) and must demonstrate its effectiveness to a visiting team.*

*The address to contact to initiate the process is Baby Friendly, USA, 8 Jan Sabastian Way #13, Sandwich, MA 02563; (508) 888-8044.

THE HISTORY OF BREASTFEEDING

The world scientific literature, predominantly from countries other than the United States, includes many tributes to human milk. Early writings on infant care in the 1800s and early 1900s pointed out the hazards of serious infection in bottle-fed infants. Mortality charts were clear in the difference in mortality risk between breastfed and bottle-fed infants.[36,37] Only in recent years have the reasons for this phenomenon been identified in terms comparable with those used to define other antiinfectious properties. The identification of specific immunoglobulins and determination of the specific influence of the pH and flora in the intestine of the breastfed infant are examples. It became clear that the infant receives systemic protection transplacentally and local intestinal tract protection orally via the colostrum. The intestinal tract environment of a breastfed infant continues to afford protection against infection by influencing the bacterial flora until the infant is weaned. Breastfed infants also have fewer respiratory infections, occurrences of otitis media, gastrointestinal infections, and other illnesses. The immunologic protection afforded by specific antibodies such as respiratory syncytial virus and rotavirus also protects the infant from illness.

Refinement in the biochemistry of nutrition has afforded an opportunity to restudy the constituents of human milk. Attention to brain growth and neurologic development emphasizes the unique constituents of human milk that enhance the growth and development of the exclusively breastfed infant. Because the human brain doubles in size in the first year of life, the nutrients provided for brain growth are critical (see Chapter 7). A closer look at the amino acids in human milk has demonstrated clearly that the array is physiologically suited for the human newborn. Forced by legislation mandating mass newborn screening for phenylalanine in all hospitals, physicians were faced with the problem of the newborn who had high phenylalanine or tyrosine levels. It became apparent that many traditional formulas provided

Fig. 1-1. Armenian woman suckling her child. (Redrawn from Wickes IG: *Arch Dis Child* 28:151, 1953.)

an overload of these amino acids, which some infants were unable to handle well.

The mysteries and taboos about colostrum go back to the dawn of civilization.[86] Most ancient primitive peoples let several days go by before putting the baby to the breast, with exact times and rituals varying from tribe to tribe. Other liquids were provided in the form of herbal teas; some were pharmacologically potent, and others had no nutritional worth. Breastfeeding positions varied as well.[86] Most cultures held their infants while seated; however, Armenians and some Asians would lean over the supine baby, resting on a bar that ran above the cradle for support (Fig. 1-1). These infants were not lifted for the purpose of burping. Many groups carried their infants on their backs and swung them into position frequently for feedings, a method that continues today. These infants are not burped either but remain semierect in the swaddling on the mother's back. The ritual of burping is actually a product of necessity in bottle feeding because air is so easily swallowed.

Although the modern woman may be selectively chastised for abandoning breastfeeding because of the ready availability of prepared formulas, paraphernalia of bottles and rubber nipples, and ease of sterilization, this is not a new issue. Meticulous combing of civilized history reveals that almost every generation has had to provide alternatives when the mother could not or would not nurse her infant. Blame cannot be placed solely on an uninformed and unsupportive medical profession or on the formula manufacturers.

Hammurabi's code, from about 1800 BC, contained regulations on the practice of wet nursing, that is, nursing another woman's infant, often for hire. Throughout Europe, spouted feeding cups have been found in the graves of infants dating from about 2000 BC. Although ancient Egyptian feeding flasks are almost unknown, specimens of Greek origin are fairly common in infant burials. Paralleling the information about ancient feeding techniques is the problem of abandoned infants. Well-known biblical stories report such events, as do accounts from Rome during the time of the early popes. In fact, so many infants were abandoned that foundling homes were started. French foundling homes in the 1700s were staffed by wet nurses who were carefully selected and their lives and activities controlled to ensure adequate nourishment for the foundling.

In Spartan times a woman, even if she was the wife of a king, was required to nurse her eldest son; plebeians were to nurse all their children.[78] Plutarch, an ancient scribe, reported that a second son of King Themistes inherited the kingdom of Sparta only because he was nursed with his mother's milk. The eldest son had been nursed by a stranger and therefore was rejected. Hippocrates is said to have written, "One's own milk is beneficial, others' harmful."

No known written works describe infant feeding from ancient times to the Renaissance.[87] In 1472 the first pediatric incunabulum, written by Paul Bagellardus, was printed in Padua, Italy. It described the characteristics of a good wet nurse and counseled about hiccups, diarrhea, and vomiting. Thomas Muffett (1584) wrote of the medicinal and therapeutic use of human milk for men and women of "riper years, fallen by age or by sickness into compositions." His writings referred to the milk of the ass as being the best substitute for human milk at any age when nourishment was an issue. The milk of an ass is low in solids compared with that of most species, low in fat and protein, and high in lactose:

	Total solids	Fat	Protein	CHO	Ash
	%	%	%	%	%
Human	12.4	3.8	1.0	7.0	0.2
Ass	11.7	1.4	2.0	7.4	0.5
Cow	12.7	3.7	3.7	4.8	0.7

CHO, Carbohydrates; *Ash,* residual after burning, includes Na, Ca, etc.

From 1500 to 1700 AD, wealthy English women did not nurse their infants, according to Fildes,[26] who laboriously and meticulously reviewed infant feeding history in Great Britain. Although breast-feeding was well recognized as a means of delaying another pregnancy, these women preferred to bear anywhere from 12 to 20 babies than to breastfeed them.[92] They had a notion that breastfeeding spoiled their figures and made them old before their time. Husbands had much to say about how the infants were fed. Wet nurses were replaced by hand feeding cereal or bread gruel from a spoon. The death rate in foundling homes from this practice approached 100%.

The Dowager Countess of Lincoln wrote on "the duty of nursing, due by mothers to their children" in 1662.[87] She had borne 18 children, all fed by wet nurses; only one of the children survived. When her son's wife bore a child and nursed it, the Countess saw the error of her ways. She cited the biblical example of Eve, who breastfed Cain, Abel, and Seth. She also noted that Job 39:16 states that to withhold a full breast is to be more savage than dragons and more cruel than ostriches to their little ones. The noblewoman concluded her appeal to women to avoid her mistakes: " . . . be not so unnatural as to thrust away your own children; be not so hardy as to venture a tender babe to a less tender breast; be not accessory to that disorder of causing a poorer woman to banish her own infant for the entertaining of a richer woman's child, as it were bidding her to unlove her own to love yours."

Fig. 1-2. Pewter pap spoon, circa 1800 AD. Thin pap, a mixture of bread and water, was placed in bowl. Tip of bowl was placed in child's mouth. Flow could be controlled by placing finger over open end of hollow handle. If contents were not taken as rapidly as desired, one could blow down on handle.

Toward the end of the eighteenth century in England, the trend to wet nursing and artificial feeding changed, partially because medical writers drew attention to health and well-being and mothers made more decisions about feeding their young.

In eighteenth-century France, both before and during the revolution that swept Louis XVI from the throne and brought Napoleon to power, infant feeding included maternal nursing, wet nursing, artificial feeding with the milk of animals, and feeding of pap and panada.[21] *Panada* is from the French *panade,* meaning bread, and means a food consisting of bread, water or other liquid, and seasoning, boiled to the consistency of pulp (Fig. 1-2). The majority of infants born to wealthy and middle-income women, especially in Paris, were placed with wet nurses. The reason given for this widespread practice was that maternal nursing was "not the custom." Mothers wished to "guard their beauty and freshness." In 1718, Dionis wrote, "Today not only ladies of nobility, but yet the rich and the wives of the least of the artisans have lost the custom of nursing their infants." As early as 1705, laws controlling wet nursing required wet

Fig. 1-3. Arnold Steam Sterilizer advertisement. (From *NY Med J* June 22, 1895.)

nurses to register, forbade them to nurse more than two infants in addition to their own, and stipulated a crib should be available for each infant, to prevent the nurse from taking a baby to bed and chancing suffocation.*[21] On the birth of the Prince of Wales (later George IV) in 1762, it was officially announced: wet nurse, Mrs. Scott; dry nurse, Mrs. Chapman; rockers, Jane Simpson and Catherine Johnson.[87]

A more extensive historical review would reveal other examples of social problems in achieving adequate care of infants. Long before our modern society, some women failed to accept their biologic role as nursing mothers, and society failed to provide adequate support for nursing mothers (Fig. 1-3). Breastfeeding was more common and of longer duration in stable eras and rarer in periods of "social dazzle" and lowered moral standards. Urban mothers have had greater access to alternatives, and rural women have had to continue to breastfeed in greater numbers.

A handful of research-oriented physicians sought a substitute for mother's milk to replace wet nursing in the mid-nineteenth century.[87] Most of the solutions were cow's milk with added sugar and water. Dr. William H. Cumming of Atlanta recognized that these solutions were low in "butter," creating a "deficiency of nerve food." He added cream and then lime water to bring the pH up and make the solution digestible. In 1884, Dr. A.V. Meigs published a surprisingly accurate comparative analysis of human and bovine milks. He then set about improving bovine milk to match human milk by adding lime water, fat, and sugar. When these preparations were boiled to sterilize them, scurvy became common.

Pierre Budin (1846-1907) is credited with creating perinatal medicine as well as with establishing the first clinics for nurslings.[79] Written when infant mortality was 288 per 1000 live births, his book *The Nursling* stated, "Favor breastfeeding by all possible means and provide mothers with advice and help in order to provide the best nutrition for the infant."

Soon, chemists entered the field of infant feeding, which had been previously limited to physicians who had mothers make the profitable mixtures and concoctions.[87] Henri Nestlé, a Swiss merchant, combined sugar and wheat flour with milk from Swiss cows fed Alpine grass. The wheat flour had been cooked with malt. Nestlé advertised his product as "scientifically correct so as to leave nothing to be desired." He directed most of his promotional efforts to mothers as he insisted that "mothers will do my publicity for me." Most infant food companies, however, advertised in medical as well as nonmedical journals. As industry took over producing human milk substitutes from physicians who had prescribed their own formulas, the mother became the target. Some concoctions contained no milk at all. Little attention was paid to the fact the product might be reconstituted with contaminated water. In 1888 the

---

*Interestingly, at the National Convention of France of 1793, laws were passed to provide relief for infants of indigent families. The provisions are quite similar to those in our present-day welfare programs.[21]

American Medical Association (AMA) subcommittee on infant feeding could not reach a consensus as to the best mother's milk substitute, although little enthusiasm existed for wet nursing.

The competition for the nonnursing mother's market was well launched by the end of the nineteenth century. Science was equated with progress. Infant-feeding concoctions were described as scientifically prepared, although the statements were never supported by any documentation. The popular lay journals of the day, such as *Babyhood* and *Ladies' Home Journal,* were the arena in which mothers could support or condemn various infant-rearing practices in light of their own limited personal experiences. Apple[2] points out that "the commercialization and medicalization of infant care established an environment that made artificial feeding not only acceptable to many mothers but also natural and necessary."

Apple[2] further states that "a combination of the ideology of scientific motherhood, confidence in the medical profession, and shrewd media presentation altered the relationship between mothers and physicians and encouraged mothers to seek out commercial and medical solutions to the problems of infant feeding." Despite a renewed interest in breastfeeding in the mid-twentieth century among mothers and physicians, the legacy of scientific motherhood lives on.

Sociologists have reviewed the reasons for the decrease in breastfeeding in the twentieth century.[20] Urbanization and technologic advances have affected social, medical, and dietary trends throughout the world.[29] The social influences include the changing pattern of family life—smaller, isolated families that are separated from the previous generation. The practice of medicine has emphasized disease and its treatment, especially as it relates to laboratory study and hospital care. The science of nutrition has developed a reliance on measurement and technology, which has led to the conclusion that prepared foods are superior because they can be measured and calculated to meet precise dietary requirements.

In the 1920s, women were encouraged to raise their infants scientifically. "Raising by the book" was commonplace. The U.S. government published *Infant Care,* referred to as the "good book," which was the bible of child rearing read by women from all walks of life. It emphasized cod liver oil, orange juice, and artificial feeding. A quote from *Parents* magazine in 1938 reflects the attitude of women's magazines in general, undermining even the staunchest breastfeeders: "You hope to nurse him, but there is an alarming number of young mothers today who are unable to breastfeed their babies and you may be one of them. . . . "[12] Apple[2] details the transition from breastfeeding to raising children scientifically, by the book, and precisely as the doctor prescribes.

There are encouraging trends, however. The acceptance or rejection of breastfeeding is being influenced in the Western world to a greater degree by the knowledge of the benefits of human milk and breastfeeding. Cultural rejection, negative attitudes, and lack of support from health professionals are being replaced by interest in child rearing and preparation for childbirth. This has created a system that encourages a prospective mother to consider the options for herself and her infant.[74] The attitude in the Western world toward the female breast as a sex object to the exclusion of its ability to nurture has influenced young mothers in particular not to breastfeed. The emancipation of women, which began in the 1920s, was symbolized by short hair, short skirts, contraceptives, cigarettes, and bottle feeding. In the second half of the twentieth century, women have sought to be well informed, and many want the right to choose how they feed their infant. Within the boundaries of medical prudence, the medical profession should be prepared with adequate information to support the mother's desire to breastfeed.

The great success of the mother-to-mother program of the La Leche League and other women's support groups in helping women breastfeed or, as with International Childbirth Education Association (ICEA), in helping women plan and participate in childbirth, is an example of the power of social relationships. Raphael[65] described the *doula* as a key person for lactation support, especially in the first critical days and weeks after delivery.

Bryant[10] explored the social networks in her study of the impact of kin, friend, and neighbor networks on infant-feeding practices in Cuban, Puerto Rican, and Anglo families in Florida. She found that these networks strongly influenced decisions about breastfeeding, bottle feeding, use of supplements, and introduction of solid foods. Network members' advice and encouragement contributed to a successful lactation experience. The impact of the health care professional is inversely proportional to the distance of the mother from her network. The health care worker must work within the cultural norms for the network. For individuals isolated from their cultural roots, the health care system may have to provide more support and encouragement to ensure lactation success and adherence to health care guidelines.[70]

The trend in infant feeding among mothers who participated in the WIC Program in the late 1970s and early 1980s was analyzed separately by Martinez and Stahl[54] from the data collected by questionnaires mailed quarterly as part of the Ross Laboratories Mother's Survey. The responses represented 4.8% of the total U.S. births in 1977 and 14.1% of the total U.S. births in 1980. WIC participants in 1977, including those who supplemented with formula or cow's milk, were breastfeeding in the hospital in 33.6% of cases. A steady and significant increase occurred in the frequency of breastfeeding to 40.4% in 1980 ($p < 0.5$).

WIC data continue to be collected, and the trends have paralleled other groups; fewer WIC mothers initiated breastfeeding in 1990 (only 33.7%) than in 1985, and only 8.9% were still breastfeeding at 5 to 6 months (Table 1-2). In 1992, however, there was an increase to 38.4% breastfeeding at birth and 10.7% still breastfeeding at 5 to 6 months. The rate of initiation was 50.4% in 1997, with 16.2% continuing to 5 to 6 months.

The Food and Consumer Service (FCS) of the U.S. Department of Agriculture (USDA) entered into a cooperative agreement with Best Start, a not-for-profit social marketing organization that promotes breastfeeding to develop a WIC breastfeeding promotion project that is national in scope and being implemented at the state level. The

TABLE 1-2	Percentage of breastfeeding among WIC participants, 1977-1997	
	In hospital	**At 5 to 6 months of age**
1977	33.6	12.5
1978	34.5	11.2
1979	37.0	12.2
1980	40.4	14.4
—	—	—
1985	40.1	12.8
1986	38.0	11.6
1987	37.3	11.5
1990	33.7	8.9
1992	38.4	10.7
1994	44.3	11.6
1995	46.6	12.7
1996	46.6	12.9
1997	50.4	16.2

From Martinez GA, Stahl DA: *Am J Pub Health* 72:68, 1982; Ryan AS, Rush D, Krieger FW et al: *Pediatrics* 88:719, 1991; Krieger FW: A review of breastfeeding trends. Presented at the Editor's Conference, New York, September 1992; Ross Laboratories Mother's Survey, unpublished data, Columbus, Ohio, 1992; Mother's Survey, Ross Products Division, Abbott Laboratories, unpublished data, 1998; and Ryan AS: *Pediatrics* 99(4):2, 1997 (electronic article).

project consists of six components: social marketing research, a media campaign, a staff support kit, a breastfeeding resource guide, a training conference, and continuing education and technical assistance. With an annual $8 million budget, the project's goals are to increase the initiation and duration of breastfeeding among WIC clients and to expand public acceptance and support of breastfeeding. Breastfeeding women are favored in the WIC priority system when benefits are limited; they can continue in the program for a year, whereas those who do not breastfeed are limited to 6 months. All pregnant WIC participants are encouraged to breastfeed.

Montgomery and Splett[58] reported the economic benefits of breastfeeding infants for mothers enrolled in WIC. Comparing the costs of the WIC program and Medicaid for food and health care in Colorado, administrative and health care costs for a formula-fed infant, minus the rebate for the first

180 days of life, were $273 higher than those for the breastfed infant. These calculations did not include the pharmacy costs for illness. When these figures are translated to large WIC programs in high-cost areas (e.g., New York City, Los Angeles) and multiplied by millions of WIC participants, the savings from breastfeeding are substantial. If the goal of 75% breastfeeding by the year 2000 were realized among WIC recipients, the cost savings could be $4 million a month for the WIC program.[58]

Frequency of breastfeeding

Data collected in the 1970s in the Ross Laboratories Mother's Survey MR77-48, which included 10,000 mothers, revealed a general trend toward breastfeeding.[53] In 1975, 33% of the mothers started out breastfeeding, and 15% were still breastfeeding at 5 to 6 months. In 1977, 43% of the mothers left the hospital breastfeeding, and 20%

were still breastfeeding at 5 to 6 months. Other studies have shown a regional variation, with a higher percentage of mothers breastfeeding on the West Coast than in the East.

A continuation of the study of milk-feeding patterns in 1981 in the United States by Martinez and Dodd[53] showed a sustained trend toward breastfeeding in 55% of the 51,537 new mothers contacted by mail. Although mothers who breastfeed continue to be more highly educated and have a higher income, the greatest increase in breastfeeding occurred among women with less education. From 1971 to 1981, breastfeeding in the hospital more than doubled (from 24.7% to 57.6%), with an average rate of gain of 8.8%. The incidence of breastfeeding at 1 week of age was 56.4%. For infants 2 months old, breastfeeding more than tripled (from 13.9% to 44.2%) in this 10-year period (Table 1-3).

The National Natality Surveys (NNS) conducted by the Centers for Disease Control in 1969

TABLE 1-3   Percentage of infants at 1 week of age receiving different milks and formulas, 1955 to 1996

	Breast milk*	Prepared infant formula	Evaporated milk	Cow's milk	Total*
1955	29.2	23.2	45.9	4.1	102.4
1960	28.4	34.9	40.0	2.8	106.1
1965	26.5	59.0	17.3	1.5	104.3
1970	24.9	74.9	3.0	0.6	103.4
1975	33.4	69.2	0.7	0.3	103.6
1978	45.1	58.6	0.5	0.1	104.3
1979	49.7	54.7	0.3	0.1	104.8
1980	54.0	50.6	0.2	0.1	104.9
1981	56.4	48.5	0.2	0.1	105.2
1985	55.4	49.8	0.1	0.1	105.4
1987	54.1	52.5	<0.1	<0.1	106.7
—	—	—	—	—	—
1990	51.5	(52.6)†	<0.1	<0.1	104.2
1992	53.9	(51.0)†	<0.1	<0.1	105.0
1994	57.4	(43.0)†	<0.1	<0.1	>100
1995	59.7	(41.0)†	<0.1	<0.1	>100
1996	59.2	(41.0)†	<0.1	<0.1	>100

Modified from *Ross Laboratories Mother's Survey* MR77-48, 1988 through 1992, and survey trends through 1996.
*Includes supplemental bottle feeding (i.e., formula in addition to breastfeeding).
†Calculated.

and 1980 included questions about infant-feeding practices after birth by married women.[28] Questionnaires were mailed at 3 and 6 months postpartum. In 1969, 19% of white women and 9% of black women were exclusively breastfeeding. The highest rate was among white women up to 34 years old, with three to six children. In 1980, 51% of white women and 25% of black women were exclusively breastfeeding, and they were more highly educated and primiparous.

The Ross Laboratories Mother's Survey remains the only national study that includes sampling of all women who give birth in the 50 states.[48] The study has been expanded to monthly mailings, with special efforts to ensure participation of low-income and less-educated mothers; 725,000 surveys are mailed annually. The results have documented the persistent decline in the number of women initially breastfeeding, from a high in 1982 of 61.9% to an apparent low in 1991 of 51%, with the decline finally involving all categories of women, including those with higher socioeconomic status and higher education. The decline in duration of breastfeeding was similar, with a peak in 1982 of 27% and a trough in 1991 at 18.5%. The data for 1992 reflected an increase that persisted through the months across all categories. In the hospital, 53.9% were breastfeeding, and 20.1% continued for 5 to 6 months, nationally.[48] By 1996 the initiation rate had risen in all categories, averaging 59.2%.[71] Duration showed a steady increase to 21.7% at 6 months. The greatest increase was seen in the groups least likely to breastfeed (e.g., low income, less education).

Although the validity of questionnaires requesting mothers to recall their feeding behaviors months later has been questioned, a study of maternal recall of infant-feeding events demonstrated that recall is accurate up to 18 months later when breastfeeding is the mode. Data on formula feeding recall were not as accurate as those for breastfeeding and solid food feeding.[50]

The social network

Scientific evaluation has established that both a theoretical basis and a strong empirical basis exist for the causal impact of social relationships on health and well-being.[41] Scientists have long noted that more socially isolated or less socially integrated individuals are less healthy psychologically and physically. They point out that unmarried and more socially isolated people have more infectious disease, accidents, and mental disorders.[70] Conversely, clinicians have noted the health-enhancing qualities of social relationships and contacts. The demographic information indicated that WIC mothers were slightly younger (18.5% less than 20 years old compared with 5.4% of those not in WIC). WIC respondents did not differ significantly from non-WIC mothers in plans for postpartum employment, although they were less educated. Of infants born to WIC mothers, 7.9% were premature; of infants born to non-WIC mothers, only 4.3% were premature. The national average was 7.1% of births.[4] The percentage of WIC mothers in 1992 who breastfed varied across the states, with a high of 61.5% in the Rocky Mountain area to a low of 25% in the East-South-Central area.[48] In 1996, 46.6% initiated breastfeeding, and 12.9% were still breastfeeding on average.

Ethnic factors

Nationally, the data by ethnicity revealed an in-hospital breastfeeding rate of 27.2% among blacks, 51.7% among Hispanics, and 59.7% among whites in 1992. The rates were even lower in South Central United States (17% among blacks) and in the mid-Atlantic states (40% among Hispanics).[48] In 1996 the rate among blacks was 37.1% and was 60.5% among Hispanics. Duration was 11.3% and 19.5%, respectively.

The international trends have received considerable attention, and data on all countries but Russia are available in *The International Breast-Feeding Compendium.*[89] Because studies vary in methodology, there is no accurate way to generalize. Breastfeeding patterns in low-income countries, as extracted from world fertility surveys and secondary sources, indicate that in all but a few countries, most children are breastfed for a few months at least, and in 53% of the 83 countries listed, the incidence is 90% or higher. Most localized trend data in both developed and Third World countries reveal increasing frequency of breastfeeding since the 1970s.

Demographic factors

The demographic factors associated with a higher incidence of breastfeeding have remained the same

since the low point in 1970.[1] The rate for well-educated, higher socioeconomic status families has been about 70% initiation at birth, although a slight decline occurred toward the end of the 1980s among these women and other groups[73] (Table 1-4). In 1992, 20.1% were still breastfeeding at 5 to 6 months of age, but the rate among blacks was

TABLE 1-4	In-hospital breastfeeding rates: all infants and selected maternal demographics								
	1988	**1989**	**1990**	**1991**	**1992**	**1993**	**1994**	**1995**	**1996**
All infants	54.3	52.2	51.5	53.3	54.2	55.9	57.4	59.7	59.2
Parity									
Primiparous	55.2	52.6	52.5	54.5	56.4	58.7	59.7	61.6	61.0
Multiparous	53.5	51.7	50.6	52.3	52.8	54.3	55.3	57.8	57.4
Education									
Grade school	31.4	31.7	31.6	35.2	35.9	37.5	38.8	43.8	46.8
High school	44.9	42.5	41.3	42.9	43.9	46.0	47.7	49.7	49.2
Non-college	44.5	42.1	41.0	42.6	43.6	45.7	47.4	49.5	49.1
College	72.2	70.7	69.8	70.2	70.9	71.9	72.9	74.4	73.8
Employment									
Employed full time	53.5	50.8	51.3	54.0	55.9	57.8	58.6	60.7	60.2
Employed part time	61.4	59.4	59.1	60.1	61.4	61.5	62.5	63.5	63.3
Total employed	56.3	53.9	54.1	56.2	57.8	59.1	59.9	61.7	61.3
Not employed	53.0	51.0	49.7	51.2	51.6	53.5	55.3	58.0	57.5
Annual income									
<$10,000	34.2	31.7	30.5	33.3	34.7	37.5	39.9	41.8	41.5
$10,000-$19,999	51.0	49.3	46.4	47.8	49.4	51.0	52.5	53.8	53.0
$20,000-$29,000	61.1	58.6	57.1	57.8	58.7	60.1	60.3	61.8	61.1
$30,000+	70.1	68.1	N/R	N/R	N/R	N/R	N/R	N/R	N/R
$30,000-$39,999	N/A	N/A	62.7	63.6	64.9	65.3	66.0	66.8	66.5
$40,000-$49,999	N/A	N/A	66.4	67.8	67.2	68.3	68.4	69.8	69.4
$50,000+	N/A	N/A	74.1	74.5	74.5	74.7	75.3	77.3	76.3
Age (yr)									
<20	31.3	30.2	30.0	32.2	33.6	36.6	39.9	42.8	43.3
20-24	48.4	45.2	44.0	45.7	46.9	49.0	51.2	52.6	52.7
25-29	61.3	58.8	57.3	57.8	58.7	60.2	61.5	63.1	62.2
30-34	66.6	65.5	64.2	65.2	65.0	65.9	66.3	68.1	67.5
35+	66.6	66.5	65.4	66.7	67.2	67.4	67.7	70.0	69.3

From Mother's Survey, Ross Products Division, Abbott Laboratories, Columbus, Ohio, 1998. Updated breastfeeding trend through 1996, *N/R*, Not reported; *N/A*, not available.

only 8.1% and among WIC participants only 10.7%. The 1996 data revealed a rate of 21.7% at 6 months overall, 12.9% among WIC mothers, and 11.3% among blacks.[71]

Study after study has confirmed the relationship of breastfeeding to education, social status, marriage, and other demographic factors. The well-educated, well-to-do groups of all races breast-feed. In a study by Wright et al[91] of 1112 healthy infants in a health maintenance organization (HMO) in Arizona, 70% were breastfed, with a mean duration of almost 7 months. Education and marriage were associated with breastfeeding. Maternal employment outside the home and ethnicity (being Hispanic rather than Anglo-American) were related to higher rates of bottle feeding. The authors suggest that effects of ethnicity are independent of those of education. New immigrants who would have breastfed in their homeland tend to bottle feed here because they think this practice is "American."

The impoverished mother is choosing to bottle feed not because she is working; statistics show she is staying home and bottle feeding. When mothers were interviewed about their infant-feeding choice at a prenatal WIC clinic, they knew mother's milk was best.[33] They said it was too difficult to breastfeed and there were too many rules. In the classes on breastfeeding given by lactation experts, the instructions on preparing the breasts and diet rules were overwhelming. The mothers said if their physician would tell them breastfeeding was important, they would do it for as long as the physician said.[33] Similar data in the Ross Laboratories Mother's Survey also indicated the power of the physician's word. Mothers trusted their physician's advice and were more successful at breastfeeding if the physician was supportive and expressed his or her views.[72,73]

Duration of breastfeeding

Coupled with concerns about the decreasing number of mothers who breastfeed their infants when they leave the hospital is the concern about duration of breastfeeding. A sharp decline occurs by age 6 months; in 1977 this decline was from 43% to 20%. Other studies have noted an appreciable decline shortly after discharge from the hospital.[42]

In 1984 the duration of breastfeeding in the United States and elsewhere was increasing. The number still breastfeeding at 6 months was 25%. This number, however, has dropped slowly to 21% in 1987[72] and to 19.7% in 1992 and rose to 21.7% in 1996.

The two types of breastfeeding, as Newton[60] points out, are unrestricted and token. *Unrestricted breastfeeding* usually means that the infant is put to the breast immediately after delivery and breastfed on demand thereafter, without rules or limitations. There may be 10 or 12 feedings a day in the early weeks, with the number gradually decreasing over the first year of life. Breast milk continues to be a major source of nourishment during infancy.

Token breastfeeding, in contrast, is characterized by constant restrictions on the time and duration of nursing. Usually the feedings are scheduled. Even the amount of mother-infant contact is limited initially, and the infant is often offered water or glucose water by bottle. The whole process is inhibited, and a secure milk supply may not be established. The duration of breastfeeding is one of the major differences between unrestricted-feeding and token-feeding groups.

In 1988 the Interagency Group for Action on Breastfeeding met to develop a set of definitions that could be used as standardized terminology for the collection of information on breastfeeding behavior. The recommendations were then reviewed extensively by researchers and providers, and a schema was finalized, as follows[49]:

1. Acknowledge that the term *breastfeeding* alone is insufficient to describe the numerous types of breastfeeding behavior.
2. Distinguish full from partial breastfeeding.
3. Subdivide full breastfeeding into categories of exclusive and almost-exclusive breastfeeding.
4. Differentiate among levels of partial breast-feeding.
5. Recognize that token breastfeeding has little or no nutritional impact.

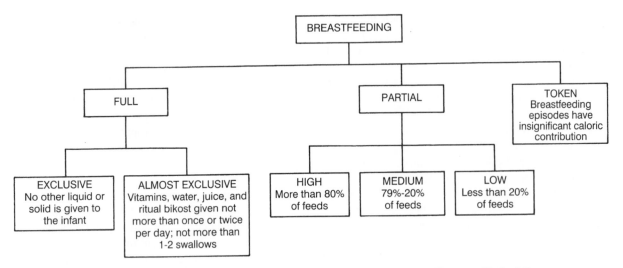

Fig. 1-4. Schema for breastfeeding definition. (Modified from Labbok M, Krasovec K: *Stud Fam Plan* 21:226, 1990.)

The group hoped that the schema and framework would assist researchers and agencies in efforts to describe and interpret breastfeeding practices accurately (Fig. 1-4).

Cultural differences also affect duration of breastfeeding. In societies not yet industrialized that maintain ancient cultural patterns of child rearing, the duration is well beyond a year. A study of 46 such societies by Ford[27] revealed that weaning at about 2 to 3 years of age occurred in three fourths of them. One fourth of the groups began weaning at 18 months of age, and one culture started at 6 months. A similar anthropologic investigation of primitive child-rearing practices found a distinct correlation between the time of weaning and the behavior of the tribes.[27] Where weaning was delayed, tribes were peaceful. In contrast, tribes that abruptly weaned their infants at 6 months of age and practiced other rigid disciplinary practices were warlike.

In the United States and Europe at the beginning of the twentieth century, more than 50% of the infants were breastfed beyond 1 year of age. The Plunket Society of New Zealand conducted three surveys to evaluate the extent and duration of breastfeeding.[19] These showed a progressive de-cline in the number of nursing mothers and in the duration of nursing (Fig. 1-5).

In 1966, fewer than one in three mothers in the United States were breastfeeding when they left the hospital. Only 5% of the nation's infants were breastfed after 6 months of age. Mothers who had successfully nursed a previous infant had a higher rate of duration success compared with the duration of breastfeeding in primiparas. The decline was attributed to a lack of appropriate advice and of support in the hospital and at home (Fig. 1-6). The differential in rates between primiparas and multiparas has been seen in the annual figures as well, with multiparas initiating breastfeeding at a slightly lower rate: 50.9% in 1980, 56.2% in 1985, and 52.2% in 1992; however, the durations were higher than those of primiparas. In 1996, primiparas initiated breastfeeding more frequently (61.0%) than multiparas (57.4%). Similarly, the duration was higher in multiparas (23.6%) than primiparas (19.7%).[59]

The most frequent reasons given for stopping were (1) not enough milk, (2) felt tired, and (3) infant's physician told mother to stop. These studies also pointed out the pivotal role for the pediatrician in the successful maintenance of

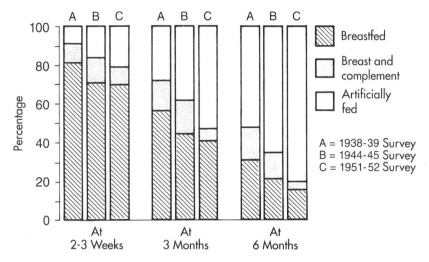

Fig. 1-5. Breastfeeding in New Zealand. Summary of results of Plunket Society's surveys of 1938 to 1939, 1944 to 1945, and 1951 to 1952. (From Deem H, McGeorge M: *N Z Med J* 57:539, 1958.)

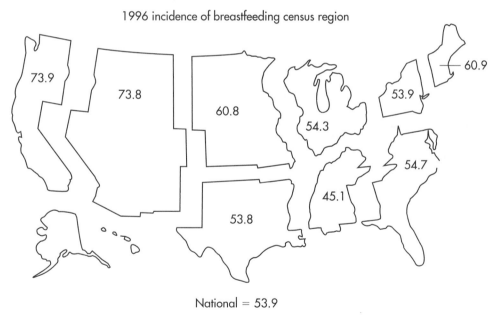

Fig. 1-6. Census breastfeeding data. (Modified from Ross Laboratories, Mother's Survey, Columbus, Ohio.)

lactation as well as the importance of the postpartum environment.[13,84]

The 1981 Milk Feeding Pattern survey by Martinez and Dodd[53] reported on the duration of breastfeeding. The rate of infants breastfed at ages 3 to 4 months was 35.2%, a fourfold increase from 1971; at 5 and 6 months of age the rate was 26.8% in 1981 and only 5.5% in 1971 (Fig. 1-7). Data collected by telephone follow-up revealed rates of 18% at 8 months, 13% at 10 months, and 9% at

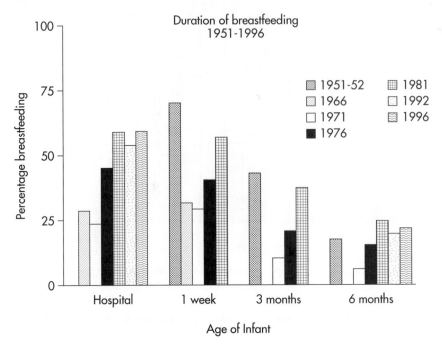

Fig. 1-7. Duration of breastfeeding, 1951 to 1981. (Data from Woo-lun M, Gussler J, Smith N, editors: *The international breast-feeding compendium,* ed 3, Columbus, Ohio, 1984, Ross Laboratories; Kreiger F: A review of breastfeeding trends. Presented at the Editor's Conference, New York, September 1992; and Ryan AS: *Pediatrics* 99(4):2, 1997 [electronic article].)

12 months in 1981.[53,54] Breastfeeding rates in the United States from 1965 to 1995 are shown in Fig. 1-8.

The maternal demographic data on duration of breastfeeding in this study further supported the trend of higher educational level and higher income for mothers breastfeeding at 6 and 12 months (Table 1-4). More multiparas than primiparas continued to breastfeed, but duration was negatively affected by maternal employment. The influence of maternal employment in this survey was significant ($p < 0.1$). For every 100 mothers employed full time and breastfeeding in the hospital, 19.8% were still breastfeeding at 6 months postpartum, whereas among mothers not employed and breastfeeding in the hospital, 50.1% were still breastfeeding at 6 months postpartum. The employed mothers in most studies tend to be in better-educated, higher socioeconomic groups than those who are unemployed. Thus it is not necessarily employment alone that deters the lower

socioeconomic group from breastfeeding.[53,54] Another study reported that duration was influenced by social class but not by the mother's age.[84]

Table 1-5 lists reasons for terminating breastfeeding. Return to work was a reason for discontinuing for only 5 of the 116 women. One hundred, or 86%, of the mothers who stopped by 22 weeks would have liked to continue but said they had insufficient milk or other unsurmountable problems. Unrelated to length of breastfeeding, a large percentage of all the survey mothers stated they could have benefited from more assistance from health care professionals.

Women at high risk for not implementing their prenatal breastfeeding intention were identified in a study of 187 women who planned to breastfeed.[11] Interviews prenatally and postnatally identified lower confidence in ability to breastfeed, less certainty in the decision to breastfeed, delayed first breastfeeding experience, and lack of rooming-in with the baby as significant predictors. The authors

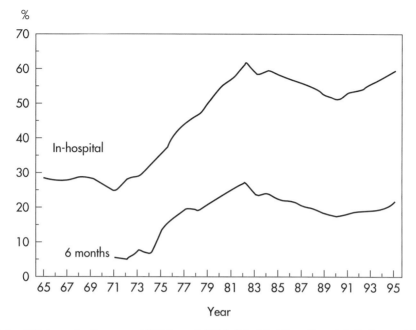

Fig. 1-8. U.S. breastfeeding rates, 1965 through 1995. (Modified from Ryan AS: *Pediatrics* 99(4):2, 1997 [electronic article].)

TABLE 1-5	Reasons for discontinuing breastfeeding			
	Duration of breastfeeding (wk)			
Reason	**<6 (n = 49)**	**6-11 (n = 39)**	**12-22 (n = 28)**	**Total (n = 116)**
Inadequate milk supply	28	18	12	58
Baby unsettled after breastfeeds	18	11	2	31
Very frequent feeds required	17	8	4	29
Breastfeeding was too tiring	13	5	2	20
Painful nipples	14	2	1	17
Baby refused the breast	9	4	2	15
Unable to go out	6	4	0	10
Too time-consuming	7	2	1	10
Illness of mother	3	6	0	9
Breast abscess	2	3	1	6
Return to work	0	3	2	5
Dislike of breastfeeding	5	0	0	5
Insufficient privacy at home	2	1	0	3
Illness of baby	2	1	0	3
Other factors*				
Anxiety, lack of confidence	6	2	1	9
Breast problems—mastitis, engorgement	1	5	0	6
Older children upset or jealous	3	0	0	3
Contraceptive pill reduced milk supply	0	1	1	2
Anticoagulant therapy	1	0	0	1

From West CP: *J Biosoc Sci* 12:325, 1980.
*Not listed but volunteered by the mothers.

TABLE 1-6	Selected demographic characteristics associated with duration of breastfeeding*		
	Group 1: never breastfed (n = 12)	Group 2: breastfed ≤7 days (n = 22)	Group 3: breastfed >7 days (n = 153)
Black	9 (75%)	10 (46%) $\chi^2 = 6.81$, $df = 2$; $p = .03$	57 (37%)
Mean years education	11.3	13.5 F = 10.14, $df = 2$; $p = .0001$	14.9
Mean age	23.3	26.7 F = 4.57, $df = 2$; $p = .01$	27.9
Married	2 (17%)	16 (73%) $\chi^2 = 25.37$, $df = 2$; $p = .001$	124 (81%)
<$10,000 income	6/10 (60%)	3/19 (16%) $\chi^2 = 27.02$, $df = 6$; $p = .001$	15/143 (10%)
First pregnancy	5 (42%)	9 (41%) $\chi^2 = .52$, $df = 2$; $p = .77$	53 (35%)

*See Table 1-7 for explanation.

of the study recommend interventions that focus on prenatal confidence building, early and continuing contact with the newborn, anticipatory guidance before discharge, and early pediatric follow-up (Tables 1-6 and 1-7).

The positive and negative emotional and physical experiences of 152 long-term breastfeeding American and Canadian women were reported by Reamer and Sugarman.[66] This sample of mothers was randomly selected from 1038 women who responded to a 1974 request for volunteers in a La Leche League newsletter. They all answered the eight-page questionnaire, which had 51 short-answer and 52 free-response questions. All the respondents were older, better educated, predominantly white, and had belonged at some time to the league. The average age was 29.4 years, age at first child was 25, 77% had more than one year of college, and 44% had four or more years of college. Far fewer were employed than the national average (13% full or part time vs. 34% nationally). The average weaning age for the 339 children represented by this study was 18 months, with a range of 3 weeks to 5 years. At the time of the study, 136 children were still being breastfed. Two mothers thought there were no positive effects of prolonged nursing on their children, but others gave more than one answer to the question (Table 1-8). Emotional security, happiness, mutual love, and future independence were the key positive outcomes of long-term nursing in the mothers' view. Good health was mentioned by 22%.

When asked to list the negative aspects of nursing longer than 6 months, 47% of mothers said there were none at 6 months, but only 26% of mothers had no negative feelings about nursing past 12 months. Perceived social hostility was the major negative effect, reported by 24% of mothers at 6 months and by 42% at 12 months (Table 1-9). Ninety percent felt there were no negative effects for the children. The social stigma has driven many well-educated, caring, dedicated mothers to conceal nursing, called "closet nursing." Unfortunately, this leads physicians and the public alike to think that breastfeeding in the United States terminates by 6 months of age.[3]

TABLE 1-7   **Probability of early cessation by selected prenatal and postpartum characteristics among women initiating breastfeeding**

	Probability	Odds ratio (95% confidence interval)
Prenatal characteristics		
Confidence in ability		
Low (n = 47)	.28*	5.05 (1.99, 6.42)
High (n = 128)	.07*	
Certainty of decision		
Low (n = 21)	.33†	4.86 (1.68, 14.01)
High (n = 150)	.09†	
Postpartum characteristics		
Timing of first breastfeeding		
Late (n = 92)	.18‡	3.44 (1.21, 9.87)
Early (n = 81)	.06‡	
Baby's daytime location		
Nursery (n = 23)	.26§	3.00 (1.03, 8.71)
Mother's room (n = 152)	.11§	

Modified from Buxton KE, Gielen AC, Faden RR et al: *Am J Prev Med* 7:101, 1991.
Early cessation is defined as breastfeeding for 7 days or less. The confidence scale was dichotomized to reflect less confident (raw scores 1-3) and more confident (raw scores 4-6).
*$\chi^2 = 13.31$, $df = 1$; $p < .001$.
†$\chi^2 = 9.85$, $df = 1$; $p < .01$.
‡$\chi^2 = 5.88$, $df = 1$; $p < .02$.
§$\chi^2 = 4.40$, $df = 1$; $p < .05$.

TABLE 1-8   **Positive consequences of long-term nursing as perceived by the mother**

Perceived consequences	Mothers (n = 130)	%*
Positive emotional effect on child—child is more secure	65	50.0
Better physical health (fewer allergies)	29	22.3
Child is loving, friendly, cheerier	27	20.8
Child can separate more easily—relative independence achieved with less stress	22	16.9
Enhanced maternal sensitivity	19	14.6
Close relationship of mother and child	18	13.8
Positive influence or education for older siblings	11	8.5
Child easily comforted during crisis, pain, or teething	10	8.0
Broad, all-encompassing positive effect	6	4.6
Incidental positive consequences	13	10.4
No positive effects perceived	2	1.5

From Reamer SB, Sugarman M: *J Trop Pediatr* 33:93, 1987.
*Mothers could give multiple responses, thus percentages add to more than 100%.

TABLE 1-9   Mothers' responses to the question "what do you think are the negative aspects of nursing past 6 months (past 1 year)?"

Negative aspects listed by mothers	Past 6 months (total responses = 132)		Past 12 months (total responses = 133)	
	No.	%	No.	%
Mother states there are no negative aspects	62	47.1	35	26.4
Social stigma—negative attitudes of others	32	24.3	56	41.9
Mother's activities are restricted	19	14.7	9	6.6
Baby is less discreet—embarrassing in public	3	2.2	13	9.6
Tiredness	7	5.1	3	2.2
Breastfeeding mother has special concerns	1	0.7	5	3.7
Intrudes upon life with husband	1	0.7	4	2.9
Breast discomfort/leaking, soreness	2	1.5	1	0.7
Sex life interrupted—less interest in sex	2	1.5	2	1.5
Mother believes she should ignore negative aspects	2	1.5	1	0.7
Intrudes upon mother's time with siblings	0	—	1	0.7
Baby care, not nursing, causes negative aspects	0	—	1	0.7

From Reamer SB, Sugarman M: *J Trop Pediatr* 33:93, 1987.

Impact of commercial discharge packs

Several studies have evaluated whether commercial discharge packs result in diminished breastfeeding duration. Unfortunately, none of the studies was so well randomized and controlled that the answer was clear. Those studies that did mention use of bottles in the hospital noted a stronger correlation between bottle use and diminished duration of breastfeeding.[9]

In New York State, regulations regarding breastfeeding support instituted in July 1984, among other things, disallowed discharge packs to breastfeeding women unless requested by the mother or prescribed by the physician. A mother who requests such a pack is usually at high risk for early termination of lactation in most investigators' experience. Giving such a packet to a vulnerable mother (young, less educated, single, poor support system) may be a message not unlike *Parents* magazine circa 1938: "You may be one of them . . . " (i.e., those who fail).[66] In a study in Virginia, Hayden et al[39] reported that most pediatricians did not know and had never been asked if they approved of the discharge packages with

samples of powders, creams, baby food, and other baby items that may or may not be appropriate for indiscriminate use. The authors suggest that pediatricians should investigate and review the procedures in their own hospitals.

Controlling discharge packs deflects attention from the real problem: inadequate counseling about breastfeeding and a system to support the mother who needs it. This point is well illustrated in a study by Feinstein et al,[24] who found that initiating breastfeeding in the first 16 hours and minimizing use of formula in the nursery correlated highly with successful lactation. The negative impact of supplementation could be overcome by frequent breastfeeding at home.

Frank et al[31] found that a gift packet of breast pads and breastfeeding information of equal monetary value to a formula packet, along with a special counselor who made five home visits in the first 28 days and three more in the next 6 weeks, resulted in longer duration of breastfeeding. Howard et al[43] showed that discharge packs did not have the same impact on duration as many other factors, including bottle feeding in the hospital and the mother's original plan about how long she would breastfeed.

A force that is difficult to measure is the public advertising of infant formula, a direct violation of the letter and the intent of the WHO Code (see earlier discussion). Some formula companies have television advertisements that include a subliminal message that their product is equal to breastfeeding, so why bother.[35] Furthermore, when the message says, "Just ask your doctor," it implies that physicians agree. Sending free samples and coupons aimed at the vulnerable woman 2 to 4 weeks postpartum, when she is fatigued and overwhelmed, can undermine the confidence of even a dedicated breastfeeding mother. In addition to the pregnant woman or new mother, the audience consists of the world of television viewers. The daily repetition of the message that bottle feeding is just as good as breastfeeding is cementing the national image that it is "American" to bottle feed.[51]

Young children, adolescents, and new immigrants all are relentlessly receiving the message. The ads are played during programs that attract low-income, less well-educated viewers who are already the least likely to breastfeed. Studies that examine television advertising of breastfeeding have measured the impact of only one viewing of the ad, not the effect of daily repetitions, which, as marketing experts know well, is more important. Greer and Apple[35] note that advertising directly to the public "will once again remove the control of infant feeding from the supervision of the physician and will likely have a negative impact on the incidence and duration of breastfeeding."

Infants in Latin America were less likely to be breastfed than infants in Africa and Asia, and the duration was 6 months compared with 12 months or more in Asia and Africa.[34] A significant increase in the Latin American rates resulted after an aggressive breastfeeding promotion program (PROALMA) was initiated and supported by the various governments.[62,63]

A study of attitudes toward breastfeeding and infant feeding among Iranian, Afghan, and Southeast Asian immigrant women in the United States reported that women discontinue breastfeeding to

return to work because (1) economics is important, (2) the workplace is hostile to nursing mothers, and (3) there is little or no maternity leave.[34] The author recommends that (1) health care workers should have greater sensitivity to cultural barriers, (2) adult language school programs coordinate infant nutrition programs with WIC, (3) workplaces encourage breastfeeding, and (4) American social customs recognize breastfeeding as normal.[34]

In an effort to identify the "real" reason women stopped breastfeeding, Ferris et al[25] followed more than 250 women who delivered in Connecticut. They tried to identify crucial biologic and sociocultural links in the chain of events that precede the change in feeding from breast to bottle.

Hospital routines influenced the early "failures." Successful breastfeeders experienced milk let-down a full day sooner than those who discontinued by 2 weeks. They had also fed their infant 5 hours earlier than those who discontinued. Mothers who nursed early had prepared themselves to insist on early feeding. Mothers who were unsure and lacked confidence turned to supplements. Providing just 1 ounce of formula per day led to ultimate discontinuation.[52] A small amount of doubt eroded confidence. The most vulnerable time was the immediate postpartum period. Women who had wanted to lose weight postpartum were disappointed that they did not lose more rapidly. The authors also identified the need for close follow-up by the pediatrician in these critical 2 weeks[25] (Table 1-10).

Attitudes of health care professionals

A 1980 survey of physicians' and nurses' medical and educational practices regarding breastfeeding was published when breastfeeding was at its zenith. A follow-up survey was completed in the summer of 1991, after several years of decline. A comparison of the results of these two surveys showed little change in the current practices of health professionals regarding breastfeeding, their attitudes toward breastfeeding, and who among them they believed to be primarily responsible for managing breastfeeding and supporting the breastfeeding mother.

TABLE 1-10	Sources of advice on breastfeeding: comparison of intent vs. action			
	Intent: at 1 week postpartum, mothers were asked:		**Action: at 10 weeks, mothers were asked:**	
Source of advice	**(1) If you have a problem with nursing, whom will you call? (n = 113)**	**(2) If you have already had a problem, whom did you call? (n = 19)**	**(1) If you had a problem with nursing, and continued nursing, whom did you go to for advice? (n = 23)**	**(2) If you stopped nursing, whom did you go to for advice? (n = 26)**
	%			
Pediatrician	36	32	65	46
Support group	24	32	5	0
Family	12	5	4	0
Friends	10	5	0	0
Obstetrician/gynecologist	6	5	0	4
Nurse/midwife	6	21	9	0
No one	0	0	17	50
Do not know	3	0	—	—

From Ferris AM, McCabe LT, Allen LH et al: *J Am Diet Assoc* 87:316, 1987.

Regarding responsibility for managing breastfeeding mothers and infants, more than 80% of pediatricians believed that medical encouragement or support of breastfeeding was primarily a responsibility of the infant's physician. Approximately two thirds of family practitioners thought that both the mother's physician and the infant's physician were responsible.

The respondents viewed mother's employment as the main reason for the decline in breastfeeding.[51]

MORBIDITY AND MORTALITY STUDIES IN BREASTFED AND ARTIFICIALLY FED INFANTS

Assessing the mortality of breastfed infants compared with bottle-fed infants is difficult today because many breastfed infants also receive supplements of formula and solid foods. The risk of death in the first year of life diminished in civilized countries in the twentieth century since the advent of antibiotics and many other advances in pediatric care.[77] Data from previous decades and other nations do show a significant difference, however.[36,37] Knodel[47] presented a complete table, including rates from cities in Germany, France, England, Holland, and the United States (Table 1-11). Mortality among breastfed infants is clearly lower than that among bottle-fed infants. Knodel pointed out that early neonatal deaths, in the first week or so of life, were excluded.

Woodbury[88] reported the trends in infant feeding (Fig. 1-9) and in another study in 1922 reported mortality of infants by type of feeding. Mortality is lower at all ages for breastfed infants. Overwhelming evidence of the impact of human milk on mortality is displayed in the widely publicized statistics currently available on Third World countries, where infant formulas are rapidly replacing human milk. The death rate is higher, malnutrition starts earlier and is more severe, and the incidence of infection is greater in formula-fed infants (Figs. 1-10 and 1-11). Data from the work of Scrimshaw et al[76] show mortality of 950 of 1000 live births in artificially fed infants and 120 of 1000 in breastfed infants. The data were collected in Punjab villages from 1955 through 1959. The deaths were predominantly caused by diarrheal disease. The Pan

TABLE 1-11 Mortality rates and survivorship to age 1 year in breastfed and artificially fed infants*

Study area	Date	Mortality (per 1000)		Survivors to age 1 yr (per 1000)		
		Breastfed	Artificially fed	Breastfed	Artificially fed	Difference
Berlin, Germany	1895-1896	57	376	943	624	319
Bremen, Germany	1905	68	379	932	621	311
Hanover, Germany	1912	96	296	904	704	200
Boston, Mass.	1911	30	212	970	788	182
Eight U.S. cities†	1911-1916	76	255	924	745	179
Paris, France	1900	140	310	860	690	170
Cologne, Germany	1908-1909	73	241	927	759	168
Amsterdam, Holland	1904	144	304	856	696	160
Liverpool, England	1905	84	134	916	866	144
Eight U.S. cities‡	1911-1916	76	215	924	785	139
Derby, England	1900-1903	70	198	930	802	128
Chicago, Ill.	1924-1929	2	84	998	916	82
Liverpool, England	1936-1942	10	57	990	943	47
Great Britain	1946-1947	9	18	991	982	9

From Knodel J: *Science* 198:1111, 1977. Copyright 1977 by the American Association for the Advancement of Science.
*Most of these rates do not include deaths in the first few days or weeks of life; mortality is therefore underestimated and survival overestimated. Only the rates for the eight U.S. cities in 1911-1916 represent mortality from birth; deaths that occurred before any feeding are proportionately allocated to the two feeding categories. The rates for Berlin, Bremen, Hanover, Cologne, and the eight U.S. cities were derived by applying life table techniques to mortality given by single months of age.
†Comparison of breastfed infants with infants artificially fed from birth.
‡Comparison of breastfed infants with all infants artificially fed in the period of observation.

American Health Organization has reported similar correlations among malnutrition, infection, and mortality. In Puffer and Serrano's[64] 1973 work in São Paulo, death rates among breastfed infants and proportions from diarrheal disease and malnutrition were also lower than among bottle-fed infants.

The incidence of illness or morbidity among artificially fed infants in Third World countries is as dramatic as the mortality. Kanaaneh's[45] observations in Arab villages in Israel showed hospitalization rates vary with method of feeding. Only 0.5% of breastfed infants required hospitalization, whereas infants fed more than 3 months but less than 6 months at the breast had a 2.9% hospitalization rate, and infants who were bottle fed had a 24.8% rate. This is a fiftyfold difference.

There is a bias against bottle feeding as sicker, smaller infants are bottle fed. Infants who die are weaned early by death. The benefits of breastfeed-

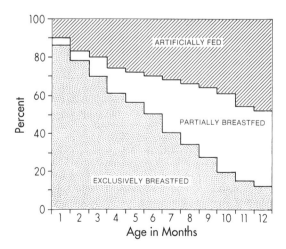

Fig. 1-9. Percentage of infants who were breastfed, partially breastfed, and artificially fed by age in months. (Modified from Woodbury RM: *Am J Hyg* 2:668, 1922.)

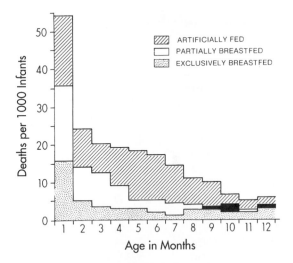

Fig. 1-10. Death rate per 100 infants by type of feeding and age in months. (Modified from Woodbury RM: *Am J Hyg* 2:668, 1922.)

ing are enhanced by these confounding variables. Habicht et al[38] point out that had there been no breastfeeding in the sample, twice as many infants would have died after the first week of life. In 1968, Lee Forrest Hill[40] articulated what many physicians have believed: "Formula feeding has become so simple, safe, uniformly successful that breastfeeding no longer seems worth the bother." This ignores the protective qualities of human milk, not only in the Third World but in industrialized nations as well. It neglects the immunologic protection.

Evidence for protection by breastfeeding against infant death from infectious diseases in Brazil in 1987 is even more persuasive, as noted in a carefully controlled study by Victora et al.[81,82] Compared with infants who were breastfed without supplementation, those who were completely bottle fed had a 14.2 greater risk of death from diarrhea and 3.6 greater risk of death from respiratory infection. Partial breastfeeding was less protective. Formula and cow's milk were equally hazardous. The greatest risk from diarrhea was in the first 2 months of life. Barros et al[6] note that birthweight influences breastfeeding and that small infants tend to be weaned sooner.

Demonstrating the differences in morbidity between breastfed and bottle-fed infants has become even more complex in industrialized countries since the resurgence of breastfeeding. Among the confounding variables are the inherent differences between mothers who choose to breastfeed and those who choose to bottle feed.[75] Although many investigators have recognized the necessity of controlling these variables, none has succeeded totally because an unavoidable factor of self-selection makes random assignment of infants impossible.[23] There is a one-way flow of infants from the breastfed group to the bottle-fed group, because a baby may change from breast to bottle but rarely from bottle to breast. Documenting breastfeeding practices is difficult when the possibility exists that some bottle feedings are included or that solid foods have been introduced.

Investigators[45,62,64,82] have reported differences between breastfed and bottle-fed infants in the incidence of morbidity associated with diarrhea, respiratory infections, otitis media, and pneumonia; they have also compared breastfed and bottle-fed infants seen in clinics and emergency rooms or hospitalized in the first year of life. This extensive material has been reviewed by Cunningham.[15-17] The majority of reports demonstrate a significant advantage for the breastfed group. The relationship between breastfeeding or bottle feeding and respiratory illness in the first year of life among nearly 2000 cohort children was reported by Watkins et al[83] in England. There was a significant advantage to breastfeeding. Mothers who smoked were less likely to breastfeed, but even when smoking was considered, the breastfeeding advantage remained. Young et al[93] reported on 1000 infants in the Yale Harvard Research Project in Tunisia who were followed from birth to 26 months and found breastfed infants had fewer infections, illnesses, and allergies.

Victora et al[81,82] investigated 127 respiratory deaths in the first year of life in Brazil in 1985. Having controlled for prematurity, congenital malformation, and socioeconomic factors, the researchers believed that 82 of the deaths could be attributed to feeding method (i.e., lack of breast-

THE MESSAGE ON BREAST-FEEDING ISN'T NEW

Fig. 1-11. "Value of Natural Feeding" poster used in 1918 to educate parents. Text explains that mortality of bottle-fed infants (Flaschenkinder) is seven times higher than that of breastfed infants (Brustkinder). (From Langstein R: *Atlas der Hygiene des Sauglings und Kleinkindes,* Berlin, 1918, Springer-Verlag.)

feeding). A number of well-controlled studies of industrialized countries in the past 15 years have shown at least a twofold relative risk of respiratory infection with bottle feeding and that the infections breastfed infants do experience are usually less severe.[44]

When Victora[80] presented his studies of the impact of early weaning on infection and disease at a workshop held by the Pontifical Academy of Sciences and The Royal Society, he stated that a 40% reduction in nonbreastfeeding would prevent up to 15% of diarrhea deaths and 7% of pneumonia deaths. He noted that even the introduction of water or herbal teas to a previously exclusively breastfed infant increases morbidity and mortality. Figures 1-12 and 1-13 illustrate the relative risks of pneumonia and otitis media.

Cunningham[15,16] undertook a study in rural upstate New York to determine the impact of feeding on infant health. Of 326 infants studied, 162 were fed proprietary formula and 164 were breastfed at birth, with only 4% still breastfed at 1 year. Breastfeeding was associated with significantly less illness during the first year of life. The protection was greatest during the early months, increased with the duration of breastfeeding, and appeared more striking for serious illness (Tables 1-12 and 1-13). Breastfeeding was associated with a higher level of parental education, but controlling for that factor, the difference in morbidity is even more significant.[80]

In the United States, diarrheal disease is uncommon in breastfed infants, and the treatment is usually to continue to breastfeed. Similarly, breast-

Fig. 1-12. Risk of pneumonia (odds ratio for incidence) in children under 2 years of age at two Brazilian sites, Porto Algere and Fortaleza, in 1993-1995 according to type of milk. (Modified from Victora CG: *Food Nutr Bull* 17:390, 1996.)

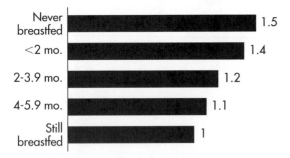

Fig. 1-13. Risk of otitis media (odds ratio for incidence in last month) in infants 6 months of age in Brazil in 1993-1994 according to duration of breastfeeding. (Modified from Victoria CG: *Food Nutr Bull* 17:390, 1996.)

TABLE 1-12   **Significant episodes of illness according to feeding mode at onset of illness (Cooperstown, NY)**

Illness	Breast	Artificial
Otitis media	3.7*	9.1
Lower respiratory infection	1.1	5.6
Diarrhea, vomiting	3.5	6.9
Hospital admissions	1.0	3.0
Total episodes of illness	8.2	21.1

From Cunningham AS: Breastfeeding and morbidity in industrialized countries: an update. In Jelliffe DB, Jelliffe EFP, editors: *Advances in international maternal and child health,* vol 1, Oxford, 1981, Oxford University Press.
*Episodes per 1000 patient weeks.

TABLE 1-13   **Significant episodes of illness, regardless of feeding mode at onset of illness (Cooperstown, NY)**

Months of life	Breastfed	Limited breast	Artificially fed
1-2	0.7*	3.8	11.8
3-4	5.9	11.3	16.0
5-6	7.4	20.0	20.5
7-8	18.5	16.3	21.5
9-10	14.1	22.5	21.2
11-12	11.9	20.0	19.8
First year	58.5	93.8	110.8

From Cunningham AS: Breastfeeding and morbidity in industrialized countries: an update. In Jelliffe DB, Jelliffe EFP, editors: *Advances in international maternal and child health,* vol 1, Oxford, 1981, Oxford University Press.
*Episodes per 100 patients.

---

fed infants have fewer episodes of respiratory illness and otitis media. When afflicted with such febrile illnesses, the breastfed infant does not become dehydrated and rapidly toxic.[23]

The issue is not as clear in Western countries because of the associated variables among bottle feeders, that is, young mothers with low socioeconomic status and less education and small, sick infants who are more likely to be bottle fed.

Despite the clear-cut data on mortality and morbidity from past generations and from cultures seemingly remote from industrialized and medically sophisticated societies, pediatricians had discounted any but the psychologic advantages of breastfeeding.[7] The current increase in illness in young infants in day-care centers is providing a new study group. To date, breastfeeding appears to be protective for the few

TABLE 1-14 **Percentage of babies with gastrointestinal illness up to 1 year of age according to duration of breastfeeding***

| Age of baby (weeks) | Duration of breastfeeding (full and partial) | | | | | | χ^2 | |
	Never (n = 246)	1-13 weeks (n = 164)	14-26 weeks (n = 49)	27-39 weeks (n = 71)	40-52 weeks (n = 60)	>52 weeks (n = 30)	Never vs. 1-13 weeks	Never vs. 14-52 weeks
0-13	15.7	16.6	2.2	3.5	6.3	7.7	0.06	11.02§
14-26	18.0	20.3	8.6	9.1	7.2	3.5	0.32	8.06‡
27-39	21.6	21.0	13.7	13.4	16.0	7.4	0.02	4.03‡
40-52	22.3	12.7	7.9	14.2	11.7	13.4	6.02†	6.70‡

From Forsyth JS: *Eur J Clin Nutr* 46(suppl 1):S19, 1992.
*Adjusted for social class, maternal age, and parental smoking.
†$p < .05$.
‡$p < .01$.
§$p < .001$.

children whose mothers continue to nurse them while in day care.

In a study in Scotland, Forsyth[30] confirmed that breastfeeding during the first 3 months (13 weeks) of life confers protection against gastrointestinal disease that persists beyond the period of breastfeeding (Table 1-14). There was a significant reduction in hospitalization in breastfed infants and a smaller but significant reduction in respiratory illness until 40 to 52 weeks of age. These data parallel the global epidemiologic review by Cunningham et al[18] that breastfeeding reduces illness in early life. Thus Forsyth[30] concludes that the answer to the question, "Is it worthwhile breastfeeding?" is a resounding *"yes!"*

SUDDEN INFANT DEATH SYNDROME AND OTHER ISSUES

Recent interest in sudden infant death syndrome (SIDS) has generated several studies investigating the position in which the infant is put down in the crib and SIDS.[22,57] The New Zealand Cot Death Study showed the prone sleeping position to be a greater risk, but not greater than the risk of not being breastfed.[57] Other investigators have shown the importance of breastfeeding as a risk-lowering factor.[22] Although breastfeeding does not eliminate SIDS, its incidence is lower among breastfed infants.

No single consistent factor has been a predictor of SIDS.[22] Prone sleeping has continued to be a cofactor in continued studies, but maternal smoking is a relative causative factor as well. Breastfeeding has shown the strongest protection. Infants of smokers who breastfeed and sleep supine have a reduced risk of SIDS. Several studies confirm a reduced risk while breastfeeding, and one study links the effect to a dose response of the amount of breastfeeding. The National Maternal and Infant Health Survey of 10,000 births and 6000 deaths of infants born in 1988 and 1989 was analyzed using a consistent "dosage definition" of breastfeeding while controlling for major confounding factors. These factors included birthweight; maternal age, race, and education; smoking; prenatal cocaine use; lack of private insurance; household smoking; daycare; and household size. In 7102 controls, 499 SIDS deaths and 584 non-SIDS deaths occurred. Fredrickson et al[32] reported that "the risk of SIDS for black infants increased by 1.19 for every month of not breastfeeding, and 2.13 for every month of not exclusively breastfeeding. Among white infants, the risk increased by 1.19 and 2.0 times, respectively. These associations remained even when deaths within the first month of life were excluded. A similar protective association existed for non-SIDS deaths."

Sleep patterns of infants have been the subject of much study.[20] In the early weeks of life, infants have REM (rapid eye movement) sleep, active body movements, and rapid, irregular heart and respiratory rates. At about 2 to 3 months of age they begin to increase the proportion of quiet sleep, which coincides with the peak incidence of SIDS. When breastfeeding decreased, the advantage of co-sleeping seemed to diminish. Child care became very organized and focused on encouraging the infant to sleep alone and through the night. Only in about the last century have Western industrialized societies considered breastfeeding and infant sleep location to be separate issues. McKenna and Bernstraw[55] and Mosko[56] describe the physiologic benefits to infants sleeping in proximity to their caregivers. They have documented the physiologic changes infants experience as they move from a solitary sleep environment to co-sleeping. They monitored a group of mother-infant pairs in the sleep laboratory, using each pair as their own control (i.e., co-sleeping and sleeping separately). Infants moved from one stage of sleep to the other more frequently when co-sleeping than when sleeping alone, even when briefly waking and increasing their heart and respiratory rates. The authors comment that modern technology, including baby monitors, breathing teddy bears, and other gadgets, has replaced traditional co-sleeping.[56]

THE MAMMARY GLAND AND SCIENCE

Newer additions to the laboratory have permitted rapid advances in the understanding of the mammary gland, especially actions of hormones and enzymes. The "knock-out mouse" is a concept using mice whose DNA (deoxyribonucleic acid) has been altered to "knock out" a specific gene that controls a specific hormone, such as one important to lactation. Observations of growth and development in these animals provide new insights into the physiology of the mammary gland. In evolutionary biology, lactogenesis is one of the most important functions for the survival of the species. Advances in molecular biology have provided biologists with a better understanding of the mechanisms that produce milk and its specific nutrient constituents. Mammary epithelial cells secrete milk. In an innovative experimental model, mammary epithelial cells are cultured in a petri dish and form a *mammosphere*, a micromodel of the mammary gland. The advantage of bioengineering the mammary gland, initially focused on the dairy species, is to advance our knowledge and understanding of human lactation in the laboratory so that more women may nurse their infants successfully.[69]

SUPPORT FOR THE BREASTFEEDING WOMEN OF THE WORLD

On May 12, 1995, His Holiness John Paul II granted a Solemn Papal Audience in the Apostolic Palace of the Vatican to the participants of the Working Group on "Breastfeeding: Science and Society." In response to the group report, the Holy Father pronounced the following discourse (in part)[61]:

> . . . The advantages of breastfeeding for the infant and the mother . . . include two major benefits to the child: protection against disease and proper nourishment. . . . This natural way of feeding can create a bond of love and security between mother and child and enable the child to assert its presence as a person through interaction with the mother. . . . Responsible international agencies are calling on governments to ensure that women are enabled to breastfeed their children for four to six months from birth and to continue this practice, supplemented by other appropriate foods, up to the second year of life and beyond.

REFERENCES

1. Andrew EM, Clancy KL, Katz MG: Infant feeding practices of families belonging to a prepaid group practice health care plan, *Pediatrics* 65:978, 1980.
2. Apple RD: *Mothers & medicine: a social history of infant feeding, 1890-1950,* Madison, 1987, University of Wisconsin Press.
3. Auerbach K: To breastfeed or not to breastfeed, *Keeping Abreast J* 1:316, 1976.
4. Baer EC: Promoting breastfeeding: a national responsibility, *Stud Fam Plan* 12:198, 1981.
5. Baghurst KI: Infant feeding: public health perspectives, *Med J Aust* 148:112, 1988.
6. Barros FC, Victora CG, Vaughn JP et al: Birthweight and duration of breastfeeding: are the beneficial effects of human milk being overestimated? *Pediatrics* 78:656, 1986.
7. Bauchner H, Leventhal JM, Shapiro ED: Studies of breastfeeding and infections: how good is the evidence? *JAMA* 256:887, 1986.
8. Baumslag N, Michels DL: *Milk, money and madness,* Westport, Conn, 1995, Bergin & Garvey.
9. Bergevin Y, Dougherty C, Kramer MS: Do formula samples shorten the duration of breastfeeding? *Lancet* 1:1148, 1983.
10. Bryant CA: The impact of kin, friend, and neighbor networks on infant feeding practices, *Soc Sci Med* 16:1757, 1982.
11. Buxton KE, Gielen AC, Faden RR et al: Women intending to breastfeed: predictors of early infant feeding experiences, *Am J Prev Med* 7:101, 1991.
12. Carroll EGC: Home from the hospital, *Parents* 13:22, 52, 1938.
13. Cole JP: Breastfeeding in Boston suburbs in relation to personal-social factors, *Clin Pediatr* 16:352, 1977.
14. Commonwealth Department of Health: Towards better nutrition for Australians, Report of the Nutrition Taskforce of the Better Health Commission, Canberra, AGPS, 1987 (catalogue no 86-1660).
15. Cunningham AS: Breastfeeding and health, *J Pediatr* 110:658, 1987.
16. Cunningham AS: Breastfeeding and illness, *Pediatrics* 73:416, 1984.
17. Cunningham AS: Breastfeeding and morbidity in industrialized countries: an update. In Jelliffe DB, Jelliffe EFP, editors: *Advances in international maternal and child health,* vol 1, Oxford, 1981, Oxford University Press.
18. Cunningham AS, Jelliffe DB, Jelliffe EFP: Breastfeeding and health in the 1980's: a global epidemiologic review, *J Pediatr* 118:659, 1991.
19. Deem H, McGeorge M: Breastfeeding, *N Z Med J* 57:539, 1958.
20. Dettwyler KA: Beauty and the breast: the cultural context of breastfeeding in the United States. In Stuart-Macadam P, Dettwyler KA, editors: *Breastfeeding: biocultural perspectives,* Hawthorne, NY, 1995, Aldine de Gruyter.
21. Drake TGH: Infant welfare laws in France in the 18th century, *Ann Med Hist* 7:49, 1935.
22. Dumas K, Pakter J, Krongrad E et al: Postnatal medical and epidemiological risk factors for the sudden infant death syndrome. In Harper RM, Hoffman HJ, editors: *Sudden infant death syndrome,* New York, 1988, PMA.
23. Fallot ME, Boyd JL, Oski FA: Breastfeeding reduces incidence of hospital admissions for infections in infants, *Pediatrics* 65:1121, 1980.
24. Feinstein JM, Berkelhamer JE, Gruszka ME et al: Factors related to early termination of breastfeeding in an urban population, *Pediatrics* 78:210, 1986.
25. Ferris AM, McCabe LT, Allen LH et al: Biological and sociocultural determinants of successful lactation among women in eastern Connecticut, *J Am Diet Assoc* 87:316, 1987.
26. Fildes V: *Breast, bottles, and babies,* Edinburgh, 1986, Edinburgh University Press.
27. Ford CS: *A comparative study of human reproduction,* Anthropology Pub No 32, New Haven, Conn, 1945, Yale University Press.
28. Forman MR, Fetterly K, Graubard BI: Exclusive breast-feeding of newborns among married women in the United States: the National Natality Surveys of 1969 and 1980, *Am J Clin Nutr* 42:864, 1985.
29. Forman MR, Graubard BI, Hoffmann HJ et al: The PIMA infant feeding study: breastfeeding and gastroenteritis in the first year of life, *Am J Epidemiol* 119:335, 1984.
30. Forsyth JS: It is worthwhile breastfeeding? *Eur J Clin Nutr* 46(suppl 1):S19, 1992.
31. Frank DA, Wirtz SJ, Sorenson JR et al: Commercial discharge packs and breastfeeding counseling: effects on infant-feeding practices in a randomized trial, *Pediatrics* 80:845, 1987.
32. Fredrickson DD, Sorenson JR, Biddle AK et al: Relationship of sudden infant death syndrome to breast-feeding duration and intensity, *Am J Dis Child* 147:460, 1993.
33. Gabriel A, Gabriel KR, Lawrence RA: Cultural values and biomedical knowledge: choices in infant feeding, *Soc Sci Med* 23:501, 1986.
34. Ghaemi-Ahmadi S: Attitudes toward breastfeeding and infant feeding among Iranian, Afghan, and South East Asian immigrant women in the United States: implications for health and nutrition education, *J Am Diet Assoc* 92:354, 1992.

35. Greer FR, Apple RD: Physicians, formula companies and advertising: a historical perspective, *Am J Dis Child* 145:282, 1991.

36. Grulee CG, Sanford HN, Herron PH: Breast and artificial feeding, *JAMA* 103:735, 1934.

37. Grulee CG, Sanford HN, Schwartz H: Breast and artificially fed infants, *JAMA* 104:1986, 1935.

38. Habicht JP, DaVanzo J, Butz WP: Does breastfeeding really save lives or are apparent benefits due to biases? *Am J Epidemiol* 123:279, 1986.

39. Hayden GF, Nowacek GA, Koch W et al: Providing free samples of baby items to newly delivered parents, *Clin Pediatr* 26:111, 1987.

40. Hill LF: A salute to La Leche League International, *J Pediatr* 73:161, 1968.

41. House JS, Landis KR, Umberson D: Social relationships and health, *Science* 241:540, 1988.

42. Houston MJ, Howie PW, Smart L et al: Factors affecting the duration of breastfeeding: early feeding practices and social class, *Early Hum Dev* 8:55, 1983.

43. Howard CR, Howard FM, Weitzman MD et al: Antenatal formula advertising: another potential threat to breastfeeding, *Pediatrics* 94:102, 1994.

44. Howie PW, Forsyth JS, Ogston SA et al: Protective effect of breastfeeding against infection, *Br Med J* 300:11, 1990.

45. Kanaaneh H: The relationship of bottle feeding to malnutrition and gastroenteritis in a preindustrial setting, *J Trop Pediatr* 18:302, 1972.

46. Konner M: The nursing knot, *Sciences* 25:10, 1985.

47. Knodel J: Breast feeding and population growth, *Science* 198:1111, 1977.

48. Krieger FW: A review of breastfeeding trends. Presented at the Editor's Conference, New York, September 1992.

49. Labbok M, Krasovec K: Toward consistency in breastfeeding definitions, *Stud Fam Plan* 21:226, 1990.

50. Launer LJ, Forman MR, Hundt GL et al: Maternal recall of infant feeding events is accurate, *J Epidemiol Community Health* 46:203, 1992.

51. Lawrence RA: Choosing to breastfeed: a national challenge. Will it become American to breastfeed? *Birth* 18:226, 1991.

52. Loughlin HH, Clapp-Channing NE, Gehlbach SH et al: Early termination of breastfeeding: identifying those at risk, *Pediatrics* 75:508, 1985.

53. Martinez GA, Dodd DA: 1981 milk feeding patterns in the United States during the first 12 months of life, *Pediatrics* 71:166, 1983.

54. Martinez GA, Stahl DA: The recent trend in milk feeding among WIC infants, *Am J Pub Health* 72:68, 1982.

55. McKenna JJ, Bernstraw NJ: Breastfeeding and infant-parent co-sleeping as adaptive strategies: are they protective against SIDS? In Stuart-Macadam P, Dettwyler KA, editors: *Breastfeeding: biocultural perspectives,* Hawthorne, NY, 1995, Aldine De Gruyter.

56. McKenna JJ, Mosko S: Evolution and infant sleep: an experimental study of infant-parent co-sleeping and its implications for SIDS, *Acta Paediatr Suppl* 389:31, 1993.

57. Mitchell EA, Scragg R, Stewart AW et al: Cot Death Supplement: results from the first year of the New Zealand Cot Death Study, *N Z Med J* 104:71, 1991.

58. Montgomery DL, Splett PL: Economic benefit of breastfeeding infants enrolled in WIC, *J Am Diet Assoc* 97:379, 1997.

59. Mother's Survey, Updated breast-feeding trend through 1996, Ross Products Division, Abbott Laboratories, Columbus, Ohio, 1998.

60. Newton N: Psychologic differences between breast and bottle feeding. In Jelliffe DB, Jelliffe EFP, editors: Symposium: the uniqueness of human milk, *Am J Clin Nutr* 24:993, 1971.

61. Pope John Paul II, Solemn Papal Audience: Breastfeeding: science and society, *Food Nutr Bull* 17:289, 1996.

62. Popkin BM, Bilsborrow RE, Akin JS: Breastfeeding patterns in low-income countries, *Science* 218:1088, 1982.

63. Popkin BM, Canahauti J, Bailey PE et al: An evaluation of a national breastfeeding promotion programme in Honduras, *J Biosoc Sci* 23:5, 1991.

64. Puffer RR, Serrano CV: *Patterns of mortality in childhood,* Scientific Pub No 262, Washington, DC, 1973, Pan American Health Organization.

65. Raphael D: *The tender gift: breast feeding,* New York, 1976, Schocken.

66. Reamer SB, Sugarman M: Breastfeeding beyond six months: mothers' perceptions of the positive and negative consequences, *J Trop Pediatr* 33:93, 1987.

67. *Report of the Surgeon General's Workshop on Breastfeeding and Human Lactation,* Pub No HRS-D-MC 84-2, Department of Health and Human Services, 1984.

68. *Report of the Second Surgeon General's Workshop on Breastfeeding and Human Lactation,* Washington, DC, National Center for Education in Maternal and Child Health, 1991.

69. Romagnob D, DiAugustine RP: The mammary gland: protein factory of the future, *Environ Health Perspect* 102:644, 1994.

70. Ruvalcaba RHA: Stress-induced cessation of lactation, *West J Med* 146:228, 1987.

71. Ryan AS: The resurgence of breastfeeding in the United States, *Pediatrics* 99(4):2, 1997 (electronic article).

72. Ryan AS, Martinez GA: Breastfeeding and the working mother: a profile, *Pediatrics* 83:524, 1989.

73. Ryan AS, Rush D, Krieger FW et al: Recent declines in breastfeeding in the United States, 1984 through 1989, *Pediatrics* 88:719, 1991.

74. Sarett HP, Bain KR, O'Leary JC: Decisions on breastfeeding or formula feeding and trends in infant-feeding practices, *Am J Dis Child* 137:719, 1983.

75. Sauls HS: Potential effects of demographic and other variables in studies comparing morbidity of breast-fed and bottle-fed infants, *Pediatrics* 64:523, 1979.

76. Scrimshaw NS, Taylor CE, Gordon JE: Interaction of nutrition and infection, *WHO Monograph,* No 29, Geneva, 1968, World Health Organization.

77. Sloper K, McKean L, Baum JD: Patterns of infant feeding in Oxford, *Arch Dis Child* 49:749, 1974.

78. Taylor J: The duty of nursing children. In Ratner H: The nursing mother: historical insights from art and theology, *Child Fam* 8(4):19, 1949.

79. Toubas PL: Forgotten lessons of the past, *Pierre Budin Perinatal Section News* 17:2, 1992.

80. Victora CG: Infection and disease: the impact of early weaning, *Food Nutr Bull* 17:390, 1996.

81. Victora CG, Smith PG, Barros FC et al: Risk factors for death due to respiratory infections among Brazilian infants, *Int J Epidemiol* 18:918, 1989.

82. Victora CG, Smith PG, Vaughan JP et al: Evidence for protection by breastfeeding against infant deaths from infectious diseases in Brazil, *Lancet* 2:319, 1987.

83. Watkins CJ, Leeder SR, Corkhill RT: The relationship between breast and bottle feeding and respiratory illness in the first year of life, *J Epidemiol Community Health* 33:180, 1979.

84. West CP: Factors influencing the duration of breastfeeding, *J Biosoc Sci* 12:325, 1980.

85. WHO/UNICEF: Protecting, promoting and supporting breastfeeding: the special role of maternity services, a joint WHO/UNICEF statement, Geneva, 1989, World Health Organization.

86. Wickes IG: A history of infant feeding. I. Primitive peoples, ancient works, Renaissance writers, *Arch Dis Child* 28:151, 1953.

87. Wickes IG: A history of infant feeding. II. Seventeenth and eighteenth centuries, *Arch Dis Child* 28:232, 1953.

88. Woodbury RM: The relation between breast and artificial feeding and infant mortality, *Am J Hyg* 2:668, 1922.

89. Woo-Iun M, Gussler J, Smith N, editors: *The international breast-feeding compendium,* ed 3, Columbus, Ohio, 1984, Ross Laboratories.

90. World Health Organization: Contemporary patterns of breast-feeding. In *Report on the WHO Collaborative Study on Breast-feeding,* Geneva, 1981, World Health Organization.

91. Wright AL, Holberg C, Taussig LM et al: Infant-feeding practices among middle-class Anglos and Hispanics, *Pediatrics* 82:496, 1988.

92. Yalom M: *A history of the breast,* New York, 1997, Knopf.

93. Young HB, Buckley AE, Hamza B et al: Milk and lactation: some social and developmental correlates among 1,000 infants, *Pediatrics* 69:169, 1982.

$\mathscr{A}$natomy of the human breast

GROSS ANATOMY

The *mammary gland,* as the breast is medically termed, received its name from *mamma,* the Latin word for breast. The human mammary gland is the only organ that is not fully developed at birth. It experiences dramatic changes in size, shape, and function from birth through pregnancy, lactation, and ultimately involution. The gland undergoes three major phases of growth and development before pregnancy and lactation: in utero, during the first 2 years of life, and at puberty.

Embryonic development

The milk streak appears in the fourth week, when the embryo is 2.5 mm long. It becomes the milk line, or ridge, during the fifth week (2.5 to 5.5 mm). Mammary glands begin to develop in the 6-week-old embryo, continuing their proliferation until milk ducts are developed by the time of birth[33] (Table 2-1). Embryologically, the mammary glands develop as ingrowths of the ectoderm into the underlying mesodermal tissue.[15] In the human embryo a thickened, raised area of the ectoderm can be recognized in the region of the future gland at the end of the fourth week of pregnancy. The thickened ectoderm becomes depressed into the underlying mesoderm, and thus the surface of the mammary area soon becomes flat and finally sinks below the level of the surrounding epidermis. The mesoderm in contact with the ingrowth of the ectoderm is compressed, and its elements become arranged in concentric layers, which at a later stage give rise to the gland's stroma. The ingrowing mass of ectodermal cells soon becomes flask shaped and then grows out into the surrounding mesoderm as a number of solid processes that represent the gland's future ducts. These processes, by dividing and branching, give rise to the future lobes and lobules and, much later, to the alveoli.

By 16 weeks' gestation, the branching stage has produced 15 to 25 epithelial strips that represent future secretory alveoli. At this time the secondary mammary anlage (primordium) develops. Elements of hair follicles, sebaceous glands, and sweat glands develop, as well as the Montgomery glands around the alveoli. Thus far, development is independent of hormone stimulation. By 28 weeks' gestation, placental sex hormones enter the fetal circulation and induce canalization.[19]

The lumina develop in the outgrowths, forming the lactiferous ducts and their branches. The lactiferous ducts open into a shallow epithelial depression known as the *mammary pit.* The pit becomes elevated as a result of the mesenchymal proliferation forming the nipple and areola. An inverted nipple is the failure of the pit to elevate.[3] A lumen is formed in each part of the branching system of cellular processes after 32 weeks' gestation. Near term, about 15 to 25 mammary ducts form the fetal mammary gland (Fig. 2-1).

Age of embryo (wk)	Crown-rump length of embryo (mean)	Developmental stage
		TABLE 2-1 Embryonic timetable of breast development in the human
4	2.5 mm	Mammary streak
5	2.5-5.5 mm	Milk line, or milk ridge
6	5.5-11 mm	Parenchymal cells proliferate
7-8	11-25 mm	Mammary disk progresses to globular stage
9	25-30 mm	Cone stage: inward growth of parenchyma
10-12	30-68 mm	Epithelial buds sprout from invading parenchyma
12-13	68 mm-5 cm	Indentation buds become lobular with notching at epithelial-stromal border
15	10 cm	Buds branch into 15-25 epithelial strips
20-24	20 cm	Solid cords canalize by desquamation and lysis
24-32	30 cm	Further canalization
32-40	35-50 cm	Lobular-alveolar development

Data from Russo J, Russo IH: Development of the human mammary gland. In Neville MC, Daniel CW, editors: *The mammary gland,* New York, 1987, Plenum.

Fetal and prepubertal development

The mammary glands of male and female fetuses of 13 to 40 weeks' gestation were studied ultrastructurally by Tobon and Salazar.[29] This work confirms morphologic developments in the fetal breast tissue in response to hormonal stimuli that are similar to those in the maternal breast. The Golgi system and abundant reticula with dilated cisternae filled with finely granular material are present in the cellular structure. Abundant mitochondria and lipid droplets are observed. Proliferation and conditioning of the epithelial cells are evident, and in the last trimester there are microvilli along the ductal lumen accompanied by large cytoplasmic protrusions.

Study of the ultrastructure of the fetal breast may help in understanding the functional lactating breast. The secretion of a fluid resembling milk may take place at birth as a result of maternal hormones that have passed across the placenta into the fetal circulation. The lactiferous sinuses appear before birth as swellings of the developing ducts.

An extensive anatomic and histologic study of the human infant breast revealed an epithelial differentiation that followed a chronologic pattern, starting with secretory changes and apparently going through a period of apocrine metaplasia before the postsecretory changes and involution.[2] The embryonic fat probably plays a role in growth and morphogenesis of the ductal system. However, no distinguishing features were found between the breasts of female and male infants.[2]

The terminal end buds, lateral buds, and lobules of three to five alveolar buds predominate in prepubertal tissue. Lobules of alveolar buds and lobules of up to 60 ductules predominate in pubertal females. In prepuberty, these are epithelial-lined ducts that will bud out to form alveoli when stimulated by hormones of menarche (Fig. 2-1).

The breast is made up of glandular tissue, supporting connective tissue, and protective fatty tissue. Immediately after birth, the newborn's breast may even be swollen and secreting a small amount of milk, known as *witch's milk.* This very common phenomenon among both male and female infants is caused by the stimulation of the infant's mammary glands by the same hormones produced by the placenta to prepare the mother's breast for lactation. This secretory activity subsides within 3 to 4 weeks, and then the mammary glands are inactive until shortly before the onset of puberty, when hormones begin to stimulate growth

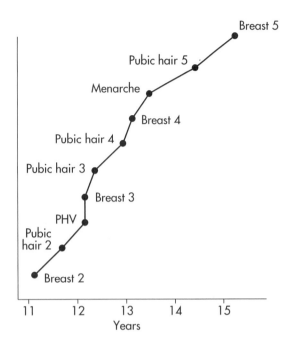

Fig. 2-2. Pubertal development in the female. The sequence and mean ages of pubertal events in females, adapted from the data of Marshall and Tanner. *PHV,* Peak height velocity. (From Root AW: *J Pediatr* 83:1, 1973.)

Fig. 2-1. Evolution of nipple. **A,** Thickening of epidermis with formation of primary bud. **B,** Growth of bud into mesenchyma. **C,** Formation of solid secondary buds. **D,** Formation of mammary pit and vacuolation of buds to form epithelial-lined ducts. **E,** Lactiferous ducts proliferate. Areola is formed. Nipple is inverted initially. (Modified from Weatherly-White RCA: *Plastic surgery of the female breast,* Hagerstown, Md, 1980, Harper & Row.)

again. During childhood (prepuberty) the gland merely keeps pace with physical growth (Figs. 2-2 and 2-3).

Pubertal development

The development of the human breast involves two distinct processes: organogenesis and milk production.[8] *Organogenesis* involves ductal and lobular

growth and begins before and continues through puberty, resulting in growth of the breast parenchyma with its surrounding fat pad. When the female is between 10 and 12 years of age, just before puberty, the ductal tree extends and generates its branching pattern, lengthening the existing ducts, dichotomously branching the growing ductal tips, and monopodially branching with the growth of the lateral buds at the sides of the ducts (Table 2-2). During this period of rapid growth, the ducts can develop bulbous terminal end buds. The formation of alveolar buds begins within a year or two of the onset of menses. The sprouting of new alveolar buds continues for several years, producing alveolar lobes.[23]

Anatomic location

The breast is located in the superficial fascia between the second rib and sixth intercostal

Fig. 2-3. Female breast from infancy to lactation with corresponding cross section and duct structure. **A, B,** and **C,** Gradual development of well-differentiated ductular and peripheral lobular-alveolar system. **D,** Ductular sprouting and intensified peripheral lobular-alveolar development in pregnancy. Glandular luminal cells begin actively synthesizing milk fat and proteins near term; only small amounts are released into lumen. **E,** With postpartum withdrawal of luteal and placental sex steroids and placental lactogen, prolactin is able to induce full secretory activity of alveolar cells and release of milk into alveoli and smaller ducts.

cartilage and is superficial to the pectoralis major muscle.[17] It tends to overlap this muscle inferiorly to become superficial to the external oblique and serratus anterior muscles. It measures 10 to 12 cm in diameter. It is located horizontally from the parasternal to midaxillary line. The central thickness of the breast is 5 to 7 cm (Fig. 2-4).

At puberty, the breasts in the female enlarge to their adult size, with the left frequently slightly larger than the right.[32] In a nonpregnant woman the mature breast weighs approximately 200 g. During pregnancy, breast size and weight increase; thus when the woman is near term, the breast weighs 400 to 600 g. During lactation the breast weighs 600 to 800 g (Fig. 2-3).

The shape of the breast varies from woman to woman, just as do body build and facial characteristics. Racial variations may be associated with discoidal, hemispheric, pear-shaped, or conical forms. Typically, the breast is dome shaped or conic in adolescence, becoming more hemispheric and finally pendulous in the parous female. Mammary glandular tissue projects somewhat into the axillary region. This is known as the *tail of Spence* (Fig. 2-6). Mammary tissue in the axilla, which is connected to the central duct system, becomes

TABLE 2-2   Phases of breast development

Phase	Age (yr)	Developmental characteristics
I	Puberty	Preadolescent elevation of nipple with no palpable glandular tissue or areolar pigmentation.
II	11.1 ± 1.1	Presence of glandular tissue in subareolar region. Nipple and breast project as single mound from chest wall.
III	12.2 ± 1.09	Increase in amount of readily palpable glandular tissue, with enlargement of breast and increased diameter and pigmentation of areola. Contour of breast and nipple remains in single plane.
IV	13.1 ± 1.15	Enlargement of areola and increased areolar pigmentation. Nipple and areola form secondary mound above breast level.
V	15.3 ± 1.7	Final adolescent development of smooth contour with no projection of areola and nipple.

Modified from Tanner JM: *Wachstun und Reifung des Menschen,* Stuttgart, 1962, Thieme-Verlag.

Fig. 2-4.   Mammary gland in longitudinal cross section showing mature, nonlactating duct system.

more obvious during pregnancy and produces milk during lactation, when it may cause various symptoms[1] (see Chapter 8). The tail of Spence is distinguished from a supranumerary gland because it connects to the normal duct system.

The three major structures of the breast are skin, subcutaneous tissue, and corpus mammae. The *corpus mammae* is the breast mass that remains after freeing the breast from the deep attachments and removing the skin, subcutaneous connective tissue, and adipose tissue.

The breasts of the adult female are always paired and develop from a line of glandular tissue found in the fetus and known as the *milk lines.* This milk streak, or *galactic band,* develops from the axilla to the groin during the fifth week of embryonic life.[19] In the thoracic region, the band develops into a ridge, and the rest of the band regresses (Fig. 2-5).

Abnormalities

In some women, additional residual of the galactic band remains as mammary tissue, which can develop anywhere along this line. *Hypermastia* is the presence of accessory mammary glands, which are phylogenic remnants of the embryonic mammary ridge resulting from incomplete regression or dispersion of the primitive galactic band (Fig. 2-5). Because of this origin, accessory nipples and glandular tissue may be found along these lines, which extend from the clavicular to the inguinal regions. Occasionally, supernumerary glands are found in the urogenital region, on the buttocks, or on the back as well.[33] The glands are derived from the ectoderm, whereas the connective tissue stroma is mesodermal in origin.

The accessory tissue may involve the corpus mammae, the areola, and the nipple.[20] From 2% to 6% of women have hypermastia. The response of hypermastia to pregnancy and lactation depends on the tissue present.

Box 2-1 defines other selected breast abnormalities. *Symmastia* is a webbing across the midline between the breasts, which are usually symmetric.[3] A more common variation is the presternal conflu-

Fig. 2-5. Sites of supernumerary nipples along milk line. Ectopic nipples, areolae, or breast tissue can develop from groin to axilla and upper inner arm. They can lactate or undergo malignant change. (Modified from Weatherly-White RCA: *Plastic surgery of the female breast,* Hagerstown, Md, 1980, Harper & Row.)

ence representing blending of breast tissue associated with large breasts. These abnormalities are ectodermal in origin and have many variations, from an empty skin web to the presence of significant glandular tissue. Little is known about their function, but several procedures exist for their surgical amelioration.[3]

Congenital absence of the breast is called *amastia,* which is rare. When a nipple is present but no breast tissue, the condition is called *amazia.* Another term for this condition when it occurs in addition to a normal breast is *hyperthelia.*

Some have suggested a relationship between *polythelia* (supernumerary nipple) and renal defect. Polythelia has also been associated with renal agenesis, renal cell carcinoma, obstructive dis-

BOX 2-1   Breast abnormalities

Accessory breast Any tissue outside the two
  major glands
Amastia Congenital absence of breast and
  nipple
Amazia Nipple without breast tissue
Hyperadenia Mammary tissue without nipple
Hypoplasia Underdevelopment of breast
Polythelia Supernumerary nipple(s) (also *hyper-
  thelia*)
Symmastia Webbing between breasts

BOX 2-2   Types of breast hypoplasia, hyperplasia, and acquired abnormalities

Unilateral hypoplasia, contralateral breast
  normal
Bilateral hypoplasia with asymmetry
Unilateral hyperplasia, contralateral breast
  normal
Bilateral hyperplasia with asymmetry
Unilateral hypoplasia, contralateral breast hyperplasia
Unilateral hypoplasia of breast, thorax, and pectoral muscles (Poland syndrome)
Acquired abnormalities caused by trauma,
  burns, radiation treatment for hemangioma
  or intrathoracic disease, chest tube insertion
  in infancy, and preadolescent biopsy

Modified from Osbourne MP: Breast development and anatomy. In
Harris JR, Lippman ME, Morrow M, Hellman S, editors: *Diseases of the
breast,* Philadelphia, 1996, Lippincott-Raven.)

ease, and supernumerary kidneys.[22] Others have described associations with congenital cardiac anomalies, pyloric stenosis, ear abnormalities, and arthrogryposis multiplex congenita.[3] After careful study of 65 patients with a supernumerary nipple, Hersh et al[12] found seven (11%) individuals who had significant renal lesions, somewhat less than the incidence reported originally. Apparently no association exists in blacks.

Poland syndrome, first described in 1841 (Box 2-2), includes absence of the pectoral muscle, chest wall deformity, and breast anomalies.[19] It is now known also to include symbrachydactyly, with hypoplasia of the middle phalanges and central skin webbing. *Hypoplasia* is underdevelopment of the breast. Although 90% of cases of breast hypoplasia are associated with hypoplasia of the pectoral muscles, 92% of women with pectoral muscle abnormalities have normal breasts. Box 2-2 lists types of breast hypoplasia, *hyperplasia* (over-development), and acquired breast abnormalities.

Hyperadenia is the presence of mammary tissue without nipples. The swelling and secretion of this tissue may produce pain during lactation. Occasionally, aberrant breast tissue can cause discomfort or embarrassment in adolescence and during menses, especially when located in the axilla.[14] Mammographic features of normal accessory axillary breast tissue were reviewed by Adler et al[1] in 13 women who were diagnosed on routine mammography. Seven of these women had a mass or fullness on physical examination; one was seen postpartum because of pain; nine were asymptomatic. They ranged in age from 31 to 67 years. Radiographically, the accessory tissue resembled the rest of the normal glandular tissue but was separate from it. It occurred on the right in 11 of the 13 women. The accessory tissue was recognized as a normal developmental variant, distinguishable from the frequent axillary tail of Spence, which represents a direct extension from the outer margin of the main mass of glandular tissue.

On mammography, accessory tissue is best visualized on oblique and exaggerated craniocaudal views. In rare cases, it may be appropriate to remove the tissue surgically, a treatment well known to experienced plastic surgeons. If treatment is not initiated before pregnancy and lactation in these women, pain and swelling will be intensified and may progress to mastitis or the necessity to terminate lactation.

Apart from physiologic variations, other conditions of abnormal anatomy include *hypomastia* (abnormally small breasts), hypertrophy, and inequality.

Corpus mammae

The mammary gland is an orderly conglomeration of a variable number of independent glands. It undergoes a series of changes that can be divided into developmental and differentiation phases. Surgical dissection of many postoperative specimens has contributed more precise information about the anatomic structure of the breast.[6] The ramifications of the lactiferous ducts and stroma were carefully studied by Hicken,[13] who reported that in 95% of women the ducts ascend into the axilla, occasionally following the brachial plexus and axillary vessels into the apex of the axilla. Ducts are found in the epigastric region in 15% of women. In rare cases, ducts cross the midline (Fig. 2-6).

The morphology of the corpus mammae includes two major divisions, the parenchyma and the stroma.[1] The *parenchyma* includes the ductular-lobular-alveolar structures. It is composed of the alveolar gland with treelike ductular branching alveoli, which are approximately 0.12 mm in diameter. The ducts are approximately 2 mm in diameter. The lactiferous sinuses are 5 to 8 mm in diameter. The lobi, which are arranged like spokes converging on the central nipple, are 15 to 25 in number. Each lobus is divided again into 20 to 40 lobuli, and each lobulus is again subdivided into 10 to 100 alveoli for tubulosaccular secretory units. The *stroma* includes the connective tissue, fat tissue, blood vessels, nerves, and lymphatics.[17]

The mass of tissue in the breast consists of the tubuloalveolar glands embedded in fat (the adipose tissue), giving the gland its smooth, rounded contour. The mammary fat pad is essential for the proliferation and differentiation of the mammary epithelium, providing the necessary space, support, and local control for duct elongation and, ultimately, lobuloalveolar proliferation. Each gland forms a lobe of the breast, and the lobes are separated by connective tissue septa. These septa attach to the skin. Each tubuloalveolar gland opens into a lactiferous duct, which leads into a more dilated area, the lactiferous sinus; there is a slight constriction before the sinus opens onto the surface of the nipple (Fig. 2-7). Extension of ducts within

Fig. 2-6. Ramification of lactiferous ducts and mammary tissue. Ducts extend onto upper medial aspect of arm, to midline, and into epigastrium. Composite drawing from mammographic studies. (Modified from Hicken NF: *Arch Surg* 40:6, 1940.)

the fat pad is orderly. An inhibitory zone exists around each duct into which other ducts cannot penetrate, and development does not normally proceed beyond the duct end-bud stage before puberty.[2]

Nipple and areola

The skin of the breast includes the nipple, areola, and general skin. The skin is the thin, flexible, elastic cover of the breast adherent to the fat-laden subcutaneous tissue. It contains hair, sebaceous glands, and apocrine sweat glands. The nipple, or *papilla mammae,* is a conic elevation located in the center of the areola at about the fourth intercostal

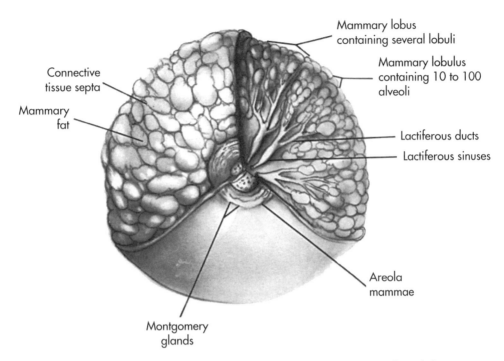

Connective
tissue septa

Mammary
fat

Mammary lobus
containing several lobuli

Mammary lobulus
containing 10 to 100
alveoli

Lactiferous ducts
Lactiferous sinuses

Areola
mammae

Montgomery
glands

Fig. 2-7. Morphology of mature breast with dissection to reveal mammary fat and duct system.

space, slightly below the midpoint of the breast. Although very different in size, the nipples and areolae of women and men are qualitatively identical.[18] The nipple contains 15 to 25 milk ducts. Each of the tubuloalveolar glands that make up the breast opens onto the nipple by a separate opening. The nipple also contains smooth muscle fibers and is richly innervated with sensory nerve endings and Meissner's corpuscles in the dermal papillae; it is well supplied with sebaceous and apocrine sweat glands, but no hair.

The nipple is surrounded by the areola, or *areola mammae,* a circular pigmented area. It is usually faintly darker before pregnancy, turning reddish brown during pregnancy, and always maintaining some darker pigmentation thereafter. The average areola measures 15 to 16 mm in diameter, although the range is great, enlarging during pregnancy and lactation. The pigmentation results from many melanocytes distributed throughout the skin and glands. The understructure of the epidermis of the areola is not as elaborate as that of the nipple but intermediate to that of the surrounding

skin. The nipple and areola are extremely elastic.

Little or no true lobuloalveolar development occurs before the first pregnancy. A framework is laid down within which the specialized secretory cells will proliferate[7] (Fig. 2-8). The framework forms a vital part of the gland's overall developmental course, and maldevelopment or trauma during fetal or juvenile life can seriously reduce the size and secretory potential of the mature gland.

Montgomery's tubercles, containing the ductular openings of sebaceous and lactiferous glands, are present in the areola,[27] as are sweat glands and smaller, free sebaceous glands. The corium (dermis) of the areola lacks fat but contains smooth muscle and collagenous and elastic connective tissue fibers in radial and circular arrangements. The Montgomery glands become enlarged and look like small pimples during pregnancy and lactation (Fig. 2-9). They secrete a substance that lubricates and protects the nipples and areolae during pregnancy and lactation. A small amount of milk is also secreted from these tubercles. After

Fig. 2-8. A, Duct end from a 15-year-old nulligravida on second day of menstruation showing typical form of puberty: a coarsely diversified system of thick, mostly well-filled ducts with round, often ball-shaped or half-ball–shaped ends. Note use of connective tissue as guiding tracts, circumvention of fat tissue, and paucity of secretory alveoli. **B,** Sagittal section through milk gland of a nulligravida 19-year-old between menses (died of skull fracture). Note massive body of connective tissue without preserved lobes of fatty tissue and richness of connective tissue with respective richness of parenchyma. Note also distribution of larger ducts in superficial parallel connective tissue septum of former subcutaneous fat tissue and smaller ducts in vertical septa. Thin section; drawing with Busch magnifying glasses. **C,** Gland of a nulligravida 19-year-old (part of a 4 mm–thick section). Bushy short sprout and duct build long sprout, with the latter in acute angled bifurcation, often lying very close to each other. This demonstrates development of ductal and secretory elements during menstrual cycle; however, connective tissue and fat are predominant. (From Dabelow A: Die Milchdrüse. In *Handbuch der Mikroskopischen Anatomie des Menschen,* vol III, part 3, Berlin, 1957, Springer-Verlag.)

lactation, these glands recede again to their former unobtrusive state.

Light microscopy has shown that Morgagni was correct in 1719 when he first described the 12 to 20 areolar glands and noted them to be sebaceous and to include lactiferous structures as well. Building on the original work, Montgomery in 1837 prepared a more detailed treatise on the tubercle itself and named it after himself. Serial sections of 35 tubercles also showed that there were lactiferous ducts from the deeper breast parenchyma ascending into the sebaceous glands of the tubercle (Fig. 2-9). The sebaceous gland itself was no different from those of the skin or those associated with the terminal lactiferous ducts

of the nipple. The mammary duct was lined with two layers of cuboidal to columnar cells. They arose from the underlying mammary lobules through the subcutaneous tissues and into the region of the sebaceous gland. The terminal portion of the mammary duct in some cases joined the duct to the sebaceous gland and in other cases opened separately but close to it. The ducts appear to be a miniature of the major mammary system. Sebaceous and mammary ductal components underlie the areolar tubercle.

The areola and nipple are darker than the rest of the breast, ranging from light pink in very fair-skinned women to very dark brown in others. The areola's darker color may be a visual signal to

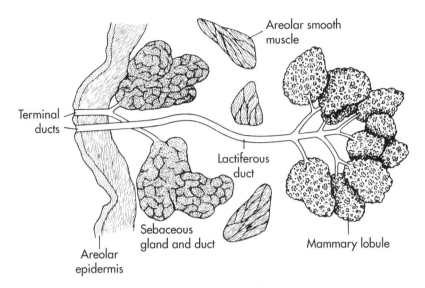

Fig. 2-9. Tubercle of Montgomery and underlying structures. Lactiferous duct may join sebaceous gland ducts and terminate at common opening in areolar epidermis as shown. (Modified from Smith DM, Peters TG, Donegan WL: *Arch Pathol Lab Med* 106:62, 1982.)

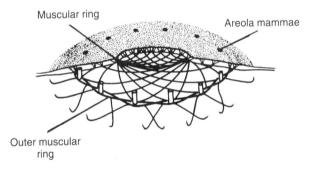

Fig. 2-10. Nipple and areola with smooth musculature structure.

newborns so that they will close their mouth on the areola, not on the nipple alone, to obtain milk. Nipple erection is induced by tactile, sensory, or autonomic sympathetic stimuli. The dermis of the nipple and the areola contains many multi-branched, free nerve fiber endings. Local venostasis and hyperemia occur to enhance the process of erection of the nipple because the nipple and areola are rich in arteriovenous anastomoses. The glabrous skin of the nipple is wrinkled, containing large papillae of the corium.

Each nipple contains 15 to 25 lactiferous ducts surrounded by fibromuscular tissue (Figs. 2-10 to 2-13). These ducts end as small orifices near the tip of the nipple. Within the nipple, the lactiferous ducts may merge. The ductular orifices therefore are sometimes fewer in number than the respective breast lobi. The milk ducts within the nipple dilate at the nipple base into the cone-shaped ampullae of milk sinuses. The ampullae function as temporary milk containers during lactation but contain only epithelial debris in the nonlactating state. The lining of the infundibular and ampullar parts of the lactiferous ducts consists of an eight- to ten-cell

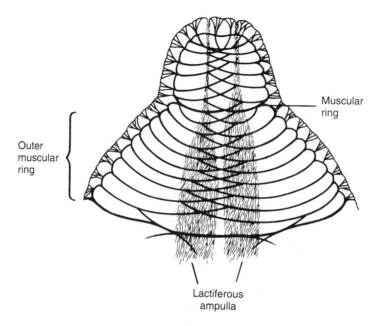

Fig. 2-11.   Smooth musculature of areola and nipple in cross section when contracted to make nipple erect.

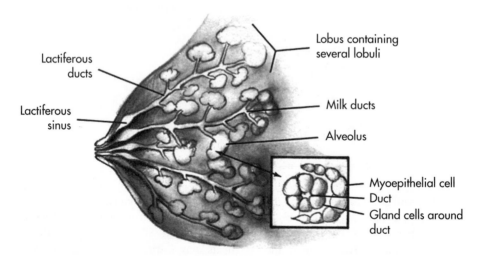

Fig. 2-12.   Simplified schematic drawing of duct system with cross section of myoepithelial cells around duct opening. Myoepithelial cells contract to eject milk.

layered squamous epithelium. The bulk of the nipple is composed of smooth musculature, which represents a closing mechanism for the milk ducts and sinuses of the nipple (Figs. 2-10 and 2-11). The milk ducts in the nipple are embedded in stretch-able and mobile connective tissue. The inner longitudinal muscular arrangements and the outer, more circular and radial arrangements do not obstruct the milk ducts. Tangential fibers also branch off from the more circular muscular fibers

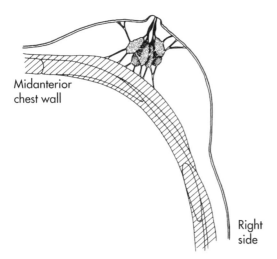

Midanterior
chest wall

Right
side

Fig. 2-13. Horizontal cross section of breast ligaments, looking from head to foot. Ligaments of Cooper suspend 15 to 20 lobes of breast within matrix of fat. They are attached to lobes, skin, and deep fascia.

of the nipple bases to the outer circular muscular range.

The functions of the muscular fibroelastic system of the areola and nipple include decreasing the surface area of the areola, producing nipple erection, and emptying the lactiferous sinuses and ducts during nursing. When the nipple erects because of tactile, thermal, or sexual stimulation, the system causes the nipple to become smaller, firmer, and more prominent (Fig. 2-11).

The mammary tissues are enveloped by the superficial pectoral fascia, and the breast is fixed by fibrous bands to the overlying skin and the underlying pectoral fascia, which are known as *ligaments of Cooper* (Fig. 2-13). The glandular part of the breast is surrounded by a fat layer that seldom extends beyond the lower border of the pectoralis major muscle. The breast is supported by the muscles attached to the ribs, the collarbone, and the bones of the upper arm near the shoulder.

Blood supply

The blood supply to the breast is from branches of the intercostal arteries and the perforating branches of the internal thoracic artery; the third, fourth, and fifth are usually most prominent. The major blood supply to the breast is provided by the internal mammary artery and the lateral thoracic artery. A small supply is obtained from the intercostal arteries and the arterial branches of the axillary and subclavian arteries, but this contribution is minimal; 60% of the total breast tissue, especially the medial and central part, receives blood from the internal mammary artery. All the mammary branches of this artery lead transversely to the nipple and anastomoses, with branches coming from the lateral thoracic artery.[6] Anastomoses with intercostal arteries are less common, but the blood supply to the nipple is extensive and close to the surface, contributing to the richer color. Many areas of the breast are supplied by two or three different arterial sources (Fig. 2-14).

The venous supply parallels the arterial supply and bears similar names. The veins drain the breast and enter the fascia, muscle layers, and intercostal spaces at the same point. The veins end in the internal thoracic and the axillary veins. Some veins may reach the external jugular vein. The veins create an anastomotic circle around the base of the papilla, called the *circulus venosis.*[4]

Lymphatic drainage

The lymphatic drainage of the breast has been the subject of considerable study because of the frequency of breast cancer, but it has significance for the lactating breast as well. The lymphatic drainage can be quite extensive. The main drainage is to axillary nodes and to the parasternal nodes along the internal thoracic artery inside the thoracic cavity. The lymphatics of the breast originate in the lymph capillaries of the mammary connective tissue, which surrounds the mammary structures, and drain through the deep substance of the breast.

The lymph drainage of the breast consists of the superficial or cutaneous section, the areola, and the glandular or deep-tissue section. Other points of drainage are to pectoral nodes between the pectoralis major and minor muscles and to the subcla-

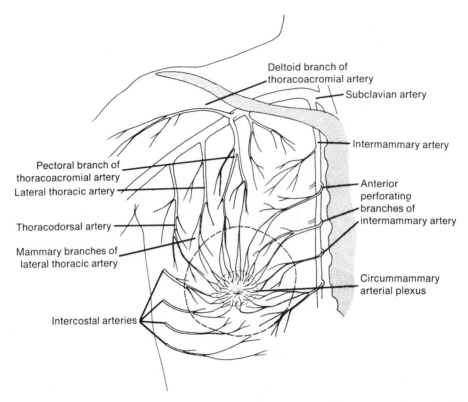

Fig. 2-14. Blood supply to mammary gland. Major blood supply is from anterior perforating branches of internal mammary artery.

vicular nodes in the neck deep to the clavicle. Some transmammary lymph drainage occurs to the opposite breast as well as to subdiaphragmatic lymphatics that lead ultimately to the liver and intraabdominal nodes (Fig. 2-15).

Innervation

The nerves of the breast are from branches of the fourth, fifth, and sixth intercostal nerves and consist of sensory fibers innervating the smooth muscles in the nipple and blood vessels. The sensory innervation of the nipple and areola is extensive and consists of both autonomic and sensory nerves. A detailed anatomic and clinical study of the nipple-areola complex showed that it is innervated from the lateral cutaneous branch of the fourth intercostal nerve, which penetrates the pos-

terior aspect of the breast at the intersection of the fourth intercostal space and the pectoralis major muscle (4 o'clock on the left breast and 8 o'clock on the right breast).[9] The nerve divides into five fasciculi, one central to the nipple, two upper, and two lower branches (always at 5 and 7 o'clock left and right side, respectively) (Figs. 2-16 and 2-17).

The innervation of the corpus mammae is minimal by comparison and predominantly autonomic. No parasympathetic or cholinergic fibers supply any part of the breast. No ganglia are found in mammary tissue. Norepinephrine-containing nerve fibers are abundant among the smooth muscle cells of the nipple and at the interface between the media and adventitia of the breast arteries. Physiologic observations demonstrate that the efferent nerves to these structures are sympathetic adrenergic.

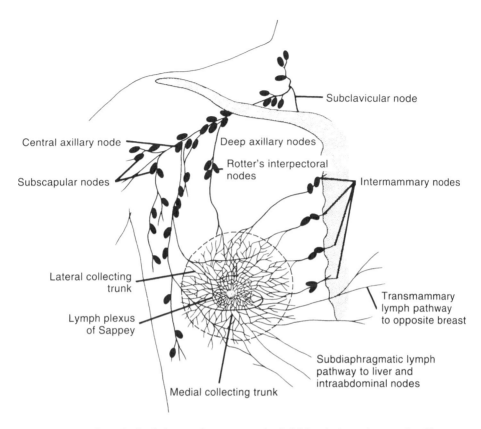

Subclavicular node

Central axillary node

Deep axillary nodes

Rotter's interpectoral nodes

Subscapular nodes

Intermammary nodes

Lateral collecting trunk

Lymph plexus of Sappey

Transmammary lymph pathway to opposite breast

Subdiaphragmatic lymph pathway to liver and intraabdominal nodes

Medial collecting trunk

Fig. 2-15. Lymphatic drainage of mammary gland. Major drainage is toward axilla.

The majority of the mammary nerves follow the arteries and arterioles and supply these structures. A few fibers from the perivascular networks course along the walls of the ducts. They may correspond to sensory fibers for sensing milk pressure. No innervation of mammary myoepithelial cells has been identified. It can therefore be concluded that secretory activities of the acinar epithelium depend on hormonal stimulation, such as that of oxytocin and other hormones, and are not stimulated via the nervous system directly.

Stimulation of the sensory nerve fibers or sensory receptors does induce the release of adenohypophyseal prolactin and neurohypophyseal oxytocin via an afferent sensory reflex pathway whereby stimuli reach the hypothalamus. Sympathetic mammary stimulation causes the contraction of the small muscles of the areola and the

nipple. The locally released norepinephrine induces stimulation of the myoepithelial adrenergic receptors, causing muscular relaxation. In the absence of parasympathetic activity, a minor physiologic catamine inhibitory effect on the mammary myoepithelium may exist, which is overcome by oxytocin release during suckling, inducing myoepithelial contraction.

The supraclavicular nerves supply the sensory fibers for innervation of the upper cutaneous parts of the breast. Branches of the intercostal nerves provide the major sensory innervation of the mammary gland. The sympathetic sensory and motor fibers are derived from the supraclavicular and intercostal nerves, respectively. Sympathetic fibers run only along the mammary gland–supplying arteries to innervate the glandular body. There is relatively restricted innervation to the epidermal

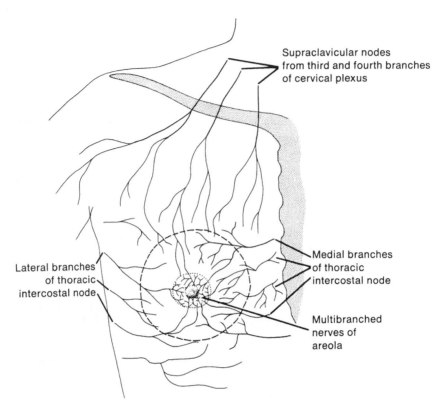

Fig. 2-16. Innervation of mammary gland. Supraclavicular nerves and lateral and medial branches of intercostal nerves provide sensory innervation. Sympathetic and motor nerves are provided by supracervical and intercostal nerves.

parts of the nipple and areola, leading to lack of superficial sensory acuity.

Breast sensation was measured in a large number of women by Courtiss and Goldwyn[5] using a device that emitted a variable current producing a burning sensation when the threshold was exceeded. The areola was shown to be the most sensitive and the nipple the least sensitive, with the skin of the breast intermediate. Thus the skin in these areas responds only to major stimuli, such as sucking. The relatively large number of dermal nerve endings provides a high mammary responsiveness toward stimuli for elicitation of the sucking reflex. The neuroreflex induces adequate release of both prolactin and oxytocin. It appears that, in addition to the hormonal actions, breast

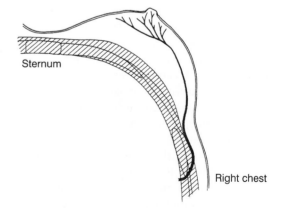

Fig. 2-17. Cross section of nerve supply of breast and nipple. Cutaneous nerves run close to deep fascia before turning outward toward skin.

nerves can also influence the mammary blood supply and milk secretion. Abnormalities of sensory or autonomic nerve distributions in the areola and nipple therefore could impair adequate lactation, especially in the functioning of the let-down reflex and the secretion of prolactin and oxytocin.

In summary, the somatic sensory cutaneous nerve supply of the breast includes the supraclavicular nerves and the thoracic intercostal nerves. The autonomic motor nerve supply of the breast is derived from the sympathetic fibers of the intercostal nerves, which supply the smooth musculature of the areola and the nipple. The autonomic supply is also derived from sympathetic fibers of the accompanying arteries, which innervate the smooth musculature of the inner glandular blood vessel walls to produce constriction. The nerve supply to the area of the areola and the nipple includes free sensory nerve endings, tactile corpuscles to the papillae of the corium of the nipple and areola, and the fibers around the larger lactiferous duct and in the dermis of the areola and peripheral breast. All cutaneous nerves run radially to the glandular body toward the nipple. The nerve supply to the inner gland is sparse and contains only sympathetic nerves accompanying blood vessels (Fig. 2-16).

MICROSCOPIC ANATOMY

After many decades of neglect since the phylogenic studies of the mammary gland in the 1800s and early 1900s, the mammary gland has become one of the most studied organs because of its usefulness as a tool in developmental biology, biochemistry, endocrinology and biology, histology, oncology, virology, and molecular biology.[26] No cell can exist independent of its surrounding cells. All cells have relations with neighboring cells and also with cells at distant sites. The interactions of the epithelial parenchyma and mesenchymal stroma are most important in primary and secondary induction in organogenesis.

The mammary gland consists of a branching system of excretory ducts embedded in connective tissue.[11] The gland is composed of two layers of epithelial cells: luminal epithelium and basal layer epithelium, along with a few basal (stem) cells. The whole structure is surrounded by a basement membrane. In the ducts, elongated myoepithelial cells make up a continuous sheath. The luminal cell interaction with the extracellular matrix is mediated by the myoepithelium.

The integrity of the normal mammary gland is maintained by several adhesion systems.[11] The mammary gland is composed of epithelial parenchyma and two types of mesenchymal stroma: dense mammary mesenchyma and fatty stroma. The dense mammary mesenchyma is present in the embryonic stage, in end buds of puberty, and in cancers. It determines mammary epithelium and fixes the ability of the epithelium to interact with the fatty stroma. The fatty stroma is essential for typical mammary gland morphogenesis.[26]

The two types of mammary stroma synthesize different extracellular matrix proteins. Dense mesenchyma makes fibronectin and tenascin. Fatty stroma makes liminin, proteoglycans, and also fibronectin.

In their structure and mode of development, the mammary glands somewhat resemble the sweat glands.[10] During embryonic life, their differentiation is similar in the two sexes. The male experiences little additional development postnatally. The female, in contrast, experiences extensive structural change paralleling her age and the functional state of the reproductive system.

Vogel et al[31] studied histologic changes in the normal human mammary gland in association with the menstrual cycle. They describe five phases: proliferative (days 3 to 7), follicular phase of differentiation (days 8 to 14), luteal phase of differentiation (days 15 to 20), secretory (days 21 to 27), and menstrual (days 28 to 2). Table 2-3 outlines the morphologic criteria for these phases. These findings illustrate the correlation of morphologic response to hormonal stimulus of the mammary gland during normal cycling.

The greatest development in the female is reached by the twentieth year. Gradual changes are correlated with the menstrual cycle, and major

TABLE 2-3   Morphologic criteria for phase assignment in menstrual cycle

	Stroma	Lumen	Cell types	Epithelium Orientation of epithelial cells	Epithelium Mitoses	Epithelium Active secretion
Phase I Days 3-7	Dense, cellular	Tight	Single predominant pale eosinophilic cell	No stratification apparent	Present, average 4/10 HPF	None
Phase II Days 8-14	Dense, cellular-collagenous	Defined	1. Luminal columnar basophilic cell 2. Intermediate pale cell 3. Basal clear cell with hyperchromatic nucleus (myoepithelial)	Radial around lumen	Rare	None
Phase III Days 15-20	Loose, broken	Open with some secretion	1. Luminal basophilic cell 2. Intermediate pale cell 3. Prominent vacuolization of basal clear cell (myoepithelial)	Radial around lumen	Absent	None
Phase IV Days 21-27	Loose, edematous	Open with secretion	1. Luminal basophilic cell 2. Intermediate pale cell 3. Prominent vacuolization of basal clear cell (myoepithelial)	Radial around lumen	Absent	Active apocrine secretion from luminal cell
Phase V Days 28-2	Dense, cellular	Distended with secretion	1. Luminal basophilic cell with scant cytoplasm 2. Extensive vacuolization of basal cells	Radial around lumen	Absent	Rare

Modified from Vogel PM, Georgiade NG, Fetter BF et al: *Am J Pathol* 104:23, 1981.
HPF, high powered field.

changes accompany pregnancy and lactation (Fig. 2-8).

Russo and Russo[24] describe the development of the mammary gland as "an asynchronous process of progressive invasion of the mammary stroma by a parenchyma composed of ductal elements in which the advancing ends are the club-shaped terminal end buds (TEBs) that progressively differentiate into alveolar buds (ABs) or regress to terminal ducts (TDs)." (Fig. 2-18.)

Mature mammary gland

The mammary gland is a compound tubuloalveolar gland containing 15 to 25 irregular lobes radiating from the nipple. Each lobe has a lactiferous duct (2 to 4 mm in diameter) lined by stratified squamous epithelium. The duct opens on the nipple and has an irregular angular outline. Beneath the areola, each duct has a local dilatation, the lactiferous sinus, and finally emerges at the end of the nipple as a 0.4- to 0.7-mm opening. Each lobe is subdivided into lobules of various orders; the smallest are elongated tubules, the alveolar ducts, covered by small saccular evaginations, the alveoli. The interlobular connective tissue is dense; however, it is more cellular, has fewer collagenous fibers, and contains almost no fat. Greater distensibility is permitted by the looser connective tissue.

The ducts and ductules of mature women consist chiefly of two cell types: the inner lining of epithelial cells and the outer lining of myoepithelial cells. A basement membrane separates these structures from the stroma. Histochemical and immunocytochemical reagents can distinguish these elements, their positions, and their infrastructures. Rudland[23] has reported on the histochemical organization and cellular composition of ductal buds in the developing human breast. This work suggests that there are cytochemical intermediates between epithelial and myoepithelial cells. The undifferentiated peripheral cap cells may be transitional forms of the cortical epithelial cells that will line the lumina and of the myoepithelial cells of the subtending duct.

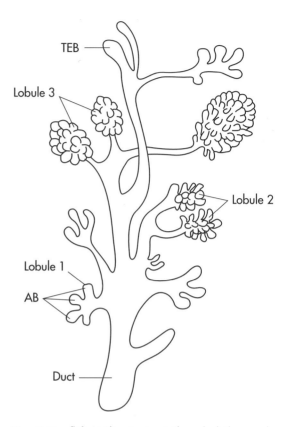

Fig. 2-18. Schematic representation depicting various topographic compartments of human mammary gland: terminal end buds *(TEB);* alveolar buds *(AB);* lobules types 1, 2, and 3; and ducts. (Modified from Russo J, Russo IH: Development of human mammary gland. In Neville MC, Daniel CW, editors: *The mammary gland,* New York, 1987, Plenum.)

Transforming growth factors (TGF-β1, 2, and 3) are potent inhibitors of cell proliferation but play an important role in mammary gland development. They exhibit overlapping patterns of expression within the epithelium of the developing gland. TGF-β3 is detected in the myoepithelial progenitor cells of the growing end buds and the myoepithelial cells in the mature duct.[21]

The secretory portions of the gland, the alveolar ducts and the alveoli, have cuboidal or low-columnar secretory cells, resting on basal laminae and myoepithelial cells. These myoepithelial cells enclose the alveoli in a loosely meshed network with their many starlike branchings. The myoepithelial cells are stimulated by oxytocin and sex steroids. The presence of myoepithelial cells has been used as evidence that the mammary gland is related to the sweat gland.

In the resting phase, epithelial structures consist of the ducts and their branches. The presence of a few alveoli budding off from the ends of ducts is still under investigation. This variance may be caused by the effect of the menstrual cycle. The swelling and engorgement accompanying the menstrual cycle are associated with hyperemia and some edema of the connective tissue. Most significant is that the gland does not have a single duct but many. Each lobe is a separate compound alveolar gland whose primary ducts join into larger and larger ducts. These ducts drain into a lactifer-ous duct. Each lactiferous duct drains separately at the tip of the nipple.

The epidermis of the nipple and areola is invaded by unusually long dermal papillae whose capillaries richly vascularize the surface and impact the richer hue. Bundles of smooth muscle, placed longitudinally along the lactiferous ducts and circumferentially within the nipple and at its base, permit the erection of the nipple. In the areola are the areolar Montgomery glands, which are intermediate in their microscopic structure between sweat glands and true mammary glands. The periphery of the areola also has sweat glands and sebaceous glands (Figs. 2-9 and 2-10).

Mammary gland in pregnancy

Changes in levels of circulating hormones result in profound changes in the ductular-lobular-alveolar growth during pregnancy (Fig. 2-19). During the first trimester there is rapid growth and branching from the terminal portion of the duct system into

Fig. 2-19. A, Milk gland of 21-year-old primigravida in second month of pregnancy. Development of small lobes has protruded almost to mammilla. Very regular development is shown over whole range of this thick section. Natural dimensions: 2.6×2.1 cm. **B,** Milk gland of same 21-year-old primigravida. Note very different forms of sprouting. Partly atypical sprouts above diagonal line are composed from same section; bifurcations below line are in natural position. Alveoli are beginning to resemble mature gland. (From Dabelow A: Die Milchdrüse. In *Handbuch der Mikroskopischen Anatomie des Menschen,* vol III, part 3, Berlin, 1957, Springer-Verlag.)

the adipose tissue. As the epithelial structures proliferate, the adipose tissue seems to diminish. During this time, increasing infiltration of the interstitial tissue occurs with lymphocytes, plasma cells, and eosinophils. The rate of hyperplasia levels off. In the last trimester, any enlargement is the result of parenchymal cell growth and distention of the alveoli with early colostrum, which is rich in protein and relatively low in lipid. Fat droplets gradually accumulate in the secretory alveolar cells. The interlobular connective tissue is noticeably decreased, and alveolar proliferation is extensive.

The histologic appearance of the gland varies. The functional state appears to vary from dilated, thin-walled lumen to narrow-lumened, thick-walled glandular tissue. Epithelial cells vary, being flat to low columnar in shape with indistinct boundaries. Some cells protrude into the lumen of the alveoli; others are short and smooth. The lumen of the alveolus is crowded with fine granular material and lipid droplets similar to those protruding from the cells.

The former concepts of mammary gland secretion indicated that the mode of release was apocrine secretion. *Apocrine secretion* is the process by which the cell undergoes partial disintegration. A fat-filled portion projects into the lumen; the fat globule constricts at the base; and the cell replaces itself. Electron microscopy has shown that the cell has two distinct secretory products, formed and released by different mechanisms. The protein constituents of milk are formed and released identically to those of other protein-secreting glands, classified as *merocrine glands.* Secretory materials are passed out through the cell apex without appreciable loss of cytoplasm in merocrine glands.

The fatty components of milk arise as lipid droplets free in the cytoplasmic matrix. The droplets increase in size and move into the apex of the cell. They project into the lumen, covered by a thin layer of cytoplasm. The droplets are ultimately cast off, enveloped by a detached portion of the cell membrane and a thin rim of subjacent cytoplasm. (See Fig. 2-3 and Chapter 3 for further discussion.)

Lactating mammary gland

The lactating mammary gland is characterized by a large number of alveoli (Fig. 2-20). The alveoli of the lactating gland are made up of cuboidal epithelial and myoepithelial cells. Only a small amount of connective tissue separates the neighboring alveoli. Under special preparations, lipid can be seen as small droplets within the cells. These droplets become larger and are discharged into the lumen.

The functioning of the mammary gland depends on the interplay of multiple and complex nervous system and endocrine factors. Some factors are involved in the development of the mammary glands to a functional state *(mammogenesis),* others in the establishment of milk secretion *(lactogenesis),* and others in responsibility for the maintenance of lactation *(galactopoiesis).*

The division and differentiation of mammary

Fig. 2-20. Part of mammary gland with significant milk obstruction in 26-year-old woman who died from food poisoning after ingesting spoiled fish 3 weeks postpartum and who had not breastfed for 48 hours before death. In upper half, formed duct and lobes are located on alternating sides. This form results from different development of two parts of a dichotomized bifurcation: one takes over production of small lobes, while the other continues the stem. Thick section; *arrow,* very primitive, undeveloped sprouts. (From Dabelow A: Die Milchdrüse. In *Handbuch der Mikroskopischen Anatomie des Menschen,* vol III, part 3, Berlin, 1957, Springer-Verlag.)

epithelial cells and presecretory alveolar cells into secretory milk-releasing alveolar cells take place in the third trimester. Stimulation of ribonucleic acid (RNA) synthesis promotes galactopoiesis and apocrine milk secretion into the alveoli. The deoxyribonucleic acid (DNA) and RNA content of the cellular nuclei increases during pregnancy and is highest at lactation (Fig. 2-3).

The ultrastructure of the human mammary gland during lactogenesis was studied by Tobon and Salazar,[30] who reviewed surgical specimens from seven lactating women, 1 day to 5½ months postpartum. They noted widespread hypertrophy and hyperplasia of the acini accompanied by dilatation and engorgement of the lumen by milk. The vascular channels were engorged. The lactogenic epithelial cells had rich cytoplasm, prominent layers of reticulum, and enlarged oval mitochondria. The Golgi apparatus was hypertrophied. The myoepithelium was stretched and thinned to contain the filled acini.

Postlactation regression of mammary gland

If milk is not removed from the breast, the glands become greatly distended and milk production gradually ceases. Part of the decrease results from the lack of stimulation of sucking, which initiates the neurohormonal reflex for maintenance of prolactin secretion. Perhaps a stronger effect is the engorgement of the breast with compression of blood vessels, causing diminished flow. The diminished blood flow results in decreased oxytocin to the myoepithelium. The alveoli are greatly distended and the epithelium flattened. The secretion remaining in the alveolar spaces and ducts is absorbed. The alveoli gradually collapse, with an increase in perialveolar connective tissue. The glandular elements gradually return to the resting state. Adipose tissue and macrophages increase. The gland does not return completely to the prepregnancy state in that the alveoli formed do not totally involute. Some appear as scattered, solid cords of epithelial cells.

Microscopically, increased autophagic and heterophagic processes occur in the first few days after weaning. Lysosomal enzymes increase, whereas nonlysosomal enzymes decrease.

Although the process of regression has been studied carefully in animals, little study has been done in the human. Slow weaning, which usually takes 3 months, probably has a very different timetable from abrupt weaning, in which marked involution has been intense and rapid over days or weeks.

REFERENCES

1. Adler DD, Rebner M, Pennes DR: Accessory breast tissue in the axilla: mammographic appearance, *Radiology* 163:709, 1987.
2. Anbazhagan R, Bartek P, Monaghan P et al: Growth and development of the human infant breast, *Am J Anat* 192:407, 1991.
3. Bland KI, Romnell LJ: Congenital and acquired disturbances of breast development and growth. In Bland KI, Copeland EM III, editors: *The breast: comprehensive management of benign and malignant diseases,* Philadelphia, 1991, Saunders.
4. Clemente CD, editor: *Gray's anatomy of the human body,* Philadelphia, 1985, Lea & Febiger.
5. Courtiss EH, Goldwyn RM: Breast sensation before and after plastic surgery, *Plast Reconstr Surg* 58:1, 1976.
6. Crafts RC: *A textbook of human anatomy,* New York, 1966, Ronald Press.
7. Dabelow A: Die Milchdrüse. In *Handbuch der Mikroskopischen Anatomie des Menschen,* vol III, part 3, Berlin, 1957, Springer-Verlag.
8. Egan RL: Breast embryology, anatomy, and physiology. In *Breast imaging diagnosis and morphology of breast diseases,* Philadelphia, 1988, Saunders.
9. Farina MA, Newby BG, Alani HM: Innervation of the nipple-areolar complex, *Plast Reconstr Surg* 66:497, 1980.
10. Fawcett DW: *Bloom and Fawcett: a textbook on histology,* ed 11, Philadelphia, 1986, Saunders.
11. Glukhova M, Koteliansky V, Sastre X et al: Adhesion systems in normal breast and in invasive breast carcinoma, *Am J Pathol* 146:706, 1995.

12. Hersh JH, Bloom AS, Cromer AO et al: Does a supernumerary nipple/renal field defect exist? *Am J Dis Child* 141:989, 1987.

13. Hicken NF: Mastectomy: a clinical pathologic study demonstrating why most mastectomies result in incomplete removal of the mammary gland, *Arch Surg* 40:6, 1940.

14. Kaye BL: Axillary breasts: a significant esthetic deformity, *Plast Reconstr Surg* 53:61, 1974.

15. Knight CH, Peaker M: Development of the mammary gland: symposium report no 19, Lactation, *J Reprod Fertil* 65:521, 1982.

16. Kreipe RE: Normal somatic adolescent growth and development, *J Pediatr* 83:1, 1973.

17. Larson BL, editor: *Lactation,* Ames, 1985, Iowa State University Press.

18. Montagna W, Macpherson EE: Some neglected aspects of the anatomy of human breasts, *J Invest Dermatol* 63:10, 1974.

19. Osbourne MP: Breast development and anatomy. In Harris JR, Lippman ME, Morrow M, Hellman S, editors: *Diseases of the breast,* Philadelphia, 1996, Lippincott-Raven.

20. Pellegrin JR, Wagner RF Jr: Polythelia and associated conditions, *Am Fam Physician* 28:129, 1983.

21. Pierce DF Jr, Johnson MD, Matsui Y et al: Inhibition of mammary duct development but not alveolar outgrowth during pregnancy in transgenic mice expressing active TGF-β1, *Genes Dev* 7:2308, 1993.

22. Rahbar F: Clinical significance of supernumerary nipples in black neonates, *Clin Pediatr* 21:46, 1983.

23. Rudland PS: Histochemical organization and cellular composition of ductal buds in developing human breast: evidence of cytochemical intermediates between epithelial and myoepithelial cells, *J Histochem Cytochem* 39:1471, 1991.

24. Russo IH, Russo J: Progestagens and mammary gland development: differentiation versus carcinogenesis, *Acta Endocrinol* 125:7, 1991.

25. Russo J, Russo IH: Development of human mammary gland. In Neville MC, Daniel CW, editors: *The mammary gland,* New York, 1987, Plenum.

26. Sakakura T: New aspects of stroma-parenchyma relations in mammary gland differentiation, *Int Rev Cytol* 125:165, 1991.

27. Smith DM, Peters TG, Donegan WL: Montgomery's areolar tubercle, *Arch Pathol Lab Med* 106:60, 1982.

28. Tanner JM: *Wachstun und Reifung des Menschen,* Stuttgart, 1962, Thieme-Verlag.

29. Tobon H, Salazar H: Ultrastructure of the human mammary gland. I. Development of the fetal gland throughout gestation, *J Clin Endocrinol Metab* 39:443, 1974.

30. Tobon H, Salazar H: Ultrastructure of the human mammary gland. II. Postpartum lactogenesis, *J Clin Endocrinol Metab* 40:834, 1975.

31. Vogel PM, Georgiade NG, Fetter BF et al: The correlation of histologic changes in the human breast with the menstrual cycle, *Am J Pathol* 104:23, 1981.

32. Vorherr H: *The breast: morphology, physiology, and lactation,* New York, 1974, Academic Press.

33. Weatherly-White RCA: *Plastic surgery of the female breast,* Hagerstown, Md, 1980, Harper & Row.

$\mathscr{P}$hysiology of lactation

Lactation is the physiologic completion of the reproductive cycle. The human infant at birth is the most immature and dependent of all mammals except for marsupials. The marsupial joey is promptly attached to the teat of a mammary gland in an external pouch. The gland changes as the offspring develops, and the joey remains there until able to survive outside the pouch. In the human, throughout pregnancy the breast develops and prepares to take over the role of fully nourishing the infant when the placenta is expelled.

The breast is prepared for full lactation from 16 weeks' gestation without any active intervention from the mother. It is kept inactive by a balance of inhibiting hormones that suppress target cell response. In the first few hours and days postpartum, the breast responds to changes in the hormonal milieu and the stimulus of the newborn infant's suckling to produce and release milk.[87]

The energy expenditure during lactation has suggested an efficiency of human milk synthesis greater than the 80% value previously hypothesized by investigators. Frigerio et al[21] suggest, from work in Gambian women and extensive review of other studies, that the energy cost of human lactation is minimal and the process functions at 95% efficiency.

This chapter provides a review of the physiologic adaptation of the mammary gland to its role in infant survival. Several major reviews are referenced that include substantial bibliographies for readers who need the detailed reports of the original investigators.* Newer scientific techniques in the study of human lactation provide more precise, more detailed, and more integrated data on which the clinician can base a physiologic approach to lactation management.

Box 3-1 lists the abbreviations for the hormones involved in lactation and discussed in this chapter.

HORMONAL CONTROL OF LACTATION

The mammary gland undergoes most of its morphogenesis postnatally in adolescence and adulthood, in contrast to most organs, which are fully developed prenatally.[56] Lactation is an integral part of the reproductive cycle of all mammals, including humans. The hormonal control of lactation can be described in relation to the five major stages in the development of the mammary gland: (1) embryogenesis; (2) mammogenesis, or mammary growth; (3) lactogenesis, or initiation of milk secretion; (4) lactation (stage III lactogenesis), or full milk secretion; and (5) involution[56] (Table 3-1).

Embryogenesis

Embryogenesis begins with the mammary band, which develops about the 35th embryonic day and progresses to a bud at the 49th day (see Chapter 2).

---

*References 16, 44, 51, 54, 57, 58, 87.

BOX 3-1   Hormone abbreviations

Adrenocorticotropic hormone	ACTH
Epidermal growth factor	EGF
Feedback inhibitor of lactation	FIL
Follicle-stimulating hormone	FSH
Growth hormone (human growth hormone)	GH (HGH)
Human growth factor	HGF, hGF
Human placental lactogen	HPL, hPL
Heregulin	NDF
Insulin-like growth factor 1	IGF-1
Prolactin	PRL
Prolactin-inhibiting factor	PIF
Thyroid-stimulating hormone	TSH
Thyrotropin-releasing hormone	TRH
Transforming growth factor beta	TGF-β

Ducts continue to elongate to form a mammary sprout, which invades the fat pad, branches, and canalizes, forming the rudimentary mammary ductal system present at birth. After birth, growth of this set of small branching ducts parallels the child's linear growth but remains limited, probably controlled by growth hormone before onset of ovarian activity.

Under the influence of sex steroids, especially the estrogens, the mammary glandular epithelium proliferates, becoming multilayered. Buds and papillae then form. The growth of the mammary gland is a gradual process that starts during puberty. The process depends on pituitary hormones. Lobuloalveolar development and ductal proliferation also depend on an intact pituitary gland.

The following six well-documented factors help explain organization of mammary growth. Much of this work has resulted since the availability of "knockout" studies in mice and associated techniques.

1. Mammary ducts must grow into an adipose tissue pad if morphogenesis is to continue. Only adipose stroma supports ductal elongation.[13] The mammary epithelium is closely associated with the adipocyte-containing stroma in all phases of development. In midgestation during human fetal development, a fat pad is laid down as a separate condensation of mesenchyma. Rudimentary ducts expand into the fat pad but do not progress.[56] At puberty the ducts elongate to fill the entire fat pad, terminating growth as they reach the margins of the fat pad.

2. Estrogen is essential to mammary growth. Ductal growth does not occur in the absence of ovaries but can be stimulated when estrogen is provided. In the ovariectomized (oophorectimized) mouse, an estrogen pellet placed in the mammary tissue stimulates growth in that gland but not in the opposite gland. When the estrogen receptor is "knocked out" in the mouse, no mammary development occurs. The increase in estrogen at puberty results in mammary development. Although estrogen is essential, it is not adequate alone.[4]

3. The exact location of the estrogen receptors in the human breast is unclear. Estrogen receptors are not in the proliferating cells and have not been located in the stroma. Cells with estrogen receptors, however, secrete a *paracrine factor* that is responsible for the proliferation of ductal cells. This paracrine factor may hold the key to understanding both normal and abnormal breast development.

4. In addition to estrogen, the pituitary gland is necessary for breast development. Kleinberg[35] has identified growth hormone (GH) as important to pubertal development and development of the terminal end buds in the breast. Prolactin could not replace GH in these experiments, but insulin-like growth factor 1 (IGF-1) could. It is produced in the stromal compartment of the mammary gland under stimulation by GH, and together with estradiol from the ovaries, IGF-1 brings about ductal development at puberty.

5. Transforming growth factor beta (TGF-β) maintains the spacing of the mammary ducts as they branch and elongate.[56] These ducts

TABLE 3-1 Stages of mammary development*

Developmental stage	Hormonal regulation	Local factors	Description
Embryogenesis	?	Fat pad necessary for ductal extension	Epithelial bud develops in 18- to 19-week-old fetus, extending short distance into mammary fat pad with blind ducts that become canalized; some milk secretion may be present at birth
Mammogenesis			Anatomic development
Puberty			
Before onset of menses	Estrogen, GH	IGF-1, hGF, TGF-β, ? others	Ductal extension into mammary fat pad; branching morphogenesis
After onset of menses	Estrogen, progesterone, ? PRL		Lobular development with formation of terminal duct lobular unit (TDLU)
Pregnancy	Progesterone, PRL, hPL	HER, ? others	Alveolus formation; partial cellular differentiation
Lactogenesis	Progesterone withdrawal, PRL, glucocorticoid	Not known	Onset of milk secretion Stage I: midpregnancy Stage II: parturition
Lactation	PRL, oxytocin	FIL	Ongoing milk secretion
Involution	PRL withdrawal	Milk stasis, ? FIL	Alveolar epithelium undergoes apoptosis and remodeling; gland reverts to prepregnant state.

Modified from Neville MC: Mammary gland biology and lactation: a short course. Presented at biannual meeting of the International Society for Research on Human Milk and Lactation, Plymouth, Mass, October 1997.
*See Box 3-1 for abbreviations.

exhibit unique behavior during growth, turning away to avoid other ducts and end buds. This avoidance behavior accounts for the orderly development of the duct system in the breast and the absence of ductal entanglements. This pattern provides ample space between ducts for later development of alveoli. TGF-β has been identified as the negative regulator and is found in many tissues, including breast tissue produced by an epithelial element. The pattern formation in ductal development depends on the localized expression of TGF-β.[14]

6. Progesterone secretion brings about the side branching of the mammary ducts.[32] The presence of progesterone receptors in the epithelial cells has been confirmed by studies in knockout mice whose mammary glands develop to the ductal stage but not to alveolar morphogenesis. Ormandy et al[62] established that prolactin is necessary for full alveolar development through prolactin receptor studies in knockout mice whose mammary glands do not develop beyond the ductal stage. This was further confirmed in murine mammary cultures when full development of the alveoli depends on prolactin.

Further, when prolactin is withdrawn, apoptosis of the alveolar cells occurs.[91]

The coordination of epithelial and stromal activity in the mammary gland is complex. Hepatocyte growth and scatter factor has been associated with the process during puberty.[62] Another growth factor, heregulin, a member of the epidermal growth factor (EGF) family has been identified in the stroma of mammary ducts during pregnancy.

Neville[56] has diagrammed the regulation of mammary development (Fig. 3-1). She notes that the concentrations of estrogen, progesterone, and lactogenic hormone in the form of prolactin or placental lactogen greatly increase, enhance alveolar development, and result in the differentiation of alveolar cells. Although many investigators have contributed pieces to the puzzle of mammogenesis, Neville has succeeded in creating the current visualization.

Mammogenesis: mammary growth
Prepubertal growth

Mammogenesis occurs in two phases as the gland responds to the hormones of puberty and later of pregnancy.[54] During the prepubertal phase the primary and secondary ducts that develop in the

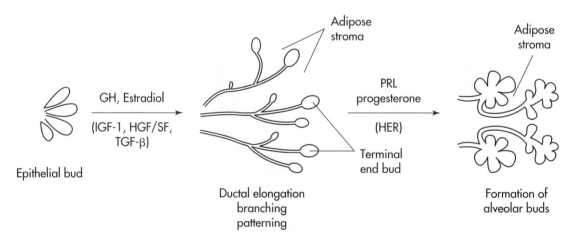

Fig. 3-1. Scheme for regulation of mammary development in the mouse. (From Neville MC: Mammary gland biology and lactation: a short course. Presented at annual meeting of the International Society for Research on Human Milk and Lactation, Plymouth, Mass, October 1997.)

fetus in utero continue to grow in both the male and the female in proportion to growth in general. Shortly before puberty, a more rapid expansion of the duct system begins in the female. The growth of the duct system seems to depend predominantly on estrogen and does not occur in the absence of ovaries. The complete growth of the alveoli requires stimulation by progesterone as well.

Studies of hypophysectomized animals have shown failure of full mammary growth even with adequate estrogen and progesterone. Secretion of prolactin and somatotropin by the pituitary gland results in mammary growth. Adrenocorticotropic hormone (ACTH) and thyroid-stimulating hormone (TSH) acting on the adrenal and thyroid glands also play a minor role in growth of the mammary gland.

Growth and development during organogenesis involve the interaction of cells with extracellular matrices and neighboring cells.[76] Necropsy breast specimens from six male and eight female infants ranging in age from 1 day to 9 months were studied to determine the process of organogenesis in the human.[1] Integrins were expressed in a pattern that correlates with morphologic and functional differentiation of the normal mammary gland. *Integrins* are transmembrane glycoproteins that form receptors for extracellular matrix proteins such as fibronectin, laminin, and collagen. Integrins are widely expressed in normal tissue and are considered critical to the control of cell growth and differentiation. This suggests integrin involvement in the functional characterization of the adhesion molecules in the breast.

Pubertal growth

When the hypophyseal-ovarian-uterine cycle is established, a new phase of mammary growth begins, which includes extensive branching of the system of ducts and proliferation and canalization of the lobuloalveolar units at the distal tips of the branches. Organization of the stromal connective tissue forms the interlobular septa. The ducts, ductules (terminal intralobular ducts), and alveolar structures are all formed by double layers of cells. One layer, the epithelial cells, circumscribes the lumen. The second layer, the myoepithelial cells, surrounds the inner epithelial cells and is bordered by a basement lamina.

Menstrual cycle growth

The cyclic changes of the adult mammary gland can be associated with the menstrual cycle and the hormonal changes that control that cycle. Estrogens stimulate parenchymal proliferation, with formation of epithelial sprouts. This hyperplasia continues into the secretory phase of the cycle. Anatomically, when the corpus luteum provides increased amounts of estrogens and progesterone, there is lobular edema, thickening of the epithelial basal membrane, and secretory material in the alveolar lumen. Lymphoid and plasma cells infiltrate the stroma. Clinically, mammary blood flow increases in this luteal phase. This is experienced by women as fullness, heaviness, and turgescence. The breast may become nodular because of interlobular edema and ductular-acinar growth.

After onset of menstruation and reduction of sex steroid levels, milk-secretory prolactin action is limited. Postmenstrual changes occur rapidly, with degeneration of glandular cells and proliferation tissue, loss of edema, and decrease in breast size. The ovulatory cycle actually enhances mammary growth in the early years of menstruation (until about age 30) because the postmenstrual regression of the glandular-alveolar growth after each cycle is not complete. These changes of ductal and lobular proliferation, which occur during the follicular phase before ovulation, continue in the luteal phase and regress after the menstrual phase, exemplifying the sensitivity of this target organ to variations in the balance of hormones.

Fowler et al[18] measured cyclic changes in composition and volume of the breast during the menstrual cycle using nuclear magnetic resonance (NMR) imaging. The T1 relaxation time (spin-lattice T1 relaxation) is a measure of the rate of energy loss from tissues after NMR excitation. This energy loss depends on the biophysical environment of the excited protons. A short T1, therefore, indicates the presence of lipids and organic structures that bind water tightly. A longer

T1 occurs with greater hydration and with the greatest amount of cellular water. This study revealed the lowest total breast volume and parenchymal volume. T1 and water content occurred between days 6 and 15 of the cycle. Between days 16 and 28, T1 rose sharply and peaked the 25th day. The rise in parenchymal volume in the second half of the cycle resulted not only from increased tissue water but also growth and increased tissue fluid, according to Fowler et al.[18]

Growth during pregnancy

Hormonal influences on the breast cause profound changes during pregnancy (Fig. 3-2). Early in pregnancy, a marked increase in ductular sprouting, branching, and lobular formation is evoked by luteal and placental hormones.[94] Placental lactogen, prolactin, and chorionic gonadotrophin have been identified as contributors to the accelerated growth. The dichorionic ductular sprouting has

been attributed to estrogen and lobular formation to progesterone.

Prolactin is essential for complete lobular-alveolar development of the gland. Almost complete growth of the mammary lobular-alveolar system can be obtained experimentally in the hypophysectomized-adrenalectomized rat if the animal receives estrogen, progesterone, and prolactin.[38] Prolactin, as with other protein hormones, exerts its effect through receptors for the initiation of milk secretion located on the alveolar cell surfaces. The induction of milk synthesis requires insulin-induced cell division and the presence of cortisol. Prolactin is secreted by the pituitary, which is negatively controlled by prolactin-inhibiting factor (PIF) from the hypothalamus.[38]

From the third month of gestation, secretory material that resembles colostrum appears in the acini. Prolactin from the anterior pituitary gland stimulates the glandular production of colostrum.

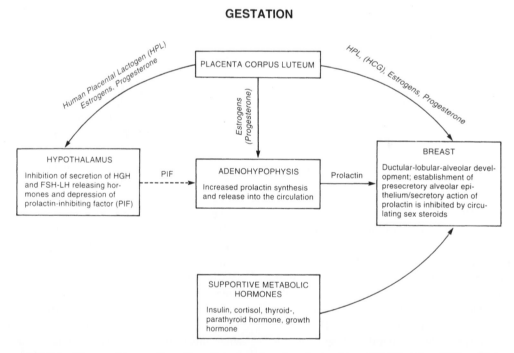

Fig. 3-2.   Hormonal preparation of breast during pregnancy for lactation. (Modified from Vorherr H: *The breast: morphology, physiology and lactation,* New York, 1974, Academic Press.)

By the second trimester, placental lactogen begins to stimulate the secretion of colostrum. A mother who delivers after 16 weeks of gestation will secrete colostrum, even though she has had a nonviable infant. This demonstrates the effectiveness of hormonal stimulation on lactation.

An estrogen-mediated increase in prolactin secretion in pregnancy may produce as much as a 10-fold to 20-fold increase in plasma prolactin. This effect may be partially controlled by lactogen from the placenta, which inhibits the production of prolactin. Hormonal regulation of the growth and proliferation of the mammary gland cells has been carefully studied in many species.

A complex sequence of events, governed by hormonal action, prepares the breast for lactation (Fig. 3-2). Estradiol-17β stimulates the ductal system of epithelial cells to elongate during pregnancy. In contrast to puberty, however, when estrogens appear to directly and indirectly stimulate breast development, estrogens have no indispensable role in mammary development during pregnancy except as a prolactin potentiator, according to Neville;[53] when estrogen levels are low in pregnancy, the breast still develops. Estrogen levels are normally high in pregnancy, but not for mammogenesis. Induced lactation in the cow is dependably reproduced with 7 days of estrogen and progesterone treatment. Progesterone, in turn, induces the specific epithelial cells of the tubular invaginations to produce distinct ducts, which branch from the main tubules. The end result of the combined actions of estrogen and progesterone is a richly branched arborization of the gland. Highly differentiated secretory alveolar cells develop at the ends of these ducts under the influence of prolactin.

Serum growth factor, which is present in normal human serum, and insulin can stimulate the stem cells of the gland to proliferate. These dividing cells are further directed to the formation of alveoli by corticosteroid hormones. At least two types of cells are identified in the epithelial layer of the gland: stem cells and secretory alveolar cells. At this point in the pregnancy, prolactin influences the production of the constituents of milk.

TGF-β influences pattern formation in the developing mammary gland and may negatively regulate ductal growth as well.[14] The pattern of mammary ductal development varies widely among species and is a function of both genotype and hormonal status. Normal human breast cells secrete TGF-β and are themselves inhibited by it, suggesting an autoregulatory feedback circuit that may be modulated by estradiol. Growth and patterning of the ductal tree are regulated in part by TGF-β operating through an autocrine feedback mechanism and by paracrine circuits associated with epithelial-stromal interactions.[14]

The high circulating levels of prolactin are not associated with milk production partly because of the progesterone antagonism of the stimulatory action of prolactin on casein messenger ribonucleic acid (mRNA) synthesis. During late pregnancy the lactogenic receptors, which have similar affinities for both prolactin and human placental lactogen (HPL), are predominantly occupied by HPL. High doses of estradiol impair the incorporation of prolactin into milk secretory cells.

Prolactin is prevented from exerting its effect on milk excretion by the elevated levels of progesterone. Following the drop in progesterone and estrogen at delivery, copious milk secretion begins. The key hormone requirements for lactation to begin are prolactin, insulin, and hydrocortisone. Prolactin stabilizes and promotes transcription of casein mRNA and stimulates synthesis of a lactalbumin that is the regulatory protein of the lactose-synthetase enzyme system.[63] Prolactin further increases the lipoprotein lipase activity in the mammary gland. Prolactin exists in three heterogenic forms of varying biologic activity. The monomer is in greatest quantity and is the most active form.

Lactogenesis: initiation of milk secretion

Hartmann[28] has described the two stages of lactogenesis. Stage I starts about 12 weeks before parturition and is heralded by significant increases in lactose, total proteins, and immunoglobulin and by decreases in sodium and chloride, and the gathering of substrate for milk production. The composition of prepartum secretion is fairly constant until delivery, as monitored by the milk protein α-lactalbumin.

Lactogenesis is initiated in the postpartum period by a fall in plasma progesterone while prolactin levels remain high (Fig. 3-3). The initiation of the process does not depend on suckling by the infant until the third or fourth day, when the secretion declines if milk is not removed from the breast.[92,93]

Stage II includes the increase in blood flow and oxygen and glucose uptake as well as the sharp increase in citrate concentration, considered a reliable marker for lactogenesis stage II. Stage II at 2 to 3 days postpartum begins clinically when the secretion of milk is copious and biochemically when plasma α-lactalbumin levels peak (paralleling the period when "the milk comes in"). The

major changes in milk composition continue for 10 days, when "mature milk" is established. The establishment of mature milk supply, once called *galactopoiesis,* is now referred to as *stage III of lactogenesis.*[93,94]

The profound changes in milk composition have been established for the period of transitional to mature milk in relationship to increase in milk volume.[54] Detailed studies of successfully lactating women were performed by Neville et al,[57] who report that a significant fall in sodium, chloride, and protein and a rise in lactose precede the major increase in milk volume during early lactogenesis. At 46 to 96 hours postpartum, copious milk production is accompanied by an increase in citrate, glucose, free phosphate, and calcium concentrations and a decrease in pH (Figs. 3-15 and 3-16).

The breast, one of the most complex endocrine target organs, has been prepared during pregnancy and responds to the release of prolactin by produc-

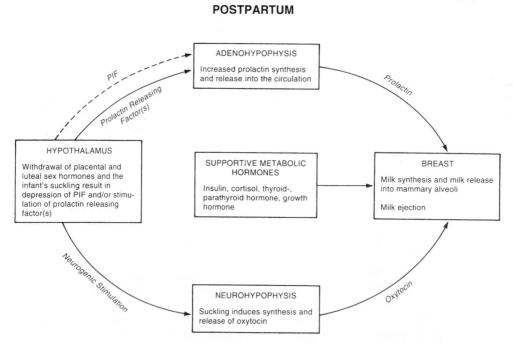

Fig. 3-3.   Hormonal preparation of breast postpartum for lactation. (Modified from Vorherr H: *The breast: morphology, physiology and lactation,* New York, 1974, Academic Press.)

ing the constituents of milk (Fig. 3-3). The lactogenic effects of prolactin are modulated by the complex interplay of pituitary, ovarian, thyroid, adrenal, and pancreatic hormones.

Prolactin

Human prolactin is a significant hormone in pregnancy and lactation.[19] Prolactin also has a range of actions in various species that is greater than any other known hormone. Prolactin has been identified in many animal species whether they nurse their young or not. Because of the original association with lactation, the term describes its action, "support or stimulation of lactation." Prolactin, however, has been shown to control nonlactating responses in other species and has been identified with more than 80 different physiologic processes. Study of prolactin was hampered until 1970, when it became possible to separate prolactin from human growth hormone (HGH) and to isolate and characterize prolactin from human pituitary glands.[84]

Before 1971, HGH and prolactin in humans were considered the same hormone. Until 1971, in fact, it was thought that prolactin did not exist in humans. HGH, however, is present in the human pituitary gland in an amount 100 times that of prolactin.

Plasma prolactin varies in relation to psychosocial stress. Utilizing four different real-life stress studies in a longitudinal design, Theorell[85] found that change situations associated with passive coping are accompanied by increased plasma prolactin levels. Change situations associated with active coping are associated with unchanged or even lowered prolactin levels. The regulation of plasma prolactin is part of a dopaminergic system (see the list of pharmacologic suppressors on p. 68).

In vitro, prolactin stimulates the synthesis of the mRNAs of specific milk proteins by binding to membrane receptors of the mammary epithelial cells. Prolactin has been demonstrated to penetrate the cytoplasm of these cells and even their nuclei. These specific actions in the gland require the presence of extracellular calcium ions. Some prolactin actually appears in the milk substrate itself,

the functional significance of which is uncertain, although it is thought to influence fluid and ion absorption from the neonatal jejunum.

The effect of the stimulation of protein synthesis by allowing the expression of milk protein genes is not a direct effect of the hormone but rather the consequence of the activation of sodium/potassium adenosinetriphosphatase (Na/K ATPase) in the plasma membrane. The intracellular concentration of potassium is kept high and that of sodium low compared with the concentrations in extracellular fluid. As a result, the Na/K ratio is high both in the milk and in the intracellular fluid. Further action of prolactin has been identified in the development of the immune system in the mammary gland and, possibly more directly, in the lymphoid tissue. In conjunction with estrogen and progesterone, prolactin attracts and retains immunoglobulin A (IgA) immunoblasts from the gut-associated lymphoid tissue for the development of the immune system for the mammary gland. A very sensitive bioassay has been developed using the in vitro biologic effect of prolactin to stimulate the growth of cell cultures for malignant niobium (Nb) rat lymphomas.

The baseline levels of prolactin are essentially the same in the normal human male and female (Table 3-2). Moreover, both male and female experience a rise in prolactin levels during sleep. At puberty the increase in estrogens causes a slight but measurable increase in prolactin. Prolactin increases during the proliferative phase of the menstrual cycle but not during the secretory phase. There is also a normal diurnal variation in levels in both male and female. A number of factors, including some that are significant for the nursing mother, such as psychogenic influence and stress, increase prolactin levels. Anesthesia, surgery, exercise, nipple stimulation, and sexual intercourse also produce increased amounts in both lactating and nonlactating females. Prolactin levels increase as serum osmolality increases.

Although prolactin levels in maternal serum are well established, less is known about prolactin levels in the milk and its role in the newborn. Prolactin in milk is biologically potent and is

TABLE 3-2   Prolactin levels*

	Range (ng/ml)	Average (ng/ml)
Males and prepubertal and postmenopausal females	2-8	
Females' menstrual life	8-14	10
Term pregnancy	200-500	200
Amniotic fluid	Up to 10,000	
Lactating women	Response to breastfeeding	
First 10 days	Baseline 200	Rise to 400
10-90 days	60-110	70-220
90-180 days	50	100
180 days-1 year	30-40	45-80

*Collation of values from multiple studies and sources.

absorbed by the newborn. In the intestine, prolactin influences fluid, sodium, potassium, and calcium transport. Prolactin content is highest in the early transitional milk just after the colostrum in the first postpartum week (levels of 43.1 ± 4 ng/ml).[99] Levels drop to 11.0 ± 1.4 ng/ml in mature milk over time until 40 weeks postpartum.

Prolactin-inhibiting factor

Prolactin-inhibiting factor (PIF) controls the secretion of prolactin from the hypothalamus. Prolactin thus is unusual among the pituitary hormones because it is inhibited by a hypothalamic substance. Catecholamine levels in the hypothalamus control the inhibiting factor, which is poured into the circulation as a result of dopaminergic impulses. Drugs and events that decrease catecholamines also decrease the inhibiting factor, causing a rise in prolactin. Dopamine itself can act directly on the pituitary gland to decrease prolactin secretion. Agents that increase prolactin by decreasing catecholamines and thus the PIF level include the phenothiazines and reserpine.

Thyrotropin-releasing hormone (TRH) is a strong stimulator of prolactin secretion, but its physiologic role is not clear, because thyrotropin levels do not rise during normal nursing. In the postpartum period, a dose of TRH will cause a marked increase in prolactin. Even the nonnursing postpartum mother will experience engorgement and milk release when stimulated with TRH. Ergot,

which is frequently prescribed for the postpartum patient, inhibits prolactin secretion either by direct inhibition or by its effect on the hypothalamus.

Prolactin response to breast stimulation in lactating women is not mediated by endogenous opioids. Neither baseline nor stimulated prolactin values were affected by naloxone.[7]

Following are factors affecting prolactin release in normal humans:

Physiologic stimuli
    Nursing in postpartum women—breast stimulation
    Sleep
    Stress
    Sexual intercourse
    Pregnancy
Pharmacologic stimuli
    Neuroleptic drugs
    TRH
    Metoclopramide (procainamide derivative)
    Estrogens
    Hypoglycemia
    Phenothiazines, butyrophenones
    Norepinephrine
    Histamine
    Acetylcholine
Pharmacologic suppressors
    L-Dopa
    Ergot preparations (2-Br-α-ergocryptine)
    Clomiphene citrate
    Large amounts of pyridoxine
    Monoamine oxidase inhibitors
    Prostaglandins E and $F_{2\alpha}$

Fig. 3-4. Prolactin levels after suckling. (From Battin DA, Marrs RP, Flaeiss PM et al: *Obstet Gynecol* 65:785, 1985.)

In pregnancy, prolactin levels begin to rise in the first trimester and continue to rise throughout gestation. In the nonnursing mother, prolactin levels drop to normal in 2 weeks, independent of therapy to suppress lactation.

At delivery, with the expulsion of the placenta, levels of placental lactogen, estrogens, and progesterone abruptly decline.

Placental lactogen disappears within hours.[58] Progesterone drops over several days, and estrogens fall to baseline levels in 5 to 6 days (see Figs. 19-2 to 19-4). Prolactin in nonlactating women requires 14 days to reach baseline. Progesterone is considered the key inhibiting hormone, and decline in plasma progesterone levels is considered the lactogenic trigger for stage II lactogenesis.[53] However, progesterone does not inhibit established lactation because breast tissue does not contain progesterone-binding sites. Estrogens enhance the effect of prolactin on mammogenesis but antagonize prolactin by inhibiting secretion of milk. After delivery, there are low estrogen and high prolactin levels. Suckling provides a continued stimulus for prolactin release. If prolactin, essential for lactation, is diminished by hypophysectomy or medication, lactation ceases. Baseline prolactin levels do eventually diminish to more normal levels months after parturition, although lactation may continue.

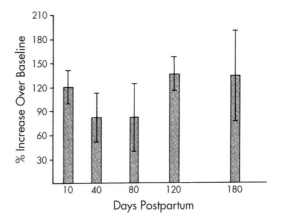

Fig. 3-5. Percent increase in prolactin over baseline after suckling. (From Battin DA, Marrs RP, Fleiss PM et al: *Obstet Gynecol* 65:785, 1985.)

The surge in prolactin over baseline levels is critical to milk production, not the baseline levels (Figs. 3-4 and 3-5). Although prolactin is necessary for milk secretion, the volume of milk secreted is not directly related to the concentration of prolactin in the plasma. Local mechanisms within the mammary gland that depend on the amount of milk removed by the infant are responsible for the day-to-day regulation of milk volume. Suckling stimulates the release of adenohypophyseal prolactin and neurohypophyseal oxytocin. These hormones stimulate milk synthesis and production of milk-ejection metabolic hormones, which are also necessary in the process of milk synthesis.[53] Thus, suckling, emptying the breast, and receiving adequate precursor nutrients are essential to effective lactation (Fig. 3-6).

When milk is not removed, secretion ceases in a few days, and the composition of the mammary secretion returns to a colostrum-like fluid. When the composition of the breast secretion of breastfeeding and nonbreastfeeding women was followed by Kulski and Hartmann,[37] it was the same for 3 to 4 days. Thereafter, the sodium and chloride concentrations in the nonbreastfeeding women increased rapidly.

The regulation of milk production in full lactation is based primarily on infant demand.[59] Maternal nutrition, age, body composition, and parity have only secondary impact. Suckling is a powerful stimulus to prolactin synthesis and secretion, and prolactin is necessary for milk secretion.[85] The pulsatile nature of prolactin secretion makes it difficult to measure over time. Milk yield is not directly correlated to prolactin levels. Evidence indicates that a proteinaceous factor in milk itself actually inhibits milk production and is associated with residual milk in the breast. This has been identified as feedback inhibitor of lactation (see p. 80).

Prolactin circadian rhythm persists throughout lactation. Prolactin levels are notably higher at night than during the day, despite greater nursing times during the day. The highest levels in Stern and Reichlin's study were when the least nursing occurred.[81]

The most effective and specific stimulus to prolactin release is nursing. The stimulation is a result of nipple or breast manipulation, especially suckling, not a psychologic effect of the presence of the infant (Fig. 3-6). The prolactin-release reflex during nipple stimulation is suppressed in some adult women, being evidenced only during pregnancy and lactation.

During human pregnancy, when serum prolactin rises steadily to 150 to 200 ng/ml at term, there is a brief drop in levels hours before delivery and then a rise again as soon as the neonate is suckled.[42,51] The response to nipple stimulation can be abolished by applying local anesthetic. On the other hand, trauma or surgery to the chest wall can initiate a prolactin rise and, in some reported cases, milk production.

Although it was initially reported that the high levels of prolactin measured in the first days and weeks of lactation dwindled to normal baseline by 6 months and showed no response to suckling stimulus, later studies clearly showed a different picture with more sensitive assays.[42] Baseline does not drop to normal, but further stimulus causes a doubling of levels over baseline at all stages of lactation through the second year (Table 3-2).

Acute prolactin and oxytocin responses were measured by Zinaman et al,[100] who compared various mechanical pumping devices with manual ex-

Fig. 3-6. Plasma prolactin measured by radioimmunoassay before, during, and after period of nursing in three mothers, 22 to 26 days postpartum. Prolactin levels rose with suckling and not with infant contact. (Modified from Josimovich JB, Reynolds M, Cobo E: Lactogenic hormones, fetal nutrition, and lactation. In *Problems of human reproduction,* vol 2, New York, 1974, John Wiley & Sons.)

pression and infant suckling. Prolactin response to mechanical expression in quantity and duration depended on the device used, with the full-size pulsatile electric pump (White River) eliciting the greatest response. This compared equally with infant suckling. There was no difference seen in oxytocin response with various devices. These data confirm that results in studies of milk production and release in humans also depend on the equipment used to stimulate the breast.[100]

Eight fully lactating women were followed through the first 6 months postpartum at 10, 40, 80, 120, and 180 days, recording serum prolactin, luteinizing hormone (LH), follicle-stimulating hormone (FSH), and estradiol (zero time only) obtained just before the initiation of suckling and during the next 120 minutes.[2] Samples were obtained at 0, +15, +30, +60, and +120 minutes. Prolactin levels were high the first 10 days (90.1 ng/ml) but slowly declined over 180 days (44.3 ng/ml). The stimulus of suckling doubled the baseline values. Mean estradiol levels were low at 10 days (7.2 pg/ml), then gradually rose to a mean of 47.3 pg/ml at 180 days postpartum in the subjects whose menses had resumed. In the amenorrheic subjects the estradiol levels remained low (4.25 pg/ml), whereas baseline prolactin remained high (63.6 ng/ml). The subjects were breastfeeding on demand, averaging 11 feedings (range 8 to 16) per day at 10 days and 8 feedings (range 5 to 12) at 120 and 180 days. All infants had stopped one night feeding, and two infants had started some solids between the third and fourth months.

The effort to relate the prolactin level to the volume of milk has not produced consistent findings.[9] Stimulating both breasts simultaneously, however, by either feeding two babies or "double pumping" (attachment to both breasts to pump via a Y tube) does produce a higher prolactin surge and a greater volume of milk totally as well as per unit of time. Howie et al[31] reported the relationship between suckling-induced prolactin response and production of milk as being imprecise, finding no close temporal correlation between prolactin concentrations and milk yield. Milk yield was measured by electronic scale weighings before

and after feedings. They calculated not only the peak prolactin level but also the area under the curve, and this latter value was consistent within the individual mother.

When specific binding sites for prolactin were looked for in the tammar wallaby, many sites were demonstrated in the lactating mammary gland but not the inactive gland.[44] Mammary prolactin receptors were also identified in the rabbit. Thus the increased binding capacity would enhance tissue responsiveness, which may explain the maintenance of full lactation in the face of falling concentrations of prolactin. Prolactin also plays a critical role in increasing maternal bile secretory function postpartum.[46]

Human placental lactogen and human growth hormone

Three main hormones are recognized in the lactogenic process: human placental lactogen (HPL), human growth hormone (HGH), and prolactin. The progressive rise in prolactin during pregnancy parallels the rise in HPL, becoming measurable at 6 weeks' gestation and increasing to 6000 ng/ml at term. This parallel action contributed to the belief that prolactin and HPL were the same. Although the principal function of HPL and prolactin in the human is a lactogenic one, no lactation appears before delivery.[79]

First described in 1962, HPL has been studied more than lactogens from any other species.[52] Extensive immunologic and structural homology exists between HGH and HPL, which probably explains their similar biologic activities. Concentrations of HPL increase steadily during gestation and decrease abruptly with the delivery of the placenta. A large-molecular-weight substance, HPL is derived from the chorion. Receptor sites that bind lactogen also bind protein and HGH.[90] HPL has been associated with mobilization of free fatty acid and inhibition of peripheral glucose utilization and lactogenic action.

HGH is secreted from the anterior pituitary eosinophilic cells. These cells have been identified by staining techniques that distinguish them from those that produce prolactin. Toward the end of pregnancy, the cells that produce prolactin are noticeably more numerous, whereas those that produce HGH are "crowded out." The role of HGH in the maintenance of lactation is poorly defined and may be synergistic with prolactin and glucocorticoids.

Prolactin, HGH, placental lactogen (PL), and chorionic somatotropin (CS) form a family of polypeptide hormones from the same ancestral gene, even though prolactin and HGH are produced by the pituitary and PL and CS by the placenta.[95] The suckling stimulus in postpartum lactation causes a rapid increase in serum HGH and prolactin. HGH and prolactin evolve from the same precursor, and although the hormones are distinct, the acute interruption of HGH secretion does not interfere with the milk secretion.

The possible role of TRH as a physiologic prolactin-releasing factor has been disproved by Gehlbach et al,[23] who state that TSH is not responsible for the brisk release of prolactin with suckling. Normal lactation is possible in ateliotic dwarf women in the absence of detectable quantities of HGH.[73] For any hormone to exert its biologic effects, however, specific receptors for the hormone must be present in the target tissue. Changes in serum concentration have no effect if receptors are not present in the mammary gland to bind the hormone.

Stage III lactogenesis (galactopoiesis): maintenance of established lactation

The maintenance of established milk secretion, originally called *galactopoiesis,* is now labeled *stage III lactogenesis,* or simply *lactation.* An intact hypothalamic-pituitary axis regulating prolactin and oxytocin levels is essential to the initiation and maintenance of lactation.[39] The process of lactation requires milk synthesis and milk release into the alveoli and the lactiferous sinuses. When the milk is not removed, the increased pressure lessens capillary blood flow, and inhibits the lactation process. Lack of sucking stimulation means lack of prolactin release from the pituitary gland. Basal prolactin levels that are enhanced by the spurts that result from sucking are

necessary to maintain lactation in the first weeks postpartum. Without oxytocin, however, a pregnancy can be carried to term, but the female will fail to lactate because she will fail to let-down.

Sensory nerve endings, located mainly in the areola and nipple, are stimulated by suckling. The afferent neural reflex pathway, via the spinal cord to the mesencephalon and then to the hypothalamus, produces secretion and release of prolactin and oxytocin. Hypothalamic suppression of earlier PIF secretion causes adrenohypophyseal prolactin release. When prolactin is released into the circulation, it stimulates milk synthesis and secretion. A conditioned milk ejection can occur in lactating women without a concomitant release of prolactin, so that indeed the releases are independent, which may be significant in treating apparent lactation failure (Fig. 3-7).

Hormonal regulation of prolactin and oxytocin

The release of prolactin is inhibited by PIF.[40] The PIF has not been described but is closely associated with dopamine. There is also evidence of either serotonin release of prolactin or catecholamine-serotonin control of prolactin release. TSH has also been shown to simulate the release of prolactin. The amount of prolactin is proportional to the amount of nipple stimulation during early stages of lactation.

Although both oxytocin and prolactin release are stimulated by nipple stimulation, some oxytocin is released by other sensory pathways, such as the visual, tactile, olfactory, and auditory.[60] Thus a woman may release milk on seeing, touching, hearing, smelling, or thinking about her infant. Prolactin, however, is released only on nipple stimulation so that milk production is not initiated by other sensory pathways. Oxytocin is also released under physical stress, such as pain, exercise, cold, heat, changes in plasma osmolality, or hypovolemia, but these responses are blunted or reversed during lactation.[60]

When suckling occurs, oxytocin is released.[11] It enters the circulation and rapidly causes ejection of milk from alveoli and smaller milk ducts into

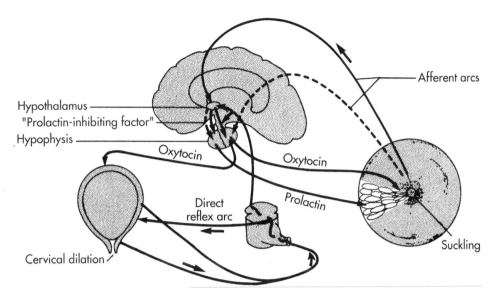

Fig. 3-7. Neuroendocrine control of milk ejection. (Modified from Vorherr H: *The breast: morphology, physiology and lactation,* New York, 1974, Academic Press.)

larger lactiferous ducts and sinuses. This is the pathway of the letdown, or ejection, reflex. Oxytocin also causes contraction of the myometrium and involution of the uterus.

The nonpeptide oxytocin is a messenger molecule with diverse physiologic actions as well as modes of delivery to its target sites. Oxytocin exerts effects as a hormone carried by the systemic circulation to distant targets in the uterus and the breast.[12] Oxytocin also serves as a hypophysiotropic factor, released from nerve terminals in the median eminence into the pituitary portal vasculature to affect anterior pituitary secretion. Its action here is as a peptidergic neurotransmitter or neuromodulator within the central nervous system, influencing a variety of neuroendocrine, behavioral, and autonomic functions. Its well-known role is related to reproduction and lactation, but it has other, less well-explored physical and metabolic roles.[12]

After suckling is initiated, the oxytocin response is transient and intermittent rather than sustained. Plasma levels often return to basal between milk ejections, even though suckling continues. Ejection can be measured by placing

a microcatheter in the mammary duct or can be noted subjectively by the mother as tingling or turgescence. The contractions last about 1 minute, with about four to 10 occurring in a 10-minute period. Corresponding pulses of oxytocin can be measured in the maternal bloodstream. The controls of oxytocin release are complex and are extensively described by Crowley and Armstrong.[12] Centrally released oxytocin in control of the milk-ejection reflex was established in 1981 by Freund-Mercier and Richard.[20] They demonstrated that intracerebroventricular administration of oxytocin greatly increased the frequency and amplitude of pulsatile oxytocin release during suckling. Administration of oxytocin antagonists produced the opposite effect and suppressed responses.[20]

The human pituitary has an excessive storage capacity and contains 3000 to 9000 mU oxytocin, but the reflex milk ejection only involves the release of 50 to 100 mU.[96] Except in extreme cases (Sheenan's syndrome), hormone depletion is rarely an issue, but hormone release and target-organ sensitivity are. Opiate and β-endorphin released during stress are known to block stimulus-secretion coupling by dissociating electrical activity at the terminal. This inhibition is naloxone reversible.

The mammary gland, from the platypus to the human, has an identical fine structure consisting of alveolar tissue that has increased its surface area 10,000-fold during gestation compared with the size of the gland.[48] It continuously produces milk throughout lactation, but the most complex issue is the release of milk. Because of the substantial surface tension forces opposing the movement of fluid in the small ducts, simple suction applied by suckling is relatively ineffective, especially in early lactation. Thus the alveolus is enveloped in a basketlike network of myoepithelial cells that respond to oxytocin by contracting and expelling the milk into larger and larger ductules until it can be removed by the infant (Fig. 3-8). This is a classic example of a neuroendocrine reflex, a process that is remarkably uniform in all mammals.

Neuroendocrine control of milk ejection

Milk ejection involves both neural and endocrinologic stimulation and response. A neural afferent pathway and an endocrinologic efferent pathway are required.[52]

The ejection reflex depends on receptors located in the canalicular system of the breast. When the canaliculi are dilated or stretched, the reflex release of oxytocin is triggered. Tactile receptors for both oxytocin and reflex prolactin release are in the nipple. Neither the negative and positive pressures exerted by suckling nor the thermal changes trigger the milk-ejection reflex. Negative pressures have a minor effect, but tactile stimulation is the most important factor.

Studies in tactile stimulation show changes in sensitivity at puberty, during the menstrual cycle, and at parturition.[74] No difference exists in sensitivity between the sexes before puberty. In the female, tactile sensitivity increases after puberty and is increased at midcycle and during menstruation. (Midcycle peak is absent in women taking oral contraceptives.) Dramatic changes occur within 24 hours of delivery after several weeks of

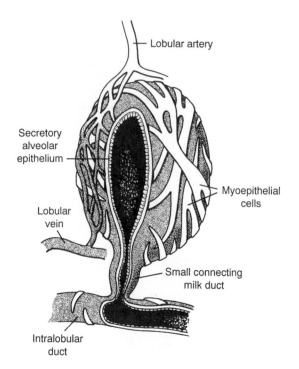

Fig. 3-8. Fundamental mammary unit at lactation, with arrangement of secretory alveoli, myoepithelial cells, and vasculature. Secretory alveolar epithelium is monolayered, and epithelial lining of milk ducts consists of two layers. Between bases of glandular epithelial cells and tunica propria, starlike myoepithelial mammary cells surround alveolus in basketlike arrangement. (Modified from Vorherr H: *The breast: morphology, physiology and lactation,* New York, 1974, Academic Press.)

complete insensitivity. The nipple is the more sensitive area to both touch and pain, followed by the areola; the least sensitive area is the cutaneous breast tissue. The increased sensitivity of the breast continues several days postpartum, even when the woman does not breastfeed. Estrogen treatment suppresses the induction of prolactin release on nipple stimulation, whereas on withdrawal of estrogen the prolactin response returns. Increased tactile sensitivity may be the key event activating the suckling-induced release of oxytocin and prolactin at delivery (Figs. 3-9 and 3-10).

The clinical study of oxytocin challenge tests for use in measuring the viability of the fetus has led to the study of breast stimulus on the uterus.

Fig. 3-9. Changes in tactile sensitivity of cutaneous breast tissue in perinatal period. Sensitivity was calculated from two-point discrimination according to formula $K - \log^e$. K is an arbitrary figure employed to portray low two-point discrimination value as peaks of sensitivity. Dramatic increase in tactile sensitivity at delivery enhances response to suckling of newborn. (From Robinson JE, Short RV: *Br Med J* I:1188, 1977.)

Fig. 3-10. Sensitivity of human mammary epithelium to oxytocin during pregnancy and lactation. Right-hand scale shows threshold dose necessary to evoke increase in intramammary pressure; left-hand scale shows maximum intramammary pressure obtained. (Modified from Caldeyro-Barcia R: Milk ejection in women. In Reynolds M, Folley SJ, editors: *Lactogenesis: the initiation of milk secretion at parturition,* Philadelphia, 1969, University of Pennsylvania Press.)

Numerous studies have confirmed that oxytocin levels rise significantly during nipple stimulation, with short bursts of oxytocin during accompanying uterine contractions.[8] When the effect of breast stimulation on prostaglandin secretion was tested at 38 to 40 weeks' gestation, uterine contractions occurred and prostaglandin metabolite levels increased in all cases. Shalev et al[77] suggest that the principal action of oxytocin is to stimulate prostaglandin synthesis in uterine tissues, which then becomes the primary cause of the uterine contractions.

The oxytocin-binding sites are located within the basement membrane of the mammary alveolus and along the interlobular ducts. A gradual 10-fold increase occurs in the concentration of oxytocin receptor sites in the mammary gland during pregnancy.[43] This contrasts sharply with the sudden 40-fold increase in oxytocin receptors in the uterus in the hours before delivery that then rapidly disappear. These changes in receptor availability may be why copious milk does not occur until shortly after delivery, because oxytocin first facilitates delivery and then promotes milk ejection sequentially. When the increase in intramammary pressure obtained with varying doses of oxytocin in nonpregnant, pregnant, and lactating women was recorded by Caldeyro-Barcia,[5] the amount of oxytocin required for a response dropped from 1000 mU in nonpregnancy to about 1 mU in late pregnancy and further to 0.5 mU in lactation.[53] (Fig. 3-10). The maximum intramammary pressure that could be evoked increased from 1 mm Hg to a peak of 10 mm Hg 5 days postpartum. Caldeyro-Barcia suggests that not only the sensitivity of the myoepithelial cells but the number of receptor sites increases as well during pregnancy.

Conflicting information exists regarding the exact nature of the release of oxytocin from the pituitary. The dose-response curve of the mammary gland has a very limited dynamic range, so that a bolus of 0.1 mU oxytocin (0.2 mg) given intravenously to a lactating rat fails to change intramammary pressure. An injection of 1.0 mU evokes an increase in pressure that begins after a delay of 10 seconds and peaks in 15 seconds at 8 to 10 mm Hg. A bolus has greater effect than a slow push, suggesting that a pulsatile pattern of hormone release would be the most effective way of utilizing oxytocin to produce milk ejection.[51]

Plasma oxytocin levels measured by Lucas et al[48] with continuous sampling every 20 seconds revealed the hormone was released in surges and persisted in the circulation for less than 1 minute. The multiparas had a greater total response, but with no difference between early (1 to 3 days postpartum) and late (5 to 7 days). When a similar study was done by Dawood et al[15] collecting samples only every 3 minutes, no pulsing was identified. Oxytocin was measurable within 2 minutes of suckling, peaked at 10 minutes, and had a bimodal curve dropping to a mean at 20 minutes comparable with that before suckling, which followed the burping and changing breasts at about 15 minutes. A secondary peak occurred at 25 minutes. They found maximum response of intramammary pressures at the fifth to seventh day. McNeilly et al[51] measured release of oxytocin in response to suckling in early and established lactation, drawing samples every 30 seconds. A catheter for blood sampling was placed in the forearm 40 minutes before lactation. Oxytocin levels increased 3 to 10 minutes before suckling in response to the baby crying or becoming restless or the mother preparing herself to feed. There was no prolactin response until suckling began.

Most results clearly showed response before tactile stimuli and then a second surge in response to suckling. The levels were pulsatile during suckling and not related to milk volume, prolactin response, or parity of the mother.

Significant elevations of the maternal oxytocin level occur at 15, 30, and 45 minutes after delivery when the infant is put skin to skin, compared with levels just before delivery during expulsion of the placenta.[61] Levels return to baseline after 60 minutes if the infant does not suckle. When oxytocin levels were measured after initiating breast stimulation with a mechanical breast pump in early lactation (10 to 90 days), midlactation (90 to 190 days), and late lactation (180 days to 12 months), baseline levels were similar in all three periods. The stimulated plasma oxytocin levels were greater in early than late lactation, but there was always a response. Thus the oxytocin secretory reflex appears to continue for at least the first year of lactation.

The release of oxytocin by neurohypophyseal responses during lactation has been evoked both by infant's suckling and by mechanical dilatation of the mammary ducts. This release of oxytocin was demonstrated to be independent of vasopressin release. Conversely, further study[39,40] demonstrated that there could be stimulation of vasopressin release independent of oxytocin release.

When the levels of HGH, vasopressin, prolactin, calcitonin, gastrin, insulin, epinephrine, norepinephrine, and dopamine were measured in six lactating women during breastfeeding, Widstrom et al[97] confirmed the rise in prolactin and demonstrated the progressive increase in insulin that may be secondary to prolactin rise and may participate in stimulating milk production. Gastrin level decreased, and there were no consistent findings for calcitonin, HGH, norepinephrine, or epinephrine and no change in dopamine and vasopressin. Vagally stimulated release of insulin and gastrin is antagonized when the tone of the sympathetic nervous system is increased, such as during stress, pain, or anxiety. Increased insulin also is known to stimulate the synthesis of casein and lactalbumin and thus secondarily milk production. It should be advantageous to breastfeed after a meal rather than before (practically, many mothers eat while feeding the infant).

Human myoepithelium, the effector tissue, is specifically stimulated by oxytocin, and this sensitivity and specificity increase throughout pregnancy. Suckling can induce milk secretion, which is under control of the adenohypophysis. In this case, oxytocin released by the neurohypophysis because of the suckling stimulus would cause both milk ejection and release of the anterior pituitary hormones responsible for milk secretion as well. This is probably the mechanism behind relactation and induced lactation in the woman who has never been pregnant. Mammary growth and lactogenesis

may be induced by suckling, massage, and breast stimulation in many species.[17]

Alcohol has a dose-related effect on the central nervous system in inhibiting milk ejection. When intramammary pressure was measured in response to suckling by the infant while the mother received measured doses of alcohol, milk ejection was inhibited in a dose-dependent manner.[9] Doses up to 0.45 g/kg body weight (blood alcohol less than 0.1%), however, had no effect on intramammary pressure. Mechanical breast stimulation for 10 minutes and concomitant administration of intravenous fluid containing normal saline, naloxone, ethanol, or a combination of ethanol and naloxone were initiated in normal nonlactating women on day 22 of the regular menstrual cycle.[10] Plasma oxytocin levels rose twofold, with breast stimulation peaking at 10 minutes. Responses were unchanged by naloxone but were completely abolished by alcohol taken orally (approximately 110 ml of whiskey). Naloxone partially reversed the inhibiting effects of ethanol. The authors concluded that naloxone-sensitive endogenous opioids do not appear to be involved in the control of the oxytocin rise induced by breast stimulation and that opioid peptides are partly involved in the alcohol action.[10] Alcohol has been used in obstetrics to suppress premature labor in humans.

Normal alert newborns have been observed to "crawl" to the nipple and latch on unassisted when placed on the maternal abdomen following a normal delivery and the clamping and severing of the umbilical cord.

Suckling brings about functional changes in the offspring. An infant who sucks on an artificial nipple quickly decreases the amount of body movement, increases mouth activity, and decreases crying. The suckling experience may affect infant behavior and mother-infant interaction. Nonnutritive sucking is observed in many species. In the human infant, nutritive sucking is shown to be a continuous stream of regular sucks with few, if any, pauses. Nonnutritive sucking has bursts of activity alternating with no sucking. Suckling can be altered by extraneous aural, visual, or olfactory stimuli.

Maternal effects of suckling

Effects of suckling on the mother include the stimulation of afferent nerves for the removal of milk.[41] Reduction in sucking stimulus produces a reduction in prolactin and in milk synthesis. The lactating glands adjust the milk supply to demand, probably because of both a local and an endocrinologic mechanism. Variations in milk secretion are rapidly reflected in anatomic changes in the mammary gland. Mammary tissue shows regression after the first week or so, if unstimulated. Tissue regression proceeds at a rate parallel to the demand for secretory tissue. Thus, when a suckling infant signals needs, the breast will respond.[75]

Effects on maternal behavior have been attributed to lactation. Maternal behavior is more easily defined in many other species, in which early nursing is initiated by the mother, who stimulates the neonate to suckle by grooming. She then presents her mammary gland to the offspring so that the nipple is located with minimal effort. All species of lactating females have a lessened response to stress. In the human, however, nursing behavior has a strong voluntary nature. When lactating women were stressed with graded treadmill exercise, significant decreases in plasma levels of ACTH, cortisol, and epinephrine were observed compared with a matched group of nonlactating women.[6] Plasma glucose levels did not increase in either group. Oxytocin pulse in the plasma in response to suckling was also accompanied by a decrease in plasma ACTH and cortisol in the lactating women.

Oxytocin administered intraventricularly to virgin rats induces maternal behavior. Local infusion of oxytocin antagonists to appropriate regions of the hypothalamus during parturition blocked the dams from pup retrieval, a measure of maternal behavior in rats.[68] Similar observations have been made in sheep.[69] The neurophysical mechanism is under study in the human. It is well established that oxytocin promotes the development of human maternal behavior and mother-infant bonding.[67] Some effects of oxytocin in the nipple and mammary gland appear to be caused by peptides released in the nipple from axon collaterals of somatosensory afferent nerves. Oxytocin is also present in neurons projecting to many areas in the brain and exerts many central actions. In addition to maternal behavior, oxytocin causes more nonspecific behavior changes, such as sedation or antistress effects, and optimizes transfer of energy to the mammary gland.[67]

Investigations of the agile wallaby, *Macropus agilis,* have revealed the let-down reflex as this species displays concurrent asynchronous lactation.[44] The young, weighing 35 g, attach to the teat at birth. The lactating gland continues to grow for 200 days, increasing 10-fold in size. At 200 to 220 days, weighing 2500 g, the young first leave the pouch. Twenty-six days later a second young is born, although the older one continues to suckle intermittently for another 160 days at the original teat. The second young attaches to an unused nipple, which begins to develop, displaying complete autonomy. Measurements of oxytocin during the initial lactation show an increase in intraductal pressure response with a decline in sensitivity over time. This permits milk ejection in response to a small release of oxytocin to be confined to the mammary gland to which the neonate is continuously attached. The release of large quantities of oxytocin in response to the suckling of the juvenile would cause release in both glands.[44]

Mammals have thus evolved diverse strategies for survival. Tandem nursing in the human has not been so carefully studied, but no known change occurs in let-down, although the milk reverts to colostrum at the birth of the new infant.

The spinothalamic tract is the most likely of the possible spinal and brainstem pathways by which the suckling stimulus reaches the forebrain. The areas of the forebrain influenced by the suckling stimulus include the hypothalamic structures that mediate oxytocin and prolactin release. The inhibition of milk ejection by visual and auditory stimuli, pinealectomy, and ventrolateral midbrain lesions in lactating rats has been studied to define further the neurohormonal pathways. In these experiments the pineal gland appeared to mediate an inhibitory visual reflex on both oxytocin release and milk ejection.[26,71]

A mechanism consisting of smooth muscle and elastic fibers acting as a sphincter at the end of the ducts in the nipple appears to prevent most unwanted loss of milk. Sympathetic control does not appear to be present in humans, although it is demonstrable in most other species.

As the end of pregnancy approaches, the breast is prepared to respond to the suckling offspring.[72] In the human this is evidenced by increased sensitivity of the breast to tactile stimulation; increased responsiveness of the ductiles to oxytocin, thus preparing to eject the milk; and increased response of the breast to signaling the release of prolactin to stimulate milk production. The signal for lactation occurs when the placenta is removed and the end organs in the breast can fully respond to the surge of prolactin resulting from suckling.[88]

Concentrations of oxytocin in milk

Human milk samples obtained by manual expression daily from the first to the fifth postpartum day were collected immediately before and after a feeding as well as 2 hours after nursing.[83] The baseline mean oxytocin concentrations were 3.3 to 4.7 mg/ml, increasing significantly with nursing. Oxytocin in milk is fairly stable compared with that in maternal serum, which is inactivated by oxytocinase in plasma, liver, and kidney. When oxytocin was administered to rat dams, it was also found in the suckling offspring's gastric contents, where it is stable in acid. Some is absorbed into the neonatal blood, where it is unstable. Levels of oxytocin in neonatal serum are produced predominantly by the neonate itself. Whether oxytocin has a physiologic role on the gut or other hormones is unknown.

Role of prostaglandins as milk ejectors

Because prostaglandins have many physiologic effects and are known to increase mammary duct pressure, Toppozada et al[86] investigated their role as milk ejectors.[61] Comparison was made among three treatments: intravenous (IV) injec-

tions of oxytocin, PGE_2, and 16-phenoxy-PGE_2 given to one group of women on the third to sixth day postpartum; IV oxytocin, 15-methyl-$PGF_{2\alpha}$, and $PGF_{2\alpha}$ tromethamine salt to a second group; and oxytocin and PGF intranasally to a third group. All combinations had some effect, with the IV route having a shorter latency period than the intranasal. $PGF_{2\alpha}$, the more potent of the prostaglandin preparations, was more potent via the nasal route than oxytocin nasally. The response lasted 25 minutes after intranasal instillation of 400 µg. PGE_2 and $PGF_{2\alpha}$ orally reduce prolactin levels and appear to be successful in suppressing lactation in the immediate postpartum period when given in large doses of 2 to 4 mg or in multiple doses up to 10 times greater. Although they are produced in larger quantities by the mammary gland in vitro and in vivo, the role of prostaglandins is still not clear, because these studies[86] are in conflict with previous results by Vorherr.[94] The practical application of this in lactation failure has not been reported.

Milk-borne prostaglandins clearly survive in the environment of the infant's gastrointestinal tract and are delivered in an active form to peripheral organs. The significance of this remains under investigation.[36]

Production of hormones by mammary gland

Hormones synthesized by the mammary gland may have endocrine, autocrine, or paracrine effects within the mother. The chemical mediators known to be synthesized by the mammary gland are epidermal growth factor (EGF), progesterone, prolactin, estrogens, and relaxin. Other hormones are transported to the gland.[65] These bioactive agents could have multiple roles in both mother and recipient infant. Insulin-like growth factors are found in high concentration in colostrum and at lower levels in mature milk. Milk factors other than nutrients are thought to control specific developmental processes in the infant. Because infants survive and grow on formula, this latter point is difficult to prove. Actions of milk regulatory substances are much more important in at-risk infants than in full-term infants.

Feedback inhibitor of lactation

The mammary gland is unique because, as an exocrine gland, it stores its secretion extracellularly. Storage within the gland's lumen suggests a local level of control on the rate of secretion.[56]

As stated earlier, milk is produced as long as it is removed from the mammary gland. Further, prolactin and oxytocin are responsible for the production and release of milk, allowing the infant to extract milk by suckling. The rate of milk secretion may differ between breasts if one breast is suckled more frequently or for a longer time. When lactating goats have an extra daily milking, the secretory rate is increased even if the milk is immediately replaced with an inert solution to maintain the gland's distention. The dilution of stored milk in the gland with an inert isotonic solution results in increased milk secretion, suggesting the dilution of a chemical inhibitor.

Identification of a factor that is produced and functions at the mammary level, called *feedback inhibitor of lactation (FIL)*, has evolved from multiple studies.[70] Wilde et al[98] described autocrine regulation of milk secretion by a previously unknown protein in the milk. When this active whey protein (FIL) was isolated and injected into the mammary gland of lactating goats, milk secretion was decreased temporarily. Similar work by Prentice et al[70] has confirmed the presence of FIL in humans. FIL is able to exert reversible concentration-dependent autocrine inhibition on milk secretion in the lactating gland. It controls secretion of all milk constituents simultaneously; that is, it affects secretion, not composition.

Maternal adaptation to lactation

Each mammalian species has evolved its own lactational strategies to meet the nutritional needs of its offspring, with influences from both genetic and environmental forces. The endocrine signals promote mammary development, inhibit milk production during gestation, and then promote development of enhanced metabolic and transport functions in adipose tissue, visceral organs, and reproductive organs.[64] Lactational adaptations of adipose tissue metabolism have been recognized in all species and may be most dramatic in seals, hibernating bears, and whales, who produce fat-rich milk from their fat stores while fasting. Lactation results in profound changes in adipose tissue metabolism to provide energy stores, modulate mammary development, affect appetite, and influence the immune system function.[89]

The substantial adaptation of the maternal intestine during lactation is the large increase in its size and complexity, which ensures adequate absorption of nutrients to meet the increased energy demand.[24] A corresponding increase occurs in liver and heart performance. In addition to extra fat demands, calcium concentration must be sufficient to maintain maternal stores while providing for the demands of milk synthesis, which are greater than those of pregnancy.[30] The estimated calcium requirement is 12 mg/kg/day in the human. The elevation in plasma dihydroxycholecalciferol $(1,25\text{-}[OH]_2D_3)$ during late gestation continues during early lactation. As lactation progresses beyond 3 months, plasma $1,25\text{-}(OH)_2D_3$ levels decline. This results in decreased calcium absorption, which is offset by greater maternal bone losses and reduced urinary calcium. Glucose requirements during lactation require major adjustments in glucose production and utilization in the maternal liver, adipose tissue, bone, muscle, and other tissues. Adaptation of folic acid metabolism is equally important, although less well studied.[64]

The mechanisms by which early pregnancy and lactation decrease the incidence of breast cancer are unclear. Close examination of the more differentiated mammary cell, which is less susceptible to the loss of growth regulation, is a next step, along with inspection of mucin, a glycoprotein and normal differentiation antigen expressed in both milk fat globules and mammary tumors.

LACTATION: SYNTHESIS OF HUMAN MILK

The function of the mammary gland is unique in that it produces a substance that makes tremendous demands on the maternal system without producing any physiologic advantage to the maternal organism. Because lactation is anticipated, the body prepares the breast anatomically and physiologically.[80] When lactation begins, the mother's metabolism changes greatly. The blood supply is redistributed, and the demand for nutrients increases, which requires an increased metabolic rate to accommodate their production. The mammary gland may need to produce milk at the metabolic expense of other organs. The supply of materials to the lactating breast for milk production and energy metabolism requires extensive cardiovascular changes in the mother. There is increased mammary blood flow, increased blood flow into the gastrointestinal tract and liver, and a high cardiac output. The mammary blood flow, cardiac output, and milk secretion are suckling dependent. Suckling induces the release of anterior pituitary hormones that act directly on breast tissue.

Milk is isosmotic with plasma in all species.[40] Human milk differs from many other milks in that the concentration of major monovalent ions is lower and that of lactose is higher; in other milks, the higher the ions, the lower the lactose, and vice versa. Many disparities in the intermediary metabolism among species of animals can be linked to evolutionary adaptations involving the digestive process.[39] Nonruminants rely on glucose, derived from carbohydrate in the diet. Ruminants, because of extensive fermentation in the rumen, absorb little glucose. The microbial fermentation products, which include acetate, propionate, and butyrate, play a significant part as energy and carbon sources for tissue metabolism. Amino acids are primary substitutes for glucose in ruminants.[40]

The biosynthesis of milk involves a cellular site where the metabolic processes occur. The epithelial cells of the gland contain stem cells and highly differentiated secretory alveolar cells at the terminal ducts. The stem cells are stimulated by HGH and insulin. Prolactin synergizes the insulin effect to stimulate the cells to secretory activity.

The cells of the acini and smaller milk ducts are active in milk synthesis and milk secretion into the alveoli and smaller milk ducts. Most milk is synthesized during the process of suckling; its production is stimulated by prolactin. Cortisol plasma levels are increased during suckling as well. The secretory cells are cuboidal, changing to a cylindric shape just before milk secretion, while cellular water uptake is increased. The cell's single nucleus is at the base in the dormant cell but migrates to the apex just before milk secretion.

The differentiated structure of the functional cell is acquired gradually during pregnancy, differing little from species to species. Very early in lactation, mammary cells show active synthesis and secretion of proteins and fat. The cells are polarized with abundant rough endoplasmic reticulum and Golgi dictyosomes above the nucleus, which is smooth and rounded with many mitochondria. The apical surface has microvilli, and the basal surface is extensively convoluted for the active transport of materials from the bloodstream into the cell. Fat droplets are in the cytoplasm and bulging at the membrane. Proteins, lactose, calcium, phosphate, and citrate are packaged into secretory vesicles and pass into the lumen of the alveolus by exocytosis.

The cytoplasm is finely granular in the resting phase but striated as milk secretion begins. As secretion commences, the enlarged cell with its thickened apical membrane becomes clublike in shape. The tip pinches off, leaving the cell intact. The protein is thus free in the secreted solution, retaining a cap of membrane (Fig. 3-11).

Function of cellular components of lactating breast

The schema of the mammary secretory cell is represented in Figs. 3-12 and 3-13.

Lipid droplet

Protein cap

Golgi apparatus

Fig. 3-11. Apocrine secretory mechanism for lipids, proteins, and lactose in milk.

Nucleus

The nucleus is essential to the duplication of genetic material and the transcription of the genetic code.[92] The nucleus is also considered a regulatory organelle in cell metabolism, transmitting the design of the cell's enzymatic profile. The deoxyribonucleic acid (DNA) and RNA content of the cellular nuclei increases during pregnancy and is highest during lactation.

Cytosol

The cytosol, which consists of the cytoplasm minus the mitochondrial and microsomal fractions, is also called the *particle-free supernatant.* The cytosol contains enzymes that involve key intermediates and cofactors essential to the process of milk synthesis.

Mitochondrial proliferation

The alveolar cell population of the mammary gland must have a greatly expanded oxidative capacity during lactation. It is supplied by an increase in size and function of the cell's mitochondrial population.[34] Mitochondria are increased in the epithelial cell at the onset of the lactation process. Mitochondrial proliferation has been observed in all cells with a high metabolic rate and high oxygen utilization.

During the presecretory differentiation phase in late pregnancy and early lactation, each mitochondrion undergoes a type of differentiation in which the inner membrane and matrix expand greatly. As with other cells, the mitochondria are key to the respiratory activity of the cell. Mitochondria control some cellular metabolism through differential permeability to certain anions. The citrate in the mitochondria is a major source of carbon for fatty acid biosynthesis. Mitochondria also supply the carbon for synthesis of nonessential amino acids.

Microsomal fraction

The microsomal fraction of the cell, which includes the Golgi apparatus, the endoplasmic reticulum, and the cell membranes, is involved in lipid synthesis. The role of the microsomal fraction is also to assemble the constituent parts (e.g., amino acids, glucose, fatty acids) into the final products of protein, carbohydrate, and fat for secretion.

Intermediary metabolism of mammary gland

The pathways identified for milk synthesis and secretion in the mammary alveolus, as described by Neville et al,[54] include four major transcellular pathways and one paracellular (Fig. 3-14):

   I. Exocytosis of milk protein and lactose in Golgi-derived secretory vesicles
  II. Milk fat secretion via the milk fat globule
 III. Secretion of ions and water across the apical membrane
 IV. Pinocytosis-exocytosis of immunoglobulins
  V. Paracellular pathway for plasma components and leukocytes

Fig. 3-12. Diagram of cycle of secretory cells from resting stage to secretion and return to resting stage. (Modified from Vorherr H: *The breast: morphology, physiology and lactation,* New York, 1974, Academic Press.)

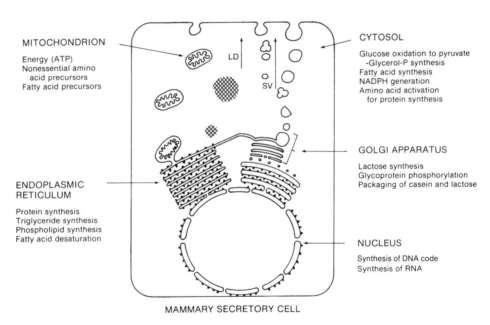

MAMMARY SECRETORY CELL

Fig. 3-13. Schema of cytologic and biochemical interrelationships of secretory cell of mammary gland. *LD,* Lipid droplet; *SV,* secretory vesicle.

Carbohydrates

The major carbohydrate for most species is lactose, a disaccharide found only in milk. In addition to lactose, more than 50 oligosaccharides of different structure have been identified in human milk. One of the most important is glucose.

Glucose metabolism has a key function in milk production.[3] Glucose serves as the main source of energy for other reactions as well as a critical source of carbon. Glucose is critical to the volume of milk produced and is used in the production of lactose. The synthesis of lactose combines glucose and galactose, the latter originating from glucose-6-phosphate.[29]

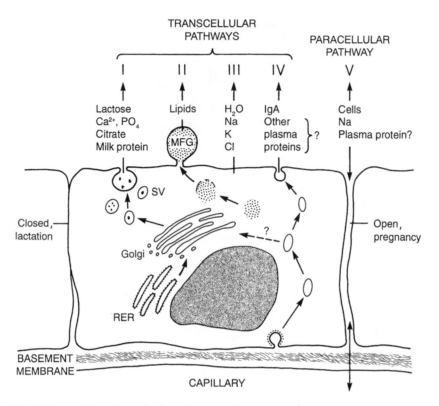

Fig. 3-14. Pathways for milk synthesis and secretion into mammary alveolus. *I,* Exocytosis of milk protein and lactose in Golgi-derived secretory vesicles. *II,* Milk fat secretion via milk fat globule. *III,* Secretion of ions and water across apical membrane. *IV,* Pinocytosis-exocytosis of immunoglobulins. *V,* Paracellular pathway for plasma components and leukocytes. *SV,* Secretory vesicle; *RER,* rough endoplasmic reticulum; *MFG,* milk fat globule. (Modified from Neville MC: *Ann NY Acad Sci* 586:1, 1990.)

Lactose synthesis is carried out by the following equations:

$$\text{UDP-galactose} + N\text{-acetylglucosamine} \quad (1)$$
$$\rightarrow N\text{-acetyllactosamine} + \text{UDP}$$

$$\text{UDP-galactose} + \text{Glucose} \rightarrow \text{Lactose} + \text{UDP} \quad (2)$$

UDP is uridine diphosphogalactose. The catalyst in equation 1 is a galactosyl transferase, *N*-acetyllactosamine synthetase. The reaction is activated by metal ions that bind to the galactosyl transferase.

Most of the intracellular glucose is derived from blood sugar. A specific whey protein, α-lactalbumin, catalyzes the lactose synthesis. It is a rate-limiting enzyme, which is inhibited by progesterone during pregnancy. In the absence of α-lactalbumin, little lactose is present. With the drop in progesterone and estrogen levels after the removal of the placenta at delivery, prolactin increases. The synthesis of α-lactalbumin becomes greater, and large amounts of lactose are produced from glucose. Progesterone regulates the onset of lactose synthesis, causing the initiation of production just as the infant is in need of nutrition.

Because lactose is synthesized only from glucose, maternal glucose utilization is increased by 30% in full lactation.[54]

Various aspects of lactose synthesis continue to be vigorously investigated.[29] The molecular mechanism of lactose synthesis is activated by metal ions, manganese (Mn), and calcium (Ca). Lactose synthesis takes place within the Golgi apparatus (Fig. 3-14). The onset of copious milk secretion depends on rapid increase of lactose synthesis. Lactose synthetase performs the rate-limiting step in lactose synthesis, which is one of the few anabolic reactions involving glucose itself rather than a phosphorylated derivative.[3] Although progesterone, thyroxine, and lactogenic hormones are important in controlling synthesis, it is not known how they act in this system. The areas available for investigation about lactose synthesis remain vast.

Fat

Fat synthesis takes place in the endoplasmic reticulum. The alveolar cells are able to synthesize short-chain fatty acids, which are derived predominantly from acetate. Long-chain fatty acids, derived chiefly from blood plasma, are used in milk fat. Triglycerides are utilized from the plasma, as well as synthesized from intracellular glucose oxidized via the pentose pathway. Synthesis of fat from carbohydrate plays a predominant role in fat production in human milk.[33]

Two enzymes, lipoprotein lipase and palmitoyl–coenzyme A (CoA) L-glycerol-3-phosphate palmitoyl transferase, increase greatly after delivery. The lipase acts at the walls of the capillaries to catalyze the lipolysis and uptake of glycerol into the epithelial cells. The transferase catalyzes the process of synthesizing glycerides to triglycerides. It is believed that the marked increase of the lipase and transferase is stimulated by prolactin. Hormonal control of the glycerol precursors and the enzymatic release of fatty acids, leading to the formation of triglycerides, have been associated not only with prolactin but also with insulin, which stimulates the uptake of glucose into the mammary cells.

Esterification of fatty acids takes place in the endoplasmic reticulum. The triglycerides subsequently accumulate into fat droplets in several cisternae. The small droplets sit on the base of the cell and coalesce to large droplets that move toward the apex of the cell. The fat droplets are engulfed in the apical membrane and project into the alveolar lumen. The discharge of fat droplets involves the bulging of the cell apex to envelop the fat globules, protein, and a small amount of cytoplasm; with the pinching off, the globule becomes detached into the lumen. The membrane of the fat globule contains all the normal plasma enzymes. The fat droplets contain predominantly polar lipid and phosphatidyl choline.

Fatty acid synthesis involves a source of substrates and associated enzymes for their conversion to acetyl-CoA and reduced nicotinamide-adenine dinucleotide phosphate (NADPH) in the cytoplasm of the cell and the conversion of acetyl-CoA to malonyl-CoA. The newly synthesized fatty acid is then released from the fatty acid–synthetase complex.

The milk-fat-globule membrane in human milk serves several roles. A layer of amphophilic (bipolar) substances at the globule/skim milk interface is required for the maintenance of emulsion stability of the fat globules.[33] This physiochemical fact applies to all emulsions and to the fat globules in the milk of all species. The globules and the milk-fat-globule membrane are compartments within the emulsion component of milk. Once in place, the components of the milk-fat-globule membrane, which is the oil-water interfacial compartment, are more or less firmly held in place by a variety of chemical and electrical forces. The stabilizing membrane acts as a reactive barrier on the interface between the globule and milk serum.[33] It is rate controlling for the binding of enzymes and trace elements, the controlled release of the products of lipolysis, the transfer of polar materials into milk serum, the maintenance of emulsion stability by the prevention of globule fission, and the availability of fatty acids and cholesterol for micellar absorption in the small intestine. All these interactions are dynamic. The envelopment mechanism involves rapid turnover of the plasma membrane lipids and proteins during milk production.

Protein

Most proteins in milk are formed from free amino acids in the secretory cells of the mammary gland. The definitive data confirming the origin of milk proteins were accumulated since 1980. The vast majority of proteins present in normal milk are specific to mammary secretions and are not identified in any quantity elsewhere in nature.[39]

The formation of milk protein and mammary enzymes is induced by prolactin and further stimulated by insulin and cortisol. De novo synthesis of protein uses both essential and nonessential plasma amino acids. Nuclear RNAs, induced by prolactin, stimulate synthesis of messenger and transfer RNA. The mRNA conveys the genetic information to the protein-synthesizing centers of the cells. The transfer RNA interprets the message to assemble the amino acids in the appropriate sequence of polypeptide chains of the specific milk proteins. The newly synthesized proteins are secreted into the milk during lactation. Casein, α-lactalbumin, and β-lactoglobulin from plasma amino acids are synthesized on the ribosomes of the endoplasmic reticulum, where they are condensed and appear as visible secretory granules moving toward the cellular apex.[50]

After some processing, the proteins pass to the Golgi complex, where they are further glycosylated and phosphorylated and then placed in secretory vesicles for export.[54] α-Lactalbumin, a protein necessary for lactose synthesis by the enzyme galactosyl transferase, is among the proteins synthesized in the mammary gland. Lactose is synthesized within the trans-Golgi complex and secreted together with the major milk proteins. The casein micelle is formed with calcium within the Golgi compartment, which presents a high concentration of calcium, phosphate, and protein via the milk. Most of the casein is bound in this manner. This pathway I (Fig. 3-14) begins in the rough endoplasmic reticulum, where the proteins are inserted through the membrane into the lumen by exocytosis.[54]

The Golgi membrane is impermeable to lactose; thus the sugar is osmotically active. Water is drawn into the Golgi apparatus.[64] Casein micelle formation begins in the terminal Golgi vesicles, adding calcium in the secretory vesicle. These secretory vesicles move to the plasma membrane and through exocytosis extrude their contents into the alveolar lumen.[47]

Human casein micelles are smaller in size (30 to 75 nm in diameter) than bovine casein (600 nm). Human milk contains only β-casein and κ-casein. Only 6% of calcium in human milk is bound to casein, compared with 65% in bovine milk. The gene for human β-casein has been cloned and sequenced.[64]

Some merocrine secretion also occurs, in which proteins and other cellular constituents are secreted, leaving the cell membrane intact. Protein caps, or signets, protruding into alveolar lumen, have been described on the outside of the apical membrane. Protein and lactose secreted into the lumen cannot be reabsorbed (Table 3-3).

The synthesis of proteins in the mammary gland follows the general pathway of all proteins under genetic control. Induction of synthesis is under hormonal control. This process involves synthesis from amino acids through the detailed system controlled by RNA and under genetic control of DNA. Glucocorticoid is required for the expression of the casein gene in the presence of prolactin. Cortisol is the limiting factor for casein gene expression.[22] Shennan[78] has reviewed the mechanisms of mammary gland ion transport.

Ions and water

Sodium, potassium, chloride, magnesium, calcium, phosphate, sulfate, and citrate pass through the

---

TABLE 3-3 Alveolar epithelial membrane permeability

Cell ↔ Alveolar lumen	Cell → Alveolar lumen
Glucose	Lactose
Water	Sucrose
Sodium	Citrate
Potassium	Proteins
Chloride	Fat
Iodine	Calcium
Sulfate	Phosphate

membrane of the alveolar cell in both directions.[57] Water also passes in both directions, predominantly from the alveolar cells but also from the interstitial fluid. Plasma water passage depends on the amount of intracellular glucose available for lactose. The aqueous phase of milk is isosmotic to plasma. The major osmole of the aqueous phase of milk is lactose. The concentrations of sodium and chloride are less than those in plasma (Figs. 3-15 and 3-16).

Human milk differs from that of many other species in that the monovalent ions are in low concentration and lactose is in high concentration.[41] The osmolarity is the same, that is, isosmotic with plasma; thus the higher the lactose, the lower the ions. It is presumed that the intracellular concentration of potassium is held high and that of sodium low by a pump on the basal membrane. The sodium and potassium ions are distributed according to the electrical potential gradient.[57] Milk is electrically positive compared with intracellular fluid. The sodium:potassium ratio is 1:3 in both milk and intracellular fluid. Vorherr[93,94] believes that lactose secretion is responsible for the potential difference across the apical membrane, thus keeping sodium and potassium ion concentration low.

The variation among species in the concentration of lactose and ions is caused by the rate of lactose synthesis, the permeability of the membrane, and the number of fixed negative charges on the membrane. The potential difference is higher in the human mammary gland than in any other species evaluated to date.

The relationship between intrastructure and function in the mammary gland changes from pregnancy to lactation. The junction between alveolar cells has attracted much interest. Cell junctions do not merely hold cells together but enable epithelia to function as permeable barriers, allowing communication between cells and coordination of activities. The three functions of cell junctions are adhesion, occlusion, and communication, which are carried out by desmosomes,

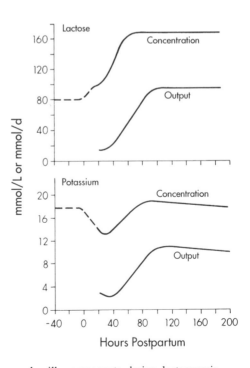

Fig. 3-15. Concentrations and secretion rates of several milk components during lactogenesis. (Modified from Neville MC, Allen JC, Archer PC et al: *Am J Clin Nutr* 54:81, 1991.)

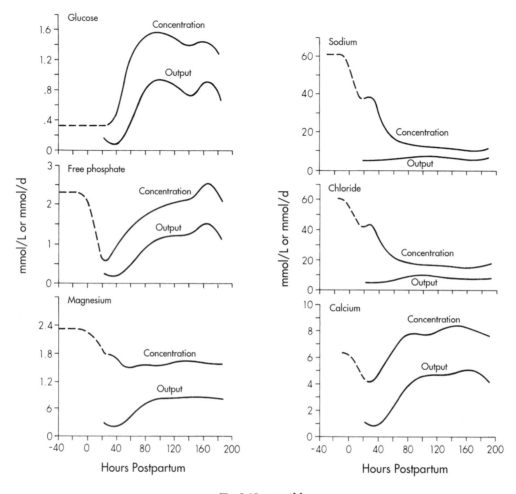

Fig. 3-15. cont'd

tight junctions, and gap junctions, respectively. Changes in tight junctions may provide the basis for a reduction in permeability between cells. For instance, at the initiation of lactation, a tight junction changing from "leaky" to very tight blocks the paracellular movement of lactose and ions. This requires transport across cells of these materials and the maintenance of control of high intracellular potassium and low intracellular sodium concentrations.[16]

Citrate is thought to be the harbinger of lactogenesis. Citrate plays a central role in the metabolism of all cells, but its significance and mode of secretion remain unknown.[66] In the final stages of lactogenesis in ruminants, the previously quiescent epithelial cells suddenly start to secrete large quantities of protein, fat, and carbohydrates. The exact lactogenic trigger is unknown, although significant hormonal changes occur. In women the onset of copious milk secretion does not begin until 3 to 4 days postpartum. Significantly, citrate levels are low at delivery and rise quickly, reaching a peak on day 4[66] (Fig. 3-16). In the cow and the goat, copious production occurs at delivery, and the citrate levels begin to rise, increasing 10 to 100 times the baseline values.

Citrate is the main buffer system of milk.[57] It is formed within the secretory cell, but how it is

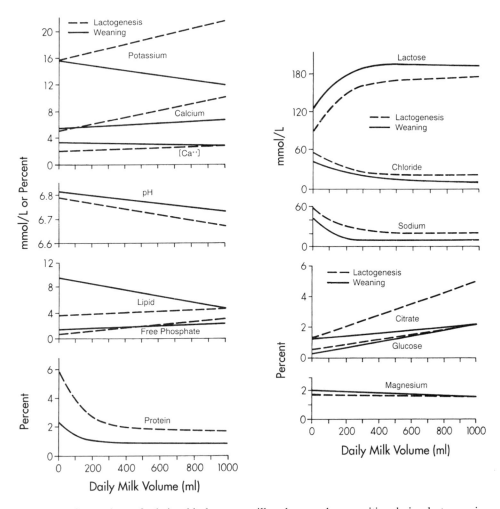

Fig. 3-16. Comparison of relationship between milk volume and composition during lactogenesis (---) and weaning (—). (Modified from Neville MC, Allen JC, Archer PC et al: *Am J Clin Nutr* 54:81, 1991.)

secreted into the milk is not clear. Citrate and lactose may be secreted by a similar route. After dilution of milk in the gland with isosmotic lactose, the equilibrium is restored across the apical membrane in experimental models by the entrance of sodium, potassium, and chloride into the milk. No citrate, calcium, or protein enters in excess of the normal secretion rate. Inorganic phosphate is the other major buffer system, but how it is secreted is also unknown (Fig. 3-15).

Calcium, much of which is bound to casein,

enters the Golgi apparatus, where it is essentially trapped with casein in the micelle, and then enters the alveolar milk by unidirectional flow.

The mammary gland is unusual among exocrine glands because the rate of secretion slows and some secretion can be stored in its ducts.[78] Direct neural control of secretion is lacking. The parenchyma of the gland also consists of ductal tissue in addition to secretory tissue. The ductal cells, however, are impermeable to the major milk ions during lactation, so they cannot modify the secretion, in contrast to the ductal cells of other exocrine glands (e.g., sweat, salivary)[45] (Fig. 3-16).

A comparison of the levels of various constituents of the milk with corresponding plasma levels demonstrates the mechanism partly responsible for that mechanism (see Table 4-17).

Milk enzymes

Some milk enzymes enter the alveolar milk from the mammary blood capillaries via the intercellular fluid. Others come from the breakdown of the mammary secretory cells. The milk enzymes, xanthine oxidase, aldolase, and alkaline phosphatase, are contained in the fat globule, membrane, and milk serum. The most significant enzyme, lipase, splits triglycerides.

Human milk contains both proteolytic enzymes and protease inhibitors.[25] Amylase facilitates digestion of polysaccharides by the infant. Sulfhydryl (SH) oxidase catalyzes oxidation of SH groups. Glutathione peroxidase facilitates the delivery of selenium to the infant. Lysozyme and peroxidase are bactericidal.

Cellular components

Human milk has been called a "live fluid" by many and "white blood" in many ancient rites. Breast milk contains up to 4000 cells/ml, which have been identified with leukocytes and enter the milk via the paracellular pathway, pathway V.[92] The cell number is particularly high in colostrum. The cells in greatest number are the macrophages, which secrete lysozyme and lactoferrin. Lymphocytes, neutrophils, and epithelial cells are also present. Lymphocytes produce IgA and interferon.

Macrophages constitute a major cellular component in milk compared with levels in blood and can survive under conditions simulating the infant's gastrointestinal tract.[27] Because they release secretory IgA in association with phagocytosis, it is believed they play a role in host defense. Macrophage colony-stimulating factor in human milk and mammary gland epithelial cells are believed to be responsible for expansion of the macrophages in milk.

INVOLUTION: WEANING AND APOPTOSIS

During weaning, significant increases in milk protein, chloride, and sodium concentrations and a decrease in lactose occur when milk volumes fall below 400 ml/day. Glucose and magnesium levels are unchanged.[56] This suggests that volume is regulated differently during weaning than during lactogenesis. No sentinel substance is a reliable predictor of volume in all stages, but normal ranges of milk components during full lactation are sodium, 3 to 18 mmol/L; chloride, 8 to 24 mmol/L; protein, 8 to 23 g/L; and lactose, 140 to 230 mmol/L. Values outside these ranges suggest mastitis or weaning. During gradual weaning, between 6 and 15 months postpartum, glucose, citrate, phosphate, and calcium levels decrease, whereas lipid, potassium, and magnesium increase[57] (Fig. 3-16).

Postlactational involution of the mammary gland is characterized by two distinct physiologic processes.[49] First, secretory epithelial cells undergo apoptosis and programmed cell death. Second, the mammary gland's basement membrane undergoes proteolytic degradation. Apoptosis is almost absent during lactation but develops within 2 days of involution. In the initial phase of involution, apoptosis of fully differentiated mammary epithelial cells occurs without visible degradation of the extracellular matrix. The second phase consists of extracellular remodeling and altered mesenchymal-epithelial interactions followed by apoptosis of cells no longer differentiating.[82] During postlactational mammary gland involution, most mammary epithelium dies and is reabsorbed.

SUMMARY

In the human, lactogenesis occurs slowly over the first few days postpartum as progesterone levels drop. Women experience "milk coming in" as a feeling of fullness between 40 and 72 hours, usually corresponding to the degree of parity, with

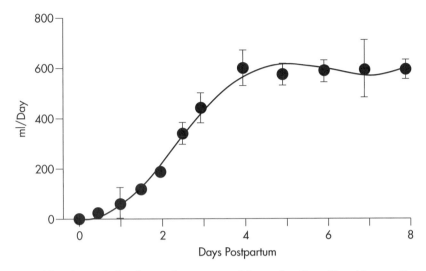

Fig. 3-17. Milk volumes during first week postpartum. Mean values from 12 multiparous Caucasian women who test-weighed their infants before and after every feeding for first 7 days postpartum. (Redrawn from Neville MC: Determinants of milk volume and composition. In Jensen RG, editor: *Handbook of milk composition,* San Diego, 1995, Academic Press.)

multiparas sensing this more quickly than primiparas. Volume of milk increases over time for the first 2 weeks, starting at less than 100 ml/day to about 600 ml/day at 96 hours (Fig. 3-17). This parallels the rise in citrate production, reflecting the metabolic activity of the mammary gland. Lactose, sodium chloride, and protein rise promptly, stabilizing at 24 hours and reflecting the closure of the pericellular pathway, which results in a decrease in direct flux into the milk. This suggests a two-step process of junctional closure followed by onset of secretory activity.

The changes in permeability of the tight junctions; rate of synthesis of lactose, lipids, and nutrient proteins; transport of glucose into the alveolar cells; transcytosis of secretory IgA; movement of immune cells into the alveolar lumen; and secretion of lactoferrin represent the distinct metabolic and cellular modifications. Neville[55] states, "The temporal sequence of these changes as they occur during lactogenesis suggests that they are either independently regulated or form part of an orderly cascade of temporally separate events." Fig. 3-18 graphically illustrates these changes.

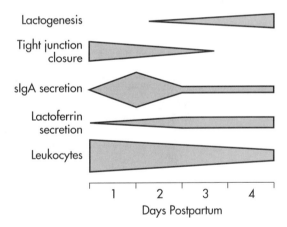

Fig. 3-18. Summary model for temporal sequence of changes in mammary gland function during lactogenesis in women. (From Neville MC: Determinants of milk volume and composition. In Jensen RG, editor: *Handbook of milk composition,* San Diego, 1995, Academic Press.)

REFERENCES

1. Anbazhagan R, Bartek J, Stamp G et al: Expression of integrin subunits in the human infant breast correlates with morphogenesis and differentiation, *J Pathol* 176:227, 1995.

2. Battin DA, Marrs RP, Fleiss PM et al: Effect of suckling on serum prolactin, luteinizing hormone, follicle-stimulating hormone, and estradiol during prolonged lactation, *Obstet Gynecol* 65:785, 1985.

3. Bell AW, Bauman DE: Adaptations of glucose metabolism during pregnancy and lactation, *J Mammary Gland Biol Neoplasia* 2:265, 1997.

4. Bochinfuso WP, Korach KS: Mammary gland development and tumorigenesis in estrogen receptor knock-out mice, *J Mammary Gland Biol Neoplasia* 2:323, 1997.

5. Caldeyro-Barcia R: Milk ejection in women. In Reynolds M, Folley SJ, editors: *Lactogenesis: the initiation of milk secretion at parturition,* Philadelphia, 1969, University of Pennsylvania Press.

6. Chiodera P, Salvarani C, Bacchi-Modena A et al: Relationship between plasma profiles of oxytocin and adrenocorticotropic hormone during suckling or breast stimulation in women, *Horm Res* 35:119, 1991.

7. Cholst IN, Wardlaw SL, Newman CB et al: Prolactin response to breast stimulation in lactating women is not mediated by endogenous opioids, *Am J Obstet Gynecol* 150:558, 1984.

8. Christensson K, Nilsson BA, Stocks S et al: Effect of nipple stimulation on uterine activity and on plasma levels of oxytocin in full term, healthy, pregnant women, *Acta Obstet Gynecol Scand* 68:205, 1989.

9. Cobo E: Effect of different doses of ethanol on the milk ejection reflex in lactating women, *Am J Obstet Gynecol* 115:817, 1973.

10. Coiro V, Alboni A, Gramellini D et al: Inhibition by ethanol of the oxytocin response to breast stimulation in normal women and the role of endogenous opioids, *Acta Endocrinol* 126:213, 1992.

11. Cowie AT, Forsyth IA, Hart IC: Hormonal control of lactation. In *Monographs in endocrinology,* vol 15, New York, 1980, Springer-Verlag.

12. Crowley WR, Armstrong WE: Neurochemical regulation of oxytocin secretion in lactation, *Endocr Rev* 13:33, 1992.

13. Daniel CW, Berger JJ, Strickland P et al: Similar growth pattern of mouse mammary epithelium cultivated in collagen matrix in vivo and in vitro, *Dev Biol* 104:57, 1984.

14. Daniel CW, Robinson S, Silberstein GB: The role of TGF-β in faltering and growth of the mammary ductal tree, *J Mammary Gland Biol Neoplasia* 1:331, 1996.

15. Dawood MY, Khan-Dawood FS, Wahi RS et al: Oxytocin release and plasma anterior pituitary and gonadal hormones in women during lactation, *J Clin Endocrinol Metab* 52:678, 1981.

16. Falconer IR, Rowe JM: Effect of prolactin on sodium and potassium concentration in the mammary alveolar tissue, *Endocrinology* 101:181, 1977.

17. Fournier PRJ, Desjardins PD, Friesen HG: Current understanding of human prolactin physiology and its diagnostic and therapeutic applications: a review, *Am J Obstet Gynecol* 118:337, 1974.

18. Fowler PA, Casey CE, Cameron GG et al: Cyclic changes in composition and volume of the breast during the menstrual cycle, measured by magnetic resonance imaging, *Br J Obstet Gynaecol* 97:595, 1990.

19. Frantz AG: Prolactin, *N Engl J Med* 298:201, 1978.

20. Freund-Mercier MJ, Richard P: Excitatory effects of intraventricular injections of oxytocin on the milk ejection reflex in the rat, *Neurosci Lett* 23:193, 1981, and *J Physiol* 352:447, 1984.

21. Frigerio C, Schutz Y, Prentice A et al: Is human lactation a particularly efficient process? *Eur J Clin Nutr* 45:459, 1991.

22. Ganguly R, Ganguly N, Mehta NM et al: Absolute requirement of glucocorticoid for expression of the casein gene in the presence of prolactin, *Proc Natl Acad Sci USA* 77:6003, 1980.

23. Gehlbach DL, Bayliss P, Rosa C: Prolactin and thyrotropin responses to nursing during the early puerperium, *J Reprod Med* 34:295, 1989.

24. Hammond KA: Adaptation of the maternal intestine during lactation, *J Mammary Gland Biol Neoplasia* 2:243, 1997.

25. Hamosh M: Enzymes in milk: their function in the mammary gland, in milk and in the infant. In Hanson LA, editor: *Biology of human milk,* Nestlé Nutrition Workshop Series 15:45, 1988.

26. Hansen S, Gummesson BM: Participation of the lateral midbrain tegmentum in the neuroendocrine control of sexual behavior and lactation in the rat, *Brain Res* 251:319, 1982.

27. Hara T, Irie K, Saito S et al: Identification of macrophage colony-stimulating factor in human milk and mammary gland epithelial cells, *Pediatr Res* 37:437, 1995.

28. Hartmann PE: Changes in the composition and yield of the mammary secretion of cows during the initiation of lactation, *J Endocrinol* 59:231, 1973.

29. Healy DL, Rattigan S, Hartmann PE et al: Prolactin in human milk: correlation with lactose, total protein, and of α-lactalbumin levels, *Am J Physiol* 238 (*Endocrinol Metab* 1):E83, 1980.

30. Horst RL, Goff JP, Reinhardt TA: Calcium and vitamin D metabolism during lactation, *J Mammary Gland Biol Neoplasia* 2:253, 1997.

31. Howie PW, McNeilly AS, McArdle T et al: The relationship between suckling-induced prolactin response and lactogenesis, *J Clin Endocrinol Metab* 50:670, 1980.

32. Humphreys RC, Lydon J, O'Malley BW et al: Mammary gland development is mediated by both stromal and epithelial progesterone receptors, *Mol Endocrinol* 11:801, 1997.

33. Jensen RG: *The lipids of human milk,* Boca Raton, Fla, 1989, CRC Press.

34. Jones DH: The mitochondria of the mammary parenchymal cell in relation to the pregnancy-lactation cycle. In Larson BL, editor: *Lactation, vol 4, The mammary gland/human lactation/milk synthesis,* New York, 1978, Academic Press.

35. Kleinberg DL: Early mammary development: growth hormone and IGF-1, *J Mammary Gland Biol Neoplasia* 2:49, 1997.

36. Koldovsky O, Bedrick A, Rao R: Role of milk-borne prostaglandins and epidermal growth factor for the suckling mammal, *J Am Coll Nutr* 10:17, 1991.

37. Kulski JK, Hartmann PE: Changes in human milk composition during the initiation of lactation, *Aust J Exp Biol Med* 59:101, 1981.

38. Kwa HG, Bulbrook RD, Wang DY: An overall perspective on the role of prolactin in the breast. In Nagasawa H, editor: *Prolactin and lesions in breast, uterus and prostate,* Boca Raton, Fla, 1989, CRC Press.

39. Larson BL, editor: *Lactation, vol 4, The mammary gland/human lactation/milk synthesis,* New York, 1978, Academic Press.

40. Larson BL, Smith VR, editors: *Lactation, vol 2, Biosynthesis and secretion of milk/diseases,* New York, 1974, Academic Press.

41. Larson BL, Smith VR, editors: *Lactation, vol 3, Nutrition and biochemistry of milk/maintenance,* New York, 1974, Academic Press.

42. Leake RD, Waters CB, Rubin RT et al: Oxytocin and prolactin responses in long-term breastfeeding, *Obstet Gynecol* 62:565, 1983.

43. Lincoln DW, Paisley AC: Neuroendocrine control of milk ejection, *J Reprod Fertil* 65:571, 1982.

44. Lincoln DW, Renfree MB: Mammary gland growth and milk ejection in the agile wallaby, *Macropus agilis,* displaying concurrent asynchronous lactation, *J Reprod Fertil* 63:193, 1981.

45. Linzell JL, Peaker M: The permeability of mammary ducts, *J Physiol* 216:710, 1971.

46. Liu Y, Hyde JF, Vore M: Prolactin regulates maternal bile secretory function postpartum, *J Pharmacol Exp Ther* 261:560, 1992.

47. Lönnerdal B, Atkinson S: Nitrogenous components of milk and human milk proteins. In Jensen RG, editor: *Handbook of milk composition,* San Diego, 1995, Academic Press.

48. Lucas A, Drewett RB, Mitchell MD: Breastfeeding and plasma oxytocin concentrations, *Br Med J* 281:834, 1980.

49. Lund LR, Rømer J, Thomasset N et al: Two distinct phases of apoptosis in mammary gland involution: proteinase-independent and -dependent pathways, *Development* 122:181, 1996.

50. Martin RH, Glass MR, Chapman C et al: Human α-lactalbumin and hormonal factors in pregnancy and lactation, *Clin Endocrinol* 13:223, 1980.

51. McNeilly AS, Robinson ICA, Houston MJ et al: Release of oxytocin and prolactin in response to suckling, *Br Med J* 286:257, 1983.

52. Meites J: Neuroendocrinology of lactation, *J Invest Dermatol* 63:119, 1974.

53. Neville MC: Regulation of mammary development and lactation. In Neville MC, Neifert MR, editors: *Lactation: physiology, nutrition, and breast-feeding,* New York, 1983, Plenum.

54. Neville MC: The physiological basis of milk secretion. Part I. Basic physiology, *Ann NY Acad Sci* 586:1, 1990.

55. Neville MC: Determinants of milk volume and composition. A. Lactogenesis in women: a cascade of events revealed by milk composition. In Jensen RG, editor: *Handbook of milk composition,* San Diego, 1995, Academic Press.

56. Neville MC: Mammary gland biology and lactation: a short course. Presented at biannual meeting of the International Society for Research on Human Milk and Lactation, Plymouth, Mass, October 1997.

57. Neville MC, Allen JC, Archer PC et al: Studies in human lactation: milk volume and nutrient composition during weaning and lactogenesis, *Am J Clin Nutr* 54:81, 1991.

58. Neville MC, Allen JC, Walters C: The mechanisms of milk secretion. In Neville MC, Neifert MR, editors: *Lactation: physiology, nutrition, and breast-feeding,* New York, 1983, Plenum.

59. Newton N: The relation of the milk-ejection reflex to the ability to breastfeed, *Ann NY Acad Sci* 652:484, 1992.

60. Newton N: The quantitative effect of oxytocin (Pitocin) on human milk yield, *Ann NY Acad Sci* 652:652, 1992.

61. Nissen E, Lilja G, Widström A-M et al: Elevation of oxytocin levels early postpartum in women, *Acta Obstet Gynecol Scand* 74:530, 1995.

62. Ormandy CJ, Binart N, Kelly PA: Mammary gland development in prolactin receptor knockout mice, *J Mammary Gland Biol Neoplasia* 2:355, 1997.

63. Ostrom KM: A review of the hormone prolactin during lactation: progress in food and nutrition, *Science* 14:1, 1990.

64. Patton S, Neville MC: Introduction: maternal adaptation to lactation, *J Mammary Gland Biol Neoplasia* 2:201, 1997.

65. Peaker M: Production of hormones by the mammary gland: short review, *Endocr Regul* 25:10, 1991.

66. Peaker M, Linzell JL: Citrate in milk: a harbinger of lactogenesis, *Nature* 253:464, 1975.

67. Pederson CA: Oxytocin control of maternal behavior, *Ann NY Acad Med* 807:126, 1997.

68. Pederson CA, Prange AJ: Induction of maternal behavior in virgin rats after intracerebroventricular administration of oxytocin, *Proc Natl Acad Sci* 76:6661, 1979.

69. Pederson CA, Caldwell JD, Walker C et al: Oxytocin activates the postpartum onset of rat maternal behavior in the ventral, tegmental and medial preoptic areas, *Behav Neurosci* 108:1163, 1994.

70. Prentice A, Addey CVP, Wilde CJ: Evidence for local feedback control of human milk secretion, *Biochem Soc Trans* 17:122, 1989.

71. Prilusky J, Deis RP: Inhibition of milk ejection by a visual stimulus in lactating rats: implication of the pineal gland, *Brain Res* 251:313, 1982.

72. Richard L, Alade MO: Effect of delivery room routines on success of first breast-feed, *Lancet* 336:1105, 1990.

73. Rimoin DL, Holzman GB, Merimee TJ et al: Lactation in the absence of human growth hormone, *J Clin Endocrinol Metab* 28:1183, 1968.

74. Robinson JE, Short RV: Changes in breast sensitivity at puberty, during the menstrual cycle, and at parturition, *Br Med J* I:1188, 1977.

75. Robyn C, Meuris S: Pituitary prolactin, lactational performance and puerperal infertility, *Semin Perinatol* 6:254, 1982.

76. Rosen JM, Humphreys R, Krnacik S et al: The regulation of mammary gland development by hormones, growth factors and oncogenes, *Prog Clin Biol Res* 387:95, 1994.

77. Shalev E, Weiner E, Tzabari A et al: Breast stimulation in late pregnancy, *Gynecol Obstet Invest* 29:125, 1990.

78. Shennan DB: Mechanisms of mammary gland ion transport, *Comp Biochem Physiol* 97A:317, 1990.

79. Sherwood LM: Human prolactin, *N Engl J Med* 284:774, 1971.

80. Smith VR: *Lactation*, vol 1, *The mammary gland/development and maintenance,* New York, 1974, Academic Press.

81. Stern JM, Reichlin S: Prolactin circadian rhythm persists throughout lactation in women, *Neuroendocrinology* 51:31, 1990.

82. Strange R, Li F, Saurer S et al: Apoptotic cell death and tissue remodeling during mouse mammary gland involution, *Development* 115:49, 1992.

83. Takeda S, Kuwabara Y, Mizuno M: Concentrations and origin of oxytocin in breast milk, *Endocrinol Jpn* 33:821, 1986.

84. Tanaka T, Shiu RPC, Gout PW et al: A new sensitive and specific bioassay for lactogenic hormones: measurement of prolactin and growth hormone in human serum, *J Clin Endocrinol Metab* 51:1058, 1980.

85. Theorell T: Prolactin: a hormone that mirrors passiveness in crisis situations, *Integr Physiol Behav Sci* 27:32, 1992.

86. Toppozada MK, El-Rahman HA, Soliman AY: Prostaglandins as milk ejectors: the nose as a new route of administration. In Samuelson B, Paoletti R, Rawell P, editors: *Advances in prostaglandin, thromboxane, and leukotrience research,* vol 12, New York, 1983, Raven.

87. Tyson JE: Mechanisms of puerperal lactation, *Med Clin North Am* 61:153, 1977.

88. Uvnäs-Moberg K, Eriksson M: Breastfeeding: physiological, endocrine and behavioral adaptations caused by oxytocin and local neurogenic activity in the nipple and mammary gland, *Acta Paediatr* 85:525, 1996.

89. Vernon RG, Pond CM: Adaptations of maternal adipose tissue to lactation, *J Mammary Gland Biol Neoplasia* 2:231, 1997.

90. Vigneri R, Squatrito S, Pezzino V et al: Spontaneous fluctuations of human placental lactogen during normal pregnancy, *J Clin Endocrinol Metab* 40:506, 1975.

91. Vonderhaar BK, Bremel RD: Prolactin, growth hormone, and placental lactogen, *J Mammary Gland Biol Neoplasia* 2:1, 1997.

92. Vorherr H: *The breast: morphology, physiology and lactation,* New York, 1974, Academic Press.

93. Vorherr H: Human lactation and breastfeeding. In Larson BL, editor: *Lactation,* vol 4, *The mammary gland/human lactation/milk synthesis,* New York, 1978, Academic Press.

94. Vorherr H: Hormonal and biochemical changes of pituitary and breast during pregnancy. In Vorherr H, editor: Human lactation, *Semin Perinatol* 3:193, 1979.

95. Wehrenberg WB, Gaillard RC: Neuroendocrine mechanisms regulating growth hormone and prolactin secretion during lactation, *Endocrinology* 124:464, 1989.

96. Weitzman RE, Leake RD, Rubin RT et al: The effect of nursing on neurohypophyseal hormone and prolactin secretion in human subjects, *J Clin Endocrinol Metab* 51:836, 1980.

97. Widstrom AM, Winberg J, Werner S et al: Suckling in lactating women stimulates the secretion of insulin and prolactin without concomitant effects on gastrin, growth hormone, calcitonin, vasopressin, or catecholamines, *Early Hum Dev* 10:115, 1984.

98. Wilde CJ, Addey CVP, Boddy LM et al: Autocrine regulation of milk secretion by a protein in milk, *Biochem J* 305:51, 1995.

99. Yuen BH: Prolactin in human milk: the influence of nursing and the duration of postpartum lactation, *Am J Obstet Gynecol* 158:583, 1988.

100. Zinaman MJ, Hughes V, Queenan JT et al: Acute prolactin and oxytocin responses and milk yield to infant suckling and artificial methods of expression in lactating women, *Pediatrics* 89:437, 1992.

$\mathcal{B}$iochemistry of human milk

The biochemistry of human milk encompasses a mammoth supply of scientific data and information, most of which has been generated since 1970. Each report or study adds a tiny piece to the complex puzzle of the nutrients that make up human milk. The answers to some questions still elude us. A question as simple as the volume of milk consumed at a feeding remains a scientific challenge. The methodology must be accurate, reproducible, noninvasive, and suitable for home use night or day and must not interrupt breastfeeding. The perfect method has not been found. On the other hand, the precision analysis available for measuring the concentration of the most minuscule of elements is remarkably accurate and reproducible in the laboratory.

Advances in analytic methods bring greater sensitivity, resolving power, and speed to the analysis of milk composition. Previously unknown and unrecognized compounds have been detected. We now know milk brings both nutrients and nonnutritive signals to the neonate. With few exceptions, all milks contain the nutrients for physical growth and new logical development. When the offspring develops rapidly, the milk is nutrient dense; when it develops slowly, the milk is more dilute. All milks contain fat, carbohydrate, and proteins, as well as minerals, vitamins, and other nutrients. The organization of milk composition includes lipids in emulsified globules coated with a membrane, colloidal dispersions of proteins as micelles, and the remainder as a true solution.[166]

The discussion in this chapter is limited to information perceived as immediately useful to the clinician. Considerable detail and species variability are eliminated to help focus attention on details directly influencing management. Extensive and exhaustive reviews are referenced to provide the reader with easy access to greater detail and validation of the general conclusions reported here.*

Human milk is not a uniform body fluid but a secretion of the mammary gland of changing composition. Foremilk differs from hindmilk. Colostrum differs from transitional and mature milks. Milk changes over time of day and as time goes by. As concentrations of protein, fat, carbohydrates, minerals, and cells differ, physical properties such as osmolarity and pH change. The impact of changing composition on the physiology of the infant gut is beginning to be appreciated. Many constituents have dual roles.

The more than 200 constituents of milk include a tremendous array of molecules whose descrip-

---

*References 33, 40, 51, 109, 120, 166, 175, 196.

TABLE 4-1   Constituents of milk (g/100 g) of specific mammals

Mammalian species in taxonomic position	Total solids	Fat	Casein	Whey protein	Total protein	Lactose	Ash
Human	12.4	3.8	0.4	0.6	—	7.0	0.2
Baboon	14.4	5.0	—	—	1.6	7.3	0.3
Orangutan	11.5	3.5	1.1	0.4	—	6.0	0.2
Black bear	44.5	24.5	8.8	5.7	—	0.4	1.8
California sea lion	52.7	36.5	—	—	13.8	0.0	0.6
Black rhinoceros	8.1	0.0	1.1	0.3	—	6.1	0.3
Spotted dolphin	31.0	18.0	—	—	9.4	0.6	—
Domestic dog	23.5	12.9	5.8	2.1	—	3.1	1.2
Norway rat	21.0	10.3	6.4	2.0	—	2.6	1.3
Whitetail jackrabbit	40.8	13.9	19.7	4.0	—	1.7	1.5

Modified from Jenness R, Sloan RE: Composition of milk. In Larson BL, Smith VR, editors: *Lactation,* vol 3, *Nutrition and biochemistry of milk/maintenance,* New York, 1974, Academic Press.

tions continue to be refined as qualitative and quantitative laboratory techniques are perfected. Resolution of lipid chemicals has advanced dramatically in recent years, but new carbohydrates and proteins have been identified as well. Some of the compounds identified may well be intermediary products in the process that occurs within the mammary cells and may be only incidental in the final product.[226] Milk includes true solutions, colloids, membranes, membrane-bound globules, and living cells.

Human and bovine milks are known in the greatest detail[84]; however, much information exists about the milk of five other species: the water buffalo, goat, sheep, horse, and pig. Miscellaneous data are available on the milk of 150 more species and no data at all on another 4000 species. Jenness and Sloan[118] have compiled a summary of 140 species from which a sampling has been extracted (Table 4-1). The constituents of milk can be divided into the following groups, according to their specificity[118]:

1. Constituents specific to both organ and species (e.g., most proteins and lipids)
2. Constituents specific to organ but not to species (e.g., lactose)
3. Constituents specific to species but not to organ (e.g., albumin, some immunoglobulins)

NORMAL VARIATIONS IN HUMAN MILK

In defining the constituents of human milk, it is important to recognize that the composition varies with the stage of lactation, the time of day, the sampling time during a given feeding, maternal nutrition, and individual variation. Many early interpretations of the content of human milk were based on spot samples or even pooled samples from multiple donors at different times and stages of lactation. Samples obtained by pumping may vary from those obtained by the suckling infant, because some variation exists in content among the various methods of pumping.

Daytime consumption of milk in a given infant has been shown by Brown et al[22] to be 46% to 58% of the total 24-hour consumption, so that reliance on less than a 24-hour sampling may be misleading. Data from samples taken every 3 hours showed a variation in milk concentration of nitrogen, lactose, and fat, as well as in the volume of milk, by time of day (Fig. 4-1). Furthermore, there were statistically significant diurnal changes in the concentration of lactose and the volume within individual subjects, but the times of those changes were not consistent for each individual. Some individuals varied as much as twofold in volume

Fig. 4-1. Mean concentrations of nitrogen, lactose, and fat in human milk by time of day. (Modified from Brown KH, Black RE, Robertson AD et al: *Am J Clin Nutr* 35:745, 1982.)

production from day to day. These investigators also found a significant difference in the concentrations of fat and lactose and in the volume of milk produced by each breast. At the extreme, the less productive breast yielded only 65% of the volume of the other breast.

The variation in the fat content has received some attention. Fat content changes during a given feeding, increasing at the end of the feeding. Fat content rises from early morning to midday; the volume increased from two to five times, as reported in early studies when feedings were controlled. Multiple studies in different countries and different decades, summarized by Jackson et al,[113] reveal that some of the variation is related to other factors. Demand feeding (Thai mothers in 1988) has a different circadian variation than scheduled feeding (U.S. mothers in 1932) (Fig. 4-2). In the later part of the first year of lactation, the fat content diminishes. Work done by Atkinson et al[13] and confirmed by other investigators has shown that the nitrogen content of the milk of mothers who deliver prematurely is higher than that of those whose pregnancies reach full term. For a given volume of milk, the premature infant would receive 20% more nitrogen than the full-term infant if each were fed his or her own mother's milk. Other constituents of milk produced

by mothers who deliver prematurely have also been studied.

An additional consideration in reviewing information available on the levels of various constituents of milk is the technique used to derive the data. In 1977, Hambraeus[83] reported that there was less protein in human milk than originally calculated. The present techniques of immunoassay measure the absolute amounts, whereas earlier figures were derived from calculations based on measurements of the nitrogen content. About 25% of the nitrogen in human milk is nonprotein nitrogen. Cow's milk has only 5% nonprotein nitrogen.

A major concern about variation in content of human milk is related to the mother's diet. Maternal diet is of particular concern when the mother is malnourished or eats an unusually restrictive diet. Malnourished mothers have approximately the same proportions of protein, fat, and carbohydrate as well-nourished mothers, but they produce less milk. Water-soluble vitamins, ascorbic acid, thiamin, and B_{12} levels are quickly affected by deficient diets.

Mother's milk is recommended for all infants under ordinary circumstances even if the mother's diet is not perfect, according to the Committee on Nutrition during Pregnancy and Lactation of the Institute of Medicine.[165]

Fig. 4-2. Circadian variation in fat concentration of breast milk from published studies. **A,** Thailand (present study)—Prefeed/postfeed expressed samples, 19 mothers studied for 24 hours each, infants aged 1 to 9 months. **B,** The Gambia (Prentice et al)—Demand feeding, pre/postexpressed samples, 16 mothers studied for 24 hours each, infants aged 1 to 18 months. **C,** Bangladesh (Brown et al)—Samples collected at scheduled intervals by total breast extraction (breast pump), seven mothers studied for 24 hours each, infants aged 1 to 9 months. **D,** United Kingdom *(UK)* (Hall)—Prefeed/postfeed expressed samples, one mother studied for 72 hours. **E,** UK[107]: (Hytten)—Samples collected by total breast extraction (breast pump). *Lower curve,* 29 mothers studied for 24 hours each, infants aged 3 to 8 days. *Upper curve,* 20 mothers studied for 24 hours each, infants aged 21 days to 4 months. **F,** United States *(USA)* (Nims et al)—Samples collected by total breast extraction (manual), three mothers studied, but values only given for one mother, for 24 hours on six occasions and 72 hours on one occasion, infant aged 6 to 60 weeks. **G,** New Zealand (Deem)—Samples collected by total breast extraction (manual), 28 mothers studied for 24 hours each, infants aged 1 to 8 months. **H,** Germany (Gunther and Stainier)—Collection of samples by total breast extraction (manual), two mothers studied for 24 hours each, six mothers studied for 52 hours each, infants aged 8 to 11 days. (Modified from Jackson DA, Imong SM, Silprasert A et al: *Br J Nutr* 59:349, 1988.)

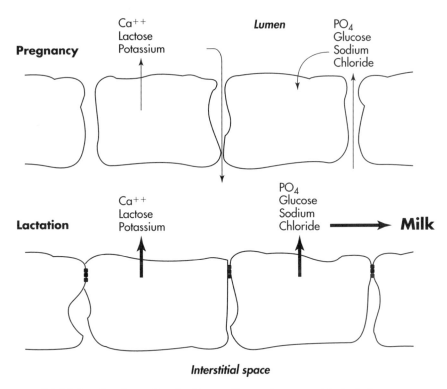

Fig. 4-3. Model for directions of major fluxes of several macronutrients during pregnancy and lactation in women. (From Neville MC: Determinants of milk volume and composition. In Jensen RG, editor: *Handbook of milk composition,* San Diego, 1995, Academic Press.)

PREPARTUM MILK

Prepartum milk is the first stage of mammogenesis and is especially conspicuous in other species such as the goat.[4] It provides evidence that the junctions between alveolar cells are "leaky" during pregnancy, allowing fluid and solutes to flow between the milk space and the interstitial fluid of the mammary gland. Fig. 4-3 illustrates the composition of this milk. The lactose concentration is directly correlated with that of potassium, but sodium and chloride are inversely related to lactose (Tables 4-2 and 4-6).

COLOSTRUM

The consistently identifiable stages of human milk are colostrum, transitional milk, and mature milk,

and their relative contents are significant for newborns and their physiologic adaption to extra-uterine life.

The first postpartum week's mammary secretion consists of a yellowish, thick fluid, colostrum. The residual mixture of materials present in the mammary glands and ducts at delivery and immediately after is progressively mixed with newly secreted milk, forming colostrum. Human colostrum is known to differ from mature milk in composition, both in the nature of its components and in the relative proportions of these components. Colostrum's specific gravity is 1.040 to 1.060. The mean energy value is 67 kcal/dl compared with the 75 kcal/dl of mature milk. The volume varies between 2 and 20 ml per feeding in the first 3 days. The total volume per day also depends on the number of feedings and is reported to average, in the first 24 hours (which is different

TABLE 4-2 Composition of prepartum human milk*

Milk component	Units	Mean ± SD (n)
Mean days prepartum		20.21 ± 12.18 (11)
Lipid	%	2.07 ± 0.98 (11)
Lactose	mM	79.78 ± 21.68 (9)
Protein	g/dl	5.44 ± 1.71 (8)
Glucose	mM	0.35 ± 0.16 (8)
Sodium	mM	61.26 ± 25.82 (10)
Potassium	mM	18.30 ± 5.67 (10)
Chloride	mM	62.21 ± 17.44 (10)
Calcium	mg/dl	25.35 ± 8.48 (10)
Magnesium	mg/dl	5.64 ± 1.44 (10)
Citrate	mM	0.40 ± 0.17 (8)
Phosphate	mg/dl	2.32 ± 0.70 (9)
Ionized calcium	mM	3.25 ± 0.84 (6)
pH		6.83 ± 0.18 (6)
Urea	mg/dl	14.87 ± 2.40 (9)
Creatinine	mg/dl	1.47 ± 0.35 (9)

From Allen JC, Keller RP, Archer P et al: *Am J Clin Nutr* 54:69, 80, 1991.
*Small samples of mammary secretion were obtained three times in prepartum period from each of 11 women. In some cases, volumes were insufficient for all analyses.

from the first day, depending on the time of delivery), 100 ml (Table 4-3). Tables 4-4 and 4-5 list the yield and composition of colostrum (1 to 5 days) and mature milk 14 days and beyond. The increased production of citrate is paralleled by the increase in volume (Figs. 4-4 and 4-5).

Dewey et al[49] clearly demonstrate that in a well-established milk supply, volume depends on infant demand, and the residual milk available at each feeding is comparable in both low-intake and average-intake dyads. Infant birthweight, weight at 3 months, and total time nursing were positively associated with intake. The volume also varies with the mother's parity. Women who have had other pregnancies, particularly those who have nursed infants previously, have colostrum more readily available at delivery, and the volume increases more rapidly.

The yellow color of colostrum results from β-carotene. The ash content is high, and the concentrations of sodium, potassium, and chloride are greater than those of mature milk. Protein, fat-soluble vitamins, and minerals are present in greater percentages than in transitional or mature milk.

The higher protein, lower fat, and lactose solution is rich in immunoglobulins, especially secretory immunoglobulin A (sIgA). The number of immunologically competent mononuclear cells is at its highest level. Fat, contained mainly in the core of the fat globules, increases from 2% in colostrum to 2.9% in transitional milk and to 3.6% in mature milk. Concentration of fat in the prepartum secretion is only 1 g/dl, and the distribution among classes of lipids differs. Prepartum milk is 93% triglycerides, increasing to 97% in colostrum, with diglycerides, monoglycerides, and free fatty acids all increasing from prepartum to postpartum secretions. Phospholipid levels decline during the same period. Prepartum secretions contain higher amounts of membrane components such as phospholipids, cholesterol, and cholesteryl esters, which decline from colostrum to mature milk.

Cholesterol appears to be synthesized in the mammary gland. The role of cholesterol in colostrum beyond its use in brain tissue development, the myelinization of nerves, and as the base of many enzymes remains elusive. Very little research has been done on cholesterol in colostrum.

Colostrum facilitates the establishment of bifidus flora in the digestive tract. Colostrum also facilitates the passage of meconium. Meconium contains an essential growth factor for *Lactobacillus bifidus* and is the first culture medium in the sterile intestinal lumen of the newborn infant. Human colostrum is rich in antibodies, which may provide protection against the bacteria and viruses that are present in the birth canal and associated with other human contact. Colostrum also contains antioxidants, which may function as traps for neutrophil-generated reactive oxygen metabolites.[23,24]

The progressive changes in mammary secretion in both breastfeeding and nonbreastfeeding women between 28 and 110 days before delivery and up to 5 months after delivery were followed by Kulski

TABLE 4-3   Average milk volume outputs (ml/24 hr) of well-nourished mothers who exclusively breastfed their infants

| | | | Month of lactation | | | | | | | | | | |
| | | | <1 | | 1-2 | | 2-3 | | 3-4 | | 4-5 | | 5-6 | |
Country	No. days measured	Gender	ml/24 hr	n	ml/24 hr	n	ml/24 hr	n	ml/24 hr	n	ml/24 hr	n	ml/24 hr	n
U.S.	2	M, F	—	—	691	3	655	5	750	3	—	—	—	—
U.S.	1-2	M, F	681	46	—	—	—	—	—	—	—	—	—	—
Canada	?	M, F	—	—	—	—	—	—	793	33	856	31	925	28
Sweden	?	M, F	558	15	724	11	752	12	—	—	—	—	—	—
U.S.	3	M, F	—	—	600	11	—	—	833	2	—	—	682	3
U.S.	3	M, F	—	—	606	26	601	26	626	20	—	—	—	—
U.K.	4	M	—	—	791	27	820	23	829	18	790	5	922	1
		F	—	—	677	20	742	17	775	14	814	6	838	4
U.S.	1	M, F	673 ± 192 SD	16	756 ± 170	19	782 ± 172	16	810 ± 142	13	805 ± 117	11	896 ± 122	11

| | | | Month of lactation | | | | | |
			7	8	9	10	11	12
U.S.	1	M, F	875 ± 142 SD	834 ± 99	774 ± 180	691 ± 233	516 ± 215	759 ± 28

Modified from Ferris AM, Jensen RG: *J Pediatr Gastroenterol Nutr* 3:108, 1984.

TABLE 4-4   **Yield and composition of human colostrum and milk from days 1 to 28**

Component	Day postpartum						
	1	2	3	4	5	14	28
Yield (g/24 hr)	50	190	400	625	700	1100	1250
Lactose (g/L)	20	25	31	32	33	35	35
Fat (g/L)	12	15	20	25	24	23	29
Protein (g/L)	32	17	12	11	11	8	9

Modified from Saint L, Smith M, Hartmann PE: *Br J Nutr* 58:87, 1984.

TABLE 4-5   **Composition of human milk from days 1 through 36 postpartum (mean ± SD), British and German donors**

Day	Component (g/dl)		
	Total protein	Lactose	Triacylglycerols
1	2.95 ± 0.86	4.07 ± 0.98	2.14 ± 0.86
3	1.99 ± 0.22	4.98 ± 0.76	3.01 ± 0.77
5	1.82 ± 0.21	5.13 ± 0.54	3.06 ± 0.45
8	1.73 ± 0.27	5.38 ± 0.97	3.73 ± 0.70
15	1.56 ± 0.42	5.42 ± 0.76	3.59 ± 0.86
22	1.51 ± 0.27	5.34 ± 0.96	3.87 ± 0.68
29	1.5 ± 0.27	4.01 ± 1.13	4.01 ± 1.13
36	1.4 ± 0.26	5.34 ± 1.31	4.01 ± 1.20

Modified from Hibberd CM, Brooke DG, Carter ND et al: *Arch Dis Child* 57:658, 1982.

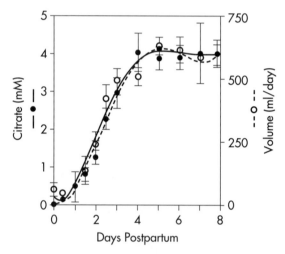

Fig. 4-4. Changes in concentration of citrate in human milk in early postpartum period compared with increase in milk volume. Data replotted from Neville et al (1991).[170] (From Neville MC: Determinants of milk volume and composition. In Jensen RG, editor: *Handbook of milk composition,* San Diego, 1995, Academic Press.)

and Hartmann[140] to study the initiation of lactation. During late pregnancy the secretion contained higher concentrations of proteins and lower concentrations of lactose, glucose, and urea than those contained in milk secreted when lactation was well established. The concentrations of sodium, chloride, and magnesium were higher and those of potassium and calcium lower in colostrum than in milk. The osmolarity was relatively constant throughout the study. The authors described a two-phase development of lactation, with an initial phase of limited secretion in late pregnancy and a true induction of lactation in the second phase, 32 to 40 hours postpartum. Comparison with the nonlactating women revealed similar secretion

during the first 3 days postpartum. This, however, was abruptly reversed during the next 6 days as mammary involution progressed. Obtaining samples in these women, however, may have served to prolong the period of production. The authors[140] point out that although breastfeeding was not necessary for the initiation of lactation in this study, it was essential for the continuation of lactation.

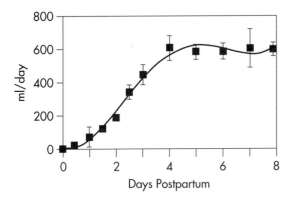

Fig. 4-5. Milk volumes during first week postpartum. Mean values from 12 multiparous Caucasian women who test-weighed their infants before and after every feeding for first 7 days postpartum. (From Neville MC, Keller R, Seacat J et al: *Am J Clin Nutr* 48:1375, 1988.)

The yield of milk has been calculated from absolute values to demonstrate the increase in output of milk constituents during lactogenesis (Fig. 4-6). Dramatic increases occurred in the production of all the milk constituents. The components synthesized by the mammary epithelium (lactose, lactalbumin, and lactoferrin) increased at a rate greater than those for IgA or proteins derived from the serum IgG and IgM. The greatest difference in yield between day 1 and day 7 postpartum was for glucose.[169]

A survey of the fatty acid components by Read and Sarrif[193] showed the lauric acid and myristic acid contents to be low in concentration the first few days. When the lauric and myristic acids increased, C_{18} acids decreased. Palmitoleic acid increased at the same rate as the myristic acid. From this it was concluded that the early fatty acids are derived from extramammary sources, but the breast quickly begins to synthesize fatty acids for the production of transitional and mature milk (Table 4-6). The total fat content may have a predictive value. In 1954, Hytten[107] showed that 90% of the women whose milk contained 20 g or more of fat per feeding on the seventh day were successfully breastfeeding 3 months later. Women who only had 5 to 10 g of fat on the seventh day had an 80% dropout rate by 3 months.

Colostrum's high protein and low fat are in keeping with the needs and reserves of the newborn at birth. Although the content of total nitrogen or any amino acid in breast milk in 24 hours is grossly related to the volume produced, the concentration in milligrams per deciliter (mg/dl) is not so related.[54] The relative distribution of the individual amino acids in each deciliter (100 ml) of milk differs in each mother. The colostrum may actually reflect a transitional maternal blood picture, which is associated with nitrogen metabolism of the postpartum period. The postpartum period is one of involution of body tissue and catabolism of protein in the mother (Fig. 4-7).

Colostrum contains at least two separate antioxidants, an ascorbate-like substance and uric acid.[23] These antioxidants may function in the colostrum as traps for neutrophil-generated, reactive oxygen metabolites. The aqueous human colostrum interferes with the oxygen metabolic and enzymatic activities of the polymorphonuclear leukocytes that are important in the reaction to acute inflammation.[24] This supports the belief that human milk is antiinflammatory.

The mineral and vitamin reserves of the newborn infant are related to the maternal diet. A fetal supply of vitamin C, iron, and amino acids is adequate because infant blood levels exceed those of the mother. Colostrum is rich in fat-soluble vitamin A, carotenoids, and vitamin E. The average vitamin A level on the third day can be three times that of mature milk. Similarly, carotenoids in colostrum may be 10 times the level in mature milk, and vitamin E may be two to three times greater than in mature milk (Fig. 4-8).

TRANSITIONAL MILK

The milk produced between the colostrum and mature milk stages is transitional milk; its content gradually changes. The transitional phase is approximately from 7 to 10 days postpartum to 2

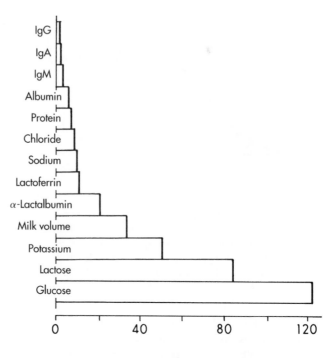

Fig. 4-6. Relative increase in yield of milk components from day 1 to day 7 postpartum. Values presented are for day 7 expressed as percentage increase over day 1. (Modified from Kulski JK, Hartmann PE: *Aust J Exp Biol Med Sci* 59:101, 1981.)

TABLE 4-6	**Fat distribution in milk**				
	Prepartum		**Postpartum**		
	Early	**Late**	**Colostrum**	**Transitional**	**Mature**
Fat (%)	—	2	2	2.9	3.6
Fat (g)	—	—	2.9	3.6	3.8
Lipid (g/dl)	1.15	1.28	3.16	3.49	4.14
Phospholipid (mg/dl)	37	40	35	31	27
Percent of total lipid	3.2	3.1	1.1	0.9	0.6
Cholesterol (mg/dl)	—	—	29	20	13.5

weeks postpartum. The concentration of immuno-globulins and total protein decreases, whereas the lactose, fat, and total caloric content increases. The water-soluble vitamins increase, and the fat-soluble vitamins decrease to the levels of mature milk.

In a study of transitional milks, breast milk samples were obtained from healthy mothers of term infants on the first, third, fifth, eighth, fifteenth, twenty-second, twenty-ninth, and thirty-

sixth days of lactation by Hibberd et al,[102] who defined the first day of lactation to be the third day postpartum. Twenty-four-hour samples were pooled for analysis and the remainder fed to the baby. The authors found a high degree of variability, not only between mothers but also within samples from the same mother. The maximum value in almost every case was more than twice the minimum. They were able to show, however, that the changes in composition were rapid before day

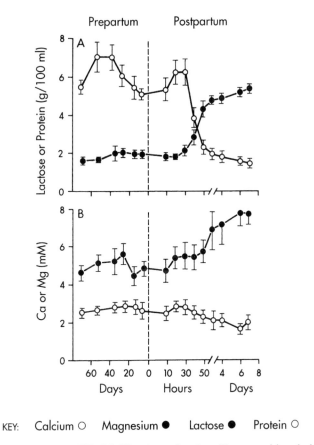

KEY: Calcium ○   Magnesium ●   Lactose ●   Protein ○

Fig. 4-7. (Modified from Dumas BR: Modifications of early milk composition during early states of lactation in nutritional adaptations of the gastrointestinal tract of the newborn. In Kretchmer N, Minkowski A, editors: *Nutritional adaptation of GI tract of the newborn,* vol 3, New York, 1983, Nestlé Vevey/Raven.)

8, and then progressively less change took place until the composition was relatively stable before day 36 (Tables 4-4 and 4-5).

MATURE MILK

Water

In almost all mammalian milks, water is the constituent in the largest quantity, with the exception of the milk of some arctic and aquatic species, who produce milks with high fat content (e.g., the

northern fur seal produces milk with 54% fat and 65% total solids) (Table 4-1). All other constituents are dissolved, dispersed, or suspended in water. Water contributes to the temperature-regulating mechanism of the newborn because 25% of heat loss is from evaporation of water from the lungs and skin. The lactating woman has a greatly increased obligatory water intake. If water intake is restricted during lactation, other water losses through urine and insensible loss are decreased before water for lactation is diminished. Because lactose is the regulating factor in the amount of milk produced, the secretion of water into milk is

Fig. 4-8. Distribution of main protein fractions *(top)* and whey protein *(bottom)* in human and bovine milk. (Modified from Dumas BR: Modifications of early human milk composition during early states of lactation in nutritional adaptation of the gastrointestinal tract of the newborn. In Kretchmer N, Minkowski A, editors: *Nutritional adaptation of GI tract of the newborn*, vol 3, New York, 1983, Nestlé Vevey/Raven.)

partially regulated by lactose synthesis. Investigations by Almroth[5] show that the water requirement of infants in a hot, humid climate can be provided entirely by the water in human milk.

Human milk is a complex fluid that scientists have studied by separating the several phases by physical forces.[120] These forces include settling; short-term, low-speed centrifugation; high-speed centrifugation; and precipitation by micelle-destroying treatments such as using the enzyme rennin (chymosin) or reducing the pH. On settling the cream floats to the top, forming a layer of fat (about 4% by volume in human milk).[105] Lipid-soluble components such as cholesterol and phospholipid remain with the fat. With a slow-speed spin, cellular components form a pellet. The high-speed spin brings the casein micelles into a separate phase or forms a pellet. On top of the protein pellet is a loose pellet referred to as the "fluff," composed of membranes.[167,168] Casein precipitation (0.2% by weight) is caused by acid

destruction of the micelles. The aqueous phase is whey, which also contains milk sugar, milk proteins, IgA, and the monovalent ions.

Lipids

Intense interest in the lipids in human milk has been sparked by the reports from long-range studies of breastfed infants that show more advanced development at 1 year,[154] 8 to 10 years,[155] and now 18 years of age[103] compared with formula-fed infants. This attention has resulted from the interest in supplementing formula with various missing factors, such as cholesterol and docosahexaenoic acid (DHA).[182] These compounds function in a milieu of arachidonic acid, lipases, and other enzymes, and no evidence indicates that they are effective in isolation or that more is better. The value of supplementing the mother's diet in pregnancy and lactation is an equally important question, because the dietary DHA levels have declined in the

TABLE 4-7 Compartments and their constituents in mature human milk*

Compartment		Major constituents	
Description	Content (%)	Name	Content (%)
Aqueous phase 　True solution (1 nm) 　Whey proteins (3-9 nm)	87.0	Compounds of Ca, Mg, PO$_4$, Na, K, Cl, 　CO$_2$, citrate, casein	0.2 as ash
		Whey proteins: α-lactalbumin, lactoferrin, 　IgA, lysozyme, serum albumin	0.6
		Lactose and oligosaccharides; 7.0 and 　1.0%	8.0
		Nonprotein nitrogen compounds: 　glucosamine, urea, amino acids; 　20% of total N	35-50 mg N
		Miscellaneous: B vitamins, ascorbic acid	
Colloidal dispersion 　(11-55 nm, 10^{16}/ml)	0.3	Caseins: beta and kappa, Ca, PO$_4$	0.2-0.3
Emulsion 　Fat globules (4 μm, 1.1^{10}/ml)	4.0	Fat globules: triacylglycerols, sterol 　esters	4.0
Fat-globule membrane 　Interfacial layer	2.0	Milk-fat-globule membrane: proteins, 　phospholipids, cholesterol, enzymes, 　trace minerals, fat-soluble vitamins	2% of total lipid
Cells (8-40 μm, 10^4-10^5/ml)		Macrophages, neutrophils, lymphocytes, 　epithelial cells	

From Jensen RG: *The lipids of human milk,* Boca Raton, Fla, 1989, CRC.
*All figures are approximate.

last half century as women avoid eggs and animal organs in their diet (see Chapter 9).

Lipids are a chemically heterogeneous group of substances that are insoluble in water and soluble in nonpolar solvents. There are many classes and thousands of subclasses of lipids. The main constituents of human milk are triacylglycerols, phospholipids, and their component fatty acids, the sterols. Jensen, a renowned milk lipidologist, et al[122] remind readers, in a comprehensive review of the lipids in human milk, of the nomenclature, such as palmitic acid (16:0), oleic acid (18:1), and linoleic acid (18:2). The figure to the left of the colon is the number of carbons and to the right the number of double bonds. Polyunsaturated fatty acids (PUFAs) have a designation for the location of the double bond; in human milk, the designation is *cis(c.),* which identifies the geometric isomer. Because milk is an exceptionally complex fluid,

Jensen et al[120,121] and other scientists have found it helpful to classify components according to their size and concentration, with solubility in milk or lack thereof as additional categories (Table 4-7). The lipids fulfill a host of essential functions in growth and development,[20,21] provide a well-tolerated energy source, serve as carriers of messages to the infant, and provide physiologic interactions, including the following[119]:

1. Allow maximum intestinal absorption of fatty acids.
2. Contribute about 50% of calories.
3. Provide essential fatty acids (EFAs) and PUFAs.
4. Provide cholesterol.

By percentage of concentration, the second greatest constituent in milk is the lipid fraction. Milk lipids provide the major fraction of kilocalories in human milk.[119,121]

BOX 4-1   Factors associated with changes in the total lipid content of human milk

Within a nursing or feed (↑)	Medication (?)
Stage of lactation, weaning (↑)	Mother's menstrual cycle or pregnancy (?)
Diurnal rhythm (variable)	Parity (↓)
Between breasts	Season (? related to diet)
Gestational age at birth, preterm vs. term	Age (?)
Diet (may occur)	Miscellaneous
Infections, metabolic disorders (usually ↓)	Individuality (adiposity ↑)

Modified from Jensen RG, Bitman J, Carlson SE: Milk lipids. A. Human milk lipids. In Jensen RG, editor: *Handbook of milk composition,* San Diego, 1995, Academic Press.
↑, Increase; ↓, decrease.

Lipids average 3% to 5% of human milk and occur as globules emulsified in the aqueous phase. The core or nonpolar lipids, such as triacylglycerols (TGs) and cholesterol esters, are coated with bipolar materials, phospholipids, proteins, cholesterol, and enzymes. This loose layer is called the *milk-lipid-globule membrane* (MLGM), which keeps the globules from coalescing and thus acts as an emulsion stabilizer.[121] Globules are 1 to 10 μm in diameter, with 1 μm globules predominating.[122]

Fats are also the most variable constituents in human milk, varying in concentration over a feeding, from breast to breast, over a day's time, over time itself, and among individuals (Box 4-1). This information is significant when testing milk samples for energy intake, fat-soluble constituents, and physiologic variation and when clinically managing lactation problems.[89] Much of the early work was based on lactation in women who "nursed by the clock" rather than tuned into infant needs. When circadian variation in fat content was studied in a rural Thai population who had practiced demand feeding for centuries, Jackson et al[113] found fat concentrations in feeds in the afternoon and evening (1600 to 2000 hours) were higher than those during the night (400 to 800 hours). Fat concentrations at start and finish of feed varied over 24 hours. The most important predictor of fat content was length of time since last feed; the longer the interval, the lower the fat concentration. Fat content at the end of a previous feed and milk intake at previous feed also influenced levels.

It is speculated that the altered posture at night, horizontal and relatively inactive, may redistribute fat. The larger the milk consumption at a feed, the greater is the increase in fat from beginning to end of the feed. Less fat change occurs during "sleep" feeds than in the daytime. Unless 24-hour samples are collected by standardized sampling techniques, results will vary. During the course of a feeding, the fluid phase within the gland is mixed with fat droplets in increasing concentration. The fat droplets are released when the smooth muscle contracts in response to the let-down reflex.

The lipid fraction of the milk is extractable by suitable solvents and may require more than one technique to extract all the lipids[144] (Table 4-8). Complete extraction in human milk is difficult because the lipids are bound to protein. From 30% to 55% of the kilocalories are derived from fats; this represents a concentration of 3.5 to 4.5 g/dl. Milk fat is dispersed in the form of droplets or globules maintained in solution by an absorbed layer or membrane. The protective membrane of the fat globules is made up of phospholipid complexes. The rest of the phospholipids found in human milk are dispersed in the skim milk fraction. Triglycerides, diglycerides, monoglycerides, free fatty acids, phospholipids, glycolipids, sterols, and sterol esters are found in human milk. Vitamin A esters, vitamin D, vitamin K, alkylglyceryl ethers, and glyceryl ether diesters are also in the lipid fraction but do not fall into the classes listed.

TABLE 4-8 **Effects of dietary cholesterol, phytosterol, and polyunsaturate (P)/saturate (S) ratio on human milk sterols**

Milk component	Maternal ad lib diet (P/S 0.53) (mg/100 g fat)	Low-cholesterol/ high-phytosterol diet (P/S 1.8) (mg/100 g fat)	High-cholesterol/ low-phytosterol diet (P/S 0.12) (mg/100 g fat)
Cholesterol	240 ± 40	250 ± 10	250 ± 20
Phytosterol	17 ± 3	220 ± 30	70 ± 10
Dietary cholesterol	450 ± 30	130 ± 5	460 ± 90
Dietary phytosterol	23 ± 8	790 ± 17	80 ± 1
Total fat (%)	3.58 ± 0.56	2.69 ± 0.17	2.66 ± 0.16

From Lammi-Keefe CJ, Jensen RG: *J Pediatr Gastroenterol Nutr* 3:172, 1984.

TABLE 4-9 **Composition of milks obtained from different mammals and growth rate of their offspring**

Species	Days required to double birthweight	Content of milk (%)			
		Fat	Protein	Lactose	Ash
Human	180	3.8	0.9	7.0	0.2
Horse	60	1.9	2.5	6.2	0.5
Cow	47	3.7	3.4	4.8	0.7
Reindeer	30	16.9	11.5	2.8	—
Goat	19	4.5	2.9	4.1	0.8
Sheep	10	7.4	5.5	4.8	1.0
Rat	6	15.0	12.0	3.0	2.0

From Hambraeus L: *Pediatr Clin North Am* 24:17, 1977.

Renewed interest in defining the constituents of human milk lipid has developed in recent years as investigators look for the causes of obesity, atherosclerosis, and other degenerative diseases and their relationship to infant nutrition (Table 4-9). A number of reports of historic value are plagued with the technical problems of sampling. Because the fat content of a feeding varies with time, spot samples give spurious results. Ferris and Jensen[62] have reviewed the literature exhaustively and describe the fractionated lipid constituents in detail.

The average fat content of pooled 24-hour samples has been reported from multiple sources to vary in mature milk from 2.10% to 5.0% (Table 4-10). Maternal diet affects the constituents of the lipids but not the total amount of fat. A minimal increase in total lipid content was observed when an extra 1000 kcal of corn oil was fed to lactating mothers. A diet rich in polyunsaturated fats will cause an increased percentage of polyunsaturated fats in the milk without altering the total fat content. When the mother is calorie deficient, depot fats are mobilized, and milk resembles depot fat. When excessive nonfat kilocalories are fed, levels of saturated fatty acids increase as lipids are synthesized from tissue stores.[111]

A 2-week crossover study of three nursing women was done by Harzer et al,[91,92] alternating high fat/low carbohydrate and the reverse. The first diet was 50% kilocalories fat, 15% protein, and 35% carbohydrate, for a total of 2500 calories. It resulted in a reduction of triglycerides (4.1% to 2.6%) and an increase in lactose (5.2% to 6.4%).

TABLE 4-10   Lipid class composition of human milk during lactation

Lipid class	Percentage of total lipids at lactation day:					Immediate extraction
	3	7	21	42	84	
Total lipid, % in milk*	2.04 ± 1.32	2.89 ± 0.31	3.45 ± 0.37	3.19 ± 0.43	4.87 ± 0.62	
Phospholipid	1.1	0.8	0.8	0.6	0.6	0.81
Monoacylglycerol	—	—	—	—	—	ND
Free fatty acids	—	—	—	—	—	0.08
Cholesterol (mg/dl)†	1.3 (34.5)	0.7 (20.2)	0.5 (17.3)	0.5 (17.3)	0.4 (19.5)	0.34
1,2-Diacylglycerol	—	—	—	—	—	0.01
1,3-Diacylglycerol	—	—	—	—	—	ND
Triacylglycerol	97.6	98.5	98.7	98.9	99.0	98.76
Cholesterol esters (mg)‡						
Number of women	39	41	25	18	8	6

From Jensen RG, Bitman J, Carlson SE: Milk lipids. In Jensen RG, editor: *Handbook of milk composition,* San Diego, 1995, Academic Press.
ND, Not done.
*Mean ± SEM.
†Total cholesterol content ranges from 10 to 20 mg/dl after 21 days in most milks.
‡Not reported, but in Bitman et al (*J Pediatr Gastroenterol Nutr* 5:780, 1986) was 5 mg/dl at 3 days and 1 mg/dl at 21 days and thereafter.

The U.S. Department of Agriculture (USDA) has reported that the average American diet now includes 156 g of fat per day, up from 141 g in 1947. The significant change is from animal to vegetable fat, which is now 39% of total dietary fats, especially resulting from the switch from butter and lard. The original studies on human milk lipids were done from 1940 to 1950.[111] A change in fatty acid content to more long-chain fatty acids and a twofold to threefold increase in linoleic acid have occurred. Except for 18:2 content in mature milk, the fatty acid composition is remarkably uniform unless the maternal diet is unusually bizarre.[144]

P/S is the ratio of polyunsaturated to saturated fats; polyunsaturated fats include $C_{18:2}$ and $C_{18:3}$, or linoleic and linolenic acid. The bovine P/S ratio is 4. The P/S ratio has shifted as a result of recent dietary changes to 1.3 from 1.35 in human milk. The P/S is significant in facilitating calcium and fat absorption. Calcium absorption is depressed by a 4:5 P/S ratio. The breast can dehydrogenate saturated and monounsaturated fatty acids in milk synthesis.

At least 167 fatty acids have been identified in human milk; possibly others are there in trace amounts. Bovine milk has 437 identified fatty acids. Major dietary changes would greatly change fatty acid composition.

Many investigators have studied essential fatty acid requirements for humans. Diets free from added fats or linoleic acid induce deficiency symptoms in infants, including skin lesions, insufficient weight gain, and poor wound healing. Low-fat diets in newborn rats have affected cerebral function. The American Academy of Pediatrics has recommended that infant formulas contain a minimum of 3.3 g of fat/100 kcal (30% of total kilocalories) and 300 mg of linoleic acid (18:2)/100 kcal (about 1.7% of total kilocalories).[39,40] It did not set a limit on linoleic content of diet, because some human milks have 8% to 10% of the fat as linoleic acid.

Milk from vegetarians (lacto-ovo) contained a lower proportion of fatty acids derived from animal fat and a higher proportion of polyunsaturated fatty acids derived from dietary vegetable fat. Women who consumed 35 g or more of animal fat per day had higher $C_{10:0}$, $C_{12:0}$, and $C_{18:3}$ but lower levels of $C_{16:0}$ and $C_{18:0}$. Finley et al[63] suggest that a maximum amount of $C_{16:0}$ and $C_{18:0}$ can be taken up from the blood and subsequently secreted into milk (Table 4-11).

TABLE 4-11   **Effects of maternal vegetarian diets on saturated and unsaturated fatty acids (wt%) in human milk lipids (mean ± SEM)**

Lipid (%)/ fatty acid	Vegetarian*	Control*	Vegan†	Vegetarian†	Omnivore†
Number	12	7	19	5	21
Saturates					
6:0	—	—	—	—	—
8:0	0.16 ± 0.03	0.22 ± 0.01	—	—	—
10:0	1.56 ± 0.13	1.57 ± 0.09	1.8 ± 0.40	1.3 ± 0.51	0.4 ± 0.23
12:0	7.07 ± 0.78	5.47 ± 0.66	6.6 ± 0.54	3.2 ± 0.49	1.7 ± 0.35
14:0	8.16 ± 1.00	6.54 ± 0.73	6.9 ± 0.58	5.2 ± 0.50	4.5 ± 0.35
16:0	15.31 ± 0.73	20.48 ± 0.64	18.1 ± 1.34	21.2 ± 1.07	25.1 ± 0.78
18:0	4.48 ± 0.37	8.14 ± 0.55	4.9 ± 0.36	7.4 ± 0.35	9.7 ± 0.68
20:0	0.54 ± 0.02	0.57 ± 0.03	—	—	—
TOTAL	37.28	42.99			
Monounsaturates					
16:1	1.66 ± 0.14	3.35 ± 0.28	4.9 ± 0.24	2.9 ± 0.37	3.4 ± 0.35
18:1	26.89 ± 1.47	34.7 ± 0.86	32.2 ± 1.06	35.3 ± 1.94	38.7 ± 1.27
TOTAL	28.55	38.06	37.10	38.2	42.1
Polyunsaturates					
N-6 series					
18:2	28.82 ± 1.39	14.47 ± 1.98	23.8 ± 1.40	19.5 ± 3.62	10.9 ± 0.96
20:2	0.72 ± 0.03	0.50 ± 0.03	—	—	—
20:3	0.62 ± 0.03	0.56 ± 0.03	0.44 ± 0.03	0.42 ± 0.07	0.40 ± 0.08
20:4	0.68 ± 0.03	0.68 ± 0.03	0.32 ± 0.02	0.38 ± 0.05	0.35 ± 0.03
TOTAL	30.84	16.21	31.4	27.5	18.4
N-3 series					
18:3	2.76 ± 0.16	1.85 ± 0.16	1.36 ± 0.18	1.25 ± 0.22	0.49 ± 0.06
22:6	0.22 ± 0.08	0.27 ± 0.08	0.14 ± 0.06	0.30 ± 0.05	0.36 ± 0.07
TOTAL	3.05	2.12	1.50	1.55	0.86

Dietary information

Vegetarian: whole cereal grains, 50%-60%; soup, 5%; vegetables, 20%-25%; beans and sea vegetables, 5%-10%; macrobiotic diet for a mean of 81 months; no meat or dairy products; occasional seafood, nuts, and fruit
Control: typical U.S. diet

Vegan: no foods of animal origin
Vegetarian: exclude meat and fish
Omnivore: typical Western diet

From Jensen RG, Bitman J, Carlson SE: Milk lipids. In Jensen RG, editor: *Handbook of milk composition,* San Diego, 1995, Academic Press.
*Modified from Specker BL et al: *J Pediatr Gastroenterol Nutr* 6:764, 1987. New England donors: vegetarians, 3-13 months postpartum; controls, 1-5 months; capillary gas-liquid chromatography (GLC) columns.
†Modified from Sanders TA, Reddy S: *J Pediatr* 120:S71, 1992. British donors: 6 weeks postpartum; packed GLC columns.

The milk of strict vegetarians has extremely high levels of linoleic acid, four times that of cow's milk (Table 4-11).[204] Some researchers include other long-chain fatty acids (e.g., $C_{20:2}$, $C_{20:3}$, $C_{24:4}$, $C_{22:3}$) as essential nutrients because they are structural lipids in the brain and nervous tissue. The effects of diet are also discussed in Chapter 9.

One important outcome of linoleic and linolenic acids is the conversion of these compounds into longer-chain polyunsaturates. These metabolites have been shown to be important for fluidity of membrane lipids and prostaglandin synthesis. They are present in the brain and retinal cells. Long-chain polyunsaturates are needed for development of infant brain and nervous system.[63] When Gibson and Kneebore[72] studied fatty acid composition of colostrum and mature milk at 3 to 5 days and later at 6 weeks postpartum, they reported that mature milk had a higher percentage of saturated fatty acids, including medium-chain acids, lower monounsaturates, and higher linoleic and linolenic acids and their long-chain polyunsaturated derivatives. The derivatives of these acids, often ignored by many investigators, have high biologic activity; thus the reporting of only linoleic acid underestimates the EFA levels in human milk.[144]

To address the issue of nutrition during brain development, it is important to consider the different periods of brain development that have been described biochemically.[213] First, cell division occurs, with the formation of neurons and glial cells, and second, myelination. Sinclair and Crawford[213] showed in the rat brain that 50% of polyenoic acids of the gray matter lipids were laid down by the fifteenth day of life. The fatty acids characteristic of myelin lipids appeared later. Gray matter is largely composed of unmyelinated neurons, whereas white matter contains a very high proportion of myelinated conducting nerve fibers. Normal brain function depends on both. The synthesis and composition of myelin can be influenced by diet in the developing rat brain.

Myelin-specific messenger ribonucleic acid (mRNA) levels are developmentally regulated and influenced by dietary fat. The neonatal response to dietary fat is tissue specific at the mRNA level.[50]

The fatty acids characteristic of gray matter ($C_{20:4}$ and $C_{22:6}$) accumulate before the appearance of fatty acids characteristic of myelin ($C_{20:1}$ and $C_{24:1}$) in the developing brain. Arachidonic acid ($C_{20:4}$) and DHA ($C_{22:6}$) are synthesized from linoleic and linolenic acids, respectively, but the latter two must be obtained in the diet.

During the first year of life the human brain more than doubles in size, increasing from 350 to 1100 g in weight. Eighty-five percent of this growth is cerebrum; 50% to 60% of this solid matter is lipid.[230] Cortical total phospholipid fatty acid composition in both term and preterm infants is greatly influenced by dietary fat intake. Phospholipids make up about one quarter of the solid matter and are integral to the vascular system on which the brain depends.[60] Brain growth is associated with an increase in the incorporation of long-chain PUFAs into the phospholipid in the cerebral cortex.[114] Extreme dietary alterations in animal experiments have demonstrated an altered PUFA composition of the developing brain.

Such studies cannot be done in humans. Farquharson et al[60] therefore examined the necropsy specimens of cerebrocortical gray matter obtained from 20 term and two premature infants, all of whom died within 43 weeks of birth. All were victims of sudden death and were genetically normal. The infants had either received exclusively breast milk or exclusively formula. The latter group was divided by formula type into three groups: mixture of formulas, SMA, or CGOST (cow's milk or osterfeed). Breastfed infants had greater concentrations of DHA in their cerebrocortical phospholipids than the formula-fed infants in all groups. A compensatory increase in n-6 series fatty acids (arachidonic, docosatetraenoic, and docosapentaenoic) occurred in the SMA group. No significant differences were seen between saturated and monounsaturated fatty acids. The two premature infants had the lowest levels of DHA.

Cerebrocortical neuronal membrane glycerophospholipids are composed predominantly (95%)

of phosphatidylcholine (PC), phosophatidyletha-nolamine (PE), and phosphatidylserine (PS).[114] After birth, neuronal membranes and retinal photoreceptor cells derive most of their phospholipid DHA from diet and liver synthesis and not from fat reserves. Neither the liver nor the retinal and neuronal cells can synthesize DHA without reserves or a dietary supply. α-Linolenic acid, an EFA, is the precursor. If the enzymes are not activated or are inactivated by an excess of n-6 fatty acids, synthesis does not take place. Human milk provides the DHA and arachidonic acid (AA).[86]

Dietary supplementation with fish oil in the latter part of pregnancy resulted in increased DHA status at birth when measured in the umbilical blood.[157] When postpartum women were supplemented with DHA by capsule in a blind study, breast milk levels of DHA ranged from 0.2% to 1.7% of total fatty acids, increasing with dose. AA levels and antioxidant status of plasma AA and levels were unaffected.

Although DHA is essential to retinal development, levels peak in the retina at 36 to 38 weeks' gestation, suggesting that the most rapid rate of retinal accumulation occurs before term.[97] This further suggests that the premature infant is especially vulnerable to dietary deficiencies of DHA.

Dietary omega-3 (ω-3) fatty acids may not be essential to life, reproduction, or growth, but they are important for normal biochemical and functional development.[195] Long-chain ω-3 fatty acids, DHA in particular, form a major structural component of biologic membranes. When the ratio of omega-6 (ω-6) is high compared to ω-3, fatty acids aggravate the deficiency. Studies in monkeys have shown that DHA deficiency affects water intake and urine excretion, as well as ω-3 acid levels in red blood cells.[195] Much remains to be learned about the effects of ω-3 fatty acids and DHA deficiency on the developing human infant.[225]

The EFAs, linoleic and linolenic acids, may have greater significance in the quality of the myelin laid down. Dick,[52] observing the geographic distribution of multiple sclerosis worldwide, noted that the disease is rare in countries where breastfeeding is common. He postulated that the development of myelin in infancy is critical to preventing degradation later. Dick investigated the difference between human milk and cow's milk in relation to myelin production in multiple sclerosis.[52]

Experimental allergic encephalitis is a demyelinating condition and can be produced by shocking animals that have been sensitized to central nervous system (CNS) antigens. Newborn rats deficient in essential fatty acids are more susceptible to this disease, which has been described as resembling multiple sclerosis pathologically.

Widdowson et al[228] analyzed the body fats of children from Britain and Holland. At birth, body fat was 1.3% linoleic acid for both groups of children. British infants received cow's milk formulas that contained 1.8% linoleic acid. The Dutch infants received corn oil formulas that were 58.2% linoleic acid. The Dutch infants had body fat that was 25% linoleic acid at 1 month of age and 32% to 37% at 4 months of age. The British infants, receiving cow's milk formulas, had 3% or less linoleic acid in their body fat. The Dutch infants had lower serum cholesterol levels. At approximately 10 years of age, the children appeared to be entirely normal.[228]

Other influences on fat content

Infections will alter milk composition. Mastitis, however, does not alter fat content but does lower volume and lactose and increase sodium and chloride.

Parity has been cited as a major influence on fat content, with primiparous women having more fat than multiparous women. Prentice et al[189] found a significant relationship between fat content and triceps skinfold thickness. The authors found seasonal changes in The Gambia, where volume and fat were lowest following the rainy season, when nutrient resources are scarce.

Hyperlipoproteinemias

Milk from women with type I hyperlipoproteinemia has been investigated.[122] Because the primary deficiency is serum-stimulated lipoprotein lipase in the plasma, resulting in reduced transfer of dietary long-chain fatty acids from blood to milk, levels of fat as fatty acids were abnormally low (about 1.5%) and the amounts of 10:0 and 14:0 higher than normal. (See Chapter 15.)

Cholesterol

Cholesterol is an essential component of all membranes and is required for growth, replication, and maintenance. Infants fed human milk have higher plasma cholesterol levels than formula-fed infants. Animal studies suggest that early postnatal ingestion of a diet high in cholesterol protects against high-cholesterol challenges later.[229]

The cholesterol content of milk is remarkably stable at 240 mg/100 g of fat when calculated by volume of fat. The range, depending on sampling techniques, is 9 to 41 mg/dl. The amount of cholesterol changed slightly over time, decreasing 1.7-fold over the first 36 days, as reported by Harzer et al,[92] and stabilizing at about the fifteenth day postpartum at 20 mg/dl. This resulted in a change in the cholesterol/triglyceride ratio. The authors found no uniform pattern of circadian variations between mothers.

Neonatal plasma cholesterol levels, on the other hand, range between 50 and 100 mg/dl at birth, with equal distribution of low-density lipoprotein (LDL) and high-density lipoprotein (HDL). Plasma cholesterol increases rapidly over the first few days of life, with LDL predominating regardless of mode of feeding.[109] In breastfed infants, however, there is a progressive increase in plasma cholesterol compared with that in infants fed low to no cholesterol and high-PUFA formulas. This may have a lasting effect on the individual's ability to metabolize cholesterol, a point yet to be confirmed.[110] Low-birthweight (LBW) premature infants are at risk for stimulation of endogenous cholesterol biosynthesis, resulting in marked elevations in plasma cholesterol as a result of intravenous nutrition.

The effect of breastfeeding on plasma cholesterol, body weight, and body length was studied longitudinally in 512 infants by Jooste et al.[127] Breastfed infants had higher plasma cholesterol than the formula-fed infants, created by a direct mechanism that persisted for as long as the infants were breastfed. Body length was similar in breastfed and formula-fed infants, but formula-fed infants weighed more.

Cholesterol has been a factor of great concern because of the apparent association with risk factors for atherosclerosis and coronary heart disease. At present, commercial formulas have high P/S ratios and little or no cholesterol compared with those of human milk. Dietary manipulation does not change the cholesterol level in the breast milk.[188] When the dietary cholesterol level is controlled, however, a fall in the infant's plasma cholesterol level is associated with an increase in the amount of linoleic acid present in the milk.[185]

Kallio et al[131] followed 193 infants from birth, measuring concentrations of cholesterol, very-low-density lipoprotein (VLDL), LDL, HDL$_2$, and, on a limited group of 36, HDL$_3$ and apoprotein B. The largest differences between exclusively breastfed and weaned infants were at 2 months (0.8 mmol/L), 4 months (0.6 mmol/L) and 6 months (0.5 mmol/L). The LDL and apoprotein B concentrations were lower in weaned infants. VLDL and HDL$_3$ were independent of diet. The authors concluded that the low intake of cholesterol and high intake of unsaturated fatty acids greatly modify the blood lipid pattern in the first year of life.[131]

In a retrospective epidemiologic study of 5718 men in England born in the 1920s, 474 died of ischemic heart disease.[59] The infant-feeding groups were divided into those breastfed but weaned before 1 year, breastfed beyond a year, and bottle fed. The first group had the lowest death rate from ischemic heart disease and had lower total cholesterol, LDL cholesterol, and apolipoprotein B than those who were weaned after a year and especially those who were bottle fed. In all feeding groups, serum apolipoprotein B concentrations were lower in men with higher birthweights and weights at 1 year.

In a study of breastfed and formula-fed baboons that ate a high-fat carnivorous diet instead of their usual vegetarian fare, breastfeeding showed no protective effect.

No long-range effect of serum cholesterol level has been identified, although Osborn[181] described the pathologic changes in 1500 young people (newborns to age 20). He observed the spectrum of pathologic changes from mucopolysaccharide accumulations to fully developed atherosclerotic plaques. Lesions were more frequent and severe in children who had been bottle-fed. Lesions were uncommon or mild in the breastfed children.

Animal investigations indicated that rats given high levels of cholesterol early in life were better able to cope with cholesterol in later life and maintained a lower cholesterol level.[50]

In a study of six breastfed and 12 formula-fed infants, ages 4 to 5 months, Wong et al[229] measured the fractional synthesis rate (FSR). The breastfed infants had higher cholesterol intakes (18.4 ± 4.0 mg/kg/day) than formula-fed infants (only 3.4 ± 1.8 mg/kg/day). Plasma cholesterol levels were 183 ± 47 versus 112 ± 22 mg/dl; LDL cholesterol levels were 83 ± 26 versus 48 ± 16 mg/dl. An inverse relationship existed between the FSR of cholesterol and dietary intake of cholesterol. The authors concluded that the greater cholesterol intake of breastfed infants is associated with elevated plasma LDL cholesterol concentrations. In addition, cholesterol synthesis in human infants may be efficiently regulated by coenzyme A (CoA) reductase when infants are challenged with dietary cholesterol.[229]

A carefully designed, well-controlled longitudinal study is needed to determine the long-range impact of cholesterol because it is a consistent constituent of human milk throughout lactation.

n-3 fatty acids

The n-3 fatty acids are important components of animal and plant cell membranes and are selectively distributed among the lipid classes. The role of DHA (22:n-3) in infantile nerve and brain tissue and retinal development has been discussed. It is also found in high levels in testis and sperm. Human milk contains DHA, and studies to evaluate the effects of "fish oil" supplements to the diet suggest an elevation of the dose-dependent levels.

Eicosapentaenoic acid (EPA, 20:5n-3) is part of another group of n-3 fatty acids, the eicosanoids, which comprise two families: the prostanoids (prostaglandins, prostacyclins, and thromboxanes) and the leukotrienes.[122] The *prostanoids* are mediators of inflammatory processes. *Leukotrienes* are key mediators of inflammation and delayed hypersensitivity. In other species, restriction of n-3 fatty acids results in abnormal electroretinograms, impaired visual activity, and decreased learning ability.

The influence of dietary n-3 fatty acids on visual activity development in very-low-birthweight (VLBW) infants was evaluated by Birch et al,[19] using visual-evoked response (VER) and forced-choice preferential-looking (FPL) procedures at 36 and 57 weeks postconception. Feeding groups were randomized to one of three diets: corn oil (only linoleic), soy oil (linoleic and linolenic), and soy/marine oil (added n-3 fatty acids). The marine oil group matched the "gold standards" of VLBW infants fed human milk. Visual activity parameters in the other infants who did not receive n-3 oils were considerably lower.

The n-3 fatty acids appear to function in the membranes of photoreceptor cells and synapses. Jensen and Jensen[119] suggest a daily intake of 18:3n-3 (about 0.5% of calories) with the inclusion of n-3 long-chain PUFA, which is available in human milk. Many studies affirm the value of n-3 fatty acids in the diet and as protection against heart disease, chronic inflammatory disease, and possibly cancer.[212]

Proteins

All milks have been evaluated for their protein contents, which vary from species to species. Proteins constitute 0.9% of the contents in human milk and range up to 20% in some rabbit species. Proteins of milk include casein, serum albumin, and α-lactalbumin, β-lactoglobulins, immunoglobulins, and other glycoproteins. Eight of 20 amino acids present in milk are essential and are derived from plasma. The mammary alveolar epithelium synthesizes some nonessential amino acids (Table 4-12). Human milk amino acids occur in proteins

TABLE 4-12	**Estimates of the concentrations of nutrients in mature human milk**		
Nutrient	**Amount in human milk**[a]	**Nutrient**	**Amount in human milk**[a]
	g/liter ± SD[b]		µg/liter ± SD
Lactose	72.0 ± 2.5	Vitamin A, RE[d]	670 ± 200 (2230 IU[e])
Protein	10.5 ± 2.0	Vitamin D	0.55 ± 0.10
Fat	39.0 ± 4.0	Vitamin K	2.1 ± 0.1
	mg/liter ± SD	Folate	85 ± 37[f]
Calcium	280 ± 26	Vitamin B_{12}	0.97[g,h]
Phosphorus	140 ± 22	Biotin	4 ± 1
Magnesium	35 ± 2	Iodine	110 ± 40
Sodium	180 ± 40	Selenium	20 ± 5
Potassium	525 ± 35	Manganese	6 ± 2
Chloride	420 ± 60	Fluoride	16 ± 5
Iron	0.3 ± 0.1	Chromium	50 ± 5
Zinc	1.2 ± 0.2	Molybdenum	NR[i]
Copper	0.25 ± 0.03		
Vitamin E	2.3 ± 1.0		
Vitamin C	40 ± 10		
Thiamin	0.210 ± 0.035		
Riboflavin	0.350 ± 0.025		
Niacin	1.500 ± 0.200		
Vitamin B_6	93 ± 8[c]		
Pantothenic acid	1.800 ± 0.200		

From Report of Subcommittee, Institute of Medicine: *Nutrition during lactation*, Washington, DC, 1991, National Academy Press.
[a]Data from *Pediatric nutrition handbook*, ed 2, Elk Grove Village, Ill, 1985, AAP, p. 363, unless otherwise indicated. Values are representative of amounts of nutrients present in human milk; some may differ slightly from those reported by investigators cited in text.
[b]Standard deviation.
[c]From Styslinger L, Kirksey A: *Am J Clin Nutr* 41:21, 1985.
[d]Retinol equivalents.
[e]International units.
[f]From Brown CM et al: *J Pediatr Gastroenterol Nutr* 5:278, 1986.
[g]From Sandberg DP, Begley JA, Hall CA: *Am J Clin Nutr* 34:1717, 1981.
[h]Standard deviation not reported; range 0.33 to 3.20.
[i]Not reported.

and peptides, as well as a small percentage in the form of free amino acids and glucosamine[2] (Table 4-13).

Tikanoja et al[223] reported that postprandial changes in plasma amion acids in breastfed infants were proportional to dietary intake and were highest for the branched-chain amino acids. This was also found to be true for most semiessential and nonessential amino acids. The blood urea levels also reflect dietary intake, with values in breastfed infants being substantially lower than levels in bottle-fed infants.[46] The sum of plasma free amino acids rose and the glycine/valine ratio

fell after a feed. When breastfed and formula-fed infants were compared by Järvenpää,[117] concentrations of citrulline, threonine, phenylalanine, and tyrosine were higher in formula-fed than in breast-fed infants. Concentrations of taurine were lower in the formula-fed infants. The peak time was different for formula-fed and breastfed infants, which points out the need to standardize sampling times.

The DARLING (Davis Area Research on Lactation Infant Nutrition and Growth) Study was the first longitudinal study to follow a large group of mother-infant dyads to 12 months.[49] The investi-

TABLE 4-13 **Free amino acid concentrations in human milk**

Amino acid	Colostral milk (μmol/dl)	Transitional milk (μmol/dl)	Mature milk (μmol/dl)
Glutamic acid	36-68	88-127	101-180
Glutamine	2-9	9-20	13-58
Taurine	41-45	34-50	27-67
Alanine	9-11	13-20	17-26
Threonine	5-12	7-8	6-13
Serine	12	6-11	6-14
Glycine	5-8	5-10	3-13
Aspartic acid	5-6	3-4	3-5
Leucine	3-5	2-6	2-4
Cystine	1-3	2-5	3-6
Valine	3-4	3-6	4-6
Lysine	5	1-11	2-5
Histidine	2	2-3	0.4-3
Phenylalanine	1-2	1	0.6-2
Tyrosine	2	1-2	1-2
Arginine	3-7	1-5	1-2
Isoleucine	2	1-2	1
Ornithine	1-4	1	0.5-0.9
Methionine	0.8	0.3-3	0.3-0.8
Phosphoserine	8	5	4
Phosphoethanolamine	4	8	10
α-Aminobutyrate	1	0.4-1.4	0.4-1
Tryptophan	5	1	. 1
Proline	—	6	2-3

From Carlson SE: *Adv Pediatr* 32:43, 1985.

gators report protein intake to be positively associated with milk lipid concentrations after 16 weeks. Milk protein concentration was negatively related to milk volume at 6 and 9 months and positively related to milk frequency at these times. Milk composition is more sensitive to maternal factors such as body composition, diet, and parity during later lactation than during the first few months.[175]

Casein

Milk consists of casein, or curds, and whey proteins, or lactalbumins. The term *casein* includes a group of milk-specific proteins characterized by ester-bound phosphate, high-proline content, and low solubility at pH of 4.0 to 5.0.[160] Caseins form complex particles or *micelles,* which are usually complexes of calcium caseinate and calcium phosphate. When milk clots or curdles as a result of heat, pH changes, or enzymes, the casein is transformed into an insoluble calcium caseinate–calcium phosphate complex. Physiochemical differences exist between human and cow caseins.[150] Casein has a species-specific amino acid composition.

When Lönnerdal and Forsum[150] originally measured the casein content of human milk by three different methods—isoelectric precipitation, sedimentation by ultracentrifuge, and indirect analysis—they consistently had three separate results.

Utilizing two newer techniques, Kunz and Lönnerdal[142] report confirming results revealing that casein synthesis is low or absent in early lactation, then increases rapidly, and then decreases. The concentration of whey proteins decreases from early lactation. The whey protein/casein ratios change accordingly from 90:10 in early milk to 60:40 in mature milk and 50:50 in late lactation. The authors suggest whey and casein are regulated by different mechanisms.[142]

Methionine/cysteine ratio. The cysteine content is high in human milk, whereas it is very low in cow's milk. Because the methionine content is high in bovine milk, the methionine/cysteine ratio is two to three times greater in cow's milk than in the milk of most mammals and seven times that in human milk. Human milk is the only animal protein in which the methionine/cysteine ratio is close to 1. Otherwise, this ratio is seen only in plant proteins.

Two significant characteristics of amino acid composition of human milk are the ratio between the sulfur-containing amino acids, methionine and cysteine, and the low content of the aromatic amino acids, phenylalanine and tyrosine. The newborn and especially the premature infant are poorly prepared to handle phenylalanine and tyrosine because of their low levels of the specific enzymes required to metabolize them.

Taurine. Taurine, 2-aminoethanesulfonic acid (so named because it was first isolated from the bile of the ox), is a third sulfur-containing amino acid that has been found in high concentrations in human milk and is virtually absent in cow's milk. It is now being added to some prepared formulas. Free taurine and glutamic acid have been measured in breast milk in high concentration. Taurine has been associated in the body at all ages with bile acid conjugation; in the newborn, bile acids are almost exclusively conjugated with taurine.

Sturman et al[220] suggest that taurine may also be a neurotransmitter or neuromodulator in the brain and retina. Taurine in the nutrition of the human infant was reviewed by Gaull,[71] who reports that evidence is accumulating that taurine has a more general biologic role in development and membrane stability.

Taurine is found in very high concentrations in the milk of cats.[192] Kittens deprived of taurine by feeding with purified taurine-free casein diets after weaning develop retinal degeneration and blind-

ness. The process can be reversed by feeding taurine, but not by feeding methionine, cysteine, or inorganic sulfate.[158] The structural integrity of the retina of the cat has been shown to be taurine dependent. The taurine levels were more severely depleted in the brain tissue, but the significance of this finding has not yet been determined.[220] Both humans and cats are unable to synthesize taurine to any degree and are therefore wholly dependent on a dietary supply. The process requires cystathionase and cysteine–sulfinic acid decarboxylase, which are enzymes that convert methionine, cysteine, or cystine to taurine.

In studies of amino acid levels, only the concentrations of taurine in plasma and urine of breastfed term infants were higher than those of preterm infants fed formula. Levels in term infants were higher than those of preterm infants fed pooled human milk at a fixed volume. The effects of feeding taurine-deficient formula to the human infant, which occurred before the addition of taurine to infant formula, are not as severe as seen in the kitten. The presence of taurine in human milk and predominance of taurine conjugates in the gut at birth suggest that bile acid conjugate status may be a controlling factor. When bile acid metabolism was measured in infants fed human milk, they consistently had higher intraluminal bile acid concentrations at all ages (1 week to 5 weeks) than did formula-fed infants with and without additional taurine. Human milk also facilitated intestinal lipid absorption.[227]

The human infant conjugates bile acids predominantly with taurine at birth but quickly develops the capacity to conjugate with glycine. Those infants fed human milk continue to conjugate with taurine, whereas those fed formulas soon conjugate with glycine predominantly. The cat, in contrast, uses only taurine throughout life.[227] In the human the various pools of taurine in the body cannot be predicted by measurement of plasma taurine alone.

Since 1968, when scientists' attention was drawn to taurine, more than a thousand reports, including reviews, have been published.[71] The physiologic actions of taurine have been reviewed exhaustively by Huxtable.[106] Nonmetabolic actions such as osmoregulation, calcium modulation, and interactions with phospholipid protein and zinc are reported. Taurine is also observed to be a product of metabolic action and a precursor of many other metabolic actions. All these actions demonstrate the careful balance in nature of a number of interdependent constituents. Taurine does not function in isolation. Because of the growing evidence for the role of taurine during development, the requirement for taurine for the neonate remains under investigation.[220]

Whey proteins

When clotted milk stands, the clot contracts, leaving a clear fluid called *whey*, which contains water, electrolytes, and proteins. The ratio of whey proteins to casein is 1.5 for breast milk and 0.25 for cow's milk; that is, 40% of human milk protein is casein and 60% lactalbumin, and cow's milk is 80% casein and 20% lactalbumin.[150]

Human milk forms a flocculent suspension with zero curd tension. The curds are easily digested. The total amount of protein has been recently measured to be 0.9%, which is lower than the previously reported 1.2%. The discrepancy is caused by recalculation of the data, in which the total amount of protein was determined by measuring the nitrogen content and multiplying by 6.25. Of the nitrogen content, 25% is nonprotein nitrogen, whereas in bovine milk, 5% of the nitrogen is from nonprotein nitrogen. Hambraeus[83] has reported the composition of the nonprotein fraction to be urea, creatine, creatinine, uric acid, small peptides, and free amino acids (Table 4-14).

Closer examination of the whey proteins shows α-lactalbumin and lactoferrin to be the chief

TABLE 4-14   Composition of protein nitrogen and nonprotein nitrogen in human milk and cow's milk*

	Human milk		Cow's milk	
Protein nitrogen	1.43	(8.9)	5.3	(31.4)
Casein nitrogen	0.40	(2.5)	4.37	(27.3)
Whey protein nitrogen	1.03	(6.4)	0.93	(5.8)
α-Lactalbumin	0.42	(2.6)	0.17	(1.1)
Lactoferrin	0.27	(1.7)	Traces	
β-Lactoglobulin	—		0.57	(3.6)
Lysozyme	0.08	(0.5)	Traces	
Serum albumin	0.08	(0.5)	0.07	(0.4)
IgA	0.16	(1.0)	0.005	(0.03)
IgG	0.005	(0.03)	0.096	(0.06)
IgM	0.003	(0.02)	0.005	(0.03)
Nonprotein nitrogen	0.50		0.28	
Urea nitrogen	0.25		0.13	
Creatine nitrogen	0.037		0.009	
Creatinine nitrogen	0.035		0.003	
Uric acid nitrogen	0.005		0.008	
Glucosamine	0.047		?	
α-Amino nitrogen	0.13		0.048	
Ammonia nitrogen	0.002		0.006	
Nitrogen from other components	?		0.074	
Total nitrogen	1.93		5.31	

Courtesy Forsum E, Lönnerdal B: Protein evaluation of breast milk and breast milk substitutes with special reference to the nonprotein nitrogen: effect of protein intake on protein and nitrogen composition of breast milk, *Am J Clin Nutr* 33:1809, 1980.
*Values refer to grams of nitrogen per liter; values within parentheses, to grams of protein per liter.

fractions, with no measurable β-lactoglobulin. β-Lactoglobulin is the chief constituent of cow's milk. The term *lactalbumin* includes a mixture of whey proteins found in bovine milk and should not be confused with α-*lactalbumin,* which is a specific protein that is part of the enzyme lactose synthetase. The α-lactalbumin content parallels lactose levels in different species. Human milk is high in both lactose and α-lactalbumin. Many investigators have continued to measure nitrogen compounds in human milk. Table 4-14 represents averages.

Lactoferrin. Lactoferrin is an iron-binding protein that is part of the whey fraction of proteins in human milk. It appears in very low amounts in bovine milk. Lactoferrin has been observed to inhibit the growth of certain iron-dependent bacteria in the gastrointestinal tract. It has been suggested that lactoferrin protects against certain gastrointestinal infections in breastfed infants. Giving iron to newborn infants appears to inactivate the lactoferrin by saturating it with iron.

Immunoglobulins

The immunoglobulins in breast milk are distinct from those of the serum. The main immunoglobulin in serum is IgG, which is present in the amount of 1210 mg/dl. IgA is found in the serum at 250 mg/dl, one-fifth the level of IgG. The reverse is true of human colostrum and milk. Colostrum has 1740 mg of IgA/dl, and milk has 100 mg/dl. Colostrum has 43 mg of IgG/dl, and milk has 4 mg/dl. The IgA and IgG in human milk are derived from serum and from synthesis in the mammary gland.

The IgA is secretory IgA (sIgA), the principal immunoglobulin in colostrum and milk. Secretory IgA contains an antigenic determinant associated with a secretory component. It is synthesized in the gland from two molecules of serum IgA linked by disulfide bonds. The sIgA levels are very high in colostrum the first few days and then decline rapidly, disappearing almost completely by the fourteenth day. Secretory IgA is very stable at low pH and resistant to proteolytic enzymes. It is present in the intestine of breastfed infants and provides a protective defense against infection by keeping viruses and bacteria from invading the mucosa. The protective qualities are further described in Chapter 5.

Nonimmunoglobulins

Human milk contains numerous nonimmunoglobulins that are being identified and their actions isolated and quantified.[231] Mucins and sialic acid–containing glycoproteins have been isolated and demonstrated to inhibit rotavirus replication and prevent experimental gastroenteritis. The rotavirus has been observed to bind to the milk mucin complex, inhibiting its replication both in vitro and in vivo. (See later discussion under oligosaccharides and glyoconjugates.)

Lysozyme

Lysozyme is a specific protein and basic polypeptide with lytic properties[96] found in high concentration in egg whites and human milk but in low concentration in bovine milk. It has been identified as a nonspecific antimicrobial factor. This enzyme is bacteriolytic against Enterobacteriaceae and gram-positive bacteria. It has been found in concentrations up to 0.2 mg/ml. Lysozyme is stable at 100° C (212° F) and at an acid pH. Lysozyme contributes to the development and maintenance of specific intestinal flora of the breastfed infant. (See later discussion under enzymes and Chapter 5.)

Polyamines

Polyamines are ubiquitous intracellular cationic amines recognized as participants in cell proliferation and differentiation in many tissues, especially those of intestinal tract development, absorption, and biologic activity, in both sucklings and adults of the species.[187] The synthesis of polyamines is an active process in the mammary gland throughout lactation.[14]

Putrescine, spermidine, and spermine have been identified and quantitated in human milk by Pollack et al.[187] They reported mean values per liter of

0 to 615 nmol putrescine, 73 to 3512 nmol spermidine, and 722 to 4458 nmol spermine. In contrast, levels in formula are low and dependent on the protein source. Levels of spermine and spermidine increase greatly during the first few days of lactation, plateauing at levels 12 and 8 times, respectively, the levels immediately postpartum.[12] These findings have been confirmed by Romain et al,[199] who noted that levels in human milk remained stable throughout lactation. They demonstrated the effects of spermine or spermidine on maturation and "gut closure" and suggest a protective effect of spermine against alimentary allergies.

Nonprotein nitrogen

Nonprotein nitrogen (NPN) accounts for 18% to 30% of the total nitrogen in human milk,[31] compared with only 3% to 5% in cow's milk. The NPN fraction of human milk is traditionally identified as the acid-soluble nitrogen remaining in the supernatant after protein precipitation or as the dialyzable nitrogen after dialysis of whole milk.[14] Because large-molecular-weight glycoproteins are also soluble in the acid, the fraction should be called *acid-soluble nitrogen* (ASN).[162]

Although these are large interindividual variations, the range is from 350 to 530 mg/L. The total nitrogen ranges from 1700 to 3700 mg/L, depend on length of gestation, duration of lactation, and maternal diet. Some of the nitrogen contributes to the pool available for synthesis of nonessential amino acids in the neonate. Those compounds having more specialized roles are peptide hormone/growth factors, epidermal growth factor, amino sugars of oligosaccharides, free amino acids, amino alcohols of phospholipids, nucleic acids, nucleotides, and carnitine. Their importance is not based on percent concentration, because they may serve roles as catalysts. Many protein factors in human milk serve roles other than growth, such as the host resistance factors (lactoferrin, sIgA, and lysozyme).

Table 4-15 presents the significance of these compounds and their relative concentrations. The wide variety of nitrogenous compounds within the fraction of human milk is only beginning to be investigated and understood. This information clearly widens the chemical gap between human milk and proprietary formulas. Increasing evidence suggests that the premature infant reaps even more benefit than the term infant from mother's milk, based on the investigations of NPN alone.[31]

Maternal milk production and the protein nitrogen (but not NPN) fraction of human milk are well preserved when lactating women are subjected to marginal dietary protein intakes in the short term.[162] In nitrogen (N) balance studies on lactating poor Mexican women, equilibrium was attained at 178.9 ± 25.8 mg N (1.1 g protein/kg body weight/day), which is close to current dietary standards.[48]

Interest in urea levels has been stimulated because women with various stages of renal failure were concerned about the effect of high serum levels of urea on their milk urea levels. Urea is 30% to 50% of the NPN in milk. Levels increase from colostrum to mature milk (3.2 g N/dl in colostrum to 1.7 g N/dl). If the original milk urea was provided solely by passive diffusion from the maternal blood, a constant level of urea nitrogen would be anticipated at all stages of lactation instead of increasing from colostrum to mature milk.[14]

Nucleotides

Increased attention has been paid to the presence and role of nucleotides in human milk as their relative absence in bovine milk has led to experimental supplementation of some infant formulas. Nucleotides have been identified as playing key roles in biochemical processes within the cell, acting as metabolic regulators and altering enzyme activities. A dietary requirement has not been established because they can be synthesized de novo in the adult. Human milk provides 20% of NPN as nucleotides; furthermore, human milk provides a larger percentage (30%) of nitrogen as NPN, three times more than other species. The daily intake from human milk is 1.4 to 2.1 mg of nucleotide nitrogen.[191] Cytidine, adenine, and uridine compose the majority of soluble nucleotides.

TABLE 4-15   Levels and significance of nonprotein nitrogen (NPN) constituents of human milk

NPN	Concentration in milk		Significance
	Under 30 days	Over 30 days	
Amino sugars			
N-Acetylglucosamine	230 mg N/L	150 mg N/L	Low oral osmotic load; control gut colonization; constituents of gangliosides for brain development
N-Acetylneuraminic acid	63 mg N/L	3-27 mg N/L	Substrate for gut epithelium
Peptides	—	60 mg N/L	
Epidermal growth factor	88 ng/ml	—	Regulates intestinal mucosal development
Somatomedin-C/insulin-like growth factor	18 ng/ml	6-8 ng/ml	Stimulates DNA synthesis and cell division in gut
Delta sleep-inducing peptide	30 ng/ml	5 ng/ml	Diurnal pattern highest at 2 PM and 8 PM; ? influence sleep/awake patterns
Insulin	21 ng/ml	2 ng/ml	? Regulates development of gut
Free amino acids			
Taurine	41-45 μmol/dl	27-67 μmol/dl	See text
Glutamic acid/glutamine	2-9 μmol/dl	13-58 μmol/dl	Improves zinc absorption; precursor to brain glutamate
Carnitine	1.0 mg N/L	0.7 mg N/L	Brain lipid synthesis
Choline and ethanolamine	7-20 mg N/L	10-20 mg N/L	Possible growth requirement
Nucleic acid	—	19 mg N/L	Pool of DNA and RNA
Nucleotides	3 mg N/L	3 mg N/L	Growth and immune advantage
Polyamines	0.1 mg N/L	0.2 mg N/L	Increase rate of transcription, translation, and amino acid activation

DNA, Deoxyribonucleic acid; *RNA*, ribonucleic acid.

Nucleotides are compounds derived from nucleic acid by hydrolysis and consist of phosphoric acid combined with a sugar and a purine or pyrimidine derivative. The level and components of acid-soluble nucleotides of several species, including humans, have been studied extensively. Work has shown a characteristic nucleotide composition in the milk that differs from that of the mammary gland. The large numbers of purine and pyrimidine nucleotides present in various tissues have a number of functions in the cell. They are part of nucleic acid synthesis and metabolism and are also part of milk synthesis. It is well known that adenosine triphosphate (ATP) supplies usable energy for biosynthetic reactions.

Human milk has been recorded to have 6.1 to 9.0 μmol of free nucleotides/dl, according to Johke.[124] The levels in colostrum and mature milk are similar. The conspicuous difference in quality and quantity of nucleotides between the mammary gland and its secretion would indicate that nucleotides are secreted from the epithelial cells of the gland into the milk. There are distinct species differences in composition and content of nucleotides as well. Cytidine monophosphate (CMP) and uracil are the nucleotides in the highest concentration in human milk, which also contains uridine diphosphate-N-acetyllactosamine and other oligosaccharides. Human milk contains only a trace of orotic acid and no guanosine diphosphate–

TABLE 4-16   **Nucleotide content of human milk**

Nucleotide	Mean* (mg/dl)
Cytidine monophosphate (CMP)	461 (17.9)
Uridine monophosphate (UMP)	179 (19.8)
Adenosine monophosphate (AMP)	175 (12.8)
Inosine monophosphate (IMP)	228 (14.5)
Guanosine monophosphate (GMP)	138 (8.5)
Uridine diphosphate (UDP)	174 (12.8)
Cytidine diphosphate (CDP)	474 (41.5)
Adenosine diphosphate (ADP)	69 (17.9)
Guanosine diphosphate (GDP)	96 (8.9)

From Hendricks K: *Semin Pediatr Gastroenterol Nutr* 2:(1)14, 1991.
Modified from Janas LM, Picciano MF: *Pediatr Res* 16:659, 1982.
*Mean nucleotide content of human milk at weeks 2, 4, 8, and 12 of lactation.

fucose. Orotic acid is the chief nucleotide of bovine milk. Nucleotide levels fall rapidly in bovine milk to minimal levels in mature bovine milk.

When the nitrogen fraction of human milk was further identified over time at 2, 4, 8, and 12 weeks by Janas and Picciano,[115] a variance was noted in the pattern of nucleotides (Table 4-16). Levels of cytidine-5'-monophosphate (CMP) and adenosine-5'-monophosphate (AMP) declined from 594 to 321 µg/dl and from 244 to 143 µg/dl, respectively, whereas levels of inosine-5'-monophosphate (IMP) increased from 158 to 290 µg/dl. The total nucleotide nitrogen remained constant, accounting for 0.10% to 0.15% of the total NPN. The average intake per day of a normal breastfed infant would be 1.4 to 2.1 mg of nucleotide nitrogen. Measurement of AMP and cyclic guanosine monophosphate (GMP) by Skala et al[214] showed variation in concentration within 15 minutes, which fluctuated over 24 hours. Milk concentration differed widely from maternal plasma levels collected at the same time.

The biologic effects of dietary nucleotides involve the immune system, the intestinal microenvironment and the absorption and metabolism of certain other nutrients (Table 4-16). They are considered "semiessential" for newborns.[73] Whether IMP contributes to the superior iron absorption is still unanswered (see discussion on p. 132).

Metabolic disturbances in nucleotide metabolism can result in abnormal accumulation of specific intermediates in cells and tissues, causing a variety of diseases.[190] An example is Lesch-Nyhan syndrome, a genetic disease characterized by mental retardation, self-mutilation, and gout, which is caused by the absence of the purine salvage enzyme. On the other hand, disturbances from lack of nucleotides in the diet have not been identified.

Nucleotides are formed by de novo synthesis by capturing or scavenging partially degraded nucleotides or completely from diet. Dietary nucleotides are absorbed by action of the microvillus membrane as nucleosides. The developing neonate has a reduced capacity to synthesize or salvage nucleotides. Exogenous nucleotides are potential stimuli, modulating not only the gene control of their own metabolism but also that of a number of functions in cardiovascular, neurologic, and immune systems.[38] Nucleotides are important as coenzymes for the processes involved in the metabolism of lipids, carbohydrates, and proteins.

Nucleotides are recognized as an integral part of the immune system, acting as the host defense against bacteria, viruses, and parasites, as well as various malignancies.[17]

Nucleotides are important in the process of protein synthesis, which is enhanced in the newborn infant by a dietary supply of nucleotides. A statistically significant increase in weight was observed by György and his colleagues[79] in 1963 when weanling rats who had been fed a low-protein diet (10% casein) were given added nucleotides as compared with controls without supplements of nucleotides. A high-protein diet (20%) did not produce significant growth increase when nucleotides were added. This may explain the satisfactory growth pattern of breastfed infants on relatively low protein intake and the more efficient protein utilization of breastfed infants.

Study of the exact role of nucleotides continues in vivo, although some effort to supplement formula has already begun.

Carnitine

Carnitine is γ-trimethylamino-β-hydroxybutyrate and is essential for the catabolism of long-chain fatty acids. Only two conditions in life have been described when carnitine is indispensable: total parenteral nutrition lasting more than 3 weeks and early postnatal life. In older individuals it is synthesized in liver and kidney from essential amino acids lysine and methionine. Carnitine serves as an essential carrier of acyl groups across the mitochondrial membrane to sites of oxidation and therefore has a central role in the mitochondrial oxidation of fatty acids in the human.[180]

The newborn undergoes major metabolic changes during transition from fetal to extrauterine life, including the rapid development of the capacity to oxidize fatty acids and ketone bodies as fuel alternatives to glucose. The fatty acids derived from high-fat milk and endogenous fat stores become the preferred fuel of the heart, brain, and tissues with high-energy demands. In addition, a dramatic increase occurs in serum fatty acids in the first hours of life. After the interruption of the fetoplacental circulation and in the absence of an exogenous supply of carnitine, neonatal plasma levels of free carnitines and acylcarnitines decrease very rapidly. Carnitine administration seems to act by increasing ketogenesis and lipolysis.[176] When serum carnitine and ketone body concentrations were measured in breastfed and formula-fed newborn infants, lower carnitine levels were found in infants fed formulas than in those fed breast milk.[205]

The levels of carnitine range from 70 to 95 nmol/ml in breast milk (up to 115 nmol/ml in colostrum) and from 40 to 80 nmol/ml in commercial formula (Enfamil). The bioavailability of carnitine in human milk may be a significant factor in the higher carnitine and ketone body concentrations in breastfed babies. In omnivorous mothers, L-carnitine levels do not vary considerably over time.[18] Levels in the milk of lacto-ovo-vegetarian mothers were always consistently lower than that of omnivores. The lower serum level of lysine in these women is a possible cause of lower carnitine.

The carnitine levels in human milk were followed for 50 days postpartum by Sandor et al,[205] who found the mean level to be 62.9 nmol/ml (56.0 to 69.8 nmol/ml range) during the first 21 days and 35.2 ± 1.26 nmol/ml until the fortieth to fiftieth day. Levels were not related to volume of milk secreted.

Carbohydrates

The predominant carbohydrate of milk is *lactose,* or milk sugar. It is present in high concentration (6.8 g/dl in human milk and 4.9 g/dl in bovine milk). Lactose is a disaccharide compound of two monosaccharides, galactose and glucose. Lactose is synthesized by the mammary gland.

A number of other carbohydrates are present in milk. They are classified as monosaccharides, neutral and acid oligosaccharides, and peptide-bound and protein-bound carbohydrates. Small amounts of glucose (14 mg/100 ml) and galactose (12 mg/100 ml) also are present in breast milk. Other complex carbohydrates are present in free form or bound to amino acids or protein, such as N-acetylglucosamine. The concentration of oligosaccharides is about 10 times greater than in cow's milk. This difference arises from biosynthetic control mechanisms yet to be described. These carbohydrates and glycoproteins possess bifidus factor activity. Fucose, which is not present in bovine milk, may be important to the early establishment of *Lactobacillus bifidus* as gut flora. The nitrogen-containing carbohydrates are 0.7% of milk solids.

In a study of carbohydrate content over the first 4 months of lactation, Coppa et al[42] observed that lactose concentrations increased from 56 ± 6 g/L on day 4 to 68.9 ± 8 g/L on day 120. Oligosaccharide levels decreased from 20.9 ± 5 g/L to 12.9 ± 3.30 g/L. Monosaccharides were only 1.2% of the total carbohydrates. The authors describe carbohydrate synthesis by the mammary gland as a dynamic process. Oligosaccharides represent a low osmolar source of calories, stimulate the growth of bifidus flora, and inhibit bacterial adhesion to epithelial surfaces, competing with cell receptors in the binding of pathogenic agents.

Lactose is hydrolyzed selectively by a brush border enzyme called *lactase* located predominantly in the tip of the intestinal villi. Digestion of lactose is the rate-limiting step in its absorption. Although lactase activity develops later in fetal life than that of other disaccharidases, it is present by 24 weeks of fetal life. Lactase concentration is greatest in the proximal jejunum. Levels continue to increase throughout the last trimester, reaching concentrations at term two to four times those levels at 2 to 11 months of age. Premature infants rapidly increase their lactase levels given a lactose challenge. A well-fed breastfed infant ingesting 150 ml of milk/kg/day receives 10 g of lactose/kg/day, which ensures the normal unstressed infant at least 4 mg/kg/min of glucose, which is considered the optimal rate.[146]

Lactose does appear to be specific, however, for newborn growth. It has been shown to enhance calcium absorption and has been suggested as being critical to the prevention of rickets, in view of the relatively low calcium levels in human milk. Lactose is a readily available source of galactose, which is essential to the production of the galactolipids, including cerebroside. These galactolipids are essential to CNS development.

Interesting correlations have been made between the amount of lactose in the milk of a species and the relative size of the brain[139] (Fig. 4-9). Because lactose is found only in milk and not in other animal and plant sources, its high level in human milk is even more significant. Lactose levels are quite constant throughout the day in a given mother's milk. Even in poorly nourished

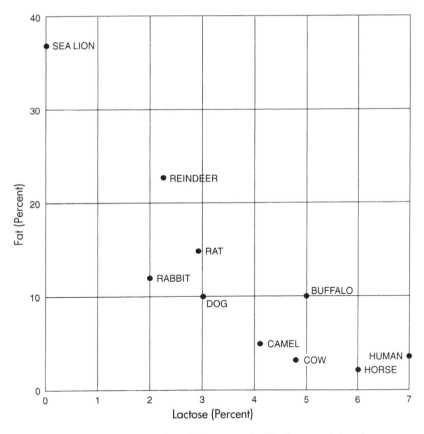

Fig. 4-9. Concentration of lactose varies with source of milk. In general, less lactose, more fat, which can also be used by newborn animal as energy source. (From Kretchmer N: Lactose and lactase, *Sci Am* 227:73. Copyright © 1972 by Scientific American, Inc. All rights reserved.)

mothers, the levels of lactose do not vary. Because lactose is influential in controlling volume, the total output for the day may be diminished, but the concentration of lactose in human milk will be 6.2 to 7.2 g/dl.[33] An adequate source of carbohydrate is important for optimal lactation, which suggests that excessive amounts of sugar substitutes may have an effect on volume.[136]

Oligosaccharides and glycoconjugates

Oligosaccharides are the third largest solid component in milk after lactose and triglyceride. Most of the milk oligosaccharides contain lactose at the reducing end of the structure and may also contain fucose or sialic acid at the nonreducing end. More than 80 neutral and acidic oligosaccharides have been identified.[173]

Glycoproteins, glycosylated major milk proteins, include lactoferrin, immunoglobulins, and mucins. Their protective characteristics have been described to act as receptor homologs, inhibiting the binding of enteropathogens to their host receptors. Research continues to link specific carbohydrate structures with protection against specific pathogens. These nonimmunoglobulin agents are also active against whole classes of pathogens.[173] The protective glyconjugates and oligosaccharides are unique to human milk and to date have not been replicated synthetically.

Minerals

Minerals represent a special category of constituents whose pathways into milk vary from simple diffusion to both positive and negative pump mechanisms. Table 4-17 records the measurements of the constituents in human milk compared with maternal serum. By examining this relationship, it can be estimated how the particular constituent reaches the milk, that is, by passive diffusion or positive or negative pump.

The total ash content of milk is species specific and parallels the growth rate and body structure of the offspring. A number of metallic elements and

organic and inorganic acids are present in milk as ions, un-ionized salts, and weakly ionized salts. Some are bound to other constituents. Sodium, potassium, calcium, and magnesium are the major cations. Phosphate, chloride, and citrate are the major anions.[35]

The monovalent ions are sodium, potassium, and chloride. The divalent ions are calcium, magnesium, citrate, phosphate, and sulfate.[12] The monovalent ions are among the most prevalent and contribute 30 mosmol, or one tenth of the total osmolarity of human milk. The sum of the concentrations of the monovalent ions is inversely proportional to the lactose content across species. Monovalent ion concentration is regulated chiefly by the secretion mechanism in the alveolar cell, with the human having the highest lactose and lowest ion content.[172] This maintains osmolality close to that of serum.

Daily intakes of calcium, phosphorus, zinc, potassium, sodium, iron, and copper from breast milk were found to decrease significantly over the first 4 months of life, with only magnesium increasing. Despite seemingly low mineral intakes, growth during this time was found to be satisfactory by Butte et al.[26] High mineral content is associated with a rapid growth rate of specific species.

Potassium and sodium

Potassium levels are much higher than those of sodium, which are similar to the proportions in intracellular fluids (Table 4-18). Although sodium, potassium, and chloride are present as free ions, the other constituents appear as complexes and compounds. Ions can pass through the secretory cell membrane in both directions and in and out of the lumen. Intracellular sodium, chloride, and potassium are in equilibrium with the ions of the plasma and alveolar milk. An apical pumping mechanism has been calculated for chloride release, whereas sodium, potassium, and intracellular chloride pass into milk because of their electrochemical gradients. The cellular pumping mechanism maintains the ionic concentrations in the extracellular fluid and alveolar milk.

The Committee on Nutrition of the American

TABLE 4-17   Difference in composition of human milk and blood plasma

	Specific gravity	Osmo-larity	pH	Calories	Water	Carbohy-drates	Fat	Protein			Iron	Na⁺	K⁺
								Albumin	Globulin				
Human mature milk	1031	295	7.3	65 kcal/dl	87.5 g%	7.0 g% (lactose)	3.7 g%	0.3 g%	0.2 g%		0.15 mg%	15 mg%	57 mg%
Blood plasma	1033	285	7.4	35 kcal/dl	92 g%	80 mg% (glucose)	200 mg%	4.5 g%	2.5 g%		125 µg%	320 mg%	18 mg%

	Ca²⁺	Mg²⁺	Cl⁻	Phosphorus	Sulfur	Vitamins						
						A*	B₁	B₂	Niacin	C	D	
Human mature milk	35 mg%	4 mg%	43 mg%	15 mg%	14 mg%	280 IU/dl	20 µg%	50 µg%	172 µg%	5 mg%	5 IU/dl	
Blood plasma	10 mg%	2.5 mg%	365 mg%	4 mg%	2 mg%	50 µg%	10 µg%	0.5 µg%	500 µg%	1 mg%	188 IU/dl	

Modified from Vorheer H: *The breasts: morphology, physiology, and lactation*. New York, 1974, Academic Press.
*1 µg of vitamin A corresponds to the activity of 3 IU of vitamin A.

Academy of Pediatrics[41] has stated that the daily requirement of sodium for growth is 0.5 mEq/kg/day between birth and 3 months of age, decreasing to 0.1 mEq/kg/day after 6 months of age (Table 4-19). To cover dermal losses, an additional 0.4 to 0.7 mEq/kg/day is needed, with little for urine and stool losses. Infants fed human milk receive enough sodium to meet their needs for growth, dermal losses, and urinary losses. Studies by Keenan et al[132] have demonstrated an apparent regulation of milk sodium and potassium concentrations by adrenocorticosteroids as well as a circadian rhythm in the levels.

Sodium levels in cow's milk are 3.6 times those in human milk (human, 7 mEq/L or 16 mg/dl; bovine, 22 mEq/L or 50 mg/dl). Hypernatremic dehydration has been associated with cow's milk feedings. Experiments with newborn rats on high salt intakes have shown that hypertension can develop.

The diurnal variation in milk electrolytes was found to vary between 22% and 80%.[132] These changes varied as the lactation period progressed but were independent of mother's diet. Sodium restriction did not influence milk levels. In a longitudinal study, Hazebroek and Hofman[94] found sodium levels fell from 20 mEq/L to 15 mEq/L in the first week. On day 8, levels were 8 mEq/L, and by the fifth week they were stabilized at 6 mEq/L. Time-dependent changes in milk composition are also reported by Allen et al[4] as a 25% or greater decrease in sodium, potassium, and citrate from 1 to 6 months. Calcium and glucose increase by 10% or more over this time. The authors suggest milk composition is always in transition.[4]

At a constant sodium intake, decreasing the sodium/potassium (Na/K) ratio in the diet by increasing potassium lowers blood pressure. The dietary Na/K ratio has an important role in determining the severity, if not the development, of salt-induced hypertension. The mechanism of po-

TABLE 4-18   Minerals in human milk and cow's milk (per deciliter)

Minerals	Colostrum	Transitional	Mature	Cow's milk
Calcium (mg)	39	46	35	130
Chlorine (mg)	85	46	40	108
Copper (µg)	40	50	40	14
Iron (µg)	70	70	100	70
Magnesium (mg)	4	4	4	12
Phosphorus (mg)	14	20	15	120
Potassium (mg)	74	64	57	145
Sodium (mg)	48	29	15	58
Sulfur (mg)	22	20	14	30
Total ash (mg)	—	—	200	700

From Food and Nutrition Board, National Research Council, National Academy of Sciences: *Recommended dietary allowances,* ed 10, Washington, DC, 1989, US Government Printing Office.

TABLE 4-19   Recommended dietary intake of electrolytes for infants

Age	Sodium (mg)	Potassium (mg)	Chloride (mg)
To 6 mo	115-350 (11.5 mg/kg)	350-925	275-700
6 mo-1 yr	250-750 (23 mg/kg)	425-1500	400-1200

From Food and Nutrition Board, National Research Council, National Academy of Sciences: *Recommended dietary allowances,* ed 10, Washington, DC, 1989, US Government Printing Office.

tassium's antihypertensive effect is unclear, but the higher potassium and lower sodium levels of breast milk appear to be physiologically beneficial.

Chloride

Little attention has been paid to the adequacy of chloride in the diet, and it has always been assumed to be sufficient until recent events focused attention on this cation.

Chloride deficiency in infants has become associated with a syndrome of failure to thrive with hypochloremia and hypokalemic metabolic alkalosis. This was first described in infants fed formula that was deficient in chloride but has also been described in a breastfed infant whose mother's milk contained less than 2 mEq/L chloride (normal is greater than 8 mEq/L).[11] This is a rare phenomenon caused by unexplained maternal production. This mother had previously successfully nourished five other infants.

Total ash

Cow's milk has three times the total salt content of human milk (Table 4-20). All the minerals that appear in cow's milk also appear in human milk.[118] The phosphorus level is six times greater in cow's milk; the calcium level is four times higher (Table 4-21).

TABLE 4-20 Principal salt constituents in bovine and human milks

Constituent	Bovine (mg/dl)	Human (mg/dl)
Calcium	125	33
Magnesium	12	4
Sodium	58	15
Potassium	138	55
Chloride	103	43
Phosphorus	96	15
Citric acid	175	20-80
Sulfur (total)	30	14 (±2.6; 4.5 mmol/L)
Carbon dioxide	20	—

From Jenness R, Sloan RE: Composition of milk. In Larson BL, Smith VR, editors: *Lactation*, vol 3, *Nutrition and biochemistry of milk/maintenance*, New York, 1974, Academic Press.

The renal solute load of cow's milk is considerably higher than that of breast milk. This is magnified by the metabolic breakdown products of the high protein content, which are in increased amounts as well. This is shown in the high urea levels in formula-fed infants (Table 4-22). Although the mean urea levels in breast milk are 37 mg/dl and only 15 mg/dl in cow's milk, the blood urea levels in breastfed infants are about 22 mg, whereas those of infants fed formula are 47 mg and those of infants fed formula plus solids are 52 mg/dl[46] (Table 4-22). The plasma osmolarity of infants fed breast milk is lower and approximates the physiologic level of plasma.

Calcium/phosphorus ratio

The calcium/phosphorus (Ca/P) ratio is considerably lower in cow's milk (1:4) than in human milk (2:2). Many investigators have studied calcium and phosphorus values in human milk and found some variation from mother to mother and from study to study. The Ca/P ratio varied from 1.8 to 2.4, with the absolute values for calcium varying from 20 to 34 mg/dl and those for phosphorus varying from 14 to 18 mg/dl. Data compiled by Forfar[66] demonstrate the variation. Fetal and newborn plasma concentrations for calcium decline sharply from 10.4 mg/dl at birth to 8.5 mg/dl by day 4. Unlike calcium, phosphorus concentrations rise in the postnatal period. The drop in serum calcium levels in the bottle-fed infants was more marked than in the breastfed infants. Infant serum phosphorus concentrations rise during the postnatal period. When gestation is prolonged or the mother has preeclampsia, the concentrations are even higher at birth.

Longitudinal studies by Greer et al,[77] measuring calcium and phosphorus in human milk and maternal and infant sera, have shown progressive increases in infant serum calcium in association with decreasing phosphorus content of breast milk and infant serum. Maternal serum calcium also increased, although the mother's dietary intake was below recommended levels for lactating women. Calcium uptake in the maternal duodenum is enhanced during lactation.

TABLE 4-21	**Recommended dietary intake of minerals for infants***					
Age	Calcium (mg)	Phosphorus (mg)	Magnesium (mg)	Iron (mg)	Zinc (mg)	Iodine (mg)
To 6 mo	400	300	40	6	5	40
6 mo-1 yr	600	500	60	10	5	50

From Food and Nutrition Board, National Research Council, National Academy of Sciences: *Recommended dietary allowances,* ed 10, Washington, DC, 1989, US Government Printing Office.
*Because there is little information on which to base allowances, these amounts are provided in the form of ranges of recommended intakes.

TABLE 4-22	**Statistical analysis by Student's t-test of blood urea levels in 61 healthy infants age 1 to 3 months**				
				Individual values >40 mg/dl	
Infant group	Number	Blood urea, mean ± SE (mg/dl)	Number	Total observations (%)	
A: breastfed	12	22.7 ± 1.6*	0	0‡	
B: artificial milk alone	16	47.4 ± 2.0†	12	75§	
C: artificial milk + solid foods	33	51.9 ± 1.8	29	88	

From Davies DP, Saunders R: *Arch Dis Child* 48:563, 1973.
*When compared with group B and group C: $p < 0.001$ ($t = 9.7$) and $p < 0.001$ ($t = 11.5$), respectively.
†When compared with group C: $p > 0.05$ ($t = 1.6$).
‡When compared with group B and group C: $p < 0.001$ ($t = 6.9$) and $p < 0.001$ ($t = 15.5$), respectively.
§When compared with group C: $p > 0.05$ ($t = 1.1$).

Although the Ca/P ratio has been stressed in the past, recent investigations have not found a statistical correlation between the calcium and phosphorus contents of plasma and corresponding breast milk Ca/P. This suggested that Ca/P ratio is not critical in the low mineral loads present in breast milk. Calcium and phosphorus decrease over time during lactation.[9] When human milk was fractionated and analyzed for distribution of calcium, whole milk contained 241.2 ± 61.9 µg/ml, with most of the calcium in the skim fraction. Significant amounts were also found in the fat; less than 4% was found in the casein. A low-molecular-weight fraction contained 34% calcium, which may explain calcium's bioavailability. The total calcium requirements for maximum growth have been questioned by those who believe the total amount of calcium is too low in breast milk. The fact that rickets has not been seen in infants totally breastfed by well-nourished mothers is supportive

circumstantial evidence. There is bone mobilization in the mother during lactation and recovery of bone mass during and after weaning.[218]

Lactating women contribute 210 mg of calcium per day in breast milk. A study of intestinal calcium absorption of women during lactation and after weaning revealed that serum calcium and phosphorus concentrations were greater in lactating compared with nonlactating postpartum women, but levels were the same after weaning.[128,129] On the other hand, calcitrol was greater in women after weaning compared with postpartum control subjects. Kalkwark et al[130] concluded that lactation stimulates increases in fractional calcium absorption and serum calcitrol after the onset of menses or after weaning. Observations of these women using bone mineral content (BMC) and bone mineral density (BMD) technology showed that lactating women lost significantly more bone throughout the body and in the lumbar spine than nonlactating

TABLE 4-23   Recommended dietary intake of trace elements for infants*

Age	Copper (mg)	Manganese (mg)	Fluorine (mg)	Chromium (mg)	Selenium (mg)	Molybdenum (mg)
To 6 mo	0.4-0.6	0.3-0.6	0.1-0.5	0.01-0.04	0.01-0.04	0.015-0.03
6 mo-1 yr	0.6-0.7	0.6-1.0	0.2-1.0	0.02-0.06	0.015-0.06	0.02-0.04

From Food and Nutrition Board, National Research Council, National Academy of Sciences: *Recommended dietary allowances,* ed 10, Washington, DC, 1989, US Government Printing Office.
*Because the toxic levels for many trace elements may be only several times the usual intakes, the upper levels for the trace elements given in this table should not be habitually exceeded.

postpartum women in the first 6 months.[130] After weaning, the lactators regained significantly more bone in the lumbar spine than nonlactating women. Early resumption of menses was associated with a smaller loss and greater increase after weaning.[44] Parathyroid hormone concentrations are reported to be higher only after weaning.

Calcium supplementation does not prevent bone loss during lactation and only slightly enhances the gain in bone density after weaning.[129] Supplementation did not affect levels in the milk. Krebs et al[138] reported that excesses of protein have a negative effect on calcium absorption in lactating women. The calcium/protein ratio appears to be critical to efficient utilization. Estradiol stimulated osteoblastic proliferation and enhanced collagen gene expression. Calcium was shown to be well absorbed in 5- to 7-month-old breastfed infants who had begun to receive beikost (solids and semisolids).

Magnesium and other salts

Magnesium is present as a free ion and in complexes with casein and phosphate in caseinate micelles or citrate complexes. Cow's milk has three times as much magnesium as human milk (12 mg/dl compared with 4 mg/dl) (Table 4-20). Magnesium was measured in human milk by Fransson and Lönnerdal,[70] who found 41.4 ± 15.4 μg/ml in whole milk samples, with most of the magnesium in the skim milk fraction but significant amounts in the fat fraction and less than 4% in the casein. The bound fraction was associated with low-molecular-weight proteins, thus enhancing bioavailability. Mineral intakes were shown to

increase between 1 and 3 months postpartum (1.15 to 1.36 mmol/L).[184]

Longitudinal magnesium concentrations were measured by Greer et al[77] in milk and maternal sera and in the infants over a 6-month period. Progressive increases in serum magnesium level were seen in the breastfed infants in association with decreasing phosphorus content of the milk. Milk magnesium levels did not change significantly between 3 and 26 weeks. The authors suggested that the rising magnesium levels in infant serum may in part be caused by a decrease in dietary phosphorus in breastfed infants.

Citrate is found in the milks of many species and is three to four times higher in cow's milk than in human milk (Table 4-20). The distribution of ions and salts differs among various milks and depends on the relative concentrations of casein and citrate.[118]

Citrate is made in the mitochondria from pyruvate and transported into the cytoplasm, where it is available for lipid synthesis and for transport into the Golgi complex.[12] Citrate levels are not often measured in human milk, although citrate may be a marker of milk production potential (Fig. 4-4). Levels are high the first few days and rise as calcium levels rise.

Most of the *sulfur* in milk is in the sulfur-containing amino acids, with only about 10% present as sulfate ion. Some organic acids are present, and they appear as anions in milk.

Trace elements

Tables 4-20 and 4-23 list the recommended daily intake of trace elements[65] for infants.

Iron. Because of the great emphasis on iron in the modern diet, and especially in the diet of the infant in the first year of life, the iron in human milk has been closely scrutinized. It has been determined that normal infants need 1500 mg of exogenous elemental iron in the first year of life, which can be translated into 8 to 10 mg/day (Table 4-22). Prepared infant formulas currently supply 10 to 12 mg/day. Human milk has 100 µg/dl, which does not meet the requirements just given. Historically, however, breastfed infants have not been anemic (Table 4-18).

In 350 samples of breast milk, there was a variation between less than 0.1 and 1.6 µg of iron/ml. Age, parity, and lactation history influenced the levels in some studies. The distribution of iron in various fractions of human milk of Swedish women was determined using multiple methods by Fransson and Lönnerdal,[70] who also found low levels, 0.26 and 0.73 ng/ml. The lipid fraction bound 15% to 46% of the iron; 18% to 56% of the iron was in the low-molecular-weight protein fraction, with only a small amount bound to lactoferrin. Feeley et al[61] studied 102 American women by stage of lactation; 96% of the women took prenatal iron supplements. A diurnal variation was observed, and a significant decrease occurred from 4 to 45 days postpartum. The authors estimated that fully breastfed infants would receive 0.10 mg/kg/day of iron.[61]

The effects of maternal iron nutrition in rats during lactation was studied by Anaokar and Garry,[7] who fed three groups of dams control amounts of 250 ppm iron, high-iron diets of 2500 ppm, and no-iron diets. Milk iron concentration decreased in all diet groups during lactation. The rate of decrease was diet dependent. Furthermore, iron levels in the dams were influenced by diet and correlated with levels in their pups.

Iron absorption from human milk is more efficient and has been noted to be 49% of iron available, whereas only 10% of cow's milk iron and 4% of iron in iron-fortified formulas are absorbed. Hematologic values of bottle-fed infants were abnormal, whereas those of breastfed infants were not. The breastfed infants had high ferritin levels, indicating a long-term adequacy of iron assimilation.

The infant who is exclusively breastfed for the first 6 months of life is not at risk for iron deficiency anemia or the depletion of iron stores during that time, according to iron depletion studies of Duncan et al.[55] These findings were confirmed in iron balance studies on exclusively breastfed infants by Schulz-Lell et al,[207] who also cautioned against supraphysiologic iron supplementation (10 to 12 mg/L), which leads to a 12- to 40-fold increase in iron retention compared with that of well-nourished, exclusively breastfed infants. Studies in adults given tagged iron in human milk and in cow's milk show better absorption from the human milk solution.

Other factors that influence iron absorption include higher amounts of vitamin C. Lactose, which promotes iron absorption, is in higher concentration in breast milk, especially compared with prepared formulas, which may not contain lactose. Calcium and phosphorus may interfere with iron absorption, as may high protein levels. Considerable doubt still exists as to whether it is physiologically sound to increase the hemoglobin of an infant with exogenous iron. All species of mammals have low iron content in their milks. All mammals investigated so far have a drop in their hemoglobin levels after birth and a gradual rise to adult levels for the species.

A study of 40 normal, full-term infants followed in an Argentinian clinic found that the exclusively breastfed infants had a 27% incidence of anemia compared with a 7% rate in those who received iron-supplemented formula.[28] There was no storage iron in the anemic breastfed infants. The average incidence of anemia in children in Argentina is 46%. The mothers had been instructed to start beef, liver, and orange juice at 6 months. Most of the iron was present in hemoglobin, the body storage iron being a small fraction of total body iron (2.05% for breastfed and 2.79% for formula-fed infants).[28]

Pisacane et al[186] studied the iron status of 30 infants breastfed until their first birthday who never received cow's milk, supplemental iron, or iron-enriched formula. Examination of their iron stores and hematocrits revealed that those exclusively breastfed for 6½ months versus 5½ months were less likely to be anemic.[186] None of the infants exclusively breastfed for 7 months was anemic and continued to have good iron status at 12 and 24 months.

The relationship between plasma concentration of ferritin and body iron stores has not been clearly established; the explanation of iron absorption and use in breastfed infants is still under study.

Absorption of iron from breast milk by 5- to 7-month-old infants receiving solid foods was studied using stable isotope [58]Fe.[1] Iron was well absorbed from human milk in older infants after the introduction of solid foods to the diet.

Zinc. Zinc has been identified as essential to the human.[93] Its chief roles described to date are as part of the enzyme structure and as an enzyme activator. Zinc has been identified as a first limiting nutrient in breast milk when anthropometric indicators of growth were correlated with zinc levels in healthy breastfed infants.[53] Zinc deficiency has been described as well, most dramatically in newborns and premature infants on hyperalimentation regimens. The chief clinical symptoms are failure to thrive and typical skin lesions. Human milk has been identified as a food with bioavailable zinc.[125]

Zinc absorption from human milk, cow's milk, and infant formula was tested in healthy adults with labeled zinc chloride, [65]Z. The absorption was 41% from human milk, 28% from cow's milk, 31% from standard infant formula, and 14% from soy formula. The dietary zinc intake of both lactating and nonlactating postpartum women was found by Moser and Reynolds[161] to be 42% of recommended allowances. No correlation was found between zinc concentrations in breast milk and maternal dietary zinc and maternal plasma and erythrocyte zinc.

Changes in hair zinc concentrations of breastfed and bottle-fed infants during the first 6 months of life were measured by MacDonald et al.[156] Only the bottle-fed males had a significant decline in hair zinc concentration. There was no decline of zinc in any breastfed infant, which supports the

concept of the superior bioavailability of zinc in breast milk.

Picciano and Guthrie[185] studied milk from 50 mothers in 350 samples. They found zinc levels to average 3.95 µg/ml and to be consistent regardless of time of day, duration of lactation, or other variables. They estimated that breastfed infants receive 0.35 mg of zinc/kg/day. They found zinc levels to decline slightly from the first to the third month postpartum (33.8 to 29.5 µmol/L). Longitudinal changes in dietary zinc requirements for infants acquiring new lean body mass through growth were studied by Krebs and Hambidge.[137] As growth velocity declines, zinc requirements decline in the male infant from a high of 780 µg/day at 1 month to 480 µg/day in the fifth through twelfth months. Meanwhile, the percentage of absorption increased over time.

Human milk was fractionated and analyzed by Fransson and Lönnerdal[70] for the distribution of zinc. Most of the zinc was found in the skim milk fraction, but significant amounts were found in the fat associated with the fat globule membrane; less than 4% was found in the casein.

Longitudinal zinc balances in breastfed and formula-fed infants revealed that the median daily zinc intake in breastfed infants decreased from 0.59 mg/kg to 0.15 mg/kg in the first 17 weeks of life.[211] Comparable values for the formula-fed infants were 0.58 mg/kg and 0.67 mg/kg. The median retention of zinc was 27% in breastfed versus 21% in bottle-fed infants. Considering the minimal urinary and fecal losses in the breastfed infants, a daily intake of zinc of 0.3 to 0.5 mg/kg is sufficient.

Khoshoo et al[133] reported zinc deficiency in a full-term, breastfed infant, previously reported in a breastfed premature infant. This case was diagnosed at 7 months of age by the characteristic perineal and perioral rash in an otherwise healthy, well-grown infant. The presumed cause was defective zinc uptake by the mammary gland, because the milk level was only 0.13 mg/L. The infant responded promptly to oral zinc supplements.

In a 9-week-old infant with an intractable diaper rash, the mother's milk was noted to have low zinc levels after the rash responded to zinc therapy.[10] She had nursed two other children without difficulty. Analyzing a small series of cases, Atkinson et al[15] concluded that lowered zinc levels in milk were caused by decreased zinc uptake by the mammary gland, because the maternal plasma levels were normal.

Cow's milk zinc is associated with high-molecular-weight fractions, and zinc in human milk is associated with low-molecular-weight fractions. The association of zinc with low-molecular-weight components of milk is related in part to protein content and composition and to the relative zinc concentration.[104] When adult females were given oral doses of zinc with human milk, cow's milk, casein hydrolysate formula, and soy-based formula, the plasma response with human milk was significantly (three times) greater than with any of the others.[36]

The low-molecular-weight ligand has been proved to be readily absorbed. Breast milk has been therapeutic in the treatment of acrodermatitis enteropathica, an inherited zinc metabolism disorder, whereas cow's milk formulas are ineffective.

Copper, selenium, chromium, manganese, molybdenum, and nickel. Trace elements constitute less than 0.01% of body weight; however, their atoms are present in large numbers and play a critical role in growth and development. The technical ability to measure these elements is expanding.[209] The effects of trace element deficiencies in fetal and neonatal development are yet to be understood.

Picciano and Guthrie[185] studied *copper* levels in human milk and noted that the content varied considerably among women and within each woman. The range was 0.09 to 0.63 µg/ml. Copper levels were higher in the morning. Dietary supplements did not alter results. Age, parity, and lactation history showed that older mothers and multiparas had higher levels. The fully breastfed infant would receive 0.05 mg of copper/kg/day (Table 4-23).

Fractionated analysis by Fransson and Lönnerdal[70] revealed whole milk concentration of copper to be 0.27 ± 0.13 µg/ml, with most of the copper in the skim milk fraction, significant amounts in the fat, and little in the casein. The predominant binding was with low-molecular-weight proteins, which would enhance bioavailability.[70]

MacDonald et al[156] studied changes in hair copper concentrations among breastfed and bottle-fed infants. Hair copper levels rose in the first 3 months in all infants and then declined, regardless of feeding or gender of infant. The authors associated this with the redistribution of copper in early infancy (Table 4-18). Copper is a component of a number of metalloenzymes.

The bioavailability of *selenium* depends on the sources and chemical form, and the quantitative significance is under investigation. Except for Keshan disease, a potentially fatal cardiomyopathy seen in infants in China, no convincingly associated clinical deficiency syndrome has been reported. Dietary recommendations have been based on those for adults. Dietary intakes less than the lower limits, however, should not be considered deficient, especially in breastfed infants.[232]

Selenium concentrations in human milk are consistent with samples collected from many parts of the world, according to work by Hadjimarkos and Shearer.[80] The mean value was 0.020 ppm, which was similar to the value from many parts of the United States, where the range was 0.007 to 0.033 ppm.

Increased selenium requirements have been observed in pregnant and lactating women. Supplementation with different compounds, such as selenium-enriched yeast and selenomethionine, significantly influenced selected indices of selenium status, including milk concentrations.[3]

Selenium is considered an essential nutrient in humans. It is an integral component of glutathione peroxidase, an enzyme known to metabolize lipid peroxides, and deficiency states have been described. Questions have been raised about the detrimental effects of high selenium intake on dentition. Smith et al[215] assessed selenium status in infants exclusively fed human milk or infant formula for 3 months. Foremilk samples had a mean concentration of 15.7 ng/ml, hindmilk mean concentration was 16.3 ng/ml, and mean formula concentration was 8.6 ng/ml. Breastfed infants have greater intakes and higher serum levels of selenium than formula-fed infants in the first 3 months (Table 4-23).

The concentration of *chromium* is highest in the organs of the newborn and declines rapidly during the first years of life. A longitudinal study of chromium in human milk was undertaken by Kumpulainen and Vuori.[141] Mothers collected samples at 8 to 18 days, 47 to 54 days, and 128 to 159 days postpartum, representing every feed during a 24-hour period with equal portions of foremilk and hindmilk. The mean concentration was 0.39 (SD = 0.15) ng/ml and the intake 0.27 (SD = 0.11) µg/day. The values did not change over time. These values are the same as those in human serum and urine. The mothers' dietary intake averaged about 30 µg/day, which is lower than the 50 to 200 µg recommended daily allowance.

When chromium metabolism was studied in 17 lactating postpartum subjects, breast milk chromium content was independent of dietary chromium intake and serum and urinary values.[8] Chromium intake did not correlate with serum or urinary chromium.

An HDL cholesterol level can be increased with chromium supplementation. Chromium also is reported to have a favorable effect on serum lipid profiles. Deficiency of chromium in infancy may be an issue with LBW infants or those with inadequate fetal stores.[141] It is present in all tissues of the body and is in high levels in nucleic acids.[209]

Mainly because of a lack of information, little is known about *manganese* in infant nutrition.[151] Manganese is a component of comparatively few metalloenzymes, including pyruvate carboxylase and mitochondrial superoxide dismutase. It does, however, activate others. Deficiencies cause impaired growth and skeletal abnormalities in all species studied. In human milk the major fraction of manganese is the 71% found in the whey, with 11% in the casein and 18% in the lipid. Levels in human milk in the first month of lactation decreased from a mean of 5.4 ± 1.6 µg/dl on day 1 to 2.7 ± 1.6 ng/ml from day 5 through day 28. The average intake of the infant in the first month was 2.0 mg/day.

The main biochemical role of *molybdenum* in mammals is as a cofactor for several enzymes.[34] Deficiencies are rare, usually occurring in those receiving total parenteral nutrition. Molybdenum levels in human milk were measured from day 1 through day 38. Levels began at 15.0 ± 6.1 µg/dl and leveled off at 1 to 2 µg/dl at 1 month.[34,35]

Nickel is generally accepted as an essential trace element for animals, but its role in humans is undefined. Levels in human milk are stable over time at 1.2 µg/dl. The average daily intake of nickel at 1 month was 0.8 µg.

Fluorine. Fluorine has been widely accepted as a significant dietary factor in decreasing dental caries (Table 4-23). The effect has been associated with the conversion of the enamel hydroxyapatite to fluorapatite with a reduction in acid solubility. The presence of fluorine during the formation of hydroxyapatite may create less soluble, more resistant crystals.

Conflicting reports of the fluorine levels in human milk had led to the belief that breastfed infants needed supplementation.[149] More accurate studies in communities where fluoride has been in the public drinking water supply show 7 µg of fluorine per liter (range 4 to 14 µg/L).[58] The American Academy of Pediatrics no longer recommends routinely supplementing breastfed infants with fluorine (see Chapter 9).

The significant development of deciduous and permanent teeth occurs after birth and depends on fetal stores, as well as on fluorine available in the diet. Studies comparing breastfed and bottle-fed infants show a distinct difference, with fewer dental caries and better dental health in breastfed infants. The role of fluorine and other factors, such as selenium, that predispose the breastfed infant to healthier teeth have yet to be defined completely. Nursing-bottle caries add to the total dental caries of the bottle-fed infant.

Iodide

Iodide levels have rarely been studied, although it was recognized that levels in the milk could be raised above those in the serum (in which radioactive iodine compounds have been examined). Mean breast milk iodide levels were 178 μg/L (range 29 to 490 μg/L), which is about four times the recommended daily allowance for infants.[78] Levels in milk were unrelated to the infant's age but directly related to maternal intake calculated in the diet.

pH and osmolarity

The pH range in human milk is 6.7 to 7.4, with a mean of 7.1. The mean pH of cow's milk is 6.8. The caloric content of both human and cow's milk is 65 kcal/dl or 20 kcal/oz. The specific gravities are 1.031 and 1.032, respectively.

The osmolarity of human milk approximates that of human serum, or 286 mosmol/kg of water, whereas that for cow's milk is higher, 350 mosmol.[45] The renal solute load of human milk is considerably lower than that of cow's milk. Renal solute load is roughly calculated by totaling the solutes that must be excreted by the kidney. It consists primarily of nonmetabolizable dietary components, especially electrolytes, ingested in excess of body needs, and metabolic end products, mainly from the metabolism of protein. Renal solute load can be estimated by adding the dietary intake of nitrogen and three minerals—sodium, potassium, and chloride. Each gram of protein is considered to yield 4 mosmol (as urea), and each milliequivalent of sodium, potassium, and chloride is 1 mosmol, according to Fomon.[64] The renal solute load of cow's milk is 221 mosmol, compared with 79 mosmol for human milk.

Dearlove and Dearlove[47] investigated osmoregulation in human lactation in an effort to determine whether fluid loading was a valid clinical maneuver. It is known that an oral hypotonic fluid load results in suppression of prolactin in adults. After an intravenous hypotonic saline infusion, a significant correlation was seen between serum osmolarity and prolactin. No changes in serum prolactin, milk yield, serum, or breast milk osmolarity were noted, however, when normal lactating women were given a hypotonic fluid load in a controlled study.

Vitamins
Vitamin A

Vitamin A content is 75 μg/dl or 280 international units (IU) in mature human milk and 41 μg/dl or 180 IU in cow's milk (Table 4-24). Thus the supply of vitamin A and its precursors, carotenoids (e.g., β-carotene), is considered adequate to meet the estimated daily requirement, which varies from 500 to 1500 IU/day if the infant consumes at least 200 ml of breast milk per day (Table 4-25). There is twice as much vitamin A in colostrum as in mature milk. During the first 6 months, retinol equivalent (RE) content of term milk in developing countries is only 330 μg RE/L compared to 660 in developed countries.[174] Retinal content of milk of mothers delivering prematurely is even higher. A single 60-mg supplement of β-carotene sustained elevated β-carotene concentrations in serum and milk longer than 1 week in normal mothers but did not affect concentrations of other major carotenoids, retinol, or tocopherol.[29] Vitamin A intake and serum vitamin A concentrations during pregnancy influence the composition of breast milk. Human milk is a vital source of vitamin A in developing countries, even beyond the first year of life.[179]

Vitamin D

Vitamin D has always been included in the fat-soluble vitamin group because that is the form in which it had been identified in nature. The levels in human milk were 0.05 μg/dl, previously reported in the fat fraction. Human milk was shown to have vitamin D in both the fat and the aqueous fractions. Investigators measured the water-soluble sulfate conjugate of vitamin D and evaluated the biologic activity of the water-soluble metabolites. When activity is calculated by an assay that measures stimulation of intestinal calcium transport, human milk is found to contain 40 to 50 IU/L of vitamin D activity. The metabolite 25-hydroxyvitamin D_3 accounts for 75% of the activity; vitamins D_2 and D_3 account for 15%. Vitamin D sulfate, or any other as yet unidentified water-soluble metabolite of vitamin D, has not been proven to have significant biologic activity.

The impact of the maternal diet content of vitamin D was measured in a double-blind study of

TABLE 4-24   **Vitamins and other constituents of human milk and cow's milk (per deciliter)**

Milk elements	Colostrum	Transitional	Mature	Cow's milk
Vitamin A (µg)	151.0	88.0	75.0	41.0
Vitamin B$_1$ (µg)	1.9	5.9	14.0	43.0
Vitamin B$_2$ (µg)	30.0	37.0	40.0	145.0
Nicotinic acid (µg)	75.0	175.0	160.0	82.0
Vitamin B$_6$ (µg)	—	—	12.0-15.0	64.0
Pantothenic acid (µg)	183.0	288.0	246.0	340.0
Biotin (µg)	0.06	0.35	0.6	2.8
Folic acid (µg)	0.05	0.02	0.14	0.13
Vitamin B$_{12}$ (µg)	0.05	0.04	0.1	0.6
Vitamin C (mg)	5.9	7.1	5.0	1.1
Vitamin D (µg)	—	—	0.04	0.02
Vitamin E (mg)	1.5	0.9	0.25	0.07
Vitamin K (µg)	—	—	1.5	6.0
Ash (g)	0.3	0.3	0.2	0.7
Calories (kcal)	57.0	63.0	65.0	65.0
Specific gravity	1050.0	1035.0	1031.0	1032.0
Milk (pH)	—	—	7.0	6.8

From Food and Nutrition Board, National Research Council, National Academy of Sciences: *Recommended dietary allowances,* ed 10, Washington, DC, 1989, US Government Printing Office.

TABLE 4-25   **Recommended daily dietary allowances of fat-soluble vitamins for infants***

Age	Weight		Height		Protein (g)	Vitamin A (µg RE)†	Vitamin D (µg)‡	Vitamin E (mg αTE)§
	(kg)	(lb)	(cm)	(in)				
To 6 mo	6	13	60	24	kg × 2.2	395	7.5	3
6 mo-1 yr	9	20	71	28	kg × 1.6	375	10	4

From Food and Nutrition Board, National Research Council, National Academy of Sciences: *Recommended dietary allowances,* ed 10, Washington, DC, 1989, US Government Printing Office.
*The allowances are intended to provide for individual variations among most normal persons as they live in the United States under usual environmental stresses. Diets should be based on a variety of common foods in order to provide other nutrients for which human requirements have been less well defined.
†Retinol equivalents. 1 RE = 1 µg retinol or 6 µg carotene.
‡As cholecalciferol, 10 µg cholecalciferol = 400 IU vitamin D.
§α-Tocopherol equivalents. 1 mg d-α-tocopherol = 1 αTE.

white mothers in a temperate climate in the winter.[200] A direct relationship was seen between maternal and infant levels of 25-OH-vitamin D$_3$ and maternal diet. An additional group of infants, whose mothers' diets were unsupplemented, received 400 IU vitamin D/day and had even higher serum concentrations of 25-OH-vitamin D$_3$. When mothers have been given large doses of vitamin D, the content of vitamin D and D$_3$ in their milk increases as it does with exposure to sunshine. The level of 25-OH-vitamin D does not change. The majority of the activity in human milk is in the form of 25-OH-vitamin D. This may be an advantage for the breastfed infant, who utilizes this form most readily. Clearly the levels vary and may be inadequate in human milk in some situations, especially in cold climates in the winter with little sunshine and for dark-skinned individuals.

Five cases of vitamin D–deficiency hypocalcemia and rickets in nonwhite infants have been reported by Chang et al[37] in exclusively breastfed infants. Serum 1,25-dihydroxyvitamin D concentrations are significantly higher in lactating compared with nonlactating women and among vegetarian compared with nonvegetarian women, reports Specker et al.[219] All lactating women in their study had elevated serum parathyroid hormone levels. The level of 40 IU/dl or 1.00 µg/dl may provide adequate amounts in the fully breastfed infant to meet the requirements of 400 IU or 10 µg/day (Table 4-25). Levels of vitamin D are also higher in colostrum than in mature milk.[143]

Vitamin E

Vitamin E has been a subject of much interest. Levels in colostrum are 1.5 mg/dl, whereas transitional milk has 0.9 mg/dl and mature milk has 0.25 mg/dl. The difference at different stages has been found to be caused by α-tocopherol, because the contents of β- and γ-tocopherol are similar. Total tocopherol in mature milk correlates with total lipid and linoleic acid contents. Significantly higher tocopherol/linoleic acid ratios are found in both colostrum and transitional milk than in mature milk.[116]

Cow's milk has 0.07 mg/dl of vitamin E (Table 4-24). Correspondingly, serum levels in breastfed infants rise quickly at birth and maintain a normal level, whereas cow's milk–fed infants have depressed levels. Vitamin E includes a group of fat-soluble compounds, α-, β-, γ-, and δ-tocopherol, and their unsaturated derivatives, α-, β-, γ-, and δ-tocotrienol. An international unit of vitamin E is equal to 1 mg of synthetic α-tocopherol or 0.74 mg of natural α-tocopherol acetate.

Vitamin E is required for muscle integrity, resistance of erythrocytes to hemolysis, and other biochemical and physiologic functions. The requirement for vitamin E is related to the PUFA content of the cellular structures and of the diet (Table 4-25). Satisfactory plasma levels are 1 mg/dl, and these can be maintained by feedings with a vitamin E/PUFA ratio of 0.4 mg/g. The requirement for infants up to age 6 months is 3 mg/day and after 6 months 4 mg/day. The requirement during lactation is 14 mg during the first 6 months and 17 mg/day after 6 months postpartum.

An estimate of the tocopherol/linoleic acid ratio in mature milk is 0.79 mg α-tocopherol equivalents/g, which is comparable to a daily requirement of 0.5 mg for term infants but may be low for premature infants, especially those receiving iron supplements.[144] Ordinarily, this would be supplied by 4 IU of vitamin E/day. Because human milk contains 1.8 mg/L or 40 µg of vitamin E/g of lipid, it supplies more than adequate levels of vitamin E.[143]

Vitamin K

Vitamin K is essential for the synthesis of blood-clotting factors, which are normal in the serum at birth. The previous levels of vitamin K reported in human milk (15 µg/dl) have been replaced with those calculated by more accurate techniques and are lower, 2.1 µg/L for mature milk and 2.3 µg/L for colostrum,[144] which is less than the recommended daily intake of 12 µg/day (Table 4-26).

The measurement of the homologs of vitamin K have been equivocal. When mothers are given a single dose of 20 mg phylloquinone (K_1), the milk level increases from 1 to 140 µg/L in 12 hours, dropping to 5 µg/L in 48 hours.[76] When infants are given 1 mg vitamin K_1 at birth, as is the practice in many countries, the concentration of K_1 in both breastfed and formula-fed infants in the first week of life remains elevated. When no neonatal prophylaxis is given, Büller et al[25] reported no

TABLE 4-26   Recommended daily dietary allowances of vitamins for infants*

Age	Vitamin K (µg)	Biotin (µg)	Pantothenic acid (mg)
To 6 mo	5 (1 µg/kg)	10	2
6 mo-1 yr	10	15	3

From Food and Nutrition Board, National Research Council, National Academy of Sciences: *Recommended dietary allowances,* ed 10, Washington, DC, 1989, US Government Printing Office.
*The allowances are intended to provide for individual variations among most normal persons as they live in the United States under usual environmental stresses. Diets should be based on a variety of common foods in order to provide other nutrients for which human requirements have been less well defined.

difference in coagulating factors among a sample of 113 breastfed, formula-fed, or combination-fed infants. They reported a case of low vitamin K levels in the milk of a mother whose infant died at 6 weeks from intracranial bleeding without neonatal prophylaxis.

Vitamin K is produced by the intestinal flora but takes several days in the previously sterile neonatal gut to be effective. Vitamin K–dependent clotting factors in normal breastfed infants were studied by Jimenez et al,[123] who reported that no infant studied had clinical evidence of bleeding. The prothrombin time and partial thromboplastin time were similar in breastfed and bottle-fed infants. The normotest and thrombotest were significantly prolonged in the breastfed group. The authors concluded that 5% of breastfed children have possible vitamin K deficiency. In several case reports,[177,178] infants exclusively breastfed with no vitamin K given at birth developed late-onset hemorrhagic disease that responded to vitamin K administration. O'Connor et al[178] note the association of vitamin K deficiency with home birth and suggest that the physician give vitamin K immediately as recommended by the American Academy of Pediatrics if it has been omitted.

At 3 months of age, 165 breastfed infants who had received 1 mg vitamin K_1 at birth had reduced serum levels of K_1. Their clotting factors were unchanged. For complete protection, Cornelissen et al[43] recommend a second oral dose of vitamin K_1 at 3 months. In a similar study, Greer et al[74] found that despite low plasma phylloquinone concentrations in the breastfed infant (less than 0.25 ng/ml) for the first 6 months, continued vitamin K_1 supplementation was not recommended. Canfield et al[30] confirm the low levels of vitamin K_1 in breastfed infants compared with those in infants fed formula containing many times the recommended daily dose (0.5 ng/day). No requirements have been set for breastfed infants. No data are available regarding the potential toxicity of excessive vitamin K.

It is recommended that all infants receive vitamin K at birth, regardless of feeding plans, to prevent hemorrhagic disease of the newborn caused by vitamin K deficiency in the first few days of life.[39]

The vitamin content of common foods has been recalculated downward so that diets of average women are probably deficient in vitamin K. Furthermore, vitamin K levels in serum of lactating women are not good markers of deficiency. Undercarboxylated prothrombin (des γ carboxy prothrombin [PIVKA]) is produced in the absence of vitamin K and is a marker of vitamin K deficiency. Greer et al[75] followed breastfed infants and found normal PIVKA at birth and 4 weeks but elevations by 8 weeks. The authors recommend maternal supplementation during lactation.

Vitamin C

Vitamin C is part of several enzyme and hormone systems, as well as of intracellular chemical reactions. It is essential to collagen synthesis (Tables 4-27 and 4-28).

TABLE 4-27	Recommended daily dietary allowances of water-soluble vitamins for infants*						
Age (yr)	Vitamin C (mg)	Thiamin (mg)	Riboflavin (mg)	Niacin (mg NE)†	Vitamin B_6 (mg)	Folacin‡ (μg)	Vitamin B_{12} (μg)
To 6 mo	30	0.3	0.4	5	0.3	25	0.3
6 mo-1 yr	35	0.4	0.5	6	0.6	35	0.5

From Food and Nutrition Board, National Research Council, National Academy of Sciences: *Recommended dietary allowances,* ed 10, Washington, DC, 1989, US Government Printing Office.
*The allowances are intended to provide for individual variations among most normal persons as they live in the United States under usual environmental stresses. Diets should be based on a variety of common foods in order to provide other nutrients for which human requirements have been less well defined.
†1 NE (niacin equivalent) is equal to 1 mg of niacin or 60 mg of dietary tryptophan.
‡The folacin allowances refer to dietary sources as determined by *Lactobacillus casei* assay after treatment with enzymes ("conjugases") to make polyglutamyl forms of the vitamin.

TABLE 4-28 Estimated secretion of nutrients in mature human milk compared with increments in Recommended Dietary Allowances (RDAs) for lactating women

A. Energy, protein, and fat-soluble vitamins

Measure	Energy, kcal	Protein, g	Vitamin A, μg RE[a]	Vitamin D, μg	Vitamin E, mg of α-TE[b]	Vitamin K, μg
Estimated secretion in milk[c]	420-700	6.3-10.5	400-670	0.3-0.6	1.4-2.3	1.3-2.1
Increment in RDAs[d,e] for following lactation periods:						
0-6 mo	500	15	500	5	4	0
6-12 mo	500	12	400	5	3	0
Comments	Estimated 80% efficiency in conversion to milk energy	Estimated 70% efficiency in conversion to milk protein	None	Increment advised in part to maintain calcium balance	Estimated 75% absorption	No increment listed because intakes usually exceed RDA

B. Water-soluble vitamins

Measure	Vitamin C, mg	Thiamin, mg	Riboflavin, mg	Niacin, mg of NE[f]	Vitamin B6, mg	Folate, μg	Vitamin B12, μg
Estimated secretion in milk[c]	24-40	0.13-0.21	0.21-0.35	0.9-1.5	0.06-0.09	50-83	0.6-1.0
Increment in RDAs[d,e] for following lactation periods							
0-6 mo	35	0.5	0.5	5	0.5	100	0.6
6-12 mo	30	0.5	0.4	5	0.5	80	0.6
Comments	Estimated 85% absorption	Increment higher than secretion because of increased energy needs	Estimated 70% utilization for milk production	Increment higher than secretion because of increased energy needs	Milk concentration used is for unsupplemented women	Estimated 50% absorption; RDA based on 50 rather than 83 μg/L	RDA based on 0.6 rather than 1.0 μg/L

c. Minerals

Measure	Calcium, mg	Phosphorus, mg	Magnesium, mg	Iron, mg	Zinc, mg	Iodine, μg	Selenium, μg
Estimated secretion in milk[c]	168-280	84-140	21-35	0.18-0.30	0.9-1.5[g] 0.3-0.5[h]	66-110	12-20
Increment in RDAs[d,e] for following lactation periods:							
0-6 mo	400	400	75	0	7	50	20
6-12 mo	400	400	60	0	4	50	20
Comments	None	Based on desired 1:1 ratio for calcium/phosphorus intake	Estimated 50% absorption	Secretion during lactation is less than menstrual loss	Estimated 20% absorption	Based on need of infant, not maternal loss in milk	Estimated 80% absorption

From Report of Nutrition During Lactation Subcommittee, Institute of Medicine: *Nutrition during lactation*, Washington, DC, 1991, National Academy Press.
[a]Retinol equivalents.
[b]α-Tocopherol equivalents.
[c]At volumes of 600-1000 ml/day, based on milk composition shown in Table 4-12.
[d]From National Research Council (NRC) (1989).
[e]Women aged 25 to 50.
[f]Niacin equivalents.
[g]0 to 6 months.
[h]6 to 12 months.

Human milk is an outstanding source of water-soluble vitamins and reflects maternal dietary intake (Table 4-25). Increased vitamin C has been measured in the milk within 30 minutes of a bolus of vitamin C being given to the mother. Human milk contains 43 mg/dl (fresh cow's milk contains up to 21 mg). Levels obtained in normal lactating women 6 months postpartum were 35 mg/L in those on normal diets and 38 mg/L in those supplemented with multivitamins containing 90 mg vitamin C.[222] Levels obtained in 16 lactating women of low-socioeconomic level were 53 mg/L for unsupplemented and 65 mg/L for supplemented mothers at 1 week postpartum and 61 mg/L and 72 mg/L, respectively, at 6 weeks postpartum. Several subjects in the unsupplemented low-socioeconomic group had levels too low to provide 35 mg vitamin C/day to their infants.

When lactating women were given 250, 500, or 1000 mg/day vitamin C for 2 days, milk levels remained within the range of 44 to 158 mg/L and did not differ significantly between dosages, even at 10 times the recommended dietary allowance (RDA).[27] Total intake of the infant through the milk ranged from 49 to 86 mg/day. These findings suggest a regulatory mechanism for vitamin C levels in milk. When women received high doses of vitamin C, levels of the vitamin excreted in the urine also increased proportionally.[183]

Vitamin B complex

Vitamin B_1. Vitamin B_1, or *thiamin,* levels increase with the duration of lactation but are lower in human milk (160 µg/dl) than in cow's milk (440 µg/dl) (Tables 4-27 and 4-28). In a study by Nail et al,[164] levels obtained by normal lactating women showed significant increases between 1 and 6 weeks postpartum, but there was no difference in levels between supplemented (1.7 mg daily) and unsupplemented women. Cases of beriberi in infants have been associated with a deficiency in the mother.

Because urinary excretion of thiamin is significantly higher in supplemented than in unsupplemented women, the amount of vitamin transferred into milk appears to be limited.[183] Malnourished women, however, do show significant increases in their milk when supplemented.[149] Thiamin is essential for the use of carbohydrates in the pyruvate metabolism (cofactor in pyruvic acid decarboxylation) and for fat synthesis. Insufficient thiamin produces insufficient carbohydrate oxidation with accumulation of intermediary metabolites such as lactic acid.

Vitamin B_2. Vitamin B_2, or *riboflavin,* is significant for the newborn in whom intestinal tract bacterial synthesis is minimal (Tables 4-27 and 4-28). Riboflavin is involved in oxidative intracellular systems and is essential for protoplasmic growth. There are 36 µg/dl in human milk and 175 µg/dl in cow's milk.

Levels obtained in normal lactating women showed significantly lower levels of riboflavin in the milk of the unsupplemented women (36.7 µg/dl) at 1 week compared with the milk of the supplemented women, who received 2 mg/day in a multivitamin (80.0 µg/dl). No significant difference was seen between 1 and 6 weeks in either group.[164]

Niacin. Niacin *(nicotinamide)* is an essential part of the pyridine nucleotide coenzymes and is part of the intracellular respiratory mechanisms. There is 147 µg/dl in human milk and 94 µg/dl in cow's milk (Tables 4-27 and 4-28). Levels respond to dietary supplementation.

Vitamin B_6. Vitamin B_6 *(pyridoxine)* forms the enzyme group of certain decarboxylases and transaminases involved in metabolism of nerve tissue. The supply of vitamin B_6 is vital to deoxyribonucleic acid (DNA) synthesis, which is needed to form the cerebrosides in the myelination of the CNS. There is 12 to 15 µg/dl of vitamin B_6 in human milk and 64 µg/dl in cow's milk (Tables 4-27 and 4-28). The principal form of B_6 in human milk is *pyridoxal* (PL), whereas pyridoxine (PN) is the principal form of vitamin B_6 fortification in infant formulas.[224] Levels of vitamin B_6 in the milk of mothers consuming more than 2.5 mg of the vitamin daily (RDA for lactating women is 2.5 mg/day) were significantly higher in the first week than were levels in the unsupplemented mothers' milk. Average maternal diets in several studies were consistently below the recommended levels of vitamin B_6.[197]

The accumulated stores of vitamin B_6 during pregnancy are significant for the maintenance of adequate vitamin B_6 status of infants during the early months of breastfeeding. For some infants, human milk alone without supplementary foods may be insufficient to meet vitamin B_6 needs after 6 months of age.[98] The recommended daily intake for infants under 6 months of age is 0.30 mg. Vitamin B_6 deficiency has been associated with CNS disorders in three breastfed infants.[134]

Long-term use of oral contraceptives has been shown to result in low levels of vitamin B_6 in maternal serum in pregnancy and at delivery and low levels in the milk of these mothers.[198] The relationship of B_6 supplements to suppression of prolactin and the treatment of galactorrhea is discussed under lactation failure (see Chapter 15). The doses used to suppress lactation (600 mg/day) far exceed the levels in multiple vitamins (1 to 10 mg) (Table 4-28).

Pantothenic acid. Pantothenic acid is part of coenzyme A, a catalyst of acetylation reactions. The reaction of coenzyme A with acetic acid to form acetyl-CoA is prime to intermediary metabolism. The levels of pantothenic acid in human milk were restudied by Johnston et al[126] because of the range of values in the literature. They found the mean to be 670 µg/dl in foremilk and hindmilk samples. No change occurred in concentrations from 1 to 6 months postpartum. They did find a positive correlation with dietary intake.

Folacin. Folacin *(folic acid)* is part of the conversion of glycine to serine. It is also involved in the methylation of nicotinamide and homocystine to methionine. It is essential for erythropoiesis (Table 4-27).

The folate (anionic form of folic acid) content of human milk produced by well-nourished women averages 80 to 130 µg/L[177] (Table 4-28). These values are substantially greater than those reported in the literature previously because of difficulty in the analysis. Folate in human milk is quantitatively bound to folate-binding proteins and presents in multiple labile forms. Folate values typically in-crease as lactation progresses and are even maintained as maternal stores begin to be depleted.

Supplementation with folic acid in deficient mothers caused prompt increase in levels in the milk. When mothers and their infants were evaluated, folate levels were two to three times higher in the breastfed infants than in their mothers, and there was a correlation between levels in the milk and in the infants' plasma.[201] Folic acid has also been identified as a critical element in deficiency states during pregnancy, being associated with abruptio placentae, toxemia, and intrauterine growth failure as well as megaloblastic anemia.

Vitamin B_{12}. Early studies reported that vitamin B_{12} is found in human milk in low concentration, 0.3 µg/dl, whereas cow's milk has 4.0 µg/ml. Well-nourished mothers on balanced diets appear to have adequate amounts for their infants. Microbiologic assay has demonstrated that very high concentrations of vitamin B_{12} appear in early colostrum but level off in a few days to those of serum. Colostric samples reported by Samson and McClelland[202] have a mean binding capacity of 72 ng/ml; in mature milk the capacity is one third of this value. Vitamin B_{12} levels were compared by Sandberg et al[203] in supplemented and unsupplemented mothers and were not significantly different. Levels were 33 to 320 ng/dl, with a mean of 97 ng/dl. When nutritionally deficient, low-socioeconomic lactating women were studied by Sneed et al,[216] supplementation with a multivitamin did result in elevated vitamin B_{12} levels. This was true for folate as well.

Although cow's milk has five to ten times more vitamin B_{12} than mature human milk, cow's milk has little vitamin B_{12}–binding capacity, which is substantial in human milk. Vitamin B_{12} functions in transmethylations such as synthesis of choline from methionine, serine from glycine, and methionine from homocysteine. It is involved in pyrimidine and purine metabolism. Vitamin B_{12} also affects the metabolism of folic acid. Megaloblastic anemia is a common symptom of vitamin B_{12} deficiency. Vitamin B_{12} occurs exclusively in animal tissue, is bound to protein, and is minimal or absent in vegetable protein.

The 1989 recommendation for the minimum daily requirement for infants is 0.3 µg/day in the first year of life, when growth is rapid (Table 4-27). Based on their data on omnivorous and vegetarian women, Specker et al[217] conclude that the current RDA for infants provides little margin for safety (Table 4-28).

Enzymes

Considerable data have been collected on the enzymatic activities of many milks. Jenness and Sloan[118] report 44 enzymes detected in bovine, human, and other milks. Xanthine oxidase, lactoperoxidase, uridine diphosphogalactose, galactosyl transferase, ribonuclease, lipase, alkaline phosphatase, acid phosphatase, and lysozyme have been isolated in crystalline form.

The role and significance of enzymes in human milk were reviewed by Hamosh,[85] who confirmed that more than 20 active human milk enzymes exist (Table 4-29). They can be categorized into three general groups by their activity: *mammary gland function,* which reflects physiologic changes occurring in the mammary gland itself during lactation; *compensatory digestive enzymes* in human milk, which have digestive functions in the neonate; and *milk enzymes,* important in stimulating neonatal development.[85] Some enzyme levels are significantly higher in colostrum than in mature milk. Most are whey proteins and contribute minimally to milk proteins. Some enzymes, like other proteins in milk, are probably produced elsewhere and transported to the breast via the bloodstream.[112]

The evidence to support the concept of local synthesis includes the demonstration of secretory

TABLE 4-29   Enzyme functions in human milk

Function	Enzyme	Process
Biosynthesis of milk components in mammary gland	Phosphoglucomutase	Synthesis of lactose
	Lactose synthetase	
	Fatty acid synthetase	Synthesis of medium-chain fatty acids
	Thioesterase	
	Lipoprotein lipase	Uptake of circulating triglyceride fatty acids
Digestive function in infant	Amylase	Hydrolysis of polysaccharides
	Lipase (bile salt dependent)	Hydrolysis of triglycerides
	Proteases	Proteolysis (not verified)
Transport	Xanthine oxidase	Carrier of iron, molybdenum
	Glutathione peroxidase	Carrier of selenium
	Alkaline phosphatase	Carrier of zinc, magnesium
Preservation of milk components	Antiprotease	Protection of bioactive proteins, i.e., enzymes and immunoglobulins
	Sulfhydryl oxidase	Maintenance of structure and function of proteins containing disulfide bonds
Antiinfective agents	Lysozyme	Bactericidal
	Peroxidase	Bactericidal
	Lipases (lipoprotein lipase, bile salt–dependent lipase)	Release of free fatty acids that have antibacterial, antiviral, and antiprotozoan actions

From Hamosh M: Enzymes in human milk: their role in nutrient digestion, gastrointestinal function and nutrient delivery to the newborn infant. In Lebenthal E, editor: *Textbook of gastroenterology and nutrition in infancy,* ed 2, New York, 1989, Raven.

tissue in the mammary gland. Amylase levels are twice as high in milk as in serum.[99,147] Casein proteins have been synthesized in vitro in cell-free mammary-derived messenger ribonucleic acid (mRNA)–enriched systems. Mammary explants from mice, monkeys, and humans have accumulated lactose synthetase B. The enzymes of possible importance in infant digestion are those with pancreatic analogs: amylase, lipases, protease(s), and ribonuclease.[208]

Amylase

Amylase, the chief polysaccharide-digesting enzyme, is not developed at birth even in full-term infants, who have only 0.2% to 0.5% of adult values. Mammary amylase is present, however, throughout lactation, with levels higher in colostrum than in mature milk. Human milk levels are 0.5 to 1.0 g/dl oligosaccharides of varying chain length. Milk levels of preterm mothers are comparable to term milk levels.

Milk levels are twice those of serum in the first 90 days and remain higher than serum over 6 months. When exposed to a pH of 5.3, this salivary-type amylase remains active; at a pH of 3.5, one half the original activity is present at 2 hours and one third at 6 hours. Amylase is stable at −20° to −70° C (−4° to −94° F) for storage and at least for 24 hours at 15° to 38° C (59° to 100° F). Much milk amylase activity remains in the duodenum after a meal of human milk. This is significant for the digestion of starch because pancreatic amylase is still low in infants. Mammary amylase may be an alternate pathway of digestion of glucose polymers, as well as of starch (Table 4-30).

Milk amylase is part of the isozyme group as

TABLE 4-30   Characteristics of milk enzymes active in infant digestion

Characteristic	Enzyme	
	Amylase	BSSL*
High parity (≥10)	Low activity	?
Malnutrition	?	Decrease in activity
Diurnal and within feed activity	Constant	Constant
Prepartum	?	Present
Presence in preterm (PT) and term (T) milk	Equal activity PT and T	Equal activity PT and T
Pattern through lactation	Colostrum greater than milk	Colostrum lower than milk
Weaning	?	Activity constant independent of milk volume
Distribution in milk	Aqueous phase	Aqueous phase
Effect of milk storage		
−20° to −70° C	Stable	Stable
15 to 38° C	Stable (at least 24 hr)	Stable (at least 24 hr)
Stability to low pH (passage through stomach)	pH >3.0	pH >3.0
Optimum pH	6.5-7.5	7.4-8.5
Enzyme characteristics	Salivary amylase isozyme	Identical with pancreatic carboxyl ester hydrolase
Evidence of activity in infant's intestine	Yes	Yes
Presence in milk of other species	?	Primates and carnivores

Modified from Hamosh M: Enzymes in human milk. In Jensen RG, editor: *Handbook of milk composition,* San Diego, 1995, Academic Press.
BSSL, Bile salt–stimulated lipase.

salivary amylase and is thought to inhibit the growth of certain microorganisms.

Lipases

Milk fat is almost completely digestible. The emulsion of fat in breast milk is greater than in cow's milk, resulting in smaller globules. Milk lipases play an active role in creating the emulsion, which yields a finer curd and facilitates the digestion of triacylglycerols (TGs). The newborn easily digests and completely uses the well-emulsified small fat globules of human milk. Free fatty acids are important sources of energy for the infant.

Lipase in human milk was first described in 1901. At least two different lipases (glycerol ester hydrolases) were described then. The lipases in human milk make the free fatty acids available in a large proportion even before the digestive phase of the intestine. The lipolytic milk-enzyme activity is similar to the activity of pancreatic lipase, breaking down triglycerides to free fatty acids and glycerol. One enzyme is present in the fat fraction and is inhibited by bile salts.[88]

Milk from underprivileged mothers may lose some of its ability to hydrolyze milk lipid esters over the course of lactation; this ability remains constant in well-nourished mothers.[56] This would have an effect on the utilization of the esters of lipid-soluble vitamins A, D, and E.

It appears that the function of this enzyme, inhibited by bile salts, is to facilitate the uptake by the mammary gland of fatty acids from circulating triglycerides for incorporation with milk lipids, because lipase in vivo depends on added serum for activity. Its presence in milk probably represents "leakage" from the mammary gland, and it is unlikely to play a major physiologic role in the lipolysis of milk triglycerides.[100]

Additional lipases in the skim milk fraction are stimulated by bile salts. *Bile salt–stimulated lipase* (BSSL) has greater activity and splits all three ester bonds of the triglyceride. This lipase is also stable in the duodenum and contributes to the hydrolysis of the TGs in the presence of the bile salts.[100]

BSSL is identical to carboxyl ester hydrolase (carboxylesterase), a pancreatic enzyme. BSSL activity is lower in colostrum than in mature milk. No correlation appears to exist between the volume of milk at various stages and the volume of enzyme secreted.[67] BSSL is present in early prepartum secretions less than 2 months before delivery and in the milk expressed during weaning. For a given well-nourished woman, levels remain stable even after prolonged lactation. BSSL activity is protective against infection by virtue of the production of free fatty acids and monoglycerides, products of fat digestion that have antiinfective properties[67] (Table 4-30).

The enzyme activity of BSSL is remarkably stable during prolonged storage up to 2 years at either $-20°$ C or $-70°$ C ($-4°$ to $-94°$ F). It has also been noted to be stable at 15°, 25°, and 38° C (59°, 77°, and 100° F).[89]

Contrary to earlier suggestions, no association exists between jaundice and increased levels of free fatty acids produced as a result of high activity of milk lipase.[67]

Investigators have continued to study the action of these lipases in the presence of bile salts.[81,82,100,101] The BSSL remains active during passage through the stomach because it is stable above pH 3.5 and only slowly inactivated by pepsin. The optimal bile salt concentration for activity is about 2 mmol/L, which is within the physiologic range in the newborn. Bile salts protect the enzyme from tryptic activity.[100]

Glucose-6-phosphate dehydrogenase

Glucose-6-phosphate dehydrogenase (G-6-PD) is rich in the milk of mothers with normal red blood cell dehydrogenase and absent in mothers with G-6-PD deficiency. Its levels depend on the increased rate of carbohydrate metabolism in the mammary gland.[208]

Lactic and malic acid dehydrogenases

Lactic and malic acid dehydrogenase levels are high in colostrum, are lower in mature milk, and increase at the end of a feeding. The levels are higher in species with small body size; thus mice and humans have more than cows.[16] Because no correlation exists with serum levels, they are thought to be synthesized in the mammary gland. A change occurs in these enzymes during lactation.

Lactose synthetase

Lactose synthetase catalyzes the synthesis of lactose from UDP-galactose and glucose. This enzyme has two components: A-protein, a glycoprotein, and B-protein, an α-lactalbumin. The control mechanism for lactose biosynthesis by the A-protein and α-lactalbumin ensures that lactose is synthesized in the mammary gland only in response to specific hormones.

Lysozyme

Lysozyme is a thermostable, nonspecific antimicrobial factor that catalyzes the hydrolysis of β-linkage between N-acetylglucosamine and N-acetylmuramic acid in the bacterial cell wall. It is bacteriolytic toward Enterobacteriaeceae and gram-positive bacteria and is considered to play a role in the antibacterial activity of milk as well as a significant role in the development of intestinal flora. It also hydrolyzes mucopolysaccharides. Human lysozyme is antigenically and serologically different from the bovine enzyme. The content in human milk is 3000 times that in bovine milk and the activity 100 times that of bovine milk. Lysozyme is considered to be a spillover product from breast epithelial cells.

Phosphatases

Acid phosphatase is similar in human and bovine milk, but alkaline phosphatase is much less active in human milk by a factor of 40. Its level increases with the increase in fat concentration and increases as the feeding progresses. In 199 samples from 20 donors, no relationship to age, nationality, or other characteristics of the donor was found, except for a tendency to increase over time. Alkaline phosphatase concentrations appeared to be related to the fat concentration in human milk. Levels increased as lactation progressed.[2] Alkaline phosphatase is a metal-carrying enzyme with four zinc molecules and two magnesium atoms. It differs from the placental alkaline phosphatase.

Proteases and antiproteases

Several enzymes have caseinolytic activity and elastase-like activity. β-Casein and V-casein and galactothermin are probably the byproducts of endogenous human milk proteolytic activity.[90] There are also small peptides of only three to eight amino acids derived from casein group called β casomorphins with specific physiologic activity. These peptides may be associated with the sleeping patterns of neonates and even have relevance to postpartum psychosis.[148]

Proteases catalyze the hydrolysis of proteins. High levels of protease are found in human milk, which suggests that enzymes may provide the breastfed infant with significant digestive assistance immediately after birth.

Antiproteases' physiologic role is not entirely clear. The main protease inhibitors in human milk are α_1-antichymotrypsin and α_1-antitrypsin.[88] Trace amounts of others have been identified. One function may be to protect the mammary gland from local proteolytic activity by leukocytic and lysosomal proteases during different stages of lactogenesis. They may prevent the breakdown of proteins in stored milk.[90] The protection of immunoglobulins that are transferred intact to the neonate and the protection of growth hormones are probably other roles of the antiproteases. The presence of such inhibitors may restrain the invading bacterial enzymes in the host tissue (breast) or secretion (milk). Thus the presence of these inhibitors may protect the mammary gland and the recipient infant from infection.

Xanthine oxidase

Xanthine oxidase catalyzes the oxidation of purines, pyrimidines, and aldehydes. Although bovine milk contains high levels, it was only after much effort that investigators were able to identify it in human milk.[233] The activity in human milk peaks on the third day after birth and decreases with the progression of lactation. It differs from that in bovine milk in that it is not of bacterial origin and its activity is correlated with protein concentration.

• • •

Many enzymes are being studied in the human and other species. See Table 4-29 for a summary of the most significant. For an extensive discussion, see Hamosh.[88]

Hormones

Protein hormones, especially prolactin, and steroid hormones, such as gestagens, estrogens, corticords, androgens, and opiate-like peptides, can be detected in human milk and in the milk of other mammals.[206] Animal studies have shown that at least some of these hormones retain physiologic activity when ingested but not when pasteurized. Although their presence was recognized in the 1930s, advances in hormone assay techniques have brought more information to light.[135] Hormones with simple structures, such as steroids and *thyroxine* (T_4), can pass easily by diffusion into the milk from circulating blood. Peptide hormones such as hypothalamic-releasing hormones, because of their small size, also would be expected to appear in milk. Of the larger-molecular-weight pituitary hormones, only prolactin has been found so far. The hormones identified in human milk include gonadotropin-releasing hormone, thyroid-releasing hormone (TRH), thyroid-stimulating hormone (thyrotropin, TSH), prolactin, gonadotropins, ovarian hormones, corticosteroids, erythropoietin, cyclic adenosine monophosphate (cAMP), and cyclic guanosine monophosphate (cGMP) (Tables 4-31, 4-32).

The concentration of hormones changes during lactation, with prolactin decreasing over time and *triiodothyronine* (T_3) and T_4 increasing. Evidence indicates that the gastrointestinal tract of suckling mammals possesses the ability to absorb various proteins with substantial preservation of their immunologic properties. The absorption of large-molecular-weight hormones has been demon-

TABLE 4-31   **Nonpeptide hormones in human milk**

Hormone	Concentration (ng/ml)
Thyroid	
Thyroxine (T_4)	1-4
	0.3-2.0
	12.0
	1.16-2.4
	0.8-2.3
Triiodothyronine (T_3)	0.02-0.40
	0.05-0.10
Reverse T_3	0.008-0.15
Adrenal gland:	
Cortisol	0.2-32.0 (5:10)*
	3.7
Sexual	
Progesterone	10-40
Pregnanediol	0-450
Estrogens	15-840 (15:60)*
Contraceptives	Biologically significant quantities

*Ratio of values in colostrum/values in mature milk.
Modified from Koldovsky O, Strbak V: Hormones and growth factors in human milk. In Jensen RG, editor: *Handbook of milk composition,* San Diego, 1995, Academic Press.

strated in suckling rats and mice, with measurable amounts appearing in serum and other tissues.

The thyroid hormones have received considerable attention because of the apparent protection of hypothyroid infants who are breastfed. TSH content was investigated by both direct ^{125}I-TSH radioimmunoassay and radioimmunoassay.[221] TSH was present in human milk in low concentrations comparable to those normally found in the serum of euthyroid adults. Experimentally, thyroidectomy of the lactating rat led to the disappearance of measurable T_4 and an increase in the level of TSH in the milk. In contrast, administration of T_3 decreased the TSH in the rat model.

Prolactin has been identified as a normal constituent of human milk. Levels are high in the first few days postpartum but subsequently decline rapidly. "Prolactin-like" biologic activity is measurable in human colostrum, with the highest levels

TABLE 4-32 **Hormonally active peptides in human milk**		
Peptide	Concentration	Ratio (colostrum/ mature milk)
Erythropoietin	Bioassay	?
Growth factors		
Epidermal growth factor (EGF)	3-107 ng/ml	2:10
Insulin	0-80 µU/ml	3:10
Insulin-like growth factor 1 (IGF-1)	1.3-7 ng/ml	2:3
Nerve growth factor (NGF)	Present	
Transforming growth factor alpha (TGF-α)	0-8.4 ng/ml	1
Other growth factors	Present	?
Gastrointestinal regulatory peptides		
Gastrin	10-30 pg/ml	2:3
Gastric inhibitory peptide (GIP)	33-59 ng/ml	1
Gastric regulatory peptide (GRP)	55-31 pg/ml 60-430 pg/ml	2:3
Neurotensin	7-15 pg/ml	2:3
Peptide histidine methionine (PHM)	3-32 pg/ml	5:10
Peptide YY (PYY)	15-30 pg/ml	2:3

Modified from Koldovsky O, Strbak V: Hormones and growth factors in human milk. In Jensen RG, editor: *Handbook of milk composition,* San Diego, 1995, Academic Press.

on day 1. Concentrations in the milk tend to parallel concentrations in the blood plasma among different species. Three stages of neuroendocrine development are theorized: placental, milk, and autonomous, in which the milk phase is the adaptation to extrauterine life.[87]

The exact mechanism by which prolactin enters the milk is unclear. Prolactin-binding sites have been identified within the alveolar cells.[95] The functional significance of prolactin also remains unclear. In rodents, milk prolactin influences fluid and ion absorption from the jejunum. It also may influence gonadal and adrenal function, as demonstrated in other species.

Endocrine responses in the neonate differ between breastfed and formula-fed infants.[152] In a study of 34 healthy, 6-day-old full-term infants who were formula fed, plasma concentrations of insulin, motilin, enteroglucagon, neurotensin, and pancreatic polypeptide changed significantly after a feeding. Similar levels were measured in 43 normal breastfed infants, and little or no change was noted. Further, the basal levels of gastric inhibitory polypeptide, motilin, neurotensin, and vasoactive intestinal peptide were also higher in the bottle-fed than in the breastfed infants. Whether pancreatic and gut hormone-release changes affect postnatal development is yet to be determined.

Prostaglandins

In the investigation of the factors in human milk that may modify or supplement physiologic functions in the neonate, the role of prostaglandins comes under review. Prostaglandins include any of a class of physiologically active substances present in many tissues and originally described in genital fluid and accessory glands. Among the many effects are those of vasodepression, stimulation of intestinal smooth muscle, uterine stimulation, aggregation of blood platelets, and antagonism to hormones influencing lipid metabolism. Prostaglandins are a group of prostanoic acids often abbreviated PGE, PGF, PGA, and PGB with numeric subscripts according to structure.

The synthesis of prostaglandins occurs when dietary linoleic acid is converted in the body by a series of steps involving chain lengthening and dehydration to arachidonic acid, the principal (but not the only) precursor of prostaglandins. Although the prostaglandins are similar in structure, the biologic effects of various prostaglandins produced from a single unsaturated fatty acid can be profoundly different and, in some cases, antagonistic.

Because of the possible beneficial effects of prostaglandins on the gastrointestinal (GI) tract of infants, several investigators[6,153,194] have measured levels in human milk. The measurements were made in colostrum, transitional milk, and mature milk with collections of both foremilk and hindmilk. PGE and PGF have been shown to be present in breast milk in more than 100 times the concentration in adult plasma (Fig. 4-10). The ratio of the principal metabolite of PGFM to PGF itself suggests a relatively long half life. Although prostaglandins occur in cow's milk, none was measurable in cow's milk–based formulas. Two inactive metabolites were found in milk in levels similar to those in the control adult plasma.

It is thought that prostaglandins play a role in gastrointestinal motility, possibly assisting peristalsis physiologically. Infantile diarrhea may occasionally be caused by excessive prostaglandin secretion into the mother's milk during menstruation, when maternal plasma levels of PGF may be raised. The difference in stool patterns between infants who are breastfed versus formula fed may be partially attributable to the presence of prostaglandins in human milk and not in formulas. The role of prostaglandins in the pathogenesis of food intolerance is also under study, because prostaglandins have a cytoprotective effect on the upper bowel and reportedly are increased in patients with abnormal peristalsis and irritable bowel syndrome.[145]

Prostaglandins E_1, E_2, and $F_{2\alpha}$ (PGE_1, PGE_2, $PGF_{2\alpha}$) were determined in milk and plasma from mothers of term and preterm infants by Shimizu et al.[210] They found the concentration of PGE_1 in milk to be similar to that in plasma and the concentrations of PGE_2 and $PGF_{2\alpha}$ to be about 1.2 to 2 times higher in milk than in plasma. On the other hand, foremilk and hindmilk levels were similar, as were term and preterm levels. Levels appeared to be constant throughout lactation. PGE_1 is credited with a variety of physiologic effects on the GI tract, including cytoprotection and a diarrhea-producing action. Other actions are expected and yet to be identified because of prostaglandins' stability throughout lactation and lack of degradation in milk and in the lumen of the gut.

Fig. 4-10.   Prostaglandins E and F (PGE, PGF) (pg/ml ± SEM) in human milk and adult plasma. (From Lucas A, Mitchell MD: *Arch Dis Child* 55:950, 1980.)

In addition, the human infant may require PGE_2 for maintenance of gastric mucosal integrity, as do adults. Therefore it is not surprising that the use of prostaglandin synthesis inhibitors, such as indomethacin for closure of a patent ductus, is associated with necrotizing enterocolitis. PGE_2 in human milk may also promote the accumulation of phospholipids in the neonatal stomach, enhancing the gastric mucosal barrier.

Relaxin

Relaxin is a hormone with a polypeptide structure similar to that of insulin. It is produced by the corpus luteum during pregnancy as well as by the decidua and the placenta. Relaxin induces cervical softening, loosens the pelvic girdle, and decreases myometrial activity during pregnancy in many species.[57] Its role in humans remains under study.

It has been postulated that human mammary tissue is a target and a source of relaxin synthesis. Relaxin was measured by specific human relaxin radioimmunoassay in milk and sera of women delivering at term, prematurely at 3 days, and at 6 weeks postpartum.[57] Sera and milk levels were similar in term and preterm mothers; however, at 6 weeks, relaxin concentrations in milk were higher in the preterm group. The presence in milk at 6 weeks suggests a nonluteal site of synthesis. The authors suggest that before lactation, relaxin may aid the growth and differentiation of mammary tissue and then in the neonate act directly on the GI tract.

Bile salts

Another limiting factor in digestion in the newborn is the decreased bile salt pool and the low concentration of bile salts in the duodenum. The presence of some biologically active substances in human milk contributes to digestion in the newborn. For this reason, the role of bile salts was investigated, and cholate and chenodeoxycholate were found in all samples of milk obtained from 28 lactating women in the first postpartum week.[68] In both colostrum and milk, cholate predominated. Samples were randomly collected, and the range of concentration was wide. The ratio of maternal serum to milk levels was 1:1 for cholate and 4:1 for chenodeoxycholate. The significance of these findings is under study.

Epidermal growth factor

Epidermal growth factor (EGF) is a small polypeptide mitogen that has been identified in many species and isolated and characterized in human milk. Of the growth factors that have been purified to date, EGF is one of the most biologically potent and best characterized as to its physical, chemical, and biologic properties. It is well established that EGF stimulates the proliferation of epidermal and epithelial tissues and has significant biologic effects in the intact mammal, particularly in the fetus and the newborn.[32] Effects verified in humans also include increased growth and maturation of the fetal pulmonary epithelium, stimulation of ornithine decarboxylase activity and DNA synthesis in the digestive tract, and acceleration of the healing of wounds of the corneal epithelium. Quite unrelated is the observation that EGF inhibits histamine- or pentagastrin-induced secretion of gastric acid. It has a maturational effect on duodenal mucosal cells and increased lactase activity and net calcium transport in suckling rats. EGF has been identified in plasma, saliva, urine, amniotic fluid, and milk. Human milk is known to be mitogenic for cultured cells. EGF is active when administered orally, stable in acid, and resistant to trypsin digestion.

Newborn puppies, fed their mother's milk, were found to have hyperplasia of the enteric mucosa as compared with formula-fed littermates. Furthermore, the intestinal weight, length, and DNA and RNA content were greater in the puppies fed their mother's milk.

Studies of EGF in human milk first reported that human milk stimulates DNA synthesis in cell cultures in which growth had been arrested.[159] The mitogenic activity of the milk was neutralized by the addition of antibody to human EGF. These findings support the concept that EGF is a major growth-promoting agent in breast milk. Actual measurements of EGF in the milk of 11 mothers who delivered at term and 20 who delivered prematurely were also done. EGF concentrations were 68 ± 19 ng/ml (mean $\pm$ SEM) in those who delivered at term and 70 ± 5 ng/ml (mean $\pm$ SEM) in the milk of those who delivered prematurely. There was no significant change over 7 weeks and no diurnal variation. The total EGF content was closely correlated with the volume of milk expressed, suggesting to the authors that EGF has a passive transport from the circulation as a function of plasma concentration.[32,159]

Using various techniques for assay, Iacopetta et al[108] found 30 to 40 ng/ml in human milk, less than 2 ng/ml in bovine milk, and none in several bovine milk–based formulas. Little change occurred with refrigeration or freezing. The role of EGF in promoting normal growth and functional maturation of the intestinal tract continues under study.

REFERENCES

1. Abrams SA, Wen J, Stuff JE: Absorption of calcium, zinc and iron from breast milk by five-to-seven-month-old infants, *Pediatr Res* 41:384, 1996.
2. Adcock EW, Brewer ED, Caprioli RM et al: Macronutrients, electrolytes and minerals in human milk: differences over time and between population groups. In Howell RR, Morriss FH, Pickering LK, editors: *Human milk in infant nutrition and health,* Springfield, Ill, 1986, Charles C. Thomas.
3. Alaejos MS, Romero CD: Selenium in human lactation, *Nutr Rev* 53:159, 1995.
4. Allen JC, Keller RP, Archer P et al: Studies in human lactation: milk composition and daily secretion rates of macronutrients in the first year of lactation, *Am J Clin Nutr* 54:69, 1991.
5. Almroth SG: Water requirements of breastfed infants in a hot climate, *Am J Clin Nutr* 31:1154, 1978.
6. Alzina V, Puig M, de Echániz L et al: Prostaglandins in human milk, *Biol Neonate* 50:200, 1986.
7. Anaokar SG, Garry PJ: Effects of maternal iron nutrition during lactation on milk iron and rat neonatal iron status, *Am J Clin Nutr* 34:1505, 1981.
8. Anderson RA, Bryden NA, Patterson KY et al: Breast milk chromium and its association with chromium intake, chromium excretion and serum chromium, *Am J Clin Nutr* 57:519, 1993.
9. Anderson RR: Variations in major minerals of human milk during the first 5 months of lactation, *Nutr Res* 12:701, 1992.
10. Ando K, Goto Y, Matsumoto Y et al: Acquired zinc deficiency in a breast-fed mature infant: a possible cause of acquired maternal decreased zinc uptake by the mammary gland, *J Am Acad Dermatol* 29:111, 1993.
11. Asnes RS, Wisotsky DH, Migel PF et al: The dietary chloride deficiency syndrome occurring in a breast-fed infant, *J Pediatr* 100:923, 1982.
12. Atkinson S, Alston-Mills B, Lönnerdal B et al: Major minerals and ionic constituents of human and bovine milks. In Jensen RG, editor: *Handbook of milk composition,* San Diego, 1995, Academic Press.
13. Atkinson SA, Bryan MH, Anderson GH: Human milk: differences in nitrogen concentration in milk from mothers of term and premature infants, *J Pediatr* 93:67, 1978.
14. Atkinson SA, Lönnerdal B: Non protein nitrogen fractions of human milk. In Jensen RG, editor: *Handbook of milk composition,* San Diego, 1995, Academic Press.
15. Atkinson SA, Whelan D, Whyte RK et al: Abnormal zinc content in human milk, *Am J Dis Child* 143:608, 1989.
16. Auricchio S, Rubino A, Mürset E: Intestinal glycosidase activities in the human embryo, fetus, and newborn, *Pediatrics* 35:944, 1965.
17. Barness LA, Carver J: Nucleotides and immune function, *Semin Gastroenterol Nutr* 2:11, 1991.
18. Barth CA, Roos N, Nottbohm B et al: L-Carnitine concentrations in milk from mothers on different diets. In Schaub J, editor: *Composition and physiological properties of human milk,* Amsterdam, 1985, Elsevier.
19. Birch EE, Birch DG, Hoffman DR et al: Dietary essential fatty acid supply and visual activity development, *Invest Ophthalmol Vis Sci* 33:3242, 1992.
20. Bitman J, Wood DL, Mehta NR et al: Comparison of the phospholipid composition of breast milk from mothers of term and preterm infants during lactation, *Am J Clin Nutr* 40:1103, 1984.
21. Bitman J, Wood DL, Neville MC et al: Lipid composition of prepartum, preterm and term milk. In Hamosh M, Goldman AS, editors: *Human lactation,* vol 2, *Maternal and environmental factors,* New York, 1986, Plenum.
22. Brown KH, Black RE, Robertson AD et al: Clinical and field studies of human lactation: methodological considerations, *Am J Clin Nutr* 35:745, 1982.
23. Buescher ES, McIlheran SM: Antioxidant properties of human colostrum, *Pediatr Res* 24:14, 1988.
24. Buescher ES, McIlheran SM: Colostral antioxidants: separation and characterization of two activities in human colostrum, *J Pediatr Gastroenterol Nutr* 14:47, 1992.
25. Büller H, Peters M, Burger B et al: Vitamin K status beyond the neonatal period, *Eur J Pediatr* 145:496, 1986.

26. Butte NF, Garza C, Smith EO: Macro- and trace mineral intakes of exclusively breastfed infants, *Am J Clin Nutr* 45:42, 1987.
27. Byerley LO, Kirksey A: Effects of different levels of vitamin C intake on the vitamin C concentration in human milk and the vitamin C intakes of breastfed infants, *Am J Clin Nutr* 41:665, 1985.
28. Calvo EB, Galindo AC, Aspres ND: Iron status in exclusively breastfed infants, *Pediatrics* 90:375, 1992.
29. Canfield LM, Giuliano AR, Neilson EM et al: Beta carotene in breast milk and serum is increased after a single beta carotene dose, *Am J Clin Nutr* 66:52, 1997.
30. Canfield LM, Hopkinson JM, Lima AF et al: Vitamin K in colostrum and mature human milk over the lactational period: a cross-sectional study, *Am J Clin Nutr* 53:730, 1991.
31. Carlson SE: Human milk nonprotein nitrogen: occurrence and possible function, *Adv Pediatr* 32:43, 1985.
32. Carpenter G: Epidermal growth factor is a major growth-promoting agent in human milk, *Science* 210:198, 1980.
33. Casey CE, Hambidge KM: Nutritional aspects of human lactation. In Neville MC, Neifert MR, editors: *Lactation, physiology, nutrition, and breastfeeding,* New York, 1983, Plenum.
34. Casey CE, Neville MC: Studies in human lactation. 3. Molybdenum and nickel in human milk during the first month of lactation, *Am J Clin Nutr* 45:921, 1987.
35. Casey CE, Smith A, Zhang PC: Microminerals in human and animal milks. In Jensen RG, editor: *Handbook of milk composition,* San Diego, 1995, Academic Press.
36. Casey CE, Walravens PA, Hambidge KM: Availability of zinc: loading tests with human milk, cow's milk, and infant formulas, *Pediatrics* 68:394, 1981.
37. Chang YT, Germain-Lee EL, Doran TF et al: Hypocalcemia in non-white breastfed infants, *Clin Pediatr* 31:695, 1992.
38. Chu SW: Nucleotides: biochemistry and metabolism, *Semin Gastroenterol Nutr* 2:11, 1991.
39. Committee on Nutrition, American Academy of Pediatrics: Vitamin K supplementation for infants, *Pediatrics* 48:483, 1971.
40. Committee on Nutrition, American Academy of Pediatrics: Nutrition and lactation, *Pediatrics* 68:435, 1981.
41. Committee on Nutrition, American Academy of Pediatrics: Sodium intake of infants in the United States, *Pediatrics* 68:445, 1981.
42. Coppa GV, Gabrielli O, Pierani P et al: Changes in carbohydrate composition in human milk over 4 months of lactation, *Pediatrics* 91:637, 1993.
43. Cornelissen EAM, Kollee LAA, DeAbreu RA et al: Effects of oral and intramuscular vitamin K prophylaxis on vitamin K_1, PIVKA-II and clotting factors in breastfed infants, *Arch Dis Child* 67:1250, 1992.
44. Cross NA, Hillman LS, Allen SH et al: Calcium homeostasis and bone metabolism during pregnancy, lactation, and post weaning: a longitudinal study, *Am J Clin Nutr* 61:514, 1995.
45. Dale G, Goldfinch ME, Sibert JR et al: Plasma osmolality, sodium, and urea in healthy breastfed and bottle-fed infants in Newcastle upon Tyne, *Arch Dis Child* 50:731, 1975.
46. Davies DP, Saunders R: Blood urea: normal values in early infancy related to feeding practices, *Arch Dis Child* 48:563, 1973.
47. Dearlove JC, Dearlove BM: Prolactin, fluid balance, and lactation, *Br J Obstet Gynaecol* 88:652, 1981.
48. DeSantiago S, Villalpando S, Ortiz N et al: Protein requirements of marginally nourished lactating women, *Am J Clin Nutr* 62:364, 1995.
49. Dewey KG, Heinig MJ, Nommsen LA et al: Maternal versus infant factors related to breast milk intake and residual milk volume: the DARLING Study, *Pediatrics* 87:829, 1991.
50. DeWille JW, Farmer SJ: Postnatal dietary fat influences mRNAs involved in myelination, *Dev Neurosci* 14:61, 1992.
51. Dial EJ, Lichtenberger LM: Gastric protective properties of human milk. In Howell RR, Morriss FH, Pickering LK, editors: *Human milk in infant nutrition and health,* Springfield, Ill, 1986, Charles C Thomas.
52. Dick G: The etiology of multiple sclerosis, *Proc R Soc Med* 69:611, 1976.
53. Dorea JG: Is zinc a first limiting nutrient in human milk? *Nutr Res* 13:659, 1993.
54. Dumas BR: Modifications of human milk composition during early states of lactation in nutritional adaptations of the gastrointestinal tract of the newborn. In Kretchmer N, Minkowski A, editors: *Nutritional adaptation of GI tract of the newborn,* vol 3, New York, 1983, Nestlé, Vevey/Raven.
55. Duncan B, Schifman RB, Corrigan JJ et al: Iron and the exclusively breastfed infant from birth to six months, *J Pediatr Gastroenterol* 4:421, 1985.
56. Dupuy P, Sauniere JF, Vis HL et al: Change in bile salt dependent lipase in human breast milk during extended lactation, *Lipids* 26:134, 1991.
57. Eddie LW, Sutton B, Fitzgerald S et al: Relaxin in paired samples of serum and milk from women after term and preterm delivery, *Am J Obstet Gynecol* 161:970, 1989.
58. Ekstrand J, Spak CJ, Falch J et al: Distribution of fluoride to human breast milk following intake of high doses of fluoride, *Caries Res* 18:93, 1984.
59. Fall CHD, Barker DJP, Osmond C et al: Relation of infant feeding to adult serum cholesterol concentration and death from ischaemic heart disease, *Br Med J* 304:801, 1992.
60. Farquharson J, Cockburn F, Patrick WA et al: Infant cerebral cortex phospholipid fatty-acid composition and diet, *Lancet* 340:810, 1992.
61. Feeley RM, Eitenmiller RR, Jones JB et al: Copper, iron, and zinc contents of human milk at early stages of lactation, *Am J Clin Nutr* 37:443, 1983.
62. Ferris AM, Jensen RG: Lipids in human milk: a review. I. Sampling, determination and content, *J Pediatr Gastroenterol Nutr* 3:108, 1984.

63. Finley DA, Lönnerdal B, Dewey KG et al: Breast milk composition: fat content and fatty acid composition in vegetarians and non-vegetarians, *Am J Clin Nutr* 41:787, 1985.

64. Fomon SJ: *Infant nutrition,* ed 2, Philadelphia, 1974, Saunders.

65. Food and Nutrition Board, National Research Council, National Academy of Sciences: *Recommended dietary allowances,* ed 10, Washington, DC, 1989, US Government Printing Office.

66. Forfar JO: Calcium, phosphorus, magnesium metabolism. In Forfar JO, editor: Aspects of neonatal metabolism, *Clin Endocrinol Metab* 5:123, 1976.

67. Forsyth JS, Donnet L, Ross PE: A study of the relationship between bile salts, bile salt stimulated lipase, and free fatty acids in breast milk: normal infants and those with breast milk jaundice, *J Pediatr Gastroenterol Nutr* 11:205, 1990.

68. Forsyth JS, Ross PE, Bouchier IAD: Bile salts in breast milk, *Eur J Pediatr* 140:126, 1983.

69. Fransson GB, Lönnerdal B: Iron in human milk, *J Pediatr* 96:380, 1980.

70. Fransson GB, Lönnerdal B: Zinc, copper, calcium and magnesium in human milk, *J Pediatr* 101:504, 1982.

71. Gaull GE: Taurine in the nutrition of the human infant, *Acta Paediatr Scand Suppl* 269:38, 1982.

72. Gibson RA, Kneebore GM: Fatty acid composition of human colostrum and mature breast milk, *Am J Clin Nutr* 34:252, 1981.

73. Gil A, Uauy R: Nucleotides and related compounds in human and bovine milk. In Jensen RG, editor: *Handbook of milk composition,* San Diego, 1995, Academic Press.

74. Greer FR, Marshall S, Cherry J et al: Vitamin K status of lactating mothers, human milk, and breastfeeding infants, *Pediatrics* 88:751, 1991.

75. Greer FR, Marshal SP, Foley AL et al: Improving vitamin K status of breastfeeding infants with maternal vitamin K supplements, *Pediatrics* 99:88, 1997.

76. Greer FR, Mummah-Schendel LL, Marshall S et al: Vitamin K_1 (phylloquinone) and vitamin K_2 (menaquinone) status in newborns during the first week of life, *Pediatrics* 81:137, 1988.

77. Greer FR, Tsang RC, Levin RS et al: Increasing serum calcium and magnesium concentrations in breastfed infants: longitudinal studies of minerals in human milk and in sera of nursing mothers and their infants, *J Pediatr* 100:59, 1982.

78. Gushurst CA, Mueller JA, Green JA et al: Breast milk iodide: reassessment in the 1980's, *Pediatrics* 73:354, 1984.

79. György P: Biochemical aspects. In Jelliffe DB, Jelliffe EFP, editors: The uniqueness of human milk, *Am J Clin Nutr* 24:970, 1971.

80. Hadjimarkos DM, Shearer TR: Selenium in mature human milk, *Am J Clin Nutr* 26:583, 1973.

81. Hall B: Changing composition of human milk and early development of an appetite control, *Lancet* 1:779, 1975.

82. Hall B, Muller DPR: Studies on bile-salt-stimulated lipolytic activity in human milk. II. Demonstration of two groups of milk with different activities, *Pediatr Res* 17:716, 1983.

83. Hambraeus L: Proprietary milk versus human milk in infant feeding: a critical approach from a nutritional point of view, *Pediatr Clin North Am* 24:17, 1977.

84. Hambraeus L, Forsum E, Lönnerdal B: Nutritional aspects of breast milk and cow's milk formulas. In Hambraeus L, Hanson L, MacFarlane H, editors: *Symposium on food and immunology,* Stockholm, 1975, Almqvist and Wiksell.

85. Hamosh M: Enzymes in human milk. In Howell RR, Morriss FH, Pickering LK, editors: *Human milk in infant nutrition and health,* Springfield, Ill, 1986, Charles C Thomas.

86. Hamosh M: Breast milk jaundice, *J Pediatr Gastroenterol Nutr* 11:145, 1990.

87. Hamosh M: Human milk composition and function in the infant, *Semin Pediatr Gastroenterol Nutr* 3:4, 1992.

88. Hamosh M: Enzymes in human milk. In Jensen RG, editor: *Handbook of milk composition,* San Diego, 1995, Academic Press.

89. Hamosh M: Lipid metabolism in pediatric nutrition, *Pediatr Clin North Am* 42:839, 1995.

90. Hamosh M, Hong MH, Hamosh P: β-Casomorphins: milk-β-casein derived opioid peptides. In Lebenthal E, editor: *Textbook of gastroenterology and nutrition in infancy,* ed 2, New York, 1989, Raven.

91. Harzer G, Dieterich I, Haug M: Effects of the diet on composition of human milk, *Ann Nutr Metab* 28:231, 1984.

92. Harzer G, Haug M, Dieterich I et al: Changing patterns of human milk lipids in the course of the lactation and during the day, *Am J Clin Nutr* 37:612, 1983.

93. Harzer G, Kauer H: Binding of zinc to casein, *Am J Clin Nutr* 35:981, 1982.

94. Hazebroek A, Hofman A: Sodium content of breast milk in the first six months after delivery, *Acta Paediatr Scand* 72:459, 1983.

95. Healy DL, Rattigan S, Hartmann PE et al: Prolactin in human milk: correlation with lactose, total protein, and α-lactalbumin levels, *Am J Physiol* 238 (*Endocrinol Metab* 1):E83, 1980.

96. Heine W, Braun OH, Mohr C et al: Enhancement of lysozyme trypsin-mediated decay of intestinal bifidobacteria and lactobacilli, *J Pediatr Gastroenterol Nutr* 21:54, 1995.

97. Heird WC, Prager TC, Anderson RE: Docosa hexaenoic acid and development and function of the infant retina, *Curr Opin Lipidol* 8:12, 1997.

98. Heiskanen K, Siimes MA, Perheentupa J et al: Risk of low vitamin B_6 status in infants breast-fed exclusively beyond six months, *J Pediatr Gastroenterol Nutr* 23:38, 1996.

99. Heitlinger LA, Lee PA, Dillon WP et al: Mammary amylase: a possible alternate pathway of carbohydrate digestion in infancy, *Pediatr Res* 17:15, 1983.

100. Hernell O, Bläckberg L: Digestion of human milk lipids: physiologic significance of sn-2 monoacylglyceral hydrolysis by bile salt–stimulated lipase, *Pediatr Res* 16:882, 1982.

101. Hernell O, Olivecrona T: Human milk lipases. II. Bile salt–stimulated lipase, *Biochim Biophys Acta* 369:234, 1974.

102. Hibberd CM, Brooke OG, Carter ND et al: Variation in the composition of breast milk during the first five weeks of lactation: implications for the feeding of preterm infants, *Arch Dis Child* 57:658, 1982.

103. Horwood LJ, Fergusson DM: Breastfeeding and later cognitive and academic outcomes, *Pediatrics* 101:e9, 1998.

104. Howell RR, Palma PA, West MS et al: Trace elements in human milk: differences over time and between population groups. In Howell RR, Morriss FH, Pickering LK, editors: *Human milk in infant nutrition and health,* Springfield, Ill, 1986, Charles C Thomas.

105. Huston GE, Patton S: Membrane distribution in human milks throughout lactation as revealed by phospholipid and cholesterol analyses, *J Pediatr Gastroenterol Nutr* 5:602, 1986.

106. Huxtable RJ: Physiological actions of taurine, *Physiol Rev* 72:101, 1992.

107. Hytten FE: Clinical and chemical studies in human lactation. VII. The effect of differences in yield and composition of milk on the infant's weight gain and duration of breastfeeding, *Br Med J* 1:1410, 1954.

108. Iacopetta BJ, Grieu F, Horlsberger M et al: Epidermal growth factor in human and bovine milk, *Acta Paediatr Scand* 81:287, 1992.

109. Innis SM: Human milk and formula fatty acids, *J Pediatr Suppl* 120:556, 1992.

110. Innis SM, Hamilton JJ: Effects of developmental changes and early nutrition on cholesterol metabolism in infancy: a review, *J Am Coll Nutr* 11:635, 1992.

111. Insull W, Ahrens EH: The fatty acids of human milk from mothers on diets taken ad libitum, *Biochem J* 72:27, 1959.

112. Isaacs CE, Wright CE, Pascal TA et al: Sulfhydryl oxidase (SHO) in human milk and induction in kidney and skin at weaning, *Pediatr Res* 15:112A, 1981 (abstract).

113. Jackson DA, Imong SM, Silprasert A et al: Circadian variation in fat concentration of breast milk in a rural northern Thai population, *Br J Nutr* 59:349, 1988.

114. Jamieson EC, Abbasi KA, Cockburn F et al: Effect of diet on term infant cerebral cortex fatty acid composition. In Galli C, Simopoulis AP, Tremoli E, editors: Fatty acids and lipids: biological aspects, *World Rev Nutr Diet Basel Karger* 75:139, 1994.

115. Janas LM, Picciano MF: The nucleotide profile of human milk, *Pediatr Res* 16:659, 1982.

116. Jansson L, Akesson B, Holmberg L: Vitamin E and fatty acid composition of human milk, *Am J Clin Nutr* 34:8, 1981.

117. Järvenpää AL, Rassin DK, Raiha NCR et al: Milk protein quantity and quality in the term infant. II. Effects on acidic and neutral amino acids, *Pediatrics* 70:221, 1982.

118. Jenness R, Sloan RE: Composition of milk. In Larson BL, Smith VR, editors: *Lactation,* vol 3, *Nutrition and biochemistry of milk/maintenance,* New York, 1974, Academic Press.

119. Jensen GL, Jensen RG: Specialty lipids for infant nutrition. II. Concerns, new developments and future applications, *J Pediatr Gastroenterol Nutr* 15:382, 1992.

120. Jensen RG: Introduction. In Jensen RG, editor: *Handbook of milk composition,* San Diego, 1995, Academic Press.

121. Jensen RG, Bitman J, Carlson SE: Milk lipids. A. Human milk lipids. In Jensen RG, editor: *Handbook of milk composition,* San Diego, 1995, Academic Press.

122. Jensen RG, Ferris AM, Lammi-Keefe CJ: Lipids in human milk and infant formulas, *Ann Rev Nutr* 12:417, 1992.

123. Jimenez R, Navarrete M, Jimenez E et al: Vitamin K–dependent clotting factors in normal breastfed infants, *J Pediatr* 100:424, 1982.

124. Johke T: Nucleotides of mammary secretions. In Larson BL, editor: *Lactation,* vol 4, *Mammary gland/human lactation/milk synthesis,* New York, 1978, Academic Press.

125. Johnson PE, Evans GW: Relative zinc availability in human breast milk, infant formulas, and cow's milk, *Am J Clin Nutr* 31:416, 1978.

126. Johnston L, Vaughn L, Fox HM: Pantothenic acid content of human milk, *Am J Clin Nutr* 34:2205, 1981.

127. Jooste PL, Roosouw LJ, Steenkamp HJ et al: Effect of breastfeeding on the plasma cholesterol and growth of infants, *J Pediatr Gastroenterol Nutr* 13:139, 1991.

128. Kalkwarf HJ, Specker BL: Bone mineral loss during lactation and recovery after weaning, *Obstet Gynecol* 86:26, 1995.

129. Kalkwarf HJ, Specker BL, Bianchi DC et al: The effect of calcium supplementation on bone density during lactation and after weaning, *N Engl J Med* 337:523, 1997.

130. Kalkwarf HJ, Specker BL, Heubi JE et al: Intestinal calcium absorption of women during lactation and after weaning, *Am J Clin Nutr* 63:526, 1996.

131. Kallio MJT, Salmenperä L, Siimes MA et al: Exclusive breastfeeding and weaning: effect on serum cholesterol and lipoprotein concentrations in infants during the first year of life, *Pediatrics* 89:663, 1992.

132. Keenan BS, Buzek SW, Garza C: Cortisol and its possible role in regulation of sodium and potassium in human milk, *Am J Physiol* 244: (*Endocrinol Metab* 7):E253, 1983.

133. Khoshoo V, Kjarsgaar DJ, Krafchick B et al: Zinc deficiency in a full term breastfed infant: unusual presentation, *Pediatrics* 89:1094, 1992.

134. Kirksey A, Roepke JLB: Vitamin B_6 nutriture of mothers of three breastfed neonates with central nervous system disorders, *Fed Proc* 40:864, 1981.

135. Koldovsky O, Strbak V: Hormones and growth factors in human milk. In Jensen RG, editor: *Handbook of milk composition,* San Diego, 1995, Academic Press.

136. Koski KG, Hill FW, Lönnerdal B: Altered lactational performance in rats fed low carbohydrate diets and its effect on growth of neonatal rat pups, *J Nutr* 120:1028, 1990.

137. Krebs NF, Hambidge KM: Zinc requirements and zinc intakes in breastfed infants, *Am J Clin Nutr* 43:288, 1986.

138. Krebs NF, Reidinger CJ, Robertson AD et al: Bone mineral density changes during lactation: maternal, dietary, and biochemical correlates, *Am J Clin Nutr* 65: 1738, 1997.

139. Kretchmer N: Lactose and lactase, *Sci Am* 227:73, 1972.

140. Kulski JK, Hartmann PE: Changes in human milk composition during the initiation of lactation, *Aust J Exp Biol Med Sci* 59:101, 1981.

141. Kumpulainen J, Vuori E: Longitudinal study of chromium in human milk, *Am J Clin Nutr* 33:2299, 1980.

142. Kunz C, Lönnerdal B: Re-evaluation of whey protein/casein ratio of human milk, *Acta Paediatr Scand* 81:107, 1992.

143. Lammi-Keefe CJ: Vitamin D and E in human milk. In Jensen RG, editor: *Handbook of milk composition,* San Diego, 1995, Academic Press.

144. Lammi-Keefe CJ, Jensen RG: Lipids in human milk: a review. 2. Composition and fat-soluble vitamins, *J Pediatr Gastroenterol Nutr* 3:172, 1984.

145. Lessof MH, Anderson JA, Youlten LJF: Prostaglandins in the pathogenesis of food intolerance, *Ann Allergy* 51:249, 1983.

146. Lifschitz CH: Carbohydrate needs in preterm and term newborn infants. In Tsang RC, Nichols BL, editors: *Nutrition during infancy,* St Louis, 1988, Mosby.

147. Lindberg T, Skude G: Amylase in human milk, *Pediatrics* 70:235, 1982.

148. Lindstrom LH, Nyberg F, Terenius L et al: CSF and plasma-casomorphine-like opioid peptides in postpartum psychosis, *Am J Psychiatry* 141:1059, 1984.

149. Lönnerdal B: Effects of maternal dietary intake on human milk composition, *J Nutr* 116:499, 1986.

150. Lönnerdal B, Forsum E: Casein content of human milk, *Am J Clin Nutr* 41:113, 1985.

151. Lönnerdal B, Keen CL, Hurley LS: Manganese binding proteins in human and cow's milk, *Am J Clin Nutr* 4:550, 1985.

152. Lucas A, Blackburn AM, Aynsley-Green A et al: Breast vs bottle: endocrine responses are different with formula feeding, *Lancet* 1:1267, 1980.

153. Lucas A, Mitchell MD: Prostaglandins in human milk, *Arch Dis Child* 55:950, 1980.

154. Lucas A, Morley R, Cole TJ et al: Breast milk and subsequent intelligence quotient in children born preterm, *Lancet* 339:261, 1992.

155. Lucas A, Morley R, Cole TJ et al: A randomised multicentre study of human milk versus formula and later development in preterm infant, *Arch Dis Child* 70:F141, 1994.

156. MacDonald LD, Gibson RS, Miles JE: Changes in hair zinc and copper concentrations of breastfed and bottle fed infants during the first six months, *Acta Paediatr Scand* 71:785, 1982.

157. Makrides M, Neumann MA, Gibson RA: Effect of maternal docosahexaenoic acid (DHA) supplementation on breast milk composition, *Eur J Clin Nutr* 50:352, 1996.

158. Malloy MH, Rassin DK, Gaull GE et al: Development of taurine metabolism in beagle pups: effects of taurine-free total parenteral nutrition, *Biol Neonate* 40:1, 1981.

159. Moran JR, Courtney ME, Orth DN et al: Epidermal growth factor in human milk: daily production and diurnal variation during early lactation in mothers delivering at term and at premature gestation, *J Pediatr* 103:402, 1983.

160. Morriss FH: Physical-chemical changes in human milk during the course of lactation. In Howell RR, Morriss FH, Pickering LK, editors: *Human milk in infant nutrition and health,* Springfield, Ill, 1986, Charles C Thomas.

161. Moser PB, Reynolds RD: Dietary zinc intake and zinc concentrations of plasma, erythrocytes, and breast milk in antepartum and postpartum lactating and nonlactating women: a longitudinal study, *Am J Clin Nutr* 38:101, 1983.

162. Motil KJ, Thotathuchery M, Bahar A et al: Marginal dietary protein restriction, reduced nonprotein nitrogen, but not protein nitrogen, components of human milk, *J Am Coll Nutr* 14:184, 1995.

163. Mott GE, Lewis DS, McGill HC Jr: Programming of cholesterol metabolism by breast or formula feeding. In *The childhood environment and adult disease, Ciba Found Symp* 156:56, 1991.

164. Nail PA, Thomas MR, Eakin R: The effect of thiamin and riboflavin supplementation on the level of those vitamins in human milk and urine, *Am J Clin Nutr* 33:198, 1980.

165. National Academy of Science: *Nutrition during lactation,* Institute of Medicine, Washington, DC, 1991, National Academy Press.

166. Neville MC: Mammary gland biology and lactation: a short course. Presented at biannual meeting of the International Society for Research on Human Milk and Lactation, Plymouth, Mass, October 1997.

167. Neville MC: Sampling and storage of human milk. In Jensen RG, editor: *Handbook of milk composition,* San Diego, 1995, Academic Press.

168. Neville MC: Determinants of milk volume and composition. In Jensen RG, editor: *Handbook of milk composition,* San Diego, 1995, Academic Press.

169. Neville MC: Volume and caloric density of human milk. In Jensen RG, editor: *Handbook of milk composition,* San Diego, 1995, Academic Press.

170. Neville MC, Allen JC, Archer PC et al: Studies in human lactation: milk volume and nutrient composition during weaning and lactogenesis, *Am J Clin Nutr* 54:81, 1991.

171. Neville MC, Keller R, Seacat J et al: Studies in human lactation: milk volumes in lactating women during the onset of lactation and full lactation, *Am J Clin Nutr* 48:1375, 1988.

172. Neville MC, Zhang P, Allen JC: Minerals, ions, and trace elements in milk. A. Ionic interactions in milk. In Jensen RG, editor: *Handbook of milk composition,* San Diego, 1995, Academic Press.

173. Newburg DS: Oligosaccharides and glycoconjugates in human milk: their role in host defense, *J Mammary Gland Biol Neoplasia* 1:271, 1996.

174. Newman V: *Vitamin A and breastfeeding: a comparison of data from developed and developing countries,* San Diego, 1993, Wellstart International.

175. Nommsen LA, Lovelady CA, Heinig MJ et al: Determinants of energy, protein, lipid, and lactose concentrations in human milk during the first 12 mo of lactation: the DARLING Study, *Am J Clin Nutr* 53:457, 1991.

176. Novak M, Monkus EF, Chang D et al: Carnitine in the perinatal metabolism of lipids. I. Relationship between maternal and fetal plasma levels of carnitine and acylcarnitines, *Pediatrics* 67:95, 1981.

177. O'Connor DL, Tamura T, Picciano MF: Pteroylglutamates in human milk, *Am J Clin Nutr* 53:930, 1991.

178. O'Connor ME, Livingston DS, Hannah J et al: Vitamin K deficiency and breastfeeding, *Am J Dis Child* 137:601, 1983.

179. Ortega RM, Andres P, Martinez RM et al: Vitamin status during the third trimester of pregnancy in Spanish women: influence on concentrations of vitamin A in breastmilk, *Am J Clin Nutr* 66:564, 1997.

180. Orzali A, Donzelli F, Enzi G et al: Effect of carnitine on lipid metabolism in the newborn, *Biol Neonate* 43:186, 1983.

181. Osborn GR: Relationship of hypotension and infant feeding to aetiology of coronary disease, *Coll Int Cont Natl Res Sci* 169:193, 1968.

182. Oski FA: What we eat may determine who we can be, *Nutrition* 13:220, 1997.

183. Picciano MF: Vitamins in milk. A. Water-soluble vitamins in human milk composition. In Jensen RG, editor: *Handbook of milk composition,* San Diego, 1995, Academic Press.

184. Picciano MF, Calkins EJ, Garrick JR et al: Milk and mineral intakes of breastfed infants, *Acta Paediatr Scand* 70:189, 1981.

185. Picciano MF, Guthrie HA: Copper, iron, and zinc contents of mature human milk, *Am J Clin Nutr* 29:242, 1976.

186. Pisacane A, DeVizia B, Valiante A et al: Iron status in breast-fed infants, *J Pediatr* 127:429, 1995.

187. Pollack PF, Koldovsky O, Nishioka K: Polyamines in human and rat milk and in infant formulas, *Am J Clin Nutr* 56:371, 1992.

188. Potter JM, Nestel PJ: The effects of dietary fatty acids and cholesterol on the milk lipids of lactating women and the plasma cholesterol of breastfed infants, *Am J Clin Nutr* 29:54, 1976.

189. Prentice A, Roberts SB, Prentice AM et al: Dietary supplementation of lactating Gambian women. I. Effect on breastmilk volume and quality, *Hum Nutr Clin Nutr* 37C:53, 1983.

190. Quan R, Barness LA, Uauy R: Do infants need nucleotide supplemented formula for optimal nutrition? *J Pediatr Gastroenterol Nutr* 11:429, 1990.

191. Quan R, Uauy R: Nucleotides and gastrointestinal development, *Semin Gastroenterol Nutr* 2:3, 1991.

192. Rassin DK, Sturman JA, Gaull GE: Taurine in milk: species variation, *Pediatr Res* 11:449, 1977.

193. Read WWC, Sarrif A: Human milk lipids. I. Changes in fatty acid composition of early colostrum, *Am J Clin Nutr* 17:177, 1965.

194. Reid B, Smith H, Friedman Z: Prostaglandins in human milk, *Pediatrics* 66:870, 1980.

195. Reisbick S, Neuringer M, Connor WE et al: Postnatal deficiency of omega-3 fatty acids in monkeys: fluid intake and urine concentration, *Physiol Behav* 51:473, 1992.

196. *Report of the Subcommittee on Nutrition During Lactation,* The Institute of Medicine, National Academy of Sciences, Washington, DC, 1991, National Academy Press.

197. Roepke JLB, Kirksey A: Vitamin B_6 nutriture during pregnancy and lactation. I. Vitamin B_6 intake, levels of the vitamin in biological fluids, and condition of the infant at birth, *Am J Clin Nutr* 32:2249, 1979.

198. Roepke JLB, Kirksey A: Vitamin B_6 nutriture during pregnancy and lactation. II. The effect of long-term use of oral contraceptives, *Am J Clin Nutr* 32:2257, 1979.

199. Romain N, Dandrifosse G, Jeusette F et al: Polyamine concentration in rat milk and food, human milk and infant formulas, *Pediatr Res* 32:58, 1992.

200. Rothberg AD, Pettifor JM, Cohen DF et al: Maternal-infant vitamin D relationships during breastfeeding, *J Pediatr* 101:500, 1982.

201. Salmenperä L, Perheetupa J, Siimes MA: Folate nutrition is optimal in exclusively breastfed infants but inadequate in some of their mothers and in formula-fed infants, *J Pediatr Gastroenterol Nutr* 5:283, 1986.

202. Samson RR, McClelland DBL: Vitamin B_{12} in human colostrum and milk, *Acta Paediatr Scand* 69:93, 1980.

203. Sandberg DP, Begley JA, Hall CA: The content, binding, and forms of vitamin B_{12} in milk, *Am J Clin Nutr* 34:1717, 1981.

204. Sanders TAB, Ellis FR, Dickerson JWT: Studies of vegans: the fatty acid composition of plasma choline phosphoglycerides, erythrocytes, adipose tissue, and breast milk, and some indicators of susceptibility to ischemic heart disease in vegans and omnivore controls, *Am J Clin Nutr* 31:805, 1978.

205. Sandor A, Pecsuvac K, Kerner J et al: On carnitine content of human breast milk, *Pediatr Res* 16:89, 1982.

206. Schams D, Karg H: Hormones in milk, *Ann NY Acad Sci* 464:75, 1986.

207. Schulz-Lell G, Buss R, Oldigs HD et al: Iron balances in infant nutrition, *Acta Paediatr Scand* 76:585, 1987.

208. Shahani KM, Kwan AJ, Friend BA: Role and significance of enzymes in human milk, *Am J Clin Nutr* 33:1861, 1980.

209. Shaw JCL: Trace elements in the fetus and young infant, *Am J Dis Child* 134:74, 1980.

210. Shimizu T, Yamashiro Y, Yabuta K: Prostaglandin E_1, E_2, and F_{2a} in human milk and plasma, *Biol Neonate* 61:222, 1992.

211. Sievers E, Oldigs H-D, Dörner K et al: Longitudinal zinc balances in breastfed and formula-fed infants, *Acta Paediatr Scand* 81:1, 1992.

212. Simopoulas AP: Omega-3 fatty acids in health and disease in growth and development, *Am J Clin Nutr* 54:438, 1991.

213. Sinclair AJ, Crawford MA: The accumulation of arachidonate and docosahexaenoate in the developing rat brain, *J Neurochem* 19:1753, 1972.

214. Skala JP, Koldovsky O, Hahn P: Cyclic nucleotides in breast milk, *Am J Clin Nutr* 34:343, 1981.

215. Smith AM, Picciano MF, Milner JA: Selenium intakes and status of human milk and formula-fed infants, *Am J Clin Nutr* 35:521, 1982.

216. Sneed SM, Zane C, Thomas MR: The effects of ascorbic acid, vitamin B_6, vitamin B_{12} and folic acid supplementation on the breast milk and maternal nutritional status of low socioeconomic lactating women, *Am J Clin Nutr* 34:1338, 1981.

217. Specker BL, Black A, Allen L et al: Vitamin B_{12}: low milk concentrations are reported to correspond to low serum concentrations in vegetarian women and to methylmalonic aciduria in their infants, *Am J Clin Nutr* 52:1073, 1990.

218. Specker BL, Tsang RC, Ho ML: Changes in calcium homeostasis over the first year postpartum: effect of lactation and weaning, *Obstet Gynecol* 78:56, 1991.

219. Specker BL, Tsang RC, Ho ML et al: Effect of vegetarian diet on serum 1,25 dihydroxy vitamin D concentrations during lactation, *Obstet Gynecol* 70:870, 1987.

220. Sturman JA, Rassin DK, Gaull GE: Taurine in the developing kitten: nutritional importance, *Pediatr Res* 11:450, 1977.

221. Tenore A, Oberkotter LV, Koldovsky O et al: Thyrotropin in human breast milk, *Horm Res* 14:193, 1981.

222. Thomas MR, Sneed SM, Wei C et al: The effects of vitamin C, vitamin B_6, and vitamin B_{12}, folic acid, riboflavin, and thiamin on the breast milk and maternal status of well-nourished women at 6 months postpartum, *Am J Clin Nutr* 33:2151, 1980.

223. Tikanoja T, Simell O, Viikari M et al: Plasma amino acids in term neonates after a feed of human milk or formula. II. Characteristic changes in individual amino acids, *Acta Paediatr Scand* 71:391, 1982.

224. Vanderslice JT, Brownlee SG, Maire CE et al: Form of vitamin B_6 in human milk, *Am J Clin Nutr* 37:867, 1983.

225. Van Houwelingen AC, Sorensen JD, Hornstra G et al: Essential fatty acid status in neonates after fish-oil supplementation during late pregnancy, *Br J Nutr* 74:723, 1995.

226. Vorherr H: *The breast: morphology, physiology, and lactation,* New York, 1974, Academic Press.

227. Watkins JB: Bile acid metabolism in the human infant: role of taurine supplementation and human milk. In Filer LJ, Fomon SJ, editors: *The breastfed infant: a model for performance,* Columbus, Ohio, 1986, Ross Laboratories.

228. Widdowson EM, Dauncey MJ, Gardner DM et al: Body fat of British and Dutch infants, *Br Med J* 1:653, 1975.

229. Wong WW, Hachey DL, Insull W et al: Effect of dietary cholesterol on cholesterol synthesis in breast-fed and formula-fed infants, *J Lipid Res* 34:1403, 1993.

230. Work Group on Breastfeeding, American Academy of Pediatrics: Breastfeeding and the use of human milk, *Pediatrics* 100:6, 1997.

231. Yolken RH, Peterson JA, Vonderfecht SL et al: Human milk mucin inhibits rotavirus replication and prevents experimental gastroenteritis, *J Clin Invest* 90:1984, 1992.

232. Young VR, Nahapetian A, Janghorbani M: Selenium bioavailability with reference to human nutrition, *Am J Clin Nutr* 35:1076, 1982.

233. Zikakis JP, Dougherty TM, Biasotto HO: The presence and some properties of xanthine oxidase in human milk and colostrum, *J Food Sci* 41:1408, 1976.

$\mathscr{H}$ost-resistance factors and immunologic significance of human milk

ROBERT M. LAWRENCE

Some of the most dramatic and far-reaching advances in the understanding of the host defenses of human milk have been made using newer techniques to observe established immunologic significance. The multifunctional capabilities of specific factors and the interactive nature of immunoglobulins, cells, and other antiinflammatory agents make human milk unique.

As early as 1892, medical literature carried data proving that milk from various species, including humans, was protective for the offspring, containing antibodies against a vast number of antigens.[50] Veterinarians have known the urgency of offspring receiving the early milk of the mother. Death rates among newborns not suckled at the breast in the Third World are at least five times higher than among those who receive colostrum and mother's milk. Evidence that lack of breastfeeding and poor environmental sanitation have a pernicious synergistic effect on infant mortality has been presented by Habicht et al[49] after studying 1262 women in Malaysia.

Lower incidence of diarrheal disease in breastfed infants is well established worldwide, even in North America, where the Native Americans and Alaskans have high risk for infection. The lowest incidence of breastfeeding in the United States is among the indigent and disadvantaged urban and rural populations, but no data on infection rate in these groups are available.[98] Day-care children are a population at extremely high risk for infection, and it is speculated these children benefit from at least partial breastfeeding. Protection against respiratory tract infections and otitis media are becoming well established for the United States because of a number of investigatory efforts.[25,28]

Using a self-administered questionnaire completed by parents in Shanghai, Republic of China, when the infant was 18 months old, Chen et al[23] studied the protective effect of breastfeeding against one or more episodes of hospitalization for infection. The definition of breastfeeding was "ever breastfed," which would bias the data against breastfeeding. However, those infants "never breastfed" were twice as likely to be hospitalized for respiratory infections and approximately one third more likely to be hospitalized for gastroenteritis or other infections in the first 18 months of life. The design of the study was clearly biased against breastfeeding, Kramer[66] points out, and still the results are clear: breastfeeding is protective.

Breastfeeding is effective in minimizing infection in infants by decreasing the exposure to enteropathogens that may contaminate other foods or formula, providing nutrition, and providing special unique protective factors, which can be loosely grouped as antibody and nonantibody.[95] The protection provided varies by the pathogen and chronologic age and maturity of the infant.[70]

As the fetus prepares for existence outside the uterus, various organ systems adjust and adapt. Protection against infection may be provided by the mother transplacentally, because it has been established that the neonate is immunologically immature at birth.

The neonate does not have sufficient innate defenses to protect against the highly contaminated environment the infant enters from the usually sterile environment of the uterus. The incidence of infection in the newborn is significant. It has been estimated that up to 10% of newborns are infected during delivery or in the first few months of life. The newborn cannot muster the same level of defense against infection that an adult is capable of developing. The diminished phagocytic function of newborn cells is an example. This maturational defect is attributed to both cellular and extracellular factors.

Ashraf et al[1] investigated potential protection of breastfeeding against neonatal sepsis in a developing country (Pakistan). Their case-control study demonstrated that even partial breastfeeding protects against neonatal sepsis in areas where the infection rate and mortality rate from neonatal sepsis are high. Winberg and Wessner[116] demonstrated protection against neonatal sepsis from breast milk in Sweden, where the incidence of neonatal sepsis is only about 3:1000 live births and the mortality is estimated at 12%.

Maternal antibody is transmitted to the fetus by different pathways in different species.[70,111] An association has been recognized between the number of placental membranes and the relative importance of the placenta and the colostrum as sources of antibodies. By this analysis, the horse, with six placental membranes, passes little or no antibodies transplacentally and relies totally on colostrum for protection of the foal. Humans and monkeys, having three placental membranes, receive more of the antibodies via the placenta and less from the colostrum. The transfer of immunoglobulin G (IgG) in the human is accomplished by active transport mechanism of the immunoglobulin across the placenta. Secretory IgA (sIgA) immunoglobulins are found in human milk and provide local protection to the mucous membranes of the gastrointestinal (GI) tract. Other investigations have established that the mammary glands and their secretion of milk are important in protecting the infant not only through the colostrum but also through mature milk from birth through the early months of life. Some information has been available for decades to support the acknowledgment of the protective role of human milk.[56] Many recent discoveries, however, have broadened this knowledge.[38]

Although the predominance of IgA in human colostrum and milk had been described, the importance of this phenomenon was not fully appreciated until the discovery that IgA is a predominant immunoglobulin present in mucosal secretions of other glands in addition to the breast. Mucosal immunity has become the subject of extensive research.[55] The data produced suggest that considerable traffic of cells may occur between secretory sites. These data support the concept of a general system of mucosa-associated lymphoid tissue (MALT), which includes the gut, lung, mammary gland, salivary and lacrimal glands, and the genital tract. This concept of MALT implies that immunization at one site may be an effective means of producing immunity at distant sites. Antibodies found in the milk have also been found in the saliva, for instance. Evidence suggests that the mammary glands may act as extensions of the gut-associated lymphoid tissue (GALT) and possibly the broncho-associated lymphoid tissue (BALT). The ability of epithelial surfaces exposed to the external environment to defend against foragers has been well established for the GI, genitourinary, and respiratory tracts.[63] The common defense is sIgA. Direct contact with the antigen and the lymphoid cells of the breast is unlikely.[87]

All mysteries of the protective value of human milk, however, have not been unraveled. The protective properties of human milk can be divided into cellular factors and humoral factors for facility of discussion, although they are closely related in vivo. A wide variety of soluble and cellular components and hormonelike agents have been identified in human milk and colostrum (Table 5-1). Although the following discussion will separate elements, it is important to emphasize that the constituents of human milk are multifunctional and interactive.

TABLE 5-1   Immunologically and pharmacologically active components and hormones observed in human colostrum and milk

Soluble	Cellular	Hormones and hormonelike substances
Immunologically specific	*Immunologically specific*	Epidermal growth factor (EGF)
Immunoglobulin	T-lymphocytes	Prostaglandins
sIgA (11S), 7S IgA, IgG, IgM	B-lymphocytes	Relaxin
IgE, IgD, secretory component		Neurotensin
	Accessory cells	Somatostatin
T-cell products	Neutrophils	Bombesin
	Macrophages	Gonadotropins
Histocompatibility antigens	Epithelial cells	Ovarian steroids
		Thyroid-releasing hormone (TRH)
Nonspecific factors		Thyroid-stimulating hormone (TSH)
Complement		Thyroxine and triiodothyronine
Chemotactic factors		Adrenocorticotropin
Properdin (factor P)		Corticosteroids
Interferon		Prolactin
α-Fetoprotein		Erythropoietin
Bifidus factor		Insulin
Antistaphylococcal factor(s)		Cytokines
Antiadherence substances		Interleukins
Epidermal growth factor (EGF)		
Folate uptake enhancer		
Antiviral factor(s)		
Migration inhibition factor (MIF)		
Gangliosides		
Nucleotides		
Carrier proteins		
Lactoferrin		
Transferrin		
Vitamin B_{12}-binding protein		
Corticoid-binding protein		
Enzymes		
Lysozyme		
Lipoprotein lipase		
Leukocyte enzymes		

Modified from Ogra PL, Fishaut M: Human breast milk. In Remington JS, Klein JO, editors: *Infectious diseases of the fetus and newborn infant,* ed 4, Philadelphia, 1995, Saunders.

CELLULAR COMPONENTS OF HUMAN COLOSTRUM AND MILK

Cells are an important postpartum component of maternal immunologic endowment. Over 100 years ago, cell bodies were described in the colostrum of animals. As with much lactation research, further study of colostral corpuscles was undertaken by the dairy industry for commercial reasons in the early 1900s. This research afforded an opportunity to make major progress in the understanding of cells in milk. Initially, it was believed that these cells represented a reaction to infection in the mammary gland and were even described as "pus cells."

It has become clear that the cells of milk are normal constituents of that solution in all species. Cells include macrophages, lymphocytes, neutrophils, and epithelial cells, and they total 4000/mm³. Cell fragments and epithelial cells were examined by electron microscope in fresh samples from 30 women by Brooker.[11] He found that the membrane-bound cytoplasmic fragments in the sedimentation pellet outnumbered intact cells. The fragments were mostly from secretory cells that contained numerous cisternae of rough endoplasmic reticulum, lipid droplets, and Golgi vesicles containing casein micelles. Secretory epithelial cells were found in all samples and, after the second month postpartum, began to outnumber macrophages. Ductal epithelial cells were about 1% of the population of cells for the first week or so and then disappeared. All samples contained squamous epithelial cells originating from galactophores and the skin of the nipple.

Living leukocytes are normally present in human milk.[63] The overall concentration of these leukocytes is of the same order of magnitude as that seen in peripheral blood, although the predominant cell in milk is the macrophage rather than the neutrophil. Macrophages compose about 90% of the leukocytes, and 2000 to 3000/mm³ are present. Lymphocytes make up about 10% of the cells (200 to 300/mm³), which is much lower than in human blood. There are large and small lymphocytes. By indirect immunofluorescence with

anti-T cell antibody to identify thymus-derived lymphocytes, it has been shown that 50% of human colostral lymphocytes are T cells. Immunofluorescence procedures to detect surface immunoglobulins characteristic of B-lymphocytes identified 34% as B-lymphocytes.

The number of leukocytes and the degree of mitogenic stimulation of lymphocytes sharply decline during the first 2 or 3 months of lactation to essentially undetectable levels, according to Goldman et al[43] (Fig. 5-1). Enumeration of the total cell numbers in milk has been difficult, but when various techniques are compared (Coulter electronic particle counter, visual cell counting with special stains, filter trapping with fluorescent detection, and automated fluorescent cell counting), stains for deoxyribonucleic acid (DNA) were superior.

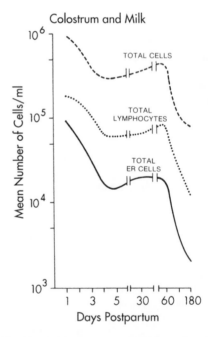

Fig. 5-1. Geometric mean concentration of total cells, lymphocytes, and E (erythrocyte) rosette-forming cells *(ER)* in colostrum and milk of 200 lactating women. (Modified from Ogra SS, Ogra PL: *J Pediatr* 92: 546, 1978.)

Macrophages

Macrophages are large-complex phagocytes that contain lysosomes, mitochondria, pinosomes, ribosomes, and a Golgi apparatus. The monocytic phagocytes are lipid laden and were previously called the *colostral bodies of Donne*. They have the same functional and morphologic features as those of other human tissue sources. These features include ameboid movement, phagocytosis of microorganisms (fungi and bacteria), killing of bacteria, and production of complement components C3 and C4, lysosome, and lactoferrin. Other milk macrophage activities include the following[95]:

Phagocytosis of latex, adherence to glass
Secretion of lysozyme, complement components
C3b-mediated erythrocyte adherence
IgG-mediated erythrocyte adherence and
    phagocytosis
Bacterial killing
Inhibition of lymphocyte mitogenic response
Release of intracellular IgA in tissue culture
Giant cell formation
Interaction with lymphocytes

Data suggest these macrophages also amplify T-cell reactivity by direct cellular cooperation or by antigen processing. The colostral macrophage has been suggested as a potential vehicle for the storage and transport of immunoglobin. A significant increase in IgA and IgG synthesis by colostral lymphocytes, when incubated with supernatants of cultured macrophages, has been reported.[97]

The macrophage may also participate in the biosynthesis and excretion of lactoperoxidase and cellular growth factors that enhance growth of intestinal epithelium and maturation of intestinal brush-border enzymes.

The mobility of macrophages is inhibited by the lymphokine migration inhibitor factor (MIF), which is produced by antigen-stimulated sensitized lymphocytes. The activities of macrophages have been demonstrated in both fresh colostrum and colostral cell culture, and certain functions are altered compared with their counterpart in human peripheral blood.

Polymorphonuclear leukocytes

The highest concentration of cells occurs in the first few days of lactation and reaches more than a million per milliliter of milk.

Colostrum (1 to 4 days postpartum) contains 10^5 to 5×10^6 leukocytes/ml, and 40% to 60% are polymorphonuclears (PMNs). Mature milk (i.e., beyond 4 days) has fewer cells (Fig. 5-2), about 10^5/ml with 20% to 30% PMNs. Beyond 6 weeks, there are few PMNs. The functions of the PMNs normally include microbial killing, phagocytosis, chemotactic responsiveness, stimulated hexose monophosphate shunt activity, stimulated nitroblue tetrazolium dye reduction, and stimulated oxygen consumption.[15] When milk PMNs are compared with those in the serum, their activity is often less than that of serum PMN cells. Whether milk PMNs actually perform a role in protection of the infant has been studied by many investigators using many techniques. Animal studies, in summary, have shown that (1) the mammary gland is susceptible to infection in early lactation, (2) a dramatic increase in PMNs occurs with mammary inflammation, and (3) in the presence of peripheral neutropenia during chronic mastitis, severe infection of the gland occurs. This implies, according to Buescher and Pickering,[15] that the primary function of milk PMNs is as defense of the mammary tissue per se and not to impart maternal immunocompetence to the newborn. This may explain the presence of large numbers of PMNs that are relatively hypofunctional early and then disappear over time.

Lymphocytes

Both T- and B-lymphocytes are present in human milk and colostrum and are part of the immunologic system in human milk. They synthesize IgA antibody. Human milk lymphocytes respond to mitogens by proliferation, with increased macrophage-lymphocyte interaction and the release of soluble mediators, including MIF. Cells destined to become lymphopoietic cells are derived from two separate influences, the thymus (T) and the bursa (B) or bursal equivalent tissues. The population of cells called *B cells* comprises the

Fig. 5-2. **A,** Longitudinal study of numbers of leukocytes. **B,** Longitudinal study of uptake of
^{3}H-thymidine in lymphocytes. Same subjects were examined during second through twelfth week
of lactation. Data are presented as means ± SD of macrophages-neutrophils (•—•) and lymphocytes
(○—○) and of stimulated (•—•) and unstimulated (○—○) lymphocytes in **B.** (From Goldman AS,
Garza C, Nichols BL et al: *J Pediatr* 100:563, 1982.)

smaller part of the total. The term *B cell* is derived
from its origination in a different anatomic site
from the thymus; in birds, it has been identified
as the bursa of Fabricius. The B cells can be
identified by the presence of surface immunoglobulin markers. The B cells in human milk
include cells with IgA, IgM, and IgG surface
immunoglobulins. B cells transform into plasma
cells and remain sessile in the tissues of the
mammary gland.

T-cell system

More rapid mitotic activity occurs in the thymus
gland than in any other lymphatic organ, yet 70%
of the cells die within the cell substance. Thymosin
has been identified as a hormone produced by
thymic epithelial cells to expand the peripheral
lymphocyte population. After emergence from the
thymus gland, T cells acquire new surface antigen
markers. The T cells circulate through the lymphatic and vascular systems as long-lived lymphocytes, which are called the *recirculating pool*. They

then populate restricted regions of lymph nodes,
forming thymic-dependent areas.[117]

The significance of the lymphocytes in human
milk in affording immunologic benefits to the
breastfed infant continues to be investigated. It is
suggested that lymphocytes can sensitize, induce
immunologic tolerance, or incite graft-versus-host
reactions. According to Head and Beer,[53] lymphocytes may be incorporated into the suckling's
tissues, achieving short-term adoptive immunization of the neonate.

Studies of the activities of lymphocytes have
been carried out by a number of investigators who
collected samples of milk from lactating women at
various times postpartum, examined the number of
cell types present, and then studied the activities of
these cells in vitro.[60,63] Ogra and Ogra[86] collected
samples from 200 women and measured the cell
content from 1 through 180 days (Fig. 5-1). They
then compared the response of T-lymphocytes in
colostrum and milk with that of the T cells in the
peripheral blood (Fig. 5-2). T-cell subpopulations

have also been shown by surface epitopes to be similar to those in the peripheral blood.

The greatest number of cells appeared on the first day, with the counts ranging from 10,000 to 100,000/mm^3 for total cells. By the fifth day, the count had dropped to 20% of the first day's count. In addition, the number of E rosette-forming cells was determined by using sheep erythrocyte-rosetting technique. The E rosette formation (ERF) lymphocytes constituted a mean 100/mm^3 on the first day and a tenth of that by the fifth day.

At 180 days, total cells were 100,000/mm^3, lymphocytes were 10,000/mm^3, and ERF lymphocytes were 2000/mm^3. The investigators compared the values with those in the peripheral blood of each mother; the levels remained essentially constant.[86]

In a similar study, Bhaskaram and Reddy[10] sampled milk over time from 74 women and found comparable cell concentrations. They examined the bactericidal activity of the milk leukocytes and found it to be comparable with that of the circulating leukocytes in the blood, irrespective of the stage of lactation or state of nutrition of the mother.

Ogra and Ogra[87] also studied the lymphocyte proliferation responses of colostrum and milk to antigens. Their data show response to stimulation from the viral antigens of rubella, cytomegalovirus, and mumps. Analysis of cell-mediated immunity to microbial antigens shows milk lymphocytes are limited in their potential for recognizing or responding to certain infectious agents as compared with cells from the peripheral circulation. This is believed to be an intercellular action and not caused by lack of external factors. On the other hand, the T cells and B cells have been shown to have unique reactivities not seen in peripheral blood.

Juto[58] studied the effect of human milk on B-cell function. Cell-free, defatted, filtered colostrum as well as mature breast milk showed an enhancing effect on B-cell proliferation and generation of antibody secretion. This was not seen with formula. Juto suggested that this could represent an important immunologic mechanism. Goldblum et al[39] were able to show a response in

human colostrum to *Escherichia coli* given orally, which was not accompanied by a systemic response in the mother. This suggests that milk provides a site for local humoral or cell-mediated immunity induced at a distant site such as the gut, with the reactive lymphoid cells migrating to the breast. This concept has been further refined to suggest that IgA and IgM in colostrum may represent migration of specific antibody-producing cells from GALT, specifically Peyer's patches, to the mammary gland. Ogra and Ogra[86,87] suggest that the cells may be selectively accumulated in the breast during pregnancy. The responses of milk cells and their antibodies are not representative of the individual's total immunity.[92] Head and Beer[53] have provided a scheme to describe this mechanism (Fig. 5-3). The diagram depicts the progeny of specifically sensitized lymphocytes that originated in GALT as they migrate to the mammary gland. As they infiltrate the mammary gland and its secretion, they supply the breast with immune cells capable of selected immune responses.

Most of these immunocompetent cells recirculate to the external mucosal surface and populate the lamina propria as antibody-producing plasma cells. A substantial number of these antigen-sensitized cells selectively home in to the stroma of the mammary glands and initiate local IgA antibody synthesis against the antigens initially encountered in the respiratory or intestinal mucosa.[10]

Colostral lymphocytes are derived from mature rather than immature T-cell subsets. The distribution of T-cell subsets in colostrum includes both T-4 and T-8 positive cells.[102] The distribution of T4 in colostrum cells is lower than in the serum, and fewer T4 cells exist than T8 cells. The percentage is higher than in the serum of either postpartum donors or normal controls. No correlation exists with length of gestation and number of cells (in normal blood there are usually twice as many T4- as T8-positive lymphocytes).[58]

Parmely et al[92] partially purified and propagated milk lymphocytes in vitro to study their immunologic function. Milk lymphocytes responded in a unique manner to stimuli known to activate T-lymphocytes from the serum. The authors found

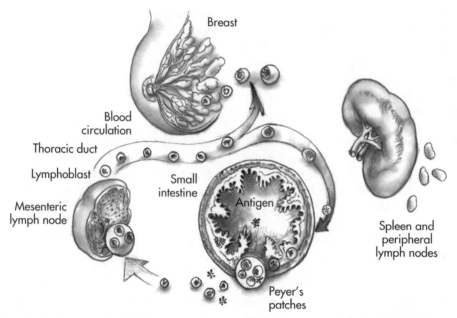

Fig. 5-3. Schema of mechanism by which progeny of specifically sensitized lymphocytes originating from gut-associated lymphoid tissue may migrate to and infiltrate mammary gland and its secretions, supplying breast with immune cells. (Modified from Head JR, Beer AE: The immunologic role of viable leukocytic cells in mammary exosecretions. In Larson BL, editor: *Lactation,* vol IV, *Mammary gland/human lactation/milk synthesis,* New York, 1978, Academic Press.)

milk lymphocytes to be hyporesponsive to nonspecific mitogens and histocompatible antigens on allogenic cells in their laboratory. They found them unresponsive to *Candida albicans.* Significant proliferation of lymphocytes occurred in response to K_1 capsular antigen of *E. coli.*[54] Lymphocytes from blood failed to respond to the same antigen. This supports the concept of local mammary tissue immunity at the T-lymphocyte level.

More recent experiments in rodents have provided evidence that T-lymphocytes reactive to transplantation alloantigens can adoptively immunize the suckling newborn. Foster nursing experiments performed in rodents have shown that newborn rats exposed to allogenic milk manifested alterations in their reactivity to skin allografts of the foster mother's strain. In animals, mothers may give their suckling newborn immunoreactive lymphocytes. The influence of maternal milk cells on the development of neonatal immunocompetence

has been demonstrated in several different immunologic contexts. Congenitally, athymic nude mice nursed by their phenotypically normal mothers or normal foster mothers had increased survival. The mothers contributed their T-cell–helper activity to the suckling newborn.

Colostral lymphocytes proliferate in response to various mitogens, alloantigens, and conventional antigens. Colostral cells survive in the neonatal stomach and in the gut of experimental animals, some remaining viable in the upper GI tract for a week. On the other hand, no evidence indicates that transepithelial migration takes place when neonatal mice are foster-nursed by newly delivered animals whose colostral cells were tagged with ^{3}H-thymidine.[15]

Cells in human milk have been studied using the same markers employed with cells in the peripheral blood. About 80% of the lymphocytes are T cells that are equally distributed between CD4 positive and CD8 positive subpopulations, and their T-cell receptors (TCRs) are principally of the α/β type. CD4 positive cells are common leukocyte cells of the helper and suppressor-inducer subsets, and CD8 positive are leukocytes of the cytotoxic and noncytotoxic subsets. T cells in human milk are presumed activated because they display increased phenotypic markers of activation. These cells are effective producers of interferon-γ, in keeping with their phenotypic features. Human milk macrophages have the morphology and motility of activated cells. The movement of these cells in a three-dimensional system is greater than that of monocytes, their counterparts in peripheral blood.[117]

The accumulated research data support the concept that lymphocytes from colostrum and milk provide the human infant with immunologic benefits. Both T- and B-lymphocytes are reactive against organisms invading the intestinal tract. Investigations on allergy, necrotizing enterocolitis, tuberculosis, and neonatal meningitis support the concept that human milk fulfills a protective function.

SURVIVAL OF MATERNAL MILK CELLS

Although it is clear that cells are provided in the colostrum and milk, the effectiveness and impact of these cells on the neonate depend on their ability to survive in the GI tract. It has been demonstrated in several species, including humans, that the pH of the stomach can be as low as 0.5, but the output of hydrochloric acid (HCl) is minimal for the first few months, as is the peptic activity. Immediately after a feeding begins, the pH rises to 6.0 and returns to normal in 3 hours. The cells from milk tolerate this. Studies have also shown that intact nucleated lymphoid cells are found in the stomach and intestines.[7] These cells, when removed from rat stomachs, are capable of phagocytosis. Lymphoid cells in milk have been shown to traverse the mucosal wall.

When human milk is stored, however, the cellular components do not tolerate heating to

63° C (145.4° F), cooling to −23° C (−9.4° F), or lyophilization. Although a few cells may be identified, they are not viable.[40]

HUMORAL FACTORS

Immunoglobulins

All classes of immunoglobulins are found in human milk. The study of immunoglobulins has been enhanced through electrophoresis, chromatographics, and radioimmunoassays. More than 30 components have been identified; of these, 18 are associated with proteins in the maternal serum, and the others are found exclusively in milk.

The concentrations are highest in the colostrum of all species, and the concentrations change as lactation proceeds.[78]

IgA, principally sIgA, is highest in colostrum. Although postpartum levels fall over the next 4 weeks, substantial levels are maintained throughout the first year, during gradual weaning between 6 and 9 months, and even during partial breastfeeding (when infant receives solid foods) in the second year of life (Figs. 5-4 and 5-5 and Table 5-2). Specific sIgA antibodies to *E. coli* persist through lactation and may even rise (Fig. 5-4).

The main immunoglobulin in human serum is IgG; IgA is only one-fifth the level of IgG. In milk, however, the reverse is true. IgA is the most important immunoglobulin in milk, not only in concentration but also in biologic activity. Of the IgA immunoglobulins, sIgA is the most significant and is likely synthesized in the mammary alveolar cells.[110]

Quantitative determinations of immunoglobulins in human milk were made from milk collected at birth up to as long as 27 months postpartum by Peitersen et al[93] and by Goldman et al.[43] The IgA content was high immediately after birth, dropping in 2 to 3 weeks, and then remaining constant. Similar observations were made on IgG levels and IgM levels. Ogra and Ogra[86,87] have compared serum and milk levels at various times postpartum. Samples obtained separately from the left and right

Fig. 5-4. Same subjects were examined during second through twelfth week of lactation. Total (•) and secretory IgA (○) data presented as mean ± SD. SIgA antibody titers to *E. coli* somatic antigens from each subject are represented by different symbols. **A,** Longitudinal study of total IgA and sIgA. **B,** Longitudinal study of reciprocal of sIgA antibody titers to *E. coli* somatic antigens in human milk. (From Goldman AS, Garza C, Nichols BL et al: *J Pediatr* 100:563, 1982.)

breasts showed similar values. The levels remained constant during a given feeding and throughout a 24-hour period. In all quantitative determinations, IgA is the predominant immunoglobulin in breast milk, constituting 90% of all the immunoglobulins in colostrum and milk.

Ogra and Ogra[86-88] studied the serum of postpartum lactating mothers and nonpregnant

matched controls and noted that the individual and mean concentrations of all Ig classes were lower in the postpartum subjects. The levels were statistically significant in IgG, being 50 to 70 mg higher in the nonpregnant women.

Immunoglobulin levels, particularly IgA and IgM, are very high in colostrum and drop precipitously in the first 4 to 6 days, but importantly, IgG does not show this decline. The volume of mammary secretion, however, increases dramatically in this same period; thus the absolute volumes are more nearly constant than it would first appear. Local production and concentration of IgA and probably IgM may take place in the mammary gland at delivery.

IgE and IgD have also been measured in colostrum and milk. Using radioimmunoassay techniques, colostrum was found to contain concentrations of 0.5 to 0.6 IU/ml IgE in 41% of samples and less in the remainder.[3] IgD was found in all samples in concentrations of 2 to 2000 μg/dl. Plasma levels were poorly correlated. The findings suggest possible local mammary production rather than positive transfer. Whether IgE or IgD antibodies in breast milk have similar specificities for antigens as the IgA antibodies in milk remains unanswered.[77] Keller et al[61] examined the question of local mammary IgD production and its possible participation in a mucosal immune system by comparing colostrum and plasma levels of total IgD with specific IgD antibodies. From their work comparing colostrum/plasma ratios for IgG, IgD, and albumin and measuring IgD against specific antigens, the authors reported evidence for IgD participation in the response of the mucosal immune system, with increases in total IgD and IgD against specific antigens found in colostrum.

To address the question of total quantities of immunologic components secreted into human milk per day and available to the infant, Butte et al[17] measured the amounts of sIgA, sIgA antibodies to *E. coli,* lactoferrin, and lysozyme ingested per day and per kilogram per day in the first 4 months of life (Figs. 5-6 to 5-10). Lactoferrin, sIgA, and sIgA antibodies gradually declined in amount ingested per day and per kilogram per day.

Fig. 5-5. Same subjects were examined during second through twelfth week of lactation. Data in longitudinal studies presented as mean ± SD. **A,** Concentration of lactoferrin progressively decreased through first 8 weeks ($r = 0.69$) (2 vs. 8 weeks; $p < 0.02$), but not thereafter. **B,** In contrast, lysozyme levels steadily increased from fourth through twelfth week ($r = 0.76$) (4 vs. 12 weeks; $p < 0.01$). (From Goldman AS, Garza C, Nichols BL et al: *J Pediatr* 100:563, 1982.)

TABLE 5-2   **Concentrations of immunologic components in human milk collected during second year of lactation**

	Duration of lactation (months)		
Component	12	13-15	16-24
IgA (mg/ml)			
Total	0.8 ± 0.3	1.1 ± 0.4	1.1 ± 0.3
Secretory (sIgA)	0.8 ± 0.3	1.1 ± 0.3	1.1 ± 0.2
Lactoferrin (mg/ml)	1.0 ± 0.2	1.1 ± 0.1	1.2 ± 0.1
Lysozyme (µg/ml)	196 ± 41	244 ± 34	187 ± 33
sIgA antibodies (reciprocal titers	5 ± 6	9 ± 10	6 ± 3
to *E. coli* somatic antigens)			

From Goldman AS, Goldblum RM, Garza C: *Acta Paediatr Scand* 72:461, 1983. Data are presented as the mean ± SD.

Lysozyme, on the other hand, rose during the same period in total amount available and amount per kilogram per day. The authors[17] suggest that production and secretion of these immunologic factors by the mammary gland may be linked to the catabolism of the components at the infant's mucosal tissues. When concentrations of SIgA, IgG, IgM, α_1-antitrypsin, lactoferrin, lysozyme, and globulins C3 and C4 were compared in relationship to parity and age of the mother, there was no consistent trend. When maturity of the pregnancy was considered, however, mean concentrations of all these proteins were higher, except for IgA, when the delivery was premature. Because several proteins in human milk have physiologic function in the infant, Davidson and Lönnerdal[26] examined the survival of human milk proteins through the GI tract. Crossed immunoelectrophoresis showed that three human milk proteins transversed the entire intestine and were present in the feces: lactoferrin, sIgA, and α_1-antitrypsin.

Miranda et al[79] reported on the effect of

Fig. 5-6. Amounts of sIgA and sIgA antibodies to *E. coli* somatic antigens in human milk ingested per day, **A,** and per kilogram per day, **B.** Data presented as mean ± SD. (From Butte NF, Goldman RM, Fehl LM et al: *Acta Paediatr Scand* 73:296, 1984.)

Fig. 5-7. Amounts of sIgA antibodies to *E. coli* somatic antigens in human milk ingested as reciprocal titers per day, **A,** per kilogram per day, **B.** Data presented as mean ± SD. (From Butte NF, Goldman RM, Fehl LM et al: *Acta Paediatr Scand* 73:296, 1984.)

maternal nutritional status on immunologic substances in human colostrum and milk. Maternal malnutrition was characterized as lower weight to height ratio, creatine/height index, total serum proteins, and IgG and IgA. The colostrum contained one third the normal concentration of IgG, less than half the normal level of albumin, and lower IgA and complement C4. Lysozyme, complement C3, and IgM levels were normal. Levels improved with development of mature milk and improvement in maternal nutrition.

Immunologic components in human milk during the second year of lactation become a significant point as more infants are nursed longer. Subjects were part of a longitudinal study, had fully breastfed their infants for 6 months to a year, and were continuing to partially breastfeed.[44] Samples were collected by fully emptying the breast by electric pump. Table 5-2 summarizes concentrations. No leukocytes were detected. Con-

centrations of total and secretory IgA, lactoferrin, and lysozyme were similar to those 7 to 12 months postpartum and during gradual weaning. sIgA antibodies to *E. coli* were produced in the second year, demonstrating significant immunologic benefit to the infant with continued breastfeeding.[44]

Immunoglobulins A, M, and G were measured in nursing women from the beginning of lactation and simultaneously in the feces of their children by Jatsyk et al[55] at the Academy of Medicine in Moscow. They reported IgA to be very high in the milk and rapidly increasing in the feces. IgG and IgM levels, however, were low in both milk and feces. In normal full-term bottle-fed infants, IgA appeared in the feces at 3 to 4 weeks of age but at much lower levels than in breastfed infants.

Savilahei et al[106] measured serum levels of IgG, IgA, and IgM in 198 infants at 2, 4, 6, 9, and 12 months of age. By 9 months, the infants exclusively breastfed had IgG and IgM levels signifi-

Fig. 5-8. Amount of total protein in human milk ingested per day, **A,** and per kilogram per day, **B.** Data presented as mean ± SD. (From Butte NF, Goldblum RM, Fehl LM et al: *Acta Paediatr Scand* 73:296, 1984.)

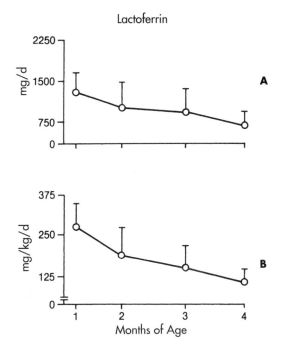

Fig. 5-9. Amount of lactoferrin in human milk ingested per day, **A,** and per kilogram per day, **B.** Data presented as mean ± SD. (From Butte NF, Goldblum RM, Fehl LM et al: *Acta Paediatr Scand* 73:296, 1984.)

cantly lower than those who had been weaned early (before 3.5 months) to formula. Six infants were still exclusively breastfed at 12 months, and their IgA levels had also lowered to levels found at 2 months with bottle feeders. Infection rates were similar. Two months after the children were weaned to formula, the IgG and IgM levels were comparable. Iron and zinc levels were the same in all children.

Stability of immunoglobulins

Preservation of human milk at $-20°$ C alters the levels of IgA, IgM, C3, C4, α_1-antitrypsin, and sIgA antibodies to *E. coli* and lactoperoxidase.[33] Heat treatments include low-temperature, short-time (LTST), 56° C for 15 minutes; Holder pasteurization (HP), 62.5° C for 30 minutes; and high-temperature, short-time (HTST), 70° C for 15 seconds. Boiling essentially destroys 100% of

immunologic activity. Secretory IgA and lysozyme activities drop by 20% with HP and by 50% at 65° C. Neither LTST nor HTST reduces the sIgA or lysozyme content. IgG and IgM are greatly reduced by HP (Table 5-3).

Secretory IgA differs antigenically from serum IgA. IgA can be synthesized in the nonlactating as well as in the lactating breast. It is a compact molecule and resistant to proteolytic enzymes of the intestinal tract and the low pH of the stomach. sIgA is manufactured by the mammary gland and by the cellular lymphocytes in milk. Levels in milk are 10 to 100 times higher than in serum. Levels in cow's milk are very low, that is, a tenth of the level in mature human milk (0.03 mg/dl). Later in life, the intestinal tract's subepithelial plasma cells secrete IgA, but this does not occur in the neonatal period.

Discussion continues as to whether any antibodies are absorbed from the intestinal tract, although

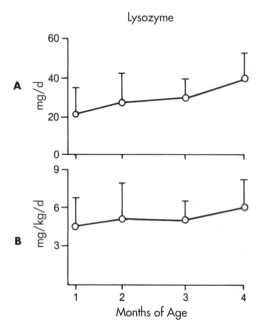

Lysozyme

Fig. 5-10. Amount of lysozyme in human milk ingested per day, **A,** and per kilogram per day, **B.** Data presented as mean ± SD. (From Butte NF, Goldblum RM, Fehl LM et al: *Acta Paediatr Scand* 73:296, 1984.)

probably 10% are absorbed. Almost 75% of ingested IgA from milk survives passage through the intestinal tract and is excreted in the feces. All immunoglobulin classes have been identified in the feces.[101] However, much evidence demonstrates the activity of the immunoglobulins, especially IgA, at the mucosal levels. These antibodies provide local intestinal protection against viruses such as poliovirus and bacteria such as *E. coli,* which may infect the mucosa or enter the body through the gut.

Bifidus factor

It has been established since the work of Tissier in 1908 on the newborn's intestinal flora that the predominant bacteria of the breastfed infant are bifid bacteria. *Bifid bacteria* are gram-positive, nonmotile anaerobic bacilli. Many observers have shown the striking difference between the flora of the guts of breastfed and bottle-fed infants. György[48] demonstrated the presence of a specific factor in colostrum and milk that supported the growth of *Lactobacillus bifidus*. Bifidus factor has been

TABLE 5-3	**Antiviral antibody in human milk**		
Factor	**Shown, in vitro, to be active against:**	**Assay***	**Effect of heat**
Secretory IgA	Enteroviruses		
	Poliovirus types 1, 2, 3	ELISA, NA, Precipitan	Stable at 56° C for 30 min;
	Coxsackievirus types A_9,	NA	some loss (0%-30%)
	B_3, B_5	NA	
	Echovirus types 6 and 9		At 62.5° C for 30 min;
	Herpesvirus		destroyed by boiling
	Cytomegalovirus	ELISA, IFA, NA	
	Herpes simplex virus	NA	
	Semliki Forest virus	IFA	
	Respiratory syncytial virus	IFA	
	Rubella	IFA, HAI	
	Reovirus type 3	ELISA, NA	
	Rotavirus		
IgM, IgG	Cytomegalovirus		Stable at 56° C for 30 min;
	Respiratory syncytial virus		IgG decreased by a third
	Rubella		at 62.5° C for 30 min

*ELISA, Enzyme-linked immunosorbent assay; NA, neutralizing assay; IFA, immunofluorescent assay; HAI, hemagglutination inhibition.

characterized as a dialyzable, nitrogen-containing carbohydrate that contains no amino acid.

In vitro studies by Beerens et al[8] showed the presence of a specific growth factor for *Bifidobacterium bifidum* in human milk, which they called BB. Other milks, including cow's milk, sheep's milk, pig's milk, and infant formulas, did not promote the growth of this species but did show some activity supporting *B. infantis* and *B. longum.* This growth factor was found to be stable when the milk was frozen, heated, freeze-dried, and stored for 3 months. Growth-promoting factors were present for the six strains studied, which varied in their resistance to physical change. Because all these factors were active in vitro, they did not require the presence of intestinal enzymes for activation. It has not been possible to show the presence of this growth factor in other mammalian milks; thus it may contribute to the implantation and persistence of *B. bifidum* in the breastfed infant's intestine.

Resistance factor

It was well known in the preantibiotic era that human milk protects the human infant throughout lactation against staphylococcal infection. György[48] identified the presence of an "antistaphylococcal factor" in experiments with young mice that had been stressed with staphylococci. This factor, with no demonstrable direct antibiotic properties, was termed a *resistance factor* and described as nondialyzable, thermostable, and part of the free fatty acid part of the phosphide fraction, probably $C_{18:2}$, but distinct from linoleic acid.

Lysozyme

Human milk contains a nonspecific antimicrobial factor, lysozyme, which is a thermostable, acid-stable enzyme. It is found in large concentrations in the stools of breastfed infants and not in stools of formula-fed infants; it thus is thought to influence the flora of the intestinal tract.

Goldman et al[43] describe an initial fall in lysozyme levels from 85 to 90 mg/ml to 25 mg/ml at 2 to 4 weeks and then a rise over 6 months to 250 mg/ml (Fig. 5-5). Lysozyme levels show an increase over time during lactation; this finding is more apparent in Indian women than in those of the Western world. Reddy et al[100] studied the levels of lysozyme in well-nourished and poorly nourished women in India and found no difference between them (Table 5-4). As shown in this study, lysozyme levels increase during lactation. Levels in human milk are 300 times the level in cow's milk. Lysozyme is bacteriostatic against Enterobacteriaceae and gram-positive bacteria.[95] Lysozyme is an enzyme that digests a bond in the cell wall proteoglycan of some gram-positive bacteria. It is secreted by neutrophils and some macrophages and is present in many body secretions in the adult.

In a study of immunologic components in human milk in the second year of lactation, Goldman et al[44] reported that concentrations of lysozyme, lactoferrin, and total and secretory IgA were similar to those in uninterrupted lactation and in gradual weaning at 6 to 9 months. sIgA antibodies to *E. coli* were also produced during the second year. The authors state that "this supports the idea that the enteromammary lymphocyte traffic pathway, which leads to the development of lymphoid cells in the mammary gland that produce IgA antibodies to enteric organisms, operates throughout lactation."[44]

When cow's milk–based formula is added to human milk, it reduces the effect of lysozyme; however, powdered human milk fortifier (Enfamil) did not inhibit the antiinfective properties.[62]

Lactoferrin

Lactoferrin is an iron-binding protein closely related to the serum iron transport protein, transferrin. A bacteriostatic effect of lactoferrin is well established for a wide range of microorganisms, including gram-positive and gram-negative aerobes, anaerobes, and yeasts. The proposed predominant mechanism of action for its bacteriostatic effect is depriving the organism of iron.

TABLE 5-4 Antibacterial factors in colostrum and mature milk in well-nourished and undernourished Indian women

Group	Hemoglobin (g/dl)	Serum albumin (g/dl)	Immunoglobulins (mg/dl)			Lysozyme (mg/dl)	Lactoferrin (mg/dl)
			IgA	IgG	IgM		
Colostrum (1 to 5 days)							
Well-nourished women	11.5 ± 0.37	2.49 ± 0.065	335.9 ± 37.39 (17)*	5.9 ± 1.58 (17)	17.1 ± 4.29 (17)	14.2 ± 2.11 (15)	420 ± 49.0 (28)
Undernourished women	11.3 ± 0.60	2.10 ± 0.081	374.3 ± 42.13 (10)	5.3 ± 2.30 (10)	15.3 ± 2.50 (10)	16.4 ± 2.39 (21)	520 ± 69.0 (19)
Mature milk (1 to 6 months)							
Well-nourished women	12.8 ± 0.43	3.39 ± 0.120	119.6 ± 7.85 (12)	2.9 ± 0.92 (12)	2.9 ± 0.92 (12)	24.8 ± 3.41 (10)	250 ± 65.0 (17)
Undernourished women	12.6 ± 0.56	3.47 ± 0.130	118.1 ± 16.2 (10)	5.8 ± 3.41 (10)	5.8 ± 3.41 (10)	23.3 ± 3.53 (23)	270 ± 92.0 (13)

From Reddy V, Bhaskaram C, Raghuramula N et al: *Acta Paediatr Scand* 66:229, 1977.
*Figures in parentheses indicate number of samples analyzed.

The biologic role of lactoferrin has been reviewed in several studies.[72,85,105] They point out that lactoferrin reversibly binds two ferric ions and that its affinity for iron is 300 times greater than that of transferrin, retaining iron down to a pH of 3. Human lactoferrin is strongly basic. Lactoferrin is normally unsaturated with iron,[16] and it is usually less than 10% saturated with iron in human milk.[35,105] Oral iron therapy for the infant can interfere with the bacteriostatic action of lactoferrin, which depends on its unsaturated state for some portion of its bacteriostatic function. Reddy et al[100] showed that giving iron to the mother did not interfere with the saturation of lactoferrin in the milk or thus its potential bacteriostatic effect. Protein energy malnutrition rather than iron supplies influences lactoferrin synthesis in the mammary gland. Malnourished but non–iron-deficient mothers are lactoferrin deficient.

The concentration of lactoferrin is high in colostrum—600 mg/dl—then progressively declines over the next 5 months of lactation, leveling off at about 180 mg/dl. Breast milk also contains small amounts of transferrin (10 to 15 μg/ml). Lactoferrin makes up about 10% to 15% of the total protein content of human milk.[72] Lactoferrin is resistant to proteolysis, especially in its iron-saturated form. Intact lactoferrin is detectable in the stool of infants, with higher proportions of lactoferrin measurable in the stool of premature infants.[29] Both intact lactoferrin and fragments have been detected in the urine of premature infants, although absorption is less likely in full-term infants.[51]

Many bacteria require iron for normal growth, and the bacteriostatic effect of lactoferrin has been ascribed to its iron-binding action. In neutrophils, lactoferrin within neutrophilic granules tightly binds iron, but neutrophils with excessive iron are inefficient at destroying bacteria. Lactoferrin does not limit the growth of all microorganisms; *Helicobacter pylori* and *Neisseria, Treponema,* and *Shigella* species all have receptors for lactoferrin, directly binding iron and allowing adequate growth.

Some evidence supports various other proposed mechanisms of action for lactoferrin's antimicrobial effect. Pepsin hydrolysate products of lactoferrin (B or H) may exert a direct bactericidal effect by binding to lipopolysaccharide of gram-negative organisms and disrupting bacterial membranes.[113] Lactoferrin may cause an increased release of cytokines by cells.[24] Others have shown that lactoferrin suppresses the release of interleukin-1 and -2 (IL-1, IL-2) and tumor necrosis factor alpha (TNF-α), which would be more of an immune-modulating effect.[73]

Several other effects have been proposed for lactoferrin, including inhibition of hydroxyl radical formation, decreasing local cell damage; lipopolysaccharide binding, also leading to a diminished inflammatory response; and DNA binding, affecting transcription and possibly regulation of the production of cell products.[85]

The exact roles and possible mechanisms of action of lactoferrin in the breastfed infant must be more specifically clarified.

Interferon

Colostral cells in culture have been shown to be stimulated to secrete an interferon-like substance with strong antiviral activity up to 150 NIH units/ml.[95] This property has not yet been identified in the supernatant of colostrum or milk. Interferon-γ has been produced by T cells from human milk when stimulated in vitro.[9] The T cells isolated from human milk were the CD45RO phenotype and have been identified as a source of interferon. Srivastava et al[109] have measured low levels of interferon-γ in not only colostrum but also transitional and mature milk. They postulated that the low level of interferon-γ (0.7 to 2 pg/ml) might be adequate to protect against infection without hyperactivation of T cells. Interferon is produced by natural killer cells and by T cells phenotypically Thy0 and Thy1. It can cause increased expression of major histocompatibility complex (MHC) molecules, increase macrophage function, inhibit IgE and IL-10 production, and produce antitumor and antiviral activity. The exact role of interferon-γ in breast milk has not been delineated.

Complement

The C3 and C4 components of complement, known for their ability to fuse bacteria bound to a specific antibody, are present in colostrum in low concentrations as compared with their levels in serum. IgG and IgM activate complement. C3 proactivator has been described, and IgA and IgE have been identified as stimulating the system. Activated C3 has opsonic, anaphylactic, and chemotactic properties and is important for the lysis of bacteria bound to a specific antibody.

Vitamin B_{12}-binding protein

Unsaturated vitamin B_{12}-binding protein of high molecular weight has been found in very high levels in human milk and in the meconium and stools of breastfed infants as compared with those levels in infant formulas and the infants who are formula-fed. The protein binding renders the B_{12} unavailable for bacterial growth of *E. coli* and *Bacteroides*.[47]

Gangliosides

Gangliosides are glycolipids found in the plasma membrane of cells, especially in cells in the gray matter of the brain. More specifically, gangliosides are glycosphingolipids that contain sialic acid, hexoses, or hexose amines as the carbohydrate component and ceramide as the lipid component of the molecule. The predominant gangliosides in human milk are GM1, GM2, GM3, and GD3, as reported by Newburg.[83]

Gangliosides appear to be responsible for blocking the activity of heat-labile enterotoxin from *E. coli* and the toxin from *Vibrio cholerae* in rat intestinal loop preparations.[89] Another toxin from *Campylobacter jejuni,* with similar binding specificity, also seems to be inhibited by GM1.[67,104] Globotriaosylceramide (Gb3), another glycolipid in human milk, is the natural cell surface receptor for the toxin from *Shigella dysenteriae* and Verotoxin released by enterohemorrhagic *E. coli*.[84] The proposed mechanism of action of these glycolipids is that by binding to the toxin, they form a stable complex that prevents the toxin from binding to the appropriate receptors on intestinal cells. Human milk gangliosides may be important in protecting infants against toxin-induced diarrhea, but this has not been specifically demonstrated in vivo (Table 5-5).[82,89]

Interleukins

Interleukins (ILs) are now considered a "subgroup" of cytokines.[71] Originally, when cytokines were first hypothesized, it was believed that they were primarily produced by leukocytes and acted on other leukocytes, and therefore they could be called *interleukins*. Although much of their effect is on lymphocyte activation and differentiation, it is now known that interleukins act on and are produced by a variety of cells.

Goldman et al[42] identified IL-1β, IL-6, IL-8, and IL-10 in breast milk (Table 5-6). Srivastava et al[109] reported measuring moderate amounts of IL-6, IL-8, and IL-10 in the different stages of breast milk. Very low amounts of IL-1β were detected, especially in comparison with the amount of IL-1 receptor antagonist (RA), which presumably could block the activity of the small amount of IL-1.

IL-6 has been identified in breast milk by other investigators, especially in the first 2 days of life.[90,103] All the authors suggest that IL-6 in human milk may augment the newborn's immune functions before the body can begin full production of cytokines. Specifically, this is accomplished by increasing antibody production, especially IgA; enhancing phagocytosis; activating T cells; and increasing $α_1$-antitrypsin production by mononuclear phagocytes.

IL-8 is a chemokine capable of attracting and activating neutrophils and attracting CD45RA+ T cells. IL-8 is produced by mammary epithelial cells.[90] Srivastava et al[109] also detected messenger ribonucleic acid (mRNA) for IL-8, suggesting that cells in breast milk were capable of producing IL-8. The exact function of IL-8 in breast milk remains to be elucidated.

IL-10 is believed to have antiinflammatory

TABLE 5-5 Nonimmunoglobulin antipathogens from human milk	
Antipathogen	**Pathogen**
Ganglioside GM$_1$	Cholera toxin
	Labile toxin of *Escherichia coli*
	Toxin of *Campylobacter jejuni*
Globotriaosylceramide (Gb3)	*Shigella* toxin I
	Shigalike toxin of *E. coli*
Fatty acids	Enveloped viruses
	Giardia lamblia
Glycoprotein (mucin)	Inhibition: rotavirus in vitro and in vivo
Glycoprotein (mucin, glycosaminoglycan)	Human immunodeficiency virus (HIV)
Mucin	Adherence: S-fimbriated *E. coli*
Glycoprotein (mannosylated)	*E. coli* intestinal adherence
Large macromolecule	Respiratory syncytial virus
Oligosaccharides	Adherence: *Streptococcus pneumoniae* and *Haemophilus influenzae* adherence of enteropathogenic *E. coli*
Fucosylated oligosaccharide	Adherence: invasion, *C. jejuni* toxicity of stabile toxin of *E. coli* (ST) in vivo

From Newburg DS: *Mammary Gland Biol Lactation Newslett* 11:10, 1992.

effects, including decreasing the production of interferon-γ, IL-12, and other proinflammatory cytokines. It has been reported to enhance IgA, IgG, and IgM synthesis.

The interaction and the direct effect of these interleukins in breast milk must be clarified. The existence of T cells bearing markers of recent activation are increased in human milk compared with the results in peripheral blood of adults. Wirt et al[117] have described a marked shift from virginal to antigen-primed (memory) T cells in human milk, which suggests certain functional capacities for these cells. The phenotypic pattern of T cells may result from T-cell–activating substances or selective homing of T cells to the breast. These activated T-cell populations (and presumably others) are transferred to the infant through breast milk and the transfer of interleukins, which may contribute to immune activation or antiinflammatory control in the infant.

Cytokines

Of the many bioactive substances that have been identified in human milk, cytokines are some of the

TABLE 5-6   Bioactivity and concentrations of cytokines in human milk

Agents	Bioactivity in milk	Concentrations*
IL-1β	±	1130 ± 478
IL-6	+	151 ± 89
IL-8	?	3684 ± 2910
IL-10	+	3400 ± 3800
TNF-α	+	620 ± 183
G-CSF	?	~358
M-CSF	+	17,120
Interferon-γ	?	?
EGF	+	~200,000
TGF-α	+	~2200-7200
TGF-β$_2$	+	130 ± 108

From Goldman AS, Chheda S, Garofalo R, Schmalstieg FC: *J Mammary Gland Biol Neoplasia* 1(3):251, 1996.

IL, Interleukin; *TNF,* tumor necrosis factor; *CSF,* colony-stimulating factor; *M,* macrophage; *G,* granulocyte; *EGF,* epidermal growth factor; *TGF,* transforming growth factor.

*The concentrations of these agents were determined by enzyme-linked immunosorbent assay (ELISA) except for IL-1β and EGF by radio-immunoassay. Concentrations are expressed as pg/ml except for M-CSF (U/ml).

most recently identified and investigated agents, although their existence has long been suspected in attempts to explain certain immunologic and protective effects of breast milk on infants. More than 40 cytokines have been described,[74] and more than 10 of these have been identified in human milk.[42,109] Cytokines are small proteins or glycoproteins that, through binding to receptors on immune and nonimmune cells, produce a broad range of effects (many still unidentified) through autocrine, paracrine, and endocrine actions. Cytokines are produced predominantly by immune cells and function in complex associations with other cytokines to stimulate and control the development and normal functioning of the immune system. The nomenclature and abbreviations used are complicated and confusing. Newer systems of classification have been established according to which cells produce them or what their general functions are[71] or based on the relative position of their cysteine residues or their receptor types (CCR, CXCR, CX3CR).[74] Box 5-1 provides a simplified list with abbreviations.

Little evidence demonstrates specific in vivo activity of the different cytokines. Based on general information on the function and interaction of the particular cytokines, as well as consideration of as yet unexplained effects of breast milk, proposed functions of the cytokines include initiation of development of host defense, stimulation of host defenses, prevention of autoimmunity, antiinflammatory effects in the upper respiratory tract and GI tract, and stimulation of the development of the digestive system, especially the mucosal immune system of the alimentary tract and the proximal respiratory tract. The maternal breast may respond to feedback stimulation or suppression by secreted cytokines, influencing growth, differentiation, and secretory function of the breast. As shown in other situations, cytokines may enhance receptor expression on cells in the respiratory and GI tracts for MHC molecules or immunoglobulins. Various cell types in the mucosal immune system may be activated or attracted to specific sites in the GI tract.

The actual measurement of cytokines in breast

BOX 5-1   Nomenclature and abbreviations for various cytokines

Interferon alpha, beta, gamma	IFN-α, -β, -γ
Granulocyte colony-stimulating factor	G-CSF
Macrophage colony-stimulating factor	M-CSF
Stem cell factor	SCF
Interleukin-1, -2, -4, -6, -8, -10	IL-1, -2, -4, -6, -8, -10
Interleukin-1 beta	IL-1β
Interleukin-1 receptor antagonist	IL-1RA
Soluble Interleukin-2 receptor	sIL-2R
Transforming growth factor beta$_2$	TGF-β_2
Tumor necrosis factor alpha	TNF-α
Transforming growth factor alpha	TGF-α
Macrophage inflammatory protein	MIP
Regulated on activation, normal T cell expressed and secreted	RANTES
Epidermal growth factor	EGF
Growth-regulated oncogene	GRO
Monocyte chemoattractant protein 1	MCP-1
Leukocyte inhibitory factor	LIF

---

milk has been complicated by a number of factors, including different assays used (bioassays, ELISA, radioimmunoassay), binding to proteins, their existence in monomeric or polymeric forms,[2] the presence of antagonists, and their varying presence in colostrum, early milk, or mature milk. Goldman et al[42] reported on the bioactivity and concentration of cytokines in breast milk from their own work and that of others (Table 5-6). Srivastava et al[109] obtained some conflicting results using different assays in colostrum, early milk, and mature milk. They confirmed the presence of M-CSF throughout lactation, as well as TGF-β_1 and -β_2, IL-1RA, GRO-α, MCP-1, RANTES, and IL-8, but reported insignificant amounts of GM-CSF, SCF, LIF, MIP-1α, IL-2, IL-4, IL-11, IL-12, IL-13, IL-15, sIL-2R, and IFN-α (see Box 5-1 for nomenclature). Srivastava et al[109] also used reverse transcriptase polymerase chain reaction (PCR) to measure the production of cytokine mRNA by cells in breast milk. They reported the presence of mRNA for MCP-1, IL-8, TGF-β_1, TGF-β_2, M-CSF, IL-6, and IL-1β, which may be another source of these cytokines in breast milk.

In their investigations of the possible antiinflammatory effects of breast milk, Buescher and Malinowska[13] examined milk for the presence of soluble receptors and cytokine antagonists. They demonstrated sICAM-1 (soluble intercellular adhesion molecule 1), sVCAM-1 (soluble vascular cell adhesion molecule 1), and sE-selectin (soluble E-selectin) in colostrum and at lower levels in mature milk, as well as high levels of sTNF-αRI (soluble tumor necrosis factor–alpha receptor I), sTNF-αRII, and IL-1RA. Also, they identified that most TNF-α did not exist "free" in breast milk but was associated with TNF receptors. The in vivo significance of these findings remains to be assessed.

Given the complex interaction and regulation of cytokine production and their relation to coordinated inflammatory and antiinflammatory responses in tissues, one should assume that the interaction of cytokines in breast milk and the effect of cytokines, cytokine receptors (soluble and expressed on various cell types), and cytokine antagonists on the infant will be equally complex. Continued investigation is essential to understanding the significance and specific effects of these substances in breast milk.

Nucleotides

Nucleotides, nucleosides, nucleic acids, and related metabolic products are essential to many biologic processes. Although they are not essential nutrients because they can be synthesized endogenously, their presence in the diet may carry significant benefits in various situations. In situations of disease, stress, rapid growth or limited dietary intake, supplementation of the diet with nucleotides may decrease energy expenditure to synthesize or salvage nucleotides, which optimizes the host response to these adverse situations.

Nucleotides exist in relatively large amounts in human milk, about 15% to 20% of the nonprotein

nitrogen (NPN), suggesting that they have some nutritional significance, although no clinical syndromes have been associated with nucleotide deficiency to date. Nucleotides are present in the natural milk of different species in varying amounts and composition. The nucleotide content and composition of bovine milk are particularly less and different from those of human milk, and subsequently the same has been true of infant formulas (see Chapter 4). Considerable debate surrounds the logic, the need, and the practical issues of adding nucleotides to formula.[94,99]

Mammalian cells contain a large variety of nucleotides and related products, which have many metabolic functions, including the following[21]:

1. Energy metabolism: adenosine triphosphate (ATP) is a major form of available cellular energy.
2. Nucleic acid precursors: the monomeric units for RNA and DNA are present.
3. Physiologic mediators: cyclic adenosine monophosphate (cAMP) and cyclic guanosine monophosphate (cGMP) serve as "messengers" for cellular processes; adenosine diphosphate (ADP) is necessary for platelet aggregation; and adenosine has been shown to affect vasodilatation.
4. Related products function as coenzymes in metabolic pathways: nicotinamide-adenine dinucleotide (NAD), flavin adenine dinucleotide (FAD), and coenzyme A (CoA).
5. Related products function as intermediate carrying molecules in synthetic reactions: uridine diphosphate–(UDP-)glucose in glycogen synthesis and guanosine diphosphate–(GDP-)mannose, GDP-fucose, UDP-galactose, and cytidine monophosphate–(CMP-)sialic acid in glycoprotein synthesis.
6. Allosteric effectors: the intracellular concentrations of nucleotides influence the progression of certain steps of metabolic pathways.
7. Cellular agonists: extracellular nucleotides influence intracellular signal transduction (e.g., cAMP and inositol-calcium pathway).

Nucleotide concentrations in cells and tissues are maintained by de novo synthesis and salvage from intermediary metabolism and diet (Fig. 5-11).[99] Nucleosides are the predominant product absorbed in the small intestine. Nucleosides are probably transported by passive diffusion and a carrier-mediated process; purines and pyrimidines are transported by passive diffusion at high concentrations and by a sodium-dependent active mechanism at low concentrations (Fig. 5-12).[99] The digestion and absorption of nucleotides, nucleosides, and pyrimidines and purines also involve polymeric and monomeric nucleotides and other adducts (nucleosides in a biologically active moiety).

In early reports on the nucleotide and nucleoside content of milk, various methods of measurement were used, and the amounts were described as either the monomeric fraction of nucleotides or the total RNA (see Chapter 4). Leach et al,[68] recognizing the complex nature of digestion and absorption of nucleotides and related products, attempted to measure the total potentially available nucleosides (TPANs) in human milk using solid-phase extraction, high-performance liquid chromatography (HPLC) analysis, and enzymatic hydrolysis of the various fractions. They analyzed breast milk samples at various stages throughout

lactation (colostrum; transitional, early, and late mature milk) from 100 European women and 11 American women. They used an aqueous TPAN-fortified solution containing ribonucleosides, 5′-mononucleotides, polymeric RNA, and nucleoside-containing adducts to estimate the accuracy of their process.

The mean ranges of TPAN values were similar for European women from different countries and American women, although broad ranges were seen and the composition of individual nucleotides varied.[68] The mean TPAN value was lowest in colostrum but did not show a consistent upward or downward trend in transitional, early, or late mature milk. The mean ranges of TPAN values were 82 to 164 μmol/L for colostrum, 144 to 210 μmol/L for transitional milk, 172 to 402 μmol/L for early mature milk, and 156 to 259 μmol/L for late mature milk (Table 5-7). Monomeric and polymeric nucleotides were the predominant forms of TPAN in pooled samples. Cytidine, guanosine, and adenosine were found mainly in these fractions, whereas uridine was found primarily as free nucleotide and adduct (Table 5-8). The methods used recovered 90% to 95% of the true TPAN values compared with the TPAN-fortified solution,

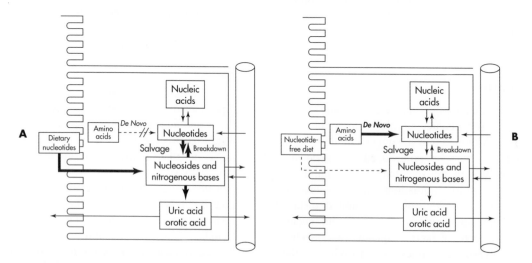

Fig. 5-11.   Metabolic regulation of cellular nucleotide pools in presence and absence of nucleotide in diet. **A,** Effect of dietary nucleotide activating salvage pathway. **B,** De novo nucleotide synthesis is enhanced with nucleotide-free diet. (From Quan R, Barness LA, Uauy R: *J Pediatr* 11(4):429, 1990.)

although the uridine and guanosine content was underestimated.

Leach et al[68] concluded that their process of estimating TPANs, including sequential enzymatic hydrolyses, and measuring the entire nucleotide fraction provides a reasonable estimate of the in vivo process and the nucleotides available to the infant from human milk.

Proposed effects of dietary nucleotides include effects on the immune system, iron absorption, intestinal flora, plasma lipoproteins, and growth of intestinal and hepatic cells. Effects on the immune system, related to nucleotide supplementation to the diet, have mainly been reported from animal studies and include increased mortality from graft-versus-host disease, improved delayed-type cutaneous hypersensitivity and alloantigen-induced lymphoproliferation, reversal of malnutrition and starvation-induced immunosuppression, increased resistance to challenge with *Staphylococcus aureus* and *Candida albicans,* and enhanced T-cell maturation and function.[94] Spleen cells of mice fed a nucleotide-free diet produce lower levels of IL-2, express lower levels of IL-2 receptors, and have decreased natural killer (NK) cell activity and macrophage activity.[20,22]

Presumably these nucleotide-associated changes are related to T-helper/inducer cells and the initial phases of antigen processing and lymphocyte proliferation.[20,114]

In vitro and in vivo experiments have documented that ingested nucleotides increased iron absorption, perhaps affecting xanthine oxidase.[99] Although in vitro studies showed that added nucleotides enhanced the growth of bifidobacteria, conflicting results have been obtained on the influence of dietary nucleotides on the fecal flora of infants receiving breast milk or nucleotide-supplemented formula.[4,99] Clinical studies in infants receiving nucleotide-supplemented formula demonstrated increased high-density lipoprotein (HDL) cholesterol, lower very low-density lipoprotein (VLDL) cholesterol, increased long-chain polyunsaturated fatty acids (PUFAs), and changes in red blood cell (RBC) membrane phospholipid composition.[99] Supplementation studies in animals have shown enhanced GI tract growth and maturation, improved intestinal repair after diarrhea, stimulation of hepatic growth, and augmented recovery from hepatectomy.[94]

Studies in human infants of the effect of dietary nucleotides on the immune system and protection

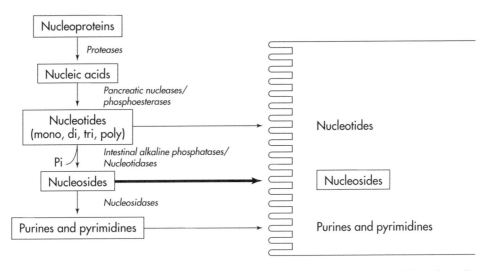

Fig. 5-12. Digestion and absorption of nucleic acids and their related products. (From Quan R, Barness LA, Uauy R: *J Pediatr* 11(4):429, 1990.)

TABLE 5-7   **Nucleotide and total potentially available nucleoside (TPAN) in pooled human milk by stage of lactation (μmol/L)***

	Uridine	Cytidine	Guanosine	Adenosine	TPAN
Colostrum					
Site 1	27	84	22	20	153
Site 2	21	33	15	13	82
Site 3	30	82	26	26	164
Site 4	24	84	20	22	150
Mean	26	71	21	21	137
Transitional milk					
Site 1	23	82	22	19	146
Site 2	33	76	19	17	144
Site 3	37	84	43	42	206
Site 4	36	100	36	38	210
Mean	32	86	30	29	177
Early mature milk					
Site 1	30	86	28	28	172
Site 2	50	79	23	21	173
Site 3	44	96	36	37	214
Site 4	67	146	91	97	402
Mean	48	102	45	46	240
Late mature milk					
Site 1	36	73	22	25	156
Site 2	58	106	29	27	219
Site 3	49	81	20	24	173
Site 4	45	124	40	49	259
Mean	47	96	28	31	202
Grand mean	38	88	31	32	189
SD	13	24	18	20	70
Range	21-67	33-146	19-92	13-97	82-402
American pool†	37	70	30	24	161

From Leach JL, Baxter JH, Molitor BE et al: *Am J Clin Nutr* 61:1224, 1995.
*Data from 100 individual samples collected at four sites and combined into 16 pooled samples (5 to 7 individual samples per site per stage of lactation). *Site 1,* Rouen and Mount Saint Aignau, France; *Site 2,* Mainz, Germany; *Site 3,* Bolzano, Italy; *Site 4,* Treviso, Italy.
†Pooled sample of milk collected from 11 American women between 2 and 4 months postpartum.

against infection are limited. Carver et al[22] compared infants receiving breast milk to those receiving commercially available infant formula and formula supplemented with nucleotides at a level of 32 mg/L. At 2 and 4 months, NK cell activity and IL-2 production were higher in the breastfed and nucleotide-supplemented groups compared with those receiving formula without nucleotide supplements. Infections occurred infrequently in all groups, but slightly less in the breastfed group. No differences were noted in hematologic profiles and plasma chemistry values, and no toxicity or intolerance was associated with nucleotide supplementation. The sample size was small, marked

TABLE 5-8   **Percentage of total potentially available nucleoside (TPAN) in pooled human milk as adducts, polymeric nucleotides, monomeric nucleotides, and nucleosides***

	Uridine	Cytidine	Guanosine	Adenosine	TPAN
Polymeric nucleotides	19 ± 7	57 ± 12	59 ± 21	47 ± 11	48 ± 8
Monomeric nucleotides	36 ± 12	37 ± 13	34 ± 14	35 ± 10	36 ± 10
Nucleosides	18 ± 14	5 ± 5	1 ± 2	5 ± 4	8 ± 6
Adducts†	27 ± 12	1 ± 1	7 ± 15	13 ± 9	9 ± 4

From Leach JL, Baxter JH, Molitor BE et al: *Am J Clin Nutr* 61:1224, 1995.
*$\bar{x} \pm$ SD. Based on the mean of entire pool of human milk collected from 100 individuals at four stages of lactation at four sites.
†Adducts are of the form nucleoside-phosphate-phosphate-X, where X is a biologically relevant moiety (e.g., uridine diphosphate–galactose or NAD).

variability was seen in the IL-2 measurements, and the differences noted at 4 months were less than at 2 months. Therefore the authors concluded that dietary nucleotides may contribute to improved immunity in breastfed infants.

Brunser et al[12] examined the effect of a nucleotide-supplemented formula on the incidence of diarrhea in infants in Chile. Although the infants receiving the supplemented formula experienced less diarrhea, the difference in the duration of diarrhea was small. The numbers were too small to comment on the causative agents of diarrhea, although there was no apparent protection against any one agent. The beneficial effect of nucleotides against diarrhea was proposed to be secondary to enhanced immune response to intestinal pathogens or improved intestinal integrity or a combination of both.

Pickering et al[94] recently published a 12-month, controlled, randomized study of 311 infants to examine the effect of added nucleotides at levels comparable to human milk on the infant's immune response to various vaccine antigens. Nonrandomized, 103 infants received breast milk for at least 2 months and then either human milk or a standard infant formula. Another 208 infants were randomized to receive either a standard infant formula or one supplemented with nucleotides. The amount and actual nucleotide content added were based on TPANs, as measured by Leach et al[68] equaling 72 mg/L. Overall growth and nutrition tolerance were similar in each group. The nucleotide group

had significantly higher geometric mean titers of Hib antibody and diphtheria antibody than the control group or the breastfed infants. No significant difference was seen between the nucleotide and control groups for the IgG response to oral poliovirus vaccine (OPV) or tetanus. Infants breastfed for longer than 6 months had significantly higher antibody responses to OPV than children breastfed for less than 6 months or either of the two formula-fed groups. No significant differences were found between the different groups with respect to total IgG, IgA, or IgE. Differences were seen in the number of children who experienced at least one episode of diarrhea: the nucleotide group (4/27, 15%) versus the control group (13/32, 41%, $p < .05$) and the breastfed group (6/27, 22%). Notably, the breastfed group was very heterogeneous relative to the amount of breast milk received and the duration of feeding, whereas the nucleotide group received supplementation for the entire 12 months.

Questions that remain concerning nucleotides and their proposed beneficial effects in an infant's diet include the following:
- What are the mechanisms of action of these proposed benefits?
- What form and concentration of nucleotides are necessary to effect these benefits?
- Is adequate information available to justify using nucleotides in infant formula in higher amounts and different compositions than are currently used?

Debate and research to answer these and other questions concerning nucleotides will continue.

Nonimmunoglobulin components

Further protective properties of human milk can be ascribed to nonimmunoglobulin components such as glycolipids, glycoproteins, and free oligosaccharides. These components are capable of inhibiting bacterial adhesion to epithelia. The protective effect of mucins present in human milk has been demonstrated as well by the agglutinations of S-fimbriated *E. coli* in the presence of human milk fat globules and lipid droplets of formula. Artificial lipid emulsions (Intralipid) had no agglutinating effect. The authors conclude that human milk fat-globule membrane inhibits bacterial adhesion to the entire intestine, thus providing protection against these infections[108] (Table 5-5).

FLORA OF INTESTINAL TRACT

As noted earlier, the normal flora of the intestinal tract of the breastfed infant is *Lactobacillus bifidus*. The gram-negative population in the gut is kept small.[119]

In a prospective study of breastfed Mayan Indian infants from birth to 3 years of age, bifid bacteria predominated and constituted 95% to 99% of the flora. Other culturable microorganisms were streptococci, bacteroides, clostridia, micrococci, enterococci, and *E. coli*. A change occurred when large amounts of solid foods were added at about 1 year of life. The solids were notably protein poor. *E. coli* progressively increased in numbers. *L. bifidus* metabolizes milk saccharides, producing large amounts of acetic acid, lactic acid, and some formic and succinic acids, which create the low pH of the stool of breastfed infants. *L. bifidus* also produces short-chain fatty acids in the course of colonization. The intestinal flora of bottle-fed infants is gram-negative bacteria, especially coliform organisms and bacteroides.

The flora of bifid bacteria is inhibitory to

certain pathogenic bacteria. Substantial clinical evidence is available to demonstrate that a resistance mechanism exists against intestinal infections from *Staphylococcus aureus, Shigella, Salmonella, Vibrio cholerae, E. coli,* rotavirus, *Campylobacter,* and protozoa.[38]

Two actions are apparent. The first encourages the growth of *L. bifidus* and thus crowds out the growth of other bacteria. In the second, the number of pathogens is also kept low by the direct action of lysozyme and lactoferrin. When the number of pathogenic bacteria is kept low, the immune antibodies can keep the growth under control and prevent the absorption of bacteria through the gut wall into the bloodstream.

EFFECTIVENESS OF HUMAN MILK IN CONTROLLING INFECTION

The properties of human milk do appear to control infection. Specific disease entities have shown a clear differential in the incidence between infants fed cow's milk and those fed human milk.[75,81]

Bacterial infection

Breast milk IgA has antitoxin activity against enterotoxins of *E. coli* and *V. cholerae* that may be significant in preventing infantile diarrhea. Antibodies against O antigen of some of the most common serotypes of *E. coli* were found in high titer in breast milk samples collected from healthy mothers in Sweden. The infants who had consumed reasonable amounts of breast milk with high titers of *E. coli* antibodies had antibodies in their stool.[50]

Protection against cholera in breastfed children by antibodies in breast milk was studied by Glass et al.[38] A prospective study in Bangladesh showed cholera antibody levels to vary in the colostrum and milk. The correlation among colonization, disease, and milk antibodies led the authors to conclude that breast milk antibodies against cholera do not protect children from colonization with *V. cholera,* but they do protect against disease.

Salmonella infection was similarly studied by France et al[34] to evaluate the immunologic mechanisms in host colostrum and milk specific for salmonellae. Vigorous responses of colostral and milk cells against these organisms and nonspecific opsonizing capacity of the aqueous phase of colostrum and milk were demonstrated.

Gothefors et al[46] showed that *E. coli* isolated from stools of breastfed infants differed from strains found in formula-fed infants in two respects. First, *E. coli* strains were more sensitive to the bactericidal effect of human serum. Second, and more often, spontaneously agglutinated bacteria from other sites, such as the prepuce or periurethral area, were less sensitive in breastfed infants. These findings support the theory that breast milk favors proliferation of mutant strains, which have decreased virulence. This mutation of bacterial strains is another way breastfeeding may protect against infection.

It has been suggested that milk immunization is a dynamic process because a mother's milk has been found to contain antibody to virtually all her infant's strains of intestinal bacteria. The mother exposed to the infant's microorganisms through either the breast or the gut responds immunologically to those microorganisms and thus automatically protects her immunologically immature infant.

The orderly review of data on the presence of antibodies in human milk has produced a substantial list of affected organisms. In addition to *E. coli,* antibodies to *Bacteroides fragilis, Clostridium tetani, Haemophilus pertussis, Diplococcus pneumoniae, Corynebacterium diphtheriae, Salmonella, Shigella, Chlamydia trachomatis, V. cholerae, S. aureus,* and several strains of *Streptococcus* (Table 5-9) have been identified.

A study in Oslo by Hanson[50] of an outbreak of severe diarrhea caused by *E. coli* strain 0111 showed that six severely ill children were formula-fed. Two infants who were breastfed had *E. coli* strain 0111 in their stools but showed few symptoms. Their mothers had no detectable antibodies for strain 0111 in their milk, which would suggest that other factors in human milk protect the infant from serious illness when there are no antibodies in the milk. Hanson[50] also showed in another study that after colonization with a specific strain of *E. coli,* mothers had large numbers of lymphoid cells in their milk with antibodies to that *E. coli.* Their serum produced no such response. This supports the concept that antigen-triggered lymphoid cells from Peyer's patches seek out lymphoid-rich tissue, producing IgA in the mammary gland. The mother is immunized in the gut at the same time as her milk. It has also been shown that *E. coli* enteritis can be cured by feeding human milk.

Schlesinger and Covelli[107] studied possible cell-mediated immunity in breastfed infants. They showed that tuberculin-positive nursing mothers had reactive T cells in their colostrum and early milk. Furthermore, 8 of 13 infants nursed by tuberculin-positive mothers had tuberculin-reactive peripheral blood T cells after 4 weeks. Cord blood had no such activity.

Viral infection

Protection against viruses has been the subject of similar studies. Breast milk contains antibodies against poliovirus, coxsackievirus, echovirus, influenza virus, reovirus, respiratory syncytial virus, rotavirus, and rhinovirus.[82] It has been confirmed that human milk inhibits the growth of these viruses in tissue culture. Nonspecific substances in human milk are active against arbovirus and murine leukemia virus, according to work by Fieldsteel.[31]

A high degree of antiviral activity against Japanese B encephalitis virus as well as the two leukemia viruses has been found in human milk. The factor was found in the fat fraction and was not destroyed by extended heating, which distinguishes it from antibodies. May[75] believes the nonimmunoglobulin macromolecule antiviral activity in human milk is caused by specific fatty acids and monoglycerides (Table 5-10).

TABLE 5-9 Nonantibody, antibacterial protective factors in human milk

Factors	Proposed mechanisms of action	Organisms affected	Effect of heat
Bifidus factor	Inhibits replication of certain bacteria in gastrointestinal tract by causing proliferation of lactobacilli	Enterobacteriaceae, including shigellae, salmonellae, and some *E. coli*	Stable to boiling
Complement components	Opsonic, chemitactic, and bacteriolytic activity	*E. coli*	Destroyed by heating at 56° C for 30 min
Lysozyme	With IgA, peroxide, or ascorbate, causes lysis of bacteria	*E. coli* Salmonellae	Same loss (0%-23%) at 62.5° C for 30 min; essentially destroyed by boiling for 15 min
Lactoferrin (nutrient binders)	Binds ferric iron	*E. coli* Candida albicans	Two-thirds destroyed at 62.5° C for 30 min
Lactoperoxidase	Oxidizes bacteria	*E. coli* Salmonella typhimurium	Presumably destroyed by boiling
Nonantibody proteins: receptor-like glycolipid or glycoprotein	Inhibit bacterial adherence	Vibrio cholerae	Stable to boiling for 15 min
Gangliosides (GM1-like)	Interfere with attachment of enterotoxin to GM1 cell membrane ganglioside receptors	*E. coli* and *V. cholerae* enterotoxins	Stable to boiling
Nonlactose carbohydrate factors	Prevent action of stable toxin (ST)	*E. coli* ST	Stable at 85° C for 30 min
Milk cells (macrophages, polymorphonuclear leukocytes, B- and T-lymphocytes)	By phagocytosis and killing: *E. coli, S. aureus, S. enteritidis*		Destroyed at 62.5° C for 30 min
	By sensitized lymphocytes: *E. coli*		
	By phagocytosis: *C. albicans* lymphocyte stimulation by *E. coli* K antigen		

Modified from May JT: *Aust Paediatr J* 20:265, 1984; and Pickering LK, Kohl S: Human milk humoral immunity and infant defense mechanisms. In Howell RR, Morriss RH Jr, Pickering LK, editors: *Human milk and infant nutrition and health*, Springfield, Ill, 1986, Thomas.

TABLE 5-10	Nonantibody, antiviral, and antiprotozoan factors in human milk		
Factors	**Proposed mechanisms of action**	**Organisms affected**	**Effect of heat**
Lipids (unsaturated fatty acids and monoglycerides)	Inactivate lipid-enveloped virus	Herpes simplex Semliki Forest Influenza Ross River	Stable to boiling for 30 min
Macromolecules	Inhibit attachment and penetration	Herpes simplex Coxsackievirus B_4 Cytomegalovirus Rotavirus	Most stable at 56° C for 30 min Destroyed by boiling for 30 min
α_2-Macroglobulin protein	Inhibits hemagglutinin activity	Influenza Parainfluenza	Stable to boiling for 15 min
α_1-Antitrypsin	Trypsin-dependent inhibition	Rotavirus	Stable to boiling for 10 min
Bile salt–stimulated lipase	May generate fatty acids and monoglycerides that inactivate organisms	Giardia lamblia Entamoeba histolytica	
Nonlipase macromolecule	Unknown	G. lamblia	Destroyed at 62.5° C for 30 min
Milk cells	Induced interferon by virus or phytohemagglutinin (PHA); induced lymphokine (LDCF) by PHA; induced cytokine by herpes simplex virus; lymphocyte stimulation by rubella, cytomegalovirus, herpes, measles, mumps		

Modified from May JT: *Aust Paediatr J* 20:265, 1984; and Pickering LK, Kohl S: Human milk humoral immunity and infant defense mechanisms. In Howell RR, Morriss RH Jr, Pickering LK, editors: *Human milk and infant nutrition and health*, Springfield, Ill, 1986, Thomas.

Specimens of human colostrum have been found to contain neutralizing activity against *respiratory syncytial virus* (RSV). RSV has become a major threat in infancy and is the most common reason for hospitalization in infancy in some developed countries. It has a high mortality rate. Epidemics have occurred in special care nurseries. Statistically significant data collected by Downham et al[30] showed that few breastfed babies (8 of 115) were among the infants hospitalized for RSV infection, compared with uninfected controls who were breastfed (46 of 167).

Fishaut et al[32] studied the immune response to RSV prospectively in 26 nursing mothers over several months. Antiviral IgM and IgG were rarely found in colostrum or milk. RSV-specific IgA, however, was identified in 40% to 75% of specimens. Two mothers with the disease had specific IgG, IgM, and IgA antibody in serum and nasopharyngeal secretions, but only IgA was found in their milk. This confirms that IgA antibody to specific respiratory tract pathogens is present in the products of lactation. Because RSV appears to replicate only in the respiratory tract, the authors suggest that viral-specific antibody activity in the mammary gland may be derived from the broncho-associated lymphoid tissue (BALT).

Necrotizing enterocolitis has been a serious threat to premature infants in acute care nurseries. Animal studies have demonstrated a protective quality to breast milk. Efforts to confirm a similar relationship in human infants have been encouraging but not conclusive. Leukocytes in milk fulfill a protective function in premature infants, possibly as a consequence of their natural transplantation, according to Beer and Billingham.[7]

In a controlled prospective study of high-risk, low-birthweight infants in India using donor human milk, there were significantly fewer infections and no major infections in the group receiving human milk, although the controls experienced diarrhea, pneumonia, septicemia, and meningitis.[81]

The relationship of *sudden infant death syndrome* (SIDS) to formula feeding is supported by circumstantial evidence and retrospective studies. The fact remains that in all series reported, SIDS is rare in breastfed infants. Whether this is related to protection against infection is not clear.

The apparent predisposition of bottle-fed infants to purulent *otitis media* as compared with the disposition of breastfed infants may result from IgA-conferred immunity in human milk. It may also be caused by the mechanics of bottle feeding. Of a group of infants with otitis media, 85% had their bottles propped up, whereas only 8% of a matched bottle-feeding control group who did not have otitis media had their bottles propped up. When an infant swallows fluid lying flat on the back, it is possible to regurgitate it into the eustachian tube.[6]

Antiprotozoan factors

In human milk, bile salt–stimulated lipase (BSSL) has been found to be the major factor inactivating protozoans (Table 5-11).[75] The mechanism by

| | Organisms affected | |
Factor	(in vitro)	Effect of heat
Bile salt–stimulated lipase	*Giardia lamblia* *Entamoeba histolytica* *Trichomonas vaginalis*	Destroyed at 62.5° C for 1 min
Nonimmunoglobulin, nonlipase macromolecule	*G. lamblia*	Stable to boiling for 20 min

TABLE 5-11 **Antiprotozoan factors in human milk**

Modified from May JT: *Aust Paediatr J* 20:265, 1984.

which lipase acts is not known, although it may generate fatty acids and monoglycerides, which inactivate enveloped bacteria, viruses, or protozoa. A nonimmunoglobulin, nonlipase, heat-stable factor has been identified in human milk that can inactivate *Giardia lamblia*.

Antiinflammatory properties

Human milk protects against many intestinal and respiratory pathogens without evidence of inflammation. Goldman et al[45] hypothesize that human milk is poor in initiators and mediators of inflammation but rich in antiinflammatory agents. Several major biochemical pathways of inflammation, they point out, including the coagulation system, the fibrinolytic system, and complement, are poorly represented in human milk. Box 5-2 outlines the antiinflammatory properties of various constituents.

The interaction of factors in the milk with one another or with host defenses cannot be entirely

---

BOX 5-2   Antiinflammatory features of human milk

A. Paucity of initiators and mediators
    1. Foreign antigens
    2. IgG antibodies
    3. Complement system
    4. Fibrinolytic system
    5. Coagulation system
    6. Kallikrein system
B. Antiinflammatory agents

1. Lactoferrin	Inhibits complement
2. Secretory IgA	Prevents bacterial adherence
	Inhibits neutrophil chemotaxis
	Limits antigen penetration
3. Lysozyme	Inhibits neutrophil chemotaxis, generation of toxic oxygen radicals
4. Catalase	Destroys hydrogen peroxide
5. α-Tocopherol	Scavengers of oxygen radicals
Cysteine	
Ascorbic acid	
6. Histaminase	Degrades histamine
7. Arylsulfatase	Degrades leukotrienes
8. α_1-Antichymotrypsin	Neutralizes enzymes that act in inflammation
α_1-Antitrypsin	
9. Prostaglandins (E$_2$, F$_{2\alpha}$)	Cytoprotective: inhibits neutrophil degranulation, lymphocyte activation
10. Pregnancy-associated α_2-glycoprotein	Inhibits lymphocyte blastogenesis
11. Oligosaccharides	Inhibits microbial attachment
12. Epidermal growth factors	Strengthens mucosal barriers

C. Special features of leukocytes
    1. No basophils, mast cells, eosinophils, or platelets
    2. T-lymphocytes respond poorly to allogeneic cells
    3. Low natural killer cell activity or antibody-dependent cytotoxicity
    4. Poor response of neutrophils and macrophages to chemoattractants

Modified from Goldman AS, Thorpe LW, Goldblum RM et al: *Acta Paediatr Scand* 75:689, 1986.

predicted by examining each factor separately. When the decreased response of human milk leukocytes to chemoattractant peptides was demonstrated by Thorpe et al,[112] the failure of the response of human milk leukocytes was not caused by alterations in maternal peripheral blood leukocytes. This suggests that inhibitors are in the milk and that the human milk leukocytes may be modified in the mammary gland to protect through noninflammatory mechanisms.[112]

The antioxidant properties of human colostrum were demonstrated by Buescher and McIlheran[14] using aqueous human colostrum on human PMNs. The colostrum significantly interfered with PMN oxygen metabolic and enzymatic activities that are important in the mediation of acute inflammation. Other antioxidants include an ascorbate-like compound, uric acid, α-tocopherol and β-carotene. Blood levels of α-tocopherol and β-carotene are higher in breastfed than unsupplemented formula-fed infants. Human milk appears to protect the recipient infant and also the mammary gland by providing antiinfective agents and by minimizing inflammation.

Mucosal barrier system

Significant differences exist between the biophysical and biochemical organization and function of the mucosal barrier system.[91] The microvillous membrane of the neonate's intestinal tract permits increased attachment of certain pathogenic enterobacteria and their toxins to epithelial cells. Growth factors in human milk, such as epidermal growth factor, lactoferrin, cortisol, and several hormones, have a stimulating effect on the neonatal gut and increase epithelial barriers. Platelet activating factor (PAF) has been associated with the pathogenesis of necrotizing enterocolitis in sick newborns.[19] A substance in the leukocytes in the aqueous phase of human milk, an acetylhydrolase that breaks down PAF, is known to have low levels in premature infants. These are important observations toward understanding the role of the antiinflammatory function of human milk.[82]

ALLERGIC PROTECTIVE PROPERTIES

In discussing the antiallergic properties of human milk, it is more difficult to identify specific protective properties. During the neonatal period the small intestine has increased permeability to macromolecules. Infants have more serum and secretory antibodies against dietary proteins than children or adults. Production of IgA in the intestinal tract is delayed until 6 weeks to 3 months of age. IgA in colostrum and breast milk prevents the absorption of foreign macromolecules when the infant's immune system is immature. Protein of breast milk is species specific and therefore nonallergic for the human infant. No antibody response has been demonstrated to occur with human milk in infants. It has also been shown that macromolecules in breast milk are not absorbed.

Indirect evidence can be inferred from a demonstration of the response to cow's milk protein. Within 18 days of taking cow's milk, the infant will begin to develop antibodies. Since the advent of prepared formulas, in which the protein has been denatured by heating and drying, the incidence of cow's milk allergy has been considered to be 1%. The most reliable means of diagnosing it is by challenging with isolated cow's milk protein. Although circulating antibodies and coproantibodies have been identified, these are not reliable techniques for the clinician involved in patient care.

The allergic syndromes that have been associated with cow's milk allergy include gastroenteropathy, atopic dermatitis, rhinitis, chronic pulmonary disease, eosinophilia, failure to thrive, and SIDS, or cot death, which has been attributed to anaphylaxis to cow's milk.[57,69] The GI symptoms have received the greatest attention and include spitting, colic, diarrhea, blood in the stools, frank vomiting, weight loss, malabsorption, colitis, and failure to thrive. Cow's milk has been associated with the GI protein and blood loss. The diagnosis is best made by elimination from diet and, when appropriate, challenge tests. Cutaneous testing is of little help.

Murray[80] showed the association of nasal secretion eosinophilia with infants freely fed cow's milk or solid foods as compared with eosinophilia in strictly breastfed infants. Of free-fed infants, 32% had high eosinophilic secretions, and only 11% of breastfed infants had eosinophils present in nasal secretions.

Not surprisingly, many different antigenic specificities are recognized when the colostrum or milk of one species is fed to or injected into another species. Cow's milk is high on the list of food allergens, particularly in children; sensitivity to cow's milk is responsible for at least 20% of all pediatric allergic conditions, according to Gerrard.[36] Evidence indicates that IgA antibodies play an important role in confining food antigens to the gut. Food antigens given to bottle-fed infants before they can make their own IgA, and when they are deprived of that in human milk and the plasma cells, may be expected to be more readily absorbed.

Glaser[37] first made the association between the drop in breastfeeding and the rise in allergy. He pioneered the theory of prophylactic management of allergy. Allergy in infancy is associated with a familial history of atopic disease and elevated cord blood IgE levels. The introduction of "foreign" proteins to the infant's diet and even to the mother's diet in the breastfeeding dyad can lead to allergic symptoms in the infant. Exclusive breastfeeding does not protect high-risk children from allergic symptoms unless the mother also adheres closely to a restrictive diet that excludes common allergens.[5]

Chapter 17 discusses the prophylactic management of the potentially allergic infant. Chapters 8 and 14 outline the management of specific syndromes such as colic and colitis.

Immunomodulating agents

Immunomodulating agents in human milk have been identified as possible explanations for the epidemiologic evidence of the lowered risk of some chronic diseases in breastfed infants, the in vivo evidence of increased levels of certain immune factors in the infant, the presence of activated leukocytes in human milk, and the presence of several cytokines in human milk.[41] As investigators pursue these avenues further, other immunomodulating agents may be identified.

Protection against infection outside the gastrointestinal tract

Although protection against GI disease while exclusively being breastfed is well recognized, protection against infections in other systems is less well known.[52] More than 1000 healthy infants followed in a health maintenance organization by Wright et al[118] were found to have significantly less lower respiratory tract infection in the first 4 months of life if they were breastfed. A study of 128 infants with urinary tract infection (UTI) and 128 matched controls confirmed protection against UTI in the ever-breastfed infant. Infants breastfed at time of study had a very low risk of UTI, but ever-breastfeeding provided some protection.[96] Several authors have reported a decreased likelihood of neonatal sepsis in breastfed infants, in both developing and developed countries.[1,116]

Protection against chronic disease in childhood

The major elements of the immune system in human milk are direct-acting antimicrobial factors, antiinflammatory factors, and immunomodulating bioactive compounds.[52] Epidemiologic studies have produced compelling information suggesting that breastfeeding for 4 months or longer can provide some immunologic protection against some childhood-onset diseases.[41,42,76]

An increase in childhood-onset diabetes was correlated with a decrease in breastfeeding in Scandinavia, retrospectively. In 1991, Viirtanen et al[115] reported a prospective long-term study among children in Finland that showed a significantly lower incidence of childhood-onset diabetes in those at-risk children who had been breastfed for 4 months or longer. These clinical observations have been supported in the laboratory by studies of diet control in diabetic mice. The isolation of a bovine albumin peptide as a possible trigger of insulin-dependent diabetes mellitus makes further study imperative.[59]

The review of the national perinatal collaborative study by Davis et al[27] showed a protective effect against development of childhood cancer by being breastfed for 4 months or longer for children followed for 10 years. The effect was greater for acute leukemia and lymphoma. The role of infant-feeding practices showed a similar effect of breastfeeding as protective in postponing the onset of Crohn's disease in childhood.[65]

Maternal renal allografts have a better survival rate in individuals who were breastfed in infancy when compared with those who were not breastfed.[18,64]

The mechanism of these immunologic observations remain unclear, although theories abound.[41]

REFERENCES

1. Ashraf RN, Jalil F, Zaman S et al: Breast feeding and protection against neonatal sepsis in a high risk population, *Arch Dis Child* 66:488, 1991.
2. Baggiolini M, Dewald B, Moser B: Human chemokines: an update, *Annu Rev Immunol* 15:675, 1997.
3. Bahna SL, Keller MA, Heiner DC: IgE and IgD in human colostrum and plasma, *Pediatr Res* 16:604, 1982.
4. Balmer SE, Hanvey LS, Wharton BA: Diet and faecal flora in the newborn: nucleotides, *Arch Dis Child* 70: F137, 1994.
5. Bardare M, Vaccari A, Allievi E et al: Influence of dietary manipulation on incidence of atopic disease in infants at risk, *Ann Allergy* 71:366, 1993.
6. Beauregard WG: Positional otitis media, *J Pediatr* 79:294, 1971.
7. Beer AE, Billingham RE: Immunologic benefits and hazards of milk in maternal-perinatal relationships, *Ann Intern Med* 83:865, 1975.
8. Beerens H, Romond C, Neut C: Influence of breastfeeding on bifid flora of the newborn intestine, *Am J Clin Nutr* 33:2434, 1980.
9. Bertotto A, Gerli R, Fabietti G et al: Human breast milk T cells display the phenotype and functional characteristics of memory T cells, *Eur J Immunol* 20:1877, 1990.
10. Bhaskaram P, Reddy V: Bactericidal activity of human milk leukocytes, *Acta Paediatr Scand* 70:87, 1981.
11. Brooker BE: The epithelial cells and cell fragments in human milk, *Cell Tissue Res* 210:321, 1980.
12. Brunser O, Espinoza J, Araya M et al: Effect of dietary nucleotide supplementation on diarrhoeal disease in infants, *Acta Pediatr Scand* 83:188, 1994.
13. Buescher ES, Malinowska I: Soluble receptors and cytokine antagonists in human milk, *Pediatr Res* 40(6): 839, 1996.
14. Buescher ES, McIlheran SM: Antioxidant properties of human colostrum, *Pediatr Res* 24:14, 1988.
15. Buescher ES, Pickering LK: Polymorphonuclear leukocytes in human colostrum and milk. In Howell RR, Morriss RH, Pickering LK, editors: *Human milk in infant nutrition and health,* Springfield, Ill, 1986, Thomas.
16. Bullen JJ: Iron-binding proteins and other factors in milk responsible for resistance to *E. coli.* In *Ciba Foundation Symposium,* no 42, New York, 1976, Elsevier North Holland.
17. Butte NF, Goldblum RM, Fehl LM et al: Daily ingestion of immunologic components in human milk during the first four months of life, *Acta Paediatr Scand* 73:296, 1984.
18. Campbell DA Jr, Lorber MI, Sweeton JC et al: Breast-feeding and maternal-donor renal allografts, *Transplantation* 37:346, 1984.
19. Caplan MS, Kelly A, Hsueh W: Endotoxin and hypoxia-induced intestinal necrosis in rats: the role of platelet activating factor, *Pediatr Res* 31:428, 1992.
20. Carver JD: Dietary nucleotides: cellular immune, intestinal and hepatic system effects, *J Nutr* 124:144S, 1994.
21. Carver JD, Walker WA: The role of nucleotides in human nutrition, *J Nutr Biochem* 6:58, 1995.
22. Carver JD, Pimental B, Cox WI et al: Dietary nucleotide effects upon immune function in infants, *Pediatrics* 88:359, 1991.
23. Chen Y, Yu S, Li W: Artificial feeding and hospitalization in the first 18 months of life, *Pediatrics* 81:58, 1988.
24. Crouch SP, Slater KJ, Fletcher J: Regulation of cytokine release from mononuclear cells by the iron-binding protein lactoferrin, *Blood* 80:235, 1992.
25. Cunningham AS: Morbidity in breast fed and artificially fed infants. II, *J Pediatr* 95:685, 1979.
26. Davidson LA, Lönnerdal B: Persistence of human milk proteins in the breast-fed infant, *Acta Paediatr Scand* 76:733, 1987.

27. Davis MK, Savitz DA, Grauford B: Infant feeding in childhood cancer, *Lancet* 2:365, 1988.

28. Dewey KG, Heinig MJ, Nommsen-Rivers LA: Difference in morbidity between breast-fed and formula-fed infants, *J Pediatr* 126:696, 1995.

29. Donovan SM, Atkinson SA, Whyte RK et al: Partition of nitrogen intake and excretion in low-birth-weight infants, *Am J Dis Child* 143:1485, 1989.

30. Downham MAPS, Scott R, Sims DG et al: Breast feeding protects against respiratory syncytial virus infections, *Br Med J* 2:274, 1976.

31. Fieldsteel AH: Nonspecific antiviral substances in human milk active against arbovirus and murine leukemia virus, *Cancer Res* 34:712, 1974.

32. Fishaut M, Murphy D, Neifert MA et al: Bronchopulmonary axis in the immune response to respiratory syncytial virus, *J Pediatr* 99:186, 1981.

33. Ford JE, Law BA, Marshall VM et al: Influences of the heat treatment of human milk on some of its protective constituents, *J Pediatr* 90:29, 1977.

34. France GL, Marmer DJ, Steele RW: Breast feeding and *Salmonella* infection, *Am J Dis Child* 134:147, 1980.

35. Fransson GB, Lönnerdal B: Iron in human milk, *J Pediatr* 96:380, 1980.

36. Gerrard JW: Allergy in infancy, *Allerg Pediatr Ann* 3:9, 1974.

37. Glaser J: The dietary prophylaxis of allergic disease in infancy, *J Asthma Res* 3:199, 1966.

38. Glass RI, Svennerholm A, Stoll BJ: Protection against cholera in breastfed children by antibodies in breast milk, *N Engl J Med* 308:1389, 1983.

39. Goldblum RM, Ahlstedt S, Carlsson B et al: Antibody-forming cells in human colostrum after oral immunization, *Nature* 257:797, 1975.

40. Goldman AS: Immunologic system in human milk, *J Pediatr Gastr Nutr* 5:343, 1986 (editorial).

41. Goldman AS: The immune system of human milk: antimicrobial, antiinflammatory and immunomodulating properties, *J Pediatr Infect Dis* 12:664, 1993.

42. Goldman AS, Chheda S, Garofalo R, Schmalstieg FC: Cytokines in human milk: properties and potential effects upon the mammary gland and the neonate, *J Mammary Gland Biol Neoplasia* 1(3):251, 1996.

43. Goldman AS, Garza C, Nichols BL et al: Immunologic factors in human milk during the first year of lactation, *J Pediatr* 100:563, 1982.

44. Goldman AS, Goldblum RM, Garza C: Immunologic components in human milk during the second year of lactation, *Acta Paediatr Scand* 72:461, 1983.

45. Goldman AS, Thorpe LW, Goldblum RM et al: Antiinflammatory properties of human milk, *Acta Paediatr Scand* 75:689, 1986.

46. Gothefors L, Olling S, Winberg J: Breast feeding and biological properties of faecal *E. coli* strains, *Acta Paediatr Scand* 64:807, 1975.

47. Gullberg R: Possible influence of vitamin B_{12} binding protein in milk on the intestinal flora in breast-fed infants. II. Contents of unsaturated B_{12} binding protein in meconium and faeces from breast-fed and bottle-fed infants, *Scand J Gastroenterol* 9:287, 1974.

48. György P: A hitherto unrecognized biochemical difference between human milk and cow's milk, *Pediatrics* 11:98, 1953.

49. Habicht J-P, DaVanzo J, Butz WP: Mother's milk and sewage: their interactive effects on infant mortality, *Pediatrics* 81:456, 1988.

50. Hanson LA: The mammary gland as an immunological organ, *Immunol Today* 3:168, 1982.

51. Hanson LA, Adlerberth I, Carsson B et al: Host defense of the neonate and the intestinal flora, *Acta Paediatr Scand Suppl* 351:122, 1989.

52. Hanson LA, Karlberg J, Ashraf R et al: *Health and human potential. Diseases. The state of health of children in the developing world,* Rome, 1992, Pontifical Academy of Sciences, The Vatican.

53. Head JR, Beer AE: The immunologic role of viable leukocytic cells in mammary exosecretions. In Larson BL, editor: *Lactation,* vol IV, *Mammary gland/human lactation/milk synthesis,* New York, 1978, Academic Press.

54. Ho PC, Lawton JWM: Human colostral cells: phagocytosis and killing of *E. coli* and *C. albicans, J Pediatr* 93:910, 1978.

55. Jatsyk GV, Kuvaeva IB, Gribakin SG: Immunological protection of the neonatal gastrointestinal tract: the importance of breast feeding, *Acta Paediatr Scand* 74:246, 1985.

56. Jelliffe DB, Jelliffe EFP: *Human milk in the modern world,* Oxford, 1978, Oxford University Press.

57. Johnstone DE, Dutton AM: Dietary prophylaxis of allergic disease in children, *N Engl J Med* 274:715, 1966.

58. Juto P: Human milk stimulates B cell function, *Arch Dis Child* 60:610, 1985.

59. Karjalainen J, Martin JM, Knip M et al: A bovine albumin peptide as a possible trigger of insulin-dependent diabetes mellitus, *N Engl J Med* 327:302, 1992.

60. Keller MA, Faust J, Rolewic LJ et al: T-cell subsets in human colostrum, *J Pediatr Gastroenterol Nutr* 5:439, 1986.

61. Keller MA, Heiner DC, Myers AS et al: IgD in human colostrum, *Pediatr Res* 19:122, 1985.

62. Kerner JA Jr, Yang CC, Stevenson DK: Effects of nutritional supplements on anti-infective factors in human milk, *Gastroenterology* 94:118, 1988.

63. Kleinman RE, Walker WA: The enteromammary immune system: an important concept in breast milk host defense, *Dig Dis Sci* 24:876, 1979.

64. Kois WE, Campbell DA Jr, Lorbert MI et al: Influence of breastfeeding on subsequent reactivity to a related renal allograft, *J Surg Res* 37:89, 1984.

65. Koletzko S, Sherman P, Corey M et al: Role of infant feeding practices in development of Crohn's disease in childhood, *Br Med J* 298:1617, 1989.

66. Kramer MS: Infant feeding, infection, and public health, *Pediatrics* 81:164, 1988.

67. Laegreid A, Otnaess A-BK: Trace amounts of ganglioside GM1 in human milk inhibit enterotoxins from *Vibrio cholerae* and *Escherichia coli, Life Sci* 40:55, 1987.

68. Leach JL, Baxter JH, Molitor BE et al: Total potentially available nucleosides of human milk by stage of lactation, *Am J Clin Nutr* 61:1224, 1995.

69. Lebenthal E: Cow's milk protein allergy, *Pediatr Clin North Am* 22:827, 1975.

70. Lewis-Jones DI, Lewis-Jones MS, Connolly RC et al: The influence of parity, age, and maturity of pregnancy on antimicrobial proteins in human milk, *Acta Paediatr Scand* 74:655, 1985.

71. Liles WC, Van Voorhis WC: Review: nomenclature and biologic significance of cytokines involved in inflammation and the host immune response, *J Infect Dis* 172:1573, 1995.

72. Lönnerdal B: Lactoferrin in milk, *Ann Nestle* 54:79, 1996.

73. Lönnerdal B, Iyer S: Lactoferrin molecular structure and biological function, *Annu Rev Nutr* 15:93, 1995.

74. Luster AD: Chemokines: chemotactic cytokines that mediate inflammation, *N Engl J Med* 338(7):436, 1998.

75. May JT: Antimicrobial properties and microbial contaminants of breast milk: an update, *Aust Paediatr* 20:265, 1984.

76. Mayer EJ, Hamman RF, Gay EC et al: Reduced risk of insulin-dependent diabetes mellitus among breast-fed children: The Colorado IDDM Registry, *Diabetes* 37:1625, 1988.

77. McClelland DBL: Antibodies in milk, *J Reprod Fertil* 65:537, 1982.

78. Michael JG, Ringenback R, Hottenstein S: The antimicrobial activity of human colostral antibody in the newborn, *J Infect Dis* 124:445, 1971.

79. Miranda R, Saravia NG, Ackerman R et al: Effect of maternal nutritional status on immunological substances in human colostrum and milk, *Am J Clin Nutr* 37:632, 1983.

80. Murray AB: Infant feeding and respiratory allergy, *Lancet* 1:497, 1971.

81. Narayanan I, Prakash K, Gujral VV: The value of human milk in the prevention of infection in the high-risk low–birth weight infants, *J Pediatr* 99:496, 1981.

82. Newburg DS: Antiviral components of human milk, *Mammary Gland Biol Lactation Newslett* 11:10, 1992.

83. Newburg DS: Oligosaccharides and glycoconjugates in human milk: their role in host defense, *J Mammary Gland Biol Neoplasia* 1:271, 1996.

84. Newburg DS, Chaturvedi P: Neutral glycolipids of human and bovine milk, *Lipids* 27:923, 1992.

85. Nuijens JH, van Berkel PHC, Schanbacher FL: Structure and biological actions of lactoferrin, *J Mammary Gland Biol Neoplasia* 1:285, 1996.

86. Ogra SS, Ogra PL: Immunologic aspects of human colostrum and milk. I. Distribution characteristics and concentrations of immunoglobulins at different times after the onset of lactation, *J Pediatr* 92:546, 1978.

87. Ogra SS, Ogra PL: Immunologic aspects of human colostrum and milk. II. Characteristics of lymphocyte reactivity and distribution of E-rosette forming cells at different times after the onset of lactation, *J Pediatr* 92:550, 1978.

88. Ogra SS, Ogra PL: Components of immunology reactivity in human colostrum and milk. In Ogra PL, Dayton DH, editors: *Immunology of breast milk,* New York, 1979, Raven.

89. Otnaess AK, Laegreid A, Ertresvag K: Inhibition of enterotoxin from *Escherichia coli* and *Vibrio cholerae* by gangliosides from human milk, *Infect Immunol* 40:563, 1983.

90. Palkowetz KH, Royer CL, Garofalo R et al: Production of IL-6 and IL-8 by human mammary gland epithelial cells, *J Reprod Immunol* 26:57, 1994.

91. Pang K, Bresson JL, Walker WA: Development of the gastrointestinal mucosal barrier. III. Evidence for structural differences in microvillus membranes from newborn and adult rabbits, *Biochem Biophys Acta* 727:201, 1983.

92. Parmely MJ, Beer AE, Billingham RE: In vitro studies of the T-lymphocyte population of human milk, *J Exp Med* 144:358, 1976.

93. Peitersen B, Bohn L, Andersen H: Quantitative determination of immunoglobulins, lysozyme, and certain electrolytes in breast milk during the entire period of lactation, during a 24-hour period, and in milk from the individual mammary gland, *Acta Paediatr Scand* 64:709, 1975.

94. Pickering LK, Granoff DM, Erickson JD et al: Modulation of the immune system by human milk and infant formula containing nucleotides, *Pediatrics* 101:242, 1998.

95. Pickering LK, Kohl S: Human milk humoral immunity and infant defense mechanisms. In Howell RR, Morriss RH Jr, Pickering LK, editors: *Human milk in infant nutrition and health,* Springfield, Ill, 1986, Thomas.

96. Pisacane A, Graziano L, Mazzarella G et al: Breastfeeding and urinary tract infection, *J Pediatr* 120:87, 1992.

97. Pitt J: The milk mononuclear phagocyte, *Pediatrics Suppl* 64:745, 1979.

98. Pittard WB III: Breast milk immunology: a frontier in infant nutrition, *Am J Dis Child* 133:83, 1979.

99. Quan R, Barness LA, Uauy R: Do infants need nucleotide supplemented formula for optimal nutrition? *J Pediatr Gastroenterol Nutr* 11(4):429, 1990.

100. Reddy V, Bhaskaram C, Raghuramula N et al: Antimicrobial factors in human milk, *Acta Paediatr Scand* 66:229, 1977.

101. Remington JS, Klein JO: Current concepts of infections of the fetus and newborn infant. In Remington JS, Klein JO: *Infectious diseases of the fetus and newborn infant,* ed 4, Philadelphia, 1995, Saunders.

102. Richie ER: Lymphocyte subsets in colostrum. In Howell RR, Morriss RH, Pickering LK, editors: *Human milk in infant nutrition and health,* Springfield, Ill, 1986, Thomas.

103. Rudloff HE, Schmalstreg FC Jr, Palkowetz KH et al: Interleukin-6 in human milk, *J Reprod Immunol* 23:13, 1993.

104. Ruiz-Palacios, Torres J, Torres E et al: Cholera-like enterotoxin produced by *Campylobacter jejuni, Infect Immun* 43:314, 1984.

105. Sánchez L, Calvo M, Brock JH: Biological role of lactoferrin, *Arch Dis Child* 67:657, 1992.

106. Savilahei E, Salmenpera L, Tainio VM et al: Prolonged exclusive breastfeeding results in low serum concentrations of immunoglobin G, A, and M, *Acta Paediatr Scand* 76:1, 1987.

107. Schlesinger JJ, Covelli HD: Evidence for transmission of lymphocyte responses to tuberculin by breastfeeding, *Lancet* 2:529, 1977.

108. Schroten H, Hanisch FG, Plogmann R et al: Inhibition of adhesion of S-fimbriated *Escherichia coli* to buccal epithelial cells by human milk fat globule membrane components: a novel aspect of the protective function of mucins in the non-immunoglobulin fraction, *Infect Immun* 60:2893, 1992.

109. Srivastava MD, Srivastava A, Brouhard B et al: Cytokines in human milk, *Res Commun Mol Pathol Pharmacol* 93(3):263, 1996.

110. Stoliar OA, Kaniecki-Green E, Pelley RP et al: Secretory IgA against enterotoxins in breast milk, *Lancet* 1:1258, 1976.

111. Telemo E, Hanson LA: Antibodies in milk, *J Mammary Gland Biol Neoplasia* 1:243, 1996.

112. Thorpe LW, Rudloff HE, Powell LC et al: Decreased response of human milk leukocytes to chemoattractant peptides, *Pediatr Res* 20:373, 1986.

113. Tomita M, Takase H, Wakabayashi et al: Antimicrobial peptides of lactoferrin, *Adv Exp Med Biol* 357:209, 1994.

114. Van Buren CT, Kulkarni AD, Fanslow WC et al: Dietary nucleotides, a requirement for helper/inducer T lymphocytes, *Transplantation* 40:694, 1985.

115. Viirtanen SE, Räsänen L, Aroa A et al: Infant feeding in Finnish children <7 yr of age with newly diagnosed insulin dependent diabetes, *Diabetes Care* 14:415, 1991.

116. Winberg J, Wessner G: Does breast milk protect against septicaemia in the newborn? *Lancet* I:1091, 1971.

117. Wirt DP, Adkins LT, Palkowetz KH et al: Activated and memory T lymphocytes in human milk, *Cytometry* 13:282, 1992.

118. Wright AL, Holberg CJ, Martinez FD et al: Breastfeeding and lower respiratory tract illness in the first year of life, *Br Med J* 299:946, 1989.

119. Yoshioka H, Isekl KI, Fujita K: Development and differences of intestinal flora in the neonatal period in breast-fed and bottle-fed infants, *Pediatrics* 72:317, 1983.

6

$\mathscr{P}$sychologic impact of breastfeeding

Although the previous chapters provide more than adequate information to support the preference for breastfeeding in almost every case, the critical impact in the return to breastfeeding in modern cultures rests with the issue of the mother's role and her perception of breastfeeding as a biologic act. The maternal influences include psychophysiologic reactions during nursing, long-term psychophysiologic effects, maternal behavior, sexual behavior, and attitudes toward men. All professionals providing support care in the perinatal period need to have a clear view not only of the biologic benefits of breastfeeding but also of their own psychologic attitudes about the breast itself.

"For men, breasts are sexual ornaments—the crown jewels of femininity."[83] This is not true worldwide, however, and other body parts (e.g., small feet, nape of neck, buttocks) are sexually charged, with much of the fascination resulting from full or partial concealment. Until the fourteenth century, the nursing Madonna was the prevailing image, but in truth, the availability of a mother's milk meant life or death for every newborn.

The breast has assumed many roles throughout history, moving from sacred, domestic, political, to erotic. The definition of the breast has been provided by moralists, historians, poets, pornographers, lovers, and women themselves. Much of the rhetoric today is about the breast in crisis: "The breast is torn between nurturance, eroticism, and the fear of cancer."[83] In the eyes of the beholder, babies see food, men see sex, physicians see disease, business sees dollar signs, religion sees spiritual symbols, and psychoanalysis places them in the center of the unconscious. The breast has a privileged place in human thought. Perhaps the love affair with science has turned women from being comfortable with their breasts as a source of infant nurturance to being uncomfortable and ashamed of breastfeeding, yet searching through science and medicine for the perfect size or shape.[83]

The breast has been regarded as a sex object in the Western world for more than a century, and its biologic benefits have been downplayed. This is clearly demonstrated by the conflicting mores that permit pornographic pictures in newspapers, movies, and nude theaters but insist on the arrest of a mother, discreetly nursing her baby in public, for indecent exposure.

Proponents of breastfeeding have generally accepted, even before the upsurge of interest and research in attachment, that the major reason to breastfeed is to provide the special relationship and closeness that accompany nursing. Conversely, the major contraindication to breastfeeding was lack of desire to do so. This was evidenced by it being considered more appropriate to present breastfeeding as a matter of personal choice with no compelling reasons to urge a mother to consider nursing. The concern over creating guilt in the mother who chose not to nurse has been significant and often resulted in a passive attitude on the part of the clinician so that the mother received no prenatal counseling about infant feeding.[42]

MOTHER-INFANT INTERACTION

The studies performed to understand bonding have largely been done without reference to breastfeeding. A supposedly comprehensive book, *Attachment and Loss* by Bowlby,[9] which reviews early other-infant interactions extensively, never mentions breastfeeding. In addition, sucking is given extensive treatment without making a distinction between bottle and breast or implying that an alternative to the bottle exists. The emphasis in the 1940s was on the effects of disrupting already-formed attachments. Separation in the neonatal period was ignored, and infant socialization was studied from 6 months of age.

Work by Spitz[73] and others has identified the devastating effects on the infant deprived of long-term maternal contact. These investigators demonstrated major deficits in both mental and motor development, as well as general failure to thrive. The impact on the mother had not yet been described. Klaus and Kennel[39] provided those data in their many writings on mother-infant interaction, which are summarized in their book, *Parent-Infant Bonding*. Evidence indicates that the maternal-infant bond is the strongest human bond when two major facts are considered: the infant's early growth is within the mother's body, and survival after birth depends on her care. Although the process had not been meticulously described yet, Budin[12] noted in 1907 that when a mother was separated from her infant and was unable to provide the early care of her sick child, she lost interest and even abandoned the infant.

The immediate emotional reactions of mothers to their newborns were studied by Robson and Kumar[68] in 193 women (two groups of primiparas, n = 112 and n = 41, and one group of multiparas, n = 40). About 40% of the primiparas and 25% of the multiparas recalled that their predominant emotional reaction when holding their babies for the very first time had been indifference. Maternal affection was more likely to be lacking if the mother had had an amniotomy or painful labor or had received more than one dose of meperidine (Pethidine) unrelated to cesarean birth or forceps delivery. The authors found no difference between breastfeeding and bottle-feeding mothers. The feelings of indifference persisted for a week or longer. This study points out that normal women may be indifferent toward their babies initially, whereas others experience great elation.

The development of positive feelings in primiparous women toward their normal newborns occurred before delivery in a third of women, immediately at birth or on the first day for 42%, and by the second or third day for an additional 19% in a study by Pascoe and French.[60] Breastfeeding mothers were more likely to express positive feelings. Labors of less than 9 hours were associated with positive feelings, but there was no association with social class, infant gender, type of delivery, or duration of initial mother-infant contact.

Klaus and Kennell[39] noted that mothers in the United States showed different attachment behavior when permitted early contact with their premature infants compared with mothers who had first contact at 3 weeks of age. Mothers of full-term infants who were allowed contact within the first 2 hours and subsequent extra contact behaved differently at 1 month and 1 year with their babies, compared with controls. Actually, Jackson et al[35] made similar observations in the Yale Rooming-In Unit from 1945 to 1955 but failed to provide control observations.

As a result of the thought-provoking work of Klaus and Kennell[39] in the 1970s, remarkable changes have taken place in labor, delivery, and postpartum services in hospitals in the United States and around the world. Mothers have been "allowed" to have their infants to hold and cuddle as soon as possible after delivery, and fathers have been "allowed" to participate in the birth experience. The take-charge attitude of health care professionals has relaxed, and gradually hospital perinatal care has been humanized. In the meantime, a number of investigators have challenged the power of bonding. In a critical review of early and extended maternal-infant contact research, Siegel[70] suggests that although many longitudinal experiences affect parenting behavior in complex ways, reasonable judgment supports early and extended contact whenever possible.

When a normal, healthy infant born to an unmedicated mother is placed on the mother's abdomen immediately after the cord is cut, the infant crawls to the breast, finds the nipple and latches on, beginning to suckle.[67] This event takes place unassisted by the mother or an attendant. The warmth of the mother maintains the infant's body temperature. This is described as a series of events beginning with the infant resting and occasionally looking at the mother, then moving toward the breast with some lip smacking and mouthing. Approaching the breast, the infant turns from one to the other before finally moving toward one nipple, bobbing over it, and grasping the areola and suckling. Experiments that involve washing one breast demonstrate the infant chooses the unwashed breast. When the mother has been medicated during labor, the infant struggles to find the breast and often fails. Infants who are left with their mothers seldom cry during this awake, alert period.[67] If unimpeded, this process takes 40 to 45 minutes, which suggests the original baby-friendly mandate of initiating breastfeeding within a half hour may have been hasty. Physiologically, the stimulus to the mother's nipple and the stimulus to the infant's mouth trigger the release of vital hormones in both mother and infant, beginning the maturation of the intestinal mucosa and enhancing nutrient absorption for both mother and infant (Fig. 6-1).

This awake, alert period immediately after delivery provides an opportunity for receiving the first measure of colostrum, which is not only nourishing but also protective from an immunologic and infectious standpoint.

When the newborn is separated from the mother in the first hours postpartum, crying occurs and stops on reunion.[37] The cry has been studied by sound spectrographic analysis in a group of infants in contact with their mothers for the first 90 minutes or kept in a crib. The separated infants cried 10 times more than the contact infants. On analysis, the cry was characterized as a discomfort cry as compared with patterns seen in cries of hunger or pain.[50]

The impact of early mother-infant interaction and breastfeeding on the duration of breastfeeding has been reported; no data appear to be available as to whether mothering is different between breastfeeding and bottle-feeding mothers in this early period.[34] Sosa et al[72] reported the effect of early mother-infant contact on breastfeeding, infection, and growth. Breastfeeding mothers who were permitted early contact but not early breastfeeding were compared with mothers without early contact who also breastfed. The mothers with early contact were observed to nurse 50% longer than the controls. The early-contact infants were heavier and had fewer infections. Sosa et al[72] conducted a similar study in Brazil, in which each mother nursed immediately on delivery and the infant was kept beside the mother's bed until they went home. At home, they had a special nurse make continual contacts to help in the breastfeeding. The control had traditional therapy, that is, contact at feeding times after an early glimpse. Infants were housed in a separate nursery. At 2 months, 77% of the early-contact mothers and only 27% of the controls were successfully nursing. The early and continued contact may have been accompanied by increased support and assistance from the nursery staff. This added support could facilitate breastfeeding and thus be the cause of the improved outcome.

An additional study by deCháteau et al[19] in Sweden investigated a group of 21 mothers with early contact and 19 control mothers, all of whom were breastfeeding in the hospital. The only difference in management was the first 30 minutes of early contact, because 24-hour rooming-in was provided for all mothers after 2 hours postpartum. The length of breastfeeding differed: for the early-contact group, 175 days, and for the controls,

Fig. 6-1. Infant crawling to breast **(A),** making mouthing and sucking movements **(B),** then taking breast **(C).** (From Righard L and Alade MO: *Lancet* 336:1105-1107, 1990.)

105 days. Follow-up observations at 3 months showed different mothering behavior. The study group displayed more attachment behavior, fondling, caressing, and kissing than the controls.

Unless heavy medication or difficult delivery intervenes, an infant experiences a period when the eyes are wide open and the infant can see, has visual preferences, turns to the spoken word, and responds to the environment.[39] Similar periods in the state of consciousness of the infant may last only a few seconds or minutes over the next 1 to 2 days.

Although some mothers begin the attachment process when the decision to have an infant is made, after conception the physiologic changes in the maternal body strengthen the developing bond.[28] During pregnancy, listening to the fetal heart and watching echocardiographic images of fetal movements are confirming factors created by modern medicine. The first picture in the infant's scrapbook may be of the infant as as 12-week fetus. The moment of delivery, the first glimpse, and the first hours are intense opportunities for further "bonding" to occur. For some, however, the process will take a day or a week before the mother feels true love for this infant. Unfortunately, studies investigating this time line do not distinguish breastfeeding from bottle-feeding women.

As in every area of medicine, new ideas and new theories invite criticism. The best type is neither partisan nor polemical and serves to repeat dispassionately the studies and confirm or disprove.[14,27] Many investigators have affirmed the "bonding" theory. Other critics,[3,14,16,26-28,41] however, have been hostile yet unable to disprove that biologic factors might play a significant role in a mother's response to her infant. A new group has called the theories "a bogus notion," reflecting medicine's need to control women and to enhance market demands and the status of medicine itself.[22] Further, it is argued that bonding is demeaning to women because it rests on the idea of instinct. These critics agree that increased contact between mother and infant in the first few days increases maternal emotional response, that early contact enhances breastfeeding, and that early extended contact decreases the incidence of child abuse, with effects solely on the parents, not the child.

Further study is needed, although randomly assigning a mother to a restricted contact control group would be difficult, if not unethical, today. Skin-to-skin versus clothed contact and hormonal components in relationship to behaviors remain to be explored. The fathers' and siblings' roles also deserve additional attention. Lamb,[41] however, has been supportive of the trend toward humanizing childbirth to provide a rich emotional experience for parents.

Sensitive periods in biologic phenomena are times when events alter later behavior. The power of attachment enables mother and father to make the many sacrifices necessary for their infant.[38] More than 30 years of investigation have confirmed the observations that the human maternal-infant bond can be facilitated, supported, and encouraged by more caring sensitive processes beginning in labor and throughout the perinatal period.

Human relationships are complex. A newborn brings joy, fear, anxiety, frustration, and triumph, reminds Richards.[66] Adaptability and compensation in the developmental processes are part of human existence. The concept of bonding has drawn attention to this period of life and begun the process of understanding the mother-infant relationship.[40]

BODY CONTACT AND CULTURAL TRADITION

If we look at other mammals, lactation behavior, including the duration and frequency of feedings, is species specific and predictable because it is a genetically controlled behavioral characteristic of the species. Only those animals kept in zoos or laboratories reject their young. Among higher primates, learning plays a significant role; monkeys reared without role models have to be taught how to groom and feed their young. In the human, breastfeeding behavior is highly variable from one culture to the next. Different cultures of the world have different sets of "rules" about lactation as they do about many other aspects of life and even death. Cultural tradition dictates the initiation, frequency, and termination of breastfeeding. Learning plays a key role in the lactation process, but the learning is focused on the beliefs, attitudes, and values of the culture.

The degree of body contact permitted by the culture is a fundamental difference among these cultures. Simpson-Herbert[71] describes the degree of mother-infant body contact as the physical and social distance that mothers keep from their babies.

The physical distance is viewed as a reflection of the social distance sanctioned by the culture.

Cultures prescribe how often infants will be held or carried and how they will be carried (e.g., in the arms, a pouch, or a sling, or on a cradle-board). How infants are clothed, where they are placed when not held, and where they spend the night are all culturally determined and also affect breastfeeding. The cultural constraints that control maternal behavior include those on the kinds and amounts of maternal clothing, acceptability of breast exposure, and beliefs on frequency and length of feedings.

The effect of increased carrying of infants was studied by Hunziker and Barr[33] in a group of primiparous breastfeeding women in Montreal. The crying pattern of normal infants in industrialized societies has been reported to increase until 6 weeks of age, followed by a decline to 4 months, with most crying occurring in the evening. The investigators had the study families increase carrying the infants either in the arms or in a carrier to a minimum of 3 hours a day, whereas control infants were placed in a crib or a seat with a mobile in view. At 6 weeks, there was significantly less (43%) crying in the "carried" infants, especially in the evening. Similar but smaller differences were noted at 4, 8, and 12 weeks.

When Cunningham et al[17] randomly provided either soft baby carriers or plastic infant seats to a group of low-income women in a clinic in New York City, they found the infants carried in a soft carrier were more securely attached than those placed in a seat when tested with the Ainsworth Strange-Situation Study. The study and control infant groups had an equal number of breastfeeders, and thus the authors found no effect of breastfeeding on study results. They concluded that in low-income groups, mother-infant relationships benefited from early use of soft carriers and "contact comfort."[17]

Although the mean length of breastfeeding was similar in both groups, the breastfeeding was not defined, that is, exclusive, partial, or minimal. Also, time spent holding to breastfeed versus time spent holding to bottle feed was not noted. There were 21 breastfeeders and 28 bottle feeders.[17] Although it is helpful to use carriers with bottle-fed infants, it should not be done to the abandonment of breastfeeding support programs.

Anthropologic studies of 60 societies by Whiting[81] considered mother-infant body contact. He classified these cultures as high or low in contact as follows:

Culture classification	Minimum distance between mother and child
High contact: ↓	1. Infant almost continuously carried by mother in the early months.
Symbiotic identification ↓	2. Little or no clothing separates the mother and infant so that they are in skin-to-skin contact.
Long breastfeeding	3. Infant sleeps with mother.
Low contact: ↓	1. Infant is separated from mother at birth.
	2. Infant is often swaddled or elaborately clothed.
Ambivalent dependency ↓	3. Infant is kept in a crib or cradle-board.
Early weaning	4. Infant does not sleep with mother at night.

Other factors influence the development of cultural mores, including climate and means of food gathering. Simpson-Herbert[71] points out that when infants are heavily clothed and swaddled, as in cold climates, they are neat packages that can be put down easily. The Eskimo is an exception, however, keeping the infant inside her parka for warmth and frequent feeding. Breastfeeding is almost axiomatic in warm climates where clothing is loose or absent, there is frequent holding and carrying, and the breast is readily accessible.

The diet of the hunter-gatherer society is not conducive to early weaning because meat, roots, nuts, and berries are difficult for infants to chew and digest, whereas the softer foods of the agricultural societies can be prepared for early infant feeding.

Study of specific world societies reveal that

North American and European women are concerned with the beliefs that it is indecent to expose the breast, it is possible to spoil an infant with too much handling, and early weaning is a sign of infant development. Western mothers keep their distance from their babies. Mothers in high–body contact societies spend at least 75% of the time in contact with their babies, whereas low-contact societies spend less than 25%.

In the 1990s, infant care in Western societies has included carrying infants in carriers close to the parent's body. Co-sleeping with the infant for easy access to the breast through the night and the concept of the family bed have emerged as more conducive to good parent-infant attachment. Their role in sudden infant death syndrome (SIDS) is being evaluated. Data on bottle feeding and co-sleeping are not available.

PSYCHOLOGIC DIFFERENCE BETWEEN BREASTFEEDING AND BOTTLE FEEDING

Professionals have spent decades reassuring mothers that they can capture the same emotional and behavioral experience by feeding an infant from a bottle as they can feeding at the breast, with the same warmth and love. Technically speaking, the same warmth is not there, because the lactating breast has been shown to be warmer than the nonlactating breast. This can be demonstrated by infrared pictures and thermograms.

Newton and Newton[57] suggest that special caution should be used in evaluating statistical associative studies that purport to study the hypothesis that breastfeeding and bottle feeding are psychologic equivalents. "Because breastfeeding involves a large measure of personal choice and because it is related to attitudinal and personality factors, no groups of breastfeeders and bottle feeders are likely to be equal in other respects. Therefore the relation of breastfeeding to any particular psychosocial measure may not be cause and effect, but simply the differences due to other uncontrolled covariables."[57] A human mother's care of her infant is derived from a complex mixture of her genetic endowment, the response of the infant, a long history of interpersonal relationships with others, her family constellation, this and previous pregnancies, and the community and culture.

The method chosen to feed a baby is but one item in a whole style of maternal-child interaction. It is unlikely that this style is determined by the method of feeding, according to Richards.[65] Breastfeeding is a very different activity when it is carried out by a small minority compared with breastfeeding that is commonplace in the community.

In a study of patterns of variation in breastfeeding behaviors, Quandt[63] offers three explanations: cultural, biologic, and biocultural. Predictions of exclusive breastfeeding duration were most accurate for women with a breastfeeding style of infrequent feedings and therefore early weaning, whereas predictions for women with a style of frequent feeding were confounded by cultural factors that independently affected supplementation.

Before reviewing specific psychologic attributes relating to breastfeeding, the distinction between styles of nursing in Western societies should be considered. The Interagency Group for Action on Breastfeeding developed a schema for breastfeeding definitions (see p. 16). Newton and Newton,[57] however, have described two distinct styles, unrestricted breastfeeding and token breastfeeding, which are important to understanding maternal choices.

Unrestricted breastfeeding

Unrestricted breastfeeding means the infant is put to the breast whenever he cries or fusses. Feeding is ad lib and not by the clock, usually leading to 10 or more feedings a day. The infant receives no bottles, and solids are not introduced until the second half of the first year. Breast milk continues to be a major source of nourishment beyond the first year of life. Interestingly, this was routine practice in the United States in the beginning of the twentieth century, as attested by writings on the subject of child rearing.

Token breastfeeding

Token breastfeeding means feeding characterized by rules and regulations. Both frequency and duration of feeding are determined by the clock. It is deemed unnecessary to permit unlimited suckling. Weaning usually occurs by the third month, if not before. Supplementary bottles and solids are not uncommon. As a result, the let-down reflex is never well established. Engorgement may occur. The infant is frequently too frantic from crying or too sleepy to feed well at the appointed times.

New definitions of breastfeeding (i.e., exclusive, partial, etc.) have been published to standardize statistical comparisons (see Chapter 1) but do not reflect the psychosocial differences between unrestricted and token breastfeeding. The American Academy of Pediatrics recommends exclusive breastfeeding for 4 to 6 months and the gradual inclusion of solids (never before 4 months), preferably at 6 months or later.

A University of Rochester study[42] of urban physicians revealed that those pediatricians who prescribed solids by 3 months or earlier also suggested supplementary bottles and had been in practice 20 years or longer. Most of the physicians in the family medicine program in the same community, however, provided no supplements and no solids until 6 months and had been in practice less than 20 years. More than 50% of mothers in that community who planned to breastfeed had made contact with some childbirth or breastfeeding program and chose their physician according to practice style.

Imprinting, pacifiers, and dummies

Scores of infants are being introduced to pacifiers or dummies shortly after birth, all too often by an impatient perinatal staff member who knows a breastfed infant should not be bottle fed. Free pacifiers are being provided as gifts by some formula companies eager to beat the competition. The UNICEF/WHO 10 steps to becoming a Baby Friendly Hospital (see Chapter 1) includes the exclusion of pacifiers from the hospital's provisions. Do pacifiers have a long-range impact on infants? For bottle-fed infants, probably not if possible dental problems are excluded; a pacifier will provide the sucking a bottle-fed infant may not receive during a feeding. For a breastfed infant, the answer may be different.

Human imprinting is little discussed in pediatric textbooks and rarely noted when discussing infant feeding, yet the human infant, as does any other mammalian newborn, recognizes the mother by the oral, tactile, and olfactory modes. "The most sensitive organ and the one over which a newborn mammal has the most control, its mouth, is the organ central to mammalian and human imprinting," states Mobbs.[51] It is believed that the imprinting process, or "stamping," as it was termed in the 1930s and 1940s, takes place for a brief period early in postnatal development when an animal seeks a particular class of stimuli (i.e., objects of particular shape).[51] Having found such an object or one resembling it, the animal responds with an unlearned pattern of attachment behavior. The process is innate. Comfort sucking and formation of nipple preference are genetically determined behaviors for imprinting to the mother's nipple. The recognition of the mother is at first through the distinctive features of the nipple. Although imprinting is multisensory and varies from species to species, it is oral/tactile for the human and other higher mammals.

Mistakes and mishaps can occur in the process when the newborn fixes on a rubber nipple (bottle), thumb, or pacifier (Table 6-1). Geese have imprinted to a man's boot. In birds, innate responses are preferentially selective to supernormal-size stimuli. Nonnutritive sucking on thumbs or pacifiers is displacement activity that would normally be directed at imprinting to mother's nipple and reflects a tendency toward supernormal size. In other species with multiple births or litters, the offspring imprints to one teat throughout the lactation period. The one nipple preference sometimes reflects emotional attachment to the object rather than a preoccupation with a need for sucking that maintains the preference; this according to Passman and Halonen,[61] who found 42% of the

TABLE 6-1 **Instinctive fixation on sucking objects in the process of oral, tactile, mother recognition**

	Objects of fixation			
	Human breast	Filled nursing bottle	Thumb/finger/ knuckles	Empty bottle/ pacifier (dummy)/ cloth
Nutritive	Yes	Yes	No	No
Animate	Yes	No	Yes	No
Non-self	Yes	Yes	No	Yes
Infant control	No	No	Yes	No

From Mobbs EJG: Human imprinting and breastfeeding: are the textbooks deficient? In Llewellyn-Jones D, Abraham S, editors: *Proceedings 16th Annual Congress, Australian Society for Psychosomatic Aspects of Reproductive Medicine,* Pokolbin, South Wales, March 1989.

interaction with the dummy to be nonsucking attachment.

Mothers of thumb-sucking infants are less likely to breastfeed successfully, as was demonstrated in a study of 93 mother-infant pairs. Those who used a dummy or pacifier breastfed a shorter period (mean of 5.5 months compared with 7.5 months). Nonnutritive sucking on objects was added to the list of causes of lactation failure by Lilburne et al[47] following this study. Margaret Mead stated that in those societies where access to the breast is unlimited and frequent suckling is accepted, there is no thumb sucking.[64]

Although the term "nipple confusion" has not yet been accepted in the medical literature, strong psychosomatic evidence suggests that human imprinting can be altered by introducing a foreign object during imprinting.

PERSONALITY DIFFERENCES BETWEEN BREASTFEEDING AND BOTTLE-FEEDING MOTHERS

Clear differences exist between mothers who practice unrestricted breastfeeding and those who bottle feed. There are even some distinctions between token breastfeeders and bottle feeders. It has been said that maternal personality is more important than either breastfeeding or bottle feed-

ing per se to the development of the infant's personality.

Experimenters looking at these factors have provided a wealth of somewhat conflicting information. Chamberlain[15] studied the differences between mothers who bottle fed and those who practiced unrestricted breastfeeding with their second child. The groups were similar in age, education, parity, intelligence, and socioeconomic status. The breastfeeding mothers were less defensive about their method of feeding, were more oriented toward home life, and had higher radicalism scores. The bottle-feeding mothers confirmed the hypothesis that they had problems in trying to breastfeed their first child because of inadequate lactation, possibly a psychosomatic reaction. They also had a greater incidence of sexual performance problems, as indicated from a higher surgency score. The breastfeeding mothers wanted their children to do things typical of children; the bottle-feeding mothers preferred their children to be conservative and other-person oriented, and urged them to be more adult.

Call[13] had studied the emotional factors favoring successful breastfeeding and noted that of 104 consecutive mothers delivering at an Air Force hospital, 42.6% of the multiparas and 50% of the primiparas chose bottle feeding. Of the breastfeeding mothers, 48% of those multiparas and 40% of the primiparas were successful beyond 3 weeks.

Failure was associated with engorgement, lack of let-down reflex, and psychologic conflict. The two conflicts seen in those who did not nurse and those who failed were as follows:

1. They had a conflict in accepting the biologic maternal role in relation to the infant versus other roles society holds for women. The maternal role is considered a general class attitude in middle-class American society.
2. They had a conflict regarding the functioning of the breast itself, that is, as an organ for nourishment of the young versus a sexual organ, affording the breast the same psychologic value as the penis in the male. Nursing thus became a "castration" threat.

PSYCHOPHYSIOLOGIC REACTIONS DURING NURSING

Newton and Newton[57] have equated psychophysiologic reactions during nursing to the degree of successful lactation. During unrestricted suckling, the gentle stroking of the nipple by undulating motion of the infant tongue occurs 3000 to 4000 times in a single feeding. This should result in an increase in temperature of the mammary skin and rhythmic contraction of the uterus. Failure to experience these signs in early lactation is related to failure to produce adequate milk.

Let-down reflex

The unrestricted breastfed infant cries, and the mother has the urge to suckle the infant because the cry has triggered her let-down reflex. The breast is turgescent and ready for the infant. Unrestricted crying is rarely seen in these infants. With token breastfeeding, such a response does not occur on schedule, and from feeding to feeding the milk supply may be little or, conversely, gushing. The infant is unable to cope with the unpredictability. Insufficient milk is rarely a problem when infants are carried and fed frequently.

The role of various hormones in inducing maternal behaviors in animals has been extensively studied. Rosenblatt[69] showed that both male and female rats, including virgin females, manifest maternal behavior after 5 to 7 days contact with foster pups. Manipulation of estrogen, progesterone, and prolactin has demonstrated that estrogen is the most potent inducer of maternal behavior, progesterone usually is inhibitory, and prolactin strangely ineffective.

More recently, evidence indicates that prolactin does have a role in stimulating maternal behaviors in the rat, but only when primed by placental lactogens that affect the maternal brain (medial preoptic area) in regard to maternal responses at birth.[11] The brain of the maternally behaving rat is altered as a result of the dam's behavior toward her pups. Morphologic changes are seen in the supraoptic nucleus, which contains oxytocinergic neurons important for lactation. The supraoptic nuclei of lactating animals have a higher incidence of dendritic bundling compared with those of nonmaternal virgin rats.[53] These experiments support the concept that maternal behavior in lactating animals can have a profound effect on the morphology and physiologic functioning of oxytocinergic neurons in the hypothalamus.

When levels were measured in 22 puerperal women, the suckling-induced oxytocin during nursing was pulsatile, with discrete, short pulses.[77] When the women were subjected to the stress of loud noise (70 dB) by earphones or to the stress of performing mathematical problems, the frequency of pulsatile release of oxytocin was significantly lower. No difference was seen in prolactin levels or milk yield. These data suggest that psychologic relaxation is necessary for a successful let-down response, confirming what Newton and Newton[57] had observed more than 30 years ago.

The induction of maternal behavior after administration of oxytocin experimentally in rats by Pedersen and Prange[62] demonstrated that estrogen priming is necessary for the effect, but oxytocin may be the triggering hormone for maternal behaviors. A strong relationship between the peptide hormones native to the central nervous system and the reproductive hormones results not only in endocrine effects but also in behavioral effects.[31]

The long-term psychophysiologic response to unrestricted nursing is a more even mood cycle than the mood swings associated with ovulation and menstruation. Unrestricted nursing is associated with secondary amenorrhea for as long as 16 months.

From studies in animals, Thoman et al[75] have noted:

> The present experiments do indicate that there is a unique buffering system which appears to protect the lactating female from large variations in responsiveness during the process of lactating. Inasmuch as there exists considerable information that indicates that maternal factors have profound and long-lasting effects on the psychophysiologic function of offspring in adulthood, the existence of such buffering systems in the lactating females would appear to be of importance in the mother-young interaction.

In relating the rate of success in breastfeeding to experiences at birth, Jackson et al[35] reported that the more difficult the labor, the less successful the breastfeeding. A direct correlation has also been made with the amount of medication and anesthetic given during labor and delivery and subsequently the sleepiness of the infant and, ultimately, the inadequacy of the suckling. Newton and Newton[57] observed that mothers who talked to their babies on the second day nursed their babies longer, that is, beyond the second month.

Modahl and Newton[52] measured mood state differences between breastfeeding and bottle-feeding mothers when feeding and not feeding. They used the Curran and Cattep questionnaire, which measures transient mood states rather than personality traits. Bottle feeders showed significantly more anxiety, stress, depression, regression, fatigue, and guilt than breastfeeders. Mothers measured while bottle feeding reported higher levels of these states and more extroversion than the control group of bottle feeders tested in a nonfeeding situation. Another control group who were lactating but also gave bottles were measured while not feeding and showed less anxiety, stress, depression, regression, fatigue, and guilt than the

average population. Measurements were taken at home with no examiner present.

The psychophysiologic responses of breastfeeding and bottle-feeding mothers to their infants' signals were measured by Wiesenfeld et al[82] using physiologic monitoring, while mothers observed previously prepared videotapes of their own infants while they smiled, were quiescent, and cried. Strikingly different response patterns characterized breastfeeding and bottle-feeding mothers across all response measures. Breastfeeding mothers were physiologically more relaxed but were more apt to want to interact with their child and expressed greater satisfaction with the feeding experience. The authors interpreted these patterns as suggesting a physiologic influence of breastfeeding rather than maternal personality factors influencing the choice of feeding mode.

When 60 primiparous mothers' maternal role adjustments were analyzed by measuring mother-infant mutuality and maternal anxiety scores, the infant-feeding method (breast, bottle, or both) was found to account for considerable variation by Virden.[79] Women who breastfed had scores indicating less anxiety and more mutuality, a central factor in maternal adjustment, than women who bottle fed. The Maternal Attitude Scale (MAS) was used. The findings are compatible with other studies showing breastfeeding to be emotionally gratifying and as stimulating a sense of emotional union between mother and infant.[45]

IMPACT OF SOCIETY, MEDICAL PROFESSION, AND FAMILY

Society

Newton[56] has pointed out that a woman's joy in and acceptance of the female biologic role in life may be an important factor in her psychosexual behavior, which includes lactation. She found that women who wished to bottle-feed also often believed that the male role was the more satisfying role. Nulliparous women who planned to breastfeed their children more often stated their satisfaction with the female role, according to Adams.[1] Breastfeeding behavior has been related to a woman's role in life as influenced by her cultural locale, education, social class, and work. Breastfeeding rates and weaning times vary in the United States by geographic area. The smaller the community, the longer is the duration of breastfeeding. Cross-cultural studies in large cities show variation in rates of nursing. These rates are influenced by education, and in the current generation, the higher the education, the higher the incidence of breastfeeding.

The attitudes of the husband, close family, and friends influence the mother's attitude toward breastfeeding. More important, these attitudes influence the rate of success and the age at weaning more negatively than positively. One study showed that a grandmother's interest did not influence the mother's decision to nurse as frequently as did a friend's (peer's) decision to bottle-feed. A woman whose husband is not supportive of breastfeeding weans early, or does not start at all.[36]

Medical profession

The enthusiastic physician can influence the number of breastfeeding mothers in the practice; this has been demonstrated. If the physician provides knowledgeable medical and psychologic support, the success rate of the patients who intended to breastfeed will increase. Some patients who had not formed an opinion or given it any thought in their preparation for motherhood will be persuaded to try. In addition, this physician will attract patients to the practice who are already successfully breastfeeding but find their own physician unable or unwilling to support their efforts.

A study was done at the University of Rochester in a small community where over 50 pediatricians practiced.[44] The pediatricians described their own practices according to the number of breastfeeding mothers (high, 75%; moderate, 50%; low, 25%). They were also asked when they started solid foods, general practice "regulations," and, finally, how their own children were fed. The physicians with a high incidence of breastfeeding

in their practices started solids after 4 months, had few rules and regulations about the office, and usually their own children had been breastfed. The physicians with a high number of bottle feeders started solids by 6 weeks, had many rules and regulations about the practice, and their own children had been bottle-fed. When asked about using lay groups to help their patients breastfeed, the female physicians were more apt than the male physicians to discredit what these lay mothers could do to help other mothers.

A national survey conducted among a representative sample of obstetricians, pediatricians, and family physicians by mailed questionnaire reinforced the observation that the physician's attitude and personal beliefs about breastfeeding influence the advice given.[42] It further confirmed that not all physicians were informed about current knowledge on human lactation, not all physicians discussed lactation with their pregnant patients, and not all believed it was worth counseling time when problems arose. Results in 1993 were similar to those of the previous decade, despite national efforts to increase the physician's knowledge base regarding breastfeeding.[43]

The family
Impact on the infant

For the infant, differences exist between breastfeeding and bottle feeding in the alleviation of hunger, the mother-infant interaction, oral gratification, activity, development, personality, and adaptation to the environment. Often mother and baby are alone together during breastfeeding, and the mother gives her full attention to the baby with stroking and fondling. Social interaction with the baby is less frequent during bottle feeding, and the mother is often in a distracting social situation or someone else feeds the infant. The breastfed infant has control of what is happening, or at least shares control, whereas the mother controls the bottle and the bouts of sucking.

In a study of newborns at 6 to 7 days of age, the effects of breastfeeding, giving breast milk by bottle, and just holding the infant were measured.[48]

Results suggest the total mother-infant interaction during breastfeeding has a positive influence on neonatal behavior. It induces a more stable state for an infant compared with that generated by giving the same human milk in a bottle and increases some sucking and holding times.

Development. Early assessment of newborns in the first and second weeks of life shows more body activity with breastfed than bottle-fed infants. They are more alert and have stronger arousal reaction. Statistics reported by Douglas[21] on age of learning to walk in Great Britain showed a distinct difference, with breastfed infants starting 2 months earlier than bottle-fed infants. The longer the infant was nursed, the more striking the differences. Thus, prolonged breastfeeding does not impede development, as has been implied by advocates of early weaning. A study in Illinois in 1929 compared children exclusively breastfed for 4 months, 9 months, and over a year with bottle-fed infants.[30] The children who were exclusively breastfed for 4 and 9 months scored significantly higher on achievement tests, but the difference was reversed beyond a year. Exclusively breastfeeding beyond a year increased morbidity as well, which is in keeping with the concept that solids should be added in the second half of the first year.

A cross-cultural study of 50 3-year-old children in Hawaii, reflecting the cultural diversity of the islands, provided periodic behavioral assessments as part of the Heptaclor study. The study, which used the McCarthy scales, showed that the duration of breastfeeding was correlated with general cognition, verbal and quantitative scores, and memory, regardless of socioeconomic status, gender, or pesticide exposure. There were no associations in this study to motor skills at 3 years of age.[6]

An extensive study by Morrow-Tlucak et al[55] investigated differences between breastfed and bottle-fed infants. Batteries of infant assessment measures and maternal interviews were conducted by trained examiners blind to the risk factors during home visits when the infant was 6, 12, and 24 months of age. The 350 children were born to women at the Cleveland Metropolitan General Hospital in 1981-1982 who were part of a study of child development and psychosocial risk factors. The Bayley scales and the Home Observation Measurement of Environment (HOME) were done. A significant difference among bottle-fed children, children breastfed 4 months or less, and those breastfed 4 months or more was found at all points, with extended breastfeeding having a positive effect.[55]

Animal research has also shown a relationship of weaning time to learning skills. Since it has become evident that species-specific proteins and amino acids exist, it is possible that the brain develops more physiologically with the precise basic nutrients. Comparisons with animal species show that the more intelligent and skillful groups within a species are nursed longer.

Personality. The personality and adjustment of infants as related to their early feeding experiences have been the subject of much discussion. The personality of the mother and the temperament of the child need to be considered. Some conflicting information is reported in studies retrospectively analyzing the effects of breastfeeding on outcome in terms of security and behavior. The emphasis has been on the duration of the breastfeeding rather than on the quality of the relationship.

In a prospective study of a birth cohort of New Zealand children followed up to the age of 8 years, both maternal and teacher assessments of conduct disorder showed a statistically significant tendency for conduct disorder scores to decline with increasing duration of breastfeeding.[24] Overall, however, the authors suggest no real evidence indicates that breastfeeding is protective against conduct disorders.

When abrupt weaning takes place, it may be psychologically very traumatic for the infant and the mother. In animals, when the mother is stressed while lactating, the nursling's plasma cortisone levels are elevated. The psychologically depressed mother may not experience postpartum depression until the infant is weaned from the breast. It has been accepted that early experience, including feeding experience, does influence later behavior in the long run. The performance in young college women on an anxiety scale questionnaire (IPAT) and a personality inventory (EPI) showed that those women who had been bottle-fed had higher anxiety scores and greater neuroticism than the women who had been breastfed, irrespective of duration of breastfeeding.[32] However, much more study must be done before the impact of nursing at the breast is truly understood in the complexity of life's events.

Impact on the father

Since the birthing process moved into the hospital setting, fathers have been moved farther from the nucleus of the new family. In recent years, this trend has been reversed. Research on interaction with the infant had focused on the mother until Parke et al[59] observed all three together. In the triadic situation, the father tends to hold the baby twice as much, touches the baby slightly more, but smiles significantly less than the mother. The father plays the more active role when both are present. The study was conducted with middle-class participants who had been to childbirth classes, but the same results were obtained among low-income families without preparation or the presence of the father in the labor and delivery room. The infant had to be relatively active and responsive to capture the father's attention. The investigators believed fathers were far more involved in and responsive toward their infants than our culture had acknowledged. Other studies have shown that when fathers were asked to undress their babies and establish eye contact with them in the first few days of life, they showed more caregiving behavior 3 months later than did controls.

Newton and Newton[57] describe the early attachments of the new family as follows:

Father	Interacts with baby	Engrossment
Mother	Interacts with baby	Bonding
Baby	Interacts with mother	Attachment

The father has been brought back into the childbirth scene as a coach. The coach role has been described as the father's role in shared childbirth. The idea of coaching has negative connotations, because a coach is one who develops the players to

work and try harder but always to win. Ideally, the father should be a partner and supporter in labor, delivery, and breastfeeding. Raphael[64] has suggested that the father may well play the role of the doula. The *doula* is one who provides psychologic encouragement and physical assistance to the newly delivered mother. Raphael further indicates that the lack of a doula to support the mother predisposes her to failure with breastfeeding.[64]

The stress placed on sharing responsibilities of parenthood implies an across-the-board division of labor. This implies that parenting is equal for women and men. There are complementary activities for fathers and mothers. Parents are not equally able to do all things. There is more to nurturing the infant than feeding. The father therefore should play a very significant role with the infant. For instance, when the infant is fussy and does not need to be fed, comforting is often best done by the father. Nonnutritive cuddling is best done by the father.

According to Waletzky,[80] the father's most common negative reaction to breastfeeding is jealousy of the physical and emotional closeness of the nursing mother and child. The degree of jealousy may reflect how much and how happily the mother breastfeeds. Actually, fathers may express distress because they have no similar way to bring food and contentment to their baby. Male envy of female sex characteristics and reproductive capacity has been identified by Lerner[46] as "a widespread and conspicuously ignored dynamic." Improving the birth experience for husbands is a significant means of helping them feel closer to their baby and better about themselves as fathers, according to Waletzky.[80]

Fathers who object to their wives' breastfeeding may do so because they do not want to share this part of their lover with an infant. Some fathers express concern that the breast will leak and destroy any sexual mystique. On the other hand, many men take great pride in the knowledge that their infants will be breastfed and support their wives in this effort. The decision to breastfeed should be made with the full involvement of the father.

Impact on siblings

Although there is some information about siblings and breastfeeding with regard to behavior patterns, no known studies compare siblings of bottle-fed and breastfed infants. Just as siblings frequently want to try the infant's bottle, they may want to nurse at the breast. The child will reflect the mother's attitude toward the breast and nursing. If the mother nurses secretly or in private and isolates herself from the family, it may cause concern in the sibling and produce feelings of shame or guilt toward the breasts.

Breastfeeding and feminism

"Breastfeeding empowers women and contributes to gender equality [and therefore] is an important feminist, human rights and women's issue," states Van Esterik.[78] Despite the Eyer's statement that the results of mother-infant research "will be shaped to address social and political agendas . . . and women inspired by feminism helped to precipitate a reform movement that actively embraces bonding,"[22] Van Esterik points out that writers on feminist theory almost always ignore the breast and ignore motherhood as well. Breastfeeding advocates have been criticized as wanting to tie women down. Van Esterik[78] makes the following suggestions for women's groups:

- Request that policy makers consult with women's groups before breastfeeding legislation is drafted.
- Recognize that breastfeeding is an emotional issue for many women, and develop strategies for framing the issue in nonjudgmental ways.
- Plan how to counter possible negative effects, such as employers threatening to fire women rather than provide maternity entitlements.
- Ensure that breastfeeding campaigns stress the welfare of both mother and child.

Intimacy and breastfeeding

Breastfeeding is an intimate activity for some women, but most health professionals tend to present it in the context of the biopsychosocial model.[20] The closeness of the mother-infant dyad is a feminine image.

According to McAdams,[49] the definition of intimacy includes 10 characteristics in the exchange between people: joy and mutual delight; reciprocal dialogue; openness; contact; union; receptivity; perceived harmony; concern for the other's well-being; surrender of manipulative control and the desire to master; and being in an encounter.

The theoretical definition for intimacy, states Timmerman,[76] is "a quality of a relationship in which the individuals must have reciprocal feelings of trust and emotional closeness toward each other and are able to openly communicate thoughts and feelings with each other. The conditions that must be met for intimacy to occur include reciprocity of trust, emotional closeness and self-disclosure."

Breastfeeding provides body contact with another and is the source of comfort, security, warmth, and nourishment for the infant and reciprocity for the mother. The mother's perception of breastfeeding as intimate describes her concept of the mother-infant relationship. The spouse's perception, however, may have the greatest effect on the success and duration of breastfeeding. Jordan and Wall[36] suggest that "supporting the father during breastfeeding may help improve the mother's satisfaction with breastfeeding, the duration of breastfeeding and adaptation of both parents to parenting."

WHY SOME WOMEN DO NOT BREASTFEED

Before the trend toward bottle feeding can be reversed, one has to understand why some women do not breastfeed. It cannot be blamed on society or the medical profession when a woman cannot accept this as part of the biologic role of a mother. A physician who does not understand the complexities of rejecting breastfeeding cannot hope to assist a mother to succeed in breastfeeding.

Exploring the question of whether body satisfaction and maternal attachment affect breastfeeding, 38 women at about 35 weeks' gestation were given the Maternal Foetal Attachment Scale, the Eating Disorders Examination, and the Body Satisfaction Scale.[26] Women who intended to breastfeed were more satisfied with their gravid shape and had higher levels of maternal-fetal attachment. The mother's age and body mass index did not differ between breastfeeders and bottle feeders. Mothers with high body dissatisfaction do not breastfeed. Not surprisingly, five mothers with a history of bulimia had difficulty breastfeeding, and three thought it was distasteful and adversely affected their appearance.[74]

Our society has assumed that no valid intellectual stimulation can occur in the company of young children. Mothers are made to feel intellectually stagnant and uncreative while breastfeeding. Indeed, they are also made to feel asexual at the peak of their sexual cycle. In response, new mothers struggle in panic to maintain their social and professional ties. They feel they must produce tangible works to be productive. Bloom[8] points out poignantly that one of the greatest intellectual voyages of our time was undertaken when Jean Piaget sat at his son's crib and observed the child's successive attempts to grasp a rattle. A nursing mother learns about her child through many internal, subjective, and kinesthetic modes that were not open to Piaget. When a mother wrote of her observations in this setting, her writing was ignored as unscientific and trivial.

Bentovim[7] has taken a systems approach to successful breastfeeding, pointing out that a range of physical, psychologic, and sociologic factors are involved. "Breastfeeding is a systemic product of many interacting factors rather than a product of individual behavior only,"[7] according to Bentovim. A good experience with breastfeeding can ensure an intense interaction and synchronous response of giving and taking. According to Brazelton,[10] this is the essence of the infant's beginning to create a secure world for the self.

Beliefs and attitudes toward breastfeeding influence the choice and the success of breastfeeding. Bentovim points out that it may be possible to restore breastfeeding as the natural choice.[7] This would depend on society finding a system in which the breast can be accepted not only as good for the infant and development, but also as the object of less ambivalent and secret pleasure. Bentovim[7] suggests, "The role of the health professionals in this area is important in that only through the right relationship with the mother will a new source of mothering be found that can act as a form of extended family for the woman to identify with and to counteract personal, family, and cultural influences." Hendrickse[29] confirms this view and states that the biggest block in the minds of women relates to feelings of shame associated with breastfeeding. More than half the women in the Newcastle survey were prevented from breastfeeding because of a sense of shame.[4] The shame is a result of relating the breast to concepts of sexuality.

Failure at breastfeeding: grief, shame, guilt, or anger

When a mother who had planned to breastfeed is unable to because of illness in herself or her baby, or when a mother begins to breastfeed and must stop, there is a grief reaction. The mother experiences a great loss. Prolonged mourning and depression may occur. Some women report feeling more distant from this child than from her other children if the others had been successfully breastfed. The stronger the commitment had been to breastfeed, the stronger is the grief reaction. Few mothers found help, according to Richards[65] in this study, from either professionals or lay support groups. Professionals failed to understand the feeling of failure or loss. The support groups tended to magnify the guilt and sense of failure.

The emotions are complex surrounding this intimate activity. Physicians who must recommend discontinuing breastfeeding for medical reasons should be aware of the impact and provide for appropriate support for the mother. A woman's choice of feeding method does not make her a good or bad mother, and her inability to produce adequate milk for her infant does not make her a bad mother. Lactation failure is often a reflection on the system and the culture rather than the person.

A random sampling of educated middle-class women in a university neighborhood revealed a number of women who had had difficulty breast-feeding. The study did not describe methodology or how it was randomized, but the report reflected much shame, guilt, and finally anger.[25] Failure at breastfeeding by a woman or her friends can be a powerful influence against deciding to breastfeed a future child.

Fear, shame, and guilt were regarded by Freud as different forms of anxiety. Objective anxiety is fear (fear of failure) and arises from external dangers; social anxiety is shame resulting from the criticisms of others; and conscience anxiety is guilt.[18] Real external dangers produce normal anxiety, but when one overreacts, this is neurotic anxiety. Defenses against guilt feelings include repression, rationalization, and projection. Any guilt can be borne more easily if someone else has had a similar experience.[23] Thus, knowing other women have failed to breastfeed successfully helps relieve the guilt.

Lasting anger following lactation failure has become more visible. The woman who writes an angry tirade against breastfeeding in a letter to the editor after a news story supporting breastfeeding deserves understanding and support. She is likely a victim of poor medical management and inadequate social support to breastfeed. Letter writing can be therapeutic, but it is never a cure for the underlying hurt.

In our clinical experience, well-educated women who have difficulty producing enough milk or who have an infant who fails to thrive are driven to find out why. The Lactation Study Center has received many calls from women who may even have had trouble feeding one or more other infants and want to be "tested" to find the cause. Testing resources are limited and reveal little more than can be identified with a good history of breast response in pregnancy and postpartum. The mother's need usually involves a desire to know that the situation is out of her control. The best management beyond ruling out simple remediable causes (positioning, timing, or reduction of fatigue) may be the therapy of a good listener and the reassurance that one is still a good mother.

Avoiding guilt as a reason not to promote breastfeeding

In many interactions with physicians, especially obstetricians, we encourage them to provide enough information about breastfeeding to a woman prenatally to allow her to make an informed choice. The response often is: "No, I don't want to make a mother feel guilty, so I say nothing."

No studies in the literature to support this position. In the dozens of reports on efforts to increase breastfeeding among many cultures, there is no report of producing guilt feelings. Women interviewed with open-ended questionnaires have not mentioned guilt feelings in response to the questioning. The only individuals who ever mention guilt are the older generation whose daughters are now choosing breastfeeding. The grandmother feels guilty because no one ever told her; no one ever encouraged her to breastfeed. "If only she had known . . . if only her doctor had told her. . . ." In the interest of good health, physicians counsel their patients about good nutrition, weight gain, smoking, drinking, and a number of detrimental personal behaviors without any concern for the guilt they might produce because of the importance of the issue. The feeding choice has an equally important impact for both mother and infant.

In a study at the University of Rochester prenatal clinic, women were randomly assigned to the group attending the Best Start program to encourage breastfeeding or to the control group spending the same time in "counseling" about pregnancy and delivery but nothing about breastfeeding.[44] After delivery, interviewed mothers in both groups were comfortable about their own infant-feeding decision. Those who received breastfeeding encouragement and chose to bottle-feed said it was right for them and denied any guilt feelings.

SUMMARY

Decades of research have shown that the breast plays an important role in the growth, development, identity, and psychologic well-being of women. Not all women have the same level of comfort with their breasts or see them in the same light with respect to their primary purpose, the nourishment of the newborn offspring. The infant, on the other hand, when given the opportunity, will find the breast, seek out and latch on, and suckle. Infants at birth are programmed to breastfeed. Their innate reflexes of rooting and suckling are designed for breastfeeding. Infants also can be taught other mechanisms for feeding. The intricacies of how women choose infant-feeding methods remain to be identified. This choice is influenced by culture, community, personal experiences, education, and the opinions of those close to the mother.

The physician can make a difference. Women indicate that they rely heavily on the messages they hear from their physicians. The issue of guilt regarding choices is no more important in choosing to breastfeed than it is in choosing to smoke, drink, abuse drugs, or give in to problems of overeating. The physician's role in the latter situations has always been clear: take a firm stand and provide guidelines for the patient. In addition to providing information and support regarding infant-feeding choices, the physician is also in a very critical position to facilitate breastfeeding in its early hours and to be supportive and constructive in ensuring its success with appropriate monitoring of progress, not only in the hospital but in the first weeks and months of the infant's life.

The impact of breastfeeding on the mother herself is more difficult to identify. Mothers who breastfeed are not different at the onset but do change in their relationship with their infant. Breastfeeding does have an impact psychologically on both mother and infant.

REFERENCES

1. Adams AB: Choice of infant feeding technique as a function of maternal personality, *J Consult Clin Psychol* 23:143, 1959.
2. Alder EM, Cox JL: Breastfeeding and post-natal depression, *J Psychosom Res* 27:139, 1983.
3. Anisfeld E, Lipper E: Early contact, social support, and mother-infant bonding, *Pediatrics* 72:79, 1983.
4. Bacon CJ, Wylie JM: Mother's attitudes to infant feeding at Newcastle General Hospital in summer 1975, *Br Med J* 1:308, 1976.
5. Barr RG, Elias MF: Nursing interval and maternal responsivity: effect of early infant crying, *Pediatrics* 81:529, 1988.
6. Bauer G, Ewald S, Hoffman J et al: Breastfeeding and cognitive development of three year old children, *Psychol Rep* 68:1218, 1991.
7. Bentovim A: Shame and other anxieties associated with breast feeding: a systems theory and psychodynamic approach. In *Ciba Foundation Symposium*, no 45, Breast feeding and the mother, Amsterdam, 1976, Elsevier Scientific.
8. Bloom M: The romance and power of breast feeding, *Birth Fam J* 8:259, 1981.
9. Bowlby J: *Attachment and loss,* London, 1969, Hogarth.
10. Brazelton TB: The early mother-infant adjustment, *Pediatrics* 32:931, 1963.
11. Bridges RS: The role of lactogenic hormones in maternal behavior in female rats, *Acta Paediatr Suppl* 397:33, 1994.
12. Budin P: *The nursling,* London, 1907, Caxton.
13. Call JD: Emotional factors favoring successful breastfeeding of infants, *J Pediatr* 55:485, 1959.
14. Campbell SBG, Taylor PM: Bonding and attachment: theoretical issues, *Semin Perinatol* 3:3, 1979.
15. Chamberlain RE: Some personality differences between breast and bottle feeding mothers, *Birth Fam J* 3:31, 1976.
16. Chess S, Thomas A: Infant bonding: mystique and reality, *Am J Orthopsychiatry* 52:213, 1982.
17. Cunningham N, Anisfeld E, Casper V et al: Infant carrying, breastfeeding and mother-infant relations, *Lancet* 1:379, 1987 (letter).
18. Davids A, Engrew T: *Introductory psychology,* New York, 1975, Random House.
19. deChâteau P, Holmberg H, Jakobsson K et al: A study of factors promoting and inhibiting lactation, *Dev Med Child Neurol* 19:575, 1977.
20. Dignam DM: Understanding intimacy as experienced by breastfeeding women, *Health Care Women Int* 16:477, 1995.

21. Douglas JWB: The extent of breast feeding in Great Britain in 1946, with special reference to health and survival of children, *J Obstet Gynaecol Br Empire* 57:335, 1950.
22. Eyer D: *Mother-infant bonding: a scientific fiction,* New Haven, Conn, 1992, Yale University Press.
23. Fenichel O: *Psychoanalytic therapy for neurosis,* New York, 1975, Norton.
24. Fergusson DM, Horwood LJ, Shannon FT: Breastfeeding and subsequent social adjustment in six- to eight-year-old children, *J Child Psychol Psychiatr* 28:378, 1987.
25. Fisher PJ: Breast or bottle: a personal choice, *Pediatrics* 72:434, 1983 (letter).
26. Foster SF, Slade P, Wilson K: Body image, maternal fetal attachment and breast feeding, *J Psychosom Res* 41:181, 1996.
27. Goldberg S: Parent-infant bonding: another look, *Child Dev* 54:1355, 1983.
28. Grossman ER: The parent-infant bonding controversy: a critique of the critics, *Dev Behav Pediatr* 15:379, 1994.
29. Hendrickse RG: *Discussion from Ciba Foundation Symposium,* no 45, Breast feeding and the mother, Amsterdam, 1976, Elsevier Scientific.
30. Hoefer C, Hardy MC: Later development of breast fed and artificially fed infants, *JAMA* 92:615, 1929.
31. Hollander E, Liebowitz MR, Cohen B et al: Prolactin and sodium lactate–induced panic, *Psychiatr Res* 28:181, 1989.
32. Hughes RN, Hawkins AB: EPI and IPAT anxiety scale performance in young women as related to breastfeeding during infancy, *J Clin Psychol* 31:663, 1975.
33. Hunziker UA, Barr RG: Increased carrying reduces infant crying: a randomized controlled trial, *Pediatrics* 77:64, 1986.
34. Hwang C-P: Aspects of the mother-infant relationship during nursing, 1 and 6 weeks after extended post-partum contact, *Early Hum Dev* 5:279, 1981.
35. Jackson EB, Wilkin LC, Auerbach H: Statistical report on incidence and duration of breast feeding in relation to personal-social, and hospital maternity factors, *Pediatrics* 17:700, 1956.
36. Jordan PL, Wall VR: Supporting the father when an infant is breastfed, *J Hum Lact* 9:31, 1993.
37. Kennell JH, Klaus MH: Bonding: recent observations that alter perinatal care, *Pediatr Rev* 19:4, 1998.
38. Kennell JH, Trause MA, Klaus MH: Evidence for a sensitive period in the human mother. In *Ciba Symposium,* no 33, Parent-infant interaction, Princeton, NJ, 1975, Excerpta Medica, Associated Scientific Publishers.
39. Klaus M, Kennell J: *Parent-infant bonding,* St Louis, 1982, Mosby.
40. Klaus M, Kennell J: Parent to infant bonding: setting the record straight, *J Pediatr* 102:575, 1983.
41. Lamb M: Early contact and maternal-infant bonding: one decade later, *Pediatrics* 70:763, 1982.
42. Lawrence RA: Practices and attitudes toward breast-feeding among medical professionals, *Pediatrics* 70:912, 1982.
43. Lawrence RA: Practices and attitudes toward breastfeeding among medical professionals: a decade after the Surgeon General's Workshop, in press.
44. Lawrence RA: Unpublished data, 1996.
45. Leifer M: Psychological changes accompanying pregnancy and motherhood, *Genet Psychol Monogr* 95:57, 1977.
46. Lerner H: Early origins of envy and devaluation of women: implications for sex role stereotypes, *Bull Menninger Clin* 38:538, 1974.
47. Lilburne AM, Oates RK, Thompson S et al: Infant feeding in Sydney: a survey of mothers who bottlefeed, *Aust Paediatr J* 24:49, 1988.
48. Maekawa K, Nara T, Hoash E: Influence of breastfeeding on neonatal behavior, *Acta Paediatr Jpn* 27:608, 1985.
49. McAdams D: *Power, intimacy, and the life story: personological inquiries into identity,* New York, 1988, Guilford.
50. Michelsson K, Christensson K, Rothgänger H et al: Crying in separated and non-separated newborns: sound spectrographic analysis, *Acta Paediatr* 85:471, 1996.
51. Mobbs EJG: Human imprinting and breastfeeding: are the textbooks deficient? In Llewellyn-Jones D, Abraham S, editors: *Proceedings 16th Annual Congress, Australian Society for Psychosomatic Aspects of Reproductive Medicine,* Pokolbin, South Wales, March 1989.
52. Modahl C, Newton N: Mood state differences between breast and bottle feeding mothers. In Carenza L, Zinchella L, editors: Emotion and reproduction, *Proc Serano Symp* 20B:819, 1979.
53. Modrey BK, Hatton GI: Maternal behaviors: evidence that they feed back to alter brain morphology and function, *Acta Paediatr Suppl* 397:29, 1994.
54. Montague A: *Touching,* New York, 1986, Harper Row.
55. Morrow-Tlucak M, Haude RH, Ernhart CB: Breastfeeding and cognitive development in the first two years of life, *Soc Sci Med* 26:635, 1988.
56. Newton N: Psychologic differences between breast and bottle feeding. In Jelliffe DB, Jelliffe EFR, editors: Symposium: the uniqueness of human milk, *Am J Clin Nutr* 24:993, 1971.
57. Newton N, Newton M: Psychologic aspects of lactation, *N Engl J Med* 277:1179, 1967.
58. Nordstrom UL, Dallas JH, Morton HG et al: Mothering problems and child morbidity amongst "mothers with emotional disturbances," *Acta Obstet Gynecol Scand* 67:155, 1988.
59. Parke RD, O'Leary S, West S: Mother-father-newborn interaction: effects of maternal medication, labor and sex of infants, *J Perspect Soc Psychol* 23:243, 1972.

60. Pascoe JM, French J: The development of positive feelings in primiparous mothers toward their normal newborns: a descriptive study, *Am J Dis Child* 142:382, 1988 (abstract).

61. Passman RH, Halonen JS: A developmental survey of young children's attachments to inanimate objects, *J Genet Psychol* 134:165, 1979.

62. Pedersen CA, Prange AJ: Induction of maternal behavior in virgin rats after intracerebroventricular administration of oxytocin, *Proc Natl Acad Sci USA* 76:6661, 1979.

63. Quandt SA: Patterns of variation in breastfeeding behaviors, *Soc Sci Med* 23:445, 1986.

64. Raphael D: *The tender gift: breastfeeding,* New York, 1976, Schocken.

65. Richards MPM: Breast feeding and the mother-infant relationship, *Acta Paediatr Scand Suppl* 299:33, 1982.

66. Richards MPM: Bonding babies, *Arch Dis Child* 60:293, 1985.

67. Righard L, Alade MO: Effect of delivery room routines on success of first breast-feed, *Lancet* 336:1105, 1990.

68. Robson KM, Kumar R: Delayed onset of maternal affection after childbirth, *Br J Psychiatry* 136:347, 1980.

69. Rosenblatt JS: Nonhormonal basis of maternal behavior in the rat, *Science* 156:1512, 1967.

70. Siegel E: Early and extended maternal-infant contact, *Am J Dis Child* 136:251, 1982.

71. Simpson-Herbert M: Breast feeding and body contact, *Populi* 7:17, 1980.

72. Sosa R, Kennell JH, Klaus M: The effect of early mother-infant contact on breast feeding: infection and growth. In *Ciba Foundation Symposium,* no 45, Breast feeding and the mother, Amsterdam, 1976, Elsevier Scientific.

73. Spitz RA: An inquiry into the psychiatric conditions in early childhood, *Psychoanal Study Child* 1:53, 1945.

74. Stein A, Fairburn C: Children of mothers with bulimia nervosa, *Br Med J* 299:777, 1989.

75. Thoman EB, Wetzel A, Levine S: Lactation prevents disruption of temperature regulation and suppresses adrenocortical activity in rats. Part A, *Community Behav Biol* 2:165, 1968.

76. Timmerman G: A concept analysis of intimacy, *Issues Ment Health Nurs* 12:19, 1991.

77. Ueda T, Yokoyama Y, Irahara M et al: Influence of psychological stress on suckling-induced pulsatile oxytocin release, *Obstet Gynecol* 84:259, 1994.

78. Van Esterik P: Breastfeeding and Feminism International, *Gynecol Obstet* 47(suppl):541, 1994.

79. Virden SF: The relationship between infant feeding method and maternal role adjustment, *J Nurse Midwifery* 33:31, 1988.

80. Waletzky LR: Husband's problems with breast feeding, *Am J Orthopsychiatry* 49:349, 1979.

81. Whiting JWM: Causes and consequences of the amount of body contact between mother and infant. In Munroe RL, Munroe RD, Whiting BB, editors: *Handbook of cross-culture human development,* New York, 1980, Garland.

82. Wiesenfeld AR, Malatesta CZ, Whitman PB et al: Psycho-physiological response of breast and bottle-feeding mothers to their infant's signals, *Psychophysiology* 22:79, 1985.

83. Yalom M: *A history of the breast,* New York, 1997, Knopf.

7

$\mathcal{M}$aking an informed decision about infant feeding*

BENEFITS OF BREASTFEEDING FOR INFANT

In any statement about breastfeeding and breast milk (human milk), it is important first to establish breast milk's distinct and irreplaceable value to the human infant.

Species specificity

Breast milk is more than just good nutrition. Human breast milk is specific for the needs of the human infant, just as the milk of thousands of other mammalian species is specifically designed for their offspring.

Nutritional benefits

The unique composition of breast milk provides the ideal nutrients for human brain growth in the first year of life. Cholesterol, desoxyhexanoic acid, and taurine are particularly important. Cholesterol is part of the fat globule membrane and is present

in about equal amounts in both cow's milk and breast milk. Maternal dietary intake of cholesterol has no impact on breast milk's cholesterol content. The cholesterol in cow's milk, however, has been removed in infant formulas. These elements are readily available from breast milk, and the essential nutrients in breast milk are readily available via the infant's bloodstream from the mother's.

The bioavailability of essential nutrients, including the microminerals, means that digestion and absorption are highly efficient. Comparison of the biochemical percentages of breast milk and infant formula fails to reflect the bioavailability and utilization of constituents in breast milk compared with modified cow's milk, from which only a small fraction of some nutrients is absorbed.

Nourishment with breast milk is a combination event, in which nutrient-to-nutrient interaction is significant. The process of mixing isolated single nutrients in formula does not guarantee the nutrient or nonnutrient benefits that result from breastfeeding. The composition of human milk is a delicate balance of macronutrients and micronutrients, each in the proper proportion to enhance absorption. Ligands bind to some micronutrients to enhance their absorption. Enzymes also contribute to the digestion and absorption of all nutrients.

---

*Taken in part from Lawrence RA: A review of medical benefits and contraindications to breastfeeding in the United States. In *Maternal and Child Health Technical Information Bulletin,* Arlington, Va, 1997, National Center for Education in Maternal and Child Health.

An excellent example of balance is the action of lactoferrin, which binds iron to make it unavailable for *Escherichia coli,* which depends on iron for growth. When the iron is bound, *E. coli* cannot flourish and the normal flora of the newborn gut, *Lactobacillus bifidus (Bifidobacterium bifidum),* can thrive. In addition, the small amount of iron in human milk is almost totally absorbed, whereas only about 10% of the iron in formula is absorbed by the infant. Examples of multiple functions of proteins in human milk include preventing infection and inflammation, promoting growth, transporting microminerals, catalyzing reactions, and synthesizing nutrients.[81]

Infection protection

Leukocytes, specific antibodies, and other antimicrobial factors protect the breastfed infant against many common infections. Protection against gastrointestinal infections is well documented.[15] Protection against infections of the upper and lower respiratory system and the urinary tract is less recognized, although those infections lead to more emergency room visits, hospitalizations, treatments with antibiotics, and health care costs for the infant who is not breastfed.[2,4]

The incidence of acute lower respiratory infections in infants has been evaluated in a number of studies examining the relationship between respiratory infections and breastfeeding or formula feeding in these infants.[5,66,84] These studies confirm that breastfed infants are less likely to be hospitalized for respiratory infection and, if hospitalized, are less seriously ill. In a study of infant deaths from infectious disease in Brazil, the risk of death from diarrhea was 14 times more frequent in the formula-fed infant, and the risk of death from respiratory illness was four times more frequent.[4,84] The association of wheezing and allergy with infant-feeding patterns has also shown a significant advantage to breastfeeding. In a report from a 7-year prospective study in South Wales, the advantage of breastfeeding persisted to age 7 years in nonatopic infants, and in at-risk infants

who were breastfed the risk of wheezing was 50% lower (after accounting for employment status, passive smoking, and overcrowding).[9] Breastfeeding is thought to confer long-term protection against respiratory infection as well.

For decades, growth in infancy had been measured according to data collected on infants who were exclusively formula fed, until the publication of data on the growth curves of infants who were exclusively breastfed.[7] The physiologic growth curves of breastfed infants show a pattern similar to that of formula-fed infants at the 50th percentile, with significantly fewer breastfed infants in the 90th percentile. This is most evident in the examination of the z scores, which indicate that formula-fed infants are heavier compared with breastfed infants.[10,19,20]

Upper and lower respiratory tract infections have been evaluated in case-control studies, cohort-based studies, and mortality studies in both clinic and hospitalized children in many countries of the developed world.[15,18,27,47] The results all show clearly that breastfeeding has a protective effect, especially in the first 6 months of life. A randomized controlled trial indicated that withholding cow's milk and giving soy milk provided no such protective effect.[9] The incidence of acute otitis media in formula-fed infants is dramatically higher than in breastfed infants,[1,3] not only because of the protective constituents of human milk but also because of the process of suckling at the breast, which protects the inner ear.[47] When an infant feeds by bottle, the eustachian tube does not close, and formula and secretions are regurgitated up the tubes. Child care exposure increases the risk of otitis media, and bottle feeding amplifies this risk.[13,47]

Immunologic protection

In addition to the protection provided by breastfeeding against acute infections, epidemiologic studies have revealed a reduced incidence of childhood lymphoma,[18] childhood-onset insulin-dependent diabetes,[85] and Crohn's disease[44] in infants who have been exclusively breastfed for at least 4 months, compared with formula-fed infants.

Allergy prophylaxis

Breastfed infants at high risk for developing allergic symptoms such as eczema and asthma by 2 years of age show a reduced incidence and severity of symptoms in early life.[9] Some studies suggest the protective effect continues through childhood.[9,25,43]

Psychologic and cognitive benefits

Newton[63] noted that children who had been breastfed were more mature, secure, and assertive, and they progressed further on the developmental scale than nonbreastfed children. More recently, studies by Lucas et al[51] and other investigators[35] have found that premature infants who received breast milk provided by tube feeding were more advanced developmentally at 18 months and at 7 to 8 years of age than those of comparable gestational age and birthweight who had received formula by tube. Such observations suggest that breast milk has a significant impact on the growth of the central nervous system. This is further supported by studies of visual activity in premature infants who were fed breast milk compared with those who were fed infant formula.[60] When similar studies were performed in term infants, visual acuity developed more rapidly in the breastfed infants.[37] Even when docosahexaenoic acid (DHA) was added to formula, the performance by the breastfed infants was still better.[36]

An 18-year longitudinal study reported by Horwood and Fergusson[31] demonstrates a small but detectable increase in childhood cognitive and educational achievement in infants who were breastfed. The effects were confirmed in a range of measures, including standardized tests, teacher ratings, and academic outcomes in high school and young adulthood. More than 1000 children in New Zealand participated. Children who were breastfed for 8 months or longer had a mean test score at age 18 that was 0.11 to 0.30 standard deviation (SD) units higher than those not breastfed.

BENEFITS OF BREASTFEEDING FOR MOTHER

Breastfeeding may provide the mother with several benefits, including reduced risk of ovarian cancer and premenopausal breast cancer.[10,52,77]

Postpartum recovery

Women who breastfeed return to prepregnancy state more promptly than women who do not, and they have a lower incidence of obesity in later life[68,81] (Box 7-1).

Empowerment

In addition to clinically proven medical benefits, breastfeeding empowers a woman to do something special for her infant.[79] The relationship of a mother with her suckling infant is considered to be the strongest of human bonds. Holding the infant to the mother's breast to provide total nutrition and nurturing creates an even more profound and psychological experience than carrying the fetus in utero.

BOX 7-1   Benefits of breastfeeding

Infant
- Species specificity
- Nutritional advantages
- Infection protection
- Immunologic protection
- Allergy prophylaxis
- Psychologic benefits

Mother
- Postpartum recovery
- Psychologic benefits, empowerment
- Improved health risks

In studies of young women enrolled in the Women, Infants, and Children (WIC) program in Kentucky who were randomly assigned to breastfeed or not to breastfeed and who were provided with a counselor/support person throughout the first year postpartum, the women who breastfed changed their behavior.[8,26] They developed self-esteem and assertiveness, became more outgoing, and interacted more maturely with their infants than did the women assigned to formula feeding. The women who breastfed turned their lives around by completing school, obtaining employment, and providing for their infants.

Decreased risk of osteoporosis

The risk of osteoporosis in later life is greatest for women who have never borne infants, somewhat less for those who have borne infants, and measurably less for those who have borne and breastfed infants.[39,40] The bone mineral loss experienced during pregnancy and lactation is temporary. Bone mineral density returns to normal following pregnancy and even following extended lactation when mineral density may exceed the original baseline.[39] Serum calcium and phosphorus concentrations are greater in lactating than in nonlactating women. Lactation stimulates the greatest increases in fractional calcium absorption and serum calcitriol after weaning.[40] Postweaning concentrations of parathyroid hormone are significantly higher than in other stages, and urinary calcium is significantly lower.[14]

Protection against ovarian cancer

There is general agreement that a woman's increasing number of pregnancies, increasing length of oral contraceptive use, and increasing duration of lactation are protective against ovarian cancer.[89] When the relationship between lactation and epithelial ovarian cancer was studied from a multinational database, short-term lactation was as effective as long-term lactation in decreasing the incidence of ovarian cancer in developed countries

where ovulation suppression may be less prolonged in relation to lactation.[70] In a study of black women, who are known to have a lower incidence of ovarian cancer, breastfeeding for 6 months or longer, as well as four or more pregnancies and oral contraceptive use, further reduced the incidence of ovarian cancer.[34]

Siskind et al[76] studied the modifying effect of menopausal status on the association between lactation and risk of ovarian cancer in 824 cancer patients and 855 community control subjects. No association was noted in women whose cancer occurred postmenopausally; however, breastfeeding was somewhat protective against ovarian cancer before menopause.

Reduced incidence of breast cancer

A mother with a new diagnosis of breast cancer should not nurse her infant in the interest of having definitive treatment immediately, because prolactin levels remain very high during lactation, and the role of prolactin in the advancement of mammary cancer is still in dispute.[30] Although endogenous prolactin by itself may not be a risk factor, it could, along with sex steroids, contribute to the acceleration of malignant growth.[82] All lumps in the lactating breast are not cancer and are not even benign tumors. The lactating breast is lumpy, and the "lumps" shift day by day. If a mass is located and the physician thinks it should be biopsied, this can be done under local anesthesia without weaning the infant.

University of Rochester (New York) surgeons have performed many such procedures following referrals in the past 35 years without postoperative complications. The diagnosis of a benign mass was made in almost all cases. Immediate surgery relieved tremendous anxiety without unnecessarily sacrificing breastfeeding. With noninvasive mammary imaging techniques such as ultrasound, computed tomography (CT) scanning, and magnetic resonance imaging (MRI), careful diagnosis can be carried out without interfering with lactation and without delaying diagnosis.

Relationship to breastfeeding

Is cancer more or less common in women who breastfeed? The answer is not easy to find, but in countries where breastfeeding is common, breast cancer is uncommon. In the United States the incidence of breast cancer has steadily risen while the frequency of breastfeeding has declined. It has been suggested that nursing protects a woman against breast cancer. This concept has been investigated in many international studies.[52] Breastfeeding does not predispose a woman to cancer and may protect her.[24]

A case-controlled study of 453 white females with breast cancer and 1365 white females without breast cancer from upstate New York showed an inverse relationship between length of breastfeeding and incidence of breast cancer in premenopausal women that has not been seen in postmenopausal women.[10] The authors found this apparent protective effect persisted throughout the childbearing years, with statistical control for age, parity, age at first pregnancy, age of menarche, and education. The women with cancer had had a higher incidence of lactation failure caused by "insufficient milk." The authors[10] suggest that the significance of this study may be that women who are unsuccessful at lactation are at increased risk for cancer rather than that breastfeeding is protective.

Kalache et al[38] studied 707 married women ages 16 to 50 years with breast cancer in eight teaching hospitals in Oxford and London. Data were collected on duration of breastfeeding of each child and on detailed medical information on study patients and 707 controls. They found no correlation between breastfeeding and cancer. The combination of low parity and late age at first birth was associated with a sevenfold increase in risk of breast cancer at ages 66 to 80 in a study by Lubin et al[50] of more than 1400 women in Canada. At all ages, the authors found an increased cancer risk associated with relative infertility, benign breast disease, and not breastfeeding.

Marriage has been established as a negative risk factor for breast cancer. Mortality rates for most causes of death are higher among single women than among ever-married women.[33]

The statistics associating pregnancy and breast cancer influence the picture. In an epidemiologic study, the risk of breast cancer had a linear relationship to the time interval between puberty and childbirth.[28] The risk was reduced by one third for women who bear their first child before 18 years of age compared with those women who have their first baby when they are older. The risk of breast cancer for women who become pregnant before age 20 was about half that of those who first become pregnant after 25 years of age. Births after the first full-term pregnancy did not influence the statistics. Women whose first pregnancy appeared after 30 to 35 years of age had a risk of breast cancer four times that of nulliparous women in the same age group.[86]

The incidence of breast cancer is low among groups who had nursed their infants, including lower economic groups, foreign-born groups, and those in sparsely populated areas.[52,56] The frequency of breast cancer in mothers and sisters of a woman with breast cancer is two to three times that expected by chance. This could be genetic or environmental. Cancer actually is equally common on both sides of the family of an affected woman. If breast milk were the cause, it should be transmitted from mother to daughter. When mother-daughter incidence of cancer was studied, no relationship was found to breastfeeding.

Unilateral breastfeeding (limited to the right breast) is a custom of Tanka women of the fishing villages of Hong Kong. Ing et al[32] investigated the question, *Does the unsuckled breast have an altered risk of cancer?* They studied breast cancer data from 1958 to 1975. Breast cancer occurred equally in the left and the right breast. Comparison of patients who had nursed unilaterally with nulliparous patients and with patients who had borne children but not breastfed indicated a highly significantly increased risk of cancer in the unsuckled breast. The authors conclude that in postmenopausal women who have breastfed unilaterally, the risk of cancer is significantly higher in the unsuckled breast. They believe that breastfeeding may help protect the suckled breast against cancer.[32]

Other authors[45] have suggested that Tanka women are ethnically a separate people and that it is possible that left-sided breast cancer is related to their genetic pool and not to their breastfeeding habits. No mention has been made of other possible influences, for instance, the impact of their role as "fishermen" or any inherent trauma to the left breast.[65]

In 1926, Lane-Claypon[46] stated that the breast that had never lactated was more liable to become cancerous. Nulliparity and absence of breastfeeding had been considered important risk factors for breast cancer. MacMahon et al[52] reported in 1970 that age at first full-term pregnancy was the compelling factor, with younger women at less risk.

Papaioannou,[65] in a collective review of the etiologic factors in cancer of the breast in humans, concludes, "Genetic factors, viruses, hormones, psychogenic stress, diet and other possible factors, probably in that order of importance, contribute to some extent to the development of cancer of the breast."

Wing[90] concluded in her 1977 review on human milk and health that "in view of the complete absence of any studies showing a relationship between breastfeeding and increased risk of breast cancer, the presence of viruslike particles in breast milk should not be a contraindication to breastfeeding." Henderson et al[28] made a similar statement in 1979, whereas Vorherr[86] concluded in 1979 that the roles of pregnancy and lactation in the development and prognosis of breast cancer had not been determined.

Gradually, studies have appeared challenging the dogma. Brinton et al,[7] McTiernan and Thomas,[55] and Layde et al[49] all showed the clearly protective effects of breastfeeding. Another example is a study conducted to clarify whether lactation has a protective role against breast cancer in an Asian people, regardless of confounding effects of age at first pregnancy, parity, and closely related factors.[94] In a hospital-based case-control study of 521 women with breast cancer and 521 women without breast cancer, statistical adjust-

ment for potential confounders and a likelihood ratio test for linear trend were done by unconditional logistic regression. Total months of lactation regardless of parity was the discriminator. Regardless of age of first pregnancy and parity, lactation had an independent protective effect against breast cancer in Japanese women.[94] Although breast cancer incidence is influenced by genetics, stress, hormones, and pregnancy, clearly breastfeeding has a protective effect. "There is a reduction in the risk of breast cancer among premenopausal women who have lactated. No reduction in the risk of breast cancer occurred among postmenopausal women with a history of lactation," according to Newcombe et al,[61] reporting a multicentered study in 1993.

Two large prospective studies[45,56] did not report a protective effect of breastfeeding. Populations of 50,274 and 89,887 identified 2130 and 459 breast cancer patients. The odds ratios indicate 1.01 (0.98 to 1.05) and 0.95 (0.86 to 1.06), respectively. As with most studies of this nature, the cancers are well defined but not the breastfeeding. No attempt was made to note exclusivity and associated amenorrhea. The studies obtained breastfeeding histories when the women were over 45 years old.

The concern for exposure to estrogen early in life has been part of breast cancer assessment. In utero exposure to estrogen is greater in twin pregnancies and when the mother is older. Estrogen levels in smokers, however, are lower. Weiss et al[88] analyzed cancer risk in a population-based case-control study in the United States (2202 with breast cancer and 2009 control subjects under 55 years of age). Twins were at greater risk than singletons, but no association with maternal age at delivery was found. A reduced breast cancer risk was seen among women who had themselves been breastfed as infants.

In an effort to understand the relationship between breastfeeding and breast cancer, Newton[62] points out that over the past two centuries, women have changed from being pregnant or lactating 60% of the time between menarche and menopause to fewer pregnancies and shorter lactation periods. Thus the amount of time a woman lives with unopposed estrogen (the proliferative phase of the menstrual cycle) was 15% in 1800 and 45% in 1996. Case-control epidemiologic studies consistently show a protective effect (Table 7-1). The most important predictors may be duration of the amenorrheal/hypoestrogenic state and the exposure to breast milk as an infant, according to Newton.[62]

Radiation therapy to breast

Ionizing radiation is carcinogenic to female mammary tissue. Women in Hiroshima and Nagasaki and those subjected to therapeutic radiation for mastitis were followed for many years.[75] The risk of cancer is 3.2 times greater in irradiated breasts, increasing over time after the irradiation. A linear relationship to radiation dose also exists.

In the late 1940s and early 1950s, radiation of the breast was performed as a treatment for mastitis. Although this approach seems irrational today, no antibiotics were readily available at that time, and women were hospitalized for mastitis. Sulfa drugs were not identified until the 1940s and penicillin shortly thereafter. The compounds were only used for life-threatening diseases. The effect of radiation on the infected breast was to clear the mastitis dramatically, stop lactation overnight, and seemingly solve the problem. The mother would continue to nurse on the other breast. The long-term follow-up of these women reveals a high incidence of cancer in the radiated breast.[75]

Radiation usually causes destruction to lobules, condensation of the cytoplasm in cells lining the ducts, and fibrosis. Successful lactation following radiation for carcinoma has been reported in a 36-year-old woman with one previous pregnancy and lactation experience 6 years previously.[16]

Protective effect of being breastfed

Davis[18] first reported the reduction of childhood-onset cancers in children who have been exclusively breastfed for at least 4 months.

The fear of cancer in the breastfed female offspring of a woman with breast cancer does not justify avoiding breastfeeding. Breastfed women have the same breast cancer experience as non-breastfed women, and no increase occurs in benign tumors. Daughters of breast cancer patients have an increased risk of developing benign and malignant tumors by merit of their heredity, not their breastfeeding history.[57,58]

The critical question remains: does being breastfed increase any child's risk of developing breast cancer, especially in female offspring? This haunting question, first posed by an experimental scientist, created tremendous publicity and genuine

TABLE 7-1	Breast cancer and lactation		
		Likelihood of breast cancer	
Study	Population	Odds ratio	(95th confidence interval)
Michels et al[56]	All	0.93	(0.83-1.03)
	BF* >2 yrs	1.11	(0.90-1.38)
Katsouyanni et al[42]	Premenopausal, BF >2 yr	0.53	(0.23-1.41)
Romieu et al[69]	All	0.39	(0.25-0.62)
Brinton et al[7]	BF >2 wk	0.87	(0.7-1.0)
Yang et al[93]	Premenopausal, failed to BF	3.0	(1.6-5.4)
Yoo et al[94]	All	0.62	(0.37-1.04)
	Premenopausal, BF >7 mo	0.39	(0.15-0.97)

Newton ER Jr: *Acad Breastfeed Med News Views* 2(2):1, 1996.
*Breastfeed

concern among physicians queried by patients. One needs to explore the available data.[73]

No documented evidence indicates that women with breast cancer have ribonucleic acid (RNA) of tumor virus in their milk. No correlation between RNA-directed deoxyribonucleic acid (DNA) polymerase activity has been found in women with a family history of breast cancer. RNA-directed DNA polymerase activity, a reverse transcriptase, is a normal feature of the lactating breast.[12,22,71,72]

CONTRAINDICATIONS TO BREASTFEEDING

In reviewing the contraindications to breastfeeding, it is important to look at the entities that put the mother or infant at significant risk and are not remedial. Contraindications are medical; the disadvantages tend to be social. The physician needs to have a clear understanding of the benefits of breastfeeding to measure the risks for a particular mother-infant dyad. The risk/benefit ratio can only be determined by the clinician in a position to weigh all the data, usually the pediatrician for the infant or the obstetrician for the mother or the family physician.

Infectious diseases

In general, acute infectious diseases in the mother are not a contraindication to breastfeeding, if such diseases can be readily controlled and treated.[13] In most cases the mother develops the infection during breastfeeding. By the time the diagnosis has been made, the infant has already been exposed, and the best management is to continue breastfeeding so that the infant will receive the mother's antibodies and other host resistance factors in breast milk.[74] This is true for respiratory infections such as the common cold. Infections of the urinary tract or other specific closed systems such as the reproductive tract or gastrointestinal tract do not pose a risk for excreting the virus or bacteria in the breast milk unless there is generalized septicemia. When the offending organism is especially

virulent or contagious (as with β-hemolytic streptococcus, group A), both mother and infant should be treated, but breastfeeding is not contraindicated[13,48] (Table 7-2).

Many agents in breast milk protect against infection, and their presence is not affected by nutritional status. Protection against infection is important in the United States, especially among infants exposed to multiple caregivers, child care outside the home, compromised environments, and less attention to the spread of organisms.[27] One of the most important and thoroughly studied agents in breast milk is secretory immunoglobulin (sIg, specifically, IgA), which is present in high concentrations in colostrum and early breast milk and in lower concentrations throughout lactation, when the volume of milk is increased.[27] Secretory IgA antibodies may neutralize viruses, bacteria, or their toxins and are capable of activating the alternate complement pathway.[13] The normal flora of the intestinal tract of the breastfed infant, as well as the offspring of all other mammalian species studied until weaning, is bifidobacteria or lactobacilli.[27] These bacteria further inhibit the growth of bacterial pathogens by producing organic acids. This is in striking contrast to the formula-fed infant, who has comparatively little bifidobacteria and many coliforms and enterococci. In addition, although the attack rates of certain infections are similar in breastfed and formula-fed infants in the same community, the manifestations of the infections are much less evident in the infants who are breastfed. This appears to result from antiinflammatory agents in breast milk.[48]

A few specific infectious diseases are capable of overwhelming the protective mechanisms of breast milk and breastfeeding[13,48] (see also Chapter 16).

Human immunodeficiency virus and acquired immunodeficiency syndrome

Clinically effective treatments for human immunodeficiency virus (HIV) and acquired immunodeficiency syndrome (AIDS) are still being developed; therefore any behavior, including breastfeeding, that increases the risk of transmitting the virus from mother to infant should be avoided in the

Problem	Breastfeeding	Conditions
Infectious diseases		
Acute infectious disease	Yes	Respiratory, reproductive, gastrointestinal infections
HIV	No	HIV positive in developed countries
Active tuberculosis	Yes	After mother has received 2 or more weeks of treatment
Hepatitis		
A	Yes	As soon as mother receives gamma globulin
B	Yes	After infant receives HBIG, first dose of hepatitis B vaccine should be given before hospital discharge
C	Yes	If no co-infections (e.g., HIV)
Venereal warts	Yes	
Herpesviruses		
Cytomegalovirus	Yes	
Herpes simplex	Yes	Except if lesion on breast
Varicella-zoster (chickenpox)	Yes	As soon as mother becomes noninfectious
Epstein-Barr	Yes	
Toxoplasmosis	Yes	
Mastitis	Yes	
Lyme disease	Yes	As soon as mother initiates treatment
HTLV-I	No	
Over-the-counter/prescription drugs and street drugs *(see Chapter 11)*		
Antimetabolites	No	
Radiopharmaceuticals		
Diagnostic dose	Yes	After radioactive compound has cleared mother's plasma
Therapeutic dose	No	
Drugs of abuse	No	Exceptions: cigarettes, alcohol
Other medications	Yes	Drug-by-drug assessment
Environmental contaminants		
Herbicides	Usually	Exposure unlikely (except workers heavily exposed to dioxins)
Pesticides		
DDT, DDE	Usually	Exposure unlikely
PCBs, PBBs	Usually	Levels in milk very low
Cyclodiene pesticides	Usually	Exposure unlikely
Heavy metals		
Lead	Yes	Unless maternal level ≥40 mg/dl
Mercury	Yes	Unless mother symptomatic and levels measurable in breast milk
Cadmium	Usually	Exposure unlikely
Radionuclides	Yes	Risk greater to bottle-fed infants

TABLE 7-2   Summary of medical contraindications to breastfeeding*

Modified from Lawrence RA: A review of the medical benefits and contraindications to breastfeeding in the United States. In *Maternal and Child Health Technical Information Bulletin,* Arlington, Va, 1997, National Center for Education in Maternal and Child Health.
*This table provides a brief summary. Each situation must be decided individually. Contraindications are rare.

United States. Even though the value of being breastfed is great, failure to breastfeed does not result in a large increase in mortality among U.S. infants. Not all infants born to U.S. HIV-infected mothers are infected at birth, but present laboratory techniques require several months to identify the newborn who has HIV.

In reviewing the role of breastfeeding in HIV infection, the following major issues continue to elude definitive answer[17]:

1. The risk of vertical transmission of HIV through breastfeeding
2. The effect of breastfeeding on HIV-infected infants
3. The effect of breastfeeding on noninfected infants of HIV-infected women
4. The effect of lactation on HIV-infected women
5. The effect of zidovudine (AZT) on transmission of HIV through breastfeeding

Advances in treatment during the perinatal period may provide the solution in the next decade. If medication can control viral shedding, breastfeeding with all its benefits may be available to the infants of HIV-infected women receiving treatment.

Studies and reports about HIV infection in the perinatal period continue to accumulate, but its association with breastfeeding is still unclear. In the United States the position of the Centers for Disease Control and Prevention (CDC) with regard to HIV-positive mothers is not to breastfeed. The World Health Organization (WHO) states that, in developing countries or areas where the risk of infant mortality from infection is great, breastfeeding is recommended even in the event of maternal AIDS.[92] This position is undergoing review and investigation, which may support or change the current recommendation. Where the risk of mortality from other infections is not great, mothers with HIV should be counseled on alternatives to breastfeeding.

Women with known AIDS who want their infant to receive human milk have two alternatives: (1) pump their own milk and have it pasteurized at a local milk bank or hospital, or (2) if that is not feasible, obtain milk from a breast milk bank, where milk is donated by screened mothers and then pasteurized.

Embryopathy associated with human T-cell lymphotropic virus type III has been described to include growth failure, microcephaly, hypertelorism, prominent forehead, flat nasal bridge, obliquity of the eyes, long palpebral fissures, blue sclerae, and patulous lips.[53] These findings are similar to those described in fetal alcohol syndrome. The greater the dysmorphism, the sooner clinical manifestations of the disease seem to appear.

About 50% of mothers of infants with congenital manifestations are still asymptomatic at birth but almost always positive for HIV antibodies. For women who are seropositive at delivery, 30% to 60% of their infants will develop AIDS or AIDS-related complex (ARC). The virus can be acquired in utero, from infected blood during delivery, or postnatally. Cesarean birth does not appear to change the rate in high-risk pregnancies. Of children under age 13 years with a parent with AIDS or a mother in the high-risk group, 80% will develop the disease. The incubation period for perinatally acquired AIDS is 6 to 8 months, compared to 28 months in adolescents and adults.

HIV has been isolated from blood, semen, vaginal secretions, saliva, tears, cerebrospinal fluid, amniotic fluid, urine, and breast milk. Only blood, semen, vaginal secretions, and possibly breast milk have been implicated in person-to-person transmission.[78] Careful study has not revealed nonsexual spread in households.

The first case of breastfeeding-associated disease was reported by Ziegler et al[95] in 1985, and attention became sharply focused on the potential of spread to infants through mothers' milk. A healthy mother delivered by emergency cesarean birth because of placenta previa and fetal distress, with a blood loss of 1500 ml. Fifteen minutes after the delivery, a two-unit transfusion was begun. The next day she received two more units. The donor of one unit was identified 13 months later as having antibody to AIDS-related virus. The infant was healthy and was successfully breastfed for 6 weeks. At 3 months of age the infant developed atopy and failure to thrive. When tested at 13 months, mother and infant had antibody to AIDS virus and later generalized adenopathy. The father and siblings tested negative.

Additional cases of AIDS in breastfeeding infants whose mothers were not at risk but received contaminated blood at delivery have been reported.[9,89]

Thoughtful consideration regarding perinatal transmission of AIDS has led the CDC and the Public Health Service to recommend that women who test positive for HIV antibody in the United States should be counseled to avoid breastfeeding to avoid postnatal transmission to a child who may not be infected.[13,83] In countries where the risk of death in the first year is 50% from diarrhea and other disease (exclusive of AIDS), breastfeeding is still the feeding of choice. Breastfeeding should be encouraged in developing countries even when the mother has hepatitis or AIDS.

As in any other clinical situation, the pediatrician and obstetrician should review all the available data in the case and facilitate the mother's (parents') informed decision in light of current clinical information and medical options.

Besides AIDS and HTLV-I, no other infection is an absolute contraindication to breastfeeding (Table 7-2). Management of other infectious diseases while breastfeeding is detailed in Chapter 16.

Human T-cell leukemia virus type I

The incidence of human T-cell leukemia virus type I (HTLV-I) has reached endemic proportions in parts of the West Indies, Africa, and southwestern Japan.[29,41,59,91]

Although HTLV-I is not increasing in the United States, trends may change. At present it is recommended in the United States that the mother with HTLV-I disease should not breastfeed.[11]

Life-threatening illnesses

Life-threatening or debilitating illness in the mother may necessitate avoiding lactation.[4] This is a clinical judgment that should be made with the mother and father, with all facts presented. Although one woman may be able to overcome all obstacles and prove she can nurse her baby, it does not necessarily mean that another patient with the same diagnosis can.[6] If the mother wants some lay reading on the subject, the clinician should be familiar with available material so any apparent inconsistencies of opinion can be discussed.

Over-the-counter/prescription drugs and street drugs
Medications

Much concern and anxiety have been expressed regarding the question of medications taken by lactating women and the risk to the suckling infant. In reality, very few drugs are contraindicated during breastfeeding.[48] Each situation should be evaluated on a case-by-case basis by the physician. The important factors include the pharmacokinetics of the drug in the maternal system and the absorption, metabolism, distribution, storage, and excretion in the recipient infant. Variables to consider in the decision include gestational age, chronologic age, body weight, breastfeeding pattern, and other dietary practices. Ultimately, the decision is made by assessing the risk/benefit ratio (i.e., the risk of a small amount of the drug compared with the tremendous benefit of being breastfed).

See Chapter 11 for a full discussion of drugs, medications, and environmental toxins. The contraindications are few but include radioactive medications, antimetabolites, and street drugs (Table 7-2) and Appendix D.

Drug abuse

Breastfeeding is contraindicated in women who are intravenous (IV) drug abusers.[81] The possibility of the infant receiving substantial amounts of drug through the milk is real; deaths have been reported in the recipient neonate. IV drug abusers have high incidences of hepatitis, HTLV-I/II, or HIV, which may be transmitted to the breastfed infant from the infected mother (see Chapter 11 and Appendix D for specific drugs of abuse).

DISADVANTAGES OF BREASTFEEDING

Disadvantages to breastfeeding are those factors perceived by the mother as an inconvenience to her, because no known disadvantages exist for the normal infant. (In the rare circumstance of galactosemia in the neonate, which involves an inability to tolerate lactose, breastfeeding is contraindicated [see Chapter 14]). In cultures where nursing in public is commonplace, nursing is not considered inconvenient because the infant and the feeding are always available.

The mother's commitment to the infant for 6 to 12 feedings a day for months may be overwhelming to a woman who has been free and independent. Motherhood itself changes a woman's lifestyle.

Guilt from failure, shame, and other anxieties are of considerable concern. Surveys evaluating the decline of breastfeeding have revealed that mothers describe feelings of shame, modesty, embarrassment, and distaste. These feelings are more common in lower social groups. Research on wider sociologic and psychologic factors regarding the feelings and attitudes toward breastfeeding can have considerable influence on the choice to breastfeed and will be helpful in dealing with these issues.

As the incidence and duration of breastfeeding increase and professionals and lay people alike are caught up in the rush to convert all parents and change all hospital routines and recommendations, a sense of balance must be maintained. It is necessary to appreciate that there are normal women who cannot or will not nurse their babies. Their babies will survive and grow normally. The sharp letter by Fisher[23] brings this to focus when she describes the frustrations and disappointments of others and dispels what she calls the myths about breastfeeding.

The popular press has drawn attention to parenting trends that divide responsibility for the infant equally between mother and father after the birth.[52] This, of course, necessitates some bottle feeding. The justification is division of labor and equal opportunity for both parents to do good things for the baby. This is probably another way of expressing breast envy and jealousy. Some husbands are jealous because they have no similar way to bring food and contentment to their infant, according to Waletzky.[87] "A certain manliness was required to foster breastfeeding in one's family when society as a whole was hostile to it," according to Pittenger and Pittenger.[67] They point out that the perinatal period is a breeding ground for marital and parental maladjustment.

Many writers, on the other hand, have described participation in childbirth as a potentially beneficial experience for men. The father's feelings are useful during labor and delivery. These experiences contribute to heightened self-concepts and better adjustments to roles as husband and father. The quality of the birth experience has been cited as the major determinant of paternal attachment. Paternal attachment has led to a greater pride in breastfeeding and a more secure, self-confident support person for the mother who is breastfeeding.

Perinatal counseling of prospective new parents may anticipate these reactions, and in turn the professional will have an opportunity to facilitate the best experience possible.

REFERENCES

1. Alho OP, Koivu M, Sorri M et al: Risk factors for recurrent acute otitis media and respiratory infection in infancy, *Int J Pediatr Otorhinolaryngol* 19:151, 1990.
2. Ando Y, Saito K, Nakano S et al: Bottle feeding can prevent transmission of HTLV-1 from mothers to their babies, *J Infect* 19:25, 1989.
3. Aniansson G, Alm B, Andersson B et al: A prospective cohort study on breastfeeding and otitis media in Swedish infants, *Pediatr Infect Dis J* 13:183, 1994.
4. Berger LR: When should one discourage breastfeeding? *Pediatrics* 67:300, 1981.
5. Beudry M, Dufour R, Marcoux S: Relation between infant feeding and infections during the first six months of life, *J Pediatr* 126:191, 1995.
6. Brewster DP: *You can breast feed your baby . . . even in special situations,* Emmaus, Pa, 1979, Rodale.
7. Brinton LA, Potischman NA, Swanson CA et al: Breastfeeding and breast cancer risk, *Cancer Causes Control* 6:199, 1995.

8. Bryant CA: Overcoming breastfeeding barriers. Presented at US Department of Health and Human Services Region IV nutrition conference, Building Support Networks for Breastfeeding, Atlanta, 1986.
9. Burr ML, Limb ES, Maguire MJ et al: Infant feeding, wheezing, and allergy: a prospective study, *Arch Dis Child* 68:724, 1993.
10. Byers T, Graham S, Rzepka T et al: Lactation and breast cancer, *Am J Epidemiol* 121:664, 1985.
11. Centers for Disease Control and Prevention, US Public Health Service Working Group: Recommendations for counseling persons infected with human T-lymphotropic virus, types I and II, *MMWR* 42(RR-9):1, 1993.
12. Chopra H, Ebert P, Woodside N et al: Electron microscopic detection of Simian-type virus particles in human milk, *Nature N Biol* 243:159, 1973.
13. Committee on Infectious Diseases, American Academy of Pediatrics: *Report of the Committee on Infectious Diseases,* ed 24, Elk Grove Village, Ill, 1997, American Academy of Pediatrics.
14. Cross NA, Hillman LS, Allen SH et al: Calcium homeostasis and bone postweaning: a longitudinal study, *Am J Clin Nutr* 61:514, 1995.
15. Cunningham AS, Jelliffe DB, Jelliffe EFP: Breast-feeding and health in the 1980s: a global epidemiologic review, *J Pediatr* 118:659, 1991.
16. David FC: Lactation following primary radiation therapy for carcinoma of the breast, *Int J Radiat Oncol Biol Phys* 11:1425, 1985.
17. Davis MK: Human milk and HIV infection: epidemiologic and laboratory data. In Mestecky J et al, editors: *Immunology of milk and the neonate,* New York, 1991, Plenum.
18. Davis MK: Review of the evidence for an association between infant feeding and childhood cancer. In International Union Against Cancer (UICC, WHO) Workshop: *Nutritional morbidity in children with cancer: mechanisms, measures and management* (in press).
19. Dewey KG, Heinig MJ, Nommsen LA et al: Growth of breast-fed and formula-fed infants from 0 to 18 months: the DARLING Study, *Pediatrics* 89(6, pt 1):1035, 1992.
20. Dewey KG, Peerson JM, Brown KH et al: Growth of breastfed infants deviates from current reference data: a pooled analysis of US, Canadian, and European data sets, World Health Organization Working Group on Infant Growth, *Pediatrics* 96(3, pt 1):495, 1995.
21. Enger JM, Ross RK, Henderson B et al: Breastfeeding history, pregnancy experience and risk of breast cancer, *Br J Cancer* 76:118, 1997.
22. Fieldsteel AH: Nonspecific antiviral substances in human milk active against arbovirus and murine leukemia virus, *Cancer Res* 34:712, 1974.
23. Fisher PJ: Breast or bottle: a personal choice, *Pediatrics* 72:435, 1983 (letter).
24. Fraumeni JF, Miller RW: Breast cancer from breast feeding, *Lancet* 2:1196, 1971.
25. Gruskay FL: Comparison of breast, cow and soy feedings in the prevention of onset of allergic disease: a 15-year prospective study, *Clin Pediatr* 21:486, 1982.
26. Gussler JD, Bryant CA, editors: *Helping mothers to breastfeed: program strategies for minority communities,* Lexington, Ky, 1984, Nutrition and Health Education division, Lexington-Fayette County Health Department.
27. Hanson LA, Adlerberth I, Carlsson B et al: Host defense of the neonate and the intestinal flora, *Acta Paediatr Scand* 351(suppl):122, 1989.
28. Henderson BE, Powell D, Rosario I et al: An epidemiologic study of breast cancer, *J Natl Cancer Inst* 53:609, 1974.
29. Hino S: Milk-borne transmission of HTLV-I as a major route in the endemic cycle, *Acta Paediatr Jpn* 31:428, 1989.
30. Hornstein E, Skornick Y, Rozin R: The management of breast carcinoma in pregnancy and lactation, *J Surg Oncol* 21:179, 1982.
31. Horwood LJ, Fergusson DM: Breastfeeding and later cognitive and academic outcomes, *Pediatrics* 101:e9, 1998 (electronic article).
32. Ing R, Ho JHC, Petrakis NL: Unilateral breast feeding and breast cancer, *Lancet* 2:124, 1977.
33. Janerich DT, Hoff MB: Evidence for a crossover in breast cancer risk factors, *Am J Epidemiol* 116:737, 1982.
34. John EM, Whittemore AS, Harris R et al: Characteristics relating to ovarian cancer risk: collaborative analysis of seven US case-control studies—epithelial ovarian cancer in black women, Collaborative Ovarian Cancer Group, *J Natl Cancer Inst* 85:142, 1993.
35. Johnson DL, Swank PR, Howie VM et al: Breastfeeding and children's intelligence, *Psychol Rep* 79:1179, 1996.
36. Jonsbo F, Jorgensen MH, Michaelsen KF: The importance of n-3 and n-6 fatty acids for visual function and development in newborn infants, *Ugeskrift Laeger* 157:1987, 1995.
37. Jorgensen MH, Hernell O, Lund P et al: Visual acuity and erythrocyte docosahexaenoic acid status in breast-fed and formula-fed term infants during the first four months of life, *Lipids* 31:99, 1996.
38. Kalache A, Vessey MP, McPherson K: Lactation and breast cancer, *Br Med J* 1:223, 1980.
39. Kalkwarf HJ, Specker BL: Bone mineral loss during lactation and recovery after weaning, *Obstet Gynecol* 86:26, 1995.
40. Kalkwarf HJ, Specker BL, Heubi JE et al: Intestinal calcium absorption of women during lactation and after weaning, *Am J Clin Nutr* 63:526, 1996.
41. Kaplan JE, Abrams E, Shaffer N et al: Low risk of mother-to-child transmission of human T lymphotropic virus type II in non-breastfed infants, *J Infect Dis* 166:892, 1992.
42. Katsouyanni K, Lipworth L, Trichopoulou A et al: A case-control study of lactation and cancer of the breast, *Br J Cancer* 73:814, 1996.

43. Kern RA: Prophylaxis in allergy, *Ann Intern Med* 12:1175, 1939.

44. Koletzko S, Sherman P, Corey M et al: Role of infant feeding practices in development of Crohn's disease in childhood, *Br Med J* 298:1617, 1989.

45. Kvale G, Heuch I: Lactation and cancer risk: is there a relation specific to breast cancer? *J Epidemiol Community Health* 42:30, 1987.

46. Lane-Claypon JE: A further report on cancer of the breast, with special reference to its associated antecedent conditions, *Report No. 32,* London, England, Reports of the Ministry of Health, 1926.

47. Lawrence R: The clinician's role in teaching proper infant feeding techniques, *J Pediatr* 126:S112, 1995.

48. Lawrence RA: A review of the medical benefits and contraindications to breastfeeding in the United States. In *Maternal and Child Health Technical Information Bulletin,* Arlington, Va, 1997, National Center for Education in Maternal and Child Health.

49. Layde PM, Webster LA, Baughman AL et al: The independent associations of parity, age at first full term pregnancy, and duration of breastfeeding with risk of breast cancer, *J Clin Epidemiol* 42:963, 1989.

50. Lubin JH, Burns PE, Blot WJ et al: Risk factors for breast cancer in women in northern Alberta, Canada, as related to age at diagnosis, *J Natl Cancer Inst* 68:211, 1982.

51. Lucas A, Morley R, Cole TJ et al: Breast milk and subsequent intelligence quotient in children born preterm, *Lancet* 339:261, 1992.

52. MacMahon B, Lin TM, Lowe CR et al: Lactation and cancer of the breast: a summary of an international study, *Bull World Health Organ* 42:185, 1970.

53. Marion RW, Wiznia AA, Hutcheon RG et al: Human T-cell lymphotropic virus type III (HTLV-III) embryopathy, *Am J Dis Child* 140:638, 1986.

54. McManus IC: Predominance of left-sided breast tumours, *Lancet* 2:297, 1977.

55. McTiernan A, Thomas DB: Evidence for a protective effect of lactation on risk of breast cancer in young women: results from a case-control study, *Am J Epidemiol* 124:353, 1986.

56. Michels KB, Willet WC, Rosner BA: Prospective assessment of breastfeeding and breast cancer incidences among 89,887 women, *Lancet* 347:431, 1996.

57. Miller RW, Fraumeni JF: Does breast feeding increase the child's risk of breast cancer? *Pediatrics* 49:645, 1972.

58. Morgan RW, Vakil DV, Chipman ML: Breast feeding, family history, and breast disease, *Am J Epidemiol* 99:117, 1974.

59. Nakano S, Ando Y, Ichijo M et al: Search for possible routes of vertical and horizontal transmission of adult T-cell leukemia virus, *Gann* 75:1044, 1984.

60. Neuringer M, Reisbick S, Janowsky J: The role of n-3 fatty acids in visual and cognitive development: current evidence and methods of assessment, *J Pediatr* 125:S39, 1994.

61. Newcombe PA, Storer BE, Longnecker MP: Lactation and a reduced risk of premenopausal breast cancer, *N Engl J Med* 330:81, 1994.

62. Newton ER Jr: Does breastfeeding protect women from breast cancer? *ABM News Views* 2(2):1, 1996.

63. Newton N: Psychological differences between breast and bottle feeding, *Am J Clin Nutr* 24:993, 1971.

64. Ory H, Cole P, MacMahon B et al: Oral contraceptives and reduced risk of benign breast diseases, *N Engl J Med* 294:419, 1976.

65. Papaioannou AN: Etiologic factors in cancer of the breast in humans: collective review, *Surg Gynecol Obstet* 138:257, 1974.

66. Pisacane A, Graziano L, Zona G et al: Breast feeding and acute lower respiratory infection, *Acta Paediatr* 83:714, 1994.

67. Pittenger JE, Pittenger JG: The perinatal period: breeding ground for marital and parental maladjustment, *Keeping Abreast J* 2:18, 1977.

68. Rebuffe-Scrive M, Enk L, Crona N et al: Fat cell metabolism in different regions in women: effect of menstrual cycle, pregnancy, and lactation, *J Clin Invest* 75:1973, 1985.

69. Romieu I, Hernandez-Avila M, Lazcano E et al: Breast cancer and lactation history in Mexican women, *Am J Epidemiol* 143:543, 1996.

70. Rosenblatt KA, Thomas DB: Lactation and the risk of epithelial ovarian cancer, The WHO Collaborative Study of Neoplasia and Steroid Contraceptives, *Int J Epidemiol* 22:192, 1993.

71. Roy-Burman P, Rongey RW, Henderson BE et al: Attempts to detect RNA tumour virus in human milk, *Nature N Biol* 244:146, 1973.

72. Sanner T: Removal of inhibitors against RNA-directed DNA polymerase activity in human milk, *Cancer Res* 36:405, 1976.

73. Sarkar NH, Charney J, Doion AS et al: Effect of human milk on mouse mammary tumor virus, *Cancer Res* 33:626, 1973.

74. Schreiner RL, Coates T, Shackelford PG: Possible breast milk transmission of group B streptococcal infection, *J Pediatr* 91:159, 1977 (letter).

75. Shore RE, Hildreth N, Woodard E et al: Breast cancer among women given x-ray therapy for acute postpartum mastitis, *J Natl Cancer Inst* 77:689, 1986.

76. Siskind V, Green A, Cain C et al: Breastfeeding, menopause, and epithelial ovarian cancer in young women, *Epidemiology* 8:188, 1997.

77. Sowers MF, Corton G, Shapiro B et al: Changes in bone density with lactation, *JAMA* 269:3130, 1993.

78. Stiehm ER, Vink P: Transmission of human immunodeficiency virus infection by breastfeeding, *J Pediatr* 118:410, 1991.

79. Stone E: A feminist fad? *Ms* 11(8):68, 1983.

80. Stuver SO, Hsieh C-C, Bertone E et al: The association between lactation and breast cancer in an international case-control study: a re-analysis by menopausal status, *Int J Cancer* 71:166, 1997.

81. Subcommittee on Nutrition During Lactation, Food and Nutrition Board, Institute of Medicine, National Academy of Sciences, Washington, DC, 1991, National Academy Press.

82. Thomas MR, Kawamoto J: Dietary evaluation of lactating women with or without vitamin and mineral supplementation, *J Am Diet Assoc* 74:669, 1979.

83. U.S. Public Health Service recommendations for human immunodeficiency virus counseling and voluntary testing for pregnant women, *MMWR* 44:(RR-7):1, 1995.

84. Victora CG, Smith PG, Vaughan JP et al: Evidence for protection by breastfeeding against infant deaths from infectious diseases in Brazil, *Lancet* 2(8554):319, 1987.

85. Virtanen SM, Räsänen L, Aro A et al: Infant feeding in Finnish children less than 7 years of age with newly diagnosed IDDM, Childhood Diabetes in Finland Study Group, *Diabetes Care* 14:415, 1991.

86. Vorherr H: Pregnancy and lactation in relation to breast cancer risk, *Semin Perinatol* 3:299, 1979.

87. Waletzky LR: Husbands' problems with breastfeeding, *Am J Orthopsychiatry* 49:349, 1979.

88. Weiss HA, Potischman NA, Brinton LA et al: Prenatal and perinatal risk factors for breast cancer in young women, *Epidemiology* 8:181, 1997.

89. Whittemore AS: Characteristics relating to ovarian cancer risk: implications for prevention and detection, *Gynecol Oncol* 55(3, pt 2):S15, 1994.

90. Wing JP: Human versus cow's milk in infant nutrition and health: update 1977, *Curr Probl Pediatr* 8(1):entire issue, 1977.

91. Wong-Staal F, Gallo RC: Human T-lymphocyte retroviruses, *Nature* 312:395, 1985.

92. World Health Organization/United National Children's Fund: *HIV and breastfeeding consensus statement,* May 1992, Geneva, Switzerland.

93. Yang CP, Weiss NS, Band PR et al: History of lactation and breast cancer risk, *Am J Epidemiol* 138:1050, 1993.

94. Yoo K-Y, Tajima K, Kuroishi T et al: Independent protective effect of lactation against breast cancer: a case-control study in Japan, *Am J Epidemiol* 135:726, 1992.

95. Ziegler JB, Cooper DA, Johnson RO et al: Postnatal transmission of AIDS-associated retrovirus from mother to infant, *Lancet* 1:896, 1985.

$\mathcal{M}$anagement of the mother-infant nursing couple

Successful nursing depends on the successful association of mother and infant, with appropriate support from the father, the family, and available medical resources. Because both mothers and infants vary, no simple set of rules in hospitals can be outlined to guarantee success. In fact, one of the difficulties has been that a rigid system was established for initiating lactation that did not fit all mother-infant couples. Furthermore, physicians do not receive formal education about breastfeeding; thus they resort to gaining information from a variety of sources and assume that this is the correct way to approach the situation.

Nowhere in medicine do one's personal interests or prejudices become more evident than in the area of counseling about childbirth and breastfeeding. Having a child does not make one an expert on the subject. Conversely, not having a child does not preclude the development of exceptional skills. Some of the world's most revered experts in human lactation have neither had a child nor nursed an infant, but they have brought to the situation the eye of a skilled observer unencumbered by emotional bias and personal prejudices and the experience of a broadly trained clinician.

Historically, rigid dogmas have directed management of lactation. In the effort to replace these with what was perceived as more rational management, new dogmas have arisen. Once there was a paucity of literature, now there is a deluge from all sources. The very careful art and science of breastfeeding are being lost in the rage of righteousness. The clinician must be careful in choosing to use the guidelines used in any other phase of medical and health care. No rules exist for breastfeeding. The clinician must adapt the recommendations to the individual patient and her circumstances.[186]

It is not ordinarily the physician's role to teach the mother how to breastfeed. Instead, all the nursing staff who interact in the perinatal period, including obstetric office nursing, labor/delivery, nursery, postpartum, birth center, and pediatric office personnel, as well as midwives, have job descriptions that include hands-on assistance for the mother in the process of breastfeeding. The physician does, however, need to understand anatomy and physiology and the basics of breastfeeding to recognize problems and their solutions. This chapter addresses the basic breastfeeding process. It is not a "how-to" manual for mothers, but the physician should be familiar with one or two good sources of information to suggest for patients, such as K. Huggins', *The Nursing Mother's Companion,* or *The Womanly Art of Breastfeeding* from La Leche League International (see Appendix K for organizations providing materials).

The references for this chapter are not an exhaustive list of all material written on the topic; rather, they are intended to assist the reader in locating research that supports the concepts described here.

The key to the management of the mother-infant nursing couple is establishing a sense of confidence in the mother and supporting her with simple answers to her questions when they arise. Good counseling also depends on understanding the science of lactation. Then, when a problem arises, a mechanism already is in place for the mother to receive help from her physician's office before the problem creates a serious medical complication.

THE SCIENCE OF SUCKLING

The ability to lactate is characteristic of all mammals, from the most primitive to the most advanced. The divergence of suckling patterns, however, makes it urgent that human patterns be studied specifically.[19] Some aquatic mammals such as whales nurse under water; others such as the seal and sea lion nurse on land. A variety of erect or recumbent postures are assumed by different terrestrial mammals.[34] Nursing may be continuous, as in the joey attached to a marsupial teat, or at widely different intervals characteristic of the species. The interval may be a half hour in the dolphin, an hour in the pig, a day in the rabbit, 2 days in the treeshrew, or a week in the northern fur seal.

Although many anatomic distinctions exist as well, the principal mechanism of milk removal common to all mammals is the contractile response of the mammary myoepithelium under the hormonal influence of oxytocin released from the neurohypophysis.[176]

The key function in all species is effective control of milk delivery to the young in the right amount and at the appropriate intervals, which requires a storage system, exit channels, a prehensile appendage, an expulsion mechanism, and a retention mechanism. The primary, secondary, and tertiary ducts form an uninterrupted channel for the passage of milk from the milk-producing alveoli to the mammary sinuses. A process of erection of the areolar region facilitates prehension by the young

during suckling. The principal object of the suction produced by the facial musculature of the young is to draw the nipple into the mouth and retain it there. Positive pressure is used to expel milk from the gland by the contractile changes in the mammary gland provided by the myoepithelial cells (see Fig. 3-7). The sympathetic nervous stimuli can oppose milk ejection by increasing vasoconstrictor tone, thereby reducing access of circulating oxytocin to the mammary myoepithelium. Sympathetic activity also can occur during conditions of apprehension or muscular exertion. The milk-ejection reflex can be blocked by emotional disturbance or reflex excitation of the neurohypophysis. The central nervous system control of milk ejection indeed suggests that restraining mechanisms exist to ensure that milk ejection can only occur under circumstances wholly conducive to the effective removal of milk by the suckling young.

In all species that have been studied, a rise in intramammary pressure and flow of milk occur as a reflex event in suckling. The excitation of the neurohypophysis results in the release of oxytocin, which is conveyed via the bloodstream to mammary capillaries, where it evokes contraction of the myoepithelium.[31] The successive ejection pressure-peaks, demonstrated in lactating women, can be duplicated more accurately by a series of separate oxytocin injections than by the same total dose as a single injection or by a continuous infusion of the hormone. This strongly suggests that oxytocin is released from the neurohypophysis in spurts. The study of suckling patterns in all species shows a high degree of ritualization, which in turn suggests a close neural connection between cognitive or behavioral and hormonal responses.

Attention has focused on the mechanisms that control suckling behavior, on its incidence, on events that precipitate and terminate it, on the effects of stress, and on how development modifies it. Suckling is characteristic of each species and is vital for survival. *Suckling* means to take nourishment at the breast and specifically refers to "breastfeeding" in all species. *Sucking* on the other hand, means to draw into the mouth by means of a partial vacuum, which is the process employed when bottle feeding. Sucking also means to consume by licking.

Although suckling has been studied in the young and the mother in other species, much human data have been collected using a rubber nipple and bottle. Other mammals suck only in the nutritive mode, whether receiving milk from the nipple or not. Human infants were noted to have two distinct patterns with rubber nipples: a nutritive mode and a nonnutritive mode.[177,178] When this work was repeated using the breastfeeding model, there was no difference between nutritive and nonnutritive suckling rates but rather a continuous variation of suckling rate in response to milk-flow rate.[20] Suckling rates in other species correlate with milk composition and species-specific feeding schedules (one suck per second in great apes and four to five sucks per second in sheep and goats).

In further experiments, a linear relationship was found between milk flow and suckling rate. Thus the higher the milk flow, the lower is the suckling rate. In human infants younger than 12 weeks of age, suckling will terminate with sleep and be reinstated on awakening, a pattern that is well described in other species.[19] In infants older than 12 weeks, suckling is not terminated by sleep.[3] At 12 to 24 weeks, infants will play with the nipple and explore the mother and not always elicit nipple attachment. Continuous measurement of milk intake during a given feeding from one breast showed a progressive reduction in intake volume per suck and an increase in the proportion of time spent pausing between bursts of sucking.

Using the miniature Doppler ultrasound flow transducer, Woolridge et al[181,184] have studied 32 normal mother-baby pairs from 5 to 9 days postpartum. Intakes during trials averaged 34.2 g ($\pm$3.7 g) on the first breast and 26.2 g ($\pm$3.5 g) on the second breast. At the start of feeds the average suck volume was about 0.14 ml/suck, which decreased to about 0.10 ml/suck or less. The mean latency for release of milk was 2.2 minutes after the infant began to suckle. The researchers also noted that on the first breast the flow increased and

stabilized after 2 minutes, with concomitant slowing and stabilizing of sucking pattern over the remainder of the feed. On the second breast the suck volume fell off dramatically toward the end of the feed (50% reduction from peak to end of feed) (Fig. 8-19).

These observations support the theory that infants become satiated at the breast and milk remains unconsumed in the breast. Over the first month of life, infants consume a given amount of fluid with decreasing investment of time.[181] The amount of fluid per suck increases over time. The control of intake appears to come under intrinsic control of the infant during the first month of life.[126]

When sucking was studied using a multisensor nipple for recording oral variables, such as lip and tongue movements and fluid flow, it was observed that fluid flow begins as the intranipple pressure decreases and tapers off as the intranipple pressure increases.[23] One flow pattern is seen in each sucking movement.

The development of the sucking response in the normal newborn with a rubber nipple transducer in a nonnutritive mode has been reported immediately after birth.[8] Pressure exerted immediately was 5 mm Hg at birth, peaking at 103 mm Hg at 90 minutes. Infants less than 24 hours old demonstrate a significantly different sucking pattern than a 3-day-old infant. The younger infants' duration of burst was longer (3.7 versus 2.8 seconds), frequency was lower in amplitude (1.7 versus 2.0 hertz), and the variability was greater. These evaluations were carried out in breastfeeding infants with a pacifier with a transducer and no nutrient reward.[56] No data are available on optimal pressures or on pressures developed with immediate breastfeeding.

The movement of the lips and tongue have been more difficult to study. A cineradiographic study of breastfeeding was done by Ardran et al[11] in 1957 and compared with a similar study of bottle feeding.[12] The nipples and areolae of 41 breastfeeding mothers were coated with a paste of barium sulfate in lanolin, and cineradiographic films were taken with the infant at breast. These were then reviewed meticulously. Box 8-1 lists the authors' conclusions in their original description. These observations are of historic interest, but newer techniques in imagery have corrected the understanding of human suckling.

In a similar study of bottle feeding by Ardran et al,[11] cineradiographic films were taken of infants, lambs, and kid goats, taking a mixture of milk and barium from a bottle. In the 1950s, when Ardran et al[11,12] made their landmark studies of bottle feeding, the rubber nipples used were different in size, shape, and consistency, so some of their observations may not pertain to present equipment. They concluded that gravity was key to the operation and that infants are not able to suck and swallow while taking a breath.

The development of real-time ultrasound improved the definition of images. Several studies have been published using this noninvasive technique to observe the action of the infant's tongue and buccal mucosa and the maternal nipple areola. Using a videorecorder that allowed frame-by-frame analysis and recorded simultaneous respiration, the pattern of suck, swallow, and breathing was documented over a period of active suckling at the breast. A *suck* was defined by Weber et al[170] as the beginning of one indentation of the nipple by the tongue to the beginning of the next. Weber et al had examined six breastfed and six bottle-fed infants between 1 and 6 days of life. Not all sucks were associated with a swallow. Box 8-2 summarizes the process.

Observations of suckling using newer techniques over time from 2 to 26 weeks showed that suckling starts with a series of fast sucking movements and then stabilizes. In a 2-week-old breastfeeding infant, sucking and breathing pattern proportions alternated smoothly at about two sucks to one breath, with swallowing occurring with every suckle. Bottle-feeding patterns were variable and sometimes asynchronous with sucking and breathing.

The process of suckling has been described as a pulsating process similar to peristalsis along the rest of the gastrointestinal tract. This undulating motion, as described by cineradiography, did not

---

BOX 8-1   Radiographic interpretation of suckling at the breast

1. The nipple is sucked to the back of the baby's mouth and a teat is formed from the mother's breast.
2. When the jaw is raised this teat is compressed between the upper gum and the tip of the tongue resting on the lower gum. The tongue is applied to the lower surface of the teat from before backwards, pressing it against the hard palate: the teat is reduced to approximately half its former width. As the tongue moves toward the posterior edge of the hard palate the teat shortens and becomes thicker.
3. When the jaw is lowered the teat is again sucked to the back of the mouth and restored to its previous size.
4. Each cycle of jaw and tongue movement takes place in approximately 1.5 seconds. The pharyngeal cavity becomes airless and the larynx closes every time the upward movement of the tongue against the teat and hard palate is completed.
5. The teat is formed from the nipple and the adjacent areola and underlying tissues.

From Ardran GM, Kemp FH, Lind J: *Br J Radiol* 31:156, 1958.

BOX 8-2   Ultrasound interpretation of suckling at the breast

1. The lateral margins of the tongue cup around the nipple, creating a central trough.
2. The suck is initiated by the tip of the tongue against the nipple followed by pressure from the lower gum.
3. There is peristaltic action of the tongue toward the back of the mouth.
4. The tongue elevation continues to move the bolus of milk into the pharynx.

Modified from Weber F, Woolridge MW, Baum JD: *Dev Med Child Neurol* 28:19, 1986.

involve stroking or friction, as was clearly pointed out by Woolridge.[179,184] The nipple should not move in and out of the infant's mouth if the breast is positioned correctly. The tip of the tongue does not move along the nipple. The positive pressure of the tongue against the teat (areola and nipple), coupled with ejection of the milk from increased intraductal pressure, evacuates the milk, not suction. The negative pressure created in the mouth holds the nipple and breast in place and reduces the "work" to refill the ampullae and ducts. Visual observations and videotapes made in our laboratory to study suckling show the undulating motion of the external buccal surfaces even in newborns. Ultrasound confirms the molding of buccal mucosa and tongue around the teat, leaving no space.

In breastfeeding the tongue action is a "roll-ing," or peristaltic, action from the tip of the tongue to the base. In the bottle feeder the tongue action is more pistonlike or squeezing. When resting between sucks, the human nipple is indented by the tongue, and the latex teat is expanded in the bottle fed (Figs. 8-1 and 8-11).

The change in nipple dimensions during suckling is detailed by Smith et al,[149,150] who also used ultrasound and examined 16 term infants ages 60 to 120 days and their mothers. They demonstrated that the human nipple is highly elastic and elongates during active feeding, including about 2 cm of areola, to form a teat approximately twice its resting length. They also showed that the infant's cheeks (buccal membranes) with their thick layer of fatty tissue, known as *sucking fat pads,* act to make a passive seal to create a vacuum (as

Fig. 8-1. Ultrasound of infant at breast. Still picture of ultrasound scan frame from videorecording. Scanner head is at bottom, with a sector view of 90 degrees. Below is artist's impression of image showing key features. Image is seen best when tilted through 45 degrees, so that infant's head is vertical. Picture corresponds to point in sucking cycle when maximum point of compression of nipple by tongue has almost reached tip of nipple. Once nipple has become fully expanded, fresh cycle of compression will be initiated at base of nipple and will then move back. (From Weber F, Woolridge MW, Baum JD: *Dev Med Child Neurol* 28:19, 1986.)

opposed to the concept that the cheeks are sucked in by the negative pressure). Milk ejection was noted to occur after maximal compression of the nipple.

Although the firm texture of the latex teat was more difficult for the infant to compress, Weber et al[170] did not observe any practical differences between breast and bottle sucking. Softer latex nipples do not readily reexpand and so do not solve the suckling problem. Ultrasound as a study tool will continue to clarify sucking patterns in neonates and can also be useful as a diagnostic tool in presumed sucking disorders before "suck training or retraining" is considered.

Coordination of suck and swallow

The ability to swallow is developed in utero during the second trimester and has been well demonstrated by fetal ultrasound. Fetal swallowing of amniotic fluid is an important part of the complex regulation of amniotic fluid. The suck is actually part of the oral phase of the swallow. Little was done to examine the role of swallowing on the suckling rate until Burke[25] studied the role of swallowing in the organization of suckling behavior, although with a bottle and solutions of 5% and 10% sucrose solution. The author reported two major observations: "First, the frequency of swallowing in newborns increased significantly as a function of increasing concentration and amount of sucrose solution given per criterion suck. Second, there was a significant difference in the duration of the sucking interresponse times which immediately followed the onset of swallowing and the duration of interresponse times not associated with swallowing." These observations explain those of previous investigators regarding nutritive and nonnutritive sucking.

The coordination of sucking and swallowing was observed by ultrasound by Weber et al[170] as a movement of the larynx. By 4 days of age, both breastfed and bottle-fed infants were swallowing with every suck. Later in the feeding the ratio of sucks to swallows changed to 2:1 or more until sucking stopped. Swallowing occurred in the end-expiratory pause between expiration and inspiration (Fig. 8-1). The change in suck/swallow ratio seemed to be a function of the availability of milk.

Factors influencing sucking

As one manages infants with difficulty feeding, a number of rituals are often initiated to enhance infant behavior. Only a few of these have been evaluated for their effect.[123] The effect of the infant's position, that is, supine or supported upright to a 90-degree angle, was found to have no influence on the sucking pattern or pressure. The effect of temperature, however, was found to be significant. Sucking pressure decreased as environmental temperature increased from 80° to 90° F (26.6° to 32.2° C), which may have application in encouraging an infant to nurse. This effect was shown to increase from the third to the fifth day of life. Higher sucking pressures have been recorded in the morning than in the afternoon.[8]

When the size of latex nipples was studied, the large nipple elicited fewer sucks and a slower sucking rate than smaller nipples, although the volume of milk delivered was the same in this study with all nipple sizes.[30] Although human nipple size cannot be altered, this knowledge may help in assessing the response of a newborn in specific situations. Increasing nipple size and decreasing sucking rate may be significant in considering using an adult finger for finger feeding.

The volume of each swallow was calculated during breastfeeding in 1905 by Süsswein,[154] who counted swallows and made test weighings. His observations have now been confirmed with elaborate electronic equipment.[180] The average swallow of a newborn is 0.6 ml, which is also the exact amount drawn from a bottle equipped with an electromagnetic flowmeter transducer and a valve that responds to negative pressure at each suck in modern studies, even though the sucking mechanism between breast and bottle is different.[144] When a conventional bottle without a valve is used, the volume is reduced to one third, to 0.19 ml/suck. The valve removes the need for the infant to suck against the negative pressure created in the bottle.

This supports the fact that a bottle-fed infant with a poor suck does better with a boat-shaped bottle, in which the distal end is kept open, or with a collapsible bag as a source of milk, such as in the Playtex nurser. The size of the hole in the nipple influences the volume of the suck only in the valved bottle. When breastfed infants were compared with a group fed by cup from birth and a group fed by bottle, the breastfed infants had a stronger suck than either of the other two groups, who did not differ from each other in sucking skill.[34,36]

Lucas et al[93] studied patterns of milk intake using electronic weighings in interrupted feeds. They reported that 50% of a feed from each breast was consumed in 2 minutes and 80% to 90% by 4 minutes, with minimal feeding from each breast in the last 5 minutes. Bottle-fed infants, evaluated with the same technique of test weighings, took 84% of the feeding in the first 4 minutes. Bottle-feeding patterns were linear, whereas the breastfed infant had a biphasic pattern when nursed on both breasts. The total intake of the two types of feeds was similar in volume in the same 25 minutes of total time.

Fat content and suckling

The high concentration of fat in breast milk toward the end of a feed was hypothesized as a satiety signal to terminate the feeding.[57] When this was studied using high- and low-fat formulas, it was found that high-fat milk did not act to cue babies to slow or stop feeding.[40,118,119] In fact, babies appeared to feed more actively on high-fat milk, sucking in longer bursts with less resting. When human milk of low- and high-fat content was fed from bottles, switching the baby from low-fat breast milk to high-fat breast milk, the babies did not alter either milk intake rate or sucking patterns.

To test the hypothesis fully, a study carefully observed infants switching from the first to the second breast and back to the first breast.[40] Infants were 2 months old and well established at exclusive breastfeeding. No significant difference was seen in the time taken to attach to the new breast and the time taken to reattach to the previously suckled breast. Mean milk intake from the first breast was 91.7 g (range 58 to 208 g), higher than that from the second breast (mean 52.5 g, range 8 to 75 g). The mean fat contents before and after nursing on the first breast were 23 g/L and 52 g/L, whereas on the second breast they were 24 g/L and 48 g/L. This shows that infants will nurse when fat content is higher, contrary to the theory that increasing fat causes satiation.[119]

Studies of 3-day-old bottle-fed infants fed sucrose and glucose solutions show that they manifest tongue movements of greater amplitude when fed stronger concentrations of carbohydrate.[118] Sensory apparatus responsible for assessing sweetness is apparently competent in the newborn.

Breathing and suckling while feeding

Breathing and sucking during feeding were addressed by Johnson and Salisbury,[77] who studied normal full-term infants from 1 to 10 days of age, measuring breathing, sucking, and flow of fluid from a feeding bottle with a flowmeter. No infant aspirated water, but 8 of 18 infants inhaled saline. Even from a bottle, breast milk was associated with more regular breathing than was formula feeding. It has been demonstrated in other species that newborns will become apneic when fed milk from species other than their own. The coordination of breathing and swallowing improves with increase in milk availability and with the maturity of the infant, according to Weber et al.[170]

Suckling patterns as indicators of problems or pathology

The behavior of the infant at birth is the first opportunity to observe the infant's adeptness at suckling. In a careful analysis of videotapes of newborns in the first 90 minutes of life, Widström and Thingström-Paulsson[174] observed a consistent pattern. Licking movements preceded and followed the rooting reflex in alert infants. The tongue was placed in the bottom of the mouth cavity during distinct rooting. The authors suggest that forcing the infant to the breast might disturb reflex

TABLE 8-1	**Duration of breastfeeding with different sucking techniques**				
	Exclusively breastfeeding 5 days	Exclusively and partly breastfeeding			
Sucking technique		1 mo	2 mo	3 mo	4 mo
No. (%) incorrect at discharge	25 (100)	16 (64)	12 (48)	11 (44)	10 (40)
No. (%) correct at discharge	57 (100)	55 (96)	48 (84)	45 (79)	42 (74)
p		<0.001	<0.01	<0.01	<0.01

From Righard L, Alade MO: *Birth* 19:185, 1992.

and tongue position. They further observe that a healthy infant should be given the opportunity to show hunger and optimal reflexes and attach to mother's nipple by itself.

Righard and Alade[137] observed that an infant placed on the mother's abdomen will self-attach to the breast and suckle correctly in less than 50 minutes.* They further reported that when the infants were separated from their mothers for delivery room procedures, the initial sucking attempts were disturbed, and many infants were too drowsy to suck at all.[137]

Righard and Alade also investigated the prognostic value of sucking technique (faulty versus correct) during the first week after birth in relation to the long-term success of breastfeeding.[138] Eighty-two healthy mother-infant pairs were observed before discharge for assessment of breastfeeding technique. The authors defined correct sucking as the infant's mouth being wide open, the tongue under the areola, and the milk expressed in slow, deep sucks. Incorrect sucking is defined as infant positioned as if bottle feeding, using the nipple as a teat. The *oral searching reflex* is defined as the infant opening the mouth wide in response to proximity of the nipple to the lips and thrusting the tongue forward in preparation to taking the breast. This reflex is a part of the normal response to circumoral stimulus resulting in rooting by the infant, who comes forward, opens the mouth wide, and extends the tongue when stimulated centrally

on the lower lip and even the upper lip. Stimulus on the side of the mouth elicits turning to that side.

In the study,[138] all the infants were assessed by the same observer before discharge from the hospital. If there was an incorrect suck, the mother-infant pairs were randomly assigned to a no-intervention group or to a group in which mothers received brief instruction on proper positioning. Telephone follow-up occurred at 2 weeks and monthly for 4 months. Switching to bottle was 10 times more common in the nipple-sucking group (9/25 or 36%) than in both the correct and the corrected group (2/57 or 3.5%). Table 8-1 lists the duration of breastfeeding in the various groups. Eighty-eight percent of the nipple-sucking group had further breastfeeding problems, with a high incidence of insufficient milk and sore nipples.[138]

Medications during labor

Newborn infants whose mothers received a single dose of 200 mg secobarbital as obstetric sedation during labor sucked at significantly lower rates and pressures and consumed less nutrient than did infants whose mothers received no medication.[81] The effect persisted for 4 days. Similar effects have been seen in Brazelton's examination.[21] The clinician must be aware of the perinatal history of medication during labor so that early identification of any effect on suckling can be made. The mother of an infant with a poor suck may need some additional stimulus by electric pump to facilitate milk production. The infant may require extra assistance in latching on and obtaining sufficient nourishment the first few days.

*Video available from Geddes Productions, 10546 McViney, Sunland, CA 91040 (818-951-2809).

Epidural anesthesia

Because of repeated concerns about the possible effect of intrapartum epidural anesthesia on the newborn infant's ability to suckle and the rising incidence of epidurals in some hospitals (more than 50% of vaginal deliveries), Rosen and Lawrence[142] investigated 83 mother-infant dyads who either exclusively breastfed or bottle-fed. The infant's ability to nurse at the breast or take the bottle was scored from multiple observations. Weight loss in the first few days was also evaluated. Epidural anesthesia had no apparent effect (although analgesics showed a relationship) on ability to feed or initial weight loss.

The question of duration of epidurals was investigated by Bader et al[15] who found that maternal venous and umbilical venous levels of fentanyl and bupivacaine were relatively constant whether the epidural lasted 1 hour or up to 15 hours. Total doses varied between 27 and 200 mg for bupivacaine and 22 to 300 μg for fentanyl. Significantly, however, bupivacaine was measurable in the umbilical venous sample of the infants $(0.15 \pm 0.06$ μg/ml). The significance of fetal tissue uptake is unclear. Umbilical artery blood gases (ABGs) and neurobehavioral scores were normal. Neonatal urine in another study had small but measurable bupivacaine metabolites 36 hours after delivery when spinal anesthesia was used for cesarean birth. It is noteworthy that usually the infant is delivered within 15 minutes of medication administration for cesearean birth.[82]

The effect on infants of different doses of meperidine given to mothers in labor was clearly demonstrated by Hodgkinson et al[66] in a double-blind comparison of neurobehaviors of 920 neonates. They used the Early Neonatal Neurobehavior Scale (ENNS), which consists of 13 assessments, including general levels of alertness, rooting, and sucking. Meperidine was associated with broad depression of most items on ENNS on both the first and the second day of life, increasing with increasing dosages of 50, 75, and 150 mg. The best scores were achieved by infants whose mothers received chloroprocaine epidural anesthesia without meperidine (280 infants whose mothers

received mean dose of 510 ± 255 mg chloroprocaine over 2.3 ± 1.1 hours; 177 mothers did not receive meperidine, and 81 did). Chloroprocaine is rapidly metabolized, whereas bupivacaine is bound to maternal plasma proteins.

The sucking rhythms of infants with a normal perinatal course were compared with those of infants with perinatal distress. The analysis showed that rhythms of nonnutritive sucking were significantly different from rhythms of normal controls even when there were no gross neurologic signs.[21,85] Subtle difficulties with feeding are sometimes the only perinatal evidence of the impact of hypoxia, as noted by low Apgar scores.

Infants whose mothers received bupivacaine epidural anesthesia were described to be less alert and have less ability to orient over the first month of life. Belfrage et al[17] have reported bupivacaine and its metabolites in the circulation of infants for the first 3 days of life whose mothers had epidural anesthesia. Murray et al[106] reported similar results using the Brazelton scale and mother-infant interaction during feeding and mothers' perception of their infants. Levels of bupivacaine were measurable in the cord blood of all these infants as well, about 100 ng/ml. More recent studies report the use of lower doses of bupivacaine and either fentanyl or sufentanil.[89] Less sufentanil appeared in the cord blood. Measurable effects on the neonate's neurobehavior were seen in the Murray et al study,[106] but not in the study by Bader et al,[15] who observed epidurals of fentanyl and bupivacaine from 1 to 15 hours of infusion and saw no signs of accumulation in the cord blood and no adverse neonatal effects, as measured by umbilical ABGs and neurobehavioral scores.

Only the Rosen and Lawrence study[142] reported the effects of epidural anesthesia on feeding ability of the neonate neonates.

Perioral stimulation

Perioral stimulation facilitated nutritive sucking abilities in high-risk newborns (29 to 30 weeks' gestation), with each subject serving as his or her own control.[85] The stimulation was applied manually with quick touch-pressure stimulus for 1 second over the buccal fat pad. Similar stimulation has been used in children with central nervous system dysfunction in an effort to facilitate better sucking and swallowing. Such studies have not been reported during breastfeeding.[46]

Sucking stimulus and prolactin

When lactating postpartum women nurse their infants, the prolactin level increases from a high baseline level to levels several times mean baseline.[5] When nursing women played with but did not feed their infants, prolactin did not rise despite the initiation of milk dripping. Substitution of a breast pump at regular intervals caused prolactin elevations similar in timing and magnitude to those induced by sucking. When normal, menstruating, nonlactating adult women were stimulated with the breast pump for 30 minutes, significant prolactin increases occurred in 7 of the 18 women. No response was obtained in normal men.

When the prolactin response was used as a measure of "success" in establishing lactation in the first week postpartum, no difference in prolactin levels was seen between women who had been considered good producers and those who were considered poor producers.[69] Mothers whose infants were in the special care unit and who were using a breast pump to establish lactation had minimal prolactin response to pumping but produced a mean of 86 g of milk per pumping. A similar study had been carried out previously, in which different responses in prolactin levels to suckling were found in good, fair, and poor producers.[68] When prolactin levels were measured after use of the breast pump at uniform settings, all three groups were similar.[10] This and the work of others[27,107] suggest that infant suckling plays a significant role in adequate milk production.

Conclusions

Knowledge about infant sucking has been accumulating rapidly, but little of it involves study of suckling at the breast. It has been established that the patterns are different mechanically. At the breast, nutritive and nonnutritive suckling vary only in rate, not in pattern. Infants can suck immediately at birth and tolerate mother's milk (colostrum) best as the pattern of respirations remains physiologic. Inadequate suckling can influence maternal production, but inadequate suckling can be improved.

•   •   •

Management of breastfeeding is best discussed in terms of the three stages: (1) prenatal period, (2) immediate postpartum, or hospital, period, and (3) postnatal, or posthospital, period.

PRENATAL PERIOD

It is most effective to prepare for breastfeeding well in advance of delivery. Prospective parents should consider feeding plans for the infant during the prenatal period, after the pregnancy is well established. Once quickening has occurred, the infant becomes more of a reality for the mother and she can relate to planning. Except in sophisticated cultures, the parents will not initiate this decision-making discussion, and it is appropriately introduced by the obstetrician, family physician, or midwife in the second trimester. Particularly with first children, it is appropriate to suggest to the parents that they select a pediatrician early. They should request a prenatal conference with the pediatrician to discuss not only feeding but also points of management and child rearing about which they might have questions. If the mother is receiving prenatal care from a family practice physician, this step is automatic.

Many studies of infant-feeding choices have been reported in the literature reviewing the reasons women breastfeed. Universally, mothers do it because it is best for the infant. Many decided long before the pregnancy, but those who chose bottle feeding admit they could have been persuaded if only someone had cared enough to tell them how important breastfeeding is to the infant. All women know mother's milk is best. Clearly, health care providers have made breastfeeding too complicated and burdened mothers with so many rules and regulations that they cannot cope and default to bottle feeding. When health care workers try to persuade a woman to breastfeed, they perpetuate the image of an impossible feat by saying, "Why not give it a try? It's not that bad," or "You'll be surprised. It isn't that hard," instead of conveying opportunity and good experience with, "It is a marvelous opportunity for you and your baby," or "It will be a special joy." Employment rarely cuts breastfeeding opportunities short, because it is usually unemployed women who are at home bottle feeding (see Chapter 13). Any time spent breastfeeding is worthwhile for the working mother and her infant.

The medical profession has been hesitant to take anything but a neutral position in discussions of breastfeeding for fear of pressuring the mother.[18] The evidence is stronger than ever that breastfeeding has distinct advantages for the infant and mother. Parents have the right to hear the data. They can make their own choice. Fear of instilling guilt is a poor reason to deprive a mother of an informed choice, especially because women do not feel guilty about their decision. After interviews with hundreds of mothers, half of whom chose to bottle feed, not one felt guilty, but some were disappointed that their physician did not discuss infant feeding.[142]

The prenatal discussion should also include any questions the parents may have about the lactation process and mother's ability to provide adequately for the infant. An examination of the breasts is part of good prenatal care and an excellent opportunity to discuss breastfeeding. If any anatomic abnormalities exist, they should be discussed. The breast tissue should be checked for lumps and cysts that might need treatment. The amount of mammary tissue is not correlated with the ability to produce milk. The more generous gland usually results from a more generous fat pad. During pregnancy the fat is replaced by proliferating acini. A woman with small breasts should not be discouraged from nursing; she may be the mother who most needs to prove herself.

Breast texture should be assessed by palpation. The inelastic breast gives the impression it is firmly knit together and the overlying skin is taut and firm so it cannot be picked up. The elastic breast is looser and the overlying skin free, and the tissue is more easily picked up. Inelastic breasts are more prone to engorgement and seem improved by prepartum massaging and close attention to prevention of engorgement (Fig. 8-2).

 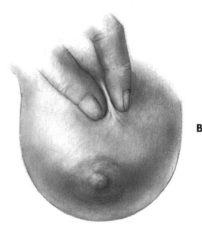

Fig. 8-2. Texture of breast tissue can be assessed by picking up skin of breast. **A,** Inelastic breast tissue. **B,** Elastic breast tissue.

Examination of the areola and nipple is equally important to identify any anatomic problems that may need attention before delivery. Gross malformations and inversion of the nipple can be easily detected, but lesser problems may go unnoticed. One must test for freedom of protrusion. When the areola is compressed and the nipple retracts, it indicates a "tied nipple" or inverted nipple caused by the persistence of fibers from the original invagination of the mammary dimple (Fig. 8-3).

The physician may provide literature on breastfeeding or suggest reading sources for the patient. One should avoid dismissing the parents' questions by merely suggesting appropriate readings because their decision making will be enhanced by open discussion with a knowledgeable professional. Although parents may have access to childbirth preparation programs in the community, they should not be put off to seek all their information from such sources. When parents have no opportunity to discuss with their care provider such issues as early infant contact, nursing the infant in the delivery room, and family-centered maternity care, they often experience tremendous disappointment and misunderstanding.

The concerns most frequently expressed by mothers considering breastfeeding are related to themselves, not the infant. Mothers who are more concerned about their own well-being have more trouble adjusting to motherhood and should be provided with more support in adapting to the role. They may be helped by selecting a doula to support them, because our modern culture tends to isolate the young couple. Raphael describes a doula as one of "those individuals who surround, interact with, and aid the mother at any time within the perinatal period, which includes pregnancy, birth and lactation."[131]

Concerns most frequently expressed prenatally include the following:

1. What is the effect on the figure? Data indicate that the breast is affected by heredity, age, and pregnancy in that order and only minimally by lactation. Women who have never borne children may "lose their figures" long before a multipara who nurses her infants. Pregnancy enlarges breasts temporarily, as does early lactation, but the effect is temporary. Poor diet and lack of exercise will destroy a figure in both the male and the female long before any other influence.

2. What is the effect on the mother's freedom? Obviously, only a mother can breastfeed the infant; however, ample data support that it is

 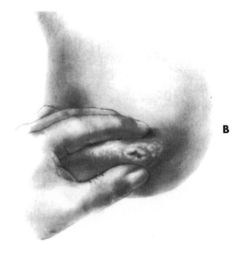

Fig. 8-3. **A,** Normal nipple everts with gentle pressure. **B,** Inverted or tied nipple inverts with gentle pressure.

possible to maintain a career, keep a job, or just get away from the house and still nurse in today's world. Actually, mothers in primitive cultures have returned to the fields or some form of productivity outside the home out of sheer necessity for generations. Mothers concerned about this often are best reassured by their peers, that is, mothers who are nursing. In communities with nursing mother groups, it is a simple referral. Employment statistics have revealed that women do successfully return to the work force and continue breastfeeding. Employment is rarely a reason for not breastfeeding, but it may influence duration.

3. Many women are concerned with exposing the breasts. Despite the constant barrage of publicity about the breast in the modern press, many women are embarrassed to consider baring their breasts. As pointed out in Chapter 6, shame is an important consideration when helping a mother accept breastfeeding. Bentovim[18] suggests that shame and anxieties arise from the influence of one's life history and current events; thus intervention is necessary at many levels. Clothes that make discreet breastfeeding possible are readily available and fashionable. Considerable body exposure is not necessary for breastfeeding. In a public survey performed in the Midwest for Surgeon General Koop in 1985, few people, male or female, in any age group considered breastfeeding embarrassing, and 82% would want their child breastfed. Universal publicity about breastfeeding in public places has created a more accepting attitude in most people, so that a nursing mother no longer needs to go and hide to feed her infant.

Preparation of the breasts

The prenatal period is a time for the couple to prepare for their new role as parents and to learn as much as possible about breastfeeding. Most mothers do no special preparation and are very successful. Carefully controlled studies do not support the contention that fair-skinned women, especially redheads, are more prone to developing cracked,

sore nipples than are others. Mothers who have had trouble with tender, cracked nipples when nursing a previous infant will need extra assistance in putting the infant to breast properly in the first few days, but elaborate rituals prenatally may actually cause problems. Nipple preparation has a negative effect on some women who are not ready to handle their breasts during pregnancy.

Bathing should be as usual, with minimal or no soap directly on the nipples and thorough rinsing. Some recommend patting the nipple dry with a soft towel, but this should not be done except after a shower or bath. Persistent removal of natural oils of the nipple and areola actually predisposes the skin to irritation. Montgomery glands in the areola secrete a sebaceous material for the cleansing and lubrication of the areola and nipple. This should not be removed by soaps or chemicals. Tincture of benzoin, alcohol, and other drying agents are contraindicated because they predispose the nipples to cracking during early lactation. Wearing protective brassieres, modern women do not experience the friction to the nipples that looser clothing provides, which may be why cracked nipples are a common problem. In Scandinavia, it is suggested that the pregnant woman get as much air and sunshine as possible directly on the breasts before delivery. Wearing a nursing brassiere with the flaps down to expose the nipples under loose clothing will serve the same purpose. However, aggressive and abrasive treatment of the nipples does not prevent nipple pain postpartum and may enhance it. Gentle love making involving the breasts is usually safe and is the most effective preparation.[62]

The use of lanolin, which is miscible with water and thus allows normal evaporation from the skin, does no apparent harm but in controlled studies also made no difference prenatally. Women allergic to wool will also be allergic to lanolin. Lanolin has been confirmed to contain insecticide residuals such as DDT and dioxins because sheep are routinely dipped in insecticides before shearing. The preparation Lansinoh is derived from natural lanolin with the contaminants and allergens removed and can be safely used if an ointment is indicated. Use of A and D ointment prophylactically also

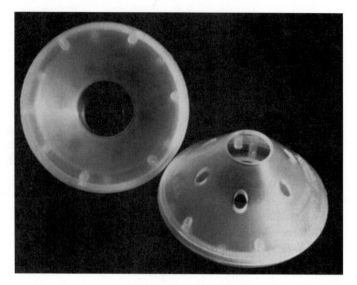

Fig. 8-4. Breast shells: vented domes worn over ring that allows nipple to evert. Shell is slipped into cup of well-fitting brassiere. Available in several styles and designs.

makes no difference, having an effect only in the treatment of fissures later. As with Lansinoh, mothers disliked the odor of this ointment. Petrolatum and other ointments made the skin more macerated and susceptible to irritation. Ointment should not be applied over the end of the nipple and the ducts.[140] It may also clog the Montgomery glands. In climates with average to high humidity, ointments are not routinely recommended for the breasts and may interfere with Montgomery gland secretion. In extremely dry climates, using ointments sparingly may be necessary.

Soap, alcohol, and tincture of benzoin have been shown to cause damage to tissue of the areola and nipple.[107]

Some believe gentle traction to the point of discomfort, but not pain, reduces perception of pain in the first week of lactation. A study carefully controlled to eliminate subjective discrepancies of interpretation revealed no significant difference in nipple sensitivity or trauma in those who practiced prenatal nipple rolling, application of breast cream, or expression of colostrum, as compared with those who had untreated breasts.[62] No increased pain or trauma was reported among the fair-skinned participants in this study, treated or untreated. Because many women are not inclined to manipulate their breasts before delivery and might be discouraged

from breastfeeding if it is implied that this must be done, physicians should prescribe treatment only when an indication exists.[178]

Preparation of the nipples

Flat nipples or inverted nipples do not preclude breastfeeding. Flat nipples respond to the same passive treatment with a breast shell that works for inverted nipples. The shells can be worn during the last trimester by women who choose to do so (Figs. 8-4 and 8-5). They should be recommended only after careful examination and discussion about advantages and disadvantages by the physician. Follow-up at subsequent prenatal visits is also appropriate.

Alexander et al[2] estimated that about 10% of pregnant women have inverted or nonprotractile nipples, which are thought to contribute to breastfeeding problems.[2] Breast shells (plastic discs with holes in the center and a domed cover) (Fig. 8-4) and Hoffman exercises (stretching and pulling of the nipple and areola) are the most common treatments suggested. Alexander et al[2] compared use of shells and no treatment and found more sustained improvement in the untreated group. The difference in use of shells/no shells was 52%/60%, which is not significant. A large multicenter trial of

Fig. 8-5. Breast shell in place inside brassiere to evert nipple.

shells, Hoffman exercises, and no prenatal treatment showed "no treatment" to be most effective.[135] Exercises have had no significant impact and are contraindicated because of their tendency to initiate uterine contractions. The most significant finding was that more women who were instructed to wear shells or do nipple exercises than controls who had no prenatal preparation never initiated breastfeeding at delivery. More women also discontinued breastfeeding by 6 weeks compared with controls. The women complained that shells caused discomfort, embarrassment, sweating, rash, milk leakage, or were conspicuous.

Such studies illustrate some of the risks of using untried methods to solve problems, although some women probably benefit by using shells. The question deserves further study. The process of assessing anatomic problems and initiating management should not be a deterrent to breastfeeding. Such assessment may best be delayed until the first few days of lactation when the mother is focused on feeding and the baby.

Inverted nipples (Fig. 8-3) can be diagnosed by pressing the areola between the thumb and the forefinger. A flat or normal nipple will protrude: a truly inverted nipple will retract. True inverted nipples are actually rare.

Treatments for inverted nipples

Exercises to evert inverted nipples are rarely successful and may be dangerous. The obstetric literature abounds with articles about the use of nipple stimulation in place of the traditional oxytocin challenge test; only a few are quoted here.[9,10,21,29,99] Using the breast pump or manual expression to produce colostrum is reported to induce labor or increase the strength of contractions in desultory labor.

Taylor and Green[156] reported a case of severe abruptio placentae after nipple stimulation. A series of patients induced labor with self-manipulation of the breasts with a 45% success rate. All patients in the series showed some ripening of the cervix with dilatation and effacement over 3 days of breast stimulation. Lipitz et al[88] and others[43,156] reported a relatively high incidence (45.5%) of exaggerated uterine activity in response to a breast-stimulation stress test, usually within 7 minutes of initiation of stimulation. Although all the cases and series cannot be reported here, it is clear that nipple stimulation in the third trimester can initiate uterine contractions and, in some, labor. Under the direction of an obstetrician, breast stimulation can be effective therapeutically, but it should not be recommended without obstetric evaluation.

Suggesting stretching (Hoffman) exercises is not advised, especially in women with a tendency to early labor. No study since Hoffman's initial report of two cases[67] has shown the process to be effective. Stretching the areola forcefully can damage the delicate Montgomery glands. Prepartum mastitis has also occurred with prenatal expression of colostrum. Whether manipulating the breast prenatally provides the mother with greater comfort in breastfeeding has not been demonstrated. Mothers who choose to bottle-feed have told us that having to "exercise" their breasts is one of the "rules" that kept them from breastfeeding.

The Hoffman exercises[67] involve placing the thumbs or forefingers opposite each other close to the base of the nipple and slowly pushing away from the areola. Done in a vertical line and then a horizontal line in the form of an imaginary cross, this is intended to stretch and break the fibers that "tie" the inverted nipple.

Pumping with a pulsatile electric pump with a soft silastin flange (White River personal or institutional model) has been shown to facilitate latch-on with flat or inverted nipples after delivery. The breast is gently pumped on low settings until the teat is drawn out and the infant offered the breast. Similar pumping is done on the second breast, when that nipple is also inverted, before placing the infant on that breast. Usually the pumping can be discontinued after a few days, or a hand pump is adequate if prefeed pumping needs to be continued at home.

A readily available, inexpensive device can be prepared in the hospital from a standard syringe, selecting the size (10 or 20 cc) that best fits the nipple's diameter. The end of the barrel of a syringe with the piston removed is cut off with a sharp blade. The piston is then replaced from the cut end. This provides a smooth surface to place over the nipple, with the piston gradually withdrawn to create gentle suction for about a minute, then repeating. Mother can comfortably do this herself, repeating the procedure before each feeding as necessary.[79]

These approaches avoid the risk of never initiating breastfeeding identified in the Alexander et al study.[2] They also provide one-on-one support from the nursing staff, which is very different from sending the mother home to use a strange plastic device.

The infant breastfeeds. The infant does not nipple-feed. If the nipples are flat or inverted, extra care is needed to provide enough areolar tissue in the infant's mouth to allow latch-on.

Surgical correction

Inverted nipples have been known to medicine for centuries, and treatment has included various exercises or use of older vigorous infants to suckle and use of adults who hired out for this purpose in difficult cases. The first surgical procedure was described in 1873. Other techniques have since been advanced.[58,132,148] A primary indication for surgical repair of the inverted nipple has been the chronic occurrence of central pockets of inflammation of the nipple, leading to spread of infection and suppurative mastitis. A simple method for correction without division of the lactiferous ducts involves using a purse-string suture and traction of holding sutures. The procedure can be done in the office under local anesthesia, according to Hauben and Mahler.[58] A truly inverted nipple may have fewer ducts. The microscopic pathology of severely inverted nipples indicates the ducts are abnormal.

Hand expression prenatally

Some breastfeeding instructions suggest handexpressing the breast to produce a few drops of colostrum every day for the last few weeks of pregnancy. Fortunately, the instructions usually suggest the patient consult her physician first. Manual or any kind of pumping of the breasts may stimulate the uterus to contract. Hand expression has no particular benefit and means that the early sequestered cells are expressed away in the drops of colostrum before delivery and are lost to the infant. Occasionally, prepartum mastitis has developed from this treatment. The risks far outweigh any seeming benefit.

Summary

1. During the first trimester, make the initial breast examination. Suggest considering how the infant is to be fed. If anatomic variations may interfere with lactation, mention them and discuss possible remedies.
2. At each prenatal visit, offer information about breastfeeding, which is part of the preparation for the birthing center, rooming-in, and discharge plans.
3. Investigate mother's knowledge of breastfeeding and document her information base to fill in the gaps and correct misinformation. Also inquire about any treatments or routines she has initiated on her own so that the total management is appropriate.
4. Once quickening has been experienced, the parents are ready to plan more concretely about the baby. Suggest a visit with the pediatrician.
5. As delivery approaches, initiate discussion about feeding the infant immediately after birth, feeding protocols, and the mother's special needs or requests.
6. Be familiar with community resources so that patients can be wisely referred for peer support or assistance unavailable from office staff.

IMMEDIATE POSTPARTUM PERIOD

Immediately after the placenta has separated, the establishment of lactation begins. This is a critical period because many mothers who do not receive the proper support in the hospital are driven to failure at breastfeeding by inept management.

Nursing at delivery

The mother will probably want to nurse her infant immediately after birth if she has read the current literature. Even if she does not ask, the obstetrician and delivery room staff should suggest and facilitate it.[87,137,175] Data confirm the view that delivery room or birthing center protocols that intercept interaction and suckling between mother and infant also impact on long-term lactation success.

Oxytocin levels at 15, 30, and 45 minutes after delivery are significantly elevated, coinciding with the expulsion of the placenta. Oxytocin has been associated with maternal bonding; thus it is appropriate to optimize mother-infant interaction at this point of high oxytocin levels by facilitating suckling.

Disease-oriented physicians who have been trained to give trials of water first, hours after delivery, are always concerned that the infant may aspirate. Clinical signs of potential for aspiration include low Apgar score, increased secretions, and polyhydramnios. Actually, most infants in the world go straight to the breast on delivery, which has a physiologic effect on the uterus, causing it to contract. Because sugar water and cow's milk formulas are very irritating if aspirated, delay in feeding has been the rule in the United States, where most infants are bottle-fed. Colostrum is not irritating, however, and is readily absorbed by the respiratory tree if aspirated.

A few possible obstacles exist to immediate nursing: (1) a heavily medicated mother, (2) an infant with a 5-minute Apgar score under 6, or (3) a premature infant under 36 weeks of gestation. The concern for the infant with a *tracheoesophageal* (TE) *fistula* is important, but a few precautions should suffice. If there is hydramnios or excess secretions at birth, a tube should be passed to the stomach to make sure the esophagus is patent. If all is well, the infant may nurse. If a TE fistula is found, it is a surgical emergency. *Choanal atresia* is another anomaly that would be of concern, but infants cannot suck on the breast or anything if they cannot breathe through the nose. Usually an infant with choanal atresia has a low

Apgar score or needs some assistance in establishing respirations.

As noted earlier, the healthy newborns placed on the mother's abdomen will find will find their way to the breast and latch on if unimpeded.[137] For this first breastfeeding, it may be best to have the mother on a bed wide enough to have the infant lie beside her. Newer delivery tables are wide enough. The infant should not be dangled in midair over the breast. The mother should be assisted to turn onto her side and the infant presented to the breast, with the ventral surface to the ventral surface of the mother. The infant should not have to turn the head toward the breast. The mother may need assistance in holding her breast so as to present the nipple squarely into the infant's mouth, which is stimulated to open by stroking the center of the lower lip with the nipple.

When the lower lip is touched by the nipple, the infant will open widely, extending the tongue under the nipple. The breast will be drawn into the mouth, the nipple and areola elongated into a teat, and the suckling reflex initiated.[138]

Both mother and infant will do better if there is an atmosphere of tranquility in the room.[133] The only other risk to the infant is thermal stress. If the room is air-conditioned, it may be necessary to provide a radiant warmer over the infant and mother, especially if the infant is naked for skin-to-skin contact. Some mothers have shaking chills following the strenuous event of labor and cannot provide adequate warmth for the infant without some external source of heat or a blanket.

Chilling an infant may set off a chain of events from hypothermia to hypoglycemia to tachypnea to mild acidosis to the extent of requiring a septic workup. Hypothermia is therefore more easily prevented than treated.

If possible, mother, father, and infant should remain together for the next hour or so. The first hour for the infant is usually one of quiet alertness, a state that will usually recur only briefly again in the next few days. It is important to delay the instillation of prophylactic eye drops until after this time spent with the mother. If the drops are put into the eyes, blepharospasm will prevent the infant from opening the eyes and will mar the eye-to-eye contact. Only if there is a known risk of gonorrhea should the drops be put in immediately. If the mother has delivered in a birthing center, early contact and nursing should be part of the routine.

Two natural hand positions for the mother to introduce the breast are used most often. With attention to a few details, either position works

Fig. 8-6. Scissor grasp, presenting breast while supporting infant.

(one is not right and the other wrong). The *scissor grasp* is the placement of the thumb and index finger above the areola and the other three fingers below the breast for support, thus allowing some compression of the areola. Care should be taken that the hand is not in the way of the infant's getting sufficient areola into the mouth (Fig. 8-6). This grip has been used for centuries and was shown in sketches and paintings even before the Christian era. If the hand is large or the breast small, it may not work as well as the palmar grasp.

The *palmar grasp* is the placement of all the fingers under the breast and only the thumb above (Fig. 8-7). This has been called the C-hold but is actually a V-hold, depending on the size of the breast and the size of the hand. This gives firm support to the breast. It permits directing the breast squarely into the infant's mouth and avoids the need to press the breast away from the infant's nose. The palmar grasp is similar to the prehensile grasp of the apes when they nurse their young.

The apes, however, are unable to assume another hand posture neurologically or anatomically. If too much pressure is exerted by the thumb, the nipple will be tipped upward (Fig. 8-8, *B*), causing abrasion of the underside. It is preferable that the nipple be directly or horizontally placed in the mouth (Fig. 8-8, *A*). Tipped down slightly is satisfactory. The palmar grasp can be used when there is nipple pain, soreness, or trauma. It is also useful when the mother's hand is too small for a large breast. The mother should be encouraged to use the most natural and comfortable hand position.

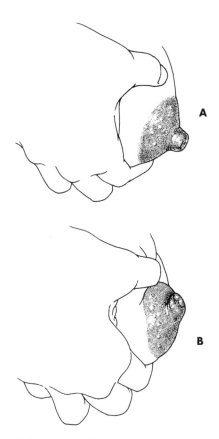

Fig. 8-8. Palmar grasp (C-hold). **A,** When palm and fingers cup breast with support and thumb rests lightly above areola, nipple projects straight ahead or slightly downward (correct). **B,** When fingers come forward and thumb presses firmly above, nipple tips up and causes improper positioning. Improper positioning is a common cause of nipple abrasion (lower half) and pain with suckling. (Modified from Higgins K: *The nursing mother's companion,* ed 2, Boston, 1990, Harvard Common Press.)

Fig. 8-7. Palmar grasp for initiating breastfeeding.

Days in the hospital

The physician should see that patients are permitted to have their infants with them as much as they wish, within the guidelines of reasonable medical care. Only the few patients with difficult deliveries, cesarean birth with medication, postpartum complications, or eclampsia need to be excluded, but the physician should make that judgment.

The influence of mode of delivery on initiation of breastfeeding was examined in 370 primiparas. Cesarean birth and other surgical delivery procedures (e.g., vacuum extraction) were associated with a sleepy infant, late start to feeding after delivery, increased incidence of bottle supplementation, less frequent night feedings, and delayed milk production in the hospital.[164] However, only 2.2% were not breastfeeding at discharge, and 52% were still breastfeeding at 6 months. Thus, despite many interventions, breastfeeding can succeed with sufficient support. An experienced nursing staff is critical to the management of the nursing mother in the first few days postpartum.[90] Advice should be reasonable and consistent, and nurses should be cautioned against interjecting their own personal opinion or experience. Too many individuals may be involved in postpartum care, and mothers are easily overwhelmed with information, especially if each person says something different.

Key points in management should include the following:

1. Help the mother find a comfortable position. No rules should exist about sitting up or lying down.
2. Help the infant to the breast. The infant should be held so that the ventral surface of the infant faces the mother.
3. Help the mother hold her breast for her baby, choosing the better grasp for the situation, and draw the baby to the breast by moving her arm toward her chest.

   NOTE: Never push the infant's head toward the breast because the infant will push back, often arching away from the breast. Pushing the infant's head has been associated with persistent arching by the infant (arching reflex).
4. Help the mother reposition the infant on the second breast if the infant is still interested after releasing the first side. Moving may be difficult for the mother immediately postpartum.
5. If the infant falls asleep after the first breast, the mother should be shown how to break the suction with her fingers. Nonnutritive suckling while asleep is especially irritating to the nipple in the first few days. The mother should wait a little, wake the baby, and then move the infant to the second side.
6. When waking an infant, unwrapping the blanket and using gentle stimulus are appropriate. Jackknifing is never appropriate and may cause regurgitation, aspiration, or trauma to vital organs.
7. The infant will nurse on the first breast until satisfied. After gentle burping, if the infant is still awake, the second side can be offered. The next feeding should be initiated on the other side. This will balance the stimulus to the breasts in the critical early days when milk production is just beginning. Stopwatch timing is not appropriate. It takes 2 to 3 minutes for the let-down reflex to produce milk in the early days, so the feeding must allow for the let-down. It is helpful for some mothers to have guidelines or estimates from which to work. Usually, infants nurse about 10 to 15 minutes per feeding in the first days. Nursing continually hour after hour may be counterproductive. Frequent small feedings will provide good stimulation to the breast without stressing the mother. The milk supply, however, is best stimulated by suckling.[126] The policy of the nursery should be to have all breastfed infants taken to their mothers when they awaken during the night,[86] if they have not roomed-in.

In keeping with the Baby Friendly Hospital Initiative (see Chapter 1), infants should be nursed on demand around the clock and receive no other food or drink. A mother should be given the infant if she so requests. On the other hand, modern hospitals are a hubbub of activity, and with liberalized visiting hours, the mother has no time to rest unless naps are scheduled. In the early days of the Rooming-In Unit at the Yale–New Haven Hospital,

Jackson insisted that all postpartum mothers have a nap after lunch. Every day the shades were drawn and traffic decreased on the unit for an hour. This is part of mothering the mother. In primitive cultures, mothers are groomed, fed, and protected after delivery, often for weeks. Furthermore, adequate rest is essential to successful lactation. In 1953, Jackson, with her colleagues Barnes et al,[16] prepared a classic description of the management of breastfeeding that remains the single most valuable source of information on the subject.

Diagnosing breastfeeding problems

To solve the problem of unsuccessful nursing, one should observe the mother feeding the infant. Often the problem is a simple one, such as a mother so uncomfortable and tense that the letdown reflex will not trigger, or perhaps an infant

with a poor suck. In these cases and others the diagnosis can be made most easily by direct observation.

Understanding the mechanism of suckling in the neonate (Fig. 8-9), however, is essential to recognizing ineffective sucking. As the breast is offered to the infant, the lips open wide and the tongue is extended as the nipple is inserted into the mouth (Fig. 8-10). In a rhythmic motion, the tongue moves up against the hard palate, drawing the nipple and areola into the mouth, creating an elongated teat. The cheeks fill the mouth because of the sucking fat pads and provide further negative pressure because they do not collapse. The tongue undulates along the teat, compressing the collecting ductules in the areola and "milking" them toward the nipple. Milk flows from the nipple and is swallowed as the swallowing reflex is triggered.

Fig. 8-9. **A,** As infant grasps breast, tongue moves forward to draw in nipple. **B,** Nipple and areola move toward palate as glottis still permits breathing. **C,** Tongue moves along nipple, pressing it against hard palate and creating pressure. Ductules under areola are milked, and flow begins as a result of peristaltic movement of tongue. Glottis closes. Swallow follows.

Fig. 8-10. Latch-on response. In response to stimulating infant's lower lip with nipple, mouth opens wide. This response has been called *oral searching reflex.* It is part of circumoral rooting reflex. (From Righard L, Alade MO: *Birth* 19:185, 1992.)

Fig. 8-11. Infant sucking on rubber nipple, which fills mouth and thus prevents tongue action and provides flow without tongue movement. Flow occurs even if lips not tight around rubber hub.

If the infant has a fluttering tongue that is discoordinate, it may not be as productive in stimulating ejection. If the infant cannot coordinate suck and swallow, choking occurs. Sometimes if ejection is strong, the first rush of milk will cause choking. Stopping and starting again should solve the problem. If the mother's milk flows abundantly with first let-down, she may need to express manually (and save) the first few milliliters to avoid choking the infant. Usually the flow moderates quickly. This problem is only temporary or is limited to times when the infant has not been nursed for an unusually long interval.

If the infant's jaw is slightly receding, the nipple may not stay in place. Gentle support from the mother's index finger at the angle of the jaw will help.

An infant who is given a bottle or rubber nipple to suck can become confused because the milking action is different (Fig. 8-11). The relatively inflexible rubber nipple may keep the tongue from its usual rhythmic action. In addition, the flow may be so rapid, even without sucking, that the infant learns to put the tongue against holes in the rubber nipple to slow down the flow. Some infants who have been breastfed gag when the relatively large rubber nipple is put in their mouths. When infants use the same tongue action needed for a rubber nipple while at the breast, they may even push the human nipple out of the mouth. When infants cannot grasp an engorged areola properly, they will clamp down on the nipple with the jaws, causing pain in the nipple and disrupting the ejection reflex. Manual expression of a little milk will soften the areola, permitting compression and an easier grasp.

When observing an infant being breastfed, take note of the following:
1. Position of mother, body language, and tension. Pillows may provide support for arms or infant.
2. Position of infant. Ventral surface should be to mother's ventral surface, with lower arm, if not swaddled, around mother's thorax. Infant cannot swallow if head has to turn to breast, and grasp of areola will be poor. Infant's head should be in crook of arm and moved toward breast by arm movement.
3. Position of mother's hand on breast not in way of proper grasp by infant

4. Position of infant's lips on areola about 1 to 1½ inches (2.5 to 3.7 cm) from base of nipple
5. Lower lip not folded in so that infant does not suck it; lips flanged
6. Actual events around presenting breast and assisting infant to latch on
7. Response of infant to lower lip stimulus by opening mouth wide (Fig. 8-10).
8. Motion of masseter muscle during suckling and sounds of swallowing
9. Mother comfortable with no breast pain

Engorgement

The best management of engorgement is prevention. The degree of engorgement lessens for a woman with each infant because the time during which the milk "comes in" seems to shorten in multiparas. The primipara suffers most from engorgement.

Breast engorgement was carefully documented by Humenick et al[70] for 14 days postpartum in 114 breastfeeding women. Four distinct patterns emerged, varying from minimal engorgement to intense engorgement and including a bell-shaped pattern and a multimodal pattern. Characteristics of mothers, infants, and feeding frequency were similar across all patterns. Engorgement in these women was increased in second-time breastfeeders, with first-time feeders peaking at about 108 hours and second-time feeders at 100 hours. Engorgement cleared more quickly the second time. Clearly, mothers' experiences differ under seemingly similar circumstances.

A number of often conflicting theories and explanations regarding engorgement have been proposed in the professional and lay literature. The dictionary defines engorgement as "swollen with blood," and pathologists define it as "congestion." Engorgement of the breast involves three elements: (1) congestion and increased vascularity, which is the physiologic response that follows removal of the placenta and does not depend on suckling; (2) accumulation of milk, also a physiologic response to placental removal; and (3) edema secondary to the swelling and obstruction of drainage of the lymphatic system by vascular increases and full-

ness of the alveoli. No parallel exists in nature because the underlying process is physiologic. Engorgement is not injury, hemorrhage, or trauma. When the physiologic process proceeds smoothly, no pain, discomfort, or excessive swelling occurs. When edema is identifiable, the surface of the breast pits with pressure; the process is out of control, and intervention is necessary.[65]

Engorgement may involve only the areola, only the body of the breast (so-called peripheral engorgement), or both. Some engorgement is normal. When the breast does not respond with "fullness," this is abnormal and requires attention.

Areolar engorgement. When the areola is engorged, it obliterates the nipple and makes properly grasping the areola impossible for the infant. If the infant sucks only the nipple, it is exquisitely painful, because this is the only area of the breast with pain fibers. In addition, the collecting ductules are not "milked" and therefore do not empty, and the infant is frustrated by lack of milk.

The treatment is directed toward reducing the engorgement so that the infant can nurse effectively, which will further reduce the overdistended ducts. Gentle manual expression by the mother usually produces a small amount of flow and softens the areola. The presence of milk on the nipple will further encourage the infant's sucking. Warm soaks just before a feeding may facilitate manual expression. A mother should be taught how to express milk manually (Fig. 8-12). Placing the thumb and forefinger at the margins of the areola and pressing back in toward the chest and then bringing the fingers together, rhythmically simulating the action of the infant's jaw, will start the flow and soften the tense tissue (see Appendix G). When the infant is put to the breast, the mother should compress the areola between two fingers to make it easier for the infant to grasp. Offering the breast this way makes it easier for any infant to grasp, especially when the infant needs encouragement to nurse (Fig. 8-13).

Peripheral engorgement. Initially the breasts increase in vascularity and begin to swell. This usually starts in the second 24-hour period after delivery. Engorgement at this stage is vascular;

Fig. 8-12. Position for manual expression of breast. Thumbs are brought toward areola, compressing areola between thumb and supporting fingers. With areola grasped, pressure is applied toward chest wall, and then pressure is released. This compression and pressure stimulate milking action (see also Appendix H).

Fig. 8-13. When breast is offered to infant, areola is gently compressed between two fingers and breast is supported to ensure that infant is able to grasp areola adequately.

thus pumping mechanically briefly to stimulate the breast when the infant is not nursing adequately is appropriate. Pumping "to relieve engorgement" will yield little milk and may traumatize the hypervascular breast.

The mother should be advised to wear a well-fitting but adjustable nursing brassiere that does not have thin straps or permanent plastic lining. She should wear it 24 hours a day. With moderately severe engorgement, the breasts become full, hard, and tender. The swelling starts at the clavicle and goes to the lower rib cage and from the midaxillary line to the midsternum. The breasts may even become hard, tense, and warm. The mother complains of throbbing and aching pain and can find no comfortable position except to lie flat on her back and very still (Fig. 8-14).

Management centers on making the mother comfortable so that she can continue to nurse and stimulate milk production as well as nourish the infant. Proper support to elevate the breasts is important. The axillae are particularly painful, probably as a result of the tension on Cooper's ligament. Cold packs reduce vascularity. Warm packs aggravate the swelling. Having the mother stand in a warm shower and manually express some milk at the same time may be the best preparation to feed the infant. Some find comfort in alternating hot and cold water. Other mothers find

Fig. 8-14. Marked mammary engorgement, predominantly vascular in nature.

leaning over a large mixing bowl of warm water just before feeding facilitates let-down and milk flow and is less disruptive than a shower.

After a feeding, cold packs reduce the swelling, edema, warmth, and pain. Acetaminophen or ibuprofen may give the mother some relief and should not bother the infant. A combination with codeine preparation can be recommended as well. The mother may need some sleep medication. Medications should be timed so that the least amount possible reaches the mother's milk and the baby. If medication is taken immediately before nursing, the pain will be relieved, but the drug will not reach the milk for more than ½ hour in the case of ibuprofen, acetaminophen, codeine, or short-acting barbiturates.

It is important to maintain drainage during this period of engorgement to prevent back pressure in the ducts from developing and eventually depressing milk production. Intraductal pressure can lead eventually to atrophy of both the secreting and the myoepithelial cells and a diminishing milk supply. The best treatment is breastfeeding frequently around the clock because suckling by the infant is the most effective mechanism for removal of milk. Relief is based on establishment of flow. The infant may have trouble grasping or may not be interested in nursing frequently in the first few days, so manual expression may also be necessary. Every

mother should be taught this technique by the perinatal nursing staff before discharge.[107]

The mother should support the breast with her fingers and place her thumbs distally and massage gently toward the areola, rotating gradually around the breast to include all quadrants. Then, once the peripheral lobules have been softened, areolar expression as previously described should be used to encourage complete emptying of the collecting ducts in the areola. This is a procedure best done by the mother, but it takes a skilled and experienced nurse to teach this technique (see Appendix G). In women with significant engorgement, it may be helpful to use an electric pump, which is very effective because of its gentle milking action (see Chapter 20). The breast should be massaged distally before and during pumping.

Hand pumps can be used but exert only negative pressure on the areola. Unless accompanied by manual expression of the distal segments, they are only temporizing.

Cabbage leaves

A favorite treatment for severe engorgement is cabbage leaves. Cabbage leaves have been used in Europe for generations to relieve edema in other body parts, including the ankles. Chopped fresh leaves are applied to ankles overnight as a poultice and wrapped with a towel. When chilled, whole cabbage leaves and chilled gel packs were compared as breast treatments for engorgement, no difference was found. Pain was relieved within 1 to 2 hours with both treatments in 68% of women. The mothers preferred the cabbage treatment.[141]

Severe engorgement occurs between the third and seventh day postpartum, and the breasts are described as full, red, hard, and warm. The literature on this therapy is sparse, but two reports have been published. An Australian study involved a series of cases where the treatment was applied.[143] There were no failures, but in several women the treatment was interrupted by other staff who applied ice and medications for pain without success. When cabbage leaves were reapplied, symptoms were relieved in 2 to 24 hours. Relief was often within 2 hours. Clinicians treated 30 patients and reported on nine in detail. Rosier[143] tried the treatment first with women who were engorged who were not nursing. No side effects have been reported.

A second randomized, controlled trial was undertaken in South Africa by Nikodem et al,[115] who studied 120 breastfeeding women. At 72 hours postpartum they were randomized to control or treatment group. Treatment was application of cool (from refrigerator) cabbage leaves to breasts, leaving just the nipple exposed. The leaves were applied after four feedings for 20 minutes or so until the leaves wilted. *Brassica oleracea L var. capitata* was used. All mothers were also taught routine breast exercises, which consisted of bending the arms at the elbow, moving the arms across the chest, with hands facing the same shoulder, so elbows touched, and swiping across the breast a total of 10 times. This exercise, known by various names, including the Johannesburg salute, is used as a preventive treatment for engorgement. Although the experimental group reported less engorgement, it was not statistically significant. Exclusive breastfeeding at 6 weeks was 76% compared with 58% among controls (p = .09). Mean duration of breastfeeding was 36 versus 30 days in controls (p = .04). However, this study had more multiparas in the control group, and engorgement is rarely a serious problem in multiparas.

Whether cabbage leaves have prophylactic value may be challenged, but their value in the therapy of severe engorgement is worth noting. Whether it is the coolness of the leaves or an innate property of cabbage itself that is therapeutic has not been proved. In Duke's *Handbook of Medicinal Herbs* (Boca Raton, Fla, 1985, CRC Press), cabbage *(Brassica oleracea)* is referred to as a *galactogogue*. The most common variety, *B. capitata,* is the one used in engorgement therapy. This handbook also lists cabbage with other angiosperms as capable of causing hypoglycemia. Cabbage is noted to contain sinigrin (allyl isothiocyanate) and rapine. Herbalists consider rapine to be an antifungal antibiotic. The text lists galactogogues and lactation suppressants found in other plants but does not mention any mammary effects of cabbage.

A new product is available on the market called Cabbage Gel (Pure Necessities, 15036 Beltway, Addison, TX 75244). This pale-green gel has a gentle odor of peppermint, is made of aloe vera, and contains peppermint oil and "herbal infusions" and apparently no cabbage. It is intended for use alone or with fresh cabbage leaves to help keep them in place and cool the engorged breast. Care must be taken to remove the gel before feeding the infant because aloe vera can be a powerful purgative.

Going home from the hospital

Currently, maternity patients are going home from the hospital in 2 to 3 days or sooner, which is certainly before lactation is well established but possibly before engorgement is full blown. When maternity floors were run so rigidly that ad lib breastfeeding was an impossible feat, it was often suggested that a mother go home and get away from the negative hospital atmosphere to a place where she could relax and concentrate on feeding the infant and resting. This is a point at which the doula, so well described by Raphael,[131] could make the difference between success and failure. It may be appropriate for the obstetrician to order the mother to have some assistance at home, whether her husband, her mother, or a friend. "The common denominator for success in breastfeeding is the assurance of some degree of help from some specific person for a definite period of time after childbirth."[131]

Raphael studied mothers in the cycle of anxiety while she became the doula for them at about 6 to 10 days postpartum. The calm that can be experienced in the presence of a confident, caring person will relax the mother. The infant senses the calm and confidence and sleeps. When feeding again, the infant nurses well. Breaking the cycle of panic that seizes a new mother when she finds herself home alone with a new infant who needs frequent feeding requires someone to instill confidence. This individual does not need to be a health professional, but should be a calm, reassuring, nonthreatening person.

Although physicians cannot be the doula, they can be sure that the family understands the need and can suggest community resources if no personal ones are available. Successful breastfeeding is not automatic, as demonstrated by the failure rate. Some problems have been generated by the disturbance of the synchronized interaction between mother and infant by rigid hospital protocol. This is continued at home when feeding is by the clock rather than by instinct. The office practice should be available by telephone. Ideally, the office nurse practitioner makes a home visit in the first week. An office visit should be scheduled within a week of birth, or sooner if a problem exists.

Most communities have a licensed, certified lactation consultant available for new mothers or any mother with a problem. The physician should be familiar with the available lactation consultants if the practice does not provide one on the staff.

Nipples

Painful nipples. Presumably the nipples will adapt to the nursing experience naturally; however, discomforts often arise. The initial grasp of the nipple and first suckles typically cause discomfort in the first few days of lactation. This is not cause for alarm but requires maternal reassurance. The sensation is created by the negative pressure on the ductules, which are not yet filled with milk. Later, when lactation is well established and the let-down reflex is experienced, mothers describe a *turgescence,* which is the increased fluid pressure being relieved by suckling. If the pain persists throughout the feeding, the situation demands attention.

Nipple pain was studied in 102 women in the first 96 hours postpartum.[86] Engorgement was most closely associated with nipple discomfort, which may be enhanced by the general discomfort of the breast. Prenatal breast preparation was unrelated to soreness. Length of time spent suckling was also unrelated. No record was kept on nonnutritive suckling, although others have found suckling without swallowing to be more stressful early in lactation. How the breast is presented to the infant is the most critical factor[48] (maternal hand position and infant squarely facing breast).

This is the time to observe the feeding, looking for malpositioning or other abnormalities.

The most common cause of painful nipples in the first few days is positioning. This should be reviewed in detail, being certain the areola is softened sufficiently to have the infant grasp adequately.[112] The infant's lower lip is checked to ensure it is flanged around the breast and not drawn into the mouth, which can abrade the nipple.

Specific areas of pain may have specific causes. Soreness on the top of the nipple or on the tip usually results from poor latch-on or tongue thrusting in an infant who is also bottle fed. Soreness can also be caused by tipping the nipple upward so that it grazes the hard palate from overzealous use of the palmar grasp or C-hold. Pain on the underside of the nipple is caused by presenting the breast with the nipple tipped up, usually because of more pressure by the mother's hand on top than below the breast, especially with the palmar grasp, so the infant "strokes" the underside of the nipple. The tip of the nipple may also graze the hard palate. The nipple may be bruised, scabbed, or blistered, depending how long the problem has continued (Fig. 8-15).

If no abnormality is found, the pain may be caused by a "barracuda baby" with a vigorous suck. The breast will gradually adapt, and this pain will not last indefinitely. Sometimes the maternal tissues are unusually tender and delicate. Brief dry heat may help between feedings. The mother should remove the waterproofing from her brassiere and expose her breasts to air briefly after each feeding.

Even more effective, especially in humid climates, is the use of an electric hair dryer, set on warm and fanned across the breast about 6 to 8 inches (15 to 20 cm) away only for 2 to 3 minutes to avoid overdrying. This brings remarkable comfort and can be done sitting, standing, or lying down. In dry climates, however, wetting the tissues is the preferred treatment. The breast will be moist with milk right after a feeding. This should not be wiped away but allowed to dry on the skin. Many primitive cultures treat irritation of the skin with human milk.[126] The surface-drying effect of the

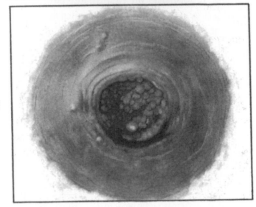

Fig. 8-15. Various types of cracks in abraded lactating nipples. **A,** Crack across nipple. **B,** Multiple cracks (stellate). **C,** Crack at lower base.

treatment helps counteract the increase in moisture experienced in the first days of lactation. This is neither necessary nor appropriate in arid climates.

Stabbing pain that radiates through the breast so that mother feels like the ducts are liquid fire is associated with *Candida* infection of the breasts, often seen after antibiotic treatment. The infant may or may not have visible thrush. This deserves special attention[41] (see Mastitis).

Ointments. The appropriate treatment of sore nipples is based on removing the cause and facilitating healing. Positioning is the most common cause, but repositioning will not heal a seriously damaged nipple without some medical intervention. The most appropriate application depends not only on cause but also on environmental conditions. With high humidity, greasy moisture-sealing ointments aggravate the skin. If the atmosphere is very dry (Denver or the desert southwest), creams may be appropriate.

All treatments are not appropriate to all lesions. Cool, wet tea bags, for instance, serve as an astringent because of the tannic acid, causing drying and cracking, and are not usually recommended. One study compared tea bag therapy with water compresses and no treatment. Both tea bags and water compresses were more effective than no treatment. Given the taste, smell, and astringent effect of the tannic acid in the tea bag, this study would further confirm that the same effect can be obtained with plain water.[84] Pugh et al[130] examined three treatments for nipple soreness: USP modified lanolin, warm water compresses, and expressed breast milk with air drying. The use of warm compresses appeared to be the most effective of the three treatments.

The routine application of ointments to the nipple, areola, or breast should be discouraged except in cases of extremely dry skin where the tissue needs to be lubricated.

Lanolin is most hazardous to anyone with a wool allergy. Lansinoh is a purified, alcohol-free, and "allergen-free" ointment, however, and should be safe if an ointment is indicated. Some ointments and creams have irritants.[60] The sebaceous and

Fig. 8-16. Nipple shield made of tasteless, odorless silicone in very thin flexible form referred to as "Mexican hat."

Montgomery glands of the areola and nipple are easily plugged by repeated applications of oily substances during pregnancy and lactation. Preparations with vitamins A and D are innocuous, but those with vitamin E or hormones are unsafe unless prescribed for a specific problem by the physician.

Moist wound healing for sore or cracked nipples has been proposed by some dermatologists as a treatment comparable to treating other areas of the body.[147] Early soreness may be caused by insufficient moisture present in the skin coupled with the friction of malpositioning.[134] Wetness on the surface caused by the milk and occlusive plastic-lined nursing pads does cause irritation. The moisture within the tissue, however, should be preserved by the application of a nonirritating ointment after a feeding when the nipple has been gently dried, according to Sharp.[147]

Local anesthetic creams should not be used because they lead to allergic reactions, but more importantly they can interrupt the let-down reflex and affect the infant by numbing the mouth and throat. The use of ice to numb the pain before feeding does not correct the cause and may interfere with the let-down reflex, which is easily intercepted by cold as well as by pain. If ice numbs the areola, it may numb the nervous response. Irritation or rash should first be treated by discon-

tinuing any ointments or other self-medicating material. This is the first step in the treatment of any dermatologic problem.

Nipple shields. A nipple shield is a device made of rubber or synthetic materials that is worn over the nipple and areola while the infant is suckling. A makeshift shield of a nursing-bottle nipple should never be used. Shields differ from the shells designed to evert nipples (Fig. 8-16). Shells should never be worn while breastfeeding, and any milk that drips into them should not be saved to feed the infant because it is heavily contaminated and of lower fat content. A study of the effect of a thin latex nipple shield on suckling showed no difference in length of suckling time and no difference in cortisol levels or prolactin levels, which were correlated with length of time suckling.[182] Wearing the shield without suckling had no effect on prolactin levels. The amount of milk received by the infant, however, was significantly reduced.

Nipple shields should not be used because it often becomes hard to wean the infant back to the bare breast. The infant becomes confused in learning the sucking routine. Glass or plastic shields with a rubber nursing nipple never work well, although the mother can see the milk through the glass or plastic. The effect of a traditional red rubber nipple shield (Fig. 8-16) was compared to a new thin latex nipple shield referred to as a "Mexican hat." Normal mothers with no problems lactating nursed their infants using the shields.[182] The red rubber shield reduced the milk transfer by 58% and increased the infants' sucking rate and time spent resting. The thin latex shield reduced milk by 22% and had no effect on sucking patterns. Many lactation experts consider the use of a breast shield a sign of failure of proper lactation guidance and a preventable situation. No medical problems have been identified when a shield is a good solution.

Small or flat nipples. When the nipples are small or flat, special attention to compress the breast and areola between two fingers to provide as much nipple as possible to the infant will assist the infant in getting a hold. Using the breast shell between feedings will help draw the nipple to greater prominence. Softening the areola before a feed to make it more compressible also helps.

Drawing the nipple out with a hospital electric pump before each feeding should help facilitate latch-on and train the infant to a proper grasp. A day or two of such preparation with the pump is usually sufficient if the infant is full term with a good suck. Once engorgement is diminished and nursing is well established, small or flat nipples are usually no longer a problem.

Large nipples. Large nipples are occasionally a problem with a small infant or an infant with an indecisive suck. The shells do not help the infant cope at first, and it is best just to work patiently with the infant. Manual expression, which softens the areola to make it more pliable before putting the infant to the breast, often helps. Preparation with an electric pump may also facilitate the infant's latch-on by drawing the nipple into a teat.

Cracked nipples. Whenever the mother complains of nipple pain on nursing, the nipple should be examined in good light to look for cracks or subepithelial petechiae, which may be the precursor to cracking.[113] Taking a thorough history about care of the breast is important to identify the use of soaps, oils, ointments, or other self-prescribed treatments. Watching the nursing process may identify abnormal positioning at the breast. The position of the crack also may identify the problem (Box 8-3).

BOX 8-3   Management of sore, painful, or cracked nipples

1. Examine the breast, nipple, and nursing scene.
2. Recommend manual expression before feeding and softening of areola.
3. Check for infant position on breast.
4. Suggest nursing on unaffected breast first with affected side exposed to air.
5. Let expressed breast milk dry on skin between feedings.
6. Recommend appropriate ointment.
7. Rarely, temporarily stop nursing on affected side and replace it with manual expression or pumping.
8. If necessary, give acetaminophen, ibuprofen, or codeine (for serious pain unresponsive to milder drugs) in short-acting preparations just before nursing (see Chapter 11).

Cracks straight across the tip of the nipple are caused by excessive dryness following original irritation of the nipple tip by poor nipple positioning against the infant's palate (Fig. 8-15, *A*). Pain may be eased by correct positioning, and healing may be promoted by application of therapeutic ointments such as A and D, purified lanolin, or a synthetic hydrocorticoid (Elocon ointment), followed by a "butterfly" bandage that brings the edges of the crack together between feedings. Local anesthetics are not appropriate, nor are nipple shields, which draw and pull the nipple. Star-shaped cracks respond to similar treatment (Fig. 8-15, *B*). Cracks at the base of the nipple (Fig. 8-15, *C*) are usually caused by sucking of the lower lip and biting, which are ultimately a result of poor positioning.

Therapy is indicated for true cracks. In the precracked stage, letting the milk dry on the skin for a few moments and applying a cream between nursing are most effective. When true fissures have developed, opening both sides of the nursing brassiere at feedings and beginning to nurse on the less painful side first will permit the initial letdown to occur "atraumatically"; then the infant can be put carefully to the affected breast. When nursing must be stopped on a given breast, it sets up a chain reaction of engorgement, reduced flow, and plugging of the ducts. Changing the infant's position, such as using a football hold, will help healing.

Hewat and Ellis[62] conducted a study comparing lanolin with dried-on milk. Mothers used one treatment on one nipple and the other treatment on the opposite breast. The authors found no correlation between pain and frequency of feedings or the mother's hair and skin color. The women reported no difference in soreness between the two treatments. Many dermatologists believe that applying two treatments to different parts on the same patient may lead to mixture of therapies and noncompliance rates higher than normal. A study of antiseptic sprays by Herd and Feeney[60] produced controversial results. Antiseptic sprays are rarely justified and may cause problems because the physiologic normal flora of the nipple and areola should not be artificially altered unless a culture has been done.[72]

In women with severe nipple cracking, the physician may prescribe synthetic topically applied corticoids, which are preferred by dermatologists. When position has been corrected and bacterial and fungal infections ruled out, application of Elocon 0.1% cream or ointment, which is antiinflammatory, antipruritic, and vasoconstrictive, can be rapidly healing. Less than 0.5% of a dose of corticoids topically is absorbed. Ultravate (halobetasol propionate) 0.05%, another synthetic corticoid ointment, is also available by prescription. Usually a 2-day treatment is adequate, and the ointment does not need to be removed before feeding. It is important to treat the underlying cause of the original trauma to the nipple.

The application of any ointment that must be removed before nursing has disadvantages because removal is traumatic. A and D ointment, which does not have to be removed, is occasionally effective. A and D ointment contains vitamins A and D from fish liver oils in a petrolatum base. An individual would have to consume several large tubes of it at one sitting even to approach toxicity.

The indiscriminate use of ointment, however, can be the cause of nipple pain, and as with many dermatologic problems, the initial treatment prescribed may be to discontinue previous treatments.[113] Some ointments suggested as breast creams contain antibiotics, astringents, bismuth subnitrate, or petrolatum, all of which are contraindicated. These creams are available over the counter without a prescription; thus the physician should inquire about their use as self-medication.

Premoistened towelettes contain benzalkonium chloride 1:750 in 20% alcohol and should not be used on a nipple or areola with or without soreness or cracks or used to cleanse. The infant could accumulate benzalkonium chloride by suckling. The infant might reject the breast because of the flavor or burning sensation in the mouth. Also, benzalkonium is usually painful for the mother.

Infant in the hospital

Feeding characteristics

Infants have been aptly classified by their feeding characteristics by Barnes and colleagues[16] as "barracudas," excited "ineffectives," procrastinators, gourmets or mouthers, and resters. These descriptions serve to demonstrate that infants are different and the management of the nursing experience will vary accordingly. Herein lies the secret to appropriate counseling: recognizing the differences among infants and responding to them.

Barracudas. When put to the breast, barracudas vigorously and promptly grasp the nipple and areola and suck energetically for 10 to 20 minutes. There is no dallying. Occasionally, this type of infant puts too much vigor into the nursing and hurts the nipple at first, but this passes.

Excited ineffectives. Some infants become so excited and active at the breast that they alternately grasp and lose the breast. Then they start screaming. The nurse or mother often must pick up and quiet the infant first, then put the infant back to the breast. After a few days the mother and infant usually become adjusted.

Procrastinators. Procrastinators often seem to put off until the fourth or fifth postpartum day what they could just as well have done from the start. They wait until the milk "comes in." They show no particular interest or ability in sucking in the first few days. It is important not to prod or force these infants when they seem disinclined. They do well once they start.

Gourmets or mouthers. Gourmets insist on mouthing the nipple, tasting a little milk, and then smacking their lips before starting to nurse. If hurried or prodded, the infant will become furious and start to scream. Otherwise, after a few minutes of mouthing the infant settles down and nurses very well.

Resters. Resters prefer to nurse a few minutes and then rest a few minutes. If left alone, they often nurse well, although the entire procedure will take much longer. They cannot be hurried.

Weight loss

Newborns usually lose some weight, which tends to be a function of whether they are appropriate, large, or small for gestational age as well as how many kilocalories they ingest in the first few days. Breastfeeding infants of multiparas often lose little weight because the milk "comes in" so quickly. On the other hand, the normal primipara may not have a full supply for 72 to 96 hours. If the weight loss is more than 5% (150 g in a 3-kg infant),

evaluate the process to identify any problems before they become serious. A 10% weight loss is acceptable if all else is going well and the physical examination is negative, but it should be justified in the record, and the infant should be seen shortly after discharge from the hospital to ensure resolution of the problem. If discharge home has taken place in 48 hours, it is imperative that the pediatrician's office keep in touch with the mother. Many have a nurse practitioner who makes the follow-up telephone calls or a home visit.

Newton and Newton[108-111] described a simple observation of breastfeeding mothers that was an accurate predictor of ultimate lactation success (Table 8-2). All the observations were related to the milk-ejection reflex (i.e., uterine pain, milk dripping on sight of baby, and relief of nipple discomfort on initiation of sucking). Successful breastfeeders had significantly more uterine pain during suckling on day 2 postpartum (after-pains), more dripping of opposite breast, more dripping on sight of infant, and cessation of nipple discomfort.[108] As a further evaluation, Newton and Newton compared the amount of milk left in the breast after feeding that was available with a dose of Pitocin (synthetic oxytocin) and pumping. Successful breastfeeders had only 27% left, and unsuccessful breastfeeders had 47% left. This techno-

TABLE 8-2 Percentage of women reporting symptoms of milk ejection with significant difference between successful and unsuccessful breastfeeders

Symptoms	Successful breastfeeders (%)	Unsuccessful breastfeeders (%)	Probability (p)
Uterine pain (cramps) during suckling: day 2	64	38	<0.05
Dripping from opposite breast during suckling: day 6	95	67	<0.01
Dripping before suckling (as oxytocin is triggered by sight or expectation of baby or other times): day 5	78	56	<0.05
Cessation of nipple pain (as milk flow counteracts negative pressure produced by suckling):			
Day 4	89	69	<0.05
Day 5	87	52	<0.01
Day 6	92	70	<0.05
All symptoms: all days	59	48	<0.01

From Newton N: *Ann NY Acad Sci* 652:484, 1992.

logic measurement is no better measure of success than the simple observations of the let-down reflex (Table 8-2).

Provision of early formula supplementation in the hospital was also associated with less successful lactation. A strong predictor of the need for supplementation was excessive time from delivery to first breastfeeding. When water and sugar water were routinely provided, there was greater weight loss in the infant and lower lactation success rate.[83]

Weighing the infant before and after feedings produces tremendous anxiety in the mother and affords little information if it is inaccurate. Weighing has been improved by the introduction of electronic digital readout scales that are accurate to 1 g and are especially helpful in the intensive care nursery for infants under 1000 g.[26] Because of the cost and the sensitivity (fragility) of the equipment, these scales are not practical for home use. Their accuracy in before-and-after weighings has been verified by several investigators using comparison techniques.[173] When ordinary scales are used, the margin of error has been shown to be greatest with the smaller volumes and is 20% in amounts less than 60 ml. Most newborn nurseries use these extremely accurate scales. Test weighings can be done when medically indicated.

Sequential breast volume measurements have been used to study short-term rates of milk synthesis.[35] Using a rapid, computerized breast measurement system, a close correlation was established between amount of milk the infant consumed and change in breast volume. The volumes measured varied between 11 and 58 ml/hour.[35] At some point this technique may be applied to clinical assessment of milk production.

This technology and the work of others have led to new insights into lactation physiology.[127] Mothers know that the breasts fill gradually to a certain degree between feedings. When feedings are delayed or missed, breasts can be very uncomfortable, with relief achieved when the infant nurses.[14] The rate of synthesis appears constant, as confirmed by topographic imaging. A factor has been identified by Prentice et al[127] that is released into the milk space and inhibits milk synthesis locally

by direct action. The action of this local inhibitory factor imposes a more phasic pattern of milk production, having its greatest effect when the breast has the least milk and slowing to a minimum as the breast fills.[14,127] "Empty breast" is a misnomer and is physiologically untenable.[180]

Vomiting blood

A breastfed baby who vomits blood should have the blood evaluated for fetal or adult hemoglobin by the Apt test (blood suspended in small amount of saline solution and equal amount of 10% sodium hydroxide added; adult hemoglobin turns brown; fetal hemoglobin stays pink). If it is adult hemoglobin, the nipple may be bleeding. Sometimes this bleeding is painless and unknown to the mother, and sometimes she is afraid to report it. If it is fetal hemoglobin, the infant demands evaluation. Breastfeeding can continue with pink milk if the infant retains it and the cause has been addressed.

Greenish or brown milk is occasionally described in the first few days if the mother is pumping or her infant vomits. It usually results from old blood in the ducts, a residual of rapid growth and vascularization during pregnancy. This milk is usually harmless and clears spontaneously in a day or two. If being pumped, it may be discarded. Breastfeeding does not need to be interrupted.

Let-down reflex

The most important single function that affects the success of breastfeeding is the let-down reflex. A mother may produce the milk, but if she does not excrete it, further production is suppressed. Much has been written on this single reflex by physiologists, endocrinologists, biochemists, pathologists, anatomists, psychologists, psychiatrists, obstetricians, and pediatricians. It is a complex function that depends on hormones, nerves, and glands, which can be inhibited most easily by psychologic block[110] (Fig. 8-17).

The hormonal mechanism of milk ejection is described in Chapter 3. The reflex stimulation of milk ejection was meticulously studied by Caldeyro-Barcia[28] while he studied intramammary

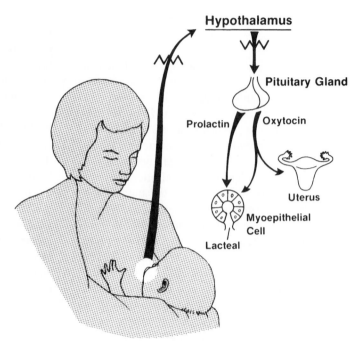

Fig. 8-17. Diagram of ejection reflex arc. When infant suckles breast, mechanoreceptors in nipple and areola are stimulated, which sends a stimulus along nerve pathways to hypothalamus, which stimulates posterior pituitary gland to release oxytocin. Oxytocin is carried via the bloodstream to breast and uterus. Oxytocin stimulates myoepithelial cells in breast to contract and eject milk from alveolus. Prolactin is responsible for milk production in alveolus. Prolactin is secreted by anterior pituitary gland in response to suckling. Stress such as pain and anxiety can inhibit let-down reflex. Sight or cry of infant can stimulate release of oxytocin but not prolactin.

pressures. The more efficient stimulus for the milk-ejection reflex is suckling the nipple. The frequency of suckling is 70 to 120 strokes per minute, and the mean pressure is −50 to −150 mm Hg. The maximum recorded was −220 mm Hg. Within 1 minute of the onset of suckling, the first contraction of the mammary myoepithelium is recorded, but it may take 2 or more total minutes for full response.

Further research by Cobo et al[31] has shown that, as in other species, the human response is undulating or spurtlike in release, although the level of oxytocin tends to reach a peak and plateau at 6 to 10 minutes during a feeding.[171] Some studies show no episodic secretion. When oxytocin levels are measured before the feeding, there is a response to the baby's crying or other anticipation of feeding. No prolactin response occurs before actual suckling (Fig. 8-18). A second release of oxytocin occurs when suckling begins.[37] No direct correlation exists between levels of oxytocin and the volume of milk released at a given feeding.[101] The average pituitary gland contains 1000 mU of

oxytocin, and only 0.5 mU is required for the let-down reflex.

Uterine contractions are also stimulated by suckling, because the oxytocin released into the bloodstream also affects the target receptors in the uterine myoepithelial cells.[116] Amplitude and frequency may increase over time during nursing. Mechanical stimulation of the nipple can produce the same effect on the breast and uterus. The milk-ejection reflex is inhibited centrally by cold, pain, and emotional stress. Ejection response can be elicited by seeing the infant or hearing the infant cry. Also, overwhelming evidence indicates that the neuropeptide oxytocin is centrally involved in activating maternal behavior at the appropriate time and plays a significant role in sustaining maternal behavior during lactation.[124]

The milk-ejection reflex can be at least partially blocked by large amounts of alcohol, which seems to have a central effect preventing the release of oxytocin, because the mammary gland and uterine response to injected oxytocin are not changed by alcohol. Studies on mothers with diabetes insipidus

Fig. 8-18. Plasma prolactin and growth hormone concentrations during nursing in postpartum women. Eight women were studied 8 to 41 days postpartum and six women 63 to 194 days postpartum. Prenursing prolactin levels in latter group were within normal range. Plasma growth hormone showed no change in any subjects during nursing. (From Noel GL, Suh HK, Frantz AG: *J Clin Endocrinol Metab* 38:413, 1974.)

suggest that the patient retains the ability to synthesize and release oxytocin despite being unable to produce antidiuretic hormone (ADH, vasopressin) in response to stimuli. Artificial cervical dilatation postpartum will also cause milk ejection. Vaginal stimulus also initiates let-down in all species.

Injection of oxytocin reproduces the effect of suckling. A rapid series of injections of 1 to 10 mU intravenously will simulate suckling. A continuous drip is less effective. Use of Pitocin as a snuff or nasal spray is the best method for home use of oxytocin to initiate let-down. The oxytocin concentration in the blood rises with suckling, which supports the hypothesis that suckling elicits the release of oxytocin.

The data on the question of ADH release during suckling are contradictory, but it would seem release of oxytocin and of ADH are independent.

The mammary myoepithelium is stimulated to contract by oxytocin, and the milk-ejection reflex results in the contraction of the myoepithelium and

the release, or let-down, of milk (Fig. 8-17). In the first weeks of lactation, the threshold dose of oxytocin to cause let-down is very low, averaging 0.65 mU from the fifth day. Thirty days after weaning it is 100 mU. Vasopressin is not as effective and requires 100 times the dosage of oxytocin to produce the same effect during lactation. Deaminooxytocin is 1.5 times as potent as oxytocin on the third postpartum day, but the difference disappears over time, probably because of the rapid breakdown of natural oxytocin by oxytocinase early in the postpartum period.

Prostaglandins (PGs) have been shown to have a number of physiologic effects, including an effect on mammary epithelium to increase mammary duct pressure.[161] In a blind crossover study, oxytocin, intravenous (IV) PG, and nasal PG were given and the intraductal pressures measured. The most effective IV PGs were 16-phenoxy-PGE$_2$ and PGF$_{2\alpha}$, which were then tried nasally, but only PGF$_{2\alpha}$ was effective nasally. The potential of nasal PGF$_{2\alpha}$ treatment in engorgement and failure of let-down is possible but is as yet unexplored clinically.[22]

Practical aspects of milk-ejection reflex

When the nipple is stimulated, the receptors in the nipple and areola are stimulated, and nervous impulses are transmitted to the hypothalamus via the somatic afferent nerves. The hypothalamus stimulates the pituitary gland to secrete prolactin, which induces the alveoli in the breast to secrete milk. The cell membranes release fat globules and protein into the lumen. This produces the hind milk, which has a higher protein and fat content. Part of the foremilk has been present since the previous nursing and is released first. It is a more dilute, less fatty solution that empties into the lactiferous sinuses awaiting the next suckling. The ejection reflex induces the holocrine excretion of milk from the cells. The posterior pituitary gland secretes oxytocin, which stimulates the myoepithelial cells to contract and eject the milk from the ducts.[162]

Early in lactation, if there is marked engorgement, the ejection reflex may be inhibited by the congested blood flow to the target organ, the myoepithelial cell. Therefore, when suckling is initiated and oxytocin is released into the bloodstream, it is delayed in reaching the myoepithelial cell with the message because of vascular congestion. Preparing the breast with warm soaks, gentle massage, and manual expression of a little milk may facilitate let-down.

Newton[110] has studied the milk-ejection reflex and clearly shows the effect of distraction on the let-down reflex. Distractions included immersing feet in ice water (reported to be the worst); being asked mathematic questions in rapid series, which resulted in electric shock if a wrong answer was given; or having painful traction on the big toe (Table 8-3). In practice, pain, stress, and mental anguish interfere with let-down in some mothers. When simple adjustments such as making the mother more comfortable, playing soft music, or leaving the mother in a quiet room do not work, other techniques should be tried.

Gentle stroking of the breast may help to decrease anxiety and stimulate flow. Use of tactile

TABLE 8-3	Milk-ejection reflex*	
Maternal disturbance	**Mean amount of milk obtained by infant (g)**
No distractions (no injection)	168
Distraction (saline injection)	99
Distraction (oxytocin injection)	153

Modified from Newton M, Newton N: *J Pediatr* 91:1, 1977.
*Interrupted milk flow can be restarted with hormone injection.

warmth as opposed to cold may improve release. Ice should not be used to make the nipple erect because it interferes with let-down. Cold is known to interrupt the neuropathway and cause vasoconstriction.[111]

Drug-enhanced lactation

The most direct therapy to enhance let-down is oxytocin. When simple supportive measures fail, this can be prescribed at home as a nasal spray. Oxytocin is no longer available as a packaged nasal spray and must be obtained by prescription as Pitocin, a synthetic oxytocin. Oxytocin is a polypeptide hormone of the posterior pituitary gland; the synthetic preparation avoids the risk of contamination with vasopressin (ADH). The hormone is destroyed by gastric juices and is not effective orally. The available preparation is intended for intramuscular (IM) or IV use and contains 10 units of oxytoxic hormone per milliliter. It is packaged in 10-ml multidose vials containing a total of 100 U. The original nasal spray, Syntocinon, contained 40 U/ml. The prescription is for a 10-ml nasal spray or nasal dropper. The dose is 1 or 2 sprays or 2 to 4 drops in the nares, followed by feeding or pumping within 2 to 3 minutes. The dose may be repeated in the other nares if let-down falters or the infant is nursed on the other breast. In most cases it is effective within one or two feedings, and the prescription rarely needs refilling. Let-down usually will continue without medication.

Aono et al[9] have suggested that sulpiride be given orally to mothers who produce less than

50 ml of total milk yield in the first 48 hours of lactation. Sulpiride is known to stimulate secretion of prolactin. In a control study of 96 normal primiparas and multiparas with poor lactation, half were given 50 mg sulpiride twice daily from the fourth to the seventh day postpartum, and half received a placebo. There was no difference in milk production in the multiparas but a significant difference in the primiparas, who had higher milk yield, higher prolactin levels, and higher percentage still breastfeeding at 1 month in the treated group. Although such medication should not be given unless routine techniques for increasing milk production have failed, occasional indications exist.

Other studies[24,42] have shown the efficacy of metoclopramide in enhancing milk production in women pumping for infants unable to nurse or in women whose infants have significant failure to thrive because of inadequate milk supply. The dose is metoclopramide 10 mg three times a day until milk volume increases (i.e., 4 to 6 days, then taper over 4 to 6 days). When the infant is actively suckling, this stimulus is usually adequate. Mothers who are pumping for a premature or ill infant may find the effect totally disappears when the drug is discontinued. The original studies did not explore long-term use. Metoclopramide is used in adults for various forms of reflux for 4 to 12 weeks. It is also used for reflux in infants, especially premature newborns (0.1 to 0.5 mg/kg body weight/day). The amount transferred to the infant through breast milk is reported as only 28 to 157 μg/L (1 to 13 μg/kg/day). Side effects are uncommon but tend to be dose related (i.e., greater than 40 mg/day in adults). Mothers may experience diarrhea, sedation, or nausea, but no symptoms have been observed in neonates. The extrapyramidal tract symptoms are associated with large doses of metoclopramide. Caution should be used in hypertensive women.

The let-down reflex has been associated with headache, which occurs transiently at time of initial let-down and then on changing breasts, related to surges in oxytocin.

Nausea has also been associated with let-down and specifically with release of oxytocin. Women compare it with the waves of nausea of pregnancy. Treatment is taking food before initiating the let-down and breastfeeding. Dry crackers work well. The symptom is more effectively prevented than cured.

Marshall et al[98] used thermal probes on the mother and infant to document hot flashes. Skin conductance increased, followed by increased skin temperature. Women also experienced night sweats and hot flashes during lactation, especially in the early weeks postpartum. They were most notable during night feedings.

Hospitals have gradually returned to "rooming-in" or birthing centers for uncomplicated deliveries.[87,138] Easy access of an infant to the mother has been shown to facilitate lactation success. The value of a well-trained, knowledgeable, empathetic nursing staff should not be underestimated. The knowledge and attitude of the staff have been one of the most important variables in successful breastfeeding.

POSTNATAL PERIOD

The family's transition from hospital to home can be stressful.[167] The parents hear the infant, who has been passive and content, wake up and cry for the first time. Because of all the procedures necessary to discharge an infant from the hospital (discharge physicals, blood tests, etc.), the well-planned discharge is often delayed and everyone is frantic, including the infant. The mother should be reassured about this and not be alarmed if she has to feed the infant frequently the first day at home.

The role of the clock

Many women today who work in demanding careers live by the clock and have trouble when advised to let a new baby give the cues. Anthropologist Millard[102] examined pediatric advice on breastfeeding and noted that major textbooks on pediatrics focus on timing. She points out that "Once the clock is seen as inherent in human behavior, adherence to the timetable becomes a

TABLE 8-4	Mammalian care patterns and composition of species milk						
	Pinnipedia: seal, sea lion	Tree shrew	Rabbit	Rat	Black rhinoceros*	Chimpanzee	Human
Infant care pattern	Return to ocean after birth	—	Cache	Carry, hibernate	—	Carry	?
Feeding interval	Once a week	48 hr	24 hr	Continuous	—	Continuous	?
Composition of milk							
Total solids (%)	62-65	20	33-40	21	8.1	11.9	12.4
Protein (%)	8-14	11	14-23	10	0.0	3.7	3.8
Fat (%)	53	6.5	18	8	1.4	1.2	1.2
Carbohydrate (%)	0-0.90	3.2	2.0	2.6	6.1	7.0	7.0

*The rhinoceros has an anatomic variation in the stomach that provides four pouches that fill during a feeding and provide a constant trickle of milk to the central groove leading to the small intestine, thus creating a constant feed.

standard for judging competence, adequacy, and normality." The clock is a central touchstone in our cultural system. Pediatric literature reinforces pressures on women regarding their infants and leads pediatricians to a role of shaping public views of infancy, motherhood, and humanity in general. In breastfeeding the pediatrician can help the mother break her bonds to timing and move to the central issues of successful breastfeeding.

Feeding frequency

Many hospital schedules are on a 4-hour feeding program based on the feedings of bottle-fed infants, whose slow emptying time of the stomach with formulas requires up to 4 hours. The emptying time for breast milk is about 1½ hours; thus frequent feedings are not unusual. Pediatric textbooks at the turn of the century described 10 to 12 feedings a day as normal.[80] Comparison of mammalian care patterns and composition of their milk shows an inverse relationship between protein content and frequency of feedings. From this it might be deduced that the human infant might need to be fed more frequently than every 4 hours (Table 8-4).[92] Infants who sleep 5 to 6 hours at a stretch at night may make up for skipped feedings during the day.

When milk intake and feeding patterns of thriving, exclusively breastfed infants were documented from birth for the first 4 months of life by Butte et al,[27] two feeding patterns emerged. In one the authors describe the feedings as distributed throughout the 24-hour day. In the other, feedings were excluded from midnight to 6 AM, although all infants were feeding ad lib. Total intake was the same in 24 hours. Milk intake per feeding decreased over the day. Frequency and duration declined over the 4-month period. Weight gain was similar in the two groups.

The pattern of intake during a feeding is different between breastfed and bottle-fed infants. A bottle-feeding infant sucks steadily in a linear pattern, receiving 81% of the feed in 10 minutes. Howie et al[69] showed that a breastfed infant has a biphasic pattern, which includes the first 4 minutes on the first breast and the first 4 minutes on the second breast (between 15 and 19 minutes into the feed). The infant receives 84% of the total volume in those 8 minutes. In another study, 50% of the feed on each breast was consumed in 2 minutes and 80% to 90% by 5 minutes.[93] Milk flow was minimal during the last 5 minutes. All these observations were made on the fifth to seventh day (Fig. 8-19).

Switch nursing is often suggested to increase

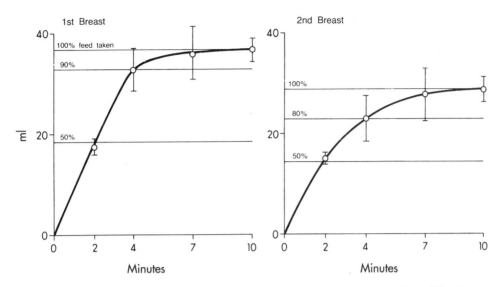

Fig. 8-19. Mother-infant pattern of milk flow. (From Lucas A, Lucas PJ, Baum JD: *Lancet* 2:57, 1979.)

total intake of an infant when milk production needs stimulating, especially if the infant is not gaining adequately (Fig. 8-19), but this may be counterproductive. When mothers fed 10 minutes on each breast (10×10), they produced the same amount of milk as they did nursing 5 minutes on a side and switching back ($5 \times 5 \times 5 \times 5$). The suckling-induced prolactin is similar with both patterns as well. A major concern of switch nursing is not feeding long enough on either breast to obtain the full calories of hindmilk. Even if volume is improved by this, total calories may be decreased. The infants do not nurse for a full 20 minutes in some cases, and the nutritive feeding time is under 15 minutes. The duration of the feeding should be determined by the infant's response and not by time.

The wide range in breast milk volume in well-nourished mothers was shown by Dewey and Lönnerdal[39] to be a variation in infant "demand" rather than an inadequacy of milk production. They stimulated milk production with postfeeding pumping for 2 weeks, but the infants failed to continue to take more than previously. Although milk production was augmented by pumping, the infants regulated their own intake.

New mothers are often most insecure and most concerned about lack of scheduling, especially if an ad lib program of feeding has been suggested. Other mothers seem to thrive on random scheduling. Some physicians continue to instruct mothers rigidly about adhering closely to a schedule designed for the bottle-fed infant. This can lead to failure of lactation unless the mother is sufficiently confident to follow her infant's demands and feed more frequently.[80]

Breastfed infants do not differ from bottle-fed infants at 3 and 5 months of age in terms of the number of night feedings. At 3 months, breastfed infants spend about 20 minutes less time at night sleeping and 20 minutes less time during the day, according to Alley and Rogers.[3]

When a mother expresses concerns about frequent feedings and worries about the adequacy of her milk (she is often disturbed that it looks so thin and blue after the luxurious color of colostrum), Jackson suggests she keep a record of feeding times and duration, as well as sleep and wakeful times.[16] If a chart is kept, the mother is usually surprised to find how quickly her infant develops a schedule. Often the infant is sleeping longer than she thought. The chart is also reassuring to the physician, especially if weight gain is marginal. In some cases it will highlight a problem not previously identified, such as a poor gainer who sleeps all night, missing several feedings. This approach serves to refocus attention on the infant and cues and not on the clock.

Milk production is influenced by the frequency, intensity, and duration of suckling by the infant, especially in the early postpartum period. Infant birthweight has been associated with the volume of milk intake. Greater suckling strength, frequency, and duration of feedings apparently play a part, according to cross-cultural studies by Prentice et al.[127] Self-regulation of milk intake has been studied by several investigators with similar conclusions. When mothers increased their milk supply by pumping after a feed, infants took a little extra milk for a few days but gradually dropped back to their previous intake. Residual milk volumes were noted by Dewey and Lönnerdal[39] to average about 100 g/day when women compared the amount extracted by pump with the infant's intake. The volume available in the second breast in a given feeding is about 60% of the volume of the first breast.

The mother's age and parity have little effect on milk production once full lactation is established. The data available from adolescent women are sparse, but healthy well-nourished adolescents produce adequate milk for normal growth of their infants. Stress and acute illness have been associated with decreased volumes, especially in relationship to poor let-down.

One-breast / two-breast feedings

The dogma of over 50 years had been that an infant should feed at both breasts at each feeding until the case report of Woolridge and Fisher[183] concerning an infant who failed to thrive when fed both breasts at each nursing. The authors demonstrated that this mother did not produce high-fat milk until well into the feeding; thus switching to the second side deprived the infant of fat-rich, calorie-rich milk. Confining the feeding to a single breast solved the problem. The authors also pointed out that consuming volumes of low-fat milk meant relatively high-lactose milk, which caused diarrhea and further calorie loss.

When a study compared the two patterns of feeding in 12 mother-infant pairs, Woolridge et al[185] found that the two patterns led to different milk volumes and mean feed-fat concentrations. The mean fat intake in 24 hours, however, was the same. Infants appeared to regulate their fat intake quickly; thus the authors recommended "baby-led" feeding. In other words, the mother should initiate feeding at one breast and continue until the infant discontinues feeding. If, after burping, the infant wants more, the mother offers the second side. The next feeding time is started on the opposite breast. Other investigators report similar findings.[139]

These studies and observations were done after the infants were 1 month of age.[139,183] When a mother is establishing her milk supply in the first days and weeks, switching to the second breast for each feed allows frequent, short stimuli to both the breasts. If an infant drifts to sleep after the first side and will not latch on the second side, the infant should be started on the "second side" when waking for the next feeding. Most successful nursing mothers adapt to their own infants' cues instead of following arbitrary rules. Switching prevents full hindmilk fat production and lowers energy content. More high-calorie milk may be produced by nursing at only one breast per feeding.

The identification of a factor that exerts a direct and local inhibitory action on further milk synthesis may explain why some women nurse only on one breast as a cultural mode. In situations where the infant rejects one breast,[127] some inhibition of milk production may precipitate the rejection. The inhibitory factor decreases the production in the "abandoned" breast while the other breast continues to function and totally sustain the infant's growth. There is no reason a woman cannot continue nursing on one breast indefinitely. This has been suggested in cases of recurrent mastitis in one breast that is unresponsive to repeated antibiotic therapy.

Van Geddren and Goosen[163] describe two cases of unilateral breastfeeding. A 41-year-old woman had nursed seven infants only on the left breast following an abscess in the right breast early with the first child. A mammogram while nursing her youngest, 18-month-old infant showed the left breast apparently lactating and the unused right breast normal and nonlactating. A 27-year-old mother was breastfeeding her second child, 2 years old, when mammography was done. The feeding breast appeared to be lactating, and the unused breast was larger and cystic. She had also nursed only on the left breast for 4 years with the first child.

Adequate rest

If nursing is not going well, a common cause of problems is maternal fatigue. The mother may need to be ordered by her physician to nap and rest. She must learn to nap when the infant is napping. This becomes more difficult with other young children, but a simultaneous nap for all the little ones and mother may have to be planned. Otherwise, she may have to go to bed with the children at night and just concentrate on resting and feeding the infant. When the need for rest is acute, the father should be assigned infant care, with the possible inclusion of bottle or cup feeding in extreme cases, while the mother sleeps undisturbed for a few hours.

Sore breasts and plugged ducts

Tender lumps in the breasts in a mother who is otherwise well are probably caused by plugging of a collecting duct. Some women on high-calcium diets have excreted grains of white sand that are thought to be calcium stones plugging a duct. The best treatment is to continue nursing. Manually massaging the area to initiate and ensure complete drainage should be recommended. Hot packs before feedings may help. If the breast is especially tender, initiating nursing on the opposite breast first permits the affected breast to let-down without the pressure of suckling. The affected breast should be completely emptied by nursing or manual expression. The brassiere may be cutting off an alveolus because of pressure from a narrow strap. Changing the infant's position may also help. Gentle persistent massage to relieve the lump usually clears the problem.

Repeated plugging

When plugging is recurrent, one needs to look for a major cause, such as exhaustion and fatigue. Several women have come to my attention who have had repeated lumps in their breasts with poor flow of milk, often as if the ducts were plugged. The condition responded fairly well to manual expression before each feeding, often with the expulsion of small plugs. These plugs were fatty, in contrast to the hard white "grains of sand." The condition dramatically improved by limiting the mother to polyunsaturated fats and adding lecithin to the diet. It was also necessary for subsequent pregnancies in all three cases. Lecithin, a lipid constituent of human milk, is an oily substance that can be used as an oil on salads or taken by spoon, 1 tablespoon per day.

Galactocele

Milk-retention cysts are uncommon and, when found, are almost exclusively a problem in lactating women. The contents at first are pure milk. Because of fluid absorption, they later contain thick, creamy, cheesy, or oily material. The swelling is smooth and rounded, and compression of it may cause milky fluid to exude from the nipple. Galactoceles are believed to be caused by the blockage of a milk duct. The cyst may be aspirated to avoid surgery but will fill up again. It can be removed surgically under local anesthesia without stopping the breastfeeding. Its presence does not require cessation of lactation. A firm diagnosis can be made by ultrasound; a cyst and milk will appear the same, whereas a tumor will be distinguishable.

Figs. 8-20 and 8-21 illustrate mammography of the lactating breast.

White bleb on nipple (white dot)

Often described as a "white dot," a white bleb on the nipple has frequently been a source of considerable discomfort for the mother and concern for the health professional. The solitary bleb appears on the surface of the nipple, usually at the opening of a duct; has a shiny, smooth surface; and is a millimeter or less in diameter. The mother usually describes exquisite pinpoint pain when the baby nurses. The bleb does not break or disappear with proper grasp and suckling. It may be "cured" or disappear when the health professional opens it with a sterile needle. It may reappear and have to

be opened again. The bleb probably represents a small pressure cyst formed at the end of the duct from milk seeping into this very elastic tissue. The bleb is different from the sucking blister that appears early in lactation associated with vigorous suckling or malposition. The blister covers a larger area and is not associated with a duct or exquisite pain. The bleb also should be distinguished from thrush, especially if there is more than one. Although a nipple with thrush usually is pink and painful with suckling, a nipple can have small caseous lesions similar to oral thrush. This requires specific treatment for *Candida albicans*.

Breast rejection

Infants have been observed to reject the breast intermittently, most often at 3 to 4 months, and then to go back after several feedings or a day or

Fig. 8-20. Normal breast tissue visualized by mammography. Tissue is one third fat and appears cystic in nature. (Courtesy Dr. Wende Logan-Young.)

so. A bottle can be substituted, or cup feedings as described in Chapter 14. Total rejection of both breasts may follow the return of menstruation. A mother will notice that the infant will reject the breast for a day or so with each period. Other infants seem unaffected. Strong foods in the diet may cause rejection of milk, which usually occurs 8 to 12 hours after ingestion and disappears by 24 hours after ingestion. Occasionally, one breast is permanently rejected so that the milk supply dwindles. One-breast nursing is done, as noted previously.

Refusal to nurse may not be a nursing strike or abrupt weaning. It may be a change in milk flavor.

Onions and garlic have been cited as culprits and vindicated by research, but a case was reported of refusal to nurse after maternal ingestion of mint candies in especially large quantity.[47] Strong flavors may pass into the milk. A dietary history including beverages and herbs is an important part of searching out problems. (Nursing strikes are discussed in Chapter 10.)

Unilateral breast rejection

Some infants prefer one breast and even refuse the other. When this occurs, manual expression or softening the nipple for easier grasp may help, thus enticing the infant to suckle. Holding the infant in

Fig. 8-21. Breast tissue during pregnancy and lactation is visualized by mammography. Fat is replaced by lactation tissue and presents a solid appearance. Tumors would be easily distinguished by this procedure in the lactating breast. Mammography is a safe, noninvasive technique that does not interfere with nursing. (Courtesy Dr. Wende Logan-Young.)

Fig. 8-22. This 38-year-old patient's craniocaudal view shows segmental duct draining a lobe in medial aspect of right breast. Ductal patterns differ among women. (From Logan-Young W, Hoffman NY: *Breast cancer: a practical guide to diagnosis,* vol 1, *Procedures,* Rochester, NY, 1994, Mt. Hope.)

TABLE 8-5	**Comparison of findings of engorgement, plugged duct, and mastitis**		
Characteristics	**Engorgement**	**Plugged duct**	**Mastitis**
Onset	Gradual, immediately postpartum	Gradual, after feedings	Sudden, after 10 days
Site	Bilateral	Unilateral	Usually unilateral
Swelling and heat	Generalized	May shift; little or no heat	Localized, red, hot, swollen
Pain	Generalized	Mild but localized	Intense but localized
Body temperature	<38.4° C (101° F)	<38.4° C	>38.4° C
Systemic symptoms	Feels well	Feels well	Flulike symptoms

the same position (i.e., on same side in same direction, so-called football hold) for the other breast may lead the infant to take the second breast. Sometimes applying syrup to the rejected nipple will help. Unilateral breastfeeding is a custom in some parts of China. Sodium and chloride levels

may rise in milk after mastitis. It is wise to taste the milk or have sodium and chloride levels measured in milk from both breasts if the problem persists to be sure no reason exists for the rejection.

Goldsmith[53] reported five cases of lactating women whose infants suddenly rejected a single breast. Weeks or months later the mother noted a mass, and biopsy revealed a malignancy. It would be wise to examine any patient who complains of unilateral breast rejection that does not respond to simple measures to rule out a tumor. Ultrasound followed by a mammogram, if necessary, can be performed without discontinuing lactation.

Mastitis

Mastitis is an infectious process in the breast producing localized tenderness, redness, and heat, together with systemic reactions of fever, malaise, and sometimes nausea and vomiting. It no longer occurs in epidemics, as once seen in hospitals before the common use of antibiotics and when hospital stays were prolonged for normal childbirth. The infection, however, may be hospital acquired if the mother or infant is colonized with virulent bacteria before leaving the hospital.

Little appears in the medical literature about mastitis because women are rarely hospitalized for the problem and are treated at home and, in some cases, over the telephone. When staphylococcal disease was a major problem on postpartum wards, lactating and nonlactating women alike developed mastitis; thus the differentiation of two types: acute puerperal mammary *cellulitis,* a nonepidemic mastitis involving interlobular connective tissue, and acute puerperal mammary *adenitis,* which was epidemic and associated with an outbreak of skin infections in infants.

The current definition of *mastitis* includes fever of 38.5° C (101° F) or more, chills, flulike aching, systemic illness, and a pink, tender, hot, swollen, wedge-shaped area of the breast[114] (Fig. 8-22). Table 8-5 lists the significant differential points among mastitis, engorgement, and plugged duct.

The portal of entry of the disease is through the lactiferous ducts to a secreting lobule, through a nipple fissure to periductal lymphatics, or through hematogeneous spread. The common organisms involved include *Staphylococcus aureus, Escherichia coli,* and (rarely) *Streptococcus.* Tuberculous mastitis does occur, and the infant often develops tuberculosis of the tonsils. In populations

where tuberculosis is endemic, it occurs in about 1% of cases of mastitis.[55]

Factors predisposing the woman to mastitis include poor drainage of a duct and then of an alveolus, presence of an organism, and lowered maternal defenses such as those associated with stress and fatigue (Figs. 8-23 and 8-24). Insufficient emptying and obstruction of ducts by tight clothing can cause plugged ducts, which can be prevented from becoming mastitis if identified early and treated vigorously with local massage, moist heat, and rest. Missing a feeding or having the infant suddenly sleep through the night may cause engorgement, plugging, and then mastitis.[140] Cracked or painful nipples may herald a problem, more because the mother avoids complete emptying on the painful side than because bacteria suddenly gain access.

Devereux[38] described 20 years of experience with 53 lactating patients who experienced 71 acute attacks of mastitis. The highest incidence was in the second and third weeks postpartum. No infant was weaned because of the mastitis. No infants were sick in association with the mastitis. All but five mothers nursed subsequent infants. Six patients had mastitis with other pregnancies. Eight of 71 patients (11.1%) developed abscesses, six of which required incision and drainage. The bacterial cause was not stated. When treatment was delayed beyond 24 hours, the abscess rate increased.

Another series of 65 cases of mastitis, reported by Marshall et al,[97] showed a 2.5% incidence of the disease among a population of 2534 lactating women. *S. aureus* was the offending organism in 23 of the 48 infected breasts that were cultured. In 19 normal (no mastitis) lactating women, only one grew this organism. Of the 65 women, 41 continued to nurse without difficulty for an average of 13 weeks longer. Three breast abscesses for a rate of 4.6% occurred in women who had chosen to wean. Onset was 5½ weeks postpartum (range 5 days to 1 year). Of the 65, nine had missed feedings or acutely weaned, eight women had noticed a fissured nipple before the infection, and the others were unanticipated. Treatment included 41 with penicillin V, 12 with ampicillin, and 8 with other antibiotics. Mastitis recurred in four of the women who continued to nurse.

Half the patients with mastitis in a series reported by Niebyl et al[114] were infected with *S. aureus,* as determined by culture. They were treated with antibiotics, continued nursing on both sides, and observed no abscesses or problems in the infant. Investigators in The Gambia[129] observed mastitis in 2.6% of women, with recurrence common. They noted the milk was deficient in immunoglobulin A, complement C3, and lactoferrin when compared with that of other lactating mothers. The authors suggested these mothers were predisposed to mastitis. Coagulase-negative staphylococci isolated from the milk of mothers with mastitis has been shown to cause experimental acute mastitis when injected into mice and should be considered a possible etiologic agent in nursing women.[160]

Although breastfed infants usually remain well during bouts of acute mastitis in their mothers, Katzman and Wald[78] reported a case of scalded skin syndrome in an infant fed by a mother with mastitis that did not respond to ampicillin for 14

Fig. 8-23. This 39-year-old patient's ductogram shows a single segmental duct *(small arrow)* draining a lobe (a segment) from medial aspect of right breast, which joins a single segmental duct *(large arrow)* draining a lobe from lateral aspect of right breast. These two segmental ducts merge to form lactiferous sinus *(open arrow* points to air bubble in lactiferous sinus). This ductogram demonstrates how five to seven lactiferous sinuses can accommodate drainage from 15 to 20 lobes (segments) in breast and suggests explanation for plugged ducts and distribution of breast infection. (From Logan-Young W, Hoffman NY: *Breast cancer: a practical guide to diagnosis,* vol 1, *Procedures,* Publishing Co., Rochester, 1994, Mt. Hope.)

days. The child responded to IV nafcillin. The mother had a lesion on her areola on the infected breast, and she was told to use breast shields, although she was to continue nursing. Breast shields have been shown to decrease breast emptying by half. This case points out the urgency of evaluating both the mother and the infant when mastitis or any breastfeeding problem occurs.

Using leukocyte counts and microbiologic counts, Thomsen et al[159] have separated breast inflammations into three clinical states: milk stasis (counts $<10^6$ leukocytes and $<10^3$ bacteria per milliliter of milk), noninfectious inflammation (counts of $>10^6$ leukocytes and $<10^3$ bacteria), and infectious mastitis (counts $>10^6$ leukocytes and $>10^3$ bacteria) (Tables 8-6 and 8-7). The authors concluded that no treatment was needed in stasis, but lack of treatment led to recurrence and lactation failure in noninfectious inflammation and abscess in mastitis. Emptying the breast (frequent feedings and pumping or hand-expressing three times a day after a feed) was sufficient in noninfectious inflammation and ameliorated the course in most cases of mastitis. However, recurrence was then inappropriately high. Mastitis requires antibiotics in addition to emptying the breast.[159]

Because cultures require time, when the bacteria count is finally available and the clinical course is clear, the noninfectious variety should already be cleared. Laboratory results are confirmatory; however, the skilled clinician can avoid the relapses and progression to abscess by close monitoring and selective aggressive treatment before the cultures are reported (Table 8-7).

Fig. 8-24.   Mastitis of right breast, upper outer quadrant.

TABLE 8-6   Categories of patients with inflammatory breast symptoms

Symptom	Leukocytes per milliliter of milk	Bacteria per milliliter of milk
Milk stasis	$<10^6$	$<10^3$
Noninfectious inflammation	$>10^6$	$<10^3$
Infectious mastitis	$>10^6$	$>10^3$

From Thomsen AC, Espersen T, Maigaard S: *Am J Obstet Gynecol* 149:492, 1984.

TABLE 8-7   Course of infectious mastitis with and without treatment

Treatment	Number of cases	Duration of symptoms (days, mean)	Result (number of cases) Normal lactation	Poor*
None	55	6.7	8	47
Emptying of breast	55	4.2	28	27
Antibiotics and emptying of breast	55	2.1	53	2

From Thomsen AC, Espersen T, Maigaard S: *Am J Obstet Gynecol* 149:492, 1984.
*Breast abscess, 6 cases; symptoms of sepsis, 12 cases; recurrence of symptoms, 21 cases; duration of >14 days, 10 cases; impaired lactation only, 27 cases.

In lactating Gambian women, unilateral breast dysfunction is not an unusual finding.[128] It has been attributed to episodes of low-grade mastitis with the production of high-sodium milk, which the infant rejects. The unused breast involutes, and the functioning breast increases production. In subsequent pregnancies, function returns to the involved breast.

The clinician must inform patients of the need to contact the office if any unusual symptoms occur so that proper management can be initiated early, because prevention is the most effective treatment. Inappropriately or inadequately treated cases of mastitis predispose the patient to chronic mastitis, which may last for months and require more antibiotics than would have been required initially. A mother should be instructed to contact her physician if she has local pain, heat, redness, or a fever while lactating. Red streaking on the breast may be inflammation of the lymphatics (Fig. 8-25).

Most series of acute mastitis clearly demonstrate that the cases that result in unfavorable outcome, including abscess and recurrent disease, had significant delay between onset of symptoms and request for medical advice.[100,159] When proper treatment is initiated promptly, the course of the

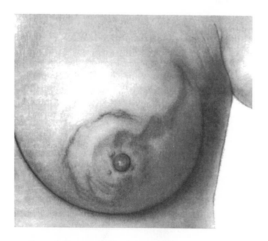

Fig. 8-25. Inflammation of lymphatics of breast demonstrating drainage of breast. Generalized infection of breast, especially staphylococcal, occasionally presents as lymph duct infection.

disease is usually brief; if treatment is delayed, prolonged antibiotics become necessary.

Recommended management regimen

1. Continue to nurse on both breasts, but start the infant on the unaffected side while the affected side "lets down." Be sure to empty the affected side by feeding or pumping.
2. Insist on bed rest (mandatory). The mother can take the infant to bed and obtain assistance for the care of other family members.
3. Choose an antibiotic that can be tolerated by the infant as well as the mother (avoid sulfa drugs when the infant is under 1 month). The decision should be based on local sensitivities and length of time since delivery or exposure to resistant flora.

Empiric therapy without cultures should consider the common organisms causing mastitis: *S. aureus* (50%), *E. coli* or other gram-negative organisms, group A streptococci, *Peptostreptococcus* species, and *Bacteroides species* (especially with abscesses). Less common organisms include *Candida albicans* and *Mycobacterium tuberculosis.* First-line antibiotics that are safe for the mother and infant include first-generation cephalosporins or dicloxacillin/oxacillin. Treatment of suspected gram-negative organisms include first-generation cephalosporins or amoxicillin/clavulanate (Augmentin). Treatment of abscesses should include some anaerobic coverage with Augmentin or clindamycin. Therapy for women with penicillin or cephalosporin allergy can include erythromycin or clindamycin. Suspected methicillin-resistant *S. aureus* (MRSA) can be treated with vancomycin, clindamycin, rifampin, or Teicoplanin, considering organism sensitivity.

An usual case of *Streptococcus pneumoniae* mastitis was reported in a 38-year-old woman who was partially breastfeeding her 9-month-old infant. Cultures of breast milk had more than 10^6 *S. pneumoniae* bacteria/ml milk. Cultures of the infant's nose and throat also grew *S. pneumoniae,* although he was asymptomatic.

Treatment was flucloxacillin. C-reactive protein was 177 mg/L at onset and 18.6 mg/L on day 6. The infant was presumed to have infected the mother.[187]

Regardless of the disease course, the antibiotic should be given for at least 10 to 14 days. Shorter courses are associated with a high incidence of relapse.

4. Apply ice packs or warm packs to the breast, whichever provides the most comfort. Experience indicates that heat provides drainage and pain relief.
5. Provide plenty of fluids for the mother.[120]
6. Give an analgesic such as acetaminophen or ibuprofen.
7. The mother should wear a supporting brassiere that does not cause painful pressure.

Recurrent or chronic mastitis and candidal infection

Recurrent mastitis is usually caused by delayed or inadequate treatment of the initial disease. If antibiotics are started, they should be continued for a minimum of 10 to 14 days. Often, because the mother feels better, she discontinues them on her own. At the first recurrence, cultures should be sent of the midstream clean-catch specimen of breast milk and the infant's nasopharynx and oropharynx. The patient should be seen and the circumstances completely reviewed. An aggressive course of rest, nourishment, stress management, and complete drainage of the breast by suckling or pumping should be initiated. The antibiotics should be carefully selected and maintained for 2 weeks. Fluids should be increased. Failure of the second treatment is usually caused by failure to complete the entire treatment, which may also mean failure to get adequate rest and build up maternal resistance.

When the mastitis continues to recur, several possible reasons exist: chronic bacterial infection, secondary fungal infection, or underlying breast disease such as a cyst or tumor. If it is chronic bacterial disease, low-dose antibiotics can be instituted for the duration of lactation (erythromy-

cin, 500 mg daily). Fungal infection is usually diagnosed by the nature of the pain, which is described as fiery throbbing pain along the duct system. Both mother and infant need treatment. If the infection is always in the same breast, examination of the breast for a unilateral unchanging lump or mass may indicate cyst, galactocele, or tumor. (The lactating breast is "lumpy," but the lumps are ever changing.) Needle aspiration or biopsy may be indicated.

A secondary complication of recurrent mastitis is invasion of the breast by a yeast infection or a fungus such as *Candida albicans* (see Chapter 16), as is frequently seen after antibiotic treatment. Mothers describe the incredible pain when the infant nurses as feeling like hot cords burning in their chest wall. This is usually fungal infection of the ducts. The best treatment is to massage nystatin cream (Mycostatin) or Mycolog, which also contains cortisone, into the nipple and areola after each feeding. The infant should also be given oral nystatin simultaneously, or the mother will be reinfected, even if the infant has no lesions. If the mother is known to have a recurrent vulvovaginitis, initiation of nystatin prophylactically should be considered when the antibiotics are begun. Although the infant may or may not have oral thrush or a diaper rash, he or she should be treated. The nipple may not look unusual despite exquisite pain.

The incidence of fungal infections has increased dramatically in the past decade, probably because of the widespread use of antibiotics, which obliterate the normal flora credited with keeping fungal growth under control.[41] Young women often have vaginal yeast infections, which serve as a reservoir of infection. Milk is an excellent culture medium for the fungi, which thrive on carbohydrates. An infant may acquire the fungus during vaginal birth, becoming colonized and inoculating the breast during breastfeeding. The disease state flares up after a course of antibiotics.

Although the problem of fungal mastitis has been well recognized in dairy cattle, reports have only recently been creeping into the medical literature. A single case of cryptococcal mastitis in a 31-year-old (para 6), formerly breastfeeding woman with a long past lactation history of painful mass in the breast has been reported.[168] Subsequent removal revealed a granuloma that showed cryptococci. She had a recurrence 4 months later in the opposite breast. She then was treated with a systemic ketoconazole after removal of the granuloma and confirmation of continuing infection.

In a review of breast infections[121] from 1969 to 1982 in 17,000 cases seen at a mammary gland disease clinic, four cases of candidal mastitis were seen, all in lactating multiparas, 14 to 24 days postpartum. Two were diabetics. Severe pruritus was described but no fever or general malaise. Cytologic and culture confirmation was made of *C. albicans*. The author treated the patients with local and oral antimycotics. Lactation was stopped with bromocriptine in these cases. Past antibiotic thrush infection has been associated with initial pruritus that degenerates to pain. Newer antifungal preparations are evolving from the azole family of antifungals. They are safer than amphotericin. Ketoconazole and miconazole have been replaced by fluconazole.[49] Fluconazole is effective against cryptococcosis, *Candida,* coccidioidomycosis, and other fungi. On the horizon are other triazoles as interest and effort in treating fungal infections have increased because of the risk in human immunodeficiency virus (HIV) infections.

Miconazole oral gel can be used for treating both the breast and the infant's mouth for at least 2 weeks. Gentian violet liquid (0.25% to 0.5%) can be used. It is applied to the nipple and areola and to the infant's mouth by swab three times a day and no longer than eight applications (3 days). It colors everything purple and masks the lesions. Clotrimazole can also be used. The prescription is for a 10-mg lozenge crushed and suspended in 5 g petrolatum or in 5 ml glycerine to make a topical ointment to be applied three times a day to the nipple and areola and orally to the infant's mouth (glycerine preparation only).[104]

Instructions to the mother should also include recommendations to treat any vaginal yeast infection with local therapy, decrease concentrated ingestion of sweets, and add yogurt or acidophils to the diet. All clothing in contact with breasts and infant must be changed daily, washed, and dried in hot temperatures.

When the microbiology of 61 lactating women with burning nipple pain was compared with that of 64 lactating women without pain and 31 nonlactators, growth of *C. albicans* in the nipple and milk was identified in 19% of those with pain and 3% of those without pain and not among the nonlactators. *S. aureus* was associated with nipple pain and nipple fissures. The authors note the difficulty in actually culturing the fungus.[6]

For recurrent fungal infection of the breast when nystatin is no longer effective, a course of fluconazole (Diflucan) can be given orally, 200 mg loading dose with 100 mg/day for 14 days. Side effects (e.g., nausea, vomiting, diarrhea) in the mother are minimal. Although fluconazole does pass into the milk, it is approved for use at 6 months of age and has a safety profile for newborns. It is currently used in neonatal intensive care units. A single dose peaks in the milk at 2 hours, and the milk/plasma (M/P) ratio is less than 1. The infant should be maintained on nystatin to avoid relapse. Freezing pumped breast milk while infected with *Candida* does not kill the fungus. The milk must be pasteurized or discarded.

Abscess formation

Abscess can also be a complication of mastitis and is usually the result of delayed or inadequate treatment. A true abscess will require surgical drainage but should be treated with antibiotics, rest, warm soaks, and complete emptying of the breast at least every few hours.

The drainage should be cultured and sensitivities determined so that antibiotics can be adjusted accordingly. The increasing number of oxacillin-resistant *S. aureus* (ORSA) cases occurring in hospitals places women recently delivered or hospitalized at risk. An infection with ORSA may require vancomycin therapy, the only antibiotic effective against it. ORSA may start as an inflammation of the lymphatics (Fig. 8-25).

The milk will remain clean unless the abscess

ruptures into the ductal system. Usually it drains to the outside. Nursing can be maintained when the breast is surgically drained as long as the incision and drainage tube are sufficiently far from the areola so that they are not involved in feeding. In any event, the breast should be manually drained of milk frequently to maintain the milk supply until feeding can resume (sufficient healing usually occurs in 4 days). The infant can continue to feed on the unaffected side. The infant should always be monitored for infection, and simultaneous therapy should be initiated, especially with staphylococcal or streptococcal disease.

Isolated cases of abscesses, which have been drained surgically but also drain milk during a feeding or pumping, have been reported to the Lactation Study Center. With adequate systemic antibiotics and careful but thorough draining of the breast by suckling or pumping, healing gradually takes place even while the mother continues to lactate. When the drain is removed, the incision can be closed and breastfeeding resumed on that breast. The mother should be instructed to press firmly over the incision with sterile gauze to keep milk from flowing from the wound during feedings. The cause of this milk drainage is a severed milk duct, an unavoidable complication of draining a deep abscess. It will heal completely within 3 to 4 weeks. Rarely is weaning from the involved breast necessary.

Laboratory findings

Cultures of the breast milk, when indicated, should be done after the breast has been cleaned with water and the mother's hands have been thoroughly washed. The milk stream should be initiated by manual expression and the first 3 ml discarded to obtain a midstream clean-catch specimen. One should check for antibody coating in the bacteria found in the milk to confirm its relationship to the disease.[158] It is important to remember that the normal cell count of uninfected human milk is 1000 to 4000/mm^3. The presence of cells should not be automatically construed as infection.

A leukocyte count greater than 10^6/ml of milk is considered diagnostic, plus a bacterial count greater than 10^3 bacteria/ml of milk (Table 8-6).

The levels of sodium and chloride in milk from mastitic breasts have been reported in the literature to be extremely elevated (Na $\geq$100 mEq/L, Cl $\geq$80 mEq/L, potassium $\leq$10).[32] Usually, electrolyte abnormalities are associated with recurrent mastitis or chronic subclinical mastitis. The quickest screen for the problem is for the mother to compare the tastes of milk from each side.

Neonatal mastitis

Neonatal mastitis occurs infrequently, although it was a common event in the 1940s and 1950s, when staphylococcal disease was rampant in the nursery. It occurs in full-term infants 1 to 5 weeks of age and in as many females as males, usually unilaterally.[169] It is unrelated to maternal mastitis and usually occurs in bottle-fed infants. Before IV antibiotic therapy, surgical incision and drainage were common. Prognosis for cure is excellent. In recent years the rare cases that occur are seen in conjunction with manipulation of the neonatal breast to express the natural secretion when the breast is engorged (witch's milk).

Other causes of nipple and breast pain

Classification of mastalgia, or breast pain, includes *cyclic* (67% of cases), *noncyclic* (i.e., not related to menstrual cycle, 26% of cases), and *Tietze's syndrome* (painful lateral costochondral junction, 7%). Mastalgia in young women may spontaneously disappear with pregnancy. This has been associated with higher basal levels of prolactin (unrelated to lactation) and low plasma levels of essential fatty acid α-linolenic acid and its metabolites, which are important components of cell membranes. Administration of α-linolenic acid improves the pain, according to Gateley and Mansel.[50] Evening primrose oil (Efamast) is a rich source of α-linolenic acid. This is a safe, even nutritional, solution to the problem.

Ankyloglossia

The common causes of nipple pain associated with lactation include poor position, nipple sucking, nipple tipped up too much because of finger pressure above nipple, infant's lower lip sucked in and irritating the underside of nipple, and taking the infant off the breast without first breaking the suction. These should be ruled out as possible causes of breast pain. Then the infant should be checked. Although rare, tongue-tie or tight-tongue frenulum may be a cause. If the infant cannot protrude the tip of the tongue over the gums and the tip is tied to the floor of the mouth by a tight cord of a thick frenulum, and the tongue becomes heart shaped when lifted up, it is known as *ankyloglossia*. When the infant tries to draw the teat into the mouth, it will not be possible and nipple biting results. The physician should consider cutting the frenulum once the diagnosis of ankyloglossia (short lingual frenulum) is confirmed by oral examination[73,117] (Box 8-4). The procedure is simple, but the cut should be carefully placed to avoid the artery, nerve, and other anatomic sites. It is usually bloodless, and the infant can be nursed immediately, now in the correct position.

Eczema

Eczema of the nipple and sometimes also the areola and breast presents as a red, dry, sore, even burning, flaking rash, the flakes often appearing as "oily potato chips." Common causes are washing nipples with soap or applying ointments that have irritants. Some creams contain peanut oil, which should be avoided by those allergic to peanuts (the

most common allergy); lanolin, for those allergic to wool; and cocoa butter, for those allergic to chocolate. The physician should instruct the mother to remove all irritants, including breast shields and plastic-backed breast pads. Lesions usually clear quickly with proper treatment and avoiding the irritant.

Nipple blanching

Blanching of the nipples may cause burning pain during suckling. A vigorous "barracuda baby" can cause blanching of the nipple from pressure. Later in lactation (i.e., after 4 months, when teething begins), infants may bite down to relieve gum pain and cause nipple blanching and burning pain. The mother should be instructed to keep her finger ready to break the suction if pain becomes extreme.

Blanching of the nipple to pure white with no apparent mechanical cause can also occur. This has been associated with some maternal medications, such as theophylline and terbutaline. Other medications that cause vasoconstriction may be associated.

Factors that control vasomotor tone in the mammary gland have not been well studied. Mammary blood vessels are exquisitely sensitive to epinephrine and norepinephrine, as well as serotonin and PGF_{20C}, as vasoconstrictive agents.

Other causes of nipple blanching are cold, especially when ice is applied, and maternal smoking. Nicotine is a vasoconstrictor, as is caffeine, especially in sensitive individuals.

In some women, warm compresses to the areola before nursing will prevent the reaction and thus the pain. Not all cases of nipple blanching have been relieved by heat; some have been relieved by cold, which is actually contrary to usual physiologic theory (see Chapter 15).

Supplementary feedings

To supplement-feed a breastfed infant continues to be controversial in pediatric circles. For the normal full-term infant it is not necessary. Evaluation of serial blood glucoses in breastfed and bottle-fed infants from birth reported by Heck and Erenberg[59]

BOX 8-4   Identification of ankyloglossia (tongue-tie)

1. When tongue protrudes, tip is anchored behind alveolar ridge.
2. When infant cries, tongue remains anchored.
3. Tongue is notched or heart shaped when protruded.
4. Tongue cannot be manually extended by examiner.
5. Frenulum is short (less than 1 cm [½ inch]), and inelastic.
6. Tongue is attached close to alveolar ridge.

demonstrated a significant number of bottle-fed infants with hypoglycemia, presumed to be a rebound phenomenon from dextrose and water feeding early in life. Some breastfed infants had a value less than 40 on the second day. No significant differences were found in serum bilirubins and weight loss between supplemented and unsupplemented breastfed infants in Herrara's study.[61] At age 3 months a significant number of supplemented infants were no longer breastfeeding (still breastfeeding, 81% unsupplemented versus 53% supplemented). Even in hot, dry climates, water supplements were not found to be necessary.[4,13,52] Urine osmolarity remained within physiologic ranges in unsupplemented breastfed infants studied by Goldberg and Adams.[52] This has been demonstrated by a number of other investigators. The supplementation with water did not influence the "coming-in" of mother's milk, according to Schutzman et al.[146] They did observe, however, that infants in the group being supplemented took very little water after nursing (less than 4 oz in the first 3 days).

Many physicians suggest to mothers that a supplementary bottle can be added any time. Actually, when lactation is going well, it is not needed, and when it is not going well, a bottle may aggravate the problem. During hospitalization, giving a substitute bottle may confuse a new infant, who may be having trouble sucking at first. Infants who are given water or glucose water in the hospital do less well and usually lose more weight. A significant relationship exists between supplements in the hospital and early discontinuation of breastfeeding. It is a marker of impending trouble and of insufficient milk production, which is best treated with frequent feedings at the breast and some intervention from an experienced support person.

In a study by Gray-Donald et al[54] the effect of formula supplementation on outcome of breastfeeding was observed in two nurseries, one used as a control and the other supplemented. Mothers could request supplements in either group, and any baby put to the breast only twice was called "breastfed." It was clear that mothers who requested formula in the hospital and requested a going-home formula package were more likely to discontinue breastfeeding. They considered this early behavior a marker of high risk for failure. These patients,[54] therefore, should have received follow-up and considerable support when identified as high risk.

In a study by Cronenwett et al,[33] when infants were randomly selected to receive one bottle feeding per day between 2 weeks and 6 weeks of age, there was little difference compared to those exclusively breastfed. The study group received five bottles a week and the control group two. At 6 months, 59% of the five-bottle group were still breastfeeding, compared with 69% of the two-bottle group. These infants had no trouble switching back and forth. The authors[33] believed their study justified a casual approach to the bottle in breastfed infants and suggested that the difference between two bottles per week and five bottles was insignificant and proved that nipple confusion did not happen.

However, the use of complementary bottles, that is, those given after a breastfeeding to "top off" the feeding, is the beginning of a downhill course that may doom lactation to failure. It would be better to take the infant to breast more often or switch back to the first breast if the baby is hungry. If the mother must be away at feeding time, she can pump a feeding ahead of time and save it in the refrigerator or freezer for someone else to give by bottle. If this is not practical, a bottle of formula can be given. It can be made up from a formula powder more economically one feeding at a time, and there is no waste. Powder preparations have a long shelf life even when open and are better tolerated by the infant because lower temperatures are required to manufacture powders; thus there is no caramelizing of the sugars or denaturing of the proteins. A powder goes quickly into solution if the water is warm when mixing is attempted. (Prepare formula powder as follows: one scoop of powder to 2 oz of warm water gives 20 kcal/oz).

Solid foods

Successful nursing mothers are rarely impatient to start the baby on solid foods, as bottle-feeding mothers frequently are. Milk, and especially human milk, supplies the appropriate nutrients. At about 6 months a normal infant begins to use iron stores, and this is probably an appropriate time to start solid foods, especially iron-containing ones. This permits the entire process of weaning to cup and solid foods to be gradual. An infant does not need teeth to eat baby food and, conversely, does not have to be weaned from the breast because teeth have erupted. By 6 months the number of feedings usually has decreased, and the timing and volume are beginning to cycle to a schedule that resembles three meals a day and some snacks. A breastfed infant should start some solids by 6 months of age.

Carrying and holding

Carrying and holding young infants have been considered by some in the era of peak bottle feeding as predisposing to spoiling the infants. In many cultures around the world, infants are carried with the mother night and day.[96] In Western cultures, infants are tightly swaddled, that is, wrapped up like a package and put down. In a randomized controlled study of primiparous breastfeeding women, Hunziker and Barr[71] showed that increased carrying reduces infant crying and colicky behavior. The authors concluded that lack of carrying predisposes to crying and colic. A study among young mothers in New York City who were given infant carriers showed that carrying the infant was more apt to influence infant crying than breastfeeding in that population.

Sleeping

Sleeping through the night has been assumed to be an important developmental milestone dependent on maturation. Twenty-six first-time parents of exclusively breastfed infants were randomly assigned to a treatment or control group.[125] The treatment group was instructed to offer a "focal feed" between 10 PM and midnight and then offer reswaddling, diapering, walking, and rocking to postpone the next feeding to 5 AM, minimizing light

and sound. By 3 weeks the treated group was sleeping significantly longer. By 8 weeks, 100% of the treated group compared with 23% of control infants were sleeping at least from midnight to 5 AM. They fed more frequently during the day, especially early morning. Milk intakes for 24 hours between the two groups were not different. The authors[125] concluded that parents can teach their breastfed infants to lengthen nighttime sleep periods. Parents should be encouraged to develop management plans that they find most comfortable. Whether they share the family bed or keep the newborn in the same room or in the next room is their decision.

Milk composition influences infant sleep latency. Tryptophan concentrations are higher in human milk than in formula. Tryptophan is known to increase sleep in adults. When breastfed and formula-fed infants were compared using formulas with different levels of tryptophan, they had shorter sleep latency with high levels of tryptophan.[153]

Colic and crying

By definition, colic is spasmodic contractions of smooth muscle causing pain and discomfort. It can be experienced in many organs, such as the gastrointestinal or genitourinary tract, and at all ages. When the term *colic* is used in reference to infants, it usually means a syndrome in which the young infant has unexplained paroxysms of irritability, fussing, and crying for a prolonged period, often at the same time of day, in the early months of life. The infant usually draws the legs up as if in pain. A myriad of remedies are directed at various possible causes, including allergy, hypertonicity, and hormone withdrawal. It may be a matter of parenting style, however, and expectations that brings a parent to complain about colic. Colic does occur in premature infants but usually not until they reach 42 weeks' adjusted gestation.[63]

Infantile colic has been reported to occur equally among breastfed (20%), formula-fed (19%), and mixed breastfed and formula-fed (21%) infants in a study of almost 1000 infants.[1] The fecal α-antitrypsin and fecal hemoglobins were not different in colicky infants. There was no evidence of dietary protein hypersensitivity in this series.[157]

Characteristically, the infant will cry and scream as if in pain from 3 to 4 hours at a stretch, often between 6 PM and 10 PM at night. The infant will nurse frequently, then scream and pull away from the breast as if in pain, only to cry out a few minutes later. Sometimes the infant can be comforted by another adult such as the father or grandmother. The infant will respond to gentle rocking when held against a warm shoulder. If the infant is put down, the screaming starts again. If the nursing mother holds the infant, he or she is frantic unless nursed and yet does not need to be fed. This may disturb a new mother, who wonders why she cannot console her infant (Is her milk weak? Does it disagree with her infant? Is she an inadequate mother?). None of these options is true, but the infant smelling her milk makes the infant behave as if needing to nurse. Anyone who is not nursing can quickly quiet the infant. Picking the infant up does not spoil the child, and rocking and cuddling are appropriate. Warm pressure is usually palliative; a warm hot water bottle or warm shoulder with some pressure or massage is comforting. The use of rhythmic incessant sounds or lights (e.g., vacuum cleaner, untuned TV) has variable success.

A carefully taken history and physical examination are always in order to rule out other pathologic conditions, such at otitis media, anal fissure, hair tourniquet, or hernia before a diagnosis of colic is made. Hunger should be ruled out. Sometimes an infant who was just fed needs to be fed again. True colic, however, is characterized by an inconsolable infant who continues to fret, fuss, and cry out. If true colic is diagnosed because of the consistency of the screaming for several hours each day at the same time, treatment is in order.

Influence of cow's milk in maternal diet

The literature is not straightforward on the issue of the effect of cow's milk in the maternal diet and infantile colic. Talbot[155] first published information on congenital sensitization to food, especially eggs and cow's milk, in humans in 1918, which was manifested as clinical allergy in the breastfed infant. Research techniques are far superior today, and information is accumulating. Gerrard and Shenassa[51] report sensitization caused by substances in breast milk thought to be due to two types of food allergy; one is immunoglobulin E (IgE) mediated and triggered by trace amounts of antigen, and the other is not IgE mediated and is triggered by large amounts of antigen. Gastrointestinal (GI) transport of macromolecules in the pathogenesis of food allergy is under investigation, as is T-cell–mediated immunity in food allergy. However, the present state of scientific knowledge has not resolved the issue of colic and cow's milk for the clinician.

Clinical studies have been done to test the association of dairy products in the mother with colic in some breastfed babies. Jakobsson and Lindberg[74] described a cause-and-effect relationship in a group of 18 mothers in 1978, which was criticized because it was not a double-blind study. Evans et al[45] then reported that they found no such relationship when they did a double-blind crossover study in which mothers received cow's milk protein for 2 days and then a placebo for 2 days. Jakobsson and Lindberg[75] have repeated their work using a double-blind crossover study design in the mother-baby pairs in which the infants had colic; 35% of the infants improved on maternal diets free of cow's milk. A torrent of mail to the journals confirmed these conclusions in small clinical practice trials as well.

Jakobsson et al[76] found bovine β-lactoglobulin in the milk of 18 of 38 mothers chosen at random. Three mothers had very high amounts, and their infants had colic that was relieved by a maternal diet free of bovine milk products. Dietary modification with a low-allergen diet should be considered in the mothers of healthy breastfed infants with colic, according to Hill et al,[64] who reported a community-based study. They also restricted the diet by eliminating artificial color, preservatives, and milk, eggs, wheat, and nuts.[64]

Colic has been investigated in breastfed and formula-fed infants by measuring breath hydrogen

(H_2) production, a product of lactose metabolism.[105] H_2 levels were significantly higher at both 6 weeks and 3 months of age in infants who developed colic. The authors suggest that increased lactose malabsorption may be related to colic. Studies using lactase to minimize the effect of lactose did not cause an improvement. On the other hand, nursing long enough to obtain high-fat hindmilk and relatively less lactose could improve colic.

Lothe et al[91] reported macromolecular absorption using human α-lactalbumin as a marker. Breastfed infants with colic had significantly higher levels of macromolecules than infants without colic. The authors conclude that gut mucosa is affected in infants with colic. Further study by this laboratory reported that there were increased levels of motilin from the first day of life in infants who later developed colic, indicating the GI tract is affected even before symptoms appear.[90]

No type of crying should go untended in a young infant. Holding and rocking do not spoil infants. Crying levels normally increase from birth to 6 to 8 weeks. Most infants spend 2 to 2½ hours a day crying at this age.[152]

With a clinical picture of colic, a history of allergy in the family, especially to cow's milk, is suggestive. A diet free of cow's milk should be tried for at least a week (2 days rarely produces significant improvement) for any case of severe colic. Usually a mother eliminates drinking milk, and for some babies that is enough. If not, all milk products are then eliminated. If mild improvement results with elimination of dairy products, elimination of all bovine protein (i.e., beef) may make a difference. For the group of infants who have a cow's milk allergy, the treatment is impressive. However, not all colic is caused by cow's milk. It may be associated with other dietary items, such as eggs or chocolate, or it may be totally unrelated to maternal food intake.

Acute 24-hour colic in a breastfed infant may result from particular items in the maternal diet. When a strong vegetable (e.g., beans, onions, garlic, rhubarb) is taken for the first time, and the infant starts to cry within a few hours and continues for 20 to 24 hours, this may be transient colic.

This colic is self-limited and needs no treatment. The colic-inducing foods are different for different infants. Mailed questionnaires to 272 mothers, when their infants were about 4 months old, asked about symptoms related to colic. A high correlation was found between 24-hour colic and the mother's consumption of cruciferous vegetables, onions, cow's milk, and chocolate and less so with beans, legumes, spicy foods, and caffeine.[95]

Management of colicky behavior

During the period of colic the infant may need frequent small feedings and much cuddling. Sometimes the infants overfeed, then vomit and settle down and go quietly to sleep, just as an overfed bottle infant does.

The distress or discomfort may be caused by tension, and "colic" has been noted to be more common in the first infants of high-strung mothers.[151] Colic has been associated with hormone withdrawal and has been treated with progesterone. In the breastfed baby this is a less likely cause because of the presence of hormones in breast milk. Colicky breastfed infants who are weaned to formula are usually much worse. Weaning is not an appropriate treatment for the colicky breastfed infant in most cases. Colic usually diminishes in the third month of life, when the infant's GI tract matures.

Type A behaviors during pregnancy were measured by a self-selected cohort of 72 primiparas.[122] After delivery their infants were assessed at 48 hours and 3 months of age. The women who were type A had infants who cried more during neurobehavioral assessment compared with infants of type B women. At 3 months the infants were more intense and less predictable in their responses to the environment. Type A women, however, were more likely to be still breastfeeding.[122]

In a thorough review of infantile colic, Miller and Barr[103] conclude colic is still poorly understood. Causes in the GI tract include sensitivity to dietary components, excessive gas, hypermotility, and hormonal factors. Social causes include normal crying behavior, atypical parenting, and problems of parent-infant interaction. The authors conclude that colicky infants are not a homogeneous group and that it is a variation of normal behavioral and biologic factors and not pathology.[103] The breastfeeding mother needs to know it is not her fault. Appropriate remedial advice should be provided.

Weizman et al[172] studied a herbal tea preparation and found it improved colic in 57% of infants, compared with only 26% of infants who received the placebo of warm glucose-flavored water. The herbal tea, however, contained chamomile, verbain (Verbena officinalis), licorice, fennel, and balm mint, several of which are not recommended for infants (see Chapter 11). Unfortunately, the dose of active ingredient is never predictable in herbal preparations, even when obtained from a reliable source.

Another explanation for colic and failure to thrive has been suggested by Woolridge and Fisher,[183] who note that when an infant is taken from the first breast and switched to the second, this may decrease the amount of fat and energy received. In addition, it will take the infant more volume to receive enough calories, which may cause symptoms of hunger with crying and fretfulness.

When mothers were randomly assigned to use only one breast or both breasts at a feeding, Evans et al[44] found that one-sided breastfeeding was associated with less colic and less postpartum engorgement. Later, most mothers felt they needed to feed on the second side to satisfy their infants' hunger.

Lower fat causes rapid gastric emptying with less digestion of lactose, thus producing diarrhea. It may be appropriate for such an infant to empty the first breast before switching. Colicky infants are often given more to eat, first one breast, then the other, which will increase volume but will also increase lactose and discomfort.

Esophageal reflux

Although less common than in bottle-fed infants, esophageal reflux can occur in breastfed infants and may be a cause of colic. The pattern of colic may be different. Crying begins at the end of the feeding, or the infant falls asleep and is put down, only to wake up crying inconsolably. Esophageal reflux also tends to occur around the clock with little relief. The diagnosis can be confirmed by an esophageal probe test for reflux or by a trial of therapy with metoclopramide.

Pacifiers

Pacifiers have become the subject of much controversy for full-term healthy infants. A bottle-fed infant may have nonnutritive sucking with a pacifier and avoid overeating. Pacifiers in breastfed infants risk interfering with proper suckling at the breast. On the other hand, some breastfed infants go back and forth with artificial nipples without a problem. Infants are born with some self-comforting mechanisms, including resuming the fetal position and sucking a thumb, finger, or fist.

When 354 children in Brazil were studied,[166] it was found that when a pacifier was used, there was a greater probability of early weaning. Mothers had introduced pacifiers to decrease crying. Victora et al[165] followed an additional 650 infants for 6 months; 85% of infants had pacifiers by 1 month of age, and some started and abandoned them. Mothers seemed anxious to introduce them to increase the interval between feeding. Intense pacifier use was associated with weaning by 6 months. Nonwhite mothers and those with infant girls seemed more confident and less concerned about feeding difficulties. The authors concluded that epidemiologic and ethnographic factors influenced the complex relationship between pacifier use and breastfeeding.

In a positive approach to pacifiers, Anderson[7] concluded that they reduced stress in the infant and did not negatively influence feeding. In another study, 602 healthy newborns in 10 centers were randomly assigned to a UNICEF group with restrictive fluids, no bottles, and no pacifiers during the first 5 days or to a control group liberalized to have bottles and pacifiers.[145] Fluid supplements by bottle, with or without use of pacifiers, were not associated with lower frequency or shorter duration of breastfeeding in the first 6 months of life. When Righard[136] studied 52 healthy mother-infant pairs with breastfeeding problems, however, he noted a clear relationship between a faulty nursing pattern and introduction of bottle feedings and pacifier use when compared with a control group who were successfully breastfeeding.

Clearly, pacifiers are a parental decision. A pacifier should not be introduced by hospital staff unless the mother requests it. Exclusion of pacifiers is part of Baby Friendly Hospital Initiative, a program initiated by UNICEF.

Stool patterns for breastfed infants

In the first week of life the pattern of an infant receiving adequate colostrum, which has a cathartic effect on the gut, is to have a stool with most feedings. All the meconium will be passed in 48 hours, and after a few transitional stools (24 hours), the stool becomes yellow. The stools are loose and seedy in consistency. Breastfed infants have a strong gastrocolic reflex and continue to have stools with feedings, with a minimum of four seedy yellow stools per day. Over the next month, a breastfed baby should have a stool every day. When this does not happen, the physician needs to confirm that all is really well. This means a check of urine output (six to eight diapers wet a day and at least one really soaked) and urine specific gravity as well as a review of breastfeeding patterns. The purpose is to identify the potential failure-to-thrive situation before it becomes serious. Many wet diapers and no stool can indicate "low-calorie, low-fat milk." This requires a minor adjustment in breastfeeding to increase the amount of high-fat hindmilk by allowing the infant to nurse until satisfied on the first breast. Ultraabsorbent diapers make assessing voiding patterns difficult and should be avoided in breastfed infants in the first few weeks of life. A tissue can be placed in the diaper to confirm voiding.

Weight gain after the first week of life should be 15 to 30 g daily (½ to 1 oz). Birthweight should be regained in 2 weeks. The mother will observe milk leaking from her breasts, especially from the opposite breast while nursing. Feedings should occur every 2 to 3 hours for 8 to 12 per day. Length of feedings will vary throughout the day, from very short and "businesslike" to dawdling and prolonged or a series of snacks. Mother and infant are symbiotic in this relationship. In most cases, the infant's cues guide the schedule. Successful breastfeeding is an infant-led process.

REFERENCES

1. Adams LM, Davidson M: Present concepts of infant colic, *Pediatr Ann* 16:817, 1987.
2. Alexander JM, Grant AM, Campbell MJ: Randomised controlled trial of breast shells and Hoffman's exercises for inverted and non-protractile nipples, *Br Med J* 304:1030, 1990.
3. Alley JM, Rogers CS: Sleep patterns of breast-fed and non breast-fed infants, *Pediatr Nurs* 12:349, 1986.
4. Almroth SG: Water requirements of breastfed infants in a hot climate, *Am J Clin Nutr* 31:1154, 1978.
5. Amatayakul K, Vutyavanich T, Tanthayaphinant O et al: Serum prolactin and cortisol levels after suckling for varying periods of time and the effect of a nipple shield, *Acta Obstet Gynecol Scand* 66:47, 1987.
6. Amir LH, Garland SM, Dennerstein L et al: *Candida albicans:* is it associated with nipple pain in lactating women? *Gynecol Obstet Invest* 41:30, 1996.
7. Anderson GC: Pacifiers: the positive side, *Matern Child Nurs* 11:122, 1986.
8. Anderson GC, McBride MR, Dahm J et al: Development of sucking in term infants from birth to four hours post birth, *Res Nurs Health* 5:21, 1982.
9. Aono T, Aki T, Koike K et al: Effect of sulpiride on poor puerperal lactation, *Am J Obstet Gynecol* 143:927, 1982.
10. Aono T, Shioji T, Shoda T et al: The initiation of human lactation and prolactin response to suckling, *J Clin Endocrinol Metab* 44:1101, 1977.
11. Ardran GM, Kemp FH, Lind J: A cineradiographic study of bottle feeding, *Br J Radiol* 31:11, 1958.
12. Ardran GM, Kemp FH, Lind J: A cineradiographic study of breast feeding, *Br J Radiol* 31:156, 1958.
13. Armelini PA, Gonzalez CF: Breastfeeding and fluid intake in a hot climate, *Clin Pediatr* 18:424, 1979.

14. Arthur PG, Jones TJ, Spruce J et al: Measuring short-term rates of milk synthesis in breastfeeding mothers, *Q J Exp Physiol* 74:419, 1989.

15. Bader AM, Fragneto R, Terui K: Maternal and neonatal fentanyl and bupivacaine concentrations after epidural infusion during labor, *Anesth Analg* 81:829, 1995.

16. Barnes GR, Lethin AN, Jackson EB et al: Management of breast feeding, *JAMA* 151:192, 1953.

17. Belfrage P, Berlin A, Raabe N et al: Lumbar epidural analgesia with bupivacaine in labor, *Am J Obstet Gynecol* 123:839, 1975.

18. Bentovim A: Shame and other anxieties associated with breastfeeding: a systems theory and psychodynamic approach. In Ciba Foundation Symposium: *Breast feeding and the mother,* No 45, Amsterdam, 1976, Elsevier Scientific.

19. Blass EM, Teicher MH: Suckling, *Science* 210:15, 1980.

20. Bowen-Jones A, Thompson C, Drewett RF: Milk flow and sucking rates during breastfeeding, *Dev Med Child Neurol* 24:626, 1982.

21. Brazelton TB: Psychophysiologic reactions in the neonate. II. Effect of maternal medication on the neonate and his behavior, *J Pediatr* 58:513, 1961.

22. Bremme K, Eneroth P, Kindahl H: 15-Keto-13,14-dihydroprostaglandin $F_{2\alpha}$, and prolactin in maternal and cord blood during prostaglandin E_2 or oxytocin therapy for labor induction, *J Perinat Med* 15:143, 1987.

23. Brenman HS, Pierce L, Mackowiak R et al: Multisensor nipple recording oral variables, *J Appl Physiol* 26:494, 1969.

24. Budd SC, Erdman SH, Long DM et al: Improved lactation with metoclopramide, *Clin Pediatr* 32:53, 1993.

25. Burke PM: Swallowing and the organization of sucking in the human newborn, *Child Dev* 48:523, 1977.

26. Butte NF, Garza C, Smith EO et al: Evaluation of the deuterium dilution technique against the test-weighing procedure for the determination of breast milk intake, *Am J Clin Nutr* 37:996, 1983.

27. Butte NF, Wills C, Jean CA et al: Feeding patterns of exclusively breast-fed infants during the first four months of life, *Early Hum Dev* 12:291, 1985.

28. Caldeyro-Barcia R: Milk ejection in women. In Reynolds M, Folley SJ, editors: *Lactogenesis,* Philadelphia, 1969, University of Pennsylvania Press.

29. Chayen B, Tejani N, Verma U: Induction of labor with an electric breast pump, *J Reprod Med* 31:116, 1986.

30. Christensen S, Dubignon J, Campbell D: Variations in intra-oral stimulation and nutritive sucking, *Child Dev* 47:539, 1976.

31. Cobo E, DeBernal MM, Gaitan E et al: Neurohypophyseal hormone release in the human. II. Experimental study during lactation, *Am J Obstet Gynecol* 97:519, 1967.

32. Conner AE: Elevated levels of sodium and chloride in milk from mastitic breast, *Pediatrics* 63:910, 1979.

33. Cronenwett L, Stukel T, Kearney M et al: Single daily bottle use in the early weeks postpartum and breastfeeding outcomes, *Pediatrics* 90:760, 1992.

34. Cross BA: Comparative physiology of milk removal, *Symp Zool Soc* 41:193, 1977.

35. Daly SEJ, Kent JC, Huynh DQ et al: The determination of short-term breast volume changes and the rate of synthesis of human milk using computerized breast measurement, *Exp Physiol* 77:79, 1992.

36. Davis HV, Sears RR, Miller HC et al: Effects of cup, bottle, and breast feeding on oral activities of newborn infants, *Pediatrics* 2:549, 1948.

37. Dawood MY, Khan-Dawood FS, Wahi RS et al: Oxytocin release and plasma anterior pituitary and gonadal hormones in women during lactation, *J Clin Endocrinol Metab* 52:678, 1981.

38. Devereux WP: Acute puerperal mastitis, *Am J Obstet Gynecol* 108:78, 1970.

39. Dewey KG, Lönnerdal B: Infant self-regulation of breast milk intake, *Acta Paediatr Scand* 75:893, 1986.

40. Drewett RF: Returning to the suckled breast: a further test of Hall's hypothesis, *Early Hum Dev* 6:161, 1982.

41. Edwards JE Jr: Should all patients with candidemia be treated with antifungal agents? *Clin Infect Dis* 15:422, 1992 (editorial).

42. Ehrenkranz RA, Ackerman BA: Metoclopramide effect on faltering milk production by mothers of premature infants, *Pediatrics* 78:614, 1986.

43. Elliott JP, Flaherty JF: The use of breast stimulation to ripen the cervix in term pregnancies, *Am J Obstet Gynecol* 145:553, 1983.

44. Evans K, Evans R, Simmer K: Effect of method of breast feeding on breast engorgement, mastitis and infantile colic, *Acta Paediatr* 84:849, 1995.

45. Evans RW, Fergusson DM, Allardyce RA et al: Maternal diet and infantile colic in breast-fed infants, *Lancet* 1:1340, 1981.

46. Fisher SE, Painter M, Milmor G: Swallowing disorders in infancy: symposium on pediatric otolaryngology, *Pediatr Clin North Am* 28:845, 1981.

47. Font L: "Incidental" maternal dietary intake and infant refusal to nurse, *J Hum Lact* 6:9, 1990.

48. Frantz K: Techniques for successfully managing nipple problems and the reluctant nurser in the early postpartum period. In Freier S, Eidelman A, editors: *Human milk: its biological and social value,* Amsterdam, 1980, Excerpta Medica.

49. Galgiani JN: Fluconazole, a new antifungal agent, *Ann Intern Med* 113:177, 1990.

50. Gateley CA, Mansel RE: Management of the painful and nodular breast, *Br Med Bull* 47:284, 1991.

51. Gerrard JW, Shenassa M: Sensitization to substances in breast milk: recognition, management and significance, *Ann Allergy* 51:300, 1983.

52. Goldberg NM, Adams E: Supplementary water for breast-fed babies in a hot and dry climate—not really a necessity, *Arch Dis Child* 58:73, 1983.

53. Goldsmith HS: Milk-rejection sign of breast cancer, *Am J Surg* 127:280, 1974.

54. Gray-Donald K, Kramer MS, Munday S et al: Effect of formula supplementation in the hospital on the duration of breastfeeding: a controlled clinical trial, *Pediatrics* 75: 514, 1985.

55. Gupta R, Gupta AS, Duggal N: Tubercular mastitis, *Int Surg* 67:422, 1982.

56. Hafström M, Lundquist C, Lindecrantzk et al: Recording non-nutritive sucking in the neonate: description of an automatized system for analysis, *Acta Paediatr* 86:82, 1997.

57. Hall B: Changing composition of human milk and early development of an appetite control, *Lancet* 1:779, 1975.

58. Hauben DJ, Mahler D: A simple method for the correction of the inverted nipple, *Plast Reconstr Surg* 71:556, 1983.

59. Heck LJ, Erenberg A: Serum glucose levels in term neonates during the first 48 hours of life, *J Pediatr* 110:119, 1987.

60. Herd B, Feeney JG: Two aerosol sprays and nipple trauma, *Practitioner* 230:31, 1986.

61. Herrara AJ: Supplemented versus unsupplemented breast-feeding, *Perinatol Neonatol* 8:70, 1984.

62. Hewat RJ, Ellis DJ: A comparison of the effectiveness of two methods of nipple care, *Birth* 14:41, 1987.

63. Hide DW, Guyer BM: Prevalence of infant colic, *Arch Dis Child* 57:559, 1982.

64. Hill DJ, Hudson IL, Sheffield LJ et al: A low allergen diet is a significant intervention in infantile colic: results of a community-based study, *J Allergy Clin Immunol* 96:886, 1995.

65. Hill PD, Humenick SS: The occurrence of breast engorgement, *J Hum Lact* 10:79, 1994.

66. Hodgkinson R, Bhatt M, Wang CN: Double-blind comparison of the neurobehavior of neonates following the administration of different doses of meperidine to the mother, *Can Anaesth Soc J* 25:405, 1978.

67. Hoffmann JB: A suggested treatment for inverted nipples, *Am J Obstet Gynecol* 66:346, 1953.

68. Horowitz M, Higgins GD, Graham JJ et al: Effect of modification of fluid intake in the puerperium on serum prolactin levels and lactation, *Med J Aust* 2:625, 1980.

69. Howie PW, McNeilly AS, McArdle T et al: The relationship between suckling-induced prolactin response and lactogenesis, *J Clin Endocrinol Metab* 50:670, 1980.

70. Humenick SS, Hill PD, Anderson MA: Breast engorgement: patterns and selected outcomes, *J Hum Lact* 10:87, 1994.

71. Hunziker UA, Barr RG: Increased carrying reduces infant crying: a randomized controlled trial, *Pediatrics* 77:641, 1986.

72. Inch S, Fisher C: Antiseptic sprays and nipple trauma, *Practitioner* 230:1037, 1986.

73. Jain E: Tongue-tie (ankyloglossia). Presented at First Annual International Meeting, Academy of Breastfeeding Medicine: Physicians and Breastfeeding: a New Alliance, Rochester, NY, October 1996.

74. Jakobsson I, Lindberg T: Cow's milk as a cause of infantile colic in breast-fed infants, *Lancet* 2:437, 1978.

75. Jakobsson I, Lindberg T: Cow's milk proteins cause infantile colic in breast-fed infants: a double-blind cross-over study, *Pediatrics* 71:268, 1983.

76. Jakobsson I, Lindberg T, Benediksson B et al: Dietary bovine β-lactoglobulin is transferred to human milk, *Acta Paediatr Scand* 74:342, 1985.

77. Johnson P, Salisbury DM: Breathing and sucking during feeding in the newborn. In Bosma JF, Showacre J, editors: *Development of upper respiratory anatomy and function,* Bethesda, Md, 1975, National Institutes of Health.

78. Katzman DK, Wald ER: Staphylococcal scalded skin syndrome in a breastfed infant, *Pediatr Infect Dis J* 6:295, 1987.

79. Kesaree N, Banapurmath CR, Banapurmath S et al: Treatment of inverted nipples using a disposable syringe, *J Hum Lact* 9:27, 1993.

80. Klaus MH: The frequency of suckling, *Obstet Gynecol Clin North Am* 14:623, 1987.

81. Kron RE, Stein M, Goddard KE: Newborn sucking behavior affected by obstetric sedation, *Pediatrics* 37: 1012, 1966.

82. Kuhnert BR, Zuspan KJ, Kuhneet PM et al: Bupivacaine disposition in mother, fetus and neonate after spinal anesthesia for cesarean section, *Anesth Analg* 66:407, 1987.

83. Kurinij N, Shiono PH: Early formula supplementation of breastfeeding, *Pediatrics* 88:745, 1991.

84. Lavergne NA: Does application of tea bags to sore nipples while breastfeeding provide effective relief? *J Obstet Gynecol Neonatal Nurs* 26:53, 1997.

85. Leonard EL, Trykowski LE, Kirkpatrick BV: Nutritive sucking in high-risk neonates after perioral stimulation, *Phys Ther* 60:299, 1980.

86. L'Esperance CM: Pain or pleasure: the dilemma of early breastfeeding, *Birth Fam J* 7:21, 1980.

87. Lindenberg CS, Artola RC, Jimenez V: The effect of early postpartum mother-infant contact and breastfeeding promotion on the incidence and continuation of breastfeeding, *Int J Nurs Stud* 27:179, 1990.

88. Lipitz S, Barkai G, Rabinovici J et al: Breast stimulation test and oxytocin challenge test in fetal surveillance: a prospective randomized study, *Am J Obstet Gynecol* 157:1178, 1987.

89. Loftus JR, Hill H, Cohen SF: Placental transfer and neonatal effects of epidural sufentanil and fentanyl administered with bupivacaine during labor, *Anesthesiology* 83:300, 1995.

90. Lothe L, Ivarsson S-A, Ekman R et al: Motilin and infantile colic, *Acta Paediatr Scand* 79:410, 1990.

91. Lothe L, Lindberg T, Jakobsson I: Macromolecular absorption in infants with infantile colic, *Acta Paediatr Scand* 79:417, 1990.

92. Lozoff B, Brittenham GM, Trause MA et al: The mother-newborn relationship: limits of adaptability, *J Pediatr* 91:1, 1977.

93. Lucas A, Lucas PJ, Baum JD: Differences in the pattern of milk intake between breast and bottle fed infants, *Early Hum Dev* 5:195, 1981.

94. Deleted in press.

95. Lust KD, Brown JE, Thomas W: Maternal intake of cruciferous vegetables and other foods and colic symptoms in exclusively breast-fed infants, *J Am Diet Assoc* 96:47, 1996.

96. Maekawa K, Nara T, Hoashi E: Influence of breastfeeding on neonatal behavior, *Acta Paediatr Jpn* 27: 608, 1985.

97. Marshall BR, Hepper JK, Zirbel CC: Sporadic puerperal mastitis, *JAMA* 233:1377, 1975.

98. Marshall WM, Cumming DC, Fitzsimmons GW: Hot flushes during breastfeeding? *Fertil Steril* 57: 1349, 1992.

99. Mashini IS, Devoe LD, McKenzie JS et al: Comparison of uterine activity induced by nipple stimulation and oxytocin, *Obstet Gynecol* 69:74, 1987.

100. Matheson I, Aursnes I, Horgen M et al: Bacteriological findings and clinical symptoms in relation to clinical outcome in puerperal mastitis, *Acta Obstet Gynecol Scand* 67:723, 1988.

101. McNeilly AS, Robinson ICA, Houston MJ et al: Release of oxytocin and prolactin in response to suckling, *Br Med J* 286:257, 1983.

102. Millard AV: The place of the clock in pediatric advice: rationales, cultural themes, and impediments to breast-feeding, *Soc Sci Med* 31:211, 1990.

103. Miller AR, Barr RG: Infantile colic: is it a gut issue? *Pediatr Clin North Am* 38:1407, 1991.

104. Montello JM, Darby MH, Faubel K et al: Clotrimazole by thumb, *N Engl J Med* 301:1005, 1979.

105. Moore DJ, Robb TA, Davidson GP: Breath hydrogen response to milk containing lactose in colicky and noncolicky infants, *J Pediatr* 113:979, 1988.

106. Murray AD, Dolby RM, Nation RL et al: Effects of epidural anesthesia on newborns and their mothers, *Child Dev* 52:71, 1981.

107. Neifert MR, Seacat JM: A guide to successful breastfeeding, *Contemp Pediatr* 3:16, 1986.

108. Newton N: Nipple pain and nipple damage: problems in the management of breast feeding, *J Pediatr* 41:411, 1952.

109. Newton N: The quantitative effect of oxytocin (Pitocin) on human milk yield, *Ann NY Acad Sci* 652:481, 1992.

110. Newton N: The relation of the milk-ejection reflex to the ability to breastfeed, *Ann NY Acad Sci* 652:484, 1992.

111. Newton M, Newton NR: The let-down reflex in human lactation, *J Pediatr* 33:698, 1948.

112. Newton M, Newton NR: The normal course and management of lactation, *Clin Obstet Gynecol* 5:44, 1962.

113. Newton NR, Newton M: Relationship of ability to breastfeed and maternal attitudes toward breast feeding, *Pediatrics* 5:869, 1950.

114. Niebyl JR, Spence MR, Parmley TH: Sporadic (nonepidemic) puerperal mastitis, *J Reprod Med* 20:97, 1978.

115. Nikodem VC, Danziger D, Gebka N et al: Do cabbage leaves prevent breast engorgement.? A randomized controlled study, *Birth* 20:61, 1993.

116. Nissen E, Lilja G, Widström A-M et al: Elevation of oxytocin levels early postpartum in women, *Acta Obstet Gynecol Scand* 74:530, 1995.

117. Notestine GE: The importance of the identification of ankyloglossia (short lingual frenulum) as a cause of breastfeeding problems, *J Hum Lact* 6:113, 1990.

118. Nowlis GH, Kessen W: Human newborns differentiate differing concentrations of sucrose and glucose, *Science* 191:865, 1976.

119. Nysenbaum AN, Smart JL: Sucking behavior and milk intake of neonates in relation to milk fat content, *Early Hum Dev* 6:205, 1982.

120. Olsen A: Nursing under conditions of thirst or excessive ingestion of fluids, *Acta Obstet Gynecol* 20:313, 1940.

121. Opri F: Mammary mycoses, *Chemotherapy* 28 (suppl): 561, 1982.

122. Parker SJ, Barrett DE: Maternal type A behavior during pregnancy, neonatal crying and early infant temperament: do type A women have type A babies? *Pediatrics* 89:474, 1992.

123. Paul K, Dittrichová J, Papousek H: Infant feeding behavior: development in pattern and motivation, *Dev Psychobiol* 29:563, 1996.

124. Pedersen CA: Oxytocin control of maternal behavior: regulation by sex steroids and offspring stimuli, *Ann NY Acad Sci* 807:126, 1997.

125. Pinilla T, Birch LL: Help me make it through the night: behavioral entrainment of breastfed infants' sleep patterns, *Pediatrics* 91:436, 1993.

126. Pollitt E, Consolazio B, Goodkin F: Changes in nutritive sucking during a feed in two-day and thirty-day-old infants, *Early Hum Dev* 5:201, 1981.

127. Prentice A, Addey CV, Wilde CJ: Evidence for local feedback control of human milk secretion, *Biochem Soc Trans* 17: 489, 1989.

128. Prentice A, Prentice AM: Unilateral breast dysfunction in lactating Gambian women, *Ann Trop Pediatr* 4:19, 1984.

129. Prentice A, Prentice AM, Lamb WH: Mastitis in rural Gambian mothers and the protection of the breast by milk antimicrobial factors, *Trans R Soc Trop Med Hyg* 79:90, 1985.

130. Pugh LC, Buchko BL, Bishop BA et al: A comparison of topical agents to relieve nipple pain and enhance breast-feeding, *Birth* 23:88, 1996.

131. Raphael D: *The tender gift: breast feeding,* New York, 1976, Schocken.

132. Rayner CR: The correction of permanently inverted nipples, *Br J Plast Surg* 33:413, 1980.

133. Reiff MI, Essock-Vitale SM: Hospital influences on early infant-feeding practices, *Pediatrics* 76:872, 1985.

134. Renfrew M, Fisher C, Arms S: *Breastfeeding: getting breastfeeding right for you,* Berkeley, Calif, 1990, Celestial Arts.

135. Renfrew MJ, McCandish R: With women: new steps in research in midwifery. In Roberts H, editor: *Women's health matters,* London, 1992, Routledge.

136. Righard L: Are breastfeeding problems related to incorrect breastfeeding technique and the use of pacifiers and bottles? *Birth* 25:40, 1998.

137. Righard L, Alade MO: Effect of delivery room routine on success of first breastfeed, *Lancet* 336:1105, 1990.

138. Righard L, Alade MO: Sucking technique and its effect on success of breastfeeding, *Birth* 19:185, 1992.

139. Righard L, Flodmark C-E, Lothe L et al: Breastfeeding patterns: single and two-breast principles vis à vis infant behavior (in press).

140. Riordan J, Auerbach KG: *Breastfeeding and human lactation,* ed 2, Boston, 1998, Jones and Bartlett.

141. Robert KL: A comparison of chilled cabbage leaves and chilled gelpaks in reducing breast engorgement, *J Hum Lact* 11:11, 1995.

142. Rosen AR, Lawrence RA: The effect of epidural anesthesia on infant feeding, *J Univ Roch Med Ctr* 6(1):3, 1994.

143. Rosier W: Cool cabbage compresses, *Breastfeed Rev* 12:28, 1988.

144. Salisbury DM: Bottle-feeding: influence of teat hole size on suck volume, *Lancet* 1:655, 1975.

145. Schubiger G, Schwarz U, Tönz O et al: UNICEF/WHO Baby Friendly Hospital Initiative: does the use of bottles and pacifiers in the neonatal nursery prevent successful breastfeeding? *Eur J Pediatr* 156:874, 1997.

146. Schutzman DL, Hervada AR, Branca PA: Effect of water supplementation of full-term newborns on arrival of milk in the nursing mother, *Clin Pediatr* 25:78, 1986.

147. Sharp DA: Moist wound healing for sore or cracked nipples, *Breastfeeding Abstracts* 12(2):19, 1992.

148. Skoog T: Surgical correction of inverted nipples, *J Am Med Wom Assoc* 20:931, 1965.

149. Smith WL, Erenberg A, Nowak A: Imaging evaluation of the human nipple during breastfeeding, *Am J Dis Child* 142:76, 1988.

150. Smith WL, Erenberg A, Nowak A et al: Physiology of sucking in the normal term infant using real-time US, *Radiology* 156:379, 1985.

151. Ståhlberg M-R, Savilahti E: Infantile colic and feeding, *Arch Dis Child* 61:1232, 1986.

152. St. James-Roberts I: Persistent infant crying, *Arch Dis Child* 66:653, 1991.

153. Steinberg LA, O'Connell NC, Hatch TF et al: Tryptophan intake influences infants' sleep latency, *J Nutr* 122:1781, 1992.

154. Süsswein J: Zur Physiologie des Trinkens beim Säugling, *Arch Kinder Heilkd* 40:68, 1905.

155. Talbot FB: Eczema in childhood, *Med Clin North Am* 1:985, 1918.

156. Taylor RN, Green JR: Abruptio placentae following nipple stimulation, *Am J Perinatol* 4:94, 1987.

157. Thomas DW, McGilligan K, Eisenberg LD et al: Infantile colic and type of milk feeding, *Am J Dis Child* 141:451, 1987.

158. Thomsen AC: Infectious mastitis and occurrence of antibody-coated bacteria in milk, *Am J Obstet Gynecol* 144:350, 1982.

159. Thomsen AC, Espersen T, Maigaard S: Course and treatment of milk stasis, noninfectious inflammation of the breast, and infectious mastitis in nursing women, *Am J Obstet Gynecol* 149:492, 1984.

160. Thomsen AC, Mogensen SC, Jepsen FL: Experimental mastitis in mice induced by coagulase-negative staphylococci isolated from cases of mastitis in nursing women, *Acta Obstet Gynecol Scand* 64:163, 1985.

161. Toppozada MK, El-Rahman HA, Soliman AY: Prostaglandins as milk ejectors: the nose as a new route of administration, *Adv Prost Thrombox Leukotr Res* 12:449, 1983.

162. Uvnas-Moberg K, Widström A-M, Werner S et al: Oxytocin and prolactin levels in breastfeeding women, *Acta Obstet Gynecol Scand* 69:301, 1990.

163. Van Geddren, Goosen A: Mammographic features of unilateral breastfeeding, *Clin Radiol* 5:134, 1996.

164. Vestermark V, Hogdall CK, Birch M et al: Influence of the mode of delivery on initiation of breastfeeding, *Eur J Obstet Gynecol Reprod Biol* 38:33, 1990.

165. Victora CG, Behague DP, Barros FC et al: Pacifier use and short breastfeeding duration: cause, consequence or coincidence? *Pediatrics* 99:445, 1997.

166. Victora CG, Tomasi E, Olinto MTA et al: Use of pacifiers and breastfeeding duration, *Lancet* 341:404, 1993.

167. Waldenstrom U, Sundelin C, Lindmark G: Early and late discharge after hospital birth: breastfeeding, *Acta Paediatr Scand* 76:727, 1987.

168. Walia HS, Abraham TK, Shaikh H: Fungal mastitis, *Acta Chir Scand* 153:133, 1987.

169. Walsh M, McIntosh K: Neonatal mastitis, *Clin Pediatr* 25:395, 1986.

170. Weber F, Woolridge MW, Baum JD: An ultrasonographic study of the organization of sucking and swallowing by newborn infants, *Dev Med Child Neurol* 28:19, 1986.

171. Weitzmen RE, Leake RD, Rubin RT et al: The effect of nursing on neurohypophyseal hormone and prolactin secretion in human subjects, *J Clin Endocrinol Metab* 51:836, 1980.

172. Weizman Z, Alkrinawi S, Goldfarb D et al: Efficacy of herbal tea preparation in infantile colic, *J Pediatr* 122:650, 1993.

173. Whitfield MF, Kay R, Stevens S: Validity of routine clinical test weighing as a measure of the intake of breast-fed infants, *Arch Dis Child* 56:919, 1981.

174. Widström A-M, Thingström-Paulsson J: The position of the tongue during rooting reflexes elicited in newborn infants before the first suckle, *Acta Paediatr* 82:281, 1993.

175. Widström A-M, Wahlberg V, Matthiesen A-S et al: Short-term effects of early suckling and touch of the nipple on maternal behavior, *Early Hum Dev* 21:153, 1990.

176. Wolff PH: Sucking patterns of infant mammals, *Brain Behav Evol* 1:354, 1968.

177. Wolff PH: The serial organization of sucking in the young infant, *Pediatrics* 42:943, 1968.

178. Woolridge MW: Aetiology of sore nipples, *Midwifery* 2:172, 1986.

179. Woolridge MW: The "anatomy" of infant sucking, *Midwifery* 2:164, 1986.

180. Woolridge MW, Baum JD: Recent advances in breastfeeding, *Acta Paediatr Jpn* 35:1, 1993.

181. Woolridge MW, Baum JD, Drewett RF: Does a change in the composition of human milk affect sucking patterns and milk intake? *Lancet* 2:1292, 1980.

182. Woolridge MW, Baum JD, Drewett RF: Effect of a traditional and of a new nipple shield on sucking patterns and milk flow, *Early Hum Dev* 4:357, 1980.

183. Woolridge MW, Fisher C: Colic, "overfeeding," and symptoms of lactose malabsorption in the breast-fed baby: a possible artifact of feed management, *Lancet* 2:382, 1988.

184. Woolridge MW, How TV, Drewett RF et al: The continuous measurement of milk intake at a feed in breast-fed babies, *Early Hum Dev* 6:365, 1982.

185. Woolridge MW, Ingram JC, Baum JD: Do changes in pattern of breast usage alter the baby's nutrient intake? *Lancet* 336:395, 1990.

186. Work Group on Breastfeeding, American Academy of Pediatrics: Breastfeeding and the use of human milk, *Pediatrics* 100:1035, 1997.

187. Wüst J: *Streptococcus pneumoniae* as an agent of mastitis, *Eur J Clin Microbiol Infect Dis* 14:156, 1995 (letter).

9

*D*iet and dietary supplements for the mother and infant

Lactation is the physiologic completion of the reproductive cycle. The maternal body prepares during pregnancy for lactation not only by developing the breast to produce milk, but also by storing additional nutrients and energy. For milk production, the transition to fully sustaining the infant should not be complex or require major adjustments for the mother. After delivery, mothers usually note an increase in appetite and thirst and a change in some dietary preferences. In simple cultures, anthropologists have noted that tradition prescribes on the birth of a baby bringing gifts of special foods—usually high in protein, nutrients, and calories—for the mother to ensure she will make good milk for the infant. This tradition may have affected some early studies in which relatively malnourished women were noted to produce milk comparable to that produced by well-nourished women in industrialized countries.

The Subcommittee on Nutrition During Lactation of the Committee on Nutritional Status during Pregnancy and Lactation of the Food and Nutrition Board of the Institute of Medicine at the National Academy of Sciences[152] published its first report in 1991 following an exhaustive study of the world's literature and current scientific evidence. The subcommittee stated that breastfeeding is recommended for all infants in the United States under ordinary circumstances. Women living under a wide variety of circumstances in the United States and elsewhere are capable of fully nourishing their infants by breastfeeding them. Furthermore, exclusive breastfeeding is preferred for the first 4 to 6 months.

Throughout the course of its investigation,[152] the subcommittee was impressed by the overwhelming evidence indicating that women are able to "produce milk of sufficient quantity and quality to support growth and promote the health of infants—even when the mother's supply of nutrients is limited." On the other hand, the depletion of mother's nutrient stores is a risk if efforts to achieve adequate food intake are not made.

Most writings for the nursing mother regarding maternal diet during lactation set up complicated "rules" about dietary intake that fail to consider the mother's dietary stores and normal dietary preferences. Thus one barrier to breastfeeding for some women is the "diet rules" they see as being too hard to follow or too restrictive.[54] Therefore the physician and nutritionist must understand the simple requirements and widely acceptable variations so that dietary guidelines make minimal demands on a woman's lifestyle. All over the world, women produce adequate and even abundant milk on very inadequate diets.[75] Women in primitive cultures with modest but adequate diets produce milk without any obvious detriment to themselves and none of the fatigue and loss of well-being that some well-fed Western mothers experience.[168,169]

IMPACT OF MATERNAL DIET ON MILK PRODUCTION

Although much has been learned about dietary requirements for lactation by studying women from many cultures[76] and various levels of poor nutrition, some of the information is conflicting, principally because of varying sampling techniques and the improvement over time in laboratory analysis. Extensive reviews of the current literature on various nutrients in human milk and the influence of maternal dietary intake have been referenced.[48,63,87,91,95,167,168] Those readers needing access to the original studies are referred to the bibliographies from these reviews, which include hundreds of items, a listing beyond the scope of this text.

Milk volume

The volume of milk produced varies over the duration of lactation from the first few weeks to 6 months and beyond but is remarkably predictable except for extreme malnutrition or severe dehydration. In periods of acute water deprivation, manifested in the healthy mother by an acute bout of vomiting and diarrhea, the volume of milk will diminish only after the maternal urine output has been significantly compromised (10% dehydration).

Malnutrition, on the other hand, is complex, and single-nutrient deficiencies are rare. Malnutrition does seem to have an effect on the total volume of milk produced. In the extreme, when famine occurs, the milk supply dwindles and ceases, with ultimate starvation of the infant. The classic study is the report of Smith[137] on the effects of maternal undernutrition on the newborn infant in the Hunger Winter in Holland in 1944-1945. It was reported that the volume of milk was slightly diminished, but the duration of lactation was not affected. The latter is a testimony to courage rather than diet.

Analysis of milk produced showed no significant deviations from normal chemical structure. Milk was produced at the expense of maternal tissue.

These data from the Dutch famine were reexamined by Stein et al,[148] who pointed out that the women who had conceived during the famine did develop some maternal stores in anticipation of lactation that were not accounted for by the fetus, placenta, or amniotic fluid, even though the fetus was a pound lighter at birth. They reported fetal weight down by 10% but maternal weight down by only 4%. This demonstrates the maternal body's strong commitment to preparing for lactation during pregnancy.

There is a wide range of volume of milk intake among healthy breastfed infants, averaging 750 to 800 g/day and ranging from 450 to 1200 g/day.[16] Any factor that influences the frequency, intensity, or duration of sucking by the infant influences the volume. The self-regulation of milk supply by the infant has been confirmed by studies by Dewey et al[38] in which additional milk was pumped after each feeding for 2 weeks, thus increasing the milk supply. The infants, however, quickly went back to baseline consumption after the pumping ceased. The residual milk supply of healthy women (i.e., that which can be extracted after a full feeding) is about 100 g/day, even when an infant consumes comparatively low volumes of milk.[38]

Prentice and Prentice[123] described "energy sparing adaptations" that were associated with normal lactation when energy intake is limited. These were decreases in basal metabolic rate, thermogenesis, and physical activity.

When well-nourished mothers reduced their intake by 32% for 1 week, consuming no less than 1500 kcal/day, there was no reduction in milk volume, although plasma prolactin levels increased. Those mothers who consumed less than 1500 kcal/day for a week did experience decreased milk volumes compared with those of the control and the group consuming more than 1500 kcal.

Exercise, manual labor, and losing weight do not usually alter milk volume. Milk production will increase with infant demand, but infant demand will only increase with growth, which depends on sufficient nourishment.[78] Supplementing the mother could improve production and stimulate the infant's appetite. Milk may contain appetite inhibitors and possibly appetite stimulants.

Energy supplementation and lactation performance

In one study, when women received supplements during the last trimester of pregnancy, no effect was noted in their milk production. This suggests that short-term supplementation may be ineffective.[157] Other studies that provided supplementation of up to 900 kcal/day for 2 weeks resulted in an increase in milk production (662 to 787 g/day).[152] There was no increase in infant weight compared with the control group's infants in this period (2 weeks).

The problem of insufficient milk supply for the baby is reported in well-nourished as well as poorly nourished populations, but in cross-cultural studies it appears to be unrelated to maternal nutrition status.[155] The effect of supplementation may be more psychologic than physiologic.

In countries where food supplies vary with the season, milk supplies drop 1 dl/day during periods of progressively greater food shortages. Studies continue on lactation performance of poorly nourished women around the world, including Burma, The Gambia, Papua New Guinea, and Ethiopia as well as among the Navajo. Results continue to reflect an impact on quantity, not quality, of milk.[15,32,84,113,135]

The interrelationship of milk volume, nutrient concentration, and total nutrient intake by the infant must be considered.[36] The reason for low protein content in a given sample may be lack of protein, lack of total energy content, or lack of vitamin B_6, a requirement of normal protein metabolism.

Of great concern, however, is the report of dietary supplementation of Gambian nursing mothers in which the lactational performance was not affected by increased calories (700 kcal/day).[126] The supplement produced a slight initial improvement in maternal body weight and subcutaneous fat but not in milk output. Whether the mothers utilized the increased energy to work harder farming or whether the infants did not stimulate increased milk production is unresolved. The Subcommittee on Nutrition During Lactation concluded that food supplementation of lactating women in areas where malnutrition is prevalent has generally had little, if any, impact on milk volume.[152] However, such supplementation, they believed, improves maternal health and is more likely to benefit the mother than the infant except where milk composition had been affected by specific deficiencies.

Protein content

Since the work of Hambraeus[62] has reestablished the norms for protein in human milk to be 0.8 to 0.9 g/dl in well-nourished mothers, figures from previous studies will have to be recalculated to consider that all nitrogen in human milk is not protein; 25% of the nitrogen is nonprotein nitrogen (NPN) in human milk, and only 5% of the nitrogen is NPN in bovine milk. The protein content of milk from poorly nourished mothers is surprisingly high, and malnutrition has little effect on protein concentration. An increase in dietary protein increases volume but not overall protein content, given the normal variations seen in healthy, well-nourished women.[44]

Observations made over a 20-month period of continued lactation showed that milk quality did not change, although the quantity decreased slightly, which Von Muralt[159] attributed to the decreasing demand of a child who is receiving other nourishment. Therefore the total protein available with the decreased volume of milk and increased weight of the child decreased from 2.2 g/kg of body weight to 0.45 g/kg. The need for additional protein sources for the child after 1 year of age becomes obvious.

In its painstaking review of the literature, the Subcommittee on Nutrition During Lactation[152] determined that the composition of human milk is maintained even with less-than-recommended dietary intake of macronutrients. The concentrations of major minerals, including calcium, phosphorus, magnesium, sodium, and potassium, are not affected by diet. Maternal intakes of selenium and iodine, however, are positively affected by diet: an increase in the diet increases the level in the milk. The proportion of different fatty acids in human milk varies with the maternal dietary intake.

Eighty-three lactating Zairian mothers with protein malnutrition were given 500 kcal (2093 kilojoules, kJ) and 18 g of protein as a cow's milk supplement for 2 months, after which their nutritional status improved significantly.[40] The volume of milk did not change (607 versus 604 ml). Their breastfed infants, however, did show significant improvement in their mean serum albumin levels, and their growth matched that of healthy infants of the same age.

The effect of very-low-protein (8% of energy) and very-high-protein (20% of energy) diets on the protein and nitrogen composition of breast milk in three healthy Swedish women "in full lactation" was significant.[50] High-protein diets produced higher production and greater concentrations of total nitrogen, true protein, and NPN. The increased NPN was caused by increased urea levels and free amino acids. The 24-hour outputs of lactoferrin, lactalbumin, and serum albumin were not significantly higher.

When marginally nourished women were provided a mixed-protein diet predominantly from plant sources up to 1.2 g/kg/day, equilibrium was achieved at 1.1 g protein/kg intake. In a study of healthy women given marginal protein intakes, Motil et al[105] reported that maternal milk production and the protein nitrogen, but not the NPN, fraction of human milk were relatively well preserved in the short term.

The practical significance, except as related to fad diets, of these results is limited because the diets were extreme and were maintained for only 4 days. The impact on human nutritional physiology, however, is significant.[50]

Taurine, an amino acid found only in animal products, is the second most abundant free amino acid in human milk. Even milk of women who have no animal foods in their diet contains some taurine at levels (35 mg/dl) that are lower than those in women who consume animal products (54 mg/dl).[128]

Of practical significance for counseling the healthy woman in the industrialized world is the work of Butte et al[16] investigating the effect of maternal diet and body composition on lactational performance. Forty-five healthy lactating women were followed for 4 months from delivery with detailed measurements of milk production, dietary intake, and maternal body composition. The overall mean energy intake was 2186 ($\pm$ 463) kcal/day. Milk production averaged 751, 725, 723, and 740 g/day for months 1, 2, 3, and 4. Average maternal weight reduction was from 64.6 kg to 59.3 kg. Energy was calculated to be sufficient for maintenance and activity, yet the mothers achieved gradual weight reduction. The authors conclude that energy intakes of approximately 15% less than those currently recommended are compatible with full lactation, full activity, and gradual weight reduction to prepregnant weight (Tables 9-1 and 9-2). Diets otherwise contained recommended daily allowances for lactation.[49] Other investigators studying the impact of weight loss noted that the rate of postpregnancy weight loss affected the level of elaidic acid in milk and of *trans* fatty acid level.[20] This is explained by the mobilization of fatty acids from adipose tissue.

Fat, cholesterol, and omega-3 fatty acids

Mature human milk contains about 50% of its energy as fat. This fat is necessary for the tremendous growth of the newborn and is essential to the structural development of the brain, retina, and other tissues. Both n-6 and n-3 fatty acids are essential components of the phospholipids of cell membranes. They are critical to the fluidity, permeability, and activity of membrane-bound enzymes and receptors. During the first 4 to 6 months of life, an infant accumulates 1300 to 1600 g of lipids.[67]

Considerable attention has been focused on the impact of dietary fat and cholesterol on the composition of human milk. Fat is the main source

---

TABLE 9-1	Milk production over first 4 months of lactation							
	Mo 1 (n = 37)		Mo 2 (n = 40)		Mo 3 (n = 37)		Mo 4 (n = 41)	
Human milk* (g/day)	751	(130)†	725	(131)	723	(114)	740	(128)
Feedings (no/day)	8.3	(1.9)	7.2	(1.9)	6.8	(1.9)	6.7	(1.8)
Total nitrogen (mg/g)	2.17	(0.30)	1.94	(0.24)	1.84	(0.19)	1.80	(0.21)
Protein nitrogen (mg/g)	1.61	(0.24)	1.42	(0.17)	1.34	(0.15)	1.31	(0.17)
Nonprotein nitrogen (mg/g)	0.56	(0.28)	0.52	(0.20)	0.50	(0.13)	0.48	(0.14)
Fat (mg/g)	36.2	(7.5)	34.4	(6.8)	32.2	(7.8)	34.8	(10.8)
Energy (kcal/g)	0.68	(0.08)	0.64	(0.08)	0.62	(0.09)	0.64	(0.10)

From Butte NF, Garza C, Stuff JE et al: *Am J Clin Nutr* 34:2216, 1981.

*At the onset of the study, milk was estimated by deuterium dilution, a technique that was later determined to be inaccurate. For this reason, data are missing at 17 time points during the first 3 months.

†Mean (SD).

TABLE 9-2	Anthropometric changes in mothers during lactation									
Parameter	Postpartum		Mo 1		Mo 2		Mo 3		Mo 4	
Wt (kg)	64.6	(9.1)*	61.3	(9.5)	60.7	(10.0)	60.2	(10.4)	59.3	(10.5)
Wt/ht (kg/cm)†	0.40	(0.04)	0.37	(0.05)	0.37	(0.05)	0.37	(0.05)	0.36	(0.06)
Wt/prepregnancy wt‡	1.16	(0.06)	1.08	(0.05)	1.07	(0.05)	1.06	(0.05)	1.05	(0.07)
Wt change (kg/mo)			−3.83	(2.26)	−0.59	(1.20)	−0.62	(1.12)	−0.80	(1.86)
Triceps (mm)	16.3	(5.1)	16.9	(4.6)	17.0	(4.7)	17.3	(5.3)	17.2	(5.2)
Subscapular (mm)	18.2	(7.1)	16.8	(6.4)	16.4	(7.4)	15.7	(7.2)	15.1	(7.3)
Biceps (mm)	7.8	(3.9)	6.9	(3.2)	6.9	(3.3)	7.3	(4.6)	6.8	(3.4)
Suprailiac (mm)	26.1	(8.5)	25.7	(6.9)	25.2	(7.6)	23.1	(8.1)	22.2	(8.0)
Sum skinfolds (mm)	68.4	(20.2)	66.3	(18.9)	65.5	(20.6)	63.4	(22.9)	61.7	(21.8)
Midarm circumference (cm)	26.9	(3.5)	26.7	(2.6)	26.8	(3.2)	26.6	(2.9)	26.7	(3.6)

From Butte NF, Garza C, Stutt JE et al: *Am J Clin Nutr* 39:296, 1984.

*Mean (SD).

†Maternal height (ht) = 163.0 (6.3 cm).

‡Prepregnancy weight (wt) gain = 14.4 (3.3 kg).

of kilocalories in human milk for the infant. The fatty acid composition of the triglycerides, which make up over 98% of the lipid compartment of human milk, can be affected by maternal diet. Diets with different lipid composition, caloric content, proportion of calories from fat, and fatty acid composition have been studied.

In a classic work that was carefully controlled, Insull et al[73] fed a lactating woman in a metabolic ward diets that differed in caloric content, proportion of calories from fat, and fatty acid composition. Neither milk volume nor total milk fat was affected by diet. When the high-calorie, no-fat diet was fed, milk triglycerides were higher in fatty acids 12:0 and 14:0 and lower in 18:0 and 18:1, which indicated that when fatty acids were synthesized from carbohydrate, there were more intermediate-chain fatty acids. When the low-calorie, no-fat diet was fed, the fatty acid composition of the milk resembled the maintenance diet and the depot fat. When corn oil was the fat source, milk levels of 18:2 and 18:3 were higher, with a major increase in linoleic acid, than when lard or butter was used. Multiple studies have shown that medium-chain fatty acids, lauric and myristic acid (12:0 and 14:0), are not affected by diet, indicating synthesis by the mammary gland.[47,91,95]

Trans fatty acids are produced in hydrogenation reactions and appear in human milk as a reflection of dietary intake, so that women who eat margarine rather than butter have high levels in their milk.[86] Elaidic acid (18:1 *trans*) is found in margarine, for instance. Because of the high level of *trans* fatty acids in hydrogenated vegetable oils such as margarine, the milk of U.S. women is high in *trans* fatty acids, whereas the milk of West German women is low in *trans* fatty acids.[47] Considerable controversy surrounds the biologic effects. The recommendations for substituting margarines was reversed in 1997. In mammals, *trans* isomers have been noted to alter permeability and fluidity of membranes, inhibit a number of enzyme reactions of lipid metabolism, and impair synthesis of arachidonic acid and prostaglandins.

The concern about fat composition in terms of the polyunsaturated fatty acid (PUFA) to saturated fatty acid ratio (P/S ratio) and the high level of cholesterol normally found in breast milk have led to monitoring mothers on altered lipid intakes. Potter and Nestel[117] studied lactating women who were placed on one of two experimental diets after a period of a study of their normal Australian diet, which includes 400 to 600 mg of cholesterol/day and fat that is rich in saturated fatty acids. Following this baseline study, the mothers were either given diet A, with 580 mg cholesterol and a high level of saturated fats, or diet B, with 110 mg cholesterol and a higher level of polyunsaturated fats from vegetable oils. A second study was carried out with the two diets high in either saturated or unsaturated fats, but the cholesterol remained the same, 345 to 380 mg/day.

The low-cholesterol diets lowered the maternal blood cholesterol but not the triglyceride levels. The cholesterol level of the milk, however, was unaffected in any diet combination.[91,92] The increase in PUFA in the diet rapidly increased the levels of linoleate in the milk to twice the previous level at the expense of myristate and palmitate. Protein levels remained the same in the milk throughout the study. Infant plasma cholesterol levels decreased in response to an increase in the concentration of linoleate in the milk. The significant dietary change seemed to depend on the consumption of high PUFA and low cholesterol to alter the levels in the milk and thus in the infant's plasma[117] (Table 9-3).

Cholesterol levels remain relatively stable throughout at least 16 weeks of lactation. The presence or absence of phytosterols influences both the accuracy of analysis (i.e., overestimate level of cholesterol) and the physiologic significance of cholesterol. *Phytosterols* are those sterols derived from plant sources. They are distinguishable from cholesterol, which is of animal origin. During a given feeding, the concentration of cholesterol in the milk may increase over 60%, although the total for the feeding is constant. The effect of maternal

TABLE 9-3   Lipid concentrations of mature human milk

Study	Diet			Lipid concentration in milk		
	Plan	Saturation of fat*	Cholesterol (mg/day)	Cholesterol (mg/dl)	Triglyceride (g/dl)	Phospholipid (mg P/dl)
I (n = 7)	A	S	580	18.1 ± 2.7†	3.42 ± 0.61	4.04 ± 0.71
	B	P	110	19.3 ± 3.6	3.57 ± 0.82	4.18 ± 0.91
II (n = 3)	C	S	380	23.3 ± 2.3	4.11 ± 0.42	
	D	P	345	21.3 ± 2.4	4.12 ± 0.56	

From Potter JM, Nestel PJ: *Am J Clin Nutr* 29:54, 1976.
*S, Rich in saturated fatty acids (P/S ratio ~ 0.07); P, rich in polyunsaturated fatty acids (P/S ~ 1.3).
†Mean ± SEM.

diet on cholesterol and phytosterol levels in human milk was measured by Mellies et al,[99] who reported no change in cholesterol but a dramatic increase in phytosterols on high-cholesterol and phytosterol diets. The level of phytosterol in infant plasma did not change, however. These observations further confirm that cholesterol is synthesized at least in part in the mammary gland, whereas phytosterol is not.

Thus there is no evidence that concentrations of cholesterol and phospholipid can be changed by diet. Milk cholesterol is stable at 100 to 150 mg/L even in hypercholesterolemic women and increases only in severe cases of pathologic hypercholesterolemia, according to Jensen.[77] The fat globule membrane contains both cholesterol and phospholipids, and their secretion rates are related to the total quantity and are not influenced by diet.

Where maternal undernutrition is commonplace, the percentage of maternal body fat may influence the concentration of fat in the milk.[123] Milk fat concentrations in Gambian women were positively correlated with maternal skinfold thickness and decreased over the course of lactation. In lactation beyond 6 months, similar correlations have been noted in the United States by Nommsen et al.[106] Women with parity of 10 and above appear to have a decreased capacity to synthesize milk fat and thus have lower milk fat concentrations in their milk.

The synthesis of fatty acids up to the carbon number of 16, as well as the direct desaturation of stearic acid into oleic acid, can take place in the mammary gland, whereas longer-chain fatty acids come directly from plasma triglycerides (see Chapter 4). The intake of both carbohydrate and fat must be taken into account when evaluating maternal diet, because high-carbohydrate diets increase lauric acid and myristic acid and moderate levels of carbohydrate influence linoleic acid.

When serum lipids are measured in African women accustomed to a low fat intake, the levels are relatively low and the women are virtually free of coronary heart disease.[3,118] Among long-lactating (1 to 2 years minimum) African mothers, the amount of fat in their daily milk is of the same order as that ingested in their habitual diet.[161] Despite this, they are not significantly hypolipidemic when compared with nonlactators.

Human milk samples obtained from women living in five different regions of China showed the great diversity of milk fatty acids.[22] The docosahexaenoic acid (DHA) concentrations in women from the marine region were twice as high as those from rural areas.[112] The milk concentrations of DHA varied greatly (0.44 ± 0.29 to 2.78 ± 1.20 g/100 g total fat), with pastoral regions being lowest and the marine region highest. Seafood consumption was high in the marine group. Similarly, arachidonic acid (AA), when stated as a ratio (AA/DHA, g/g), was 2.77 in pastoral areas and 0.42 in the marine region. AA has been associated with infant growth and DHA with brain and retinal growth. Similar findings are reported in Alaskan Eskimos who had a diet high in fish and fish oil. When women's diet was supplemented with fish and fish oils, the blood concentrations of DHA in the maternal plasma and red blood cells (RBCs) were increased.[26] Infants showed a 35% DHA increase in RBCs and 45% in plasma, which supports the concept that maternal diet can influence the DHA levels in the newborn.

Guthrie et al[60] have provided data on the fatty acid patterns of human milk in correlation with the current American diet, which has a high P/S ratio. Compared with studies conducted in 1953, 1958, and 1967, there was a shift toward higher levels of $C_{18:2}$ fatty acids, linoleic acid, and $C_{18:3}$ linolenic acid. *Depot fat* reflects dietary fatty acid patterns and thus the pool for mammary gland synthesis of milk fats. The mammary gland can dehydrogenate saturated and monosaturated fatty acids.

Using newer methodologies of stable isotopes, Hachey et al[61] confirmed the work of early investigators showing that diet composition affects milk fat synthesis. They demonstrated that when a woman is in energy balance, the fatty acids from the diet account for about 30% of the total fatty acids in her milk.

The habitual diet of healthy primiparas in Finland was associated with breast milk containing 3.8% fat.[160] Their diet was 16% protein, 39%

fat, and 45% carbohydrate. Half the fatty acids of the diet and the milk were saturated, and one third were monoenoic. PUFAs were 15% of the diet and 13% of the breast milk, with a P/S ratio of 0.3 for both. The maternal diet had no effect on total fat content of the milk except for the low level of oleic acid, which is apparently peculiar to Finnish breast milk.

A word of caution on the lowering of fats in the diet inordinately: evaluation of the effects of a low-fat maternal diet on neonatal rats by Sinclair and Crawford[136] is pertinent. They made the distinction between two types of lipid in animals: storage and structural. This is correlated with histologic findings of visible and invisible fats. *Visible (storage) fats* are triglycerides found in body depots. *Invisible (structural) fats* include phosphoglycerides, sphingolipids, and some neutral lipids, including cholesterol. The structural fats are key constituents of cellular membranes, certain enzymes, and myelin. The brain contains more structural lipids than protein.

Sinclair and Crawford[136] found that neonatal rats born to mothers raised on low-fat diets had a higher mortality, and survivors had smaller body, brain, and liver weights than controls. The lipid content of the body, brain, and liver was significantly less than controls. During life, the rat pups had depended entirely on their mother's milk for nutrition.

DHA, a long-chain fatty acid (22:6, omega-3) has attracted attention because deficiency has been associated with visual impairment in offspring of rhesus monkeys.[95] Human milk contains consistent levels; formulas contain little or none. DHA can be synthesized from linoleic acid, but high levels of linoleic acid suppress production. Fish oil is an excellent dietary source of DHA, and women who consistently eat fish have higher levels in their milk. Vegetarians have higher DHA levels in their milk than omnivore controls.[47]

A strong association exists between body fat of the mother and lipid in her milk. The best predictor of milk lipids was overall "fatness" rather than the distribution of that fat. Dietary fat was not associated with milk fat in the "fat" women (27% or

more body fat) but was positively correlated with diet in lean women (less than 27% body fat).[97]

When healthy pregnant women are supplemented with fish oil capsules from the 30th week of gestation, the fatty acid compositions of the phospholipids isolated from umbilical plasma and umbilical vessel walls differ from those of unsupplemented mothers, with more n-3 and less n-6 fatty acids.[156] This suggests that DHA status can be altered at birth.

A group of lactating women were given supplements of different doses of fish oil concentrates rich in omega-3 (ω-3) fatty acids, including DHA.[64] Receiving 5 g/day for 28 days, 10 g/day for 14 days, and 47 g/day for 8 days, each experienced significant dose-dependent increases in DHA in their milk and plasma. Baseline levels in milk were 0.1% of total fatty acids, and levels rose from 0.8% to as high as 4.8% on the 47 g/day diet. This suggests that relatively small supplements of DHA can enhance levels in the milk. Preformed dietary DHA is known to be better synthesized into nervous tissue than that synthesized from linolenic acid, and other essential fatty acids can inhibit this transformation to DHA.[64]

Studies of linoleic acid supplementation from 20 weeks' gestation in normal women showed that levels increased in those with low linoleic acid levels to match those with high levels.[1] The neonatal linoleic acid status did not change. Linoleic acid supplementation did result in slightly but significantly higher total amounts of n-6 long-chain polyenes in umbilical plasma. Linoleic acid (18:2, n-6) is essential to the maintenance of the epidermal water barrier and is the ultimate dietary precursor of eicosanoids, which include leukotrienes, prostaglandins, and thromboxanes. Linoleic acid is not synthesized by humans and must be supplied by diet.

A diet deficient in ω-3 fatty acids leads to a triad of signs in the rhesus monkey: visual impairment, electroretinographic abnormalities, and polydipsia. Profound biochemical changes in fatty acid composition of the membranes of the retina, brain, and other organs are seen experimentally. Low concentrations of ω-3 fatty acids occur at birth in the placenta, RBCs, and neural tissues when the mothers are fed deficient diets. Studies in monkeys confirm that the most critical period of life for providing ω-3 fatty acids is during pregnancy and during lactation in early infancy.[26] In humans, supplementation of the maternal diet with fish and fish oils has increased the levels of ω-3 fatty acids, especially DHA. Humans can synthesize DHA from linolenic acid, but this is limited in both infants and adults. Supplementing with linolenic acid does not significantly increase DHA in the blood.[22] No evidence suggests that supplements in normal women with good diets are beneficial. Excesses of DHA affect AA levels and interfere with the AA/DHA ratio.

Lactose

In human milk the principal carbohydrate is lactose, present at about 70 g/L and second only to water as a major constituent. The milk of all species is isotonic with maternal plasma, and 60% to 70% of the osmotic pressure is created by lactose. Lactose provides twice the energy value per molecule or unit of osmotic pressure. Because milk volume is driven by available lactose, its concentration is very stable.[38] Changes in the carbohydrate levels in the diet have been studied. Comparison of mothers on diets with three different levels of carbohydrate shows that the amounts of protein, fat, and carbohydrate in their milk are similar. The Subcommittee on Nutrition During Lactation believes there is no evidence to indicate that dietary manipulations affect lactose.[152]

Water

No data support the assumption that increasing fluid intake will increase milk volume. Conversely, restricting fluids has not been shown to decrease milk volume.[71,109] Forcing fluids, on the other hand, has been shown by Dusdieker et al[42] to affect milk production negatively in a controlled crossover-design study of breastfeeding mothers. Thus women taking excessive fluids produced less milk, suggesting that drinking to thirst and heeding

body cues is more physiologic than prescribing a specific amount of fluid a day. This observation was first demonstrated in a 1939 study by Olsen,[109] who concluded, "Forced, excessive drinking is therefore neither necessary nor beneficial as far as the nursing is concerned and may even be harmful." He had studied great variations in quantity of fluids taken and also noted that "hypogalactia cannot be arrested by forced drinking beyond the natural dictates of thirst." Urine output in these studies was proportional to intake. Illingworth and Kilpatrick[72] did a similar study in 210 postpartum mothers, half of whom drank ad lib, taking an average of 69 oz daily; the other half were forced to take 6 pints and averaged 107 oz daily. The mothers forced to drink beyond thirst produced less milk, and their babies gained less well.

From a practical standpoint, mothers have an increased thirst, which usually maintains a need for added fluid intake. When fluids are restricted, mothers will experience a decrease in urine output, not in milk. On the other hand, sharply decreasing fluids to prevent engorgement in the mother who is not lactating is ineffectual and only adds another inconvenience and discomfort.[41]

Kilocalories

The caloric content, sample by sample, of milk from well-nourished mothers does vary somewhat but averages about 75 kcal/dl. Because fat is the chief source of kilocalories, the fat content has the greatest impact on total kilocalories, with lactose and protein also contributing to the total. Thus in malnourished mothers the caloric content may be reduced.

Body fat increases during pregnancy and decreases during lactation. Changes in the adipose depot primarily result from a change in fat cell size, not number. Adipose tissue fatty acid synthesis remains low throughout lactation, as does lipoprotein lipase activity. Mammary lipoprotein lipase activity, on the other hand, increases and remains high during lactation.[150]

How does this correlate with the caloric needs of the mother to produce milk? The calculations for energy requirements have been made by comparing the energy intakes of nursing mothers and nonnursing mothers who were matched for other variables. English and Hitchcock[45] found that nursing mothers consumed 2460 kcal daily and nonnursing mothers consumed 1880 kcal, a net difference of 580 kcal.

Lactation will not produce a net drain on the mother if the amount of energy available and the requirement of any given nutrient are replaced in the diet. There is a small energy cost of milk production, because the breast does work at re-

Fig. 9-1. Energy utilization during lactation, showing availability of body stores and dietary sources.

markable efficiency. During pregnancy, fat and other nutrients are stored for the fetus and in preparation for lactation. Lactation is subsidized, as is fetal growth, by maternal stores, even though the diet on any given day may be relatively deficient in a specific nutrient. This can be clarified by Fig. 9-1, which shows that diet and stores are available for milk, as well as for maintenance of the mother.

A study of 26 healthy, normotensive, nonsmoking, euthyroid women—12 of whom were breastfeeding, 7 bottle feeding, and 7 nonpregnant, nonlactating controls—was reported by Illingworth et al.[71] Energy expenditure at rest and in response to a meal and to an infusion of noradrenaline was measured. During lactation the resting metabolic rate was unaltered, but there was a reduced response to infusion of noradrenaline and to a meal. These responses returned to normal control values in these women postlactation. Bottle feeders were similar to control subjects. The woman's metabolic efficiency is greatly enhanced during lactation and results in a reduction in the nonlactational component of maternal energy expenditure (Fig. 9-2).

When comparing dietary intake during lactation at 6 weeks postpartum to the intake of a comparable group of nonpregnant women and a group of

Fig. 9-2. Metabolic response to test meal while breastfeeding compared with response of bottle feeders and nonpregnant controls. (From Illingworth PJ, Jung RT, Howie PW et al: *Br Med J* 292:437, 1986.)

nonlactating but postpartum women using a 7-day food diary and questionnaire, total daily intakes and meal patterns were not different between body weight–matched lactators and nonlactators. The lactating women, however, consumed a significantly smaller percentage of the recommended daily allowances (RDAs) per day and were much more calm both before and after meals. Because the lactating women did not increase their daily intake over their prepregnancy diet, Heck and deCastro[65] suggest that they catabolize the weight gain during pregnancy faster and/or increase their metabolic efficiency.

The Subcommittee on Nutrition During Lactation[152] stated that "the total amount of nutrients that the lactating mother secretes in her milk are directly related to the extent and duration of lactation." Furthermore, lactating women who consume a well-balanced diet with adequate calories (2700 kcal/day) also meet the RDA for all nutrients with the exception of calcium and zinc, according to assessments of the average American diet for young women. The subcommittee based its assumption on nutrient density (nutrient intake per 1000 kcal) of the average woman's diet in the United States (see Appendix B). Nutrient densities for proteins, minerals, and vitamins were determined from nationally representative samples of women aged 19 to 50 years of age. The nutrient values at three different levels of energy have been calculated (nutrient density × kcal of energy = total intake). The levels of energy used are 2700 kcal, the recommendation for lactating women; 2200 kcal, as reported by lactating women as actual consumption; and 1800 kcal, the minimal level a lactating woman should consider in a restricted diet. The relative nutrient deficiencies are identified next.

For the lactating woman, a 2700-kcal diet may be deficient in calcium and zinc; the 2200-kcal diet is deficient in calcium, magnesium, zinc, thiamin, vitamin B_6, and vitamin E; and the 1800-kcal diet is deficient in all the previously mentioned nutrient levels plus riboflavin, folate, phosphorus, and iron unless special attention is paid to intake of these nutrients (Table 9-8).

The subcommittee[152] recommends that women be encouraged to follow dietary guidelines, especially in terms of fruits, vegetables, and whole grains; calcium-rich dairy products; and protein-rich foods. Vitamin and mineral supplements are not recommended for lactating women. If, however, dietary review suggests intake is lower than recommended, the woman should be encouraged to consume more foods rich in those nutrients. A woman with serious dietary problems leading to low intake of one or more nutrients should be encouraged by counseling to correct her dietary deficiencies. Nutrient supplements are recommended only as a last resort.

Diets of adolescents have been noted to be low in iron and vitamin A (1500 IU/1000 kcal instead of 1950 IU/1000 kcal). Black women consume 30% less calcium, 20% less magnesium, and 20% less vitamin A than white women. Appendix B lists recommendations for culturally acceptable diets, and Table 9-4 suggests measures for improving nutrient intake of women with restrictive eating patterns. Overt signs of deficiency are rare in the United States, even for the nutrients with small safety margins.

Vitamins

Water-soluble vitamins

Water-soluble vitamins move with ease from serum to milk; thus their dietary fluctuation is more apparent. Levels of water-soluble vitamins in milk are raised or lowered by change in the maternal diet. The body's requirement for vitamin C increases under stress, including lactation. Furthermore, the vitamin C content of human organs at autopsy is much higher in the neonate than at any other time of life. This is true of all the major organs, including the brain.

The influence of maternal intake of vitamin C on the concentration of vitamin C in human milk and on the intake of vitamin C by the infant was carefully measured by Byerley and Kirksey[17] in 25 well-nourished lactating women. Supplements ranged from 0 to 1000 mg (10 times the RDA) vitamin C daily. Concentrations in milk ranged

TABLE 9-4   **Suggested measures for improving nutrient intake of women with restrictive eating patterns**

Type of restrictive eating pattern	Corrective measures
Excessive restriction of food intake, i.e., ingestion of less than 1800 kcal of energy per day, which ordinarily leads to unsatisfactory intake of nutrients compared with amounts needed by lactating women	Encourage increased intake of nutrient-rich foods to achieve energy intake of at least 1800 kcal/day; if mother insists on curbing food intake sharply, promote substitution of foods rich in vitamins, minerals, and protein for those lower in nutritive value; in individual cases, it may be advisable to recommend a balanced multivitamin-mineral supplement; discourage use of liquid weight loss diets and appetite suppressants
Complete vegetarianism, i.e., avoidance of all animal foods, including meat, fish, dairy products, and eggs	Advise intake of regular source of vitamin B_{12}, such as special vitamin B_{12}–containing plant food products or a 2.6-μg vitamin B_{12} supplement daily
Avoidance of milk, cheese, or other calcium-rich dairy products	Encourage increased intake of other culturally appropriate dietary calcium sources, such as collard greens for blacks from southeastern United States; provide information on appropriate use of low-lactose dairy products if milk is being avoided because of lactose intolerance; if correction by diet cannot be achieved, it may be advisable to recommend 600 mg of elemental calcium per day taken with meals
Avoidance of vitamin D–fortified foods, such as fortified milk or cereal, combined with limited exposure to ultraviolet light	Recommend 10 μg of supplemental vitamin D per day

From the Subcommittee on Nutrition During Lactation, Committee on Nutritional Status during Pregnancy and Lactation, Food and Nutrition Board, Institute of Medicine, National Academy of Sciences: *Nutrition during lactation,* Washington, DC, 1991, National Academy Press.

from 44 to 158 mg/L and were not correlated significantly with maternal intakes, which ranged from 156 (0 mg supplement) to 1123 (1000 mg supplement). Dietary vitamin C had no effect on the volume of milk produced. Maternal excretion of vitamin C in urine was correlated with maternal intake. Regardless of the level of maternal intake of vitamin C, the mean vitamin C concentration in breast milk was twice that recommended for infant formula. Vitamin C levels in milk did not increase in response to increasing maternal intake despite tenfold increases, whereas urinary excretion did suggest that mammary tissue becomes saturated.

The investigators[17] postulate a regulatory mechanism to prevent an elevation in concentra-

tion of vitamin C beyond a certain level in milk. Vitamin C levels were at the same or higher levels in exclusively breastfed infants at 6 months and 9 months of age than levels of supplemented bottle-fed controls.[133] Levels were dependent on maternal nutrition and vitamin C levels in milk. Byerley and Kirksey[17] found 6% of well-nourished healthy mothers had low levels of vitamin C. In malnourished women, tissue stores may take time to replenish, which explains why 35 mg/day supplementation failed to increase low plasma levels.[138] Data from multiple studies suggest that there is a level above which further vitamin C supplementation will not affect milk vitamin C levels.[95]

The level of *B vitamins,* also water soluble,

reflects dietary intake. The levels are affected acutely by maternal diet. Infantile beriberi is not unheard of in seemingly normal infants nursed by apparently well-nourished mothers with thiamin-deficient diets. The influence of maternal diet has been pointed out dramatically in reported cases of megaloblastic anemia and methylmalonic aciduria and homocystinuria in the breastfed infants of strict vegetarians. *Vitamin B_{12}* exists in all animal protein but not in vegetable protein. A strict vegetarian would require B_{12} supplements during pregnancy and lactation.[56,68,103] B_{12} deficiency in infants has also been seen in New Delhi, where mothers produced B_{12}-deficient milk. These infants also had megaloblastic anemia.[32]

Specker et al[142] have noted that infants of vegetarians who have low B_{12} serum and milk levels have methylmalonic acid in their urine inversely proportional to their B_{12} levels, even though they are asymptomatic. Other authors[56,68,103] have concluded that the current RDA for infants provides little margin of safety: 0.3 μg/day or 0.05 μg/kg body weight is close to the intake below which infant urinary methylmalonic acid measures are elevated.

Thiamine (B_1) has been studied infrequently, but maternal supplementation does not increase milk levels beyond a certain limit. Urinary excretion of thiamine is significantly higher in supplemented compared with unsupplemented women. In malnourished women, evidence indicates that supplementation does increase thiamine levels in milk. The Subcommittee on Nutrition During Lactation[152] recommends that thiamine intake be at least 1.3 mg/day (the RDA for nonpregnant, nonlactating women of 1.1 mg/day plus an increment for milk secretion of 0.2 mg/day) when the calorie intake is less than 2200 kcal/day.

Riboflavin (B_2) requirements of lactating women in The Gambia in a controlled study showed the minimum to be 2.5 mg/day to maintain normal biochemical status in the mother and adequate levels of B_2 in her milk.[12] This level is higher than that recommended in the United States and the United Kingdom. The pantothenic acid content of human milk does not vary appreciably with dietary variations in well-nourished mothers, but the overall intake over time does influence milk levels.[80]

Niacin (B_3) content of human milk has been reported to parallel dietary intake. In unsupplemented diets, low B_3 levels usually parallel low levels of other B vitamins and low protein intakes.

Pyridoxine (B_6) intake and milk levels were studied in healthy lactating women by West and Kirksey.[167] They found marked diurnal variations of B_6 levels, with peaks occurring in those mothers taking supplements 3 to 5 hours after a dose. Those taking less than 2.5 mg/day had much lower milk levels (129 μg/L). Vitamin B_6 concentrations in human milk change rapidly with maternal intake.[6] When supplemented, the level in the milk is a direct reflection of amount ingested. Plasma pyridoxal-5'-phosphate (PLP) levels and birthweight are the strongest predictors of infant growth.[82,151]

When lactating mothers received supplements of B_6 ranging from 0 to 20 mg pyridoxine hydrochloride, the levels of B_6 measurable in the milk paralleled the intake, with levels peaking 5 hours after ingesting the supplement.[5] When maternal intakes of vitamin B_6 approximated 2.0 mg/day, breastfed infants were unlikely to receive the current RDA of 0.3 mg vitamin B_6 per day when intake was calculated from morning B_6 levels in milk and daily volume was assumed to be 850 cc. The American Academy of Pediatrics (AAP) Committee on Nutrition[24] recommends a minimum of 0.35 mg vitamin B_6/100 kcal milk from birth to 12 months. The RDA for B_6 for lactating women is 0.5 mg daily. B_6 is the vitamin most likely to be deficient, and pyridoxine levels in milk are closely influenced by dietary intake.[6,82] Supplementing with an additional 2.5 mg/day results in levels twice as high as in unsupplemented women. On the other hand, as reported in two studies, infants of unsupplemented lactating women in the United States had no clinical symptoms of vitamin B_6 deficiency, although infant plasma PLP levels were lower than those in comparable bottle-fed infants.

None of the women had used oral contraceptives in the previous 5 years.[6] The increment in the RDA for B_6 in lactation is more than five times the estimated secretion of this vitamin in milk,[152] which varies between 0.01 and 0.02 mg/L early in lactation to 0.10 to 0.25 mg/L in mature milk. The recommendation is to advise diets rich in B_6, such as poultry, meat, fish, and some legumes, and reserve supplementation for special-risk cases.

Pantothenic acid levels in milk are strongly correlated with maternal intake for the preceding day. Johnston et al[80] have suggested that some pantothenic acid is stored in the body. Studies of malnourished women show increased levels in milk after supplementation.

Biotin is reported in few studies, but the findings are consistent that levels range from 5 to 12 µg/L, with supplementation even up to 250 µg/day having little effect except when levels are significantly below this range.[125,126]

Pregnant and lactating women are at risk for suboptimal *folate* status because of the increased dietary requirement to facilitate enhanced anabolic activity. Until megaloblastic anemia develops, no validated quick, nonintrusive tests exist to assess functional folate status. Milk folate levels are maintained at the expense of maternal reserves, thereby protecting the nursling. O'Connor[107] provides an extensive review of the issues.

Folate supplementation in well-nourished women does not affect the level of folate in the milk, although studies involving women with low folate (less than 60% RDA) show they responded to supplementation with an increased level in their milk. Differences in assay methods have produced inconsistencies among studies. Milk levels normally range between 40 and 70 µg/L and increase slightly in the early weeks of lactation. Supplementation is 0.8 to 1.0 mg/day in those with chronic deficiency.[95]

Deodhar and Ramakrishnan[32] studied the effect of the stage of lactation on levels of vitamins B_1, B_2, B_3, B_6, B_{12}, and ascorbic acid. The values remained fairly constant throughout, except for those of B_3, which increased slightly over time. The relationship to socioeconomic group showed an increase in B_3 and B_6 levels with increased status. B_1 was higher in poorer mothers. Tables 9-5 and 9-6 summarize the effect of diet on vitamin levels in maternal milk.

Fat-soluble vitamins

Fat-soluble compounds are generally transported into milk via the fat, and levels are less easily improved by dietary change. Because A and D are stored in tissues, the impact of dietary supplement is more difficult to measure. Milk levels do not change until a certain level is achieved in the

TABLE 9-5   Water-soluble vitamins in human milk

Vitamin	Recognizable clinical deficiency in infant	Effect of maternal supplements		Effect of dietary intake on milk content
		In malnourished	In well-nourished	
Ascorbic acid (C)	Rare	Yes	Minimal	Limited at 50 mg/L
Thiamin (B_1)	Yes	Yes	Limited	Yes, up to 200 µg/L
Riboflavin (B_2)	Yes	Yes	Yes	Yes
Niacin (B_3)	Unknown	Yes	Yes	Yes
Pantothenic acid	Unknown	Yes	No	Yes
Pyridoxine (B_6)	Yes	Yes	Yes	Yes
Biotin	Yes	Yes	No	Limited
Folate	Unknown	Yes	No	No
Cyanocobalamin (B_{12})	Rare	Yes	No	Yes

Prepared from Subcommittee on Nutrition During Lactation,[152] Committee on Nutritional Status during Pregnancy and Lactation, Food and Nutrition Board, Institute of Medicine, National Academy of Sciences: *Nutrition during lactation*, Washington, DC, 1991, National Academy Press.

stores. High dietary levels of β-carotene do not appear to result in excessive levels of either vitamin A or β-carotene. Increase in vitamin A in the diet of undernourished women does increase its level in milk.

When malnourished mothers were given a single oral megadose of 209 μmol of vitamin A and the control subjects given none, serum retinol (vitamin A_1) levels increased in the supplemented mothers and remained significantly higher for at least 3 months.[132] Breast milk levels were higher (11.3 μmol/L versus 2.9 μmol/L) and remained so for 6 months. An associated observation was the reduction in the duration of respiratory tract infections and febrile illnesses in the infants.

Most women have very adequate *vitamin D* levels.[152] Vitamin D was considered to be at a stable level in milk; however, studies involving maternal supplementation have demonstrated increased milk levels.[69] When mothers were given 0, 500, and 2500 IU ergocalciferol daily, they produced milk with 39, 218, and 3040 mg/ml vitamin D. The effect on levels of 25-hydroxyvitamin D (25-OHD) was less dramatic. The physiologic significance to the infant is disputed, however, because the major source of antirachitic sterols seems to be sunlight, not milk. The role of water-soluble vitamin D in human milk has not been confirmed.[143,145] Infants born to mothers with inadequate vitamin D stores need a regular supply of vitamin D through diet, supplements, and exposure to ultraviolet light.[152]

Multiple studies have demonstrated that maternal 25-OHD levels can be raised by supplementation.[29] In women at risk, this supplementation should begin in pregnancy and continue through lactation to ensure adequate levels in their milk. Supplementing mothers is preferred to supplementing the breastfed infant because the mother is also in deficit.[111,140]

Dark-skinned infants reared in climates where sunlight is minimal may be at significant risk for rickets when breastfed unless attention is given to the possible need for supplements of vitamin D.[10] Although rickets was considered a disease of the past, the disease has reemerged since the 1980s partially because of the high risk of premature infants, especially micropremature infants, but also because of the increase in breastfeeding, especially by women who avoid dairy products, which are the major source of food vitamin D supplementation.[29]

The emphasis has been on the rare cases of deficiency in breastfed infants, but accidents of oversupplementation with vitamin D have appeared since mass supplementation has been mandated as a public health policy. A recent report of a dairy adding 70 to 600 times the recommended amount of vitamin D resulted in exposure to a large population, with variable subclinical effects.[134]

Specker et al[144,145] estimated that 30 minutes of sunlight per week wearing only a diaper or 2 hours a week fully clothed (no hat) would maintain serum 25-OHD concentrations above lower limits of normal.

Vitamin E has not been the focus of study of maternal dietary supplements except in the report by Kramer et al[87] that sunflower oil replacing lard

---

TABLE 9-6   Fat-soluble vitamins in human milk

| Vitamin | Recognizable clinical deficiency in infant | Effect of maternal supplements | | Effect of dietary intake on milk content |
		In malnourished	In well-nourished	
D	Yes	Yes	Yes	Yes
K	Yes	Yes	Variable	Probable
A	Unknown	Yes	Minimal	Yes
E	Unknown	Unknown	Yes	Unknown

Prepared from Subcommittee on Nutrition During Lactation,[152] Committee on Nutritional Status during Pregnancy and Lactation, Food and Nutrition Board, Institute of Medicine, National Academy of Sciences: *Nutrition during lactation*, Washington, DC, 1991, National Academy Press.

in the diet resulted in a 50% increase in vitamin E levels in the milk. On the other hand, the liberal use of vitamin E creams by health enthusiasts may well expose an infant to large doses by maternal absorption as well as directly when the creams are applied to the breast. α-Tocopherol levels are highest in the colostrum, when the neonate is most dependent on its physiologic effect as an antioxidant, and in the prevention of hemolytic anemia attributed to vitamin E deficiency. Maternal vitamin E intake can influence the levels of E in the milk. However, no evidence indicates that vitamin E deficiency occurs in individuals with normal fat absorption.[152]

The most critical need for vitamin K is during the birth process and in the first few days of life, when the risk of bleeding, especially intracranial bleeding, is greatest.[58] Maternal dietary intake, on the other hand, is most critical during the last trimester. Transplacental passage of *vitamin K* is slow. Cord blood levels are almost imperceptible. The synthesis of menaquinones by bacteria in the breastfed infant gut is minimal because lactobacillus does not synthesize them. Studies on supplementation of lactating women have shown that small doses are inadequate to raise the maternal plasma level and subsequently the levels in the milk.[115] Newer technology has forced a recalculation of maternal vitamin K intakes. Greer et al[57] have shown that the average woman's intake is now 0.8 to 1.03 μg/kg/day.

PIVKA (undercarboxylated prothombin produced in the absence of vitamin K) levels are a marker of K deficiency. The cord blood of full-term infants often has high PIVKA levels (0.1 AU/ml) correlating with low vitamin K. Levels in the infant are undetectable at 4 weeks after intramuscular (IM) vitamin K administration at birth, but in some infants they become elevated by 8 weeks. This has led to the recommendation that mothers be supplemented with 5 mg of vitamin K daily through the first 3 months of lactation.[57]

The consensus is that late vitamin K deficiency bleeding should be prevented by prophylaxis (Box 9-1). After a study of different oral schedules in Australia, Germany, the Netherlands, and Switzer-

---

BOX 9-1   Vitamin K recommendations

1. Vitamin K_1 should be given to all newborns as a single, intramuscular dose of 0.5 to 1 mg.
2. Further research on the efficacy, safety, and bioavailability of oral formulations of vitamin K is warranted.
3. An oral dosage form is not currently available in the United States but ought to be developed and licensed. If an appropriate oral form is developed and licensed in the United States, it should be given at birth (2.0 mg) to all infants and should be administered again at 1 to 2 weeks and at 4 weeks of age to breastfed infants. If diarrhea occurs in an exclusively breastfed infant, the dose should be repeated.
4. Data from the United States and elsewhere suggest that additional cohort studies are unlikely to be helpful.

From Report of Ad Hoc Task Force on Vitamin K, American Academy of Pediatrics, *Pediatrics* 91:1002, 1993.

---

land, it was confirmed that oral doses of 1 mg vitamin K for the infant are less effective than IM dosing. Further, Cornelissen et al[28] reported that the most effective regimen was an initial dose of 1 mg followed by 25 μg vitamin K orally for breastfed infants. The new mixed micellar preparation remains under investigation. The least invasive method would be to increase the milk levels by supplementing the mother. In the 1950s, efforts to increase vitamin K and prothrombin levels at birth by giving mothers a large dose of K in labor failed to change the incidence of hemorrhagic disease in newborns. However, maternal supplementation during lactation is effective.

Although the amount of vitamin K available in infant formulas is very high, no toxicity has yet been demonstrated.

Summary

Although dietary supplements improve the milk quality and quantity in malnourished women, a balanced diet without excessive supplementation is the most physiologic and economic way to ensure good milk. Nutrients, especially vitamins, are only excreted in the urine when taken in excess.

Minerals

Calcium

Calcium has been associated with bone growth, and concern has been expressed because the total calcium in breast milk is low. The available information is inadequate to determine the true requirement for lactation. Studies with radioactive calcium in the nonpregnant adult have shown that losses occur into the gut and through the kidney. Absorption and retention also depend on the reserves in the body. Long-term shortage causes economy of utilization, and the apparent requirement is lower.[18] During lactation the absorption and retention are greater.

Serum calcium and phosphorus concentrations are greater in lactating women compared with non-lactating women.[81] Lactation stimulates increases in fractional calcium absorption and serum calcitrol. This is most apparent after weaning. Alterations in absorption, metabolism, and excretion may conserve calcium during lactation. Women with low calcium intakes have no direct benefit from supplementation as a protective mechanism to maintain breast milk calcium or maternal bone mineral content.[120,121] Urinary calcium is higher in the supplemented group. Of significance, however, is the presence of risk factors: positive family history of osteoporosis, fair complexion, lower body mass and height, not breastfeeding their infants, smoking, and fat deposits have greatest predictability for osteoporosis.[81]

Atkinson and West[9] showed by scanning transmission techniques that lactating women mobilize about 2% of their skeletal calcium over 100 days of nursing. The calcium content of milk appears to be maintained despite greatly deficient intake, probably because of skeletal stores. The milk calcium levels are the same in mothers of rachitic and non-rachitic infants. This is most important for women under age 25 because calcium content of bones is expected to increase until age 25.[94] Peak bone mass is achieved during the childbearing years.

Estradiol concentrations are related to bone mineral density (BMD) because it stimulates osteoblastic proliferation and enhances collagen gene expression. The relatively low estrogen levels during lactation increase bone mobilization. Prolonged amenorrhea is associated with increased mobilization, and the greatest reduction in bone mass occurs early in lactation. Prolactin has a synergistic effect on mobilization. The ratio of dietary calcium to dietary protein has also been identified as important; that is, women with high-protein diets must also have high calcium intake. Recovery after weaning is reported to be negatively affected by parity.[90]

The RDAs for calcium and vitamin D are higher for women under age 25, even when prepregnant, than for older women (1200 mg calcium compared with 800 mg recommended for nonpregnant women over age 25). Calcium status is only one of many possible factors in the etiology of osteoporosis. Dietary guidance during lactation should include recommendations for the replacement of stores. Women who have lactated are not more prone to osteoporosis than nonlactators or nulliparas, and they may be less prone.[18,37,150]

The additional requirement for calcium in the lactating woman's diet is 400 mg daily above normal levels, or 1200 mg total, which is not easily achieved without milk products and may require special attention by the physician.[58] When dietary calcium intake is greater than the RDA for lactating women, bone mineral content is not diminished during at least the first 6 weeks of lactation.

Sodium, potassium, and chlorine

The concentration of sodium is the most variable of all the minerals, fluctuating as much as tenfold during normal lactation and diurally, separate from the effects of mastitis, emotional stress, or involution. Maternal sodium or potassium intake has no immediate influence, either high or low, on postprandial milk sodium or potassium concentrations.[46] Dietary potassium may influence milk potassium more significantly. With increasing numbers of women with cardiac and renal disease choosing to lactate, potassium levels in the diet would be of significance, in addition to concerns about necessary medications.[83]

Chlorine level in the breast milk is not believed to be affected by maternal diet. Chlorine deficiency reported in a breastfed infant was associated with normal maternal serum and dietary intake[8] but with deficit levels in the milk (less than 2 mEq/L). Normal is greater than 8 mEq/L.

The concentration of electrolytes (sodium, potassium, chloride) in milk is determined by an electrical potential gradient in the secretory cell rather than by maternal nutritional status.[150]

Iron

The iron content of milk is not readily affected by the iron content of the diet or the maternal serum iron level. Increases in dietary iron that increase serum levels do not increase iron in the milk. It is important, however, for the mother to replace her iron stores postpartum.[114] It has not been established that increases in tissue iron are advantageous. Iron that is added to human milk will bind to lactoferrin and may interfere with its function. Infants exclusively breastfed for 7 months or longer were not found to be anemic at 12 or 24 months.[116] Half the infants breastfed for a shorter period were anemic at 12 months if additional dietary iron from solids was not provided.

Phosphorus, magnesium, zinc, and copper

Phosphorus, magnesium, zinc, and copper levels in milk are not affected by dietary administration of these elements.[88] Again, however, it is important for the mother to replenish her stores.[114]

According to the RDA, many lactating women are receiving marginal amounts of magnesium.[105] The amount recommended for lactation is two to three times the amount estimated to be in the milk.

Zinc has an RDA increment during lactation 4 to 13 times higher than the amount estimated to be in the milk on the basis that it is poorly adsorbed (20%).[49] Studies done with stable isotopes in lactating women show that absorption was 59% to 84% of intake. Zinc absorption during pregnancy increases dramatically and during lac-

tation decreases slightly but is double the prepregnant rates, presumably in response to the demand by the breast for milk synthesis.[53] Milk levels are unaffected by supplementation and gradually decline over time from 2 mg/day.[89] Supplementation does result in increased maternal absorption and increased plasma levels. Although no major health risks have been associated with low zinc intakes, zinc is known to be important to immune function.[74]

Iron supplementation has no significant effect on levels of copper, selenium, and zinc in mother's serum and breast milk.[7]

Selenium

A correlation exists between selenium in human milk and maternal dietary intake.[93] Maternal plasma levels vary with the form of selenium supplementation (selenomethionine or selenium-enriched yeast).[98] The original source of selenium is the soil, and levels vary geographically. It is transferred to plants and works up the food chain. Breastfed infants are known to have higher intake and utilization than infants fed formula or cow's milk because of the bioavailability.[2] Many selenoproteins have been identified, but glutathione peroxidase is involved with producing a variety of organic hydroperoxides or reactive oxygen radicals in the liver. Although selenium toxicity is possible, deficiency from low intake is a problem.[93] Two diseases described are Keshan disease and Kashin-Beck disease, which are associated with accumulation of lipid peroxides. Dietary studies have shown that intake can affect the mother's plasma and milk levels.[2]

Chromium

Breast milk levels of chromium are reported to be 3.54 ± 40 nmol/L (0.18 ng/ml) and independent of dietary intake.[4] Total absorption for lactating women was 0.79 ± 0.08 µmol/dl, which was greater than that of nonlactators. Serum levels were correlated with urinary chromium excretion, a good indicator of serum levels. The estimated RDA for breastfed infants is 10 µg, which is much greater than the levels measured in this study. The

TABLE 9-7	Minerals in human milk		
Mineral	Concentration throughout lactation	Facilitated bioavailability	Effect of maternal mineral intake on milk content
Sodium	Varies	Unknown	None
Calcium	Unchanged	Unknown	None
Iron	Unchanged	Facilitated	None
Zinc	Declines	Facilitated	None
Copper	Unchanged	Unknown	None
Manganese	Declines	Unknown	Yes
Selenium	Diet dependent	Facilitated	None
Iodine	Declines	Unknown	Yes
Fluoride	Stable	Unknown	Yes

Modified from the Committee on Nutrition, American Academy of Pediatrics: *Pediatrics* 68:435, 1981.

RDA for adults is 50 μg; most adults achieve 50% to 60% of this level. RDAs for chromium may need to be reevaluated.

Iodine

Iodine in milk does depend on dietary content. The breast is able to raise the concentration of iodine in the milk above that in the blood, and thus there is an increased danger in giving radioactive iodine to the lactating woman. With iodized salt, bread dough conditioners, and common use of iodine-containing cleansers, there is actually a risk of excessive iodine intake. Milk iodine concentrations are higher now than were reported in the 1930s. Mean breast milk iodide levels ranged from 29 to 490 ng/L, averaging 178 ng/L, above the RDA for infants.[59]

Fluorine

Human milk contains 16 ± 5 μg fluoride/L and reflects to some degree the level in the water supply. The risk of excessive fluoride has been pointed out by Walton and Messer,[166] who report dental mottling and milk fluorosis in supplemented breastfed infants. The AAP Committee on Nutrition therefore has stated, "It may not be necessary to give fluoride supplements to breastfed infants who are living in an area where water is adequately fluoridated."[25]

Fluoride concentrations of infant foods and drinks have been found to vary widely, ranging from 0.01 to 0.72 mg/kg, so that no need exists for supplementation when solid foods are initiated if the diet is well balanced.[158]

Summary

Table 9-7 summarizes mineral levels in maternal milk and dietary effect.

MATERNAL NUTRITION: IMMUNOLOGIC SUBSTANCES AND LEUKOCYTE ACTIVITY

Substances in colostrum and mature milk confer important infection protection on the breastfed infant. Maternal malnutrition was associated with lower levels of immunoglobulins G and A (IgG, IgA) in a group of Colombian women studied by Miranda et al.[104] The colostrum contained only one-third the normal levels of IgG and less than half the normal albumin. Significant reductions in IgA and complement C4 were observed in colostrum, but lysozyme, C3, and IgM were normal. Titers against respiratory syncytial virus were unaffected by nutritional status. The protective deficiencies improved in mature milk over time and with improvement of nutritional status. The total leukocyte concentrations as well as their bactericidal capacity were similar in well-nourished and undernourished women.[13]

Prentice et al[124] measured breast milk antimicrobial factors of rural Gambian mothers. The concentrations and daily secretions of all immunoproteins, except lysozyme, decreased during the first year and then remained steady. Compared with those in Western women, levels of IgG, IgM, C3, and C4 were higher in Gambian women; IgA and lactoferrin were similar; and lysozyme was lower. Dietary supplement in Gambian women did not raise the breast milk immunoproteins in this study.

The Subcommittee on Nutrition During Lactation has concluded that the effects of maternal nutritional status on the immunologic system in human milk are controversial.[152] Some studies suggest that malnutrition decreases the production and secretion of some components of the immunologic system, but further investigation clearly is necessary.

RECOMMENDATIONS FOR NUTRITIONAL SUPPORT DURING LACTATION

The previous section noted that the quantity, protein content, and calcium content of milk are relatively independent of maternal nutritional status and diet. Amino acids, lysine and methionine, certain fatty acids, and water-soluble vitamin contents vary with intake. It is important to point out that stores of calcium, minerals, and fat-soluble vitamins need to be replenished.[169] Much of the data collected have varied, depending on the method used in collection. The daily intakes believed necessary for infants were determined by feeding infants processed human milk in a bottle, which is not a physiologic standard. It is known, for example, that putting the entire sample in one container removes the natural variation in fat from beginning to end of the feeding.

The Subcommittee on Nutrition During Lacta-

tion[49,152] has recommended a balanced diet comparable to one for the nonlactating postpartum mother, with a few additions. Although the calculated caloric cost of producing 1 L of milk is 940 kcal, during pregnancy most women store 2 to 4 kg of extra tissue in the physiologic preparation for lactation. Thus it is probably necessary to add only 500 kcal to the diet, except in women with known high metabolic rates.

Preparation for lactation begins in pregnancy, if not before. The major daily increases for pregnancy are 300 kcal; 20 g of protein; a 20% increase in all vitamins and minerals except folic acid, which is doubled; and a 33% increase in calcium, phosphorus, and magnesium. In comparing the RDA[49] for lactating women with that for nonlactating adult women, the increases suggested should provide ample nutrition and replace stores (Table 9-8).

When dietary supplements are suggested (Table 9-9), concern arises about increased costs. Cost increases are modest for the standard diet and minimal for the low-budget diet, as demonstrated by Worthington-Roberts.[170] Although one rarely chooses breastfeeding or bottle feeding on the basis of cost, the price of a few extra maternal kilocalories versus the cost of formula feeding makes a reassuring comparison. Hypoallergenic formulas are even more costly, estimated to be more than $3 per day.

Following the report of the Subcommittee on Nutrition During Lactation,[152] an additional report was prepared, *Nutrition During Pregnancy and Lactation: an Implementation Guide.* Its purpose is to offer practical guidance to the primary care provider by including a sample nutrition screening questionnaire, indications for supplementation, nutritional assessment guidelines, and how and when to refer to a registered dietitian.[153] It provides a chart for estimating body mass index (BMI) (Fig. 9-3).

The subcommittee did not propose a food guide because it recognized that diverse ways are available to meet nutrient needs and that culturally appropriate foods are important, especially in

TABLE 9-8	**Estimated mean nutrient intakes by U.S. women at three energy levels compared with the recommended dietary allowances (RDAs) for lactation**

A. Protein and fat-soluble vitamins

Measure	Protein (g)	Vitamin A (μg of RE)	Vitamin D (μg)	Vitamin E (mg of α-TE)	Vitamin K (μg)
Average nutrient density of diets of U.S. women ages 19 to 50 yr* (nutrient content per 1000 kcal)	40	805	NR	5	NR
Nutrient intake assuming average nutrient density at:					
2700 kcal	108	2174	NA	14	NA
2200 kcal	88	1771	NA	11	NA
1800 kcal	72	1449	NA	9	NA
RDA for lactation†					
0-6 mo	65	1300	10	12	65
6-12 mo	62	1200	10	11	65

B. Water-soluble vitamins

Measure	Vitamin C (mg)	Thiamin (mg)	Riboflavin (mg)	Niacin (mg of NE)	Vitamin B$_6$ (mg)	Folate (μg)	Vitamin B$_{12}$ (μg)
Average nutrient density of diets of U.S. women ages 19 to 50 yr* (nutrient content per 1000 kcal)	56	0.7	0.9	11.2	0.8	13.7	2.9
Nutrient intake assuming average nutrient density at:							
2700 kcal	151	1.9	2.4	30.2	2.2	370	7.8
2200 kcal	123	1.5	2.0	24.6	1.8	301	6.4
1800 kcal	101	1.3	1.6	20.2	1.4	247	5.2
RDA for lactation†							
0-6 mo	95	1.6	1.8	20	2.1	280	2.6
6-12 mo	90	1.6	1.7	20	2.1	260	2.6

From Subcommittee on Nutrition During Lactation, Committee on Nutritional Status during Pregnancy and Lactation, Food and Nutrition Board, Institute of Medicine, National Academy of Sciences: *Nutrition during lactation,* Washington, DC, 1991, National Academy Press.
RE, Retinol equivalents; *α-TE,* α-tocopherol equivalents; *NR,* not reported; *NA,* not applicable.
*From Continuing Survey of Food Intake by Individuals, Report No 86-1, Hyattsville, Md, 1987, Department of Agriculture.
†Assumes 2700 kcal of energy per day, from Food and Nutrition Board, National Research Council: *Recommended dietary allowances,* ed 11, Washington, DC, 1994, National Academy Press. *Continued*

TABLE 9-8 **Estimated mean nutrient intakes by U.S. women at three energy levels compared with the recommended dietary allowances (RDAs) for lactation—cont'd**

c. Minerals

Measure	Calcium (mg)	Phosphorus (mg)	Magnesium (mg)	Iron (mg)	Zinc (mg)	Iodine (µg)	Selenium (µg)
Average nutrient density of diets of U.S. women ages 19 to 50 yr* (nutrient content per 1000 kcal)	397	645	143	7.0	5.8	145‡	3.5‡
Nutrient intake assuming average nutrient density at:							
2700 kcal	1072	1742	386	18.9	15.7	392	95
2200 kcal	873	1419	315	15.4	12.8	319	77
1800 kcal	715	1161	257	12.6	10.4	261	63
RDA for lactation†							
0-6 mo	1200	1200	355	15	19	200	75
6-12 mo	1200	1200	340	15	16	200	75

‡Estimated from the Total Diet Study; Pennington JAT, Young BE, Wilson DB: *J Am Diet Assoc* 89:659, 1989.

TABLE 9-9 **Extra daily nutrient allowances for lactation over baseline**

Nutrient	Nonpregnant, nonlactating	Lactating	Increase
Energy (kcal)	2100	2700	500
Protein (g)	40	65	25
Retinol (µg)	800	1300	500
Vitamin D (µg)	7.5	10	3
Vitamin E (mg)	8	11	3
Vitamin C (mg)	60	100	40
Riboflavin (mg)	1.3	1.8	0.5
Nicotinic acid (mg)	14	20	6
Vitamin B_6 (mg)	2.0	2.5	0.5
Folate (µg)	40	280	240
Thiamin (mg)	1.1	1.6	0.5
Calcium (mg)	800	1200	400
Iron (mg)	18	18	18
Zinc (mg)	15	25	10

From Food and Nutrition Board, National Research Council: *Recommended dietary allowances,* ed 11, Washington, DC, 1994, National Academy Press.

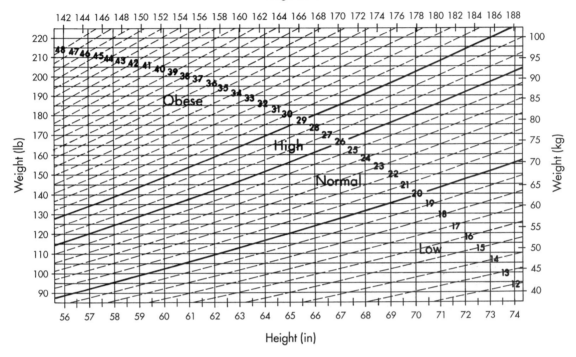

Fig. 9-3. Chart for estimating body mass index (BMI) category and BMI. To find BMI category (e.g., obese), find point where woman's height and weight intersect. To estimate BMI, read bold number on the dashed line that is closest to the point. (From Subcommittee on Nutrition During Lactation, Committee on Nutritional Status during Pregnancy and Lactation: *Nutrition during pregnancy and lactation: an implementation guide,* Washington, DC, 1992, National Academy Press.)

the perinatal period. It did offer the following recommendations[153]:

- Avoid diets and medications that promise rapid weight loss.
- Eat a wide variety of breads and cereal grains, fruits, vegetables, milk products, and meats or meat alternates each day.
- Take three or more servings of milk products daily.
- Make a greater effort to eat vitamin A–rich vegetables or fruits often. Examples of foods high in vitamin A include carrots, spinach or other cooked greens, sweet potatoes, and cantaloupe.
- Be sure to drink when you are thirsty. You will need more fluid than usual.
- If you drink coffee or other caffeinated bever-

ages, such as cola, do so in moderation. Two servings daily are unlikely to harm the infant. Caffeine passes into the milk.

Malnutrition: Special supplementation for the lactating woman

It has been suggested that supplementing the diet of malnourished mothers with a special formula would be the best way to achieve ideal nourishment for mother and child. The infant will then gain the additional advantages of human milk, such as protection against infection.[85] Such formulas have been devised. Sosa et al[139] tried this approach in Guatemala.

With the ready availability of well-balanced

nutrition supplements today in both supermarkets and drugstores in the form of stable powders, it should not be difficult to initiate a high-protein, vitamin-enriched diet supplementation that is also palatable for the occasional mother who is at nutritional risk. With the inclusion of breastfeeding as a goal in the Women, Infants, and Children (WIC) program, dietary counseling and supplementation are available for mothers at poverty level to encourage these mothers to breastfeed and give them nutritional support while doing so. Infants in the WIC programs will receive the greatest benefit from being breastfed. Present WIC supplements focus on improved diet.

Because studies have revealed a negative effect of malnutrition on infection protection properties as well as on galactopoietic hormones (corticosteroids are greatly increased and prolactin decreased), nourishing the mother is the most effective way of benefiting the infant rather than supplementing the infant to meet growth standards.[95]

The impact of dietary supplementation on lactating women with restricted diets has been reported to be inconsistent with respect to lactational amenorrhea.[35] Most recently, a study in Sri Lankan women did not show an effect on menstruation or ovulation with supplementation. However, the study did result in a longer duration of full breastfeeding in the supplemented women, which may have had an effect in suppressing ovulation. No difference was seen between supplemented and unsupplemented women in regard to lactational amenorrhea.[154]

Allergy

In families with a strong history of allergy, a hypoallergenic diet avoiding the common allergens such as wheat and eggs should be recommended. Interest in the transfer of cow's milk proteins to the infant via breast milk has increased as case reports appear of breastfed infants' reaction to cow protein. β-Lactoglobulin has been identified in breast milk and appears to be related to long-term exposure to cow's milk products.[51] Controlling intake has also been reported to reverse the presence of β-lactoglobulin in the milk. Ovalbumin has been identified in human milk in only a fraction of mothers tested, although the average intake was four eggs per week. (See Chapter 17).

Vegetarian diet

The growing interest in vegetarianism has necessitated a better understanding of the several types of diets and their potential for adequate nutrients and growth as well as the motivation for these diets (Table 9-10). In general, serious vegetarians usually have a greater knowledge of and commitment to good nutrition.[21]

Reports of malnutrition among breastfed infants of vegetarians usually focus on the very strict groups such as vegans and those on macrobiotic diets. The dietary risks involved are chiefly with the B vitamins because these vitamins are usually associated with protein, which is also proportionally lower from vegetable sources.[127] An additional concern is the availability of various amino acids in specific concentrations to utilize them for protein synthesis. The *net protein utilization* (NPU) of a food may be considerably lower than total protein content; therefore it is important when using vegetable sources of protein to use foods with "complementary protein" at the same meal. Vegetarian cookbooks emphasize this.[130] Throughout history, culturally traditional meals have ensured complementary proteins. Concentrations of PCBs (polychlorinated biphenyls) are lower in milk of vegetarians.

Vitamin B_{12} deficiency has been described in vegans because of the absence of animal protein.[171] It is advisable in these cases to supplement diets of the pregnant or lactating woman, as well as of an infant or growing child, with up to 4 mg/day of B_{12}. It has been shown that fermented soybean foods do contain B_{12}, as do the single-cell proteins such as yeast. In a study of vegetarian mothers and their infants, a large proportion of the infants had elevated methylmalonic acid levels, indicative of vitamin B_{12} deficiency.[141] A significant number of vegetarian women, both lactators and nonlactators,

TABLE 9-10   **Vegetarianism and associated risks**

Type of vegetarian	Diet includes	Diet avoids	Risks
Semivegetarian	Vegetables, milk products, seafood, poultry	Red meat	Minerals*
Ovo-lacto-vegetarian	Vegetables, milk products, eggs	Flesh foods (meat, seafood, poultry)	Minerals* esp. zinc
Lacto-vegetarian	Vegetables, milk products	Flesh foods, eggs	Minerals* esp. zinc, protein†
Ovo-vegetarian	Vegetables, eggs	Flesh foods, milk products	Minerals* esp. iron and zinc, protein,† riboflavin, vitamin D, B_{12}
Vegan	Only vegetables	Flesh foods, milk products, eggs	Minerals,* protein,† riboflavin, vitamin D, B_{12}
Macrobiotic	Gradual progression to a diet of only cereals		Advanced stage nutritionally inadequate

*Excessive dietary phytates and dietary fiber inhibit absorption of minerals such as iron, zinc, and calcium. *Phytates* are organic chemicals present in many vegetables and unleavened bread that bind with minerals.
†Diets not using complementary proteins may be deficient in net protein because the net protein utilization (NPU) is low.

had elevated methylmalonic acid levels and low B_{12} levels.

As noted previously, vegetarians had higher levels of DHA.[129] On comparison of umbilical cord vessels and cord blood of infants born to South Asian vegetarian women, there was less DHA in the plasma and cord artery phospholipids of those born to omnivores.[129] Early onset of labor, incidence of cesarean birth, lower birthweight, head circumference, and length, after adjusting for maternal height, duration of gestation, parity, smoking, and gender of infant, were also related.

Reports of growth curves in vegetarian children over the first few years show them to be shorter and leaner than standard, with the greatest effect among those on the most restricted diets.[43] Studies of children from birth to 10 years in the Netherlands reared in macrobiotic tradition showed the greatest growth retardation with fat and muscle wasting and slower psychomotor development between 6 and 18 months of age.[30] Breast milk of their mothers, who breastfed an average of 13.6 months, contained less vitamin B_{12}, calcium, and magnesium compared with matched omnivorous controls.[31] Breastfed vegetarian infants are usually on the norms for growth with the exception of those receiving minimal vitamin D and calcium, as

reported in dark-skinned mothers in cloudy climates. The mean serum 1,25-dihydroxyvitamin $D(1,25\text{-}OH_2D)$ concentrations were 37% higher in lactating vegetarian women than nonvegetarian women.[143] The serum parathyroid hormone was elevated in all lactators compared with the nonlactators. It is postulated that the low calcium in the vegetarian diet stimulates the elevated $1,25\text{-}OH_2D$, and this in turn stimulates the increased absorption of calcium to meet the needs of milk production.[142]

A study of the milk from vegetarian mothers compared with that from nonvegetarian mothers looked at fat and fatty acid composition.[31] Those fats and fatty acids produced de novo by the breast were not different.[146] The precursors of AA were higher in the vegetarians, yet the AA level in the milk was lower and continued to decrease the longer the vegetarian diet was maintained. Linoleic acid was greater among vegetarians. The amounts of DHA were not different. Among 34 breastfed infants at 7 months in the Tufts study, three infants were below the tenth percentile for height and weight, one had low weight for length, and three had high weight for length, whereas of the 51 who were not breastfed, six were below the tenth percentile, two had low weight for length, and four had high weight for length.[52]

Four vegetarian children between 8 months and 24 months of age were reported by Hellebostad et al[66] to have vitamin D–deficient rickets (three with tetany and seizures) and vitamin B_{12} deficiency. All the infants were initially breastfed by mothers whose diets were low in vitamin D, high in fiber and phytate (which interferes with enterohepatic circulation of vitamin D), and low in calcium and phosphate.

General recommendations for lactating vegetarian women are as follows[152]:

1. Supplement with soy flour, molasses, and nuts.
2. Use complementary protein combinations.
3. Avoid excessive phytates and bran.
4. Watch protein and iron intake. Calcium should be supplemented if bone mineralization decreases as the milk will be adequate.
5. Supplement vitamin D with adequate sunshine.
6. Know that vitamins B_{12} and B_2 (riboflavin) are low in vegetarian diets and should be supplemented. If the mother does not supplement, the infant must be supplemented.

Supplementation of the breastfed infant's diet

For the newborn infant, human milk is the ideal food containing all the necessary nutrients. In establishing dietary norms for infants fed cow's milk, many nutrients identified as being needed in the diet were found to exist in greater amounts in cow's milk than in human milk. This does not consider the probability that the nutrient may be in a more bioavailable form in human milk. The specific items in question are protein, sodium, iron, vitamin D, and fluorine.

When a breastfed infant must be supplemented with formula, it is preferable that a formula low in iron be used to avoid providing excessive iron that will bind with lactoferrin and interfere with its protective activity.

The AAP Committee on Nutrition[23] has noted that iron deficiency is rare in breastfed infants and attributes this to increased absorption and the absence of microscopic blood loss into the gastrointestinal tract, which is seen in bottle-fed infants. The committee recommends a source of iron in solid foods (fortified infant cereal) at 6 months of age for breastfed infants.

Because rickets have been described in breastfed infants, consideration should be given to the maternal intake of vitamin D and the exposure of the infant to sunshine, as discussed previously. The Subcommittee on Nutrition During Lactation[152] recommends that if the infant's exposure to sunlight appears to be inadequate, the infant should be given 5 to 7.5 μg supplement of vitamin D daily. Individual discretion is appropriate, because infants of healthy mothers have not been observed to have rickets.

The AAP no longer recommends fluoride supplements in all breastfed infants.[25] Many breastfed infants have done without fluorine supplementation and have had no adverse dental problems, but the decision should be based on individual determinants, including family dental history and level of fluoride in the water supply, which is ideally between 0.7 and 1.0 ppm. If the level is less than 0.3 ppm, 0.25 mg of daily fluoride should be given.

Exercise while breastfeeding

There are usually no contraindications to exercise in moderation during lactation. The greatest obstacle is usually having sufficient time. The availability of home exercise equipment does offer an option for home programs. Exercise baby carriages, which have large wheels for greater speed and rough terrain, are another option. Because they tip somewhat easily, the infant may need a helmet. A safety strap that attaches to the runner's wrist prevents the vehicle from getting away. These carriages are excellent for brisk walks as well.

The impact of programmed exercise on milk volume, milk composition, and ultimately milk acceptability has been studied.[34] Women who exercise excessively, especially jogging, may have trouble maintaining milk supply. This difficulty has been attributed to any activity that results in persistent motion of the breasts and excessive friction of clothing against the nipples. A firm athletic brassiere made of cotton will reduce this effect. No data are available on the impact of jogging with or without support on later breast sagging.

The production of lactic acid while exercising has been studied in relationship to lactation by Wallace et al,[163,165] who had mothers report whether their infants refused to nurse or fussed when breastfed postexercise. The study demonstrated that seven healthy lactating women who normally spent over 30 minutes in aerobic activity (jogging, running, swimming, biking, and aerobics), as well as some who did calisthenics and racket sports, had an increase in their blood lactic acid levels postexercise. When a standardized treadmill exercise was used to maximal voluntary effort, blood lactic acid level increased at 10 minutes compared with that of the resting sample, but the level at 30 minutes had returned almost to the resting level. Milk samples at 10 and 30 minutes continued to have elevated lactic acid, although wide variation was seen among subjects.[165]

In a larger sample, when 26 women between 2 and 6 months postpartum who normally exercised during pregnancy and postpartum were exercised on a standardized treadmill to maximal voluntary effort, the levels of lactic acid were correlated to infant acceptance of the milk.[163] The breast was wiped with a dry towel before collection. Milk samples collected before exercise and at 10 and 30 minutes postexercise revealed an increase in lactic acid levels over baseline at both 10 and 30 minutes. In a double-blind order of samples, the infants were offered milk by dropper and were less likely to accept samples with high lactic acid. The authors[163] noted that the levels of lactic acid were high enough for adults to detect when offered water solutions at the same concentrations (1.6 mmol). Human milk is very sweet, but lactic acid is known to be bitter sour. Infants have been noted to make a puckering facial expression to a sour taste as early as a few hours of age.[149] Studies of sucking in newborns have shown more rapid rates with sweet than sour, with some change in heart rate, respiratory rate, and sucking patterns.[79] The lactic acid level can remain elevated in the milk for as long as 90 minutes, according to Wallace and Rabin.[165]

When exercise studies were again undertaken by Wallace et al[162,164] comparing the effects of a typical workout and a standard maximal exercise regimen, significant differences were noted. The milk lactate level before exercise was 0.61 ± 0.14 mM and after typical exercise was 1.06 ± 33 mM. After maximal exercise in the same women, the level was 2.88 ± 0.80 mM. Seventeen percent of the subjects had lactate levels above the reported adult taste threshold of 1.5 mM.[164] Milk rejection probably is a function of lactate concentration in the milk and the infant's sensitivity to taste. Women who exercised with full breasts developed a peak postexercise lactate concentration at 10 minutes, whereas women who exercised with empty breasts did not peak until 30 minutes.[162] Many of the studies reported may have not measured peak lactate when samples were only collected at 10 minutes.

Mothers have reported that their infants may reject their milk after the mother had exercised. Women have reported to the Lactation Study Center that their infants have been fussy and colicky for as long as 4 to 6 hours after the mother's strenuous exercise. Exercise generates sweat high in sodium and chloride, and lactic acid may change the pH. While these studies are being expanded, the following precautions might be recommended when breastfeeding after strenuous exercise:

- Shower, or at least wash the breast of perspiration.
- Manually express 3 to 5 ml of milk from each breast and discard.
- If infant displays puckering facial expression, postpone feeding or replace feeding with previously pumped milk.

Levels of prolactin and adrenal activation have been studied in eumenorrheic and amenorrheic women who exercise regularly. Prolactin levels following exercise are elevated for 20 to 40 minutes.[34] The effect appears to be unrelated to anaerobiosis. The hypothalamic-pituitary-adrenal

(HPA) axis is known to be activated under the influence of various forms of stress, including exercise. How this activation might affect milk production or oxytocin-stimulated milk let-down after exercise has yet to be determined.

Serum prolactin and growth hormone increased severalfold during prolonged acute exercise in normal women and runners with and without menses, demonstrating that a threshold of exercise intensity must be reached for this reaction to occur.[19] There was no correlation to their menstrual dysfunction.

When the lactation performances of eight physically fit, exercising women were compared with those of sedentary controls, there were no significant differences in milk volume or composition despite wide variations in energy intake and expenditure.[96] Exercising women compensated by increasing energy intake; thus no net difference was seen between the groups. It has been reported that lactating women exercising on a regular basis expend an average of 2630 kcal/day exclusive of milk energy output, compared with the 1800 to 1900 kcal/day expenditures of women who did not exercise.[152]

Dewey et al[39] studied the impact of regular exercise on the volume and composition of breast milk and further confirmed that breastfeeding women can safely exercise. Whereas previous studies were done on exercising fit women, this study randomly assigned sedentary women to exercise with supervised aerobic exercise to 60% to 70% of the heart rate reserve for 45 minutes per day, 5 days a week for 12 weeks. The control group remained breastfeeding but sedentary. Measurements of energy expended, dietary intake, body composition, and milk volume and composition were collected at 6 to 8 weeks, 12 to 14 weeks, and 18 to 20 weeks postpartum. Maximum oxygen uptake and plasma prolactin response over 2 hours postnursing were measured at the first and last assessment times. No significant differences were seen in maternal weight and fat losses, volume or composition of milk, infant weight gain, or plasma prolactin response between exercising and sedentary women. No women reported difficulty nursing

Fig. 9-4. Percent increase in breast milk volume and energy output and absolute increase in infants' weight in exercise and control groups during a 12-week study. Values shown are means +SE. To convert kilocalories to megajoules, multiply by 0.004186. None of the differences between the groups was significant. The 95% confidence intervals were as follows: for the percent change in milk volume, 2% to 17% for the exercise group and −1% to 16% for the control group ($p = 0.66$); for the percent change in energy output in breast milk, −2% to 15% for the exercise group and −1% to 12% for the control group ($p = 0.85$); and for infant weight gain, 1871 to 2279 g for the exercise group and 1733 to 2355 g for the control group ($p = 0.86$). (Modified from Dewey KG, Lovelady CA, Nommsen-Rivers LA et al: *N Engl J Med* 330:449, 1994.)

after moderate exercise. The authors[39] did note that the 300 kcal/day mean extra energy expenditure of the exercise group at midpoint in the study decreased toward the end as they cut back on other activities to compensate. This suggests that high levels of energy expenditure may be difficult to sustain while lactating because of fatigue and time limitations (Figs. 9-4 and 9-5).

Lovelady et al[97] further evaluated this same study group, randomly assigned to exercise or remain sedentary. Exercise marginally increased high-density lipoprotein (HDL) cholesterol levels but did not affect other lipid concentrations. Further, resting metabolic rate did not change over time. Weight and percent body fat declined similarly in both groups. No difference was found between exercising and sedentary groups regarding insulin, glucose, or thermal response. The authors

Fig. 9-5. Plasma prolactin response to nursing in control and exercise groups at beginning and end of study. Values shown are mean +SE. Study began 6 to 8 weeks postpartum and ended 18 to 20 weeks postpartum. Change in the area under the curve from beginning to end of the study was not significantly different between the two groups ($p = 0.38$). (Modified from Dewey KG, Lovelady CA, Nommsen-Rivers LA et al: *N Engl J Med* 330:449, 1994.)

concluded that sedentary women can initiate moderate exercise programs during lactation but that exercise does not increase weight loss or fat loss without dietary control, that is, avoiding compensatory increased intake. In a similar randomized study of 33 women, Prentice[119] reported that moderate exercise sufficient to improve cardiovascular fitness without marked changes in energy expenditure, dietary intake, and body weight and composition does not jeopardize lactation performance.

Dieting while breastfeeding

The Subcommittee on Nutrition During Lactation[152] stated in its report that the average rate of weight loss postpartum while maintaining adequate milk volume is 0.5 to 1.0 kg (1 to 2 lb) per month. In individuals who are significantly overweight, a weight loss of up to 1 to 2 kg (about 4 to 5 lb) per month should not affect milk volume, although weight gain and feeding pattern in the infant should be monitored. The subcommittee[152] considers rapid weight loss, that is, more than 2 kg

per month after the first month, inadvisable. In addition, because no data exist about curtailing maternal energy intake during the first 2 to 3 weeks postpartum, dieting immediately postpartum is not recommended and could be associated with poor milk supply. Energy intake must be balanced with the level of physical activity. The subcommittee does not recommend intakes less than 1500 kcal/day; however, brief fasts, perhaps for religious reasons, of less than a day are unlikely to affect milk supply. Liquid diets or weight loss medications are not recommended.

Studies of weight loss during lactation are scarce. Many women in developed countries experience an appetite surge with lactation and may experience no weight loss in the first months beyond that lost with the first weeks. They may not return to prepregnancy weight for 6 months. Women who are prone to gaining weight may be more apt to gain on an unregulated diet. Maternal nutrition status in the United States, as measured by anthropometric indices prenatally and postpartum, is unrelated to milk volume, according to studies of Butte et al[16] and Dewey et al.[38] Total energy expenditure of sedentary women, including those housebound with a new baby, averages 1800 kcal/day, exclusive of the energy put into the milk produced.[96]

No consistent relationship was reported in a study of 411 postpartum women between mode of feeding and postpartum weight loss.[118] Despite the energy deficiency of breastfeeding women, the trend was to greater weight loss in nonlactators. Women who gained more during pregnancy lost more postpartum regardless of their pregnancy weight. No dietary intake was recorded because the data were collected retrospectively.

The Stockholm Pregnancy and Weight Development Study prospectively investigated trends in eating patterns, physical activity, and sociodemographic factors in relation to postpartum body weight development, following 1423 pregnant women.[108] Weight retention 1 year postpartum was greater in women who increased their energy intake during and after pregnancy. Weight retention also increased in those who not only increased their snacking to three or more times a day but also decreased their lunch frequency. Sedentary lifestyle was correlated with 5 kg or more weight gain over prepartum weight. The authors summarized their findings as being related most closely to a change in lifestyle after pregnancy.

The tremendous variability in women's responses to the stress of reproduction and lactation suggests that there is very low stress per unit time. Thus many different variables exist during the perinatal period to rebalance the energy equation, according to Prentice et al.[122] Some women are energy sparing and some energy profligate. Although generally beneficial, the interaction between exercise and skeletal integrity is influenced by hormonal status and many exercise variables.

Dietary advice for women who choose to diet while lactating should include the following[152]:

- Diet must include balanced, varied foods rich in calcium, zinc, magnesium, vitamin B_6, and folate.
- Minimum energy intake should be 1800 kcal.
- Calcium and multivitamin-mineral supplements may be necessary to replace stores if diet is marginal.

Foods to avoid

The concern about gassy foods causing gas in the breastfed baby has no scientific basis. The normal intestinal flora produce gas from the action on fiber in the intestinal tract. Neither the fiber nor the gas is absorbed from the intestinal tract, and they do not enter the milk, even though they may cause the mother some discomfort. The acid content of the maternal diet also does not affect the milk because it does not change the pH of the maternal plasma. Essential oils are present in such foods as garlic, and some spices that have characteristic odors and flavors may pass into the milk, and an occasional infant objects to their presence.

Studies by Mennella and Beauchamp[100] show that the diet of the lactating woman alters the sensory qualities of her milk. They found that garlic ingestion significantly and consistently increased

the intensity of the milk odor as perceived by blinded adult panelists. The odor was not apparent at 1 hour, peaked at 2 hours, and decreased thereafter. Similar observations have been made in other species. Garlic is one of the most potent of the volatile sulfur-containing foods (onions, broccoli, etc.). Garlic consumption by the mother increased the length of time spent suckling and the rate of suckling of the next feeding. This behavior is usually associated with a tendency of the breast to make more milk. The authors suggest that the mouth movements made during sucking facilitated the retronasal perception of the garlic volatile oils in the milk. This study reports only the first 4 hours postingestion and makes no reference to the period between 4 and 24 hours postingestion, a time occasionally associated with colic in the breastfed infant after ingestion of certain foods by the mother.

When these mothers and infants were tested over an 11-day period, those infants who had garlic previously showed no response to reexposure; that is, suckling pattern and volume ingested were unchanged.[101] Garlic odor of amniotic fluid has been noted when the mother consumed garlic. These investigators also report that alcohol, mint, and cheese flavors are transmitted to milk. When mothers were fed carrot juice while lactating, the infant subsequently preferred cereal mixed with carrot juice rather than with plain formula or milk.[102]

Animal studies show that odors in utero and early in life are associated with a preference for them after birth. Breastfed infants actually experience a wide variety of odors and flavors during lactation, which may enhance their weaning to solid foods. Conversely, it suggests that infants fed standard formulas experience a constant set of flavors, thus missing significant sensory experiences. In experiments with rats, Galef and Sherry[55] found a mother's milk contains gustatory cues reflecting the flavor of the mother's diet and that these cues are sufficient to influence dietary preferences at weaning.

Extensive clinical experience suggests, however, that some infants do not tolerate certain foods in the mother's diet, predominantly specific vegetables and fruits. Garlic and onions may cause colic in some infants. Cabbage, turnips, broccoli, or beans may also bother others, making them colicky for 24 hours. The same has been said of rhubarb, apricots, and prunes. If a mother questions the effect of a food, she should avoid it or document its effect carefully by watching for colic in the 24 hours following ingestion. In the summer, a heavy diet of melon, peaches, and other fresh fruits may cause colic and diarrhea in the infant. Chocolate rarely lives up to its reputation and can be consumed in moderation without causing colic, diarrhea, or constipation in most infants.

Red pepper, which contains capsaicin and related compounds, has been reported to cause dermatitis in the breastfed infant within an hour of milk ingestion.[27] The rash can last 12 to 48 hours and differs from the contact dermatitis known to occur from capsaicin applied directly. When hot peppers are prepared with bare hands, an intensely painful reaction can occur. In countries where red pepper dishes such as Gimchee (Korea) are common, a perianal rash has long been seen in breastfed infants whose mothers ingested these hot dishes.

Food additives

Artificial sweeteners are the most common food additives. Saccharin and cyclamate are not known to be tetratogenic, but the remote relationship to cancer in rats has led to the recommendation that they be used in moderation. The same pertains during lactation. Cyclamate is a cyclohexylamine, an indirectly acting sympathomimetic amine that has been banned from use.

Aspartame is a dipeptide sweetener, aspartyl-phenylalanine methyl ester, that metabolizes to phenylalanine and aspartic acid. Thus it poses a risk to those with phenylketonuria. Normal individuals can consume 50 mg/kg/day without adverse effects. In large doses of 75 mg/kg/day, individuals increase their excretion of formate and methanol. When given aspartame, lactating women were noted to have elevated phenylalanine levels four times normal in their plasma.[147] Milk levels of phenylalanine and tryrosine were only slightly

elevated. Aspartame in moderation during lactation is presumed safe.

Color of milk and maternal diet

The color of mature human milk is bluish white (foremilk), initially changing to creamy white (hindmilk). The color of colostrum is yellow to yellow orange. Mothers occasionally report changes in the color of their milk. Most of these reports can be traced to pigments consumed in the diet, medications, or herbal remedies. The infant's urine may also turn color.

Pink or pink-orange milk

Pink-orange milk was traced to Sunkist orange soda, which contains red and yellow dyes. A case of a breastfed infant with pink to orange urine was reported by Roseman.[131] This combination of food dyes is also used in other brands of soda, fruit drinks, and gelatin desserts.

Green milk

Several cases of green milk have been reported to our study center. A careful search of the diet for the offending substance was made in each case. The effect of ingestion of the identified culprit and its avoidance were then tested to confirm the association with the milk's color. Several items have been clearly identified. Gatorade (the green beverage), kelp and other forms of seaweed (especially in tablet form), and natural vitamins from health food sources each have been associated with one or more cases of green milk and usually green urine.

Black milk

Minocycline hydrochloride therapy was associated with black milk galacorrhea in galactorrhea in a 24-year-old woman who had received the compound for pustulocystic acne for 4 years.[11] Examination of the fluid revealed that the macrophages contained hemosiderin, thus causing the black color. This drug is known to cause black pigmentation of the skin. A second case was reported in a 29-year-old female who had weaned but could express black milk 3 weeks after beginning oral minocycline therapy. Hunt et al[70] found iron-staining pigment particles in the mac- rophages and suggested it was an iron chelate of minocycline.

REFERENCES

1. Al MD, Houwelingen AC, Badart-Smook A et al: Some aspects of neonatal essential fatty acid status are altered by linoleic acid supplementation of women during pregnancy, *J Nutr* 125:2822, 1995.
2. Alaejos MS, Romero CD: Selenium in human lactation, *Nutr Rev* 53:159, 1995.
3. Alexander RP, Walker BF, Bhamjee D: Serum lipids in long-lactating African mothers habituated to a low-fat intake, *Atherosclerosis* 44:175, 1982.
4. Anderson RA, Bryden NA, Patterson KY et al: Breast milk chromium and its association with chromium intake, chromium excretion, and serum chromium, *Am J Clin Nutr* 57:519, 1993.
5. Andon MB, Howard MP, Moser PB et al: Nutritionally relevant supplementation of vitamin B_6 in lactating women: effect on plasma prolactin, *Pediatrics* 76:769, 1985.
6. Andon MB, Reynolds RD, Moser-Veillon PB et al: Dietary intake of total and glycosylated vitamin B_6 and the vitamin B_6 nutritional status of unsupplemented lactating women and their infants, *Am J Clin Nutr* 50:1050, 1989.
7. Arnaud J, Prual A, Preziosi P et al: Effect of iron supplementation during pregnancy on trace element (Cu, Se, Zn) concentrations in serum and breast milk from Nigerian women, *Ann Nutr Metab* 37:262, 1993.
8. Asnes R, Wisotsky DH, Migel PF et al: The dietary chloride deficiency syndrome occurring in a breastfed infant, *J Pediatr* 100:923, 1982.
9. Atkinson PJ, West RR: Loss of skeletal calcium in lactating women, *J Obstet Gynecol Br Commonwealth* 77:555, 1970.
10. Bachrach S, Fisher J, Parks JS: An outbreak of vitamin D deficiency rickets in a susceptible population, *Pediatrics* 64:871, 1979.
11. Basler RS, Lynch PJ: Black galactorrhea as a consequence of minocycline and phenothiazine therapy, *Arch Dermatol* 121:417, 1985.
12. Bates CJ, Prentice AM, Watkinson M et al: Riboflavin requirements of lactating Gambian women: a controlled supplementation trial, *Am J Clin Nutr* 135:701, 1982.
13. Bhaskaram P, Reddy V: Bactericidal activity of human milk leukocytes, *Acta Paediatr Scand* 70:87, 1981.
14. Blaauw R, Albertse EC, Beneke T et al: Risk factors for development of osteoporosis in a South African population, *South Afr Med J* 84:328, 1994.
15. Butte NF, Calloway DH, Van Duzen JL: Nutritional assessment of pregnant and lactating Navajo women, *Am J Clin Nutr* 34:2216, 1981.
16. Butte NF, Garza C, Stuff JE et al: Effect of maternal diet and body composition on lactational performance, *Am J Clin Nutr* 39:296, 1984.
17. Byerley LO, Kirksey A: Effect of different levels of vitamin C intake on the vitamin C concentration in human milk and vitamin C intakes of breastfed infants, *Am J Clin Nutr* 41:665, 1985.
18. Byrne J, Thomas MR, Chan GM: Calcium intake and bone density of lactating women in their late childbearing years, *J Am Diet Assoc* 87:883, 1987.
19. Chang FE, Dodds WG, Sullivan M et al: The acute effects of exercise on prolactin secretion: comparison between sedentary women and women runners with normal and abnormal menstrual cycles, *J Clin Endocrinol Metab* 62:551, 1986.
20. Chappell JE, Clandinin MT, Kearney-Volpe C: Trans fatty acids in human milk lipids: influence of maternal diet and weight loss, *Am J Clin Nutr* 42:49, 1985.
21. Christoffel K: A pediatric perspective on vegetarian nutrition, *Clin Pediatr* 20:632, 1981.
22. Chulei R, Xiaofang L, Hongsheng M et al: Milk composition in women from five different regions of China: the great diversity of milk fatty acids, *J Nutr* 125:2998, 1995.
23. Committee on Nutrition, Academy of Pediatrics: Iron supplementation for infants, *Pediatrics* 58:765, 1976.
24. Committee on Nutrition, American Academy of Pediatrics: Nutrition and lactation, *Pediatrics* 68:435, 1981.
25. Committee on Nutrition, American Academy of Pediatrics: Fluoride supplementation, *Pediatrics* 77:758, 1986.
26. Connor WE, Lowensohn R, Hatcher L: Increased docosahexaenoic acid levels in human newborn infants by administration of sardines and fish oil during pregnancy, *Lipids* 31:5183, 1996.
27. Cooper RL, Cooper MN: Red pepper–induced dermatitis in breast-fed infants, *Dermatology* 193:61, 1996.
28. Cornelissen M, vonKries R, Loughnan P et al: Prevention of vitamin K deficiency bleeding: efficacy of different multiple oral dose schedules of vitamin K, *Eur J Pediatr* 156:126, 1997.
29. Daaboul J, Sanderson S, Kristensen K et al: Vitamin D deficiency in pregnant and breastfeeding women and their infants, *J Perinatol* 17:10, 1997.

30. Dagnelie PC, van Staveren WA: Macrobiotic nutrition and child health: results of a population-based, mixed-longitudinal cohort study in the Netherlands, *Am J Clin Nutr* 59(suppl):1187S, 1994.

31. Dagnelie PC, van Staveren WA, Roos AH et al: Nutrients and contaminants in human milk from mothers on macrobiotic and omnivorous diets, *Eur J Clin Nutr* 46:355, 1992.

32. Deodhar AD, Ramakrishnan CV: Studies on human lactation. II. Effect of socioeconomic status on vitamin content of human milk, *Indian J Med Res* 47:352, 1959.

33. DeSantiago S, Villalpando S, Ortiz N et al: Protein requirements of marginally nourished lactating women, *Am J Clin Nutr* 62:364, 1995.

34. DeSouza MJ, Maguire MS, Maresh CM et al: Adrenal activation and the prolactin response to exercise in eumenorrheic and amenorrheic runners, *J Appl Physiol* 70(6):2378, 1991.

35. Dewey KG: Does maternal supplementation shorten the duration of lactational amenorrhea? *Am J Clin Nutr* 64:377, 1996.

36. Dewey KG, Finley DA, Lönnerdal B: Breast milk volume and composition during late lactation (7-20 months), *J Pediatr Gastroenterol Nutr* 3:713, 1984.

37. Dewey KG, Finley DA, Strode MA et al: Relationship of maternal age to breastmilk volume and composition. In Hamosh MH, Goldman AS, editors: *Human lactation: maternal and environmental factors,* New York, 1986, Plenum.

38. Dewey KG, Heinig MJ, Nommsen LA et al: Maternal vs infant factors related to breast milk intake and residual milk volume: The Darling Study, *Pediatrics* 87:829, 1991.

39. Dewey KG, Lovelady CA, Nommsen-Rivers LA et al: A randomized study of the effects of aerobic exercise by lactating women on breast-milk volume and composition, *N Engl J Med* 330:449, 1994.

40. Donnen P, Brasseur D, Dramaix M et al: Effects of cow's milk supplementation on milk output of protein deficient lactating mothers and on their infants' energy and protein status, *Trop Med Int Health* 2:38, 1997.

41. Duckman S, Hubbard JF: The role of fluids in relieving breast engorgement without the use of hormones, *Am J Obstet Gynecol* 60:200, 1950.

42. Dusdieker LB, Booth BM, Stumbo PJ et al: Effect of supplemental fluids on human milk production, *J Pediatr* 106:207, 1985.

43. Dwyer JT, Palombo R, Thorne H et al: Preschoolers on alternate lifestyle diets, *J Am Diet Assoc* 72:264, 1978.

44. Edozien JC, Khan MAR, Waslien CI: Human protein deficiency: results of a Nigerian village study, *J Nutr* 106:312, 1976.

45. English RM, Hitchcock NE: Nutrient intakes during pregnancy, lactation and after the cessation of lactation in a group of Australian women, *Br J Nutr* 22:615, 1968.

46. Ereman RR, Lönnerdal B, Dewey KG: Maternal sodium intake does not affect postprandial sodium concentrations in human milk, *J Nutr* 117:1154, 1987.

47. Finley DA, Lönnerdal B, Dewey KG et al: Breast milk composition: fat content and fatty acid composition in vegetarians and non-vegetarians, *Am J Clin Nutr* 41:787, 1985.

48. Fomon SJ: Breastfeeding and evolution, *J Am Diet Assoc* 86:317, 1986.

49. Food and Nutrition Board, National Research Council: *Recommended dietary allowances,* ed. 11, Washington, DC, 1994, National Academy Press.

50. Forsum E, Lönnerdal B: Effect of protein intake on protein and nitrogen composition of breast milk, *Am J Clin Nutr* 33:1809, 1980.

51. Fukushima Y, Kawata Y, Onda T et al: Consumption of cow milk and egg by lactating women and the presence of β lactoglobulin and ovalbumin in breast milk, *Am J Clin Nutr* 65:30, 1997.

52. Fulton JR, Hutton CW, Sitt KR: Preschool vegetarian children, *J Am Diet Assoc* 76:260, 1980.

53. Fung EB, Ritchie LD, Woodhouse LR et al: Zinc absorption in women during pregnancy and lactation: a longitudinal study, *Am J Clin Nutr* 66:80, 1997.

54. Gabriel A, Gabriel KR, Lawrence RA: Cultural values and biomedical knowledge: choices in infant feeding: analysis of a survey, *Soc Sci Med* 23:501, 1986.

55. Galef BG, Sherry DF: A medium for transmission of cues reflecting the flavor of mother's diet, *J Comp Physiol Psychol* 83:374, 1973.

56. Gambon RC, Lentze MJ, Rossi E: Megaloblastic anaemia in one of monozygous twins breast fed by their vegetarian mother, *Eur J Pediatr* 145:570, 1986.

57. Greer FR, Marshall SP, Foley AL et al: Improving the Vitamin K status of breastfeeding infants with maternal vitamin K supplements, *Pediatrics* 99:88, 1997.

58. Greer FR, Tsang RC, Levin RS et al: Increasing serum calcium and magnesium concentrations in breast-fed infants: longitudinal studies of minerals in human milk and in sera of nursing mothers and their infants, *J Pediatr* 100:59, 1982.

59. Gushurst CA, Mueller JA, Green JA et al: Breast milk iodide: reassessment in the 1980s, *Pediatrics* 73:354, 1984.

60. Guthrie HA, Picciano MF, Sheehe D: Fatty acid patterns of human milk, *J Pediatr* 90:39, 1977.

61. Hachey DL, Thomas MR, Emken EA et al: Human lactation: maternal transfer of dietary triglycerides labeled with stable isotopes, *J Lipid Res* 28:1185, 1987.

62. Hambraeus L: Proprietary milk versus human breast milk in infant feeding: a critical approach from the nutritional point of view. In Neumann CG, Jelliffe DB, editors: *Symposium on nutrition in pediatrics, Pediatr Clin North Am* 24:17, 1977.

63. Hanafy MM, Morsery MRA, Seddick Y et al: Maternal nutrition and lactation performance, *J Trop Pediatr Environ Child Health* 18:187, 1972.

64. Harris WS, Connor WE, Lindsey S: Will dietary omega-3 fatty acids change the composition of human milk? *Am J Clin Nutr* 40:780, 1984.

65. Heck H, deCastro JM: The calorie demand of lactation does not alter spontaneous meal patterns, nutrient intakes, or moods of women, *Physiol Behav* 54:641, 1993.

66. Hellebostad M, Markestad T, Halvorsen KS: Vitamin D deficiency rickets and vitamin B_{12} deficiency in vegetarian children, *Acta Paediatr Scand* 74:191, 1985.

67. Hernell O: The requirements and utilization of dietary fatty acids in the newborn infant, *Acta Paediatr Scand Suppl* 365:20, 1990.

68. Higginbottom MC, Sweetman L, Nyhan WL: A syndrome of methylmalonic aciduria, homocystinuria, megaloblastic anemia and neurologic abnormalities in a vitamin B_{12} deficient breastfed infant of a strict vegetarian, *N Engl J Med* 299:317, 1978.

69. Hollis BW, Pittard III WB, Reinhardt TA: Relationships among vitamin D, 25-hydroxyvitamin D, and vitamin D-binding protein concentrations in the plasma and milk of human subjects, *J Clin Endocrinol Metab* 62:41, 1986.

70. Hunt MJ, Salisbury ELC, Grace J et al: Black breast milk due to minocycline therapy, *Br J Dermatol* 134:943, 1996.

71. Illingworth PJ, Jung RT, Howie PW et al: Diminution in energy expenditure during lactation, *Br Med J* 292:437, 1986.

72. Illingworth RS, Kilpatrick B: Lactation and fluid intake, *Lancet* 2:1175, 1953.

73. Insull W, Hirsch J, James T et al: The fatty acids of human milk. II. Alterations produced by manipulation of caloric balance and exchange of dietary fats, *J Clin Invest* 38:443, 1959.

74. Jackson MJ, Giugliano R, Giugliano LG et al: Stable isotope metabolic studies of zinc nutrition in slum dwelling lactating women in the Amazon valley, *Br J Nutr* 59:193, 1988.

75. Jelliffe DB, Jelliffe EFP: *Human milk in the modern world*, New York, 1978, Oxford University Press.

76. Jelliffe EFP: Maternal nutrition and lactation. In Ciba Foundation Symposium, no 45, *Breast feeding and the mother*, Amsterdam, 1976, Elsevier Science.

77. Jensen RG: *The lipids of human milk*, Boca Raton, Fla, 1989, CRC.

78. Jensen RG: Miscellaneous factors affecting composition and volume of human and bovine milks. In Jensen RG, editor: *Handbook of milk composition*, San Diego, 1995, Academic Press.

79. Johnson P, Salisbury DM: Preliminary studies on feeding and breathing in the newborn. In Weiffenbach JM, editor: *Taste and development: the genesis of sweet preference*, Bethesda, Md, 1977, US Public Health Service, National Institute of Health, US Department of Health, Education and Welfare Publication (NIH).

80. Johnston L, Vaughn L, Fox HM: Pantothenic acid content of human milk, *Am J Clin Nutr* 34:2205, 1981.

81. Kalkwarf HJ, Specker BL, Herbi JE et al: Intestinal calcium absorption of women during lactation and after weaning, *Am J Clin Nutr* 63:526, 1996.

82. Kang-Yoon SA, Kirksey A, Giacoia G et al: Vitamin B-6 status of breastfed neonates: influence of pyridoxine supplementation on mothers and neonates, *Am J Clin Nutr* 56:548, 1992.

83. Keenan BS, Buzek SW, Garza C et al: Diurnal and longitudinal variations in human milk sodium and potassium: implications for nutrition and physiology, *Am J Clin Nutr* 35:527, 1982.

84. Khin-Maung-Naing, Tin-Tin-Oo, Kywe-Thein et al: Study on lactation performance of Burmese mothers, *Am J Clin Nutr* 33:2665, 1980.

85. Kliewer RI, Rasmussen KM: Malnutrition during the reproductive cycle: effects on galactopoietic hormones and lactational performance in the rat, *Am J Clin Nutr* 46:926, 1987.

86. Koletzko B, Gwosdz M, Bremer HJ: Trans isomeric fatty acids in human milk lipids in West Germany. In Schaub J, editor: *Composition and physiological properties of human milk*, Amsterdam, 1985, Elsevier Science.

87. Kramer M, Szöke K, Lindner K et al: The effect of different factors on the composition of human milk and its variations. III. Effect of dietary fats on the lipid composition of human milk, *Nutr Diet* 7:71, 1965.

88. Krebs NF, Hambidge KM, Jacobs MA et al: The effects of a dietary zinc supplement during lactation on longitudinal changes in maternal zinc status and milk zinc concentrations, *Am J Clin Nutr* 41:560, 1985.

89. Krebs NF, Reidinger CJ, Hartley S et al: Zinc supplementation during lactation: effects on maternal status and milk zinc concentrations, *Am J Clin Nutr* 61:1030, 1995.

90. Krebs NF, Reidinger CJ, Robertson AD et al: Bone mineral density changes during lactation: maternal, dietary, and biochemical correlates, *Am J Clin Nutr* 65: 1738, 1997.

91. Lammi-Keefe CJ, Jensen RG: Lipids in human milk: a review. II. Composition and fat-soluble vitamins, *J Pediatr Gastroenterol Nutr* 3:172, 1984.

92. Lammi-Keefe CJ, Jensen RG, Clark RM et al: Alpha tocopherol total lipid and linoleic acid contents of human milk at 2, 6, 12, and 16 weeks. In Schaub J, editor: *Composition and physiological properties of human milk*, Amsterdam, 1985, Elsevier Science.

93. Levander OA, Moser PB, Morris VC: Dietary selenium intake and selenium concentrations of plasma, erythrocytes, and breast milk in pregnant and post partum lactating and non-lactating women, *Am J Clin Nutr* 46:694, 1987.

94. Lipsman S, Dewey KG, Lönnerdal B: Breastfeeding among teenage mothers: milk composition, infant growth, and maternal dietary intake, *J Pediatr Gastroenterol Nutr* 4:426, 1985.

95. Lönnerdal B: Effects of maternal dietary intake on human milk composition, *J Nutr* 116:499, 1986.

96. Lovelady CA, Lönnerdal B, Dewey KG: Lactation performance of exercising women, *Am J Clin Nutr* 52:103, 1990.

97. Lovelady CA, Nommsen LA, McCrory MA et al: Relationship of human milk lipid concentration to maternal body composition and dietary fat intake, *FASEB J* 7:A200, 1993.

98. McGuire MK, Burgent SL, Milner JA et al: Selenium status of lactating women is affected by the form of selenium consumed, *Am J Clin Nutr* 58:649, 1993.

99. Mellies MJ, Ishikawa TT, Gartside P et al: Effects of varying maternal dietary cholesterol and phytosterol in lactating women and their infants, *Am J Clin Nutr* 31:1347, 1978.

100. Mennella JA, Beauchamp GK: Maternal diet alters the sensory qualities of human milk and nursling's behavior, *Pediatrics* 88:737, 1991.

101. Mennella JA, Beauchamp GK: The effects of repeated exposure to garlic-flavored milk on the nursling's behavior, *Pediatr Res* 34:805, 1993.

102. Mennella JA, Beauchamp GK: The early development of human flavor preferences. In Capaldi ED, editor: *Why we eat what we eat: the psychology of eating,* Washington, DC, 1996, American Psychological Association.

103. Michaud JL, Lemieux B, Ogier H et al: Nutritional vitamin B_{12} deficiency: two cases detected by routine newborn urinary screening, *Eur J Pediatr* 151:218, 1992.

104. Miranda R, Saravia NG, Ackerman R et al: Effect of maternal nutritional status on immunological substances in human colostrum and milk, *Am J Clin Nutr* 37:632, 1983.

105. Motil KJ, Thotathuckery M, Bahar A et al: Marginal dietary protein restriction reduced nonprotein nitrogen, but not protein nitrogen components of human milk, *J Am Coll Nutr* 14:184, 1995.

106. Nommsen LA, Lovelady CA, Heinig MJ et al: Determinants of energy, protein, lipid and lactose concentrations in human milk during the first 12 mo of lactation: The Darling Study, *Am J Clin Nutr* 53:457, 1991.

107. O'Connor DL: Folate status during pregnancy and lactation, *Adv Exp Med Biol* 352:157, 1994.

108. Ohlin A, Rossner S: Trends in eating patterns, physical activity and sociodemographic factors in relation to postpartum body weight development, *Br J Nutr* 71:457, 1994.

109. Olsen A: Nursing under conditions of thirst or excessive ingestion of fluids, *Acta Obstet Gynaecol Scand* 20:313, 1940.

110. Olson CM: Promoting positive nutritional practices during pregnancy and lactation, *Am J Clin Nutr* 59(suppl): 525S, 1994.

111. Park MJ, Namgung R, Kim DH et al: Lower serum 25-hydroxy Vitamin D, but similar bone mineral content by dexa in human milk–fed versus cow milk–based formula-fed infants. *Pediatr Res* 35:205A, 1994.

112. Parkinson AJ, Cruz AL, Heyward WL et al: Elevated concentrations of plasma ω^3 polyunsaturated fatty acids among Alaskan Eskimos, *Am J Clin Nutr* 59:384, 1994.

113. Paul AA, Muller EM, Whitehead RG: The quantitative effects of maternal dietary energy intake on pregnancy and lactation in rural Gambian women, *Trans R Soc Trop Med Hyg* 73:686, 1979.

114. Picciano MF, Calkins EJ, Garrick JR et al: Milk and mineral intakes of breastfed infants, *Acta Paediatr Scand* 70:189, 1981.

115. Pietschnig B, Haschke F, Vanura H et al: Vitamin K in breast milk: no influence of maternal dietary intake, *Eur J Clin Nutr* 47:209, 1993.

116. Pisacane A, DeVizia B, Vallante A et al: Iron status in breast-fed infants, *J Pediatr* 127:429, 1995.

117. Potter JM, Nestel PJ: The effects of dietary fatty acids and cholesterol on the milk lipids of lactating women and the plasma cholesterol of breast-fed infants, *Am J Clin Nutr* 29:54, 1976.

118. Potter S, Hannum S, McFarlin B et al: Does infant feeding method influence maternal postpartum weight loss? *J Am Diet Assoc* 91:441, 1991.

119. Prentice A: Should lactating women exercise? *Nutr Rev* 52:358, 1994.

120. Prentice A: Maternal calcium requirements during pregnancy and lactation, *Am J Clin Nutr* 59(suppl):477S, 1994.

121. Prentice A, Landing MAJ, Cole TJ et al: Calcium requirements of lactating Columbian mothers: effects of a calcium supplement on breast milk calcium concentration, maternal base content, and urinary calcium excretion, *Am J Clin Nutr* 62:58, 1995.

122. Prentice AM, Poppitt SD, Goldberg GR et al: Energy balance in pregnancy and lactation, *Adv Exp Med Biol* 352:11, 1994.

123. Prentice AM, Prentice A: Energy costs of lactation, *Annu Rev Nutr* 8:63, 1988.

124. Prentice A, Prentice AM, Cole TJ et al: Breast milk antimicrobial factors of rural Gambian mothers. I. Influence of stage of lactation and maternal plane of nutrition, *Acta Paediatr Scand* 73:796, 1984.

125. Prentice AM, Roberts SB, Prentice A et al: Dietary supplementation of lactating Gambian women. I. Effect on breast milk volume and quality, *Hum Nutr* 37C:53, 1983.

126. Prentice AM, Whitehead RG, Roberts SB: Dietary supplementation of Gambian nursing mothers and lactational performance, *Lancet* 2:886, 1980.

127. Rana SK, Sanders TAB: Taurine concentrations in diet, plasma, urine, and breast milk of vegans compared with omnivores, *Br J Nutr* 56:17, 1986.

128. Rassin DK, Sturman JA, Gaull GE: Taurine and other free amino acids in milk of man and other mammals, *Early Hum Dev* 2:1, 1978.

129. Reddy S, Sanders TAB, Obeid O: The influence of maternal vegetarian diet on essential fatty acid status of the newborn, *Eur J Clin Nutr* 48:358, 1994.

130. Robertson L, Flinders C, Godfrey B: *Laurel's kitchen: a handbook for vegetarian cookery and nutrition,* Petaluma, Calif, 1976, Nilgiri.

131. Roseman BD: Sunkissed urine, *Pediatrics* 67:443, 1981, (letter).

132. Roy SK, Islam A, Molla A et al: Impact of a single megadose of vitamin A at delivery on breastmilk of mothers and morbidity of their infants, *Eur J Clin Nutr* 51:302, 1997.

133. Salmenpera L: Vitamin C nutrition during prolonged lactation: optimal in infants while marginal in some mothers, *Am J Clin Nutr* 40:1050, 1984.

134. Scanlon KS, Blank S, Sinks T et al: Subclinical health effects in a population exposed to excess Vitamin D in milk, *Am J Public Health* 85:1418, 1995.

135. Schutz Y, Lechtig A, Bradfield RB: Energy expenditures and food intakes of lactating women in Guatemala, *Am J Clin Nutr* 33:892, 1980.

136. Sinclair AJ, Crawford MA: The effect of a low-fat maternal diet on neonatal rats, *Br J Nutr* 29:127, 1973.

137. Smith CA: Effects of maternal undernutrition upon newborn infants in Holland (1944-1945), *J Pediatr* 30:229, 1947.

138. Sneed SM, Zane C, Thomas MR: The effects of ascorbic acid, vitamin B_6, vitamin B_{12} and folic acid supplementation on the breast milk and maternal nutritional status of low socioeconomic lactating women, *Am J Clin Nutr* 34:1338, 1981.

139. Sosa R, Klaus M, Urrutia JJ: Feed the nursing mother, thereby the infant, *J Pediatr* 88:668, 1976.

140. Specker BL: Do North American women need supplemental Vitamin D during pregnancy or lactation? *Am J Clin Nutr* 59(suppl):484S, 1994.

141. Specker BL: Nutritional concerns of lactating women consuming vegetarian diets, *Am J Clin Nutr* 59(suppl): 1182S, 1994.

142. Specker BL, Black A, Allen L et al: Vitamin B_{12}: low milk concentrations are related to low serum concentrations in vegetarian women and to methylmalonic aciduria in their infants, *Am J Clin Nutr* 52:1073, 1990.

143. Specker BL, Tsang RC, Ho M et al: Effect of vegetarian diet on serum 1,25-dihydroxyvitamin D concentrations during lactation, *Obstet Gynecol* 70:870, 1987.

144. Specker BL, Tsang RC, Hollis BW: Effect of race and diet on human milk vitamin D and 25-hydroxy vitamin D, *Am J Dis Child* 139:1134, 1985.

145. Specker BL, Valanis B, Hertzberg V et al: Sunshine exposure and serum 25-hydroxy vitamin D concentration in exclusively breastfed infants, *J Pediatr* 107:372, 1985.

146. Specker BL, Wey HE, Miller D: Differences in fatty acid composition of human milk in vegetarian and nonvegetarian women: long-term effect of diet, *J Pediatr Gastroenterol Nutr* 6:764, 1987.

147. Stegnink LD, Filer LJ, Baker GL: Plasma erythrocyte and human milk levels of free amino acids in lactating women administered aspartame or lactose, *J Nutr* 109:2173, 1979.

148. Stein ZA, Susser MW, Saenger G et al: *Famine and human development: the Dutch Hunger Winter of 1944-45,* New York, 1975, Oxford University Press.

149. Steiner JE: Facial expressions of the neonate indicating the hedonics of food-related chemical stimuli. In Weifferbach JM, editor: *Taste and development: the genesis of sweet preference,* Bethesda, Md, 1977, US Public Health Service, National Institute of Health, US Department of Health, Education and Welfare Publication (NIH).

150. Steingrimsdottir L, Brasel JA, Greenwood MRC: Diet, pregnancy, and lactation: effects on adipose tissue, lipoprotein lipase, and fat cell size, *Metabolism* 29:837, 1980.

151. Styslinger L, Kirksey A: Effects of different levels of vitamin B_6 supplementation on vitamin B_6 concentrations in human milk and vitamin B_6 intakes of breastfed infants, *Am J Clin Nutr* 41:21, 1985.

152. Subcommittee on Nutrition During Lactation, Committee on Nutritional Status During Pregnancy and Lactation, Food and Nutrition Board, Institute of Medicine, National Academy of Sciences: *Nutrition during lactation,* Washington, DC, 1991, National Academy Press.

153. Suitor CW, Olson C, Wilson J: Nutrition care during pregnancy and lactation: new guidelines from the IOM, *J Am Diet Assoc* 93:478, 1993.

154. Tennekoon KH, Karunanayake EH, Seneviratne HR: Effect of skim milk supplementation of the maternal diet on lactational amenorrhea, maternal prolactin and lactational behavior, *Am J Clin Nutr* 64:238, 1996.

155. Tully J, Dewey KG: Private fears, global loss: a cross-cultural study of insufficient milk syndrome, *Med Anthropol* 9:225, 1985.

156. Van Houwelingen AC, Sorensen JD, Hornstra G et al: Essential fatty acid status in neonates after fish-oil supplementation during late pregnancy, *Br J Nutr* 74:723, 1995.

157. vanSteenbergen WM, Kusin JA, VanRems MM: Lactation performance of Akamba mothers, Kenya breastfeeding behavior, breast milk yield, and composition, *J Trop Pediatr* 27:155, 1981.

158. Vlachou A, Drummond BK, Curzon MEJ: Fluoride concentrations of infant foods and drinks in the United Kingdom, *Caries Res* 26:29, 1992.

159. Von Muralt A: Maternal nutrition and lactation. In Ciba Foundation Symposium, no 45, *Breast feeding and the mother,* Amsterdam, 1976, Elsevier Scientific.

160. Vuori E, Kiuru K, Makinen M et al: Maternal diet and fatty acid pattern of breast milk, *Acta Paediatr Scand* 71:959, 1982.

161. Walker ARP, Walker BF, Bhamjee D et al: Serum lipids in long-lactating African mothers habituated to a low fat intake, *Atherosclerosis* 44:175, 1982.

162. Wallace JP, Ernsthausen K, Inbar G: The influence of the fullness of milk in the breasts on the concentration of lactic acid in post exercise breast milk, *Int J Sports Med* 13:395, 1992.

163. Wallace JP, Inbar G, Ernsthausen K: Infant acceptance of post exercise breast milk, *Pediatrics* 89:1245, 1992.

164. Wallace JP, Inbar G, Ernsthausen K: Lactate concentrations in breast milk following maximal exercise and a typical workout, *J Women's Health* 3:91, 1994.

165. Wallace JP, Rabin J: The concentration of lactic acid in breastmilk following maximal exercise, *Int J Sports Med* 12:328, 1991.

166. Walton JL, Messer LB: Dental caries and fluorosis in breast-fed and bottle-fed children, *Caries Res* 15:124, 1981.

167. West KD, Kirksey A: Influence of vitamin B_6 intake on the content of the vitamin in human milk, *Am J Clin Nutr* 29:961, 1976.

168. Whitehead RG: Pregnancy and lactation: nutrition and growth, aging and physiologic stress. In Shils ME, Young VR, editors: *Modern nutrition in health and disease,* ed 7, Philadelphia, 1988, Lea & Febiger.

169. World Health Organization: *Handbook on human nutritional requirements,* Geneva, 1974, World Health Organization.

170. Worthington-Roberts BS: Lactation, human milk, and nutritional considerations. In Worthington-Roberts BS, Williams SR, editors: *Nutrition in pregnancy and lactation,* ed 6, Madison, Wis, 1997, Browne Benchmark.

171. Zmora E, Gorodischer R, Bar-Ziv J: Multiple nutritional deficiencies in infants from a strict vegetarian community, *Am J Dis Child* 133:141, 1979.

$\mathcal{W}$eaning

What does *weaning* mean? The textbooks on pediatrics and the mother's manuals all imply that it is the process by which one changes from one method of feeding to another. Raphael[49] states that the very first introduction of solid foods is the true beginning of weaning. The term *weaning* is derived from the Anglo-Saxon *wenian,* which means "to become accustomed to something different." It does not mean the total cessation of breastfeeding but the addition of other things.[51] If one consults the dictionary, however, one learns that to *wean* is to transfer the young of any animal from dependence on its mother's milk to another form of nourishment or to estrange from former habits or associations. A *weanling* is a child or animal who is newly weaned. If one likens breastfeeding to the continuation of intrauterine life, weaning is a "second birth."

Weaning from a physiologic point of view is a complex process involving nutritional, microbiologic, immunologic, biochemical, and psychologic adjustments. Boys tend to be weaned earlier than girls, possibly because the energy intakes of boys at all ages are greater and the male rate of growth is more rapid. Psychosocial pressures also trend toward the earlier weaning of male infants.[14]

INFANT'S NEED

When discussing the process of weaning the human infant, one might say it is the transfer of the infant from dependence on mother's milk to other sources of nourishment. If one were to determine the appropriate time for this to take place, it would be based on nutritional needs and developmental goals. Observations among other mammals suggest that achievement of a degree of maturity that allows the pup to forage for food is a trigger for initiating weaning by the mother.

A search for the appropriate weaning time for the human infant has produced a number of extremes, from the regimen of J.R. Sackett in 1953 of introducing solids on the second day of life to withholding all solid foods until the infant had sufficient teeth to chew thoroughly, a method described by Bartholomaus Mettinger, a German physician, in 1473.[11] The birth of the infant food industry began with German chemist Justis von Leitbig in 1867. He marketed "the perfect infant food" to the public at the turn of the twentieth century, a mixture of wheat flour, malt flour, and cow's milk. Jacobi, the father of modern pediatrics, advised no solids for a year and no vegetables before 2 years of age. Thus the winds of weaning varied by culture, ethnic group, medical intervention, and financial resources.

Acknowledging that humans are primates, Dettwyler[14] recognized that lactation and weaning occur according to certain regular patterns in nonhuman primates. She searched for a natural age of weaning uninfluenced by culture and trends. Evaluating various "rules of thumb" for determining weaning age by biologic references, she found them inappropriate. Breastfeeding from an anthropologic point of view is both a biologic process and a culturized activity. In primitive cultures, age of weaning is between 2 and 5 years, averaging 3 to 4 years.

If the definition of weaning is used to mean the cessation of all feedings at the breast, the age at weaning in nonhuman primates and other mammals is a function of genetics and instinct. Primates have a longer gestation, greater infant dependency, longer life spans, and larger brains per unit of body size than other mammals. Dettwyler[14] suggests that a possible formula for weaning is the ratio of present weight to birthweight as 4 to 1; that is, the offspring weans when four times the birthweight is achieved, usually between 2 and 3 years for well-fed healthy human infants.

If weaning according to attainment of one third the adult weight is used as the rule of thumb, Dettwyler[14] notes the variations in size of human adults by ethnic and cultural groups. With averaging, adult female weight is 54 kg (119 lb), then one third is 18 kg (39½ lb), a weight achieved between 4 and 7 years for girls; 59 kg (130 lb) is average for adult males, and one third is 19.3 kg (42½ lb). This would mean boys would be nursed longer. The present tendency for obesity in the developed world would accentuate these calculations. The average female weight in the United States is 55 kg (121 lb). Harvey and Clutton-Brock[27] suggest the following equation for calculation of weaning age:

$$\text{Weaning age (days)} = 2.71 \times \text{Adult female weight (g)}$$

Thus, modern infants whose mother weighed 55 kg would be weaned at 1228 days, or 3.36 years. For small, medium, and large women this would range from 2.8 to 3.7 years.

When length of gestation is used as the determinant for weaning time, the weaning/gestation ratio can be determined. According to the work of Harvey and Clutton-Brock,[27] the ratio across primate species varies from 0.41 in the *Galago demidovii*, a small-bodied primate, to 6.40 in the *Pan* troglodytes (chimpanzee). The former nurses less than half the length of pregnancy (11 of 45 days), whereas the chimpanzee nurses 1460 days (228-day gestation). The gorilla nurses for 1583

days (256-day gestation). Because the human is closest to the chimpanzee and gorilla, six times the gestation period might be a more physiologic norm: 54 months, or 4½ years.

When the eruption of the first permanent molar is used as the indicator for complete weaning, it estimates weaning at 5½ to 6 years in humans.[14] Tooth eruption is genetically controlled and comparatively unaffected by diet or disease. Six years is also identified as the time of achieving adult level of immunocompetence in the human.

The range of calculated ages for weaning derived from these formulations ranges from 2.3 years to 6 or 7 years. Before the widespread availability of foods suitable for infants and of artificial formulas, infants were traditionally breastfed for 3 to 4 years.

Other species gradually introduce other foods and teach their offspring how to obtain them on their own. Usually the mothers in most species make the determination for final termination and no longer permit the young to nurse (Fig. 10-1). Studies on the milk-borne factors that might cue the initiation of weaning in other species have not shown any cause and effect. The rat undergoes a "weaning crisis" during which the anatomy of the gut changes; some enzymes appear and others disappear. Chapter 3 discusses the enzymatic adaptations of the human infant.

Among humans, many cultural influences mandate weaning time and process. Public and social pressures have influenced weaning for some families in industrialized society. Very few traditional societies wean under 1 year, and some do not begin until 2 years of age.[28] In the Moslem world, especially Africa and the Sudan, however, weaning of children is by the teaching of the Koran, which advises complete weaning by 2 years of age. Before 1979 the average time of complete cessation worldwide was 4.2 years. Hervada and Newman[30] provide a historic review of weaning that also presents recent concerns about iron deficiency and other problems more common to formula-fed infants.

Breastfeeding benefits for an older infant have also been evaluated. In the developing world,

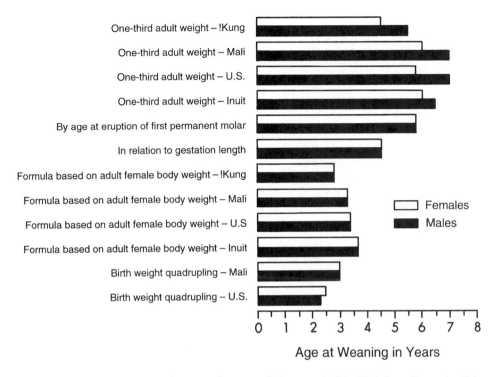

Fig. 10-1. Natural age at weaning according to technique used. (Modified from Dettwyler KA: A time to wean. In Stuart-MacAdam P, Dettwyler KA, editors: *Breastfeeding: biocultural perspectives,* New York, 1995, Aldine de Gruyter.)

breastfeeding continues for at least 1 to 2 years after introduction of solid foods. Major benefits include not only the nutrients but also protective, digestive, and trophic agents that extend the period of infertility in the mother[52] and reduce the incidence and severity of infectious diseases for the infant. A review of middle-class infants between the ages of 16 and 30 months in the United States revealed a decrease in the number of infections and improved overall health compared with those children no longer breastfed.[24]

Nutritionally, it is appropriate to begin iron-containing foods at 6 months, the time the stores from birth are being diminished. The requirement at this age exceeds that supplied by human milk. An additional source of protein becomes necessary toward the end of the first year of life because the grams of protein per kilogram of body weight

supplied by milk decrease as the infant grows heavier. The content of protein in the milk begins to drop slightly after 9 months of lactation. A human infant also needs bulk, or roughage, in the diet. The exact time this need becomes apparent is not known, but it may well be by the end of the first year.

Developmentally, the infant is ready to learn to chew solids instead of suckle liquids at about 6 months. Illingworth and Lister[34] have suggested a "critical period of development" during which infants can and must learn to chew. Chewing is an entirely different motion of the tongue and mouth from sucking. The sucking fat pads in the cheeks begin to disappear at the end of the first year. The rooting reflex has been lost. Even though the teeth are not all in, the development of good dentition requires chewing exercise.

ROLE OF DEVELOPMENT IN INITIATION OF WEANING

Although the developmental milestones of infant behavior are noted to influence the introduction of weaning foods, the development of the gastrointestinal tract plays an equal role. Even the taste buds, which can be identified at the seventh week of fetal life as collections of elongated cells on the dorsal surface of the tongue, are fully innervated over the next weeks. The fetus is known to suck and swallow in utero; sucking is discussed in Chapter 8.

When taste becomes a factor in feeding is not known, although a lack of discrimination has been noted in the first weeks of life: infants have consumed formula with high salt or absence of chloride with morbid results.[18] Because of the variation in the composition of mother's milk over a feeding, over a day, and from time to time according to maternal dietary intake, the breastfed infant has had a richer range of experience in tasting than the formula-fed infant. Breastfed infants are therefore more accustomed to new taste experiences. Similarly, feeding problems in infants are rare in breastfed infants.*

Both sucking and chewing are complex, having reflexive as well as learned components. The development of the chew-swallow reflex is necessary for the successful introduction of solids. Schmitz and McNeish[51] hypothesized that this skill develops sequentially with neuronal development, then is a learned behavior conditioned by oral stimulation. Before this point, when a spoon is introduced, the infant purses the lips and pushes the tongue against the spoon. By 4 to 6 months, the tongue is depressed in response to the spoon and the food accepted, and by 7 to 9 months, rhythmic biting movements occur regardless of the presence of teeth. Biting and masticatory strength and efficiency progress through infancy. If a stimulus is not applied when the neural development is taking place, Merchant[42] believes that the chewing reflex will not develop and the infant will always be a poor chewer. There is a relationship between

---

*References 4, 7, 25, 40, 51, 57, 59, 60.

prolonged sucking without solids and poor eating. The clinical model for this is the child sustained on parenteral feedings or gastrostomy beyond a year who has tremendous difficulty accepting solids.

For the human infant, there is also the role of nursing as a comfort and emotional support, a mechanism often referred to as "comfort nursing." Inadequate nipple contact may lead to thumb sucking or the substitute use of a pacifier. Young monkeys and apes in the wild do not suck their thumbs, but they do in captivity when bottle-fed.[27] Infants of the !Kung tribe in Africa do not suck their thumbs.[14]

In summary, the infant is ready to explore new feeding experiences at around 6 months. Feeding is an important social as well as nutritional encounter. Eating solids and learning to drink from a cup are important social achievements as well. That does not mean the infant is taken from the breast, but the diet is expanded and now includes solid foods, other liquids, and breast milk. Although there are a range of qualitative, quantitative, and temporal practices, the optimal approach matches the needs and requirements of a given child with the functions and capacities of the body.

Introduction of solids

The American Academy of Pediatrics (AAP) Committee on Nutrition[9] made recommendations on the feeding of supplemental foods to infants. The committee described three overlapping stages of infant feeding: the nursing period, during which breast milk or infant formula is the source of nutrition; a transitional period, during which solid foods are introduced; and the modified adult period, during which most of the nutrition is similar to the family's. It further stated that no nutritional advantage results from the introduction of supplemental foods before 4 to 6 months of age. Similar statements have been made by the World Health Organization (WHO), the Canadian Pediatric Society, the Paediatric Society of New Zealand, and similar groups in England and Scotland.[7,13,63] They all emphasize weaning is not the termination of breastfeeding but the addition of solids.

The Subcommittee on Nutrition During Lactation of the National Academy of Sciences[57] points out that the intake of supplementary foods may add nutrients in a less bioavailable form, decrease the bioavailability of nutrients in human milk, and decrease the intake of other important factors in human milk. Investigators have shown that when solid foods are introduced in the diet of breastfed infants, energy intake per kilogram of body weight does not increase.[46] Solid foods displaced energy intake from human milk in 6-month-old infants even though they were breastfed on demand.

The AAP Committee on Nutrition states, "By 4 to 5 months of age, the extrusion reflex of early infancy has disappeared and the ability to swallow nonliquid foods has become established. By 5 to 6 months of age, the infant will be able to indicate a desire for food by opening his or her mouth and leaning forward, and to indicate disinterest or satiety by leaning back and turning away."[10]

When new foods are added to the breastfed infant's diet, this is called *complementary feeding*. The appropriate timing was studied by a consultation group on Maternal and Young Child Nutrition of the United Nations/American College of Cardiology (U.N./A.C.C) subcommittee on Nutrition.[59] Although practice depends on many biologic, cultural, social, and economic factors, when mother's milk fails to meet the energy and nutrient needs of an infant, inadequate growth and development threaten the child's health and survival. In general, the subcommittee declared that children who are not receiving complementary feeding beyond 6 months do not maintain adequate growth but that infants should not receive it before 4 months. In an extensive review of the world literature and careful recalculation of infant requirements, Whitehead[61] states that a typical volume of breast milk of 800 ml/day is sufficient to meet the needs of a female infant to 16 weeks of age, not the 8 weeks reported by 1973 U.N. Food and Agriculture Organization (FAO)/WHO recommendations.[63] Many mothers produce 1000 ml/day, and this would sustain an average female infant to age 24 weeks and a very large male to 12 weeks. Whitehead finds these calculations compat-

ible with introducing solid foods at 4 to 6 months while continuing to breastfeed fully[61] (Fig. 10-2).

The duration for which exclusive breastfeeding is adequate was studied in a cohort of infants in Amman, Jordan, a well-nourished community.[31] The norms used for comparison were those determined by Fomon in the United States in 1974 using well-nourished formula-fed infants and indicated 4 to 6 months as the maximum time for exclusive breastfeeding. If these data are compared with information collected by Dewey et al[15] in 1994 on well-nourished breastfed infants, no "faltering" in growth pattern would be identified. In a review of protein and energy during weaning, Axelsson and Räihä[2] conclude that 1.65 g/kg/day from 5 to 9 months and 1.48 g/kg/day from 9 to 12 months are appropriate. Dewey et al[16] reported that growth of exclusively breastfed infants from 4 to 6 months of age matched or exceeded that of randomly selected breastfed infants given 20% added protein. The exclusively breastfed group received 0.98 g/kg/day, whereas the supplemented group received 1.18 g/kg/day. Thus protein intake is not a limiting factor with respect to growth that would mandate weaning from the breast. On review of protein requirements for infants and children established by WHO in 1985, Dewey et al[16] determined they

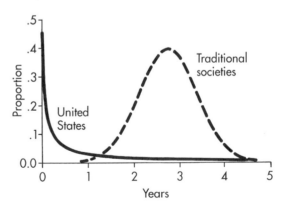

Fig. 10-2. Comparison of age at weaning in United States and 64 traditional societies. (Modified from Dettwyler KA: A time to wean. In Stuart-MacAdam P, Dettwyler KA, editors: *Breastfeeding: biocultural perspectives,* New York, 1995, Aldine de Gruyter.)

were higher than necessary for the breastfed infant. Formula-fed infants require more protein because of comparatively poor utilization.[10]

The infant's first flavor experiences probably occur in utero. When garlic was ingested by mothers before amniocentesis or delivery, the amniotic fluid smelled of garlic.[41] The normal fetus ingests amniotic fluid in utero and thus experiences those flavors. When breastfed, the infant continues to experience those flavors as a bridging experience to solid foods.[40] Not surprisingly, breastfed infants consume cereal prepared with their mother's milk more eagerly and in greater volume than when it is prepared with water. In a carefully controlled experiment, infants were fed by their mothers, who wore facial masks but no perfume to avoid affecting the infant's interest in the food.[41] The infant's interest was reflected in opening of the mouth sooner, fewer negative facial expressions, and greater intake. Mennella and Beauchamp[41] suggest that from the perspective of flavors, weaning means "to accustom," which actually describes what occurs with breastfeeding: the flavors in the milk accustom the infant to new flavors in the transition to solid foods. Putting mother's milk in the bland cereal is part of the bridging. Infants whose mothers have a more varied diet during pregnancy and lactation tend to adapt to solid foods more readily, according to these investigations.

Weaning to a cup is a natural transfer because infants learn to drink from a cup by 7 to 9 months. The use of fruit juice in the cup was originally encouraged for its vitamin C content. Fruit juice may be replacing milk, however, in the diets of young children.[12] This is a concern because milk is an important source of protein and calcium, whereas nutrients in fruit juices are limited predominantly to carbohydrates, calories, and varying amounts of vitamin C. Juices are also replacing fruit in the diet. Excessive fruit juice consumption reportedly leads to short stature and failure to thrive in some infants, chronic diarrhea in some, and obesity in others.[39] The trend often begins when fruit juice is put in a nursing bottle. The pediatrician should be alert to the exact content of the weaning foods, ensuring adequate protein, cal-

cium, vitamins, and fiber, as well as the development of feeding skills, including feeding from a cup and from a spoon.

MOTHER'S RIGHTS

In practice, human mothers are often the determinants of weaning time, as is true for other species. Some mothers want to nurse for a few weeks and wean to a bottle to go to work. Other mothers wean at 3 months to be free again.[44,45] Certainly any time spent breastfeeding is to the infant's advantage. The critical point in weaning is to make it a gradual adjustment for both mother and infant. The year-2000 health goals for the United States recommend that mothers nurse at least 6 months.[43]

A study of the psychosocial factors influencing weaning time in primigravidas was conducted when the 81 participants were 8 months postpartum.[33] Maternal worries about the demands of breastfeeding had a negative effect on the duration. If mothers worried about the demands of breastfeeding, they were more likely to perceive problems with scheduling breastfeeding when they returned to work. Mothers who worried about lack of family support to breastfeed were more apt to worry about the demands of breastfeeding. On the other hand, those women who saw the practical advantages of breastfeeding did not perceive returning to work as presenting a problem and nursed longer. Medical illness, sore nipples, fatigue, or breast infections were not influential in weaning. Work and scheduling have a larger role in most mothers' decision to wean.[30]

WEANING PROCESS

Gradually replacing one feeding at a time with solids or a bottle or cup, depending on the infant's age and stage of development, is usually preferable.[3] After the adjustment has been made to one substitute feeding, a second feeding is replaced with a substitute, usually at the opposite time of day. This process is continued until only the morning and night feedings remain. Then these two are gradually stopped. The morning and night feedings can be maintained for some months, and often an infant may be nursed beyond the second year, especially at these times. Mothers who wish to wean partially as early as 3 months may continue the morning and night nursing. This is especially suited to the working mother. The decline in lactation and the regression of the mammary gland occur slowly with gradual weaning.

When an infant is fully breastfeeding and solids are initiated, a feeding of solids is given during the day and breastfeeding continues on demand. As solids are increased and a three-meals-a-day schedule is reached, breastfeeding still continues on demand, although nursings may be fewer or briefer. No nursings need to be intentionally omitted in this scheme.

The composition of milk during abrupt weaning, carefully analyzed by Hartmann and Kulski,[26] revealed that the secretory capability of the mammary gland of women changed dramatically after complete cessation of breastfeeding but that the involuting gland remained partially functional for 45 days. After termination that occurred in 1 day, sample collections were attempted for each breast by manual expression at the same time on days 1, 2, 4, 8, 16, 21, 31, 42, and 45. The concentrations of lactose and potassium decreased, while sodium, chloride, fat, and total protein increased progressively over 42 days. The milk becomes notably salty. Infants continue to drink the salty fluid.[18] The increase in protein was related to increases in the concentrations of lactoferrin, immunoglobulin A (IgA), IgG, IgM, albumin, lactalbumin, and casein. Concentrations from each breast were similar throughout. One woman in the study breastfed for 39 days; six women fully lactated an average of 332 days (251 to 443 range).

The involution in other species is rapid. For example, complete resorption occurs in 7 days in cows. Caldeyro-Barcia[6] showed that the threshold dose of oxytocin required to elicit milk ejection increased progressively for at least 30 days after termination of breastfeeding. It is believed that a psychologic nursing stimulus contributes to this effect in humans because they continue contact with their infants, whereas other species are separated. Experimental animals given oxytocin postweaning also show a delay in involution.

Emergency weaning

Occasionally, sudden weaning is necessary because of severe illness in the mother or some prolonged separation of mother and infant. (Sudden illness in the infant does not require weaning, and, in fact, weaning would be contraindicated.) This is difficult for both. After abrupt weaning the mammary glands remain partially functional for more than a month.

Depending on the infant's age and flexibility, a patient surrogate mother may need a feeding or two to switch the infant to a bottle. In other cases the infant may take only solids and refuse other liquids for days. The mother may have considerable discomfort. Engorgement may be significant if it is only 4 to 6 weeks postpartum. The mother may experience *milk fever* at any time there is abrupt weaning. This illness is characterized by fever, chills, and malaise, resembling a flulike syndrome. It is believed to be caused by the sudden resorption of milk products into the system. Milk fever usually lasts 3 to 4 days and should not be confused with more serious illness.

The hormonal change resulting from sudden weaning early in lactation is more definitive because the prolactin levels from suckling are higher immediately postpartum (see Chapter 3). The hormone-withdrawal syndrome may be more marked with early weaning. Prolactin has been associated with a feeling of well-being; thus its decrease may be associated with relative depression. Patients with psychiatric disorders have been observed to cope postpartum until they wean the infant from the breast. It is important to provide an adequate social support system during weaning for the mother who is prone to depression.

The normal, well-adjusted mother may experience some depression and sadness at the reality of the last feeding. It may be very difficult to face this experience. It is important to recognize this as a physiologic phenomenon as well as an emotional one. If a mother is forced by circumstances beyond her control to wean early, she may need much understanding and encouragement to cope with the disappointment. If she has had pressure from friends or relatives to breastfeed, she may need to face what she considers failure and recognize that one can bottle feed and still mother very well.

Historically, weaning has varied from strict to permissive schedules with cultural styles.[11] Rigid feeding schedules were associated with early weaning. Weaning has varied from early denial to slow and gentle withdrawal. In the twentieth century the time considered proper for weaning has gradually shortened from 2 or 3 or 4 years to as soon as 6 to 8 months, or less for some mothers and infants. Public opinion has overlooked the infant's needs in favor of what are considered the mother's rights. It is not necessary to have clearly in mind a specific plan for weaning in the early weeks of nursing unless there are some constraints on the mother's time. Weaning should be done with the infant's needs as a guide. If an infant under 1 year of age rejects the breast, it is unusual but not abnormal and should not be considered by the mother as a personal rejection. Some bottle-fed infants throw down the bottle at 9 months as well.

Studies of weaning practices are few. In a study of primigravidas, they introduced solids because their infant seemed hungry and less satisfied and woke more frequently. The average time to introduce nonmilk food in bottle-fed infants was 3 months and in breastfed infants, 5 months. Most observations are done on duration of feeding when the success rate is low. Jackson et al[36] studied weaning times in mothers participating in a rooming-in project from 1942 to 1951 as compared with mothers who received traditional postpartum care at the New Haven Hospital during the same period. Rooming-in meant mother and infant were together in a special unit designed to accommodate both mothers and infants and managed as a pair by the same nursing staff. Infants were with their mothers as much as each mother wished. The rooming-in mothers nursed significantly longer.[35] They averaged 3.5 to 3.8 months, whereas the controls weaned at 1.8 to 2.5 months postpartum.

TABLE 10-1   Main reasons for premature weaning

Reason	N	%
Not enough, inadequate, or "weak" milk	307	30.9
Child refused breast	177	17.8
Illness of child	159	16.0
Mother needed to go to work	149	15.0
"Correct age for bottle feeding"	139	14.0
Other reasons	64	6.3
TOTAL	995	100.0

From Gunn TR: *N Z Med J* 97:360, 1984.

The incidence of breastfeeding decreased as the difficulty of the delivery increased. The number who breastfed their infants did not differ by age, education, or race. Older mothers, better-educated mothers, and black mothers who breastfed, however, nursed longer.

The reasons given why women in Dunedin, New Zealand, elected to wean their infants early included concern about their milk supply and other maternal problems.[32] One of the most significant factors in lactation termination was mismanagement of breastfeeding by health professionals. A similar study in Sweden reported that 66% of the mothers weaned because they thought their milk was drying up.[54]

Sousa et al[55] studied the patterns of weaning in southern Brazil. Brazil was also experiencing a decline in breastfeeding. The study was undertaken to understand the causes of early weaning to develop better means of encouraging longer breastfeeding and delaying weaning. The bottle was introduced at birth by 24% of women, by 2 months by 72.6%, and by 6 months by 88.0%.

Table 10-1 lists the main reasons given for weaning. A third of the mothers believed their milk was weak. Table 10-2 lists the reasons the mothers thought their milk was thin. Gunn[25] believed these data supported the hypothesis that the mothers did not understand the value of human milk and were influenced by advertisements about formulas and therefore compared their milk with formulas. In general, most studies of weaning practices indi-

TABLE 10-2   Reasons for "milk inadequacy"

Reason	N	%
Milk is weak, thin, translucent	189	61.0
Infant cries after being breastfed	59	18.7
Infant needs to be fed very often	35	11.2
Breast not adequately full	24	9.1
TOTAL	307	100.0

From Gunn TR: *N Z Med J* 97:360, 1984.

cated that most weaning is mother initiated, most often because she thinks her milk is no longer adequate. The primary cause of failing milk supply reported by most investigators is inadequate help or instructions about milk production from medical personnel. Those who breastfeed longer tend to be older than 25 years, well-educated, middle class, and self-educated about lactation and to enjoy breastfeeding.[25]

The problem of recall bias when reporting breastfeeding duration was investigated by Huttly et al,[33] who compared responses given at 11, 23, and 47 months postpartum by the mothers of 1000 children; 24% misclassified weaning time at 23 months and 30% at 4 years. Those in the better-educated, higher socioeconomic group were more apt to report longer breastfeeding.

In worldwide epidemiologic studies, Edmonston[17] pointed out that interruption of breastfeeding because of pregnancy may play a significant role. He estimated the mean monthly bias introduced was to reduce breastfeeding by 2 months. In Third World countries, infant death also lowers the duration of breastfeeding inversely to the mother's education, that is, the less educated the mother, the greater the risk of death from infection and accident.

Infant-initiated weaning

Infant-initiated weaning in the first year of life was investigated by Clarke and Harmon,[8] who studied 50 healthy breastfed infants who were totally weaned; 46% of the group of infants initiated the weaning. This is often mistakenly referred to as "self-weaning." The onset was usually between 5

to 9 months of age, with a median age of 6 months. Mothers described the behavior as an increased interest in exploring the environment and in other foods with a decreased interest in breastfeeding. Brazelton[5] described a similar phenomenon and reported three ages in the first year during which the infant exhibits a lagging interest in breastfeeding as a direct or indirect result of developmental events: 4 to 5 months, 7 months, and 9 to 12 months.

The duration of infant-initiated weaning is about 1 month and is an interactive process that requires "at a minimum maternal complicity."[21] It can lead to relatively easy mutual weaning. It can usually be reversed, however, by the mother's efforts to continue breastfeeding.

Refusal to breastfeed: "nursing strike"

Sudden onset of refusal to nurse can occur at any time and often is taken as a personal rejection by the mother, who promptly follows through by weaning completely. Often these mothers consider the refusal to mean that they do not have enough milk or that something is wrong with their milk. This behavior has been called "nursing strike" and has been noted to be temporary.[21] The various causes associated with this abrupt behavior include the following:
1. Onset of menses in the mother
2. Dietary indiscretion by the mother
3. Change in maternal soap, perfume, or deodorant
4. Stress in the mother
5. Earache or nasal obstruction in the infant
6. Teething
7. Episode of biting with startle and pain reaction by the mother

If a reason is identified that is possibly associated and can be changed, nursing will resume. It may take extra effort to reestablish the relationship. Suggestions that may be made to the mother include the following:
1. Make feeding special and quiet, with no distractions and no other people.
2. Increase amount of cuddling, stroking, and soothing the baby. Walk with the infant cradled in the arms or an infant sling.

3. Offer the breast when the infant is very sleepy.
4. Do not starve the child into submission.
5. If simple remedial steps do not result in a return to nursing, the physician should see the child to rule out otitis media, fever, infection, thrush, and so on.
6. If biting was the associated event, keep finger ready to break suction should it occur again to avoid startling the infant.

Weanling diarrhea and malnutrition

Most writings on weaning refer to the problems in underdeveloped countries when infants are weaned early to overdiluted cow's milk or to artificial formulas that do not contain the antiinfective properties of human milk for the human infant.[53] Weanling diarrhea is well described by Gordon et al[23] as the clinical syndrome (weanling diarrhea is a collection of diseases) associated with weaning from the breast. In 1900 in New York City, the death rate from dysentery, diarrhea, and enteritis in children in the first year of life was 5603 in 100,000 infants. This was largely attributed to weaning from the breast. Diarrheas are strongly associated with weaning not only because of the introduction of other foods but also because of the loss of the protective properties of human milk.

The diarrheas contribute to the malnutrition seen in underdeveloped countries because of the resultant lack of appetite and increased metabolic losses. In Third World countries, morbidity and mortality in infancy rise sharply at the time of weaning from human milk because of the rapid onset of infections. Malnutrition is also a major threat to the weanling in the developing world.[48] Rickets, iron deficiency, and protein energy malnutrition are the three major threats. Close behind are the risks of zinc deficiency, allergy, and obesity, which affect a wider group of children.[60]

In well-nourished mothers and their infants, diarrhea does not occur from controlled gradual weaning unless the infant has a milk allergy or metabolic disorder.

Changes in milk composition during gradual weaning

Changes in the nutrient composition of human milk during gradual weaning were studied by Garza et al[20] in six fully lactating women recruited at 5 to 7 months postpartum (Table 10-3). The weaning consisted of decreasing the frequency and duration of breastfeeding by one third each month for a period of 3 months. Milk was collected at 2-week intervals. Volume decreased to 67%, 40%, and 20% of baseline each month. The concentrations of protein and sodium were increased to 142% and 220% of baseline, respectively, by the twelfth week of weaning. Changes in fat composition were linear through the tenth week but at the twelfth week were similar to baseline. Iron was increased 172%, calcium was unchanged, and zinc fell to 58%. Similar observations have been made

---

TABLE 10-3   Nutrient density (mg/100 kcal) of milk during weaning

	Week								
	0	2	4	6	8	10	12	PTM*	R†
Protein	1.5	1.2	1.3	1.0	1.3	1.2	1.9	1.8	2.7
Na	24.0	17.0	20.0	13.0	24.0	25.0	46.0	25.0	53.0
Ca	38.0	30.0	33.0	21.0	30.0	26.0	38.0	34.5	140.0
Zn	0.21	0.17	0.19	0.09	0.10	0.10	0.11	3.8	0.5

From Garza C, Johnson CA, Smith E et al: *Am J Clin Nutr* 37:61, 1983.

*Nutrient densities of milk from delivering premature infants.

†Nutrient densities calculated to achieve intrauterine growth rates assuming that the caloric requirement of low-birth-weight infants is 130 kcal/kg.

in bovine milk. Milk produced during either rapid or gradual weaning is characterized by a decreasing concentration of lactose. Fat accounts for an increasing percentage of calories (up 80%) and protein a stable 6% of calories.

The immunologic components in human milk were also measured, and the concentrations of certain components of the immunologic system are maintained during gradual weaning.[22] The effect of gradual weaning differs from that of abrupt weaning, in which the concentrations of all components rise dramatically. Measurements at 4 weeks, 8 weeks, and 12 weeks showed a decrease in the milk volume of 67%, 40%, and 20% as the levels of IgA and secretory IgA rose slightly. Lysozyme and lactoferrin rose slightly.

Lipase activities in human milk during weaning were studied by Freed et al.[19] Bile salt–stimulated lipase (BSSL) slowly decreased throughout weaning, whereas lipoprotein lipase (LPL) became substantially lower or absent as compared with colostrum. Lipase activity continues but decreases with the decrease in milk volume.

Studies in other species suggest that gut maturation observed at normal weaning time is not dependent on components in the milk but is triggered by thyroxine and corticosterone in the plasma of the offspring.[29] The anatomic changes in the breast during weaning are discussed in Chapter 2.

The caloric needs for infants have been overestimated in the past. Continued growth occurs on lower volumes of human milk than formula, with breastfed infants refusing additional milk even when a woman increases her volume by pumping.[47] The energy requirement is 115 kcal/kg/day in the first 2 months, after which requirements decline rapidly, reaching a low of 85 kcal/kg/day at 6 months. Between 6 and 12 months of age, requirements gradually increase with increased activity to 100 kcal/kg/day. These figures are a radical departure from those recommended in the past.[62] Most studies of energy intakes show, at all ages, that boys have greater intake and greater rates of growth than girls and are usually weaned sooner.[56] Further, the effects of infection and social deprivation are important to consider; chil-dren in supportive, loving environments have been noted to grow on fewer calories than the deprived child.

Physician's role

The physician's responsibility is the initiation of the appropriate solid foods, which probably should begin at 6 months of age.

Introduction of a cup as a developmental step should usually begin by 7 months.

Eating finger foods and learning self-feeding are the next steps for the child.

None of the above means the termination of breastfeeding but rather the gradual developmental progression of feeding. Breastfeeding continues "on demand." As other foods are introduced and feeding begins to cluster into three meals and some "snacks," breastfeedings will be decreased eventually to two or three per day in the second year.

The nourishment value is not a key issue of continued nursing after 1 year if other foods are adequate, although very valuable nutrition and immunoprotection continue to be provided.[53] The physician's role is to ensure adequate nutrition and be available for advice for as long as breastfeeding continues.

There is no known detriment to nursing, and some indication that nursing a few times a day or during times of stress is beneficial to the mother-infant relationship when the child is over a year of age. The objections raised are usually based on custom or personal taste. It is important for the clinician to avoid judgmental counseling based only on personal biases. Lay publications on the subject may help the mother who is nursing a toddler.

The physician may need to help the mother work through her own feelings about nursing her infant beyond the first year. Many women have been overwhelmed by friendly advice from lay experts about the infant who nurses for several years. Beyond a year, weaning is rarely child initiated until age 4. The child may not lose interest, so that the final steps in termination may require maternal intervention if weaning is desired sooner. A mother is not a poor parent if she begins to feel resentful toward nursing. Planning appropriate alternatives to the breastfeeding session that is to be eliminated is helpful in turning the child's attention toward the new event instead of toward the loss of an old and cherished one, a feeding at the breast. The mother may need to be helped to see how to avoid situations that easily predispose to nursing. She needs to know that it is acceptable to set some rules and to have some limitations and control over the breastfeeding.

If the mother becomes pregnant, she should decide when she wants to wean or whether she will continue to nurse through pregnancy and then tandem-nurse the new baby (see Chapter 18). For the child, it is important to avoid abrupt weaning or weaning to make room for the new baby, who will now take the child's place. Weaning well before delivery is usually less traumatic for the child than at delivery time. At delivery, however, the new infant is fed first.

Motivation to wean

The motivation to wean the infant may be multifactorial and often is suggested by the father, grandmother, or members of the mother's social circle. The physician should not initiate weaning except for medical reasons but may initiate discussion about it, to ensure that the mother has given it some thought. Parents may find nursing an older baby or a toddler distasteful. When mothers are encouraged to anticipate their weaning plans, it can be gradual, taking advantage of developmental progress and new interests of the toddler. It is wise to avoid associating sleeping with a feeding as the time to wean approaches, or it may be more difficult to make the break. The father can play a vital role in nonnutritive cuddling, beginning from birth, and can be especially helpful in easing an infant through weaning, particularly when night feedings have become the custom. Not all parents perceive weaning, night feedings, and bringing an infant to the parents' bed in the same light. Not all physicians view these matters equally, but they should avoid imposing personal views on patients.

When weaning in developing countries, the decision was thought to be made on the basis of traditional beliefs, nutritional status of the child, or similar reasons. When the reasons for termination were studied in West Africa, however, illness in the child, a new pregnancy, and illness in the mother were found to be the most common causes.[37] Health workers should be aware of this in order to counsel mothers appropriately.

CLOSET NURSING

The physician should be fully informed about breastfeeding physiologically and psychologically. The trusted physician communicates well with patients and is kept informed by the parents. Unfortunately, many mothers are driven to "closet nursing" by insensitive, uninformed relatives and friends and even physicians. Closet nursing is nursing privately at home in secret and propagates ignorance about breastfeeding duration. This not only influences other mothers but also physicians who are unaware and custody court judges who are led to believe extended nursing is abnormal. Thousands of normal, healthy children are breastfed until they are 3 or 4 years old. The benefits of human milk continue. Research documents health protection and improved development for at least 2 years. It has not been evaluated beyond that except for the positive emotional and bonding experience associated with long-term nursing.[38,48,50,58]

WORKING MOTHER

Some mothers return to work. Whether the reason is money, career, or personal satisfaction is not relevant to management. It takes tremendous commitment to work and breastfeed, but it can be done, it has been done, and it will be done. Usually the biggest problem a mother faces is coping with people who do not understand why she bothers. An understanding physician who provides the reassurance and support necessary to manage is a great asset. A mother may go home for a feeding in the middle of the day, pump milk to leave for the infant to have from a bottle, or give a substitute bottle. If there are occasional bottles of formula, the powder preparations are more economical and require only warming the water before adding the powder to ensure rapid solution. Chapter 20 offers suggestions for collecting milk.

Some infants quickly learn the mother's schedule and will sleep while she is away and feed more frequently during the evening and night to make up for it. It takes some personal adjustment to plan ahead and a babysitter who is patient and cooperative. Many infants are cared for in day-care centers, which requires packing up and transporting the infant to other surroundings.

A mother needs to be alert to the infant's needs as well and may need to leave feedings ready when she is away, even if she had hoped the infant would sleep through the day. If a mother works long hours or an inflexible schedule, it may be necessary to wean the infant to morning and night feedings at the breast. However, this arrangement still provides the special benefits of human milk as well as the closeness that an infant needs; thus it is worth the effort. Chapter 13 discusses maternal employment.

LEGAL ISSUES

In the present turmoil of family life in which parents are separating when the children are still young, several custody cases have been based on weaning times or, more accurately, on the time breastfeeding is totally terminated. A number of cases in the United States have come to my attention in which the father has sought custody on the basis of prolonged breastfeeding, when the child nursed for comfort to about age 4. In most cases the judge found in favor of the mother. In one case in Rochester, NY, the judge found in favor of the father when an expert witness, a local psychologist, declared that "you have to be crazy to nurse that long." No amount of scientific evidence could counter this inappropriate remark.

Other issues of parental rights have surfaced in cases of child custody and visitation rights when the child is under 2 years of age and breastfeeding. Usually the argument over separation of mother from her breastfeeding infant is part of a larger problem. Physicians called on to give expert testimony need to review carefully all the issues because rarely is the breastfeeding question the only problem. Right and wrong have not been established for all circumstances. It would seem appropriate also that judges review the entire case and qualifications of the respective parents and refrain from basing their decision on personal biases and emotional testimony. It is also advisable for expert witnesses to be fully informed on a subject about which they will testify, and avoid extending their comments beyond their area of expertise.

Developmental psychologist Ainsworth[1] has studied the maturation of the child and summarized the literature, which shows that infants with a strong attachment to the mother through breastfeeding are psychologically independent at 2 years of age. These children have more mastery of themselves at age 5 and less anxiety entering school than bottle-fed children.

REFERENCES

1. Ainsworth MA: The development of infant-mother attachment. In Caldwell BM, Ricciuti HN, editors: *Review of child development research,* Chicago, 1973, University of Chicago Press.

2. Axelsson IEM, Räihä NCR: Protein and energy during weaning, *Adv Pediatr* 39:405, 1992.
3. Barnes GR, Lethin AN, Jackson EB et al: Management of breast feeding, *JAMA* 151:192, 1953.

4. Birkbeck JA, Chairman: The age of weaning: a statement of the infant nutrition subcommittee of the Paediatric Society of New Zealand, *N Z Med J* 95:584, 1982.

5. Brazelton TB: *Infants and mothers: differences in development,* New York, 1969, Delacorte.

6. Caldeyro-Barcia R: Milk ejection in women. In Reynolds M, Folley SJ, editors: *Lactogenesis: the initiation of milk secretion at parturition,* Philadelphia, 1969, University of Pennsylvania Press.

7. Canadian Pediatric Society Nutrition Committee: Infant feeding: a statement, *Can J Public Health* 70:376, 1979.

8. Clarke SK, Harmon RJ: Infant-initiated weaning from the breast in the first year, *Early Hum Dev* 8:151, 1983.

9. Committee on Nutrition, American Academy of Pediatrics: On the feeding of supplemental foods to infants, *Pediatrics* 65:1178, 1980.

10. Committee on Nutrition, American Academy of Pediatrics: Supplemental foods for infants. In Barness LA, editor: *Pediatric nutrition handbook,* Elk Grove Village, Ill, 1993, American Academy of Pediatrics.

11. Cone TE Jr: *History of American pediatrics,* Boston, 1979, Little, Brown.

12. Dennison BA: Fruit juice consumption by infants and children: a review, *J Am Coll Nutr* 15:45, 1996.

13. Department of Health and Social Security: *Present day practice in infant feeding: studies on health and social subjects,* London, 1977, The Department.

14. Dettwyler KA: A time to wean: the hominid blueprint for the natural age of weaning in modern human populations. In Stuart-MacAdam P, Dettwyler KA, editors: *Breastfeeding: biocultural perspectives,* New York, 1995, Aldine de Gruyter.

15. Dewey KG, Beaton G, Fjeld C et al: Protein requirements of infants and children, *Eur J Clin Nutr* 50(suppl 1):5119, 1996.

16. Dewey KG, Cohen RJ, Rivera L et al: Do exclusively breast-fed infants require extra protein? *Pediatr Res* 39:303, 1996.

17. Edmonston B: Interruption of breastfeeding by child death and pregnancy, *Soc Biol* 37:233, 1990.

18. Finberg L, Kiley J, Luttrell CN: Mass accidental salt poisoning in infancy, *JAMA* 184:121, 1963.

19. Freed LM, Neville MC, Hamosh M: Lipase activities in human milk during weaning, *Pediatr Res* 25(pt 2):290A, 1989.

20. Garza C, Johnson CA, Smith E et al: Changes in the nutrient composition of human milk during gradual weaning, *Am J Clin Nutr* 37:61, 1983.

21. Goldfarb J, Tibbetts E: *Breastfeeding handbook,* Hillside, NJ, 1980, Enslow.

22. Goldman AS, Goldblum RM: Immunologic components in human milk during weaning, *Acta Paediatr Scand* 72:133, 1983.

23. Gordon JE, Chitkara ID, Wyon JB: Weanling diarrhea, *Am J Med Sci Prev Med Epidemiol* 245:345, 1963.

24. Gulick EE: The effects of breastfeeding on toddler health, *Pediatr Nurs* 12:51, 1986.

25. Gunn TR: The incidence of breastfeeding and reasons for weaning, *N Z Med J* 97:360, 1984.

26. Hartmann PE, Kulski JK: Changes in the composition of the mammary secretion of women after the abrupt termination of breastfeeding, *J Physiol* 275:1, 1978.

27. Harvey PH, Clutton-Brock TH: Life history variations in primates, *Evolution* 39(3):559, 1985.

28. Helsing E, King FS: *Breast-feeding practice,* New York, 1980, Oxford University Press.

29. Henning SJ: Role of milk-borne factors in weaning and intestinal development, *Biol Neonate* 41:265, 1982.

30. Hervada AR, Newman DR: Weaning: historical perspective, practical recommendations, and current controversies, *Curr Probl Pediatr* 22:223, 1992.

31. Hijazi SS, Abulaban A, Waterlow JC: The duration for which exclusive breastfeeding is adequate, *Acta Paediatr Scand* 78:23, 1989.

32. Hood LJ, Faed JA, Silva PA et al: Breast feeding and some reasons for electing to wean the infant: a report from the Dunedin Multidisciplinary Child Development Study, *N Z Med J* 88:273, 1978.

33. Huttly SRA, Barros FC, Victora CG et al: Do mothers overestimate breastfeeding duration? An example of recall bias from a study in Southern Brazil, *Am J Epidemiol* 132:572, 1990.

34. Illingworth RS, Lister J: The critical or sensitive period, with special reference to certain feeding problems in infants and children, *J Pediatr* 65:839, 1964.

35. Jackson EB: Pediatric and psychiatric aspects of the Yale Rooming-In Project, *Conn State Med J* 14:616, 1950.

36. Jackson EB, Wilkins LC, Auerbach H: Statistical report on incidence and duration of breast feeding in relation to personal-social and hospital maternity factors, *Pediatrics* 17:700, 1956.

37. Jacobsen MS, Sodemann M, Molbak K et al: Reason for termination of breastfeeding and the length of breastfeeding, *Int J Epidemiol* 25:115, 1996.

38. Kendall-Tackett KA, Sugarman M: The social consequences of long-term breastfeeding, *J Hum Lact* 11:179, 1995.

39. Lifshitz F: Weaning foods . . . the role of fruit juice in the diets of infants and children, *J Am Coll Nutr* 15:15, 1996.

40. Mennella JA, Beauchamp GK: Maternal diet alters the sensory qualities of human milk and the nursling's behavior, *Pediatrics* 88:737, 1991.

41. Mennella JA, Beauchamp GK: Mother's milk enhances the acceptance of cereal during weaning, *Pediatr Res* 41:188, 1997.

42. Merchant SM: Neural development for sucking, swallowing and chewing. In Ballabriga A, Rey J: *Weaning: why, what and when?* Workshop Series, vol II, New York, 1987, Vevey/Raven.

43. National Health Goals, *Am J Public Health Suppl* 43:142, 1978.

44. Newton N: Breast feeding, *Psychol Today* 98:68, 1971.

45. Newton N: The role of the oxytocin reflexes in three interpersonal reproductive acts: coitus, birth and breast-feeding. In Carenza L, Pancheri P, Zichella L, editors: *Clinical psycho neuro endocrinology in reproduction, Proceedings of the Serono Symposia,* vol 22, London, 1978, Academic Press.

46. Nommsen LA, Lovelady CA, Heinig MJ et al: Determinants of energy, protein, lipid and lactose concentrations in human milk during the first 12 months of lactation: the Darling Study, *Am J Clin Nutr* 53:457, 1991.

47. Poskitt EME: Energy needs in the weaning period. In Ballabriga A, Rey J, editors: *Weaning: why, what and when?* New York, 1987, Vevey/Raven.

48. Prentice A: Breastfeeding and the older infant, *Acta Paediatr Scand Suppl* 374:78, 1991.

49. Raphael D: *The tender gift: breastfeeding,* New York, 1976, Schocken.

50. Reamer SB, Sugarman M: Breastfeeding beyond six months: mothers' perceptions of the positive and negative consequences, *J Trop Pediatr* 33:93, 1987.

51. Schmitz J, McNeish AS: Development of structure and function of the gastrointestinal tract: relevance for weaning. In Ballabriga A, Rey J, editors: *Weaning: why, what and when?* Workshop Series, vol 11, New York, 1987, Vevey/Raven.

52. Short RV: The biological basis for the contraceptive effects of breastfeeding. In Jelliffe DP, Jelliffe EFP, editors: *Advances in international maternal and child health,* vol 3, Oxford, 1983, Oxford University Press.

53. Short RV: Breastfeeding, *Sci Am* 250(4):35, 1984.

54. Sjölin S, Hofvander Y, Hillervik G: Factors related to early termination of breastfeeding, *Acta Paediatr Scand* 66:505, 1977.

55. Sousa PLR, Barros FC, Pinheiro GNM et al: Patterns of weaning in South Brazil, *J Trop Pediatr Environ Child Health* 21:210, 1975.

56. Stuff JE, Nichols BL: Nutrient intake and growth performance of older infants fed human milk, *J Pediatr* 115:959, 1989.

57. Subcommittee on Nutrition during Lactation, Committee on Nutrition Status during Pregnancy and Lactation, Food and Nutrition Board, Institute of Medicine, National Academy of Sciences: *Nutrition during lactation,* Washington, DC, 1991, National Academy Press.

58. Sugarman M, Kendall-Tackett KA: Weaning ages in a sample of American women who practice extended breast-feeding, *Clin Pediatr* 34:642, 1995.

59. Underwood BA, Hofvander Y: Appropriate timing for complementary feeding of the breastfed infant, *Acta Paediatr Scand Suppl* 294:5, 1982.

60. Wharton BA: Food for the weanling: the next priority in infant nutrition, *Acta Paediatr Scand Suppl* 323:96, 1986.

61. Whitehead RG: Infant physiology, nutritional requirements, and lactational adequacy, *Am J Clin Nutr,* 41:447, 1985.

62. Widdowson EM: Mental contentment and physical growth, *Lancet* 1:1316, 1952.

63. World Health Organization: *Joint WHO/UNICEF meeting on infant and young child feeding,* Geneva, 1979, WHO.

$\mathcal{D}$rugs in breast milk

Despite the overwhelming advantages of human milk and the advantages of being breastfed, at times the physician must consider the risk of a maternal medication to the nursing infant. Even when the data about the medication include the milk/plasma ratio, the physician has to consider several factors related to each infant and each situation before deciding if breastfeeding can be initiated or continue. The more complicated the mother's medical problems, the greater is the possibility that the infant also has complications of prematurity or illness that will alter the ability to excrete medication. This situation requires scientific information and experienced clinical judgment to appraise the problems and determine the therapeutic regimen. The clinician must determine the risk/benefit ratio of continued breastfeeding. The data are still meager and sometimes conflicting, yet maternal medication is the single most common medical problem in managing breastfeeding patients.

There are a number of general reviews of drugs in breast milk and hundreds of articles about the effect of a specific medication in a particular infant.* The American Academy of Pediatrics (AAP)[21,22] Committee on Drugs has published a list of drugs and other chemicals that transfer into human breast milk. The list, which is continually updated, is divided into those that are contraindicated, those that require temporary interruption of breastfeeding, and those that are compatible with breastfeeding. Concern about this issue of drugs in

breast milk has spread. The U.S. Department of Health and Human Services (DHHS) and Food and Drug Administration (FDA) have proposed a standard warning on all nonprescription drugs that are absorbed by the body: "As with any drug, if you are pregnant or nursing a baby, seek professional advice before using this product." Because studies of pregnant women have shown that they take five to eight medications on their own during pregnancy and postpartum, the clinician's education of these patients needs to continue.

A study of more than 14,000 pregnant women in 148 hospitals in 22 countries revealed that 79% of women received an average of 3.3 drugs.[20] The drugs most often given were analgesics and anesthetics. Of the 91% of women who initiated breastfeeding, 36% received methylergonovine and 5% antibiotics. Another study of 885 women 3 to 5 months postpartum in Oslo showed that breastfeeders took fewer medications (daily dose/1000 women/day) than nonbreastfeeders.[83] The most common medication in the latter group was oral contraceptives. Colds, dyspepsia, hemorrhoids, and breast infections were the disorders that precipitated the use of albuterol (Salbutamol), clemastine fumarate (Tavist), dexchlorpheniramine maleate (cold preparations), phenylpropanolamine hydrochloride (Comtrex, Dimetane), cromolyn sodium, and methotrimeprazine hydrochloride (levomepromazine).[83]

No substitute exists for specific knowledge. It is as equally inappropriate to discontinue breastfeeding when it is not medically necessary to do so as

---

*References 3, 13, 14, 22, 46, 53, 69, 90, 94, 101, 143.

it is to continue breastfeeding while taking contra-indicated drugs.

Consideration of the pharmacokinetics contributes to the understanding of the problems involved. Some data reported have been extrapolated from experiments performed on cows, goats, and rodents. Bovine experiments have been conducted using continuous infusions, which provide data on the passage of a drug into milk under certain pH and plasma levels. In an effort to explain and clarify the issues involved, the literature has oversimplified the problem so that individuals lacking a background in pharmacology or pediatrics have misused the published data in drawing unwarranted conclusions.

Factors that influence the passage of a drug into the milk in humans include the size of the molecule, its solubility in lipids and water, whether it binds to protein, the drug's pH, and diffusion rates. Following is a summary of these factors:

I. Drug
   A. Route of administration
      1. Oral (PO)
      2. Intravenous (IV)
      3. Intramuscular (IM)
      4. Transdermal drug delivery system (TDDS)
   B. Absorption rate
   C. Half-life or peak serum time
   D. Dissociation constant
   E. Volume of distribution
II. Size of molecule
III. Degree of ionization
IV. pH of substrate
   A. Plasma 7.4
   B. Milk 6.8
V. Solubility
   A. In water
   B. In lipids
VI. Protein binding more to plasma than to milk protein

Passive diffusion is the principal factor in the passage of a drug from plasma into milk. The drug may appear in an active form or as an inactive metabolite.

Finally, a most important factor that has re-ceived relatively little attention is the infant. Will the infant absorb the chemical from the intestinal tract? If the infant absorbs the chemical, can the infant detoxify and excrete it, or will minimal amounts in the milk build in the infant's system? Is the infant premature, small for gestational age, or high risk because of complications of the pregnancy or delivery? Is the drug a material that could be safely given to an infant directly, and at what risk? What dosages and blood levels are safe? These latter two questions are more critical than the pharmacokinetic theory. The ultimate question faced by the physician is, Can this infant be safely exposed to this chemical as it appears in breast milk without a risk that exceeds the tremendous benefits of being breastfed? Almost any drug present in mother's blood will appear to some degree in her milk.

CHARACTERISTICS OF DRUGS

Protein binding

Drugs entering the circulation become protein bound or remain free in the circulation. The protein-bound component of the drug serves as an inactive reservoir for the drug that is in equilibrium with the free drug. Most drugs enter the mammary alveolar cells in the unbound form (Fig. 11-1).

At term, plasma proteins may be reduced and the fatty acid and hypoprotein fraction slightly increased in the mother, which results in the displacement of some drugs from plasma proteins.[32] During the early postpartum period for 5 to 7 weeks the free fraction of some drugs increases and therefore more readily crosses into milk (e.g., salicylate, phenytoin, diazepam).

For most drugs, more drug will be found in the plasma than in the milk. Only the small free fraction of drug can cross the biologic membrane. The total concentration in milk is only minimally influenced by binding of drugs in milk proteins (milk protein concentration is 0.9% in mature milk). Only those drug molecules that are free in solution can pass through the endothelial pores, either by

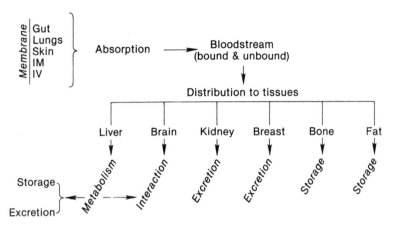

Fig. 11-1. Distribution pathways for drugs, once absorbed during lactation. (Modified from Rivera-Calimlim L: *Clin Perinatol* 14:51, 1976.)

diffusion or by reverse pinocytosis. *Pinocytosis* is the process whereby drug molecules dissolved in the interstitial fluid attach to receptors located at the surface of the cell membrane.[106,107] The cell membrane invaginates at the site of the drug attachment, bringing the drug into the cell. The membrane is pinched off, and the drug, surrounded by membrane, remains in the cell. Then the membrane is dissolved, leaving the drug molecule free in the cell.

Reverse pinocytosis is the process by which the apical membrane evaginates after fusion of the intracellular membrane-bound secretion granules with the plasma membrane. The granules include lipids, proteins, lactose, drug molecules, and other cellular constituents. The evagination of the plasma membrane is pinched off and released into the alveolar lumen. Within the extravascular space the drug may be bound to proteins in the interstitial fluid. Some agents in free solution can pass into the alveolar milk directly by way of the spaces between the mammary alveolar cells. These paracellular areas account for a major portion of the fluid changes across the epithelium. These spaces between adjacent alveolar cells serve to carry water-soluble drugs from the tissue into the milk.

The intercellular junctions are "open" at delivery as lactation is being established and gradually "tighten" over the next few days. The amount of drug passed into milk on day 1 is greater than on day 3 or later. The composition of the milk changes as well from colostrum to mature milk, altering the amount of protein and fat, which could also influence milk levels of the drug. It is always important to know when plasma and milk samples were measured in relationship to the onset of lactation. Furthermore, some studies have been done on nonlactating women by pumping enough milk to measure the drug. These "weaning samples" provide only misinformation.

Ionization

Drugs that are nonionized are excreted in the milk in greater amounts than are ionized compounds. Depending on the pH of the solvent and the drug *dissociation constant* (pK_a), many weak electrolytes are more or less ionized in solution. Blood plasma and interstitial fluid are slightly alkaline (pH 7.4). Drugs that are weak acids are ionized to a greater extent in alkaline solution and are more extensively bound to protein. The amount of drug excreted from plasma (pH 7.4) to milk (pH 6.8 to 7.3, average 7.0) depends on the pH of the compound. Thus a weakly acidic compound has a higher concentration in plasma than in milk. Conversely, weakly alkaline compounds are in equal or higher levels in the milk than in the plasma.

The degree of drug ionization changes with the pH of the plasma and milk. Weak bases become more ionized with decreasing pH; thus the ionized component will increase in milk. The concentration in plasma and milk for the nonionized fraction will be the same, but the total amount of drug in the milk will be greater than in plasma. The sulfonamides demonstrate the effect of the pK_a on the concentration of drug that reaches the milk. Sulfacetamide, with a low pK_a (5.4), has a low milk/plasma (M/P) ratio (0.08), whereas sulfanilamide has a pK_a of 10.4 and an M/P ratio of 1.00 (Table 11-1).

The studies done in cows and goats with constant infusions demonstrate this principle more dramatically because the pH of bovine plasma is 7.4 to 7.5 and of bovine milk 6.5. Under normal circumstances, however, concentrations of drugs are rarely constant, and there is a delay in achieving a new equilibrium. During periods of rapidly decreasing blood levels, some back diffusion occurs into the plasma.

Molecular weight

The passage of molecules into the milk also depends on the size of the molecule, or the molecular weight (mol wt, in daltons). Water-filled membranous pores permit the movement of molecules of less than 100 mol wt. Because of action similar to the limitation of transport of certain large-molecular-weight chemicals across the placenta,

insulin and heparin are not found in human milk either, presumably because of the molecule's size.

Solubility

The alveolar epithelium of the breast is a lipid barrier that is most permeable in the first few days of lactation, when colostrum is being produced. The solubility of a compound in water and in lipid is a determining factor in its transfer. Nonionized drugs, which are lipid soluble, usually dissolve and descend in the lipid phase of the membrane. The solubility is closely linked to the manner in which the drug crosses the membranes (Table 11-2). The membrane of the alveolar epithelial cells is composed of lipoprotein, glycolipid, phospholipid, and free lipids, as described in Chapter 3. The transfer of water-soluble drugs and ions is inhibited by this hydrophobic barrier. Water-soluble materials pass through pores in the basement membrane and paracellular spaces. Low lipid solubility of an nonionized compound will diminish its excretion into milk.

Lipid solubility affects the profile of the drug in the milk and plasma. A drug with high lipid solubility will have parallel elimination curves in the plasma and the milk. A drug with low lipid solubility will clear the plasma at a constant rate, but the clearance curve for the milk will peak lower and later, and the drug will linger in the milk.

TABLE 11-1 Association between milk/plasma (M/P) ratios and dissociation constants (pK_a) of sulfonamides

Sulfonamide	Milk/plasma ratio	pK_a
Sulfacetamide	0.08	5.4
Sulfadiazine	0.21	6.5
Sulfathiazole	0.43	7.1
Sulfamethazine	0.51	7.4
Sulfapyridine	0.85	8.4
Sulfanilamide	1.00	10.4

Modified from Gaginella TS: *US Pharm* 3:39, 1978.

TABLE 11-2 Predicted distribution ratios of drug concentrations in milk and plasma

General drug type	Milk/plasma (M/P) ratio
Highly lipid-soluble drugs	~1
Highly protein-bound drugs in maternal serum	<1
Small (mol wt <200) water-soluble drugs	~1
Weak acids	≤1
Weak bases	≥1
Actively transported drugs	>1

Modified from Gaginella TS: *US Pharm* 3:39, 1978.

A prolonged terminal elimination phase may exist when time between feedings is long.[32]

Mechanisms of transport

Drugs pass into milk by simple diffusion, carrier-mediated diffusion, or active transport, as follows:

Simple diffusion: concentration gradient decreases

Carrier-mediated diffusion: concentration gradient decreases

Active transport: concentration gradient increases

Pinocytosis

Reverse pinocytosis

Pharmacokinetic principles relate to the specific variation with time of the drug concentration in the blood or plasma as a result of its absorption, distribution, and elimination. Ultimately, by extrapolation of these factors, one determines the effect of the drug. The most elementary kinetic model is based on the body as a single compartment. Distribution of the drug in the compartment is assumed to be uniform and rapidly equilibrated. In the single-compartment model, the volume of distribution of a drug is considered to be the same as that of the plasma, assuming a rapid uniform distribution.[40] The volume of distribution is

$$V_d = \frac{\text{Total amount of drug in body}}{\text{Concentration of drug in plasma}}$$

The absorption and elimination are considered to be exponential or first-order kinetics. A two-compartment model of drug kinetics takes into account the phase of decreasing drug concentration as drug distributes into the tissues. Initially, concentrations fall rapidly as the drug distributes, then first-order elimination follows. When considering the pharmacokinetics of drugs in breast milk, one must also consider that elimination in the breast is then by two potential routes: excreted with the milk to the infant and back diffusion into the plasma to reequilibrate with the falling level in the plasma.

With access to the volume of distribution of the drug in question, the amount of the dose, and the weight of the mother, the concentration of drug in breast milk could be theoretically calculated as follows[102]:

$$\text{Concentration in breast milk} = \frac{\text{Dose}}{\text{Volume of distribution}}$$

The average total body store of drug at the plateau is approximately equal to 1.5 times the amount administered per one-half time of elimination.[102] The effect of a single dose of the drug is characterized by latency, time of peak effect, magnitude of peak effect, and duration. As dosage is increased, latency is reduced, and peak effect is increased without changing the time. Repeated dosage is usually calculated on one half-times of elimination, assuming four half-times are required for complete elimination. When the drug is given in less time, the drug accumulates. Accumulation continues, in first-order kinetics, until the rate of elimination equals the rate of administration. A constant fraction of the drug is eliminated per unit of time. In general terms, maximal accumulation occurs after four half-times, and at this time the rate of elimination is equal to the rate of administration.[145]

Three-compartment and other models

To account for the relationship of the maternal body, the breast, the milk, and the infant, Wilson and his colleagues[143-145] have proposed a three-compartment model of kinetics to describe the drug excretion in breast milk. In this model a deep compartment, the third compartment, exists in the breast (Fig. 11-2). When the infant is feeding, the rate constant is zero-order kinetics, and when no milk is being removed, drug accumulates in the deep compartment and begins to transfer back. *Compartment 1* represents the central compartment, which receives the drug directly after dosing. This compartment connects to *compartment 2,* as seen in two-compartment models by a reversible transport process of interstitial and intracellular water. The breast milk, which is *compartment 3,* is in equilibrium with compartment 2. Drug is eliminated from the mother's body at a constant rate (K_{10}) and from the breast milk by an infant-

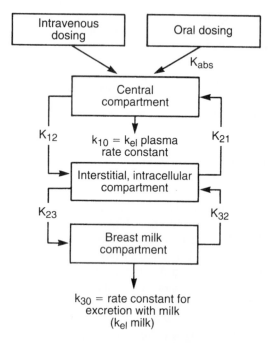

Fig. 11-2. Three-compartment model. See text for rate descriptions. (Modified from Wilson JT: *Drug Metab Rev* 14:619, 1983.)

modulated rate constant (K_{30}). It is zero order during feeding, and therefore the rate is feeding dependent. Between feedings, however, K_{30} is zero; that is, no drug leaves via the milk. The rate constants differ for different drugs.[143-145]

Other models have been developed for measuring the amount of drug that reaches the infant when the M/P ratio is not known. Using a stepwise linear regression for acidic and basic drugs, based on the drug's pK_a, the plasma protein binding value, and the octanol/water partition coefficient, an M/P ratio can be calculated. In a study of several proposed equations, Begg et al[6] demonstrated that the error is lowest for the drugs with the highest M/P ratio, that protein binding is the most important single predictor, and that the M/P ratios for basic drugs are more accurately predictable.

The concentration of the drug in the circulation of the mother depends on the mode of administration: PO, IV, IM, or TDDS. Absorption through the skin, the lungs (inhalants), or vaginally may also need to be considered.

A newer route, the *transdermal drug delivery system* (TDDS), depends on absorption through the skin; it has become a significant route of administration for certain medications. The delivery rate is determined by diffusion of drug from the reservoir matrix through the epidermis. This method offers some advantages, including convenience of dosing, reduced dosing frequency, ease of reaching a steady state, increased patient compliance, avoidance of first-pass hepatic biotransformation, and reduction of side effects through heightened selectivity of drug action.[117] The level in the plasma remains constant during the drug's anticipated life span while the patch is in place. TDDS patches are available for scopolamine, nicotine, clonidine, fentanyl, and other drugs (Table 11-3).

The levels in the blood depend on the route of administration. The curves produced by bolus IV medication peak high and early and taper sharply, thus making avoiding peak plasma levels more feasible. Absorption from IM dosing is less rapid but follows a similar but less sharp curve. PO dosing depends on other factors, such as whether the medication is taken between or during meals. Depending on the curve of uptake and removal of drug from the plasma, the area under the curve varies. Single doses are simple area-under-the-curve calculations, but calculations for multiple doses or chronic use vary with the steady state of the drug in the body.

Nonelectrolytes such as ethanol, urea, and antipyrine enter the milk by diffusion through the lipid membrane barrier and may reach the same concentrations in the milk as in the plasma, regardless of the pH. The main entrance site of molecules is at the basement laminal membrane, where water-soluble materials pass through the alveolar pores. Nonionized drugs cross the membrane more easily than ionized ones because of the structure of the membrane. The nonionized drugs pass through the membrane by diffusion. When simple diffusion takes place, the M/P ratio is 1.0. Passive diffusion provides the same ratio regardless of the plasma concentrations of the drug or the volume of milk secreted. Different M/P ratios depend on the binding to protein and are a measure of the protein-free fraction. The dissimilar ratios for the sulfa drugs

TABLE 11-3   Representative transdermal drug delivery systems (TDDS)

Drug	Total amount in patch (mg)	Delivery rate (duration of use)	Approximate postuse drug residue (mg)	Pediatric dose
Scopolamine	1.5	0.5 mg/D (3 D)	0	Therapeutic*: 6 µg/kg
Nicotine				
Habitrol	52.5	29 µg/cm^2/hr (24 hr)	21.5	**Toxic†** (mg/kg)
30 cm^2				**Severe** (1.4-1.9)
Nicoderm	114.0	40 µg/cm^2/hr (24 hr)	83.0	**Mild** (0.2-1.8)
22 cm^2				
Prostep	30.0	130 µg/cm^2/hr	8.0	
7 cm^2				
Clonidine				
Catapres-TTS-1	2.5	0.1 mg/24 hr (7 days)	0.5-1.9	**Toxic‡**: 0.025 to 3 mg
Catapres-TTS-3	10.5	0.3 mg/24 hr (7 days)	2.1-7.9	
Fentanyl				
Duragesic-75	10.0	100 µg/hr (24 hr)	6.5	Surgery: 1-3 µg/kg§

From Sangalli BC: *Hudson Valley Poison Center Toxicol Newslett* 2:1, 1992.

*IM, IV, or SC.

†PO, based on nicotine content of cigarettes.

‡PO.

§IM or IV.

(Table 11-1) partly result from the difference in protein binding, and partly from ionization.

Large molecules depend on their lipid solubility and ionization to cross the membrane, because they pass in a lipid-soluble nonionized form. The M/P ratio is determined when there is equilibrium in the amount of nonionized drug in the aqueous phase on both sides of the membrane. When drugs are only partially ionized, the nonionized fraction determines the concentration that crosses the membrane. The drugs whose nonionized fraction is not very lipid soluble will pass only in limited degree into breast milk.

Passive drug transport may occur in the form of *facilitated diffusion.* The active compound is transported across the cell membrane by a carrier enzyme or protein. The gradient is toward a lesser or equal concentration in both simple diffusion and facilitated diffusion and is controlled by chemical activity gradients. Facilitated diffusion usually involves a water-soluble substance too large to pass through the membrane pores.

Active transport mechanisms provide a process whereby the gradient is "uphill," or higher, in the milk. The process is similar to facilitated diffusion except that metabolic energy is required to overcome the gradient. Examples of substances actively transported include glucose, amino acids, calcium, magnesium, and sodium. Pinocytosis and reverse pinocytosis, as described previously, are involved in the transport of very large molecules and proteins. Chloride ions are secreted into milk via an active apical membrane pump, whereas sodium and potassium are diffused by electrical gradient. Because the level of sodium is kept low, an active return of sodium may occur into the plasma, referred to as a *reverse pump.*

A summary of the steps in the passage of drugs into breast milk follows:

1. Mammary alveolar epithelium represents a lipid barrier with water-filled pores and is most permeable for drugs during colostral phase of milk secretion (first week postpartum).

2. Drug excretion into milk depends on the drug's degree of ionization, molecular weight, solubility in fat and water, and relation of pH of plasma (7.4) to pH of milk (7.0).

3. Drugs preferably enter mammary cells basally

in the nonionized, non-protein-bound form by diffusion or active transport.

4. Water-soluble drugs of mol wt below 200 pass through water-filled membranous pores.

5. Drugs leave mammary alveolar cells apically by diffusion or active transport.

6. Drugs may enter milk via spaces between mammary alveolar cells.

7. Most ingested drugs appear in milk; drug amounts in milk usually do not exceed 1% of ingested dosage, and levels in the milk are independent of milk volume.

8. Drugs are bound much less to milk proteins than to plasma proteins.

9. Drug-metabolizing capacity of mammary epithelium is not understood.

EFFECT ON NURSING INFANT

Absorption from gastrointestinal tract

Although concern surrounds the amount of a given agent in the breast milk, of greater importance is the amount absorbed into the infant's bloodstream. No accurate way exists to measure this because other factors also affect the level in the infant's bloodstream. The tolerance of the chemical to the pH of the stomach and the enzymatic activity of the intestinal tract are significant. The volume of milk consumed is a factor as well. Some drugs are not well absorbed with food (see discussion of food-drug interactions). Oral bioavailability of a compound is a major factor in risk to the infant.

Infant's ability to detoxify and excrete agent

Any drug given to an infant by any route has to be evaluated according to the infant's ability to detoxify or conjugate the chemical in the liver and/or excrete it in the urine or stool. Some compounds that appear in milk in very low levels are not well excreted by the infant and therefore accumulate in the infant's system to the point of toxicity.

Drugs that depend on the liver for conjugation, such as acetaminophen, are theoretic risks because of the limited reserve of the neonatal hepatic detoxification system. When actual measurements were made of neonates given acetaminophen, they were noted to handle it well because they conjugate it in the sulfhydryl system as an alternative pathway used only to a small extent in adult metabolism of acetaminophen. When a single dose of a drug is given to a mother and the level is measured in her milk and in her infant, it does not give a clear picture of the potential for accumulation in the infant's system. The competition for binding a drug to protein is also important. Some drugs, such as sulfadiazine, compete for binding sites that might normally bind bilirubin in the first week or so of life. This puts the infant in jeopardy of kernicterus at a given bilirubin level because of an increase in the fraction of bilirubin left unbound for lack of binding sites. The indirect bilirubin level may even appear to be below the dangerous level. Some other compounds that displace bilirubin from albumin-binding sites include salicylic acid (aspirin or acetylsalicylic acid breaks down to salicylic acid), furosemide, and phenylbutazone.

The maturity of the infant at birth is an extremely important factor during the first few months of life; thus the gestational age at birth should be established. Clearly, the less mature the infant, the less well tolerated is the drug, not only because of the immaturity of the organ systems but also because of differences in body composition (Fig. 11-3). The less mature the infant, the greater are the water content of the body and the proportion of extracellular water. Although the percentage of body weight taken up by protein is similar for all newborns (i.e., 12%), the absolute amount of protein for binding is less the smaller the infant. The amount of body fat is also low, by percentage of body weight and in absolute values. The distribution of highly lipid-soluble drugs therefore will be more apt to deposit in the brain of a 1000-g infant with 3% body fat by weight than in a 3500-g full-term infant with 12% body fat. This may explain the more sedating effect of a drug on the central nervous system of a younger and less mature infant. The relative lack of plasma protein-binding sites in the small premature infant compared with the more mature and older infant results in more

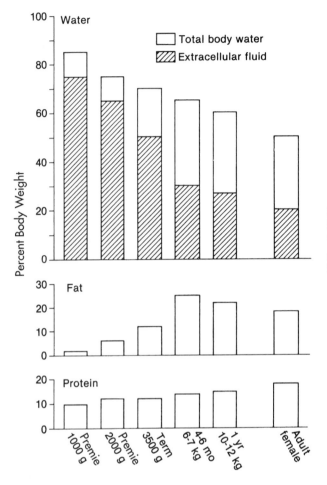

Fig. 11-3. Comparative body composition of infants and adults. (Redrawn from Pencharz PB: In Walker WA, Watkins JB, editors: *Nutrition in pediatrics: basic science and clinical application,* Boston, 1985, Little, Brown.)

free (unbound) active drug in circulation. Complications of premature birth such as acidosis and hypoxia also contribute to the unavailability of albumin-binding sites and thus result in more unbound drug.

The inability of the liver to metabolize drugs effectively results in the accumulation of some compounds that might be readily cleared by an older infant. At about 42 weeks' conceptual age, an infant's liver is able to metabolize most drugs competently. Renal clearance similarly is less effective with decreasing maturity, which increases the risk of drug accumulation. The need to dose a premature infant only once or twice a day is common to many drugs, such as antibiotics, caffeine, and theophylline, and confirms that a small premature infant does not clear drugs well.

Special problems in the neonate in addition to the presence of jaundice or low serum albumin may require special consideration. Low Apgar scores at birth signifying some degree of stress, hypoxia, or acidosis may alter binding-site availability but may also alter metabolism and excretion of a drug. Continuing respiratory distress requiring ventilatory support, sepsis, and renal failure demand special consideration when determining if a sick neonate can receive the mother's milk when she is being treated with certain medications. Prescribing for such a mother should be done in consultation with the neonatologist if the woman is providing her milk for her infant.

The age of the infant makes a difference in the total volume of milk consumed; in the older child, the diet includes other items so that milk does not compose the total intake. Age makes a difference because the more mature infant can metabolize drugs more effectively; thus sulfa drugs, for instance, can be given to infants after the first month of life.

If the agent is fat soluble, the fat content of the milk may be a significant variable. The fat content at any feeding increases over time; thus the so-called foremilk is low in fat and the hindmilk is four to five times richer in fat toward the end of a feeding. The total amount of fat in a given feeding is less in the morning, peaks at midday, and drops off in the evening even though the total amount of fat will be about the same in each 24-hour period. The coefficient of lipid solubility for a nonionized drug determines both its penetration of the biologic membrane to gain entrance to milk and its concentration in milk fat.[143] Sulfonamides with low fat solubility are in the aqueous and protein fraction of milk, whereas many barbiturates are in the lipid fraction. An inverse relationship exists between a drug's lipid solubility and the amount that appears in the skim fraction. The concentrations in fat differ for each member of the barbital family. Pentobarbital and secobarbital are found in the lipid phase, whereas phenobarbital is found in the aqueous phase.

The agent may appear in low levels in a mother's serum, but mammary blood flow during lactation is 500 ml/minute and a mother produces between 60 and 300 ml of milk/hour. The agent that appears in minimal concentrations in the milk may present a significant problem when one considers that 1000 ml of milk may be consumed in a day by an infant. Even though the volume is low, during the colostral phase of lactation, the breast is more permeable to drugs.

BREAST MILK / PLASMA RATIO FOR DRUGS

The M/P ratio for drugs has been measured and reported for many medications. This ratio can be helpful to the clinician in making a decision about a medication during lactation.[144] By definition,

M/P ratio is the concentration of the drug in the milk versus the concentration in maternal plasma (serum) at the same time. It presumes that the relationship between the two concentrations remains constant, which in most cases it does not. If it were a constant, it would allow the estimation of the amount of drug in the milk from any given plasma level in the mother.

An inaccurate ratio or one determined under variable circumstances produces erroneous estimates of the amount of drug in the milk, as pointed out by Wilson et al,[145] who state that a pharmacokinetic model is a requisite foundation for studies of drugs in breast milk. A single-point-in-time M/P ratio or an average ratio calculated with single-dose, area-under-the-curve data does not work for all drugs. Neither ratio accounts for the importance of time-dependent variations of drug concentration in milk.

The M/P ratio is most valuable if obtained when the infant would be nursed. If the ratio is 1:0, it only means the levels are equal. If the level is minimal in the mother's plasma because of the large volume of distribution, and if the milk level is also low, the M/P ratio is 1:0. If levels are drawn at peak plasma level and are equal, the M/P is still 1:0, but the infant receives a large dose. Thus the M/P ratio is only valuable when the time of the measurement is known in relationship to dosing of the mother. Dose strength, duration of dosing, maternal variation in drug disposition, maternal disease, drug interactions and competition of additional drugs for metabolism or binding sites, and racial variations in drug metabolism all influence the M/P interpretation. The characteristics of the drug and the dosing pattern are essential to the interpretation of the M/P ratio.[145]

EVALUATING DRUG DATA

The paucity of carefully controlled studies on large enough samples to validate the results when such a large number of variables are active has been lamented by many authors. Some data collected are not pharmacokinetically sound. The clinician needs to understand these variables as well as pharmacokinetic principles to make a reasonable judgment about a given case.

Interethnic and racial differences in drug responsiveness are well established. The increased heterogeneity of national populations has brought increased awareness of genetic diversity. Plasma binding, especially with drugs dependent on glycoproteins for binding, often varies greatly between Caucasian and Chinese subjects, for example.[152] Such differences contribute to the differences in drug disposition and pharmacologic response.

It should be theoretically possible to determine how much of a specific drug reaches the infant in the mother's milk by knowing all the properties of the drug, including its volume of distribution, ionization, pK_a, lipid solubility, protein-binding activity, and rate of detoxification in the maternal system. Sufficient variation in the levels that reach the infant and in how the infant deals with the agent, however, makes it necessary to have specific data about a specific drug. Thus a few simple questions in the decision-making process are helpful in determining risk.

Safety for infant

Is this a drug that can be given to the infant directly if necessary? Antibiotics (e.g., penicillin) that one could give the infant are in this category, whereas an antibiotic such as chloramphenicol, which one would not give the infant under ordinary circumstances, should be avoided in the nursing mother. The toxicity of chloramphenicol in the infant is dose related and associated with an unpredictable accumulation of the drug. Also, an idiosyncratic reaction occurs with chloramphenicol, which is unrelated to dose but is capable of causing pancytopenia.

If the drug in question can be given to the infant, is there any risk to the infant in the amount in the milk? Phenobarbital can be given to infants for various reasons; thus the question is whether enough will reach the infant to cause difficulty. The infant should be watched for symptoms of lethargy

or sleepiness, such as a change in feeding or sleeping pattern. If the infant is sleeping long periods and feeding less than usual (specifically, fewer than five or six times a day), the medication may be at fault. Phenobarbital is a significant drug for the mother with seizures; therefore a careful review of the risk/benefit ratio to the mother as well as to the infant should be undertaken. Barbiturates vary in their effect in young infants. The newborn does not handle the short-acting barbiturates well because they are dependent on detoxification in the liver, whereas phenobarbital depends more on the kidney for excretion.

If the drug was taken during pregnancy, as in epilepsy, the infant already has the drug in his system via the placenta at a steady state that the infant will have to begin to excrete on his own after delivery.[99] On the other hand, enzyme induction may have taken place in the neonate because of exposure to the drug in utero; phenobarbital hastens maturation of the fetal liver.[108] Enzyme induction of the hepatic oxygenase system by phenobarbital, phenytoin, primidone, and carbamazepine is well established. Valproate, however, does not induce enzyme activity.

If one can safely give the drug to an infant, administration becomes a question of watching for any symptoms of excessive accumulation that might develop. The age of the infant affects the ability to clear the drug.

When the drug in question is one not normally given to an infant at that particular age, weight, or degree of maturity, decision making is more difficult. Specific information about the amount of the drug that appears in the milk is essential in decision making. Often, conflicting information is available. Many lists of drug-milk levels have perpetuated the same errors in calculation; thus having more than one reference report the same information may not provide confirmation as to its accuracy.

If the medication will have to be taken for weeks or months, as with cardiovascular drugs, the drug has greater potential impact than when taken only for a few days. If the drug exposure has gone on for 9 months in utero already, some think it is less of a problem; on the other hand, it may compound the problem.

To determine the dose delivered to the infant, the following formula is used:

Dose/24 hours = Concentration of drug in milk
$\times$ Weight (kg) of infant
$\times$ Volume of milk per kg ingested in 24 hours

Dose/24 hours = $C_{milk} \times$ Weight $\times$ Volume/kg/24 hr

Sensitization

Is there risk of sensitization, even in the small dosages of a drug that might pass into the milk? This question arises most frequently with the use of antibiotics, and use of penicillin is most frequently questioned. Certainly, if the family has a strong history of drug sensitization, it should be considered. In that case, however, it should be questioned for the mother as well. Whether infants are put at risk of developing resistant strains of bacteria in their systems by small amounts of antibiotic in their feedings is a serious question. It also is pertinent for the dairy and meat industries as well as for the humans who consume those food products that have a small amount of antibiotic because of administration to livestock.

Correlation of drug safety in pregnancy and lactation

Very rarely is valid information on the appearance of a drug in milk available on the package insert, because the pharmaceutical companies usually merely indicate that it should not be taken during pregnancy and lactation. Agents that may be safe in pregnancy may not be so in lactation. During pregnancy the maternal liver and kidney are serving as detoxification and excretion resources for the fetus via the placenta, whereas during lactation the infant has to handle the drug totally on his own once it has reached his circulation. The infant in utero receives the drug in greater quantity via the circulation, whereas the nursing infant receives only what reaches the milk. One should be cautious about translating data pertaining to these two states back and forth.

Oral bioavailability

The dose of a drug delivered via the milk to the infant is significantly affected by the oral bioavailability, which is the percentage of the drug absorbed into the infant's system via the gut.[111]

Oral bioavailability is the rate and extent to which an active drug is absorbed and enters the general circulation. Absolute oral bioavailability compares the oral route with the IV route. To reach the general circulation, the oral dose must pass through the wall of the gut, liver, or lungs.[123] First-pass metabolism or elimination in the tissues of these three organs may reduce the drug's bioavailability. It is possible for a drug to be absorbed 100% and be destroyed or eliminated and have 0% bioavailability, because it is so rapidly metabolized.

These values are provided in Table D-1, Appendix D. If a compound is poorly absorbed, it is of less concern than one with 100% bioavailability. Most drugs administered by injection (e.g., insulin, heparin) only are not orally bioavailable.

Food-drug interactions

When drugs are taken with meals, numerous opportunities exist for food-drug interactions to occur.[97] Because the breastfed infant receives all maternal medications excreted in the milk "with food," this is an important consideration in the discussion of drugs in milk. The effects of food may reduce gastrointestinal irritation. Mechanisms of food-drug interactions can be summarized as follows[97]:

Physiologic
1. Changes in gastric emptying
2. Increased intestinal motility
3. Increased splanchnic blood flow
4. Increased bile, acid, and enzyme secretion
5. Induction and inhibition of drug metabolism
6. Competition in active transport .

Physiochemical
1. Food as a mechanical barrier to absorption
2. Altered dissolution of drugs
3. Chelation and adsorption

Pharmacodynamic
1. Altered enzyme activity
2. Changes in homeostasis

MINIMIZING EFFECT OF MATERNAL MEDICATION

If a mother needs a specific medication and the hazards to the infant are minimal, the following important adjustments can be made to minimize the effects:

1. Do not use the long-acting form of the drug because the infant has even more difficulty excreting such an agent, which usually requires detoxification in the liver. Accumulation in the infant is then a genuine concern.
2. Schedule the doses so the least amount possible gets into the milk. Check the usual absorption rates and peak blood levels of the drug. Having the mother take the medication immediately after breastfeeding is the safest time for the infant with most, but not all, drugs.
3. Watch the infant for any unusual signs or symptoms, such as change in feeding pattern or sleeping habits, fussiness, or rash.
4. When possible, choose the drug that produces the least amount in the milk (Tables 11-1 and 11-2).

Classification systems

A drug classification system for information regarding drug use during pregnancy and breastfeeding was devised in 1978 by the National Swedish Board of Health with the help of the drug manufacturers' trade organizations.[7,118] The system classifies drugs into categories regarding pregnancy (Categories A, B, C, or D), and the following four groups to describe drugs during lactation:

Group I   Active ingredients do not enter the milk.
Group II Active ingredients enter the milk but in such small amounts that there is no risk to the infant.
Group III Active ingredients enter the milk in sufficient quantities to represent a risk to the child even at therapeutic levels.
Group IV Not known whether active ingredients enter the milk.

Of 960 drugs registered and reviewed, 5% were in Group I, 32% in Group II, 12% in Group III, and 50.8% in Group IV.

The transfer of drugs and other chemicals into human milk has been published as a statement by the AAP Committee on Drugs in 1983, 1989, and 1994.[22] The list includes only those drugs about which there is published information, and it does not provide the pharmacologic properties of the compounds. The 1994 list is divided into seven new categories, grouping drugs by their risk factors in relationship to breastfeeding. Category 8 is a list of generic names and corresponding trade names. The categories are the following:

1. Drugs contraindicated during breastfeeding
2. Drugs of abuse: contraindicated during breastfeeding
3. Drugs that require temporary cessation of breastfeeding
4. Drugs whose effect on nursing infants is unknown, but may be of concern
5. Drugs that have been associated with significant effects on some nursing infants and should be given to nursing mothers with caution
6. Maternal medications usually compatible with breastfeeding
7. Food and environmental agents: effect on breastfeeding
8. Trade names of generic drugs

The list of more than 300 items is not inclusive. Further, the committee encourages physicians to report adverse effects in the infant consuming milk of a mother taking a specific drug to the committee at the American Academy of Pediatrics.[22]

The Breastfeeding and Human Lactation Study Center at the University of Rochester continually updates its database on drugs, medications, and contaminants in human milk. More than 3000 references pertain to drugs in the database. The tables in Appendix D have been prepared from this information. In addition to information gleaned from reports of specific levels in breast milk, the tables include the ratings by the AAP and the Swedish classification when available. In addition, other drugs typically used by women in their childbearing years about which there are no specific milk levels are listed with their oral bioavailability for the infant, peak serum time in the mother, volume of distribution for the drugs, and other pharmacologic information (pH, solubility, protein binding, metabolism) obtained from a host of resources. With this information, the physician should be able to determine relative risk and thus select the best compound and adjust the dose and the time of and association to the breastfeeding.

Further information is available from the Finger Lakes Regional Poison and Drug Information Center at 716-275-3232 or 800-333-0542. For hearing-impaired persons, TDD (716-273-3854) services are available 24 hours a day every day. This service is staffed by physicians, nurses, pharmacists, and clinical toxicologists. The Breastfeeding and Human Lactation Center is available limited hours (8 to 4 PM EST, Monday to Friday) for more complex questions (716-275-0088).

SPECIFIC DRUG GROUPS

Analgesics

Drugs such as heroin have been known for decades to appear in milk, and at one time withdrawal symptoms in the neonate were prevented or treated by breastfeeding and then gradual weaning. Codeine and meperidine (Demerol) appear in milk at low levels. The pharmacokinetics of IV *meperidine* in neonates and infants under 5 months has shown great interindividual variability in elimination half-life, median clearance, and volume of distribution.[90,103] For example, a breastfed newborn was transferred to the special care nursery at Rochester because of unusual floppiness and poor muscle tone. His mother was taking dextropropoxyphene (Darvon) every 4 hours. Temporarily stopping the nursing until the mother's drug level dropped and discontinuing use of the drug produced dramatic improvement, which persisted when the infant went back to nursing.

Diazepam (Valium) taken in multiple doses has caused sleepiness, mild depression, and decreased intake in some infants and tends to accumulate in the neonate, especially in the first weeks of life. However, an occasional diazepam is not contraindicated.

The dose schedule for analgesics is usually single dose, especially in the postpartum period. A mother should not be subjected to great discomfort when a dose or two of analgesics would improve her well-being.[38] *Aspirin* on a single-dose schedule is quite safe, although it is known to pass into her milk. The case of metabolic acidosis reported in a nursing infant occurred when the mother took 10 grains of aspirin every 4 hours for arthritis.[18] A serum salicylate level in the infant on the third day of hospitalization with no breastfeeding was still 24 mg/dl. This demonstrates the tendency of salicylate to accumulate in the neonate. Acetylsalicylic acid, not the metabolite salicylate, is responsible for the platelet aggregate abnormalities, so there should be no concern about aspirin in this regard, because it is the metabolite salicylate that appears in the milk. *Acetaminophen* is remarkably well tolerated by the neonate and can be given to a nursing mother. Although it does reach the milk in small amounts, the neonate metabolizes it well.

Prescription *ibuprofen* has been extensively used in 600- to 800-mg doses as an antiinflammatory, especially in the treatment of arthritis. Since it became available in over-the-counter preparations of 200-mg tablets, ibuprofen has become widely used by the public for pain. Pediatricians are using it liberally for fever and myalgia and generalized aches and pains. It is widely used for postpartum pain of episiotomy or cesarean birth.

Because of the initial concern about adverse effects of prostaglandin synthetase inhibiting drugs on the neonate, as well as a report of negligible (less than 0.05 µl/ml) levels in the milk of a woman after 17 days of therapy (400 mg twice a day), a careful study of ibuprofen was undertaken.[136,137] Twelve post–cesarean birth women had serum and milk samples collected at intervals for 34 hours following 400 mg ibuprofen every 6 hours for five doses. Serum half-life was 1.5 hours. No measurable amounts (capable of detecting 1 µg/ml) of ibuprofen were found in breast milk. The authors concluded that under normal dosing, a nursing infant would be exposed to less than 1 mg of ibuprofen per day.[137]

Fentanyl citrate is frequently used to provide analgesia or anesthesia to women during the postpartum period. It is a potent synthetic phenylpiperidine with extremely high lipid solubility and high pK_a but a large volume of distribution, suggesting a predisposition to appear in breast milk but clear rapidly. In a study of postpartum lactating women receiving fentanyl, concentrations were higher in colostrum than in the serum, peaked at 45 minutes after administration, and were undetectable 6 to 10 hours later. The oral bioavailability of less than 50% is reduced by food, which makes the risk to the infant minimal, via the mother's milk.

The use of *epidural anesthesia* during delivery and its continuation post–cesarean birth for pain has provided considerable relief to parturient women. Despite epidurals during labor having become commonplace; the effects of this procedure on the neonate's ability to breastfeed are still disputed. The obstetric literature clearly shows that epidurals in early labor result in an increased rate of interventions, including forceps use, vacuum extraction, and cesarean delivery.[92] These in turn result in increased postpartum complications and an increase in the length of hospital stay. When women who had cesarean delivery were followed prospectively, those who had epidural anesthesia breastfed sooner and continued longer than those women who had general anesthesia.[74] The challenging question, however, is whether an epidural affects the infant's ability to suckle and initiate breastfeeding in women who have a vaginal delivery (see infant suckling discussion in Chapter 8).

Although labor pain relief is superior with epidural analgesia compared with meperidine, labor is prolonged, uterine infection increased, and the number of operative deliveries increased, all of which interfere with successful initiation of suckling in the neonate.[92] Meperidine is widely used during labor, as are other short-acting analgesics such as nalbuphine (Nubain).[98] A study of butorphanol and nalbuphine demonstrated that receiving no medication or receiving a dose less than 1 hour before delivery was associated with earlier initiation of breastfeeding and establishment of effective feeding significantly earlier compared with mothers who received the drug more than an hour before delivery.[105] Righard and Alade[110] also observed the impact of meperidine on neonatal behavior. When he observed infants left on the maternal abdomen to find the breast and latch on, the nonmedicated infants were suckling in 20 minutes, but the medicated infants were unable to locate the breast and latch on and, in several cases, were unable to locate the breast after 40 minutes of trial.

Ketorolac tromethamine has been used for maternal pain in the first few days postpartum, especially in cesarean delivery patients. The concern has been the safety of breastfeeding during that time because ketorolac is an acidic pyrrolo-pyrrole, prostaglandin synthetase inhibitor with a pK_a of 3.54 and 99.2% plasma protein binding. Would the drug get into the milk and interfere with the physiologic closing of the infant's ductus arteriosus? Wischnik et al[146] examined this question in 10 women who received the drug 2 to 6 days after delivery. The mothers were pumping and discarding the milk because of illness in both mother and baby. Ketorolac 10 mg was given four times a day for 2 days. Plasma and milk samples were collected and levels measured; limits of detection were 10 ng/ml^{-1}. The range was 5.2 ng/ml to 7.9 ng/ml in milk, although four patients never had measurable amounts in the milk. The M/P ratio was 0.015 to 0.037. The authors estimated that a maximum dose for an infant would be 3.16 to 7.9 mg/day. They assumed 400 to 1000 ml of milk was consumed, an improbable amount in the first few days. At maximum, it was 0.16% to 0.40% of total daily maternal dose. Clinically, the authors concluded that significant sequelae from ketorolac are unlikely. The AAP rates ketorolac a category 6 drug, usually compatible with breastfeeding.[146]

Antibiotics

Levels of antibiotics in milk vary with the concentration of the drugs in plasma and their pK_a. The risks vary among groups of antibiotics. Penicillins are not usually toxic but theoretically can cause sensitivity. *Sulfa drugs* should not be used in the first month of life because they can interfere with the binding of bilirubin to protein. The risk diminishes with age, and infants are given sulfa drugs directly at 4 to 6 weeks of age. Infants with glucose-6-phosphate dehydrogenase (G6PD) deficiency should never receive sulfa drugs directly or via the breast milk. *Chloramphenicol* is contraindicated in nursing very young infants because of the risk of accumulation of the drug even from small amounts in milk and the potential for idiosyncratic reaction.

Tetracycline causes staining of teeth and abnormalities of bone growth when given directly to children for a week or more. Infants breastfed by mothers taking tetracycline for mastitis may have stained and mottled first and second teeth when therapy exceeds 10 days. The amount in milk is half that in the mother's plasma. Tetracycline should be given mothers only for life-threatening infections.

Erythromycin appears in higher amounts in milk than in plasma. When given intravenously to the mother, the levels are 10 times higher. When the infant is old enough to receive erythromycin directly, the mother can take it as well. The major concerns regarding erythromycin pertain to its cross-effects with other medications, especially the potential to increase terfenadine (Seldane) levels, possibly resulting in increased QT intervals. Terfenadine pharmacokinetics has been studied in breast milk.[14] The estimated total amount available to the neonate after a standard dose is less than 0.45% of the maternal dose. Terfenadine is not detected in milk or plasma, only the active metabolite. With dosing every 12 hours, the peak M/P levels occur between 2 and 3 hours after dosing. Seldane has been removed from the market. Erythromycin also has the potential for decreasing the clearance of carbamazepine, cyclosporine, digoxin, triazolam, theophylline, anticoagulants, and drugs metabolized by the P-450 system.

Aminoglycosides are common constituents of postpartum antibiotic therapy and are given parentally. They readily appear in the milk but, as with kanamycin, are not readily absorbed from the gastrointestinal (GI) tract; therefore under usual circumstances they pose no problem to the neonate, who will not absorb them. Newborns are given aminoglycosides directly.

Metronidazole (Flagyl) does appear in milk at levels equal to those in serum. Most researchers consider the risk to the infant sufficient to suggest alternative therapy for the mother. Symptoms include decreased appetite and vomiting and, occasionally, blood dyscrasia.

An alternative treatment regimen is 2 g metronidazole in a single dose. When milk concentrations are measured with a 2-g dose, the highest concentrations are found at 2 and 4 hours postingestion and decline over the next 12 hours to 19.1 µg/ml and to 12.6 µg/ml at 24 hours.[31,45] The dose to the infant is calculated to be 21.8 mg over the first 24 hours and only 3.5 mg in the second 24 hours. It has been recommended that the single-dose regimen be used in nursing mothers, which necessitates that a mother pump and discard milk for only 24 hours. Metronidazole in gel or cream form contains only 0.75% of the medication and is poorly absorbed because the purpose is to work on tissues locally. As a result, maternal plasma levels are 1/50 of levels from comparable oral dosing. Use of the drug in this form would probably result in undetectable amounts in the milk. Normally the gel or cream is applied in small amounts twice daily. Peak absorption could be avoided. Metronidazole is often the only drug that works in a serious trichomoniasis, giardiasis, or amebiasis infection[31] when all other treatments have failed.

Amoxicillin, cephalexin, and cefadroxil, when given orally in a single dose, peak in the milk at 4 to 6 hours.[55] Cephalothin, cephapirin, and cefotaxime, when given in a bolus IV injection, peak at 2 hours. Cefadroxil reached the highest levels (1.64 ± 0.73 µg/ml) at 6 hours.

Cephalosporins are weak acids with variable protein binding. Third-generation cephalosporins may affect the flora of the gut. Sterilization of the gut often leads to diarrhea. In general, cephalosporins are considered safe during lactation.[23] Breastfed infants rapidly recolonize the gut with lactobacillus.

The serum half-lives of parenterally administered cephalosporins are three to four times longer in the neonate than the serum half-lives in the mother. The half-life of ceftriaxone in the milk is

12 to 17 hours, compared with the maternal serum half-life of 6 hours. The M/P ratio at 8 hours was 0.05 and at 24 hours, 0.1. The neonate can be given cephalosporins directly.

Chloroquine, oxacillin, and paraaminosalicylic acid are reported by O'Brien[99] to be safe because they are not excreted in milk. Additional antibiotics are listed in Appendix D.

Because antibiotics are the most frequent medication prescribed for lactating women, it is noteworthy that the compliance is low. Maternal noncompliance was measured by Ito et al[51] in 203 breastfeeding women who consulted the Motherisk Program for information about antibiotics. Despite reassuring advice, one in five women either did not initiate therapy or did not continue breastfeeding. This has serious implications for recurrent infections, especially mastitis. Mastitis represents another situation in which termination of breastfeeding is not indicated.

Anticholinergics

Anticholinergic drugs include atropine, scopolamine (hyoscine), and synthetic quaternary ammonium derivatives, some of which are available in over-the-counter medications. Some *atropine* does enter the milk. Infants are particularly sensitive to this drug; therefore the infant involved should be watched for tachycardia and thermal changes, which are more easily measured in infants. The most important consideration is that milk secretion may decrease in the mother. Constipation and urinary retention may occur in the infant with repeat doses. The *quaternary anticholinergics* should not appear in milk to any degree because, as anions, they do not pass into the acidic milk. Both O'Brien[99] and Gaginella[37] have reported that mepenzolate methylbromide (Cantil) does not appear in milk.

Scopolamine is available by dermal patch for motion sickness and causes maternal mucous membrane dryness, which could affect milk production. Only a small amount appears in milk. The AAP rates it and atropine as category 6 drugs, usually compatible with breastfeeding, although the scopolamine patch, which provides a constant level, has not been tested.

Gastrointestinal medications

Cimetidine (Tagamet), a potent H_2-receptor antagonist, is used for conditions associated with acid peptic digestion in the GI tract, especially elevated gastric acidity. Cimetidine excretion into breast milk has resulted in concentrations higher than in the corresponding plasma sample.[127] Levels were highest at 1 hour after a single dose. Chronic-dose studies revealed variable M/P ratios, all of which were higher than the single-dose ratio. The authors suggest an active transport mechanism for this medication. The maximum amount of cimetidine ingested by an infant was calculated at 6 mg for 1 L of milk (or 1.5 mg/kg).

The neonatal dose is 10 to 20 mg/kg/24 hours for severe gastroesophageal reflux or gastric ulcer, conditions that are rare in a breastfed infant. The half-life in a neonate is 1.1 to 3.4 hours. It is contraindicated when either infant or mother is receiving cisapride because of the risk of precipitating cardiac arrhythmias.[150] Caution is recommended with nursing when taking cimetidine until more is known of its side effects, especially antiandrogenic features.[32] Although previously rated as contraindicated during breastfeeding and put in category 1 by the AAP, cimetidine is now category 6, compatible with breastfeeding, although levels may be higher in milk than in serum.[22]

Sulfasalazine treatment of ulcerative colitis and Crohn's disease during breastfeeding has been widely discussed on theoretic grounds because the compound splits to sulfapyridine and 5-aminosalicylic acid (5-ASA). The sulfapyridine is absorbed from the colon and is metabolized in the liver. The 5-ASA is partly absorbed and rapidly excreted in the urine, so serum concentrations are low. The sulfapyridine and its metabolites do appear in the milk in lower concentrations than in the serum. A dose of 2 g/day of drug to the mother would produce 4 mg/kg of sulfapyridine in the milk, about 40% of maternal levels. The oral absorption from the milk is low, so the actual amount in the infant's plasma is minimal. The risk of recurrent ulcerative colitis if medication is withdrawn outweighs the risk of sulfasalazine to the infant.[60] The AAP rates it a 5 (i.e., use with caution and close observation of the infant).[22]

Anticoagulants

Heparin, regular or unfractionated, is a large-molecular-weight molecule that does not pass into breast milk. Because it is not absorbed from the GI tract, its use in the breastfeeding mother is acceptable.

Low-molecular-weight (LMW) heparins are glycosaminoglycans consisting of chains of alternating residues of D-glucosamine and uronic acid. The regular or unfractionated heparin is a heterogeneous mixture of polysaccharide chains ranging from 3000 to 30,000 mol wt. LMW heparin has a mean mol wt of about 5000 daltons (2000 to 8000), with slight variation among brand names ardeparin (Normiflo), dalteparin (Fragmin), enoxaparin (Lovenox), nadroparin (Fraxiparine), reviparin (Clivarin), and tinzaparin (Innohep). Both unfractionated and LMW heparins cause anticoagulation by activating antithrombin. LMW heparins produce a more predictable anticoagulant response because of their better bioavailability, longer half-life, dose-independent clearance, and decreased tendency to bind to plasma proteins and endothelium. They are less likely to interfere with platelets. They are considered safer and more effective in the treatment of venous thromboembolism, can be given subcutaneously without laboratory monitoring, carry less risk of thrombocytopenia and osteoporosis, and can be given at home.[139]

No studies are reported of LMW heparin use in pregnancy or lactation. Because mol wt is greater than 2000 and only a molecule of less than 1000 mol wt crosses the placenta or into the milk, these molecules are unlikely to cross. These LMW compounds are not orally bioavailable and would not be absorbed by the infant. They are considered safe during lactation.

Analysis of the milk of mothers using *warfarin* by Orme et al[101] did not reveal any drug in the milks or in the infants. The infants' prothrombin times remained normal. This has been further confirmed by McKenna et al,[84] who followed two breastfed infants whose mothers were anticoagulated before delivery and maintained on warfarin postpartum. They found no immediate or delayed biologic effect on coagulation in 56 and 131 days of follow-up. From this, it has been suggested that warfarin is the drug of choice in the lactating mother who requires anticoagulant therapy and wants to continue breastfeeding. If surgery is contemplated or unusual trauma occurs, a review of the infant's coagulation status is indicated as a precautionary measure.

Antithyroid drugs

Iodide has been known for generations to pass into the milk in levels higher than in the maternal plasma. It has been reported to cause symptoms in infants when used not only for hyperthyroidism but also in asthma preparations and cough medicines. Iodides have been noted to be goitrogenic and to sensitize the thyroid gland to other drugs, such as lithium, chlorpromazine, and methylxanthines.

Thiouracil is actively transported into the milk and appears in higher concentration in milk than in blood or urine, being reported at levels 3 to 12 times higher in milk than in blood. It has the potential of causing goiter-suppressing thyroid activity or agranulocytes. Thiouracil is contraindicated during lactation and labeled category 1 by the AAP.

Methimazole (Tapazole) presents risks to the nursing infant similar to those seen with thiouracil (i.e., thyroid suppression, goiter). Giving 0.125 grain of thyroid extract may not adequately protect the infant, and careful monitoring of neonatal thyroid function is mandatory. Measurements of amounts of methimazole in milk and serum when a mother received 2.5 mg every 12 hours were found to be similar. Tegler and Lindström[133] found 7% to 16% of the maternal dose in the milk; thus a dose of 5 mg four times daily might provide the infant with 3 mg daily. Studies of carbimazole using ^{38}S-labeled compound show a similar trend, with

0.47% of the dose appearing in the milk. Studies were done on a single dose of 10 mg carbimazole.

Propylthiouracil (PTU) has been investigated by several groups with similar results reported, showing that little of the compound is excreted in the milk (0.025% to 0.077% of total dose) in single-dose studies.[56] An infant followed 5 months on maternal doses of 200- to 300-mg PTU daily showed no neonatal thyroid symptoms and normal triiodothyronine (T_3), thyroxine (T_4), and thyroid-stimulating hormone (TSH). On the strength of these reports, others have proceeded to use PTU and permit breastfeeding. The availability of microdeterminations for T_3, T_4, and TSH improves the quality of monitoring, and all infants given PTU via the milk should be followed closely. The AAP lists PTU in category 6, compatible with breastfeeding.[22]

Caffeine and other methylxanthines

Caffeine ingestion has been singled out for discussion because it is a frequent concern, but the data provided in most reviews are misleading. With a given dose of caffeine that is comparable to that in a cup of coffee, the level in the milk is low (1% of level in mother), and the level in the infant's plasma is also low. However, caffeine does accumulate in the infant.

Before the availability of the laboratory test for caffeine, cases were managed on clinical symptoms alone. Many clinicians recognized and the Rochester series[111] of nursing mothers documented that wakeful, hyperactive infants were often the victims of caffeine stimulation. If a mother drank more than 6 to 8 cups of any caffeine-containing beverage in a day's time, her infant could accumulate symptomatic amounts of caffeine. Soft drinks such as colas and other carbonated drinks (e.g., Mountain Dew) often contributed to the caffeine buildup. When the situation was identified—a wide-eyed, active, alert infant who never slept for long—it was suggested that the mother try caffeine-free beverages, both hot and cold. Often the infant settled down to a reasonable sleep pattern after a few days with no caffeine.

Since information on milk and plasma levels has become available, researchers have identified three cases of caffeine excess in breastfed infants, one of which Rivera-Calimlim[111] reported. The infants all had measurable levels of caffeine in the plasma, which disappeared over a week's time after the caffeine was discontinued. The corresponding milk levels were as previously reported, about 1% of the mother's level, which supports the hypothesis that caffeine accumulates in the infant. The infants do not need to be hospitalized, and verification of blood caffeine levels is helpful but not mandatory because a clinical trial will suffice. Smoking has been observed to augment the caffeine effect.

With an increasing number of women with asthma wanting to breastfeed, a question arises about the impact of theophylline. The methylxanthines have also been used in apnea of prematurity, so information has been generated regarding dose, clearance, and toxicity in the neonate.[8] In addition, microdeterminations of blood levels are readily available.

Several studies of *theophylline* in mothers receiving regular doses have shown that the serum levels are lowest just before the oral dose and that M/P ratio is 0.60 to 0.73, with milk levels paralleling serum levels.[9,128,151] The infant receives an estimated 1% of the maternal dose. Data on IV and PO medication are similar in terms of M/P ratio. Maximum exposure was estimated at 7 to 8 mg/24 hours.

Dyphylline is a compound introduced clinically as a bronchodilator because of its lack of side effects.[52] It is excreted renally with little biotransformation. The M/P ratio was determined to be 2.08 ± 0.52, and the biologic half-life was 3.21 hours. Although this is considerably greater than that of theophylline, it is not yet known how this would affect the infant.

Theobromine, which occurs in chocolate and cocoa, has been studied as well to evaluate its possible cumulative effects when taken with caffeine or theophylline.[8] A very small amount was detected in the milk, with a potential dose to the infant after one chocolate bar (1.2 oz) of 0.44 to

1.68 mg. No theobromine was found in the infant's urine.[9]

The management of asthma has shifted in recent years to steroids, antibiotics, and inhalants. *Steroids* are excreted in the milk in low doses that have not presented a problem to the nursling, who is automatically weaned as the mother is weaned. Antibiotics are well tolerated, as discussed previously. *Inhalants* are unique because they act at the level of the bronchial mucosa and are poorly absorbed. *Albuterol* is a β_2-adrenergic agonist that is rapidly effective when inhaled, peaking within 30 minutes. The potential for drug levels in the milk is minimal, and no adverse reactions have been reported in nurslings. The PO albuterol dose for infants with asthma is 0.1 to 0.3 mg/kg every 6 to 8 hours.

Drugs of abuse and alcohol

The AAP Committee on Drugs[22] has assigned a special category to drugs of abuse: category 2, which they consider contraindicated during breastfeeding. The list is short: amphetamine, cocaine, heroin, marihuana, nicotine, and phencyclidine hydrochloride (angel dust, PCP). They strongly state further that these compounds and all other drugs of abuse are hazardous not only to the nursing infant, but also to the mother's physical and emotional health. Obviously, the latter is also true for bottle-feeding mothers. (See Chapter 15 for further discussion of nicotine and smoking.) Nicotine's inclusion in category 2 is controversial, especially because the data are clear that children of smoking mothers do better if breastfed in regard to general health, respiratory illness, and risk of sudden infant death syndrome (SIDS).

The consumption of alcohol during lactation also deserves careful consideration because of the wide range of effects and the wide range of dosages.[59] Beer and wine are standard beverages in many parts of the world and have been recommended to enhance lactation, especially when the mother is stressed with worldly chores. Some forms of alcohol have also been used as an aperitif to encourage a woman to eat heartily while lactating. The AAP listing is category 6.[22]

Alcohol is one of the most rapidly absorbed compounds. Maximum blood levels are achieved in 15 minutes in adults. Lactating and nonlactating women handle alcohol differently. Lactators tend to peak at lower levels and clear the drug more quickly. Alcohol passes quickly between blood and milk, however, with peak levels in milk at 30 to 60 minutes and at 60 to 90 minutes when taken with food. Studies in males and nonlactating women show an increase in serum prolactin with alcohol.[24,87] This has not been tested in lactators. The impact of alcohol on oxytocin is dose related. No effect is seen on ingesting 0.5 g/kg or less, and varying effects are reported in different women as dose is increased.[24] At least a partial decrease in milk let-down is seen at 1.0 to 1.5 g/kg, and all women have significant to complete block in milk ejection at 1.5 to 2.0 g/kg.[19] Alcohol blocks the release of oxytocin rather than blocking the response of the breast. The amount of alcohol excreted into milk with doses less than 1 g/kg of absolute alcohol usually does not affect the infant.[71]

Experimental prolactin studies in lactating rats show that acutely administered alcohol does not affect basal plasma prolactin but does inhibit suckling-induced prolactin for about 2 hours. This effect is manifest at a blood alcohol level of 0.65%.[132] When alcohol levels were 0.20% (inebriated), extended suckling overcame the effect. The amount of milk consumed in experimental and control rats was the same in 3 hours, and growth rate over 21 days did not differ.

Many investigations have measured the pharmacologic impact of alcohol consumption.* Alcohol appears quickly in both foremilk and hindmilk at a level equivalent to or higher than corresponding maternal blood samples. Although levels are high in the blood, no acetaldehyde is found in the milk. Levels in milk drop in parallel to those in the blood because alcohol is not stored in the breast. In a study by Lawton,[71] milk levels were very low despite that the participating mothers drank as much as they could as quickly as possible, averaging between 43 and 90 ml of absolute alcohol.

---

*References 16, 35, 54, 59, 86, 148.

Levels were drawn every half hour for 4 hours in this study.

When women served as their own controls in an experiment to observe feeding behavior and volume of milk consumed by the infant with and without maternal alcohol, there was significant and uniform intensity of odor to their milk, peaking between 30 and 60 minutes postingestion.[86] The odor paralleled the concentration of alcohol (0 to 32 mg/dl). Infants sucked more frequently but consumed less milk in the presence of alcohol (120.4 ± 9.5 ml vs. 156.4 ± 8.2 ml). When a similar study was done with beer and nonalcohol beer, the findings were similar: the infants sucked less well with the alcohol beverage.[16] Mothers, however, were unaware of the differences and felt they had experienced let-down and their infants had nursed well. This work has precipitated considerable response because of the belief that a little beer or wine enhances mother's release of milk.

Although this work suggests that a little alcohol may not enhance milk volume received by the infant, the alcohol was taken in a research setting and consumed in 10 minutes. When the mother takes a little wine, it is usually to create a different ambience and help her relax and improve her ejection reflex. In addition, many women who enjoy sipping an occasional beer or wine may well be discouraged from breastfeeding if they think wine or beer would be forbidden.

The report of Little et al[77] regarding the effect of alcohol on the nursing infant implies that alcohol causes developmental delay. The drinking would be classified as heavy in this group, whose infants had slight gross motor delay at 1 year. Furthermore, the infants were subjected to the alcohol in utero as well. Heavy drinking should not be condoned; however, it will be very important to follow the children in all the cohorts for at least 7 years until their higher learning centers are testable.

Infants spent significantly less time sleeping during the 3.5 hours after consuming alcohol-flavored breast milk by bottle (56.8 minutes) compared with plain breast milk by bottle (78.2 minutes). The authors concluded that short-term exposure to small amounts of alcohol in breast milk produces distinctive changes in the infant's sleep-wake pattern.[87]

A study in Mexico following 32 infants born to mothers who drank a mild Mexican alcoholic beverage called *pulque* (3% alcohol, up to 2 L per day) throughout pregnancy produced no infants with fetal alcohol syndrome, but there was a higher incidence of low birthweight (less than third percentile).[35] Relative risk was 3.39. The infants were followed during lactation as well. Ethanol found in the milk accounted for 40 mg/day available to the infant. Postnatal growth was similar in both groups at 6 months. Developmental studies were not reported.

The recommendation regarding alcohol requires the physician to avoid prescribing or proscribing it and assist the mother in appropriately adjusting her alcohol consumption in both timing and volume.

When a nursing mother does have "a drink or two," she should avoid breastfeeding for at least 2 hours. Pumping and discarding milk does not hasten the removal from the milk because the level in the milk matches that in the plasma at the time of the feeding.

Herbs and herbal teas

Use of herbs and herbal teas has increased, especially among those interested in natural foods.[122] As is well known to all students of pharmacology, many effective medications originated from these natural products. In the early part of the twentieth century, many compounds were still being dispensed in their natural form, including foxglove leaves for digitalis. The natural product was unpredictable because one leaf or plant contains more or less active principle than another, so careful dose control was impossible and results were often unpredictable. Much of the interest in herbal teas has evolved as individuals seek a beverage that does not contain caffeine; what they receive is another compound instead, often one more potent and frequently one about which considerably less is known (Table 11-4). Contamination, adulteration, and misidentification contribute to the problems associated with use.

TABLE 11-4   Psychoactive substances used in herbal preparations

Labeled ingredient	Botanical source	Pharmacologic principle	Suggested use and reported effects
African yohimbé bark; yohimbine	Corynanthe yohimbé	Yohimbine	Smoke or tea as stimulant; mild hallucinogen
Broom; scotch broom	Cytisus spp.	Cytisine	Smoke for relaxation; strong sedative-hypnotic
Buckthorn	Hiptothae rhamnoides	Anthraquinones	Tea; cathartic toxin, severe watery diarrhea
Burdock root	Arctium minus	Atropine	Tea; anticholinergic blockade, anaphylactic shock
California poppy	Eschscholtzia californica	Alkaloids and glucosides	Smoke as marihuana substitute; mild euphoriant
Catnip	Nepeta cataria	Nepetalactone	Smoke or tea as marihuana substitute; mild hallucinogen
Chamomile	Chamomilla recutita Chamaemelum nobile	Antigens of Compositae family	Tea; contact dermatitis (in patients sensitive to ragweed, asters, chrysanthemum)
Cinnamon	Cinnamomum camphora	?	Smoke with marihuana; mild stimulant
Comfrey	Symphytum officinale	Pyrrolizidine alkaloids	Tea; venoocclusive disease, hepatic failure, ?hepatocarcinogen
Foxglove tea	Digitalis purpurea	Digitalis	Tea; malignant arrhythmias, cardiac arrest
Gordolobo, groundsel	Senecio longilobus Senecio vulgaris Senecio spartoides	Pyrrolizidine alkaloids	Tea, venoocclusive disease, hepatic failure
Hops	Humulus lupulus	Lupuline	Smoke or tea as sedative and marihuana substitute; none
Hydrangea	Hydrangea paniculata	Hydrangin, saponin, cyanogens	Smoke as marihuana substitute; stimulant
Jimson tea	Datura stramonium	Atropine, scopolamine, hyoscyamine, stramonium	Tea; ?PNH-like defect, anticholinergic blockade; CNS intoxication, hallucinations, ataxia, blurred vision
Juniper	Juniper macropoda	?	Smoke as hallucinogen; strong hallucinogen
Kavakava	Piper methysticum	Yangonin, pyrones	Smoke or tea as marihuana substitute; mild hallucinogen
Kola nut; gotu kola	Cola spp.	Caffeine, theobromine, kolanin	Smoke, tea, or capsules as stimulant; stimulant
Lobelia	Lobelia inflata	Lobeline	Smoke or tea as marihuana substitute; mild euphoriant
Mandrake	Mandragora officinarum	Scopolamine, hyoscyamine	Tea as hallucinogen

Common name	Latin name	Constituents	Effects
Maté	Ilex paraguensis	Caffeine, pyrrolizidine	Tea as stimulant; ?stimulant, venoocclusive disease
Mormon tea	Ephedra nevadensis	Ephedrine	Tea as stimulant; stimulant
Nutmeg	Myristica fragrans	Myristin	Hallucinogen, MAD inhibitor; hallucinogen, CNS intoxicant
		Myristin	?Hepatic damage
Oleander	Nerium oleander	Cardiac glycosides, Digitogenin, Nerioside, Oleandroside	Malignant arrhythmias, cardiac arrest
Passion flower	Passiflora incarnata	Harmine alkaloids	Smoke, tea, or capsules as marihuana substitute; mild stimulant
Periwinkle	Catharanthus roseus	Indole alkaloids	Smoke or tea as euphoriant; hallucinogen
Pokeroot, pokeweed	Phytolacca americana, Phytolacca decandra	Saponins, Pokeweed mitogen	Gastroenteritis, blood diarrhea; ?Respiratory depression, ?mitogenic alterations
Prickly poppy	Argemona mexicana	Protopine, berberine, isoquinilines	Smoke as euphoriant; narcotic-analgesic
Sassafras	Sassafras albidum	Safrole	Tea or cold beverage; hepatocarcinogen
Senna	Cassia acutifolia, Cassia angustifolia	Antraquinones	Tea; cathartic toxin, severe watery diarrhea
Snakeroot	Rauwolfia serpentina	Reserpine	Smoke or tea as tobacco substitute; tranquilizer
Thorn apple	Datura stramonium	Atropine, scopolamine	Smoke or tea as tobacco substitute or hallucinogen; strong hallucinogen
Tobacco	Nicotiana spp.	Nicotine	Smoke as tobacco; strong stimulant
Valerian	Valeriana officinalis	Chatinine, valerine alkaloids	Tea or capsules as tranquilizer
Wild lettuce	Lactuca sativa	Lactucarine	Smoke as opium substitute; mild narcotic-analgesic
Woodruff	Galium odoratum	Coumarin	Hemorrhagic diathesis, prolonged prothrombin time
Wormwood	Artemisia absinthium	Absinthin	Smoke or tea as relaxant; narcotic-analgesic
Yohimbe bark	Corynanthe yohimbé	Yohimbine	α_2-Sympathetic (presynaptic) blockade

Modified from Siegel RK: *JAMA* 236:473, 1976, Copyright 1976, American Medical Association; and Ridker PM: *Arch Environ Health* 42:135, 1987.

PNH, Paroxysmal nocturnal hemoglobinuria; *CNS*, central nervous system; *MAD*, major affective disorder.

BOX 11-1   Herbal teas considered safe during lactation

Tea	Origin/use
Chicory	Root/caffeine-free coffee substitute
Orange spice	Mixture/flavoring
Peppermint	Leaves/flavoring
Raspberry	Fruit/flavoring
Red bush tea	Leaves, fine twigs/beverage
Rose hips	Fruits/vitamin C

Herbal teas are available that are prepared carefully, using only herbs for essence (e.g., Celestial Seasonings brand tea) and avoiding heavy doses of herbs with active principles. However, the strength of any tea depends on how it is made. An ordinary teabag with hot water run over it will contain little caffeine and theobromine; however, when the tea is steeped for 5 minutes, the potency is increased tenfold. Some of the preparations are benign or even nutritious, such as rose hips tea, which contains a large amount of vitamin C. Other teas are made from plants known to the toxicologist as poisonous. Isolated reports of toxicity from these preparations are appearing in the medical literature; many others probably go undiagnosed.[121] Use of these preparations is certainly an important part of a medical and dietary history.

Box 11-1 lists herbal teas that are safe for the infant and mother during lactation.

Mother's milk tea

Mother's milk tea is a blend of plants handed down for many generations as a galactagogue; it contains a mixture of fennel seeds, coriander seeds, chamomile flowers, lemongrass, borage leaves, blessed thistle leaves, star anise, comfrey leaves, and fenugreek seeds[131] (Table 11-5). It is promoted as containing no caffeine. Although not all the constituents have pharmacologic actions, several do and were used medicinally for centuries. These popular teas have the same potential for problems as do the common popular beverages coffee and cola. The euphoric effects are the most prominent.[122]

Comfrey and pyrrolizidine alkaloids

Considerable concern is mounting over the use of comfrey leaves (Symphytum officinale) in the United States, and they have been banned in Canada and Germany. The leaves have been used in teas, salads, and poultices. The use of comfrey has been associated with venoocclusive disease and hepatotoxicity. Comfrey is also rich in hepatotoxic pyrrolizidine alkaloids.[48,109] The highest level of toxin occurs in the roots, which can be obtained in powder form in capsules. Comfrey has been recommended for use to cure various pregnancy, labor, and postpartum symptoms and appears in many home remedy handbooks. It has the greatest potential for toxicity in the fetus and the suckling infant, with fatal fetal venoocclusive disease reported.[1] It is also known to have carcinogenic properties. All credible references caution against its use topically, orally, or in any form.[29,138]

Another herb associated with venoocclusive disease and even death is Senecio longilobus, commonly known as thread-leafed groundsel.[48,109] As with comfrey, it contains hepatotoxic pyrrolizidine alkaloids. Seven cases of hepatitis have been reported resulting from use of Teucrium chamaedrys (germander), a member of the mint family. Botanical identification is essential; sometimes the packet contains substances other than the label indicates.

Pyrrolizidine alkaloids have been identified in an herbal tea used in the Southwest that was responsible for several deaths of children who were given the tea when they were ill. The alkaloid is excreted within 24 hours, but symptoms may not appear for several days or weeks. Death results from liver failure.

Sassafras and coumarins

Sassafras contains an aromatic oil, safrole, which has been shown to cause cancer in mice; it is therefore no longer permitted as a commercial flavoring, but it appears in herbal teas. It causes central nervous system (CNS) symptoms in mice, including

TABLE 11-5   Possible ingredients and effects of mother's milk tea

Plant	Constituents	Effects	Toxicity
Fennel seed	Volatile oil, anisic acid	Weak diuretic stimulant	CNS disturbances
Coriander seed	Volatile oil, coriandrol	Increases flow of saliva and gastric juice	
Chamomile flower	Volatile oil, bitter glycoside	Sudorific, antispasmodic, used to lighten hair	Vomiting, vertigo
Lemongrass	Lemon flavor		
Borage leaf	Volatile oil, tannin, mineral acids	Diuretic, sudorific, euphoric	Possible
Blessed thistle leaf	Volatile oil, bitter principle	Aperitif, galactagogue, diaphoretic	Strongly emetic
Star anise	Volatile oil, anethole, resin, tannin	Stimulant, mild expectorant	
Comfrey leaf (*Symphytum officinale*)	Protein, vitamin B_{12}, tannin, allantoin, choline, pyrrolizidine alkaloids	Used as mucilage to knit bones, weak sedative, demulcent, astringent	Venoocclusive disease Hepatotoxic
Fenugreek seed (Greek hayseed) (coffee substitute and natural dye)	Mucilage, trigonelline, physterols, celery flavor	Digestive tonic, galactogogue, uterine stimulant, reduces blood sugar	Hypoglycemia, can induce labor
Other beverages			
Coffee plant	Volatile oil, caffeine, tannin	Stimulant, diuretic, coloring	Insomnia, restlessness
Blue cohosh	Saponin, glucoside that affects muscles	Oxytocic, potent, acts on voluntary and involuntary muscles	Irritant, causes pain in fingers and toes

ataxia, ptosis, and hypothermia.[121] It is also thought to interfere with the action of other medications. Noted herbalists state that sassafras has no really significant medical or therapeutic use.[29,138] The oil, along with many other volatile oils, does have mild counterirritant properties on external application. It has a pleasant flavor without use but many harmful qualities. Although banned by the FDA, sassafras also appears in other natural food products. Belladonna alkaloids are common in some teas used to create euphoria or ease pain.

A hemorrhagic diathesis was described in a woman who drank quarts of herbal tea that contained tonka beans, melilot (sweet clover), and woodruff, all of which contain natural coumarins.[47] She narrowly avoided gynecologic surgery for excessive hemorrhaging before the history was obtained. The tea also included hawthorn, which contains cardioglucosides that cause hypotension.

Licorice

Licorice, the dry root of *Glycyrrhiza glabra,* has been used for medicinal purposes for millennia; stores of licorice were found in the tombs of Egyptian pharaohs, including that of King Tut. Its history is carefully reviewed by Davis and Morris.[25] The active principle is a glycoside of a triterpene called *glycyrrhizic acid.* Licorice continues to be used as a flavoring agent in drinks, drugs, and candies. In addition to its universal role as an expectorant and demulcent and in ointments for various skin disorders, it has been used for peptic ulcers. Its most perplexing properties are those that cause the retention of water, sodium, and chloride and the increased excretion of potassium, mimicking the effects of large doses of desoxycorticosterone. Because licorice is used to flavor chewing tobacco, chewing has been associated with hypertension, sodium retention, and hypokalemia. Licorice derivatives have been found to reroute the metabolism of aldosterone, desoxycorticosterone, and glucocorticoids.[25] Excessive amounts of licorice should be avoided by the lactating woman. Its use to lose weight should be discouraged. Some licorice candy contains little or no licorice, and the flavor is provided by anise, which is probably harmless. An occasional stick of licorice should not be a risk.[115,135]

Echinacea

Echinacea is used for the common cold and when "immune system enhancement is desired."[138] A lipophilic fraction of the root and leaves contains the most potent immunostimulating compounds, some yet to be identified. It is used topically to stimulate wound healing and orally to enhance immune response. The public seeks it out for the common cold. No data exist about its entry into milk. It has no known side effects, however, even when injected in high doses. Echinacea may even be safer in modest amounts than the polypharmacy available for the common cold.

Fenugreek

Fenugreek is the dried ripe seeds of a small southern European herb known as *Greek hayseed,* which contains about 40% mucilage. In addition to being used for poultices and ointments, it is used in teas and syrups and has a faint flavor similar to maple syrup. It is soothing, flavorful, and possibly nutritious. It is available as a spice, flavoring, and tea.

Studies continue in animal models to evaluate fenugreek's ability to reduce blood sugar.[70] The maple syrup smell was noted in a child hospitalized for possible maple syrup disease. He had been receiving fenugreek tea and did not have a metabolic disorder. Several coumarin compounds have been identified in the seeds, although no hemorrhaging has been reported.

In moderate use, fenugreek is considered harmless. As with all things in pregnancy and lactation, moderation is appropriate. Transport into milk is not documented, but the milk might smell like maple syrup. Fenugreek has been touted as a galactagogue, but no scientific reports support or refute this claim. Because it is in the same botanical family as peanuts and chick peas, a potential for allergy exists. It is also recognized to aggravate symptoms of allergy.

Ginseng

Ginseng is one of the oldest, most widely recognized, and most documented Oriental herb. It enjoys a reputation for increased capacity for mental work and physical activity and also "antistress" effects. The plant of origin is *Panax schinseng* (Chinese) or *P. quinquefolius* (American), two species of the Araliaceae family. *Panax* is derived from the Greek meaning "all healing."[70]

The root contains dozens of steroidlike glycosides (ginsenosides), which vary with the species, age, location of growth, and harvest time. It contains sterols, coumarins, flavonoids, and polysaccharides. Although animal studies suggest increased strength and stamina, Engels and Wirth[30] reported that in a carefully blinded and controlled study of 31 healthy men randomized to take 200 mg/day, 400 mg/day, or a placebo, no difference was found in any physiologic or psychologic parameter. They measured oxygen consumption, blood lactic acid, and heart rate while the subjects worked at maximum effort on stationary bikes.

Products available are numerous and variable, and more than half are worthless according to independent studies, and 25% contain no ginseng, which is extremely expensive ($20 per ounce). It is reported to have estrogen-like effects on some women, with mastalgia common with extended use and mammary nodularity also reported. Although animal experimentation has been considerable, there are no extensive human data, no liable or standardized preparations, no information on dosage, and no accurate recording of side effects. Ginseng is a medical enigma with no proven efficacy for humans, according to Tyler.[138] General side effects include excitement, nervousness, inability to concentrate, hypertension, hypoglycemia, and skin rash. A case of ginseng use during pregnancy and lactation is reported because the infant showed excessive hirsutism and androgen effect, which cleared when breastfeeding was discontinued at 2 weeks of life.[63] Because of the reported breast effects and occasional reports of vaginal bleeding, it is considered problematic during lactation.

St. John's wort

St. John's wort is being touted in Europe and the United States as an antidepressant and anxiolytic and is now sold in supermarkets as well as health food stores. It comes from an aggressive perennial weed in meadows and roadsides noted for its spotted leaves and numerous yellow-orange flowers with black spots and the capsular fruit. It contains 10% tannin and hypericin, a reddish dianthrone pigment, and other hypericum-like substances (0.2% to 0.5%) as well as a number of volatile oils. The extract is sold as tablets, capsules, drops, transdermal patches, oils, and teas.

The pharmacology of the extract includes inhibition of the neurotransmitters serotonin, norepinephrine, and dopamine; it also binds to γ-aminobutyric acid (GABA) receptors in vitro. When the extract is taken orally, hypericin peaks in serum in 5 hours and reaches steady state with continued dosing in 4 days. The half-life in plasma is 25 hours.[70]

Studies of varying quality abound, and some are reported on the Hypericum Home Page. Some are carefully controlled and include standardized testing of depression and mood before and after 3 to 6 weeks of treatment with St. John's wort versus placebo or treatment versus standard antidepressant medication. In their overview and meta-analysis, Linde et al[76] conclude evidence indicates that extracts of hypericin are more effective than placebo and equally effective as standard antidepressants for mild to moderately severe depressive disorders. Side effects of dry mouth, dizziness, constipation, and confusion occurred in about 20% of subjects receiving hypericin and 53% taking standard antidepressants. The doses, duration, and

assessment tools varied widely in these 23 studies and 1757 outpatients.

Adverse effects with chronic high doses (more than 30 mg/day) include photosensitivity, abdominal symptoms, rarely tachycardia, tachypnea, fever, and fatigue. Because hypericin inhibits dopamine β-hydroxylase, which leads to increased dopamine, increased prolactin inhibitory factor, and suppression of prolactin, it could decrease lactation. No clinical study has investigated this pharmacologic potential. "Better, longer studies are needed to establish the effectiveness and safety of St. John's Wort for treatment of depression. The active ingredients, potency and purity of preparations sold in the USA are all unknown."[85] It is licensed in Germany but is considered a dietary supplement in the United States and has not been evaluated by the FDA.

Product identification

The clinician needs to inquire about all foods and beverages when taking a history. If the mother is consuming an excessive amount of any herbal product, its contents should be checked. The regional poison control center may be able to identify active principles if the plant constituents of the tea are known (Table 11-6).

Cardiovascular drugs and diuretics

Digitalis is given to infants, but only for serious reasons. Measurements of digitalis in the milk in mothers maintained on digitalis throughout pregnancy and lactation showed concentrations of 0.825 nmol/L, which was 59% of the maternal plasma level in one study[17] and 75% in another.[33] If one calculates the predicted level of digitalis using the higher volume of distribution, 7.5 L/kg, the infant would receive 1.1 ng/ml in the milk of a 60-kg (132-lb) mother receiving 0.5 mg dose of digoxin.[102] Authors agree that digoxin levels would be low and the dosage to the infant low, but the long-range effects are not known.[17,33,80] There is sufficient experience accumulated to date, however, to conclude that mothers taking sustaining doses of digitalis preparations may nurse their

TABLE 11-6	Herbal teas and their side effects		
Herb/parts used	Common uses	Method of application	Side effects
Aconite (monkshood, wolfsbane)	Aconitine, hypaconitine, aconine, mesaconitine	Tea	Nausea, vomiting, hypersalivation Perioral paresthesia, progressing rapidly to neuromuscular weakness, seizures, coma Cardiac effects: Bradycardia and hypotension (most common), supraventricular or ventricular tachycardia, ventricular fibrillation, asystole
Aloe vera/pure gel from leaves	Burns Constipation Ulcers Canker sores Immunostimulant HIV infections	Gel applied topically or taken internally several times daily Doses not standardized	Diarrhea, gastric cramping when taken internally Contact dermatitis from related species, *Aloe arboresce*
Chamomile/ flowers	Calming, sedating Aromatherapy Antispasmodic Colic Antiinflammatory Soothe diaper rash, chickenpox, poison ivy	Tea (in infants) or tinctures Essential oil used in aromatherapy or added to bath	Allergic reactions One case of botulism in infant given tea from homegrown plant
Comfrey	Pyrrolizidine Demulcent Sedative Astringent	Tea Poultice Ointment	Hepatic venoocclusive disease marked by severe abdominal pain and vomiting, which may be followed by hepatomegaly and abdominal distention with ascites Hepatic necrosis leading to cirrhosis *Not recommended*
Echinacea/ leaves, stalks, roots	Immunostimulant Colds, ear and sinus infections HIV infections	Tincture, capsules, or tablets taken internally as immunostimulant Doses not standardized	None reported

Modified from Mack RB: *Pediatrics* 15:49, 1998; and Kemper KJ: *Contemp Pediatr* 13:79, 1996.
HIV, Human immunodeficiency virus; *CNS,* central nervous system.

infants without any harm to the infant. The AAP rates digitalis a 6, compatible with breastfeeding.

Propranolol, a beta blocker, was found in the milk of mothers but does not appear to accumulate in the infant. Thus, experienced cardiologists have permitted mothers taking propranolol to nurse their infants without any ill effect observed in the infants. In 1973, Levitan and Manion[73] reported significant quantities of propranolol in breast milk.

Propranolol and its major metabolites were measured in milk and found by Smith et al[126] to provide the infant with a maximum dose of less than 0.1% of the maternal dose or approximately 7 µg/dl. The half-life of elimination from the milk was over 6 hours.[5] β-Adrenergic blockade effects, including hypoglycemia, have been described in an infant breastfed by a mother taking propranolol. Because the reports are conflicting, it is necessary

TABLE 11-6   Herbal teas and their side effects—cont'd

Herb/parts used	Common uses	Method of application	Side effects
Ephedra (ma huang)/leaves, stalks	Decongestant Asthma, allergy Weight loss "Natural high"	Generally taken internally	Hypertension, tachycardia Toxic psychosis Death *Not recommended*
Feverfew/fresh or dried leaves	Migraine prophylaxis Rheumatoid arthritis Insect repellent Menstrual pain	1-3 fresh leaves, 25-50 mg capsules, or crushed, dried leaves twice a day to prevent migraine	Allergic reactions Mouth ulcers Rebound headache if discontinued abruptly
Goldenseal/ roots	Diarrhea Antiseptic, antimicro- bial for acne, conjunc- tivitis, eczema, ear infections Possible immuno- stimulator Antiarrhythmic	¼-½ tsp of tincture or ⅛ tsp of fluid extract 3 or 4 times a day for diarrhea Can be mixed with 4 oz water or juice	Hypotension, hypertension Local irritation Nausea, vomiting, diarrhea Displaces bilirubin from albumin *Not recommended for infants*
Pennyroyal	Pulegone	Tea Oil	Hepatotoxicity, hepatic failure, nausea, vomiting, abdominal pain Renal failure Delirium, confusion, restlessness, dizzi- ness, seizures, alternating lethargy and agitation Abortion *Not recommended*
Tea tree oil/ essential oil from leaves	Minor skin infections Fungicide Acne Vaginitis	Applied topically 2-4 times a day	Contact dermatitis if applied to broken or irritated skin As little as 10 ml PO can affect CNS function and cause muscle weakness *Not for internal use*

to monitor the breastfed infant carefully when the mother is taking propranolol. Monitoring plasma levels of the infant may be helpful if there is any question.

The antihypertensive drugs atenolol (Tenormin), metoprolol tartrate (Lopressor), and nadolol (Corgard, Corzide) have been evaluated in human milk.[26,27,75,84] *Metoprolol* had a peak level in blood of 713 ng/dl at 1.1 hours and in milk of 4.7 ng/dl at 3.8 hours. The data suggest that metoprolol appears minimally in milk and is probably safe for breastfeeding neonates.[27] *Nadolol* appears in serum at 77 ng/dl and in milk at 357 ng/dl.[26] *Atenolol* levels in milk are also higher than in the maternal serum.[86] Of this group, metoprolol would be the safest. These drugs are rated 6 (AAP) and II (Swedish system). Serum levels of atenolol in one breastfed infant reached 0.16 μmol/L.

A number of effective antihypertensive medications are available. The clinician should review the properties and amount excreted in breast milk when choosing the best drug for the mother.

Reserpine has been reported to cause nasal stuffiness, bradycardia, and respiratory difficulty with increased tracheobronchial secretion and is contraindicated in both pregnancy and lactation, because safer drugs are available.[99]

Most *diuretics* are weak acids and little passes into milk. Use of diuretics, however, requires careful observation because they have the potential for causing a diuresis in the neonate that could be extremely dehydrating.[2] Although diuretics such as furosemide (Lasix) are given to neonates, this is done only when fluid and electrolyte levels can be followed closely. Oral diuretics were used to suppress lactation in a study by Healy[44] in 40 postpartum women who chose not to breastfeed. *Bendroflumethiazide* (Naturetin) was used, 5 mg twice daily for 5 days. He found it more effective than estrogens, with fewer side effects. Milk volume may be reduced by the thiazides.

Reports document the interaction of three diuretics with bilirubin-albumin complexes.[140] *Chlorothiazide* presented the greatest risk for producing free bilirubin, with ethacrynic acid and furosemide producing considerably less. The latter two are clinically effective in lower doses as well. The levels of chlorothiazide and hydrochlorothiazide in milk are less than 100 ng/ml.[88,93] For most infants, these are safe; however, these findings certainly suggest caution is necessary if the infant is jaundiced or very immature.

Chlorthalidone (Hygroton) appears in milk.[141] A term baby might receive 180 µg per day. The half-life is 60 hours.

Furosemide has been shown by several techniques not only to displace bilirubin from albumin in the newborn, but also to be slowly excreted by the newborn, with only 84% excreted in 24 hours. Mofenson and Caraccio[90] reported that furosemide is not excreted into breast milk and is poorly absorbed orally.

A mother who is lactating may actually require substantially less medication, particularly diuretics. Close monitoring of the mother during lactation to try to reduce her medications may provide a therapeutic balance that is good for the mother and safe for the infant. With the short half-life of most diuretics, dosing can be timed to avoid peak plasma levels during feedings.

Central nervous system drugs

Phenobarbital can be given to infants and is usually safe, but careful observation of the infant for variation in sleeping and feeding habits is important.[66]

Phenytoin in the breast milk has been associated with vomiting, tremors, rash, blood dyscrasia (rarely), and methemoglobinemia, but not with drowsiness and lethargy. Many mothers have nursed without apparent incident while taking phenobarbital and phenytoin.[129] Phenytoin levels in milk of mothers treated for epilepsy have been measured, and levels in the infant have been calculated to provide less than 5% of the therapeutic dose for infants.[95] *Valproic acid* in maternal milk is low (3% of maternal serum concentrations), but the mean half-life is 47 hours, four times that in adults, so there is risk of accumulation (Table 11-7).[96,129] The AAP rating for valproic acid and phenytoin is 6.

A single case of *carbamazepine* exposure during pregnancy and breastfeeding is reported to have caused cholestatic hepatitis, diagnosed when the infant was 3 weeks of age.[36] The mother did not develop hepatic symptoms and continued the drug. Breastfeeding was discontinued, and the hepatitis resolved. Diagnosis was confirmed by liver function studies and liver biopsy. Carbamazepine hepatitis has been described in children and adults as a rare complication of therapy.

Poor weight gain after birth of infants whose mothers received antiepileptic medication during pregnancy has been reported by Kaneko et al.[57] They also report inadequate suckling and high incidence of vomiting immediately after birth with difficulty establishing lactation. The drug continues to be provided through the milk, and the poor suckling becomes protracted. Table 11-7 lists levels of drug in the milk. When newborn levels are high, the authors suggest giving mixed feedings

TABLE 11-7	Anticonvulsant concentrations in maternal serum and milk				
Drug (half-life in neonate)	Maternal serum (µg/ml)	Milk (µg/ml)	Day 1	Milk/serum day 7	Day 30
Diphenylhydantoin (9-56 hr)	3.0	0.7	18 ± 15	19 ± 4	13 ± 6
Phenobarbital (156 ± 29 hr)	12.0	5.0	30 ± 16	36 ± 7	30 ± 5
Primidone (23 ± 8 hr)	4.0	2.1	141 ± 9	56 ± 15	46 ± 7
Carbamazepine (13-36 hr)	4.0	1.8	41 ± 16	38 ± 8	—
Valproic acid (47 hr)	123 µmol/L	3 µmol/L	0.01 to 0.16	—	—

Modified from Kaneko S, Suzuki K, Sato T et al: In Janz D, Dam M, Richens A et al, editors: *Epilepsy, pregnancy, and the child,* New York, 1982, Raven.

for the first few days postpartum until the level of drug in the milk drops and the infant is able to clear the drug that was in the system transplacentally from birth. The clinician should observe these infants closely to be sure they receive adequate calories until they can suck vigorously. The mother should supplement the infant's suckling stimulus to the breast with a breast pump. With proper management in the first few days, the adjustment can be smooth and the infant can go on to nurse effectively and safely.[12] When infant plasma level determinations are available, it might be advisable to check the plasma level after 1 or 2 weeks of nursing, providing an opportunity to evaluate possible accumulation.

Psychotherapeutic agents

Lithium is the one drug in the psychotherapeutic group with a clear risk of toxicity in the neonate and clear evidence that it reaches the breast milk. Lithium is contraindicated in pregnancy as well as in lactation. Infants have been reported to be hypotonic, flaccid, and "depressed" when the nursing mother is taking lithium.

After a careful review of the clinical data, Schou[119] states that accumulating evidence points strongly to the beneficial effects of breastfeeding while taking lithium for both infant and mother, mentally and physically. Lithium concentrations in the breastfed infant have been measured at one tenth to one half of the concentration in the mother's blood.[120] Such concentrations are considered harmless in adults, but their risk is unknown in a child. Schou[119] also states that supported by

husband and physician, the mother should make her own choice. Initiating lithium therapy after delivery or when the breastfeeding infant is several months old greatly minimizes the theoretic risks. The Lactation Study Center has been contacted about several infants being breastfed by mothers taking lithium with the psychiatrist's and pediatrician's consent. No symptoms were apparent. No long term follow-up is yet available on these children.

Chlorpromazine or *phenothiazine* appears in the milk in small amounts, even at doses of 1200 mg, but apparently does not accumulate.[4] Doses of 100 mg/day do not appear to cause symptoms in the infants. *Diazepam* (Valium) has been detected in milk and in breastfed infants' serum and urine. It has caused depression and poor feeding with weight loss in the infant. *Chlordiazepoxide* (Librium) and *clorazepate* (Tranxene) do reach the milk and may cause drowsiness and poor suckling. These substances' metabolites are also active, and therefore the half-life of therapeutic activity is prolonged. *Meprobamate* (Miltown, Equanil) has an M/P ratio greater than 1 and has been identified in milk. Infants whose mothers are taking meprobamate may become drowsy, but dosage adjustment may be indicated if there is significant benefit for the mother to breastfeed.[4]

Tricyclic antidepressants such as imipramine are lipid soluble and have been identified in the breast milk; thus cautious use may be appropriate.[22] In an extensive study of tricyclic antidepressants in pregnancy and lactation, Misri and Sivertz[89] found that an attitude of informed and cautious encouragement regarding the growing information suggests it is safe to breastfeed while taking such medication.

When Yoshida et al[149] investigated the pharmacokinetics and possible adverse effects in infants exposed to tricyclic antidepressants in breast milk, they found no reason to prevent mothers who are taking established tricyclic antidepressants from breastfeeding. The drugs were imipramine, amitriptyline, clomipramine, and dothiepin. They had compared infants breastfed by mothers medicated with a tricyclic antidepressant with infants bottle-fed by medicated mothers. In addition, they measured the drugs in all maternal plasma and urine and in foremilk and hindmilk of the lactators. Infant plasma and urine levels were also measured. Levels in the mother and her milk were correlated with the dose. The daily dose of drug via the breast milk was about 1% of the maternal dose per kilogram of weight. Amounts were barely detectable in the infant's plasma and urine. The 30-month follow-up detected no differences in growth and development.

The *serotonin reuptake inhibitors* are a class of drugs developed as antidepressants and also used in the treatment of panic attacks, obsessive-compulsive disorder, obesity, substance abuse, sleep disorders, chemotherapy-induced nausea and vomiting, migraine, and appetite suppression. Serotonergic dysfunction has been implicated in these illnesses. This group of drugs has antidepressant actions and selectively blocks the reuptake of serotonin into presynaptic neurons (Box 11-2).

These agents undergo extensive metabolism to clinically inactive compounds, have large volumes of distribution, and are highly bound to maternal plasma proteins, suggesting little transfer into milk. The elimination half-lives in the mother range from 15 to 26 hours. Reports of isolated cases have recorded maternal plasma and milk levels of a few of the compounds, but no long-term follow-up of the nurslings. In general, no symptoms have been reported in the infants. One case of severe colic and crying in a 6-week-old infant was reported to clear when the infant was weaned when the mother was taking fluoxetine (Prozac) (Box 11-2).[72] The available pharmacology can be found in Appendix D.

The clinician must weigh the risk/benefit ratio of each drug, keeping in mind that being cared for by a depressed mother is not beneficial for the infant. Some mothers have been medicated with antidepressants during their pregnancies, and the withdrawal experienced when the infant is not breastfed may go undiagnosed and be attributed to colic, fussiness, or other disorders. If a mother is to begin medication during lactation, a baseline for the infant should be established by the pediatrician so that any effects of the medication received via the milk can be detected. The age of the infant and the feeding pattern are very important issues in the decision.

Fluoxetine (Prozac), a common and usually effective therapy for depression and other neuro-psychiatric disorders, is reported to have few side effects. Pharmacologically, it is chemically unrelated to the antidepressants, has few autonomic effects, and is considered an alternative to standard antidepressant therapy. Its peak plasma time is 6 to 8 hours, and it is highly protein bound.[15,50] Case studies on lactating women taking fluoxetine have reported no changes in the infant. Maternal blood and milk samples have one-fifth to one-quarter as much drug (i.e., M/P = 0.20 to 0.25) when fluoxetine and the active metabolite norfluoxetine are measured.[50] Total ingestion by the infant per day was no more than 15 to 20 μg/kg, a low exposure when mother had received 20 mg at bedtime for 53 days. The reported levels in milk depend on sampling and lipid content of the milk and range from 47 to 469 ng/mL.[15]

BOX 11-2   Serotonin (5-HT) reuptake inhibitors (brand names)

Fenfluramine (Ponderax, Pondimin)
Fluoxetine (Prozac)
Fluvoxamine (Faverin)
Nefazodone (Serzone)
Paroxetine (Paxil, Seroxat)
Sertraline (Lustral, Zoloft)
Trazodone (Desyrel)
Venlafaxine (Effexor)

In the AAP report of the Committee on Drugs in 1994, a special category 4 was developed for drugs whose effects on nursing infants is unknown but may be of concern.[22] The AAP considers the psychotropic drugs to be of special concern because they are taken for a long time. Although no adverse effects have been published, the drugs do appear in milk and could conceivably alter short-term and long-term CNS function. These drugs clearly require the physician's careful consideration of the benefits of breastfeeding and the therapeutic risks in each case.[91]

Methadone maintenance and risks of breastfeeding

Methadone maintenance treatment for heroin and other addictions has had a significant impact on the recovery of many addicts. When first introduced, it was hoped it would be an ideal treatment for neonatal withdrawal syndrome. It was not. It was also hoped that withdrawal from methadone for the infant born to a woman receiving maintenance therapy would be negligible, but it is not. When pregnant women were maintained on 25 mg/day or less, neonatal withdrawal rarely required treatment. Present regimens during pregnancy typically are for maternal doses up to 100 mg/day. Neonatal withdrawal from this level is substantial, requiring treatment with tincture of opium (Paregoric) for 6 to 8 weeks. A frequent question to the Lactation Study Center is, Can a woman on 50 to 60 mg of methadone per day nurse her infant? The AAP has indicated that 20 mg/day is a safe level for breastfeeding under supervision. The data are sparse, and the literature has reported little since the late 1970s.

Geraghty et al[39] present two cases with multiple maternal blood and milk samples. At a single daily dose of 73 mg, plasma levels peaked at 1 hour and milk levels at 1 to 5 hours. The M/P ratio varied over time and reflected the slow drop in the plasma level and slower drop in the milk level, but the differences as a ratio are negligible. A second mother took 30 mg at 9 AM and 30 mg at 6 PM. Her plasma levels were steady over time while milk levels dropped from a high of 0.25 mg/L to 0.11 mg/L at 14 hours, giving an M/P ratio of 1.53 at

peak milk level 2 hours after the second dose and the lowest ratio of 0.91 at 14 hours. This demonstrates that an M/P ratio is of little value unless levels are known. It does suggest that peak plasma level is at about 1 to 2 hours and peak milk level under five hours. Ranges were not different between a total of 60 mg and 73 mg.

One of the infants died of SIDS at 3½ months, and no methadone was detected at autopsy. He had been partially breastfed. Under the controlled circumstances of a methadone maintenance program with careful surveillance, an infant can be breastfed if the mother is maintained on levels below 75 mg/day and if the infant remains symptom free.

Ten women were studied by Blinick et al,[10,11] who collected milk and plasma for 3 to 10 days after delivery. Their doses varied from 10 to 80 mg/day. Levels in the breast milk ranged for 0.05 to 0.57 µg/ml, with an average M/P ratio of 0.83. Higher doses resulted in higher levels, but the relationship was not linear. Pond et al[104] reported two women who had M/P ratios that remained constant at 0.32 and 0.61, and the infants received a calculated 0.01 to 0.03 mg of methadone per day. Kreek[64] estimated daily infant intake from a mother taking 50 mg daily, assuming consumption of almost a liter of breast milk a day as a maximum of 0.112 mg/day. Kreek et al[65] also noted peak levels in the milk at 4 hours after dosing. Pumping and discarding the milk at 3 to 4 hours after dosing has been suggested as a method of reducing exposure.

In 1977 Smialek et al[125] reported an infant death at 5 weeks of age as apparent SIDS. The mother's maintenance dose was not reported. Postmortem examination noted congenital anomalies and malnutrition. The infant's postmortem methadone level was 0.4 mg/L, much higher than in any woman reported in any published reports.

Pesticides and pollutants

Monitoring chemical exposure in the breastfed infant is at the mercy of the epidemiologist and the chemist.[124] Human milk has been known to contain insecticides. *Chlorinated hydrocarbons* such as DDT and its metabolites dieldrin, aldrin, and related compounds are the best known. The major reason these compounds appear in breast milk is that they are deposited in body lipid stores and move with lipid. The fetus receives the greatest dose in utero, and adult body fat has approximately 30 times the concentration in milk.

Polychlorinated biphenyls (PCBs) in heavily contaminated pregnant Japanese women produced small-for-gestational-age infants who had transient darkening of the skin ("cola babies"). *Polybrominated biphenyls* (PBBs) are similar compounds associated with a heavy exposure to farm animals and contaminated cattle fed in the lower Michigan Peninsula. The women in the United States who have the greatest risk of high exposure to PCBs or PBBs are those who have worked with or eaten in excess the fish caught by sports fishing in contaminated waters.

Studies have refuted earlier observations of concern. No information is available in the United States on the levels of polychlorinated dibenzodioxins (PCDDs) or dibenzofurans (PCDFs) in anglers who consume a great deal of fish.[61] Others at high risk are those who live near a waste disposal site or have been involved in environmental spills. Unless there is heavy exposure, however, no contraindication exists to breastfeeding. The state health department can be consulted for specific advice or to measure plasma and milk levels. The epidemiologists are usually aware of the risks in a given geographic area and whether it is necessary to measure milk levels once lactation is fully established. If this sampling is planned in advance during the pregnancy, little time need be lost. Unless there is a unique and excessive exposure, the infant can breastfeed until levels are returned from the laboratory. Risk has diminished as environmental cleanups continue.

In most cases the levels of pesticides in human milk have been less than those in cow's milk. The accumulated amounts have not usually exceeded safe allowable limits. Several extensive reviews explore the dilemma of pollutants in human milk.[113,114,142,147] In a 1997 review of world reports on occurrence and toxicity, Rogan[112] has re-

affirmed that breastfeeding should be recommended despite the presence of chemical residues. He further states that the benefits of breastfeeding outweigh the risks of pollutants. It has been suggested that the body burden at birth can be added to by exposing the infant to small levels in the milk that may indeed exceed the exposure limits allowable for daily intake set by the World Health Organization (WHO).[130] Human milk levels are used epidemiologically as markers of human exposure in a community exposure because of a close correlation between milk levels and the levels in fat stores. Unselected mothers in the Great Lakes region were tested by the State of New York in 1978, and no chemical (PCB, PBB) was found in any milk in random sampling of residents. Thus unless the circumstances are unusual, breastfeeding should not be abandoned on the basis of insecticide contamination.

Agent Orange, the best known of the dioxins, was identified in Vietnam as a powerful teratogen. *Dioxin* has been found in human milk from pooled samples from high-risk women with known exposure. No evidence suggests that the population at large is at risk. Women working in dry-cleaning plants, viscose rayon plants, photographic laboratories, and chemical industries where proper precautions are not taken have been noted to absorb tetrachloroethylene, carbon disulfide, and bromides.[41]

Heavy metals that have been found in milk include lead, mercury, arsenic, and cadmium.[100] Whenever maternal exposure occurs, the breastfed infant and the milk should be tested. The intake of lead and cadmium by breastfed infants, as reported by the WHO study, is the same as or somewhat lower than that of infants fed formula mixed with local water.[68] Levels in milk of these heavy metals, however, are lower than would be predicted from maternal levels (see Appendix E). Most common air pollutants are not found in human milk.

Lead has become a significant issue because of the number of mothers testing positive for lead on routine screens for lead in family members of young infants.[134] The Centers for Disease Control and Prevention (CDC) has revised the standards for treatment downward (Table 11-8). The first step is always to clean up the environment and identify the source. The level of lead in milk depends on its ionization and tight binding to the red blood cells. The M/P ratio is 0.2. A lead level of 40 µg/dl or lower in a nursing mother is considered below the level of transfer through the breast milk. In addition to environmental sources of lead (e.g., old paint, contaminated ground, lead batteries), diet should be reviewed. In some cities the water supply is a significant source, especially in formula making. Herbs and herbal teas may also be a source.

TABLE 11-8 Classes and management of lead levels in blood

Blood lead level (µg/dl)	Class	Management
<10	I	Not considered lead poisoning
10-14	IIA	Many children (or large proportion of children) with blood lead levels in this range should trigger community-wide childhood lead poisoning prevention activities. Children in this range may need to be re-screened more frequently.
15-19	IIB	Nutritional and educational interventions and more frequent screening; if level persists in this range, environmental investigation and intervention recommended
20-44	III	Environmental evaluation and remediation and a medical evaluation; possible pharmacologic treatment of lead poisoning
45-69	IV	Both medical and environmental intervention, including chelation therapy
>69	V	Medical emergency; immediate medical and environmental management

Modified from Centers for Disease Control and Prevention: *MMWR* 43(30):545, 1994.

Organic mercury is another heavy metal that is being increasingly identified in food around the world. Fish is a major source, as are herbs and tonics. When the source of the methylmercury is from breast milk, the developmental scores exceed those of formula-fed infants, suggesting that the advantages of breastfeeding are significant in a study in the Faroe Islands by Grandjean et al.[42] A similar, more extensive study in the Seychelles Islands of mothers and children from birth followed over 5 years suggests that the value of a fish diet over time and during breastfeeding is significant despite measurable mercury levels.[82] Almost all the infants in the Seychelles are breastfed for at least 6 months and meet or exceed international developmental scores.[81] Acute exposures to methylmercury from industrial or environmental sources should be evaluated on a case-by-case basis, although it appears breastfeeding is safe.

Chemicals that are lipophilic, biologically stable, nonionized at a physiologic pH, and of low molecular weight transfer easily into maternal milk. Ten to 20 times more of the mother's body burden of persistent organohalogens are transferred via the milk than via the placenta, according to Jensen and Slorach,[53] who have published an extensive review of chemical contaminants in human milk. They further caution that the absolute amount transferred depends on the structure of the chemical. PCBs, for instance, are highly chlorinated and transfer more easily than less chlorinated PCBs. There is no difference in placental and milk transfer of heavy metals.

If extractable fat is measured, the levels of persistent organohalogens are about the same in milk, blood, adipose tissue, and muscle. Mobilization from fat stores is greater than that from dietary intake during lactation.[53]

Well water

Drinking well water has been a concern because of varying levels of minerals and especially of *nitrate*. More than 18% of wells in the state of Iowa are reported to exceed the maximum contaminant level of 45 mg of nitrate/L or 10 mg NO_3^--N/L. Infants under 6 months of age are especially susceptible to *methemoglobinemia,* which can lead to anoxic injury and death. It reportedly occurs at nitrate concentrations greater than 100 mg/L. Although this is a major issue for formula-fed infants, Dusdieker et al[28] explored the question, Does increased nitrate ingestion elevate nitrate levels in human milk? Carefully studying 20 healthy mothers with breastfeeding infants over 6 months old subjected to 47, 168, and 270 mg of nitrate/day, urine spot tests rose from 36 mg day 1 to 660 day 2 and 84 mg day 3. Nitrate concentrations of their milk on days 1, 2, and 3 were 4.4, 5.1, and 5.2 mg/L, respectively. The authors conclude that "women who consume water with a nitrate concentration of 100 mg/L or less do not produce milk with elevated nitrate levels."[28]

Chemicals in the workplace

An increasing number of women return to the workplace after birth of an infant, and an increasing number are breastfeeding their infants. The need for information regarding the transfer of chemicals in the workplace to human milk is an increasing problem.

Volatile chemicals in the workplace represent an important but little understood hazard, especially in paint shops, repair shops, garages, and the chemical industry. Fisher et al[34] developed a physiologically based pharmacokinetic model for a lactating woman to estimate the amount of chemical that the nursing infant ingests for a given nursing schedule and maternal occupational exposure. The two major factors are the blood/air partition coefficient, a thermodynamic factor that governs the body burden that may be achieved from inhalation of a chemical, and the pharmacokinetics of the chemical, which determines the length of time a chemical remains in the systemic circulation and is available to transfer into milk. Because milk fat is available, preferential uptake of lipophilic chemicals occurs. Of the 19 chemicals simulated in the study, the authors consider bromochloromethane, perchloroethylene, and 1,4-dioxane exposure at highest risk for the infant based on U.S. Environmental Protection Agency (EPA) drinking water guidelines (Table 11-9). Protective gear is the most practical way of minimizing exposure to both mother and infant.

The Occupational Health and Safety Act of the province of Quebec has mandated the establishment and maintenance of a *Toxicological Index* that provides information on chemical and biologic contaminants potentially present in the workplace.[41] Information can also serve as a basis for the protective reassignment of pregnant or breastfeeding employees. The *Infotox* database has information about 5500 chemicals. Of the substances in the database, 2.2% (153 of 5736) show evidence of milk transfer and pose relative risks to the breastfed infant.[41] (See Appendix D.)

Psychologic impact of toxin in milk

The psychologic reactions of a group of nursing mothers from the lower Michigan Peninsula whose breast milk was contaminated with a toxic fire-retardant chemical, PBB, were studied.[43] Every tenth woman who had had her milk tested for PBB was contacted for the study (a sample of 200 women); 139 responded and received a questionnaire, and 97 (70%) filled out the questionnaire. The subjects knew their own level and that the range for all mothers was from undetected to 0.46 ppm with an average of 0.1 ppm. The testing was voluntary and cost $25. Of those tested, 96% had measurable amounts.

The data were collected in a six-page questionnaire. Two modes of coping emerged: denial and mastery. In general, the findings indicated that the greater the level of toxic contamination of PBB reported in a mother's milk, the greater the denial, to the point of not having correct information, even about her own level. Ambivalence toward nursing was correlated with guilt in both groups (only 15% discontinued breastfeeding). The "draw-a-baby" test showed an unusual amount (94%) of distortion and expressions of anguish. These findings were consistent throughout all the test modalities; thus they were not thought to be a function of personality.[43]

TABLE 11-9 **Predicted amount of chemical ingested by nursing infant (AMILK) over 24-hour period and EPA drinking water health advisory values**

Chemical	Threshold limit value (TLV, ppm)	AMILK (mg)	EPA health advisory intake* (mg/day)
Benzene	10	0.053	0.20†
Bromochloromethane	200	2.090	1.00
Carbon tetrachloride	5	0.055	0.07
Chlorobenzene	10	0.229	—
Chloroform	10	0.043	0.1
Methylchloroform	350	3.51	40.0
Diethylether	400	1.49	—
1,4-Dioxane	25	0.559	0.4†
Halothane	50	0.232	—
n-Hexane	50	0.052	4.0
Isoflurane	50‡	0.336	—
Methylene chloride	50	0.213	2.0†
Methyl ethyl ketone	200	12.08	—
Perchloroethylene	25	1.36	1.0
Styrene	50	0.650	2.0
Trichloroethylene	50	0.496	0.6§
1,1,1,2-Tetrachlorothane	100‡	4.31	0.9
Toluene	50	0.460	2.0
o,p,m-Xylenes	100	6.590	40.0

From Fisher J, Mahle D, Bankston L et al: *Am Ind Hyg Assoc J* 58:429, 1997.
*Modified from EPA Health Advisory values for chronic ingestion of contaminated water by 10-kg (22-lb) children, assuming ingestion of 1 L of water per day. These Health Advisory concentrations for chemicals in water are thought to be protective of adverse health effects for chronic exposure.
†Modified from 10-day Health Advisory values for ingestion of contaminated water by 10 kg children, assuming ingestion of 1 L of water per day. These Health Advisory values for contaminated water are thought to be protective of adverse health effects for a 10-day period.
‡No TLV; concentration value was assigned.
§Lifetime Health Advisory value for ingestion of 2 L water per day in adults.

Radioactive materials

Because of the increasing number of diagnostic tests that use radioactive materials, a nursing mother may have such a procedure done.

Radioactive iodine (^{125}I and ^{131}I) passes into milk at levels as high as 5% of the dose. When this is used for diagnostic purposes, breastfeeding should be discontinued until milk is clear. The excretion by the breast may alter the validity of the test result. If radioactive iodine is to be used therapeutically, breastfeeding must be discontinued until the iodine has cleared the system, which may be 1 to 3 weeks. A carefully collected sample of milk can be tested for radioactivity so that the period that the infant is off the breast is not unnecessarily long. If a 30 μCi dose of ^{131}I is used, 24 hours may be adequate to pump and discard. If the infant is older and receiving other foods, time can be altered accordingly. A lung scan (300 μCi dose) requires 7 days and 2 days for renography of pumping and discarding the milk.[58]

Gallium-67 citrate appears in significant amounts in the milk. It does clear the body quickly and is relatively safe for use in patients. Breastfeeding should be discontinued for at least 72 hours.

Technetium 99m (^{99m}Tc) is reported to clear the milk in 6 to 48 hours. The stage of lactation, whether the breast is emptied before receiving the dose, and the method of clearing the breast may be responsible for the inconsistent results. Discontinuing breastfeeding for at least 24 hours is advisable.

The amount of radioactivity excreted in breast milk after administration of ^{99m}Tc hexakis 2-methoxyisobutyl isonitrile (MIBI) in a single dose was reported by Rubow et al.[116] The measurement was highest in the first sample at 3.3 hours, 0.488 kilobecquerel (kBq)/ml, with negligible amounts thereafter (less than 0.180 kBq/ml). Less than 2.96 kBq/ml is considered safe. Only the first sample needs to be discarded.[116]

With the advent of ultrasound examination, computed tomography scanning, magnetic resonance imaging, and other techniques, alternatives exist in many situations to use of radioactive material during lactation. (See Appendix E.)

IMMUNIZATIONS

Immunizing the breastfed infant

Questions often arise as to whether a breastfed infant should be immunized on a different schedule because of the protective maternal antibodies that might interfere with the infant's response to antigen stimulation. Following are some brief guidelines on the more common situations of concern[23]:

1. Vaccinations for diphtheria-pertussis-tetanus (DPT) are not altered by breastfeeding, and the regular schedule should be followed for the infant.
2. Because oral poliovirus vaccine (OPV) is a live virus vaccine, there was concern that the maternal antibodies would inactivate the live virus. However, the CDC recommendation is that the same schedule be followed. The current scientific literature indicates that for infants older than 6 weeks, which is the earliest age of vaccination recommended, no indication exists for withholding breastfeeding in relationship to OPV administration, and no need exists for extra doses of vaccine. Furthermore, antibody responses to parenteral and oral vaccines are better in breastfed than formula-fed infants.

The same is true for diphtheria and tetanus toxoid.[153]

3. Rubella, mumps, and measles vaccines should be given at the regularly scheduled times.[23]
4. A *Haemophilus influenzae* type B vaccine is available for infants. The *H. influenzae* type B conjugate vaccines should be given at 2 months of age or as soon as possible thereafter, following the AAP *Red Book* guidelines in the Report of the Committee on Infectious Disease. No modification of the immunization schedule is necessary for breastfed infants. Furthermore, data suggest breastfed infants ultimately have higher antibody titers than formula-fed infants.

Immunizing the nursing mother
Smallpox

Smallpox vaccination is inadvisable for the mother of any infant under 1 year of age, nursing or not. The personal contact, not the breastfeeding, causes the risk; therefore no advantage exists to weaning if vaccination is necessary. This vaccination is not given routinely and is rarely indicated.

Rh immune globulin

Only rare trace amounts of anti-Rh are present in colostrum and none in mature milk of women given large doses of Rh immune globulin immediately postpartum. No adverse response was noted, even with these high dosages. Any Rh antibodies in the mother's milk are thought to be inactivated by the gastric juices. Rh immune globulin or Rh sensitization is not a contraindication to breastfeeding.

Rubella

Following are the recommendations with respect to rubella[23]:

1. Approximately 85% to 90% of the adult female population are thought to have a high level of naturally acquired immunity, and only 10% to 15% are considered to be susceptible to rubella infection.
2. Vaccination of pregnant women is contraindicated under all circumstances.

3. No woman of childbearing age should be vaccinated without having been first tested for immunity.
4. If the test is negative, the woman may be vaccinated if there is reasonable assurance that she will not become pregnant for at least 2 months.

The rubella virus was found in the milk of 69% of the women immunized with live attenuated rubella (HPV-77 DE5 or RA 27/3 strains).[78,79] A virus-specific immunoglobulin A (IgA) antibody response was seen in milk of all the women. Infectious rubella virus or virus antigen was recovered from the nasopharynx and throat of 56% of the breastfed infants and none of the nonbreastfed infants. No infant had disease in this study, but 25% of the breastfed group had seroconversion transiently.[79] Infants given early strains of the virus via the milk were reported to develop mild symptoms.[13,62,67,79] Although the attenuated virus may appear in the milk, this should not dissuade one from vaccinating a breastfeeding mother at the safest time, that is, immediately postpartum.

REFERENCES

1. Abbott PJ: Comfrey: assessing the low-dose health risk, *Med J Aust* 149:678, 1988.
2. Aranda JV, Lambert C, Perez J et al: Metabolism and renal elimination of furosemide in the newborn infant, *J Pediatr* 101:777, 1982.
3. Arena JM: Drugs and breast feeding, *Clin Pediatr* 5:472, 1966.
4. Ayd F: Excretion of psychotrophic drugs in human breast milk, *Int Drug Ther Newslett* 8:33, 1973.
5. Bauer JH, Pape B, Zajicek J et al: Propranolol in human plasma and breast milk, *Am J Cardiol* 43:860, 1979.
6. Begg EJ, Atkinson HC, Duffull SB: Prospective evaluation of a model for the prediction of milk: plasma drug concentrations from physicochemical characteristics, *Br J Clin Pharmacol* 33:501, 1992.
7. Berglund F, Flodh H, Lundborg P et al: Drug use during pregnancy and breastfeeding, *Acta Obstet Gynecol Scand Suppl* 126:1, 1984.
8. Berlin CM: Excretion of methylxanthines in human milk, *Semin Perinatol* 5:389, 1981.
9. Berlin CM, Daniel CH: Excretion of theobromine in human milk and saliva, *Pediatr Res* 15:492, 1981.
10. Blinick G, Inturrisi C, Jerez E et al: Methadone assays in pregnant women and progeny, *Am J Obstet Gynecol* 121:617, 1975.
11. Blinick G, Wallach R, Jerez E et al: Drug addiction in pregnancy and the neonate, *Am J Obstet Gynecol* 125:135, 1976.
12. Bossi L: Neonatal period including drug disposition in newborns: review of the literature. In Janz D, Dam M, Richens A et al, editors: *Epilepsy, pregnancy and the child,* New York, 1982, Raven.
13. Bowes WA Jr: The effect of medications on the lactating mother and her infant, *Clin Obstet Gynecol* 23:1073, 1980.
14. Briggs GG, Freeman RK, Yaffe S: *Drugs in pregnancy and lactation,* ed 5, Baltimore, 1998, Williams & Wilkins.
15. Burch KJ, Wells BG: Fluoxetine/norfluoxetine concentrations in human milk, *Pediatrics* 89:676, 1992.
16. Carlson HE, Wasser HL, Reidelberger RD: Beer-induced prolactin secretion: a clinical and laboratory study of the role of Salsolinol, *J Clin Endocrinol Metab* 60:673, 1985.
17. Chan V, Tse TF, Wong V: Transfer of digoxin across the placenta and into breast milk, *Br J Obstet Gynecol* 85:605, 1978.
18. Clark JH, Wilson WG: A 16-day-old breastfed infant with metabolic acidosis caused by salicylate, *Clin Pediatr* 20:53, 1981.
19. Cobo E: Effect of different doses of ethanol on milk-ejecting reflex in lactating women, *Am J Obstet Gynecol* 115:817, 1973.
20. Collaborative Group on Drug Use in Pregnancy: Medication during pregnancy: an intercontinental cooperative study, *Int J Gynaecol Obstet* 39(3):185, 1995.
21. Committee on Drugs, American Academy of Pediatrics: Psychotropic drugs in pregnancy and lactation, *Pediatrics* 69:241, 1982.
22. Committee on Drugs, American Academy of Pediatrics: The transfer of drugs and other chemicals into human milk, *Pediatrics* 72:375, 1983; 84:924, 1989; 93:137, 1994.
23. Committee on Infectious Disease: Report of the Committee on Infectious Disease. In *The Red Book,* ed 23, Elk Grove, Ill, 1994, American Academy of Pediatrics.
24. daSilva VA, Malheiros LR, Moraes-Santos AR et al: Ethanol pharmacokinetics in lactating women, *Braz J Med Biol Res* 26:1097, 1993.
25. Davis EA, Morris DJ: Medicinal uses of licorice through the millennia: the good and plenty of it, *Mol Cell Endocrinol* 78:1, 1991.
26. Devlin RG, Duchin KL, Fleiss PM: Nadolol in human serum and breast milk, *Br J Clin Pharmacol* 12:393, 1981.
27. Devlin RG, Fleiss PM: Captopril in human blood and breast milk, *J Clin Pharmacol* 21:110, 1981.

28. Dusdieker LB, Stumbo PJ, Kross BC et al: Does increased nitrate ingestion elevate nitrate levels in human milk? *Arch Pediatr Adolesc Med* 150:311, 1996.

29. Ellenhorn MJ: *Ellenhorn's medical toxicology: diagnosis and treatment of human poisoning,* ed 2, Baltimore, 1997, Williams & Wilkins.

30. Engels HJ, Wirth JC: No erogenic effects of ginseng during graded maximal aerobic exercise, *J Am Diet Assoc,* 97(10):1110, 1997.

31. Erickson SH, Oppenheim GL, Smith GH: Metronidazole in breast milk, *Obstet Gynecol* 57:48, 1981.

32. Feldman S, Pickering LK: Pharmacokinetics of drugs in human milk. In Howell RR, Morris FH, Pickering LK, editors: *Human milk, infant nutrition and health,* Springfield, Ill, 1986, Thomas.

33. Finley JP, Waxman MB, Wong PY et al: Digoxin excretion in human milk, *J Pediatr* 94:339, 1979.

34. Fisher J, Mahle D, Bankston L et al: Lactational transfer of volatile chemicals in breast milk, *Am Ind Hyg Assoc J* 58:425, 1997.

35. Flores-Huerta S, Hernández-Montes H, Argote RM et al: Effects of ethanol consumption during pregnancy and lactation on the outcome and postnatal growth of the offspring, *Ann Nutr Metab* 36:121, 1992.

36. Frey B, Schubiger G, Musy JP: Transient cholestatic hepatitis in a neonate associated with carbamazepine exposure during pregnancy and breastfeeding, *Eur J Pediatr* 150:136, 1990.

37. Gaginella TS: Drugs and the nursing mother-infant, *US Pharm* 3:39, 1978.

38. George DI, O'Toole TJ: A review of drug transfer to the infant by breastfeeding: concerns for the dentist, *J Am Dent Assoc* 106:204, 1983.

39. Geraghty B, Graham EA, Logan B et al: Methadone levels in breast milk, *J Hum Lact* 13:227, 1997.

40. Gilman AG, Rall TW, Nies AS et al, editors: *Goodman and Gilman's The pharmacological basis of therapeutics,* ed 8, New York, 1990, Macmillan.

41. Giroux D, Lapointe G, Baril M: Toxicological index and the presence in the workplace of chemical hazards for workers who breastfeed infants, *Am Ind Hyg Assoc J* 53:471, 1992.

42. Grandjean P, Wiehe P, White RF: Milestone development in infants exposed to methyl mercury from human milk, *Neurotoxicology* 16:27, 1995.

43. Hatcher SL: The psychological experience of nursing mothers upon learning of a toxic substance in their breast milk, *Psychiatry* 45:172, 1982.

44. Healy M: Suppressing lactation with oral diuretics, *Lancet* 1:1353, 1961.

45. Heisterberg L, Branebjerg PE: Blood and milk concentrations of metronidazole in mothers and infants, *J Perinat Med* 11:114, 1983.

46. Hervada AR, Feit E, Sagraves R: Drugs in breast milk, *Perinat Care* 2:19, 1978.

47. Hogan RP III: Hemorrhage diathesis caused by drinking an herbal tea, *JAMA* 249:2679, 1983.

48. Huxtable RJ: The myth of beneficent nature: the risks of herbal preparations, *Ann Intern Med* 117:165, 1992.

49. Illingworth RS, Finch E: Ethyl discoumacetate (Tromexan) in human milk, *J Obstet Gynecol Br Empire* 66:487, 1959.

50. Isenberg KE: Excretion of fluoxetine in human breast milk, *J Clin Psychiatry* 51:169, 1990.

51. Ito S, Koren G, Einarson TR: Maternal noncompliance with antibiotics during breastfeeding, *Ann Pharmacother* 27:40, 1993.

52. Jarboe CH, Cook LN, Malesic I et al: Dyphylline elimination kinetics in lactating women: blood to milk transfer, *J Clin Pharmacol* 21:405, 1981.

53. Jensen AA, Slorach SA: *Chemical contaminants in human milk,* Boca Raton, Fla, 1991, CRC.

54. Jones AW: Alcohol in mother's milk, *N Engl J Med* 326:766, 1992.

55. Kafetzis DA, Siapas CA, Georgakopoulos PA et al: Passage of cephalosporins and amoxicillin into breast milk, *Acta Paediatr Scand* 70:285, 1981.

56. Kampmann JP, Johansen K, Hansen JM et al: Propylthiouracil in human milk, *Lancet* 1:736, 1980.

57. Kaneko S, Suzuki K, Sato T et al: The problems of antiepileptic medication during the neonatal period: is breastfeeding advisable? In Janz D, Dam M, Richens A et al, editors: *Epilepsy, pregnancy, and the child,* New York, 1982, Raven.

58. Karjalainen P, Penttilä IM, Pystynen P: The amount and form of radioactivity in human milk after lung scanning, renography and placental localization by ^{131}I labelled traces, *Acta Obstet Gynecol Scand* 50:357, 1971.

59. Kesäniemi YA: Ethanol and acetaldehyde in the milk and peripheral blood of lactating women after ethanol administration, *J Obstet Gynecol Br Commonwealth* 81:84, 1974.

60. Khan AKA, Truelove SC: Placental and mammary transfer of sulphasalazine, *Br Med J* 2:1533, 1979.

61. Kimbrough RD: Consumption of fish: benefits and perceived risk, *J Toxicol Environ Health* 33:81, 1991.

62. Klein EB, Byrne T, Cooper LZ: Neonatal rubella in a breast-fed infant after postpartum maternal infection, *J Pediatr* 97:774, 1980.

63. Koren G, Randor S, Martin S et al: Maternal ginseng use associated with neonatal androgenization, *JAMA* 264:2866, 1990.

64. Kreek MJ: Methadone disposition during the perinatal period in humans, *Pharmacol Biochem Behav* 11:7, 1979.

65. Kreek MJ, Schecter A, Gutjahr CL et al: Analyses of methadone and other drugs in maternal and neonatal body fluids: use in evaluation of symptoms in a neonate of mother maintained on methadone, *Am J Drug Alcohol Abuse* 1:409, 1974.

66. Kuhnz W, Koch S, Helge H et al: Primidone and phenobarbital during lactation period in epileptic women: total and free drug serum levels in the nursed infants and their effects on neonatal behavior, *Dev Pharmacol Ther* 11:147, 1988.

67. Landes RD, Bass JW, Millunchick EW et al: Neonatal rubella following postpartum maternal immunization, *J Pediatr* 97:465, 1980.

68. Larsson B, Slorach SA, Hagman U et al: WHO Collaborative Breastfeeding Study. II. Levels of lead and cadmium in Swedish human milk, 1978-1979, *Acta Paediatr Scand* 70:281, 1981.

69. Lawrence RA, Friedman LR: Drugs and contaminants in human milk. In Jensen RG, editor: *Handbook of milk composition,* San Diego, 1995, Academic Press.

70. *Lawrence review of natural products,* St Louis, 1996, Facts and Comparisons.

71. Lawton ME: Alcohol in breast milk, *Aust NZ J Obstet Gynaecol* 25:71, 1985.

72. Lester BM, Cucca J, Andreozzi L et al: Possible association between fluoxetine hydrochloride and colic in an infant, *J Am Acad Child Adolesc Psychiatry* 32:1253, 1993.

73. Levitan AA, Manion JC: Propranolol therapy during pregnancy and lactation, *Am J Cardiol* 32:247, 1973.

74. Lie B, Jurel J: Effect of epidural versus general anesthesia on breastfeeding, *Acta Obstet Gynaecol Scand* 67:207, 1988.

75. Liedholm H, Melander A, Bitzen PO et al: Accumulation of atenolol and metoprolol in human breast milk, *Eur J Clin Pharmacol* 20:229, 1981.

76. Linde K, Ramirez G, Mulrow CD et al: St. John's wort for depression: an overview and meta-analysis of randomised clinical trials, *Br Med J* 313:253, 1996.

77. Little RE, Anderson KW, Ervin CH et al: Maternal alcohol use during breastfeeding and infant mental and motor development at one year, *N Engl J Med* 321:425, 1989.

78. Losonsky GA, Fishaut JM, Strussenberg J et al: Effect of immunization against rubella on lactation products. I. Development and characterization of specific immunologic reactivity in breast milk, *J Infect Dis* 145:654, 1982.

79. Losonsky GA, Fishaut JM, Strussenberg J et al: Effect of immunization against rubella on lactation products. II. Maternal-neonatal interactions, *J Infect Dis* 145:661, 1982.

80. Loughnan PM: Digoxin excretion in human breast milk, *J Pediatr* 92:1019, 1978.

81. Marsh DO, Clarkson TW, Cox C et al: Fetal methyl mercury poisoning, *Arch Neurol* 44:1017, 1987.

82. Marsh DO, Clarkson TW, Myers GJ et al: Seychelles study of fetal methylmercury exposure and child development: introduction, *Neurotoxicology* 16(4):583, 1995.

83. Matheson I, Kristensen K, Lunde PKM: Drug utilization in breastfeeding women: a survey in Oslo, *Eur J Clin Pharmacol* 38:453, 1990.

84. McKenna R, Cole ER, Vasan U: Is warfarin sodium contraindicated in the lactating mother? *J Pediatr* 103:325, 1983.

85. *Medical Letter on Drugs and Therapeutics,* St. John's wort, 36(1014):107, 1997.

86. Mennella JA, Beauchamp GK: The transfer of alcohol to human milk, *N Engl J Med* 325:981, 1991.

87. Mennella JA, Gerrish CJ: Effects of exposure to alcohol in mother's milk on infant sleep, *Pediatrics* 101:e2, 1998.

88. Miller ME, Cohn RD, Burghart PH: Hydrochlorothiazide deposition in a mother and her breast-fed infant, *J Pediatr* 101:789, 1982.

89. Misri S, Sivertz K: Tricyclic drugs in pregnancy and lactation: a preliminary report, *Int J Psychiatry Med* 21:157, 1991.

90. Mofenson HC, Caraccio TR: Drugs, breast milk and infants, *Pediatr Ther Toxicol* 2(suppl):S1, 1988.

91. Mortola JF: The use of psychotropic agents in pregnancy and lactation, *Psychiatr Clin North Am* 12:69, 1989.

92. Morton SC, Williams MS, Keeler EB et al: Effect of epidural analgesia for labor on the cesarean delivery rate, *Obstet Gynecol* 83:1045, 1994.

93. Mulley BA, Parr GA, Pau WK et al: Placental transfer of chlorthalidone and its elimination in maternal milk, *Eur J Clin Pharmacol* 13:129, 1978.

94. Nation RL, Hotham N: Drugs and breastfeeding, *Med J Aust* 146:308, 1987.

95. Nau H, Rating D, Hauser I et al: Placental transfer at birth and postnatal elimination of primidone and metabolites in neonates of epileptic mothers. In Janz D, Dam M, Richens A et al, editors: *Epilepsy, pregnancy , and the child,* New York, 1982, Raven.

96. Nau H, Rating D, Koch S et al: Valproic acid and its metabolites: placental transfer, neonatal pharmacokinetics, transfer via mother's milk and clinical status in neonates of epileptic mothers, *J Pharmacol Exp Ther* 219:768, 1981.

97. Neuvonen PJ, Kivistö KT: The clinical significance of food-drug interactions: a review, *Med J Aust* 150:36, 1989.

98. Nissen E, Matthiesen LG, Ransjo-Arvidsson A-S et al: Effects of maternal pethidine on infant's developing breastfeeding behavior, *Acta Paediatr* 84:140, 1995.

99. O'Brien TE: Excretion of drugs in human milk, *Am J Hosp Pharm* 31:844, 1974.

100. Ong CN, Phoon WO, Law HY et al: Concentrations of lead in maternal blood, cord blood and breast milk, *Arch Dis Child* 60:756, 1985.

101. Orme ML, Lewis PJ, DeSwiet M et al: May mothers given warfarin breast-feed their infants? *Br Med J* I:1564, 1977.

102. Peterson RG, Bowes WA Jr: Drugs, toxins and environmental agents in breast milk. In Neville MC, Neifert MR, editors: *Lactation, physiology, nutrition, and breastfeeding,* New York, 1983, Plenum.

103. Pokela M-L, Olkkola KT, Koivisto M et al: Pharmacokinetics and pharmacodynamics of intravenous meperidine in neonates and infants, *Clin Pharmacol Ther* 52:342, 1992.

104. Pond SM, Kreek MJ, Tong TG: Altered methadone pharmacokinetics in methadone-maintained pregnant women, *J Pharmacol Exp Ther* 233:1, 1985.

105. Ramin SM, Gambling DR, Lucas MJ et al: Randomized trial of epidural versus intravenous analgesia during labor, *Obstet Gynecol* 86:783, 1995.

106. Rasmussen F: Mammary excretion of benzyl penicillin, erythromycin and penethamate hydriodide, *Acta Pharmacol Toxicol (Kbh)* 16:194, 1959.

107. Rasmussen F: Mammary excretion of antipyrine ethanol and urea, *Acta Vet Scand* 2:151, 1961.

108. Rating D, Jäger-Roman E, Koch S et al: Enzyme induction in neonates due to antiepileptic therapy during pregnancy. In Janz D, Dam M, Richens A et al, editors: *Epilepsy, pregnancy, and the child,* New York, 1982, Raven.

109. Ridker PM: Toxic effects of herbal teas, *Arch Environ Health* 42:133, 1987.

110. Righard L, Alade MO: Effect of delivery room routines on success of first breast-feed, *Lancet* 336(8723):1105, 1990.

111. Rivera-Calimlim L: The significance of drugs in breast milk, *Clin Perinatol* 14:51, 1987.

112. Rogan WJ: Pollutants in breast milk, *Arch Pediatr Adolesc Med* 150:981, 1997.

113. Rogan WJ, Bagniewska A, Damstra T: Pollutants in breast milk, *N Engl J Med* 302:1450, 1980.

114. Rogan WJ, Gladen B: Monitoring breast milk contamination to detect hazards from waste disposal, *Environ Health Perspect* 48:87, 1983.

115. Rosti L, Nardini A, Bettinelli ME et al: Toxic effects of an herbal tea mixture in two newborns, *Acta Paediatr* 83:683, 1994.

116. Rubow SM, Ellmann A, LeRoux J et al: Excretion of technetium ^{99}m hexakis methoxyisobutyl isonitrile in milk, *Eur J Nucl Med* 18:363, 1991.

117. Sangalli BC: The hazard (potential hazard) with transdermal drug delivery systems (TDDS), A.K.A. drug patches, *Hudson Valley Poison Center Toxicol Newslett* 2:1, 1992.

118. Sannerstedt R, Berglund F, Flodh H et al: Medication during pregnancy and breastfeeding: a new Swedish system for classifying drugs, *Int J Clin Pharmacol Ther Toxicol* 18:45, 1980.

119. Schou M: Lithium treatment during pregnancy, delivery and lactation: an update, *J Clin Psychiatry* 51:410, 1990.

120. Schou M, Amdisen A: Lithium and pregnancy. III. Lithium ingestion and children breastfed by women on lithium treatment, *Br Med J* 2:138, 1973.

121. Segelman AB, Segelman FP, Karliner J et al: Sassafras and herb tea, *JAMA* 236:477, 1976.

122. Siegel RK: Herbal intoxication: psychoactive effects from herbal cigarettes, tea and capsules, *JAMA* 236:473, 1976.

123. Sietsema WK: The absolute oral bioavailability of selected drugs, *Int J Clin Pharmacol Ther Toxicol* 27:179, 1989.

124. Sim MR, McNeil JJ: Monitoring chemical exposure using breastmilk: a methodological review, *Am J Epidemiol* 136:1, 1992.

125. Smialek JE, Monforte JR, Aronow R et al: Methadone deaths in children, *JAMA* 238:2516, 1977.

126. Smith MT, Livingstone I, Hooper WD et al: Propranolol, propranolol glucuronide, and naphthoxylactic acid in breast milk and plasma, *Ther Drug Monit* 5:87, 1983.

127. Somogyi A, Gugler R: Cimetidine excretion into breast milk, *Br J Clin Pharmacol* 7:627, 1979.

128. Stec GP, Greenberger P, Ruo TI et al: Kinetics of theophylline transfer to breast milk, *Clin Pharmacol Ther* 28:404, 1980.

129. Steen B, Rane A, Lonnerholm G et al: Phenytoin excretion in human breast milk and plasma in nursed infants, *Ther Drug Monit* 4:331, 1982.

130. Stephens RD, Rappe C, Hayward DG et al: World Health Organization International Intercalibration Study on dioxins and furans in human milk and blood, *Anal Chem* 104:3109, 1992.

131. Stuart M, editor: *The encyclopedia of herbs and herbalism,* New York, 1979, Crescent.

132. Subramanian MG, Chen XG, Bergeski BA: Pattern and duration of the inhibitory effect of alcohol administered acutely on suckling-induced prolactin in lactating rats, *Clin Exp Res* 14:771, 1990.

133. Tegler L, Lindström B: Antithyroid drugs in milk, *Lancet* 2:591, 1980.

134. Tellier L, Aronson RA: Lead in breast milk: should mothers be routinely screened? *Wis Med J* 71:257, 1994.

135. Thorley V: *Breastfeed Rev* 4:82, 1996 (letter).

136. Townsend RJ, Benedetti TJ, Erickson SH et al: A study to evaluate the passage of ibuprofen into breast milk, *Drug Intell Clin Pharm* 16:482, 1982.

137. Townsend RJ, Benedetti TJ, Erickson SH et al: Excretion of ibuprofen into breast milk, *Am J Obstet Gynecol* 149:184, 1984.

138. Tyler VE: *The new honest herbal,* Philadelphia, 1987, Stickley.

139. Weitz JI: Low-molecular-weight heparins, *N Engl J Med* 337:688, 1997.

140. Wennberg RP, Rasmussen LF, Ahlors CE: Displacement of bilirubin from human albumin by three diuretics, *J Pediatr* 90:647, 1977.

141. Werthmann MW, Krees SV: Excretion of chlorothiazide in human breast milk, *J Pediatr* 81:781, 1972.

142. Wickizer TM, Brilliant LB: Testing for polychlorinated biphenyls in human milk, *Pediatrics* 68:411, 1981.

143. Wilson JT: *Drugs in breast milk,* Balgowlah, Australia, 1981, ADIS.

144. Wilson JT: Determinants and consequences of drug excretion in breast milk, *Drug Metab Rev* 14:619, 1983.

145. Wilson JT, Brown RD, Hinson JL et al: Pharmacokinetic pitfalls in the estimation of the breast milk/plasma ratio for drugs, *Annu Rev Pharmacol Toxicol* 25:667, 1985.

146. Wischnik A, Manth SM, Lloyd J et al: The excretion of ketorolac tromethamine into breast milk after multiple oral dosing, *Eur J Clin Pharmacol* 36:521, 1989.

147. Wolff MS: Occupationally derived chemicals in breast milk, *Am J Ind Med* 4:259, 1983.

148. Wright P: Learning experiences in feeding behaviour during infancy, *J Psychosom Res* 32:613, 1988.

149. Yoshida K, Smith B, Craggs M et al: Investigation of pharmacokinetics and of possible adverse effects in infants exposed to tricyclic antidepressants in breast-milk, *J Affect Disord* 43:225, 1997.

150. Young TE, Mangum OB: Neofax A. In *Manual of drugs used in neonatal care,* ed 10, Raleigh, NC, 1997, Acorn.

151. Yurchak AM, Jusko WJ: Theophylline secreted into breast milk, *Pediatrics* 57:518, 1976.

152. Zhou H-H, Adedoyin A, Wilkinson GR: Differences in plasma binding of drugs between Caucasians and Chinese subjects, *Clin Pharmacol Ther* 48:10, 1990.

153. Zoric-Hahn M, Fulconis F, Minoli I et al: Antibody responses to parenteral and oral vaccines are impaired by conventional and low protein formulas as compared to breast-feeding, *Acta Paediatr Scand* 79:1137, 1990.

$\mathcal{N}$ormal growth, failure to thrive, and obesity in the breastfed infant

NORMAL GROWTH

The growth of exclusively breastfed infants has become the focus of much interest among pediatricians, researchers, and nutritionists. A number of long-range follow-up studies have been initiated to address the issues of growth during the critical first year of life, when brain growth is greater than it ever will be again in postnatal life. An interest in height and weight increments and ratios is only part of the concern about obesity and the long-range issues of adiposity. Does breastfeeding protect against adult obesity? Does human milk protect against cholesterol "intolerance" in adult life? The questions are clear, but the answers are not unless one assumes the teleologic approach: human milk is ideal for the human infant with its low protein, controlled calories, and persistent unchangeable cholesterol.

The question is actually, Is it safe to overfeed an infant with formula? Is it safe to deprive an infant of cholesterol during a period of critical brain growth when brain growth depends on cholesterol? When infants are deprived of cholesterol in early infancy, are they less able to tolerate it later?

Antiquated data and anthropometric standards have led to the belief that the growth curves and tables of normal height and weight do not reflect the growth of most healthy, well-fed breastfeeding infants.[85] Reliability of weight gain as a measure of growth has developed because it is a measurement easily obtained.[77] Measurement of length, however, is considered a better standard.[90] Weight gain and linear growth are not always correlated. Furthermore, during infancy and childhood the lower leg grows at a higher rate than the rest of the body. Knee-heel length expressed as a percentage of total length increases with age: 25% at birth, 27% at 12 months, and 31% in adult life. During several decades of formula feeding, "normal" growth curves were developed based only on formula-fed infants. Furthermore, whole cow's milk is fortunately almost totally abandoned, and the recommendations for introduction of solid food beyond 4 or even 6 months have been universally adopted by nutrition-conscious physicians and parents. New growth curves are being developed based on breastfed or formula-fed infants on delayed solids.

Bottle-fed infants gain more rapidly in weight and length during the first months of life than do breastfed infants.[28] Therefore evaluating an infant's physical growth by standards set by bottle-fed infants predisposes one to the diagnosis of failure to thrive. Fomon et al[36] reported a longitudinal study of breastfed and bottle-fed infants during the first few months of life that demonstrated the tenth and ninetieth percentile values for weight and length of the two groups were similar at birth, and the tenth percentile values of the two groups were similar at age 112 days. The significant difference was in the values for the ninetieth percentile. Bottle-fed infants were above this percentile in substantially greater numbers. These differences were attributed to caloric intake rather than the difference in composition of the diet. Fomon et al[36] have shown that the bottle-fed infant not only gains more in weight and length, but also gains more weight for a unit of length. This reflects the overfeeding of the bottle-fed infants. Whether this contributes to subsequent obesity is an important issue.

Most studies of growth in breastfed infants have been plagued with the problem of variation in supplementation and the occurrence of partial weaning. The growth of the exclusively breastfed infant was investigated in 1980 by Ahn and MacLean,[1] who conducted a retrospective study of enthusiastic and successful La Leche League mothers and their infants in the Baltimore–Washington, DC, area. Mothers who had exclusively breastfed for 6 months or longer were randomly selected, and all agreed to participate. They were educated, middle-income, married women. Growth records were obtained from the mothers and from their pediatricians' records. The weight and length curves of these infants remained above the National Center for Health Statistics (NCHS) fiftieth percentile through at least the sixth month.[85] In those infants who were exclusively breastfed longer, all were above the twenty-fifth percentile through the ninth and tenth months of life. Vitamin and mineral supplements were taken by 75% of all mothers and given to 35% of the infants. This study does demonstrate that under optimal circumstances, exclusive breastfeeding does support growth in the first 6 months or longer that matches norms set by formula-fed infants.

When the growth of healthy, exclusively breastfed infants was evaluated in the first 6 months of life in Australia, the weight increments in the first 3 months compared favorably with standards from the Ministry of Health in Great Britain.[52] The weight increment for the second 3 months was significantly less. The data from Great Britain have been accumulated from a mixed sample of breastfed and bottle-fed infants in the 1950s, when most infants were fed cow's milk with a high solute load.

The growth pattern of full-term infants in the United States followed prospectively from birth showed no significant differences in mean growth measurements (weight, crown-rump length, head circumference, skinfold thickness) between infants fully breastfed and those fed whey-predominant formula. Plasma amino acid concentrations, including those for taurine, were similar at 3 days and 2, 8, and 16 weeks of age in both groups.[104]

The effects on growth of specific protein and energy intake in 4- to 6-month-old infants who were either breastfed or formula-fed with high and low protein were measured by Axelsson et al.[4] No significant differences were found in the growth rate of crown-heel length and head circumference or weight gain. The authors concluded that the differences in protein intake between breastfed and formula-fed infants without differences in growth indicate that the formulas may provide a protein intake in excess of the needs. When milk intake and growth in 45 exclusively breastfed infants were carefully documented in the first 4 months by Butte et al,[12] energy and protein intakes were substantially less than current nutrient allowances. Infant growth progressed satisfactorily when compared with NCHS standards, despite that energy dropped from 110 ± 24 kcal/kg/day at 1 month to 71 ± 17 kcal/kg/day at 4 months.[12] Similarly, protein intake decreased from 1.6 ± 0.3 g/kg/day at 1 month to 0.9 ± 0.2 g/kg/day at 4 months. Axelsson et al[4] urge reevaluation of protein and energy requirements as they are currently set.

Weight-for-length and weight gain were significantly correlated with total energy intake but not with activity level during the first 6 months of life in breastfed infants studied by Dewey et al.[22-24,27] Energy intake was considerably lower than recommended, 85 to 89 kcal/kg/day, when compared with the 115 kcal/kg/day recommended dietary allowances (RDAs) of the National Academy of Sciences in 1980.[17] Those infants who consumed the most breast milk became the fattest.

The physical growth of normal, healthy, breast-fed and formula-fed infants from birth to 2 years was reported by Czajka-Narins and Jung[19] at a university hospital in the Midwest. Although breastfed males were lighter at 6 and 12 months, at 24 months the differences were not significant. Using height-to-weight indices, fewer infants who were breastfed longer were categorized as obese. These data suggest that longer breastfeeding affects weight but not length. Pomerance[94] followed 128 breastfed and 3084 formula-fed infants from birth through infancy and again from 3 to 12 years. A comparison of the two groups, both given additional foods with similar timing, revealed no significant differences in growth velocity for weight or for length/height, either during the first 3 years or from age 3 to age 12.

When patterns of growth are examined in the infants of marginally nourished mothers, weight gain is comparable to a reference population but does not permit recovery of weight differential at birth, which was significantly small for gestational age.[10] The intakes of energy and protein by individual infants were reflected in their weight gain but were below internationally recommended norms. Maternal milk alone, when produced in sufficient amounts, can maintain normal growth up to the sixth month of life. Exclusive breastfeeding in Chilean infants of low-middle and low socio-economic families produced the highest weight gain and practically no illness or hospitalization.[59]

In the Copenhagen Cohort Study, exclusively breastfed term infants had a mean intake of 781 and 855 ml/24 hours at 2 and 4 months, respectively.[78] The median fat concentration of human milk was 39.2 g/L and was positively associated with maternal weight gain during pregnancy. This supports the concept that maternal fat stores laid down during pregnancy are easier to mobilize during lactation than other fat stores. This may limit milk fat when pregnancy fat stores are exhausted.

The effect of prolonged breastfeeding on growth has been an issue of concern, especially in developing countries.[38] In a review of 13 studies, Grummer-Strawn[43] pointed out that eight reported a negative relationship, two had a positive relationship, and three had mixed results. Grummer-Strawn identified the flaws in study design and suggested that until better information is available, women should nurse as long as possible because the benefits to infant health exceed the risks in these geographic areas. Pomerance[94] studied a breastfed and formula-fed group of infants who were given solids at 6 months. No significant difference was found in growth velocity for weight or length/height, either during the first 3 years or during the period from 3 to 12 years.

While recognizing the importance of genetic, metabolic, and environmental influences in producing significant differences in growth patterns, Barness[6] suggests that recommendations for nutrition of healthy neonates may be too high for some and too low for others. However, the benchmark for nutritional requirements of the full-term infant remains milk from the infant's healthy, well-nourished mother. Dietary energy intakes are substantially lower than most recommendations, according to Whitehead and Paul[107] and Whitehead et al,[108] who reviewed infant-feeding practices. Both studies indicate that diet-related growth faltering in breastfed infants rarely occurs in developing countries until later than would be suggested by growth standards currently in use.

Gain in physical growth is not as critical as gain in brain growth, but measurements of brain growth are only indirectly implied from growth of the head. In evaluating any infant's progress, head circumference is an important consideration, especially in the first year of life. Deceleration in the rate of increase in head circumference occurs over the first year. The head circumference increases about 7.5 cm (3 inches) in the first year of life and another 7.5 cm in the next 16 years of life. When growth failure includes failure of head growth, the failure is severe. However, many other factors independent of body growth influence head growth.

A weight loss of 5% is usually accepted as the

norm for bottle-fed infants in the first week of life, although information in pediatric textbooks is meager.[93] A loss of 7% is average for breastfed infants, but when this occurs in the first 72 hours of life, the clinician should be alert to breastfeeding problems and review the process. A loss of 10% is maximum for a breastfed infant. The clinician should confirm that positioning and latch-on are correct and that the breasts have responded with some engorgement and milk production. The mother-infant dyad with this problem will need close observation and support. Referral to a lactation consultant may be appropriate if the pediatric office does not have a trained staff member available (nurse practitioner with lactation training).

Initially after birth, the normal infant loses 5% of body weight before starting to gain, whether breastfed or bottle-fed. In a study of infants at the University of Rochester, breastfed infants who were given added water or added formula to force fluids in the first few days of life lost more weight and were less likely to start gaining by the fourth day than infants who were exclusively breastfed or who were bottle-fed.

The time at which an infant regains birthweight is equally unclear. In their extensive study of breastfed and formula-fed infants, Nelson et al[88] summarize weight at 8 days for 1139 infants by stating, "Most formula fed but not most breastfed infants have exceeded their birth weights by age 8 days." They also report that gains in weight and length were greater by males than by females in the age intervals of 8 to 42 days, 42 to 112 days, and 8 to 112 days. These authors provide weights and lengths for the critical first 112 days. These data and the gains in grams/day are provided in Appendix J. The mean values are provided in Tables 12-1 and 12-2.

According to the NCHS, birthweight is doubled between the 50th and 75th percentiles at 4 months of age and tripled at 12 months.[47] When doubling and tripling times were studied by type of feeding as well as birthweight, gender, and race by Czajka-Narins and Jung,[19] they concurred with doubling time but found tripling time to be 412 days for black males and 484 days for white females, with no significant difference between breast or bottle feeders. They found obese infants with higher weight/length ratios tripled their weight sooner, suggesting that rapid tripling time may be an indicator of obesity. Black infants in general doubled and tripled their weights sooner, but more blacks were bottle-fed in this study.[19]

Growth charts for breastfed infants

Dewey et al[22-24,27] have suggested that new, separate growth charts are needed for breastfed infants. The DARLING (Davis Area Research on Lactation, Infant Nutrition, and Growth) Study collected data prospectively on growth patterns, nutrient intake, morbidity, and activity levels of matched cohorts of infants who were either exclusively breastfed or bottle-fed during the first 12 months of life. Measurements were followed beyond 12 months to 18, 21, 24, and 36 months as well. Growth in length and head circumference did not differ significantly between the two groups; however, weight gain was slower among breastfed infants after about 3 months of age. These weight gain differences continued even after solid foods were added at 6 months in both groups. Breastfed infants were leaner than their counterparts. The slower growth rates and lower energy intake of the breastfed infants were associated with normal or accelerated development and less morbidity from infectious illnesses. The authors[22,23] concluded that it is normal for breastfed infants to gain at this pace, which is less rapid than that indicated by the scales developed for bottle-fed infants.

When the growth patterns of a large sample of breastfed infants were pooled from the United States, Canada, and Europe, Dewey et al[21] reported that results were consistent across studies. Breastfed infants grew more rapidly in weight during the first 2 months and less rapidly during 3 to 12 months. Head circumference was well above the World Health Organization/Centers for Disease Control and Prevention (WHO/CDC) median throughout the first year. Length for age did

TABLE 12-1   **Weights and lengths of breastfed and formula-fed infants at selected ages**

	Feeding							
	Breastfed				Formula-fed			
	203 males		216 females		380 males		340 females	
Age (days)	Mean	SD	Mean	SD	Mean	SD	Mean	SD
Weight (g)								
8	3457	425	3355	406	3585	437	3396	387
14	3660	434	3545	413	3790	438	3575	390
28	4245	493	4058	453	4393	460	4081	396
42	4780	524	4504	496	4940	487	4529	430
56	5237	562	4879	534	5426	526	4935	461
84	5956	622	5512	593	6248	597	5642	536
112	6559	677	6085	661	6920	685	6262	607
Length (mm)								
8	512	18	506	17	514	18	504	17
14	521	18	515	17	523	18	513	17
28	539	18	533	18	542	18	530	17
42	556	18	549	17	559	19	546	17
56	570	18	562	17	576	19	562	17
84	598	19	588	18	605	19	589	18
112	623	20	611	18	631	20	612	18

From Nelson SE, Rogers RR, Ziegler EE et al: *Early Hum Dev* 19:223, 1989.
SD, Standard deviation.

not decline as did the weight for age and weight for length scores as breastfeeding increased in duration.

Since 1983 the reference standard for growth has been the WHO/CDC report *Measuring Change in Nutritional Status.*[111] This report used the anthropometric indications of nutritional status proposed by the WHO working group. When Garza et al[40] reviewed growth patterns of breastfed infants, breastfed infants clearly consumed less energy than recommended by WHO in the second 3-month period by choice and not because the mother could not produce more milk.[112] Dewey and Lönnerdal[25] first pointed this out when they had mothers pump to increase their production, and the infants self-regulated to the original intake measured before the pumping program.[25]

Tables 12-1 and 12-2 provide the growth charts that are currently used as the standard for following breastfed infants. Close monitoring of length measurements, which should match the current growth charts, is one important parameter.

Impact of weaning foods on growth

The timing of initiation of weaning foods before 6 months of age has shown that as energy intake increases from solid foods, energy intake from breast milk decreases. The downward trend of weight/age and weight/length ratio continues with the addition of solids, which would not be expected if growth faltering were the basis for the decline.[40] Breastfed infants apparently self-regulate when offered solids and also leave some solids uneaten.

TABLE 12-2   Gains in weight and length during selected age intervals in relation to gender and type of feeding

	Feeding							
	Breastfed				Formula-fed			
	203 males		216 females		380 males		340 females	
Gain	Mean	SD	Mean	SD	Mean	SD	Mean	SD
Weight (g/day)								
8-42	38.9	9.7	33.8	9.3	39.8	7.7	33.3	7.4
42-112	25.4	6.2	22.6	6.3	28.5	6.4	24.7	5.2
8-112	29.8	5.8	26.2	5.6	32.2	5.6	27.5	4.9
Length (mm/day)								
8-42	1.29	0.22	1.24	0.22	1.33	0.22	1.25	0.19
42-112	0.96	0.17	0.89	0.13	1.03	0.12	0.94	0.11
8-112	1.07	0.12	1.01	0.11	1.13	0.11	1.04	0.09

From Nelson SE, Rogers RR, Ziegler EE et al: *Early Hum Dev* 19:223, 1989.
SD, Standard deviation.

When breastfed infants were given solids between 4 and 7 months, their weight for age and weight for length were consistently lower than those for infants introduced to solids at 8 months or older. Length for age was similar between the two groups.

Does the growth rate of exclusively breastfed infants reflect a need for higher protein?[49] This question has challenged the wisdom of exclusive breastfeeding. A group of exclusively breastfed infants were matched with a second group who received preprepared solid foods, including egg yolk, beginning at 4 months of age.[26] Neither weight gain nor length gain from 4 to 6 months differed between the groups. The solid-food group received 20% higher protein intake as well as higher intakes of iron, zinc, calcium, vitamin A, and riboflavin. The authors concluded that protein intake is not a limiting factor in the growth of breastfed infants.[49]

Similarly, Cohen et al[16] demonstrated that breastfed infants given solids at 4 months self-regulated so that the energy intake and protein intake were the same in both the supplemented group and the unsupplemented group. Furthermore, when Motil et al[82] calculated the gross efficiency of nutrient utilization for each infant in a longitudinal study of breastfed and bottle-fed infants, length and weight gains and lean body mass and body fat accretion during the first 24 weeks of life were similar. The formula-fed infants had received significantly higher nitrogen and energy. The gross efficiency of dietary energy utilization for lean body mass deposition was two times greater in breastfed than bottle-fed infants. No association was found between lean body mass deposition and dietary protein intake. This confirms previous studies that human milk protein does not limit growth.[82]

Prolonged breastfeeding

Considerable controversy surrounds the question of prolonged breastfeeding. Although the value of prolonged breastfeeding has not been challenged in industrialized countries, it has in developing countries. Some studies showed that small, undergrown infants are breastfed longer.[14,57] Careful assessment reveals that larger infants are weaned earlier. A cautious review of available studies suggests that prolonged breastfeeding does not cause malnutrition; rather, the small and undergrown infants are kept at the breast longer. Child size appears to be related to the decision to wean so that, in general, large healthy infants are weaned completely from the breast earlier.[14] Thus smaller infants being breastfed longer is not the cause of the undergrowth.

Catch-up growth in small-for-gestational-age infants

Small-for-gestational-age (SGA) infants have been identified at risk for continued growth failure in extrauterine life, learning difficulties, and behavioral problems. Lucas et al[70] explored by the influence of early nutrition on growth in the first year of life in full-term SGA infants, comparing those receiving breast milk and those receiving formula. This was a subset of a study on early carnitine supplementation. An equal number of breastfed and formula-fed infants received carnitine. Additional demographic, social, clinical, and anthropometric data were collected. Breastfeeding was associated with a greater increase in weight at 2 weeks and 3 months of age, which persisted beyond the actual breastfeeding period. The authors reported greater catch-up growth in head measurement and a greater increase in body length. They suggest that breastfeeding promotes faster catch-up growth, and breastfed infants have the potential for improved catch-up growth in developmental parameters as well.[70]

In a study designed to examine the role of zinc supplementation in catch-up growth in SGA infants, Castillo-Duran et al[13] reported that infants who were exclusively breastfed had increased growth over those who were formula-fed and supplemented with zinc.

Cognitive and motor development

Cognitive development in the first 7 years of life was related to breastfeeding practices of a birth cohort in New Zealand.[32] The researchers took into account maternal intelligence, maternal education, maternal training in child rearing, childhood experiences, family socioeconomic status, birthweight, and gestational age. The breastfed children had slightly higher test scores on the Peabody Picture Vocabulary Test, the 5-year measure on the Stanford Binet Intelligence Scale, and the 7-year measure on the Weschler Child Intelligence Scale. Measures of language development were equally influenced. This very small improvement in scores persisted when all variables were taken into account. The scores were also influenced by length of breastfeeding less than and longer than 4 months.

An additional study on the same birth cohort was done to assess breastfeeding and subsequent social adjustment in 6- to 8-year-old children. Fergusson et al[33] studied prospectively 1024 children who were part of the Christ Church Child Development Study. They used the maternal and teacher ratings of childhood conduct disorders. There was a statistically significant tendency for conduct disorder scores to decline with increasing duration of breastfeeding; that is, breastfed children were less prone to conduct disorders than bottle-fed children. Breastfed children, however, tended to come from slightly more socially advantaged, economically privileged homes that were more stable. The analysis failed to examine early mother-infant interaction patterns.

This cohort of 1000 individuals has now been reported as an 18-year longitudinal study by Horwood and Fergusson.[55] There continued to be a small but detectable increase in child cognitive and educational achievement in the children who had been breastfed as infants. The results were confirmed in standardized tests, teacher ratings, and academic outcomes in high school and young adulthood.

De Andraca and Uauy[20] reviewed the factors in human milk and the breastfeeding process that affect optimal mental and visual development. The complex relationships point to a clear advantage to breastfeeding.

Another group of children was followed in New

Zealand to evaluate the effects of infant feeding, birth order, paternal occupation, and socioeconomic status on speech in 6-year-old children. Controlling for the demographic effects, the association of breastfeeding with clear speech was different for the genders, being negligible for girls and strongly positive for boys.[32]

The relationship of infant-feeding practices and dependent variables to the subsequent cognitive abilities were reported by Young et al[114] from the Yale Harvard Research Project in Tunisia. Within the underprivileged group they found that breastfeeding promoted not only physical growth but also sensory motor development as assessed by Bayley motor and mental scales. There were no great differences in the ability to sit alone or to take first steps, but especially among males in the lower socioeconomic group, there was significant superiority of breastfed infants at 8, 14, and 16 months of age in Bayley mental scales. In this study, all infants were from the same social and intellectual strata.

The question of whether breastfeeding influences a child's developmental outcome has appeared in modern literature since Hoefer and Hardy[53] first reported that breastfed infants were more active and achieved their motor milestones earlier than bottle-fed infants in 1929. These authors described enhanced learning ability and higher intelligence quotient (IQ) scores at 7 to 13 years of age, as well as in children exclusively breastfed for 4 to 9 months. Although socioeconomic status and mother's education were not reported, it is an interesting historic note that it was the well-educated, higher socioeconomic mothers who could afford to bottle-feed in the 1920s and 1930s and into the 1940s. In an attempt to clarify the relationship to maternal status, Taylor and Wadsworth[103] took the negative hypothesis but were unable to eliminate the possibility that breastfeeding had a positive effect on intellectual development. In a national study (England, Scotland, and Wales) of 13,135 children, a positive correlation was found between duration of breastfeeding and performance in tests of vocabulary and visuomotor coordination; these behavior scores

remained steady when tested against intervening social and biologic variables.

The advantage of human milk for at-risk infants has been investigated by Lucas et al,[71,72] who raised public awareness when their results were reported in newspapers internationally in 1992. The initial cohort of 771 infants whose birthweight was less than 1850 g were given their mother's milk; these infants had a mean 8-point advantage on the Bayley Mental Developmental Index over infants of mothers choosing not to do so.[71] Both groups received nutrition by feeding tube for the first month of life. A 4.3-point advantage remained when outcome was adjusted for demographic and perinatal factors. The same advantage was found using an IQ equivalent test, which is a fundamentally different test. The same group of infants was tested regularly, and results at age 7½ to 8 years showed a 10-point advantage in IQ testing even when controlled for maternal social class and education.[113]

This report precipitated a torrent of responses from other investigators,[56,80,91] who provided support for and against the conclusion that breast milk is effective in improving the outcome of high-risk infants.

Breastfeeding and cognitive development were studied prospectively between 1978 and 1982 by Rogan and Gladen.[98] They followed 788 children longitudinally through early school. There were small but statistically significant increases in scores on the Bayley and McCarthy tests among breastfed infants at all times. The infants were 95% white and all came from similar middle-class families, so the study population was a homogeneous one. There were higher scores with increasing length of breastfeeding.

To determine the effect of breastfeeding on optimal visual development, Birch et al[8] studied term and preterm infants fed human milk or corn oil–based formula with no ω-3 essential fatty acids. Visual testing using visual-evoked potential and forced-choice preferential looking activity was performed at 4 months' adjusted age; infants given human milk scored better. This was confirmed at 36 months using random dot stereo acuity and letter-matching ability. Results correlated with a measure of dietary ω-3 sufficiency index from the infants' red blood cells (RBCs) at 4 months.

FAILURE TO THRIVE

Definition

Failure to thrive is actually a symptom and not a diagnosis. The causes of failure to thrive in children have been associated with malfunctions of many organ systems as well as with nutritional, environmental, social, and psychologic factors. Failure to thrive while breastfeeding has often been inappropriately considered in the same terms as failure associated with other sources of nourishment and involving other age groups. Failure to thrive while breastfeeding is a phenomenon associated with the first year of life and more likely under 6 months. Exclusive breastfeeding is appropriate for the first 6 months, and then solids should be added, along with the gradual addition of other liquids by cup after 7 months. Therefore the symptom is no longer exclusively associated with lactation, except in rare cases where the infant is breastfed beyond 9 months with no solids added.

The term *failure to thrive* has been loosely used to describe all infants who show some degree of growth failure. It is a syndromic classification that has been used to describe infants whose gain in weight or length or both fails to occur in a normal progressive fashion. For the breastfed infant, it may be a matter of comparing a slower gainer to the excessive weight-gain patterns of the bottle-fed infant. The definition offered by Fomon[35] states that "failure to thrive [should] be defined as a rate of gain in length and/or weight less than the value corresponding to two standard deviations below the mean during an interval of at least 56 days for infants less than five months of age and during an interval of at least three months for older infants." Fomon further suggests that infants gaining in length and weight at rates less than the tenth percentile values be suspected of failing to thrive.[35] Certainly in managing the breastfed in-

fant, more careful and frequent medical evaluation should be provided for the infant who drops to the tenth percentile for weight, fails to gain weight, or continues to lose after the tenth day of life, rather than waiting for 56 days to establish the trend unquestionably.

In our work in Rochester, NY, the disorder is defined as failure to thrive when the infant continues to lose weight after 10 days of life, does not regain birthweight by 3 weeks of age, or gains at a rate below the tenth percentile for weight gain beyond 1 month of age. Unlike the bottle-fed infant, who can then be placed in the hospital where professionals can feed him, the breastfed infant needs to be evaluated in the home setting, nursing at the breast, unless it is an emergency.

A more serviceable measure of failure to thrive than percentiles is proposed by Frank et al,[39] who suggest the use of a percentage of the median values for the age on the growth chart. Thus normal is greater than 90% of median weight, mild malnutrition is 75% to 90% of median, moderate is 60% to 74% of median, and severe is less than 60% of median weight. Similar percentages are applied to height and weight for height. Thus a 1-month-old infant whose median for age would be 5000 g and who is only 3800 g is 75% of median, or mildly malnourished (Table 12-3).

Human growth has been considered a continuous process, characterized by changing velocity with age. Lampl et al[62] made serial measurements

TABLE 12-3 **Daily weight gain and recommended allowances**		
Age	Median daily weight gain (grams)	Recommended daily allowance (kcal/kg/day)
0-3 mo	26-31	108
3-6 mo	17-18	108
6-9 mo	12-13	98
9-12 mo	9	98

From National Research Council, Food and Nutrition Board, National Academy of Sciences: *Recommended daily allowances,* ed 10, Washington, DC, 1989, US Government Printing Office.

of normal infants weekly, semiweekly, and daily during their first 21 months. They show clearly that growth in length occurs by discontinuous, aperiodic, saltatory spurts. Furthermore, these bursts were 0.5 to 2.5 cm (⅕ to 1 inch) during intervals separated by no measurable change (2 to 63 days duration). The authors suggest that 90% to 95% of normal development during infancy is growth free.[62] Length accretion is distinctly a saltatory process of incremental bursts punctuating background stasis. Thus evaluation of length requires more than one measurement and the careful consideration of an experienced physician familiar with growth parameters.

As more and more women breastfeed, increasing numbers of cases of failure to thrive appear in the literature, although it is a rare phenomenon. No statistical data on incidence rates are available because no large prospective study has been done.[65] Only in extreme cases are infants hospitalized, but the number of these is increasing as well, partly because of a failure to recognize the disorder and refer the infant to medical care promptly.

Diagnosis

The problem of slow or inadequate weight gain has confounded even the physicians most committed to breastfeeding. It should be approached with the same orderly diagnostic process that one uses to attack any medical problem. Thus a complete history, including the details of the breastfeeds, a physical examination of the infant, an examination of the maternal breast, observation of the feeding, and appropriate laboratory work are indicated. Organizing the data amassed by this process will help identify the facts that do appear under maternal and infant causes separately.

Slow gaining versus failure to thrive

Some helpful distinctions exist between the breastfed infant who is slow to gain weight and the infant who is failing to thrive while breastfeeding.[63,64] These parameters should be included in the routine "well baby" evaluation of all breastfed infants, beginning with the first visit (Table 12-4). With early discharge often occurring less than 48 hours after birth, the first visit may need to be within 48 hours of discharge from the hospital, depending on the infant's gestational age, weight loss before discharge, a history of jaundice, and the mother's experience. The pediatric office or clinic should have a fail-safe system of follow-up for all newborns that includes access by telephone. In the absence of a telephone in the home, visiting nurse involvement may be appropriate. Although many hospitals provide breastfeeding warm lines that mothers can call for information and help, the family must make the transition from the birthplace to the primary care provider promptly, especially for parents of a first baby who have no previous office contact.

The feeding pattern of the infant with slow

TABLE 12-4 Parameters for evaluation of breastfed infants	
Infant who is slow to gain weight	Infant with failure to thrive
Alert healthy appearance	Apathetic or crying
Good muscle tone	Poor tone
Good skin turgor	Poor turgor
At least six wet diapers/day	Few wet diapers
Pale, dilute urine	"Strong" urine
Stools frequent, seedy (or if infrequent, large and soft)	Stools infrequent, scanty
Eight or more nursings/day, lasting 15-20 minutes	Fewer than eight feedings, often brief
Well-established let-down reflex	No signs of functioning let-down reflex
Weight gain consistent but slow	Weight erratic; may lose

weight gain is usually frequent feedings with evidence of a good suck. The mother's breasts are full before feeding, and she can describe a let-down during the feeding. There are at least six wet diapers a day, urine is pale and dilute, and stools are loose and seedy. Weight gain is slow but consistent. If the infant is gaining extremely slowly but is alert, bright, and responsive and developing along the appropriate level, the infant is a "slow gainer." In contrast, the infant with true failure to thrive is usually apathetic or weakly crying with poor tone and poor turgor. There are few wet diapers (none is ever soaked) and "strong" urine. Stools are infrequent and scanty. Feedings are often by schedule but always fewer than eight per day and brief. There are no signs of a good let-down reflex. True failure to thrive is potentially serious; early recognition is essential if the integrity of both brain growth and breastfeeding is to be safely preserved.

Although slow gaining may be familial or genetic (small parents), it is always appropriate to be sure the process of breastfeeding is optimized.[11] Attention to adequate fat in the milk is important, especially because mothers have often been encouraged to "switch nurse," that is, switch back and forth between breasts to build up an adequate milk supply. The switch-nursing process interrupts the release of fat and the production of fat-rich hindmilk. If the mother is interrupting the feeding to go to the other side, a period of feeding exclusively on one breast each feeding may change the gaining pattern. If necessary, the level of fat in the milk can be checked by doing a "creamatocrit," comparing milk before and after the timing change (see Chapter 20).

In a schema for classifying failure to thrive at the breast, the causes associated with infant behavior and problems are distinguished from those related to maternal problems (Fig. 12-1). The causes in the infant can be further evaluated by looking at net intake, which may be associated with poor feeding, poor net intake from additional losses, or high energy needs. The maternal causes

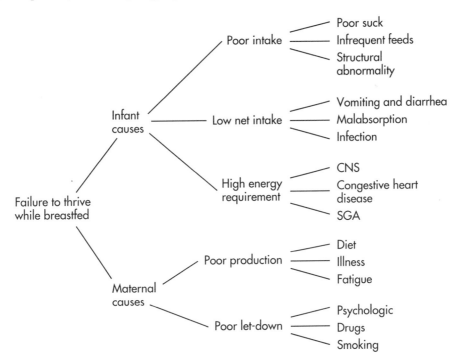

Fig. 12-1. Diagnostic flowchart for failure to thrive.

can be divided into poor production of milk and poor release of milk. When a poor let-down reflex continues long enough, it will eventually cause a decrease in milk production. Several factors may affect the outcome, and thus more than one management change may be indicated.

Evaluation of infant

Examination of the infant should suggest any underlying physical problems, such as hypothyroidism, congenital heart disease, mechanical abnormalities of the mouth (e.g., cleft palate), or major neurologic disturbances.[7] The infant's ability to root, suck, and coordinate swallowing should be observed. There is a greater risk today of missing subtle structural problems because infants spend much of their hospital life out of the newborn nursery away from the watchful eyes of experienced nurses and then are discharged before problems become manifest.

The routine observation of a feeding by the infant's physician should be part of the discharge examination from the hospital. If this is not practical, such an examination should be incorporated into the first office or clinic visit within the first week of life. The focus should be the positioning of the mother and the infant, placement of the mother's hands, and initiation of latch-on (see Chapter 8). A small number of infants will be identified with physical abnormalities that need medical attention (Table 12-5).

Lukefahr[73] identified 38 infants under 6 months of age in a suburban pediatric practice as having failure to thrive while breastfeeding. Only 2 of 28 infants (7.1%) who presented in the first 4 weeks had underlying illnesses (salt-losing adrenogenital syndrome and congenital hypotonia), whereas 5 of the 10 brought in between 1 and 6 months had underlying disease (all of whom actually presented with a problem by 4 months). This report stresses the importance of ruling out underlying disease and the urgency of having the pediatrician evaluate the child when the symptom of poor weight gain is first suspected, thus avoiding the serious complications of dehydration and metabolic disorders that may result when "home remedies" for lactation problems are used.

TABLE 12-5   Conditions associated with or causing disorders of sucking and swallowing

Absent or diminished suck	Mechanical factors interfering with sucking	Disorders of swallowing mechanism (not including esophageal abnormalities)
Maternal anesthesia or analgesia	Macroglossia	Choanal atresia
Anoxia or hypoxia	Cleft lip	Cleft palate
Prematurity	Fusion of gums	Micrognathia
Trisomy 21	Tumors of mouth or gums	Postintubation dysphagia
Trisomy 13-15	Temporomandibular ankylosis or	Palatal paralysis
Hypothyroidism	hypoplasia	Pharyngeal tumors
Neuromuscular abnormalities		Pharyngeal diverticula
Kernicterus		Familial dysautonomia
Werdnig-Hoffmann disease		
Neonatal myasthenia gravis		
Congenital muscular dystrophy		
Central nervous system infections		
Toxoplasmosis		
Cytomegalovirus infection		
Bacterial meningitis		

From Behrman RE, Driscoll JM Jr, Seeds AE, editors: *Neonatal-perinatal medicine: diseases of the fetus and infant,* ed 2, St Louis, 1977, Mosby.

Oral motor problems: feeding skills disorder.
Growth failure secondary to feeding skills disorder is the terminology proposed by Ramsay et al[96] to replace nonorganic failure to thrive (NOFTT). The authors describe a series of children who were referred for NOFTT who had displayed subtle problems since birth. The criteria include early abnormal feeding-related symptoms present shortly after birth, such as impaired oral function, suggesting the infants are minimally neurologically abnormal. Difficulties during earlier stages of feeding development not only may interfere with the development of more mature feeding skills, but also may contribute eventually to difficulties in mother-infant interaction. The common finding among all infants with failure to thrive was underlying feeding-related symptoms that were neurophysiologic but manifest in different degrees of oral sensorimotor (and pharyngeal) impairment. The neurologic impairment may vary from obvious cerebral palsy to symptoms that are inapparent on casual observation, but lead to abnormal feeding-related symptoms in early life. When the mother copes and adapts, the disorder goes unnoticed until solid foods are added. Diagnosis requires oral sensorimotor assessments and a neurologic examination sensitive enough to measure minimal neurologic impairment in an apparently healthy child who is failing to gain. Early history is also critically important.

Small-for-gestational-age infant. The SGA infant will be identified if gestational age and birthweight are scrutinized. This infant is small at birth despite full gestation time in utero. The SGA infant has a large nutritional deficit to make up from intrauterine failure to grow. The cause of the intrauterine problem should be assessed: placental insufficiency, maternal disease, toxemia, heavy smoking, or intrauterine infection such as toxoplasmosis.

SGA infants are difficult to feed initially by any method and often require tube feedings for a few days. Their caloric needs parallel the needs of an infant of appropriate weight for gestation rather than their actual low weight. SGA infants should be placed on frequent feedings, every 2 to 3 hours by day and every 4 hours at night. They should be awakened for feedings if they sleep long periods. If they have not been nursing well, the breast has not been stimulated to produce to its full capability. The mother may need to express milk manually or mechanically pump milk to enhance her production. Her milk may then be given by a passive means such as a tube, a small cup, or the lactation supplementing device, which provides stimulus to the breast while providing the extra calories needed (see Appendix F and Chapter 18).

An infant who is sufficiently starved in utero may have a degree of inanition that prevents active suckling at first, predisposing to further starvation. The successful nursing of an SGA infant may require extended efforts by the mother to ensure adequate growth. Such efforts are well worth the trouble if one considers the impact of intrauterine growth failure on the central nervous system (CNS). It would be to the infant's advantage to have the critical amino acids such as taurine and the lipids of human milk with which to "catch up" brain growth. As noted earlier, SGA infants are more likely to close the growth gap more rapidly if breastfed.

Jaundice. An infant with an elevated bilirubin level from any cause may be depressed and lethargic and therefore may not nurse well. If the infant appears jaundiced, laboratory evaluation to determine the cause and its appropriate treatment should be undertaken. Visible jaundice under 24 hours of age requires a full evaluation and is not related to breastfeeding. When an infant is taken from the breast at 2 or 3 days of age because of jaundice, this interferes with the establishment of lactation at a critical time, especially for a primipara. Management of the jaundiced infant depends on adequate calories and the active passage of stools, which is the means by which the body excretes the bilirubin in meconium.

"Breastfeeding jaundice" does not develop until the infant is 3 or more days old, so other causes must be sought. In addition, care must be taken to help the mother continue to stimulate production with manual expression or pumping to avoid inducing iatrogenic lactation failure. (See Chapter 14 for discussion of hyperbilirubinemia.)

Metabolic screen. Most hospitals provide, often because the law mandates it, screening for metabolic disorders, including galactosemia, phenylketonuria (PKU), maple sugar urine disease, and disorders of metabolism of other amino acids. If these simple screening tests were not performed or their validity is in doubt, they should be done again. Usually the service is available in the state or county laboratory. Thyroid screening for abnormal thyroxine (T_4) and/or thyroid-stimulating hormone (TSH) should also be performed. Mass screening programs for neonatal thyroid disease have identified cases of deficiency that, even in retrospect, show none of the characteristic findings of hypothyroidism in the infant, such as thick coarse features, hoarse cry, slow pulse, macroglossia, umbilical hernia, or jaundice. In the neonate, hypothyroidism is often associated with failure to thrive, if undiagnosed.

Galactosemia. Galactosemia, which is a hereditary disorder of the metabolism of galactose-1-phosphate, is manifest by renal disease and liver dysfunction after ingestion of lactose. The lack of galactose-1-phosphate uridyltransferase activity may be relative or partial. The clinical symptoms may be fulminating, with severe jaundice, hepatosplenomegaly, weight loss, vomiting, and diarrhea, or may be more subtle. Cataracts are not invariably present. In mild cases, failure to thrive may be the presenting symptom. A urine screen for reducing substances (by Clinitest and not just Dextrostix, which will only identify glucose) should be done on all infants who fail to thrive, especially if there is hepatomegaly or jaundice.

The definitive diagnosis is the identification of absence or near absence of galactose-1-phosphate uridyltransferase activity in RBC hemolysates. A urine screen should be considered even though an initial metabolic screen for galactosemia was done on the second or third day of life by hospital routine. The treatment is a lactose-free diet, which would mandate prompt weaning from breast milk to prevent further insult to the liver, kidneys, and brain. This is one of the few indications for prompt weaning from human milk. A formula free of lactose (e.g., Isomil, Nutramigen) is indicated. No

medical indications exist, however, to use a lactose-free formula for a normal breastfeeding infant either to supplement or to wean from breast milk, which contains lactose. (Refer to pediatric texts on neonatal metabolic disorders for a full description of galactosemia; see Chapter 14.)

Vomiting and diarrhea. Vomiting and diarrhea are very unusual in a breastfed infant. Spitting up small amounts of milk after feedings is sometimes observed in otherwise normal infants and is of no consequence if it does not affect overall weight gain. Although pyloric stenosis is reportedly less common in breastfed infants, this phenomenon should be ruled out in any infant who vomits consistently after feeding, has diminished urine and stools, shows no weight gain or actually loses weight, and has reverse peristalsis. Usually these infants do well initially, then the vomiting becomes progressive.

Vomiting may be a presenting symptom for various metabolic disorders. Thus metabolic disorders should be considered in the differential diagnosis. Not all possible metabolic disorders, such as congenital adrenal hyperplasia, are routinely screened. These infants may present with vomiting and weight loss in the first week or two of life or with an acute episode of sepsis. The usual causes of vomiting, as well as the causes peculiar to breast milk, should be considered. Maternal diet should be checked for unusual foods. In families at high risk for allergy, intake by the mother of known family food allergens may cause symptoms in the infant. Diarrhea may be caused by foods in the mother's diet or her use of cathartics such as phenolphthalein.

Chronic infections. Chronic fetal infection in utero, which predisposes an SGA infant to intrauterine growth failure, may continue to cause growth problems in the presence of adequate kilocalories. Chronic viral infections include cytomegalovirus (CMV), hepatitis, acquired immunodeficiency syndrome (AIDS), or other less common viruses (see Chapter 16).

Acute infections. An infant who is not growing well may have an infection in the gastrointestinal tract; therefore the nature of the stools is important.

The urinary tract may be another site of infection not readily identified. If, however, the initial evaluation includes a urinalysis with microscopic evaluation and a white blood cell (WBC) count and differential count, this can usually be ruled out.

High energy requirements. When the metabolic rate of the infant is increased, the weight gain will be diminished or absent. When the infant is hyperactive with a strong startle reflex and sleeps poorly, consideration should be given to stimulants present in the milk as well as to neurologic disorders. When a mother drinks coffee, tea including herbal teas, cola, or other carbonated beverages with added caffeine, the accumulated caffeine may be sufficient to make the infant very irritable and hyperactive. The best treatment is to replace the caffeine-containing beverages (see Chapter 11). Some CNS disorders are associated with hyperactivity. Infants with severe congenital heart disease are constantly exercising to breathe and oxygenate and have greatly increased metabolic rates. For management of these special infants at the breast, see Chapter 14.

Observation of nursing process

In addition to establishing that no obvious physical or metabolic reasons exist for the failure to gain weight, the infant should be observed suckling at the breast. Does the infant get a good grasp and suck vigorously? If not, what interferes? A receding chin, a weak suck, lack of coordination, the breast obstructing breathing, and mouthing of the nipple or other ineffectual sucking techniques are some of the possibilities. If the problem is the suckling process, the infant may need assistance. This cause is more common with infants who have had some experience with bottles or rubber nipples or who use a pacifier. Small or slightly premature infants who were started on bottle feedings have trouble relearning the proper sucking motion with the tongue (see Figs. 8-6 to 8-10).

Bottle feedings and pacifiers may have to be discontinued until the infant is more experienced at the breast. This will require a program of manually expressing milk to soften the areola, having milk at the nipple to entice the infant, and gently offering the nipple and areola well compressed between two fingers. If the infant has a receding chin or a relaxed jaw, it may help to have the mother hold the lower jaw forward by supporting the angle of the jaw with her thumb. The physician should examine the infant carefully to be sure the jaw is not dislocated, especially if a vertex delivery was done in the posterior position ("sunny side up"). The physician can easily move the jaw forward to relocate it.

Positioning infants for the breast so they directly face the breast, straddling the mother's leg in a semiupright position, may work best. This is the position twins may assume when nursing simultaneously when they are 3 to 4 months old. Although it is not recommended routinely, for an infant with a receding chin or a cleft, having the mother lean slightly forward for latch-on may help. She should then bring infant upward as she sits back for the feeding.

It may be necessary to assist both mother and baby. If the infant by 2 weeks of age cannot maintain the breast in the mouth without the mother holding it there, it is an indication of improper suckling. In that situation the infant may need to be repositioned with the ventral surface squarely facing the mother's chest wall, that is, tummy to tummy, and the breast presented by the mother with her hand positioned with thumb on top and fingers below the breast. (See discussion in Chapter 8.)

A good check of adequate let-down is to observe the opposite breast as the baby nurses to see if milk flows. It can also be tested by seeing if milk is flowing when nursing is interrupted abruptly. If there has been a good let-down, milk will continue to flow, at least drop by drop, for a few moments from the breast being suckled. The mother can also be trained to listen for the infant's swallowing. During proper sucking, the masseter muscle is in full view and is contracting visibly and rhythmically. Occasionally, infants do not suck vigorously at the breast but occasionally use rapid shallow sucks called "flutter sucking." These infants can be gradually taught to suck effectively. Correct positioning of the breast directly in the infant's mouth and holding the breast firmly in position with all the fingers under the breast and only the thumb above allow the infant to grasp properly without sucking the tongue or lower lip. Nipple shields make the situation worse and should be avoided.

The most productive part of the diagnostic workup is often observation of the baby at the breast. For this reason, this critical responsibility should not be passed on to others but should be performed personally by the physician.

The five general types of nursing patterns described in Chapter 8 should be kept in mind. If the mother understands that it is acceptable for the infant to drop off to sleep and snack later, she may not hesitate to follow this lead, thus providing a more adequate feeding.

Some infants will not settle down and nurse well if there is too much activity or noise. Some need to be tightly swaddled; others fall asleep and need to be unwrapped and stimulated to provide adequate suckling time. Frequent feedings, using both breasts, may be the answer in some cases. In others, there may be too many ineffective feedings, which are wearing the mother out; a change that lengthens the time between feedings but also lengthens the time at the breast may help. Concentrating on using one breast at a feeding to increase the fat content may be the most effective change.

Nonorganic failure to thrive

In the study of undernutrition in bottle-fed infants and infants beyond the suckling age, terminology has received more attention than the underlying issues. Thus the emphasis has been on "organic" versus "nonorganic" failure to thrive. Unfortunately, the term *nonorganic failure to thrive* (NOFTT) has been equated with a disorder of maternal/infant bonding and has become synonymous with maternal deprivation. *Reactive attachment disorder* has been the term substituted for NOFTT and essentially suggests the mother is guilty until proven innocent. In most cases, utilizing the approach of most "failure-to-thrive" man-

agement teams is rarely appropriate in cases associated with breastfeeding in the early months of life. It is important to have a source of breastfeeding information as well as an expert in failure to thrive.

When an infant does not have an organic disorder that explains the growth failure, the patient is diagnosed as having NOFTT. The typical psychosocial and nutritional pattern reported in NOFTT includes evidence of a chaotic family life, emotional deprivation, and inadequate nutrition, as pointed out by Weston et al.[106] These authors reported four children ages 13 to 19 months with NOFTT who were breastfeeding. They had exclusively breastfed for at least 12 months, reportedly refusing solid foods. Failure to gain was noted at 9 months, followed by weight loss increasing at 12 months. Children were all from middle-class families, and parents had at least high-school educations or more. The children all were first-born and scored "advanced" on the Bayley scales. They were active and alert but difficult to control. They all separated only briefly from their mothers in the clinic and initiated nursing for comfort when anxious. Total dietary energy intakes were below levels for growth. These children were not typical NOFTT in any of their demographics but had missed a critical developmental task of learning to eat. The authors interpreted this as being part of these mothers' need to keep the child close. Treatment included having someone else teach these children to eat solids.

Prolonged exclusive breastfeeding may occasionally result in a unique deficit in the developmental process of eating.[106] Exclusive breastfeeding is not nutritionally adequate in the second half of the first year, especially beyond 12 months, although nursing can safely continue for several years when combined with adequate solids and other fluids.[92]

The syndrome of the breastfed infant in the second 6 months of life, with very frequent breastfeedings, poor intake of complementary foods, and poor growth, has been labeled a manifestation of "vulnerable child syndrome" by O'Connor and

Szekely.[89] These children are described to have good weight gain for 5 to 6 months of age, and by 8 months their weight/height score has decreased dramatically. The intake of solid foods is minimal. These infants refuse solids, aggressively spitting food out. The breastfeeding pattern is usually every 1 to 2 hours during the day and frequently at night. Further investigation revealed numerous household stressors and usually the mother's need to maintain control by breastfeeding.

Parental misconception and health beliefs concerning what constitutes a normal diet for infants has been reported by Pugliese et al[95] as a cause for NOFTT as well. They report seven infants from 7 to 22 months of age with poor weight gain and linear growth who received only 60% to 90% of minimum caloric intake for their age and gender. The parents explained that they wanted to avoid obesity, atherosclerosis, or junk food habits. It has also been shown that parental health beliefs and expectations have led to short stature and delayed puberty in older children.

Maternal causes

Questions about the mother's health, dietary habits, sleep pattern, smoking habits, medication intake, the events that occur during nursing, and the psychosocial atmosphere in the home are an important part of the history (Fig. 12-2).

Fruit juice excess

The custom of excess use of fruit juices in recent decades has replaced the use of water for additional fluids after 6 months of life when the infant is learning to drink from a cup or a straw. The attractive packaging has contributed to this trend. Excessive fruit juice diminishes appetite, resulting in decreased dietary intake of nutrient-dense foods and a decrease in weight gain and ultimately in linear growth. An excess of fruit juice may be a cause of failure to thrive in older infants. Decrease in total high energy intake is combined with malabsorption of fructose and diarrhea from sorbitol, thus compounding the problem.[100]

Anatomic causes

Lactation failure from insufficient glandular development of the breast has been described by Neifert and Seacat[86] and Neifert et al,[87] who report three cases in which the breast tissue was asymmetric. Transillumination confirmed a minimally active gland. One family showed a history of similar failure. All three women benefited psychologically from the diagnosis and chose to continue to breastfeed and supplement. The authors have since

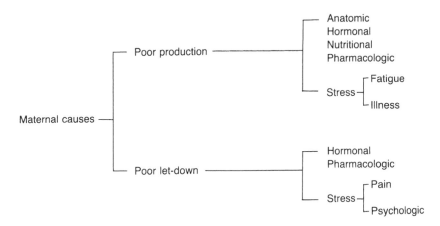

Fig. 12-2. Maternal causes of failure to thrive.

identified 14 more women who had anatomic deficiency but normal prolactin levels and failed to respond to a thorough team approach to lactation support.[86] Retained placenta is also a cause of early lactation failure that is quickly identified by a complete history of postpartum breast change and patterns of lochia that the obstetrician associates with retained tissue (see Chapter 15).

One-breast versus two-breast feeding

After an initial report by Woolridge et al[110] describing an infant whose failure to thrive was traced to inadequate fat intake associated with using both breasts, each feed resulting in low fat (and relatively high lactose by comparison), the debate regarding one or two breasts each feeding has raged. When this infant was fed at one breast per feeding, the low-density feeding changed to high-fat feeding, resulting in decreased stooling and increased weight gain. Since that time the authors[110] have continued to investigate the hypothesis that some women require longer time to release fat into the milk and that limiting the feed to one breast enhances fat content. In some cases this is true, which is further verified by the infant having many loose stools because of the high lactose and considerable gassy discomfort that also resolves with the change to single-breast feeds. No report of reducing substances in the stools has been published.

In early lactation, when milk supply is being established, mothers are encouraged to nurse on both breasts at each feed to provide frequent stimulus. The case report[110] in favor of one breast does not change that recommendation. The clinician, however, should obtain a thorough history of feeding frequency and distribution between breasts, especially when the infant is well hydrated, has many stools, may or may not be fussy, but fails to gain weight, remaining under birth weight for several weeks. The need for higher fat content in the feeding may be a consideration in the slow-gaining baby as well. An adjustment in feeding to enhance the fat content should be tried. Usually limiting each feeding to one breast will do that (see Chapter 8).

Poor milk production

Diets. Although it has been demonstrated that malnourished mothers can produce milk for their infants, marginal diets in Western cultures do affect some mothers' ability to nourish an infant. A case is reported of failure to thrive in a breastfed infant associated with maternal dietary protein and energy restriction.[81] The mother at 8 months postpartum independently reduced her dietary energy to 20 kcal/kg/day and her protein to 0.7 g/kg/day to treat cholecystitis medically and avoid surgery. At 12 months her infant's growth curves had fallen below the fifth percentile in both weight and length, although the infant had been receiving solid foods since 24 weeks of age. The authors concluded the failure to thrive was directly related to severe maternal restriction.[81]

Dietary analysis and maternal anthropometry showed that women who gained adequate weight and skin thickness during pregnancy had increased milk production and weight gain in their infants for the first 6 months of life.[31]

If the mother is restricting intake deliberately or inadvertently, she should be instructed to meet the dietary requirement for lactating women (see Chapter 9). She does not have to drink milk, but the necessary dietary constituents should be in the diet through cheese, eggs, ice cream, or other sources of calcium and protein. It may not be the nutrition itself but the calming effect of a nourishing beverage while breastfeeding that facilitates nursing. Studies of hormones triggered while eating have shown that more milk is produced if a mother eats just before or during breastfeeding. Prescribing brewer's yeast as a dietary supplement has been observed to provide improvement in milk production beyond that accounted for by mere addition of the same nutrients. Some mothers report a feeling of well-being from taking yeast that they do not obtain from taking daily vitamins. Concern has been expressed regarding the effect of increased vitamin B_6 on prolactin production, but doses that suppress lactation are 60 times the therapeutic dose.

Maternal illness. The presence of infection or other illness in the mother may affect milk production, and the cause of the illness should be identified and treated. Urinary tract infection, endometritis, or upper respiratory infection may need treatment with antibiotics. The antibiotic prescribed should be appropriate for the infant as well because it will pass into the milk. Metabolic disorders such as thyroid disease should also be considered. Postpartum hypothyroid disease is increasingly being recognized as screening tests of T_4 and TSH are being done when a mother complains of severe "baby blues" or fatigue. Adequate treatment will result in increased milk supply.

Fatigue. The most common cause of inadequate milk supply is fatigue. Fatigue may be lack of sleep because the infant demands considerable attention at night, but generally it is more subtle. The pressures of the rest of the family for meals or services or the self-inflicted demands of a job, career, or social commitments may be the cause. The mother must be placed on a medically mandated strict rest regimen that is respected by family and friends. In the first month, while lactation is being established, fatigue is devastating to milk production. The infant then becomes hungry more often, cries, and demands more frequent feeding; thus the vicious cycle is established. In later months of lactation, a mother becomes quickly aware of the impact of protracted fatigue on the nursing experience and usually will take steps to increase her rest.

Poor release of milk. Interference with the let-down reflex may cause a well-nourished lactating mother to fail to satisfy her infant. The collecting ducts may be full, but if the let-down or ejection reflex is not triggered, the process will be at a standstill. The infant becomes frustrated and pulls away crying or screaming. Interference with the ejection reflex is predominantly iatrogenic and rarely hormonal (see Fig. 8-17).

Smoking may interfere with the let-down reflex. Mothers should be discouraged from ever smoking in the same room with the infant because of the occurrence of early and frequent respiratory infections in infants of smokers. Smokers are less likely to breastfeed, and if they do choose to breastfeed, they tend to wean earlier because of insufficient milk. Trouble with milk production may be related to the nicotine itself. Extensive studies of smoking mothers have demonstrated a clear relationship between smoking and the amount of milk produced.[54] The infants of these mothers grow more slowly. Avoiding smoking for 2 hours before a feeding will improve the let-down reflex and minimize the amount of nicotine in the milk. Given the value of breastfeeding to the infant, especially in reducing the risk of sudden infant death syndrome (SIDS), it is important that smokers try to reduce the smoke exposure but still breastfeed (see Chapter 15).

Experimentally, *alcohol* has been shown to interfere with oxytocin release in laboratory animals, but the dosage used correlates with moderate to heavy drinking in humans. Studies following the offspring of women who drink heavily have shown some delay in gross motor activity at 1 year using the Bayley developmental scales.[69] Other studies have suggested that alcohol changes the flavor of the milk and that infants nurse less well at a feeding immediately after the mother has had a drink.[66,76] This is contrary to observations over the years in countries where wine and beer are common beverages and are considered galactagogues (see Chapter 11).

The clinician should consider the impact of smoking or alcohol use in the context of reviewing inadequate milk production.

Medications that the mother may be taking should be evaluated. Although L-dopa and ergot preparations are known to inhibit prolactin release, other medications less well identified may have the same effect (see Chapter 11).

The most common cause for the failure of the ejection reflex is *psychologic inhibition.* In a few cases the cause of the psychologic stress may be obvious, such as a husband or mother who openly disapproves of breastfeeding, but in most cases the nursing mother has already considered this possibility and reassures the physician that she is relaxed and calm. It will require carefully assessing the mother's history to "tease out" the source of stress. This is the time when a home visit by the nurse practitioner from the physician's office or an experienced public health nurse will be valuable.

The nurse may observe what is overlooked by the mother: construction of a new building next door, incessant barking from the neighbor's dog, or marital discord. Home observation may lead to the key to the problem.

No obvious cause

Even though no obvious cause for failure to thrive is identified, the treatment may have to include establishing a positive attitude. Jelliffe and Jelliffe[58] have often referred to nursing as a "confidence game." It becomes necessary to instill confidence rather than fear in the mother. Threatening the mother with stopping breastfeeding and switching to formula does not instill confidence. The physician should prescribe a positive plan for number and length of feedings, suggest diet and rest for the mother, and set reachable goals for infant growth.

If the let-down reflex is the crux of the problem and simple adjustments have not changed the ejection quality, oxytocin as a nasal spray (Pitocin) can be prescribed (see Chapters 8 and 18). It is available only by prescription and should be used under the physician's guidance because of possible side effects in some women (e.g., headache, vasoconstriction), although it is not dangerous. Oxytocin nasal spray does not affect the milk or the infant. It is contraindicated only in pregnancy or hypersensitivity.

Seven mothers whose breastfed infants were contented but starving were given metoclopramide (or chlorpromazine in one) in various dosages.[45] Only one mother thought it was not helpful. The authors did not describe how effective appropriate supportive breastfeeding management was and when the medication was started or how long it was maintained. All the infants gained weight, and breastfeeding was continued for 2 to 12 months.

Other authors have reported the recovery of lactation failure and high sodium levels in the milk of mothers taking metoclopramide (10 mg three times a day).[11] Gupta and Gupta[44] report a 67% success rate in those with no milk and 100% recovery in those with an inadequate supply. The effect continued after the drug was discontinued.

Such a medication is useful only when accompanied by appropriate instructions for proper breastfeeding and assistance in using a breast pump for additional stimulus to increase the supply of milk mechanically. A medication should be prescribed only when routine methods fail.

Measurement of prolactin levels is readily available in most laboratories, but the appropriate clinical protocol has not been confirmed by controlled study. Given the information about baseline and response to stimuli (see Chapter 3), it would be advisable to obtain a baseline level, which should be above normal for the laboratory, and a second value after 15 minutes of breastfeeding. Using a heparin lock with venous line placed well before the baseline specimen is drawn and before feeding ensures the least disturbance to lactation. The intrafeeding value should show a significant increase over baseline (twice baseline).

A group of women diagnosed with lactational insufficiency by history were given thyrotropin releasing hormone (TRH).[46] Four received 5 mg every 12 hours for 5 days. There was a consistent 50% increase in prolactin concentrations. Both milk production and let-down were increased. Nine women received 20 mg twice a day, and basal prolactin was significantly elevated. The women all reported subjective and objective increases in breast engorgement and milk let-down, and all returned to full nursing. Two women were given 40 mg TRH daily for 5 days and developed clinical signs of thyrotoxicosis by the seventh day, which disappeared by the tenth day. The investigators[46] had previously given TRH to fully lactating women in a controlled study to demonstrate prolactin response, which did occur within 60 minutes. There was no change in the milk volume or quality in these fully lactating women and no side effects. When Hall and Kay[46] gave 200 μg TRF and followed prolactin and milk production for 6 hours, there were no dramatic changes in milk production, although the prolactin levels rose. There is no indication that the mothers received more than 1 day's dose.

The rare infant who does not respond to management adjustment may have a malabsorption or metabolic disease as yet undiagnosed that will not become overt until formula or cow's milk is introduced. Infants with a strong family history of cystic fibrosis, milk allergy, or malabsorption should have a careful diagnostic workup before abandoning human milk, which may be the most physiologic feeding available for the infant.

Dehydration, hypernatremia, or hypochloremia

A few cases of severe disease have been reported in the literature.* These infants have been hospitalized because of dehydration and evidence of more severe metabolic disturbance. They serve to illustrate the outcome if anticipatory care or palliative home management is unsuccessful. The mothers are usually but not always primiparas, new at breastfeeding and child rearing. When the record is reviewed, one often sees that the early danger signs were present at discharge from the hospital. The mother may have a history of difficult delivery or taking medication for pain that leads to a less vigorous baby and, secondarily, inadequate stimulus for lactation. Supplementary bottles of water or milk are initiated in the hospital instead of directing attention toward the lactation process.

As a precautionary measure, the physician should see all breastfeeding dyads promptly. At this visit, review of the weight, feeding history, number of wet diapers, stool pattern, and physical findings should alert the physician to impending difficulties. Observation of the infant at the breast should be part of the assessment. A problem in monitoring breastfed infants is the use of ultraabsorbent diapers, which makes it impossible to detect the number of voidings or volume of urine passed. No specimen can be wrung from the diaper for specific gravity or other analysis. It is recommended that infants under 2 months not use ultraabsorbent diapers, especially when breastfed, until a better monitoring device is developed. If, on the other hand, the patient is not seen in the office until there is significant dehydration, it is urgent that laboratory studies be obtained, including

*See References 2, 3, 15, 41, 42, 50, 92.

sodium, chloride, potassium, pH, blood urea nitrogen (BUN), and hematocrit (bilirubin when indicated). An assessment of the degree of dehydration should be made based on skin and tissue turgor and tone.

When the breastfed infant has abnormal electrolyte levels, the physician should also obtain levels of sodium, chloride, and potassium from mother's milk, being certain to sample each breast separately. Collecting a few milliliters before and after the feeding and mixing the two samples from a single breast is a good technique. The infant may have occult loss of electrolytes, such as that seen in abnormal renal wasting or retention, cystic fibrosis, hyperaldosteronism, or pseudohyperaldosteronism. The simplest approach is to measure milk electrolytes and infant urine levels to rule out high milk sodium as a cause of the infant's hypernatremia.

In reported cases, infants with hypernatremic failure to thrive are no different at initial presentation from infants with normal sodium levels.[15,64] They may even have a negative neonatal history. At home they develop a poor suck, sleep for long intervals, cry infrequently, and feed infrequently. When observed at the breast, they may be labeled as having a sucking disorder. On examination, however, the lethargy, dehydration, and malnutrition are obvious to the skilled clinician. In the extreme, the infant may have cardiovascular collapse with hypothermia and hypoglycemia. Elevated serum BUN, creatinine, and hematocrit and urinary specific gravity confirm the diagnosis. Hypernatremia has been observed in approximately half the reported cases of severe dehydration in breastfed infants.[97,99] Although milk sodium levels were not reported in all cases, several cases of elevated milk sodium are reported. Sodium, chloride, and lactose are the prime constituents that control the osmolarity of the milk. Because the sodium chloride and lactose have a reciprocal relationship, inadequate lactose production ultimately results in elevated sodium levels.

Elevated sodium in the milk may be a cause or an effect of insufficient milk. When the breast is inadequately stimulated, it begins to involute and produces "weaning milk," which is high in sodium. Milk pumped from nonlactators in the postpartum period has high sodium. On the other hand, maternal sodium intake excesses do not result in elevated sodium levels in the milk.[29] Sodium enters the milk by a controlled mechanism independent of maternal levels in normal women.

Hypernatremic dehydration is an emergency that requires hospitalization.[63,64] The mother should room-in if at all possible. Most pediatric units provide this option. It is preferable to maintain lactation in most cases. The treatment of the illness after the dehydration has been treated with intravenous (IV) fluids depends on the etiology of the hypernatremia. The sodium of the infant's serum and mother's milk should be followed until normal. Increasing maternal milk output with appropriate lactation counseling, including mechanical pumping between feedings to increase volume, usually normalizes the sodium. The oral feedings for the infant should be limited to breastfeeding while the IV fluids are tapered. To provide increased caloric resources to the infant and an appropriate sodium load, the Lact-Aid supplementer (see Chapter 18 and Appendix F) may also be used to stimulate the breast and to avoid bottle feeding and inadequate intake until the breast increases production.

Chloride deficiency has received attention because of a highly publicized formula-manufacturing error. This syndrome is characterized by failure to thrive with anorexia, hypochloremia, and hypokalemic metabolic alkalosis. Chloride deficiency syndrome has also been reported in an infant whose mother had only 2 mEq/L chloride in her milk (normal 8 mEq/L).[50] The mother had successfully nourished her previous five infants. The infant had done well until 3 months of age and then had gradually slipped below the third percentile for weight at 6 months. The infant was severely dehydrated and hypotonic with plasma sodium of 123 mEq/L, chloride of 72 mEq/L, potassium of 2.9 mEq/L, and blood pH of 7.61. There were no abnormal urinary losses. When the breastfeeding infant has clinical dehydration, it is important to check not only the sodium but also the chloride content of the infant's serum and urine and the mother's milk.

Human infants younger than 3 weeks of age do not respond to inappropriate solutions by not suckling. This finding is also observed in studies in other species in which pups continue to suck when the solution is unphysiologic.[9] A natural experiment occurred in a newborn nursery in the 1960s, when six infants died of hypernatremia after receiving many feedings of formula made from salt rather than sugar.[34] The infants who were less than 1 week old did not reject the feedings.

Lactation failure

Occasionally, failure to thrive is actually caused by lactation failure. Historically, sudden complete cessation of lactation was described in the late 1800s after coaching accidents and other great trauma. Advocates of breastfeeding have tended to dismiss this as a possibility and struggle frantically to reverse the situation. Some women who cannot make milk have primary hypoprolactinemia, and others have secondary hypoprolactinemia, as in Sheehan's syndrome (see Chapter 15). Because it is now possible to identify these women by obtaining prolactin levels[105] that confirm the diagnosis, when reasonable efforts at stimulation are ineffective and the mother is unable to do without the Lact-Aid providing almost a full feeding volume, evaluation of the mother is appropriate. Some mothers prefer to discontinue efforts to breastfeed before they have been completely stripped of their egos by total failure.

If one explores the animal literature, one finds no similar situations in other species. Lactation failure in nursing animals is rare because it is not a trait that is transmitted from generation to generation, because the offspring do not survive. Interferences with milk ejection can be identified and treated in other mammals. A syndrome in sows involves agalactia associated with mastitis and metritis.[18] Mammalian lactation failure is attributed to nutritional, pharmacologic, and "emotional stress" causes in animals. Aside from gross dietary deficiency, there is depression or inhibition of the anterior pituitary gland, which is responsible for synthesis in the alveolar cells, and inhibition of transport and discharge of synthesized products from alveolar cells to the lumen. Certain plant alkaloids have been noted in other species to inhibit lactation. Ergot derivatives are best known, but colchicine, vincristine, and vinblastine are also causative. Some plant lectins such as concanavalin interfere with transport and discharge phases of milk production.

Understanding lactation failure is increasing among clinicians as the diagnostic resources expand.[105] Some herbs may inadvertently suppress lactation. A thorough history of herbal use is always appropriate.

MATERNAL AND INFANT OBESITY AND BREASTFEEDING

It is generally recognized that women who breastfeed return to their prepregnancy weight more quickly and in greater numbers than do bottle-feeding mothers.[102] In studies in rats, pregnancy without subsequent lactation results in increased adipose tissue stores and increased fat cell numbers. Studies in humans date back to 1949 and 1952 but do not include relevant variables or the duration and degree of lactation.[79]

When lactation performance was examined, Hilson et al[51] reported that overweight or obese women had less success initiating breastfeeding than their normal-weight counterparts. The rates of discontinuance of exclusive breastfeeding in overweight and obese women were also higher, even when socioeconomic status and maternal education were controlled. The authors conclude that excessive fatness in the reproductive period may inhibit lactational performance.

Discussion of the impact of adiposity is rarely undertaken without including a discussion of cholesterol levels. Obesity and atherosclerosis in developed societies constitute a major public health issue. Does breastfeeding in infancy protect against obesity and atherosclerosis in adult life? This remains an open question. Energy requirements for infants receiving formula have been overestimated.[12] Breastfed infants require and receive 110 kcal/kg/day at 1 month and 70 kcal/day at 4 months. The low energy intakes are not caused by limitations in maternal milk production

as previously assumed but represent physiologically regulated intakes. Breastfed infants deposit less fat than formula-fed infants despite that the two diets appear similar on paper. Although the breastfed infant appears protected against obesity in infancy, the effect appears to be lost after 3 years of age.[48]

A prospective cohort study of 462 healthy full-term infants observed from birth to 12 months was done by Kramer et al.[61] Their goal was to overcome methodologic defects in previous studies of the etiologic determinants of childhood obesity that failed to control for confounding factors. At 6 and 12 months, measurements of height, weight, body mass index (BMI, weight/height^2), and skinfold were taken and correlated with duration of breastfeeding, introduction of solids, and parental heights and weights. Significant determinants of BMI were birthweight, duration of breastfeeding, and introduction of solid foods. Breastfeeding and delayed introduction of solid foods offered some protective effect against obesity at 1 year.

The effect of breastfeeding on plasma cholesterol and weight in young adults was studied longitudinally by Marmot et al[74] in a sample of people born in 1946. The infant-feeding history was obtained. At age 32, women who had been breastfed had significantly lower mean plasma cholesterol than women who had been bottle-fed. The difference for men was smaller, and the breastfed male had higher mean weight and skinfold thickness (Fig. 12-3). Multiple studies, both short- and long-range, with small populations and conflicting results have been reported in humans, although animal studies strongly suggest that species-specific milk makes a difference in obesity and cholesterol.

McGill[75] reviewed dietary cholesterol effects on serum cholesterol and atherosclerosis in humans, as did the report of the Conference on Blood Lipids in Children: Optimal Levels for Early Prevention of Coronary Artery Disease.[109] Indices of fatness and serum cholesterol at age 8 years in relation to feeding and growth during early infancy were reported by Fomon et al[37] from their detailed longitudinal nutrition project involving 469 children born between 1966 and 1971. In infancy the

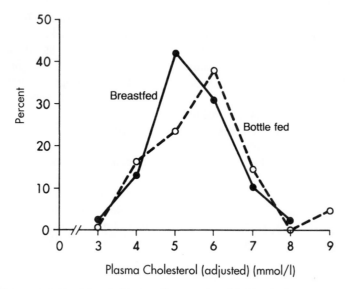

Fig. 12-3. Plasma cholesterol in adults according to type of infant feeding. (From Marmot MG, Page CM, Atkins E et al: *J Epidemiol Community Health* 34:164, 1980.)

formula-fed children had more rapid gains in height and weight, which were attributed to greater food intake. At age 8, there were no differences in indices of fatness related to mode of feeding during infancy and no significant differences in serum cholesterol concentrations. Fomon et al[37] suggest that childhood and adolescence are too early to detect possible beneficial effects of breastfeeding on cholesterol homeostasis in later life in the human.

Serum cholesterol may be too insensitive a quantitation to detect early changes and classify lipoprotein classes, and apoprotein concentrations may be necessary.[48] The effects of breastfeeding versus formula feeding are not attributable to differences in cholesterol intake. According to Mott et al,[84] varying the cholesterol content of infant formulas has not reduced long-lasting differences in serum cholesterol or lipoprotein concentrations or in cholesterol metabolism. Lack of control of genetic differences and sampling under uncontrolled dietary conditions have limited the interpretation of many human studies. Mott et al[83,84] performed a long-term study with 83 baboons to determine the effects of infant diet (breastfeeding

versus formula feeding and the level of cholesterol in the formula). The type of dietary fat and level of dietary cholesterol as well as gender and heredity were reviewed. The progeny of 6 sires and 83 dams were randomly assigned to diet groups of breastfeeding or formula with 2, 30, or 60 mg, respectively, of cholesterol/dl. The 30 mg/dl milk resembled baboon milk. They were weaned to controlled juvenile diets. The differences in cholesterol content of the formula did not lead to later differences in serum cholesterol, lipoprotein concentrations, or cholesterol metabolism. Breastfeeding (species-specific milk), however, affected the subsequent cholesterol metabolism, with absorption of a higher percentage of cholesterol and lower cholesterol production rates as juveniles. The baboons were bred for high or low serum cholesterol concentrations, and in both groups the breastfed animals had higher very-low-density lipoprotein (VLDL) and low-density lipoprotein (LDL) cholesterol levels from 6 months to 3 years than formula-fed animals and higher serum cholesterol from 6 months to 2 years (Fig. 12-4). Baboons are vegetarian, however, and the weaning diet was not.

Fig. 12-4. Cholesterol, very-low-density *(VLDL)* and low-density *(LDL)* lipoprotein in baboons: breastfed vs. formula fed. *Open circle,* Serum cholesterol; *closed circle,* VLDL plus LDL cholesterol; *solid line,* formula fed; *dashed line,* breastfed. (From Mott GE: In Report of 91st Ross Conference on Pediatric Research: *The breastfed infant: a model performance,* Columbus, Ohio, 1986, Ross Laboratories.)

Overfeeding was a variable in a study of preweaning food intake influences on the adiposity of young adult baboons reported by Lewis et al.[67] Overfeeding did not have a major effect on the fat cell number. Overfed male baboons had a greater fat mass in four of ten fat depots at necropsy at age 5. Overfed female baboons had significantly greater fat depot mass in general primarily because of fat cell hypertrophy. Underfeeding in the preweaning period did not affect body weight or adipose mass in either gender in the juveniles.

In guinea pigs, stimulation of cholesterol catabolism by feeding cholestiramine after birth rather than cholesterol feeding can influence the response to dietary cholesterol in the adult.[68] The efficient handling of dietary cholesterol in the cholestiramine-fed guinea pigs is directly associated with significantly higher levels of cholesterol

17α-hydroxylase as sensitive to high dietary cholesterol during lactation.[50] Mott[83] suggests that the long-term effects of breastfeeding on cholesterol metabolism are not likely to result from the differences in neonatal cholesterol intake but rather from other components of breast milk, such as fatty acid composition, immunoglobulins, and hormones that might affect cholesterol metabolism.[83]

The best definition of obesity should be based on the percentage of body weight accounted for by fat. What percentage would be detrimental and how it could easily be measured are not known. Fomon[35] suggests that until that is possible, a clinical definition that circumvents clinical impressions would be useful. He suggests that "values greater than +2 standard deviation value for triceps and subscapular skin-fold thickness be considered evidence of obesity." Fomon[37] also recognizes the difficulty of obtaining skinfold measurements on young infants and offers as a less satisfactory alternative the relation of body weight to stature (Table 12-6).

The infant with a heavy bone structure and musculature but without excessive fat may appear to be obese based on Table 12-6. Infants who are overfed also grow in height and may be in an advanced percentile for height. The infant who is born with a weight in the 80th percentile (weight for age) and remains there may not be obese, but the infant who is born with a weight in the 50th percentile and crosses percentiles over time to the 80th percentile may be at risk for long-term obesity. Therefore some discretion is advised when using these criteria for obesity.

Restraint of growth and development during critical periods of fetal life and infancy has an important effect on the development of cardiovascular disease, as reported by Barker[5] in a long-range study of 6500 men born between 1911 and 1930 in England. Ninety-five percent of the men were breastfed and 20% of these for more than a year. Barker notes the significance of fetal growth and growth in the first year of life being unrelated to social class and cardiovascular disease in adult life when most infants had the advantage of breastfeeding.

TABLE 12-6   Tentative definition of infant obesity*

Age (mo)	Males Length (cm) less than	Males Weight (kg) more than	Females Length (cm) less than	Females Weight (kg) more than
1	51.8	4.2	51.5	4.0
	53.0	4.5	52.2	4.3
	54.2	4.7	53.5	4.6
	55.2	5.1	54.6	4.8
3	58.0	6.0	57.1	5.6
	59.2	6.4	58.0	5.9
	60.2	6.9	59.2	6.2
	61.5	7.3	60.5	6.6
6	65.6	7.7	63.3	7.5
	66.5	8.2	65.2	8.0
	67.8	9.0	66.3	8.4
	69.2	9.6	67.8	8.9
9	70.0	9.1	68.2	8.9
	70.9	9.7	69.5	9.4
	72.3	10.7	71.1	9.9
	73.6	11.2	73.1	10.4
12	73.6	10.2	72.5	9.9
	74.7	10.9	73.2	10.5
	76.4	11.6	75.1	11.1
	78.0	12.5	76.9	11.6
18	80.0	11.6	78.7	11.1
	81.7	12.6	80.2	11.8
	83.2	13.3	82.0	12.7
	85.3	14.4	84.2	13.2
24	85.0	12.8	84.2	12.3
	87.3	13.9	85.8	13.1
	88.8	14.5	87.5	14.2
	90.9	16.0	90.3	14.9
36	93.4	14.8	92.1	14.3
	95.3	15.7	94.2	15.3
	97.3	16.8	96.2	17.0
	100.6	18.6	99.0	17.7

From Fomon SJ: *Infant nutrition,* ed 2, Philadelphia, 1974, Saunders. Table is based on data of Fomon et al (1970, 1971, 1973) for ages 1 and 3 months, and on the data of Karlberg et al (1968) for subsequent ages. At each age, values for length for each gender are the 10th, 25th, 50th, and 75th percentiles, and values for weight are the 50th, 75th, and 90th percentiles, with the mean +2 standard deviations.

Serum cholesterol levels (total and LDL) at ages 60 and 70 were higher in those men who had been bottle-fed or exclusively breastfed beyond 1 year. These data and other studies were reviewed by Fall,[30] who also concludes that adult serum cholesterol concentrations and death rates from ischemic heart disease are related to method of feeding and age at weaning. Exclusive breastfeeding (i.e., no weaning foods or solids beyond a year) is not recommended.

In a 7-year longitudinal study of children at the Slovak Academy of Sciences, the obesity rates in children breastfed for less than 3 months were substantially higher than those in children who had been breastfed longer.[101] Total serum cholesterol increased with age at weaning. The atherogenic index in 6-year-old children was best in those who were breastfed more than 1 month but not over 3 months. The authors also report breastfeeding advantages for respiratory disease, gastrointestinal disease, and thyroid levels.[101]

In a study of adiposity in 4-year-old Anglo- and Mexican-Americans, genetic and environmental factors other than infant-feeding practices had the greater influence.[115] Before age 4, breastfeeding and delayed introduction of solids to 6 months appeared to be associated with normal lean body mass and skinfold thickness.

No benefits are derived from infantile obesity. The concern for obesity rests with the long-range outcome as an obese adult. The problem is that obesity in infancy predisposes the child to immobility and inactivity; thus an obese infant lags on the developmental curve or at least has delayed gross motor skills. The question of whether obesity in infancy predisposes the child to obesity in adult life has not been resolved satisfactorily. Retrospective studies support both sides of the question. A prospective study of 403 newborns in Canada was done measuring weight, length, and subcutaneous fat, but an infant was considered "breastfed" if the infant received any breastfeeding for 2 months and early solids.[60] Food feeding was defined as beginning solids by 2 months of age. Kramer[60] believed the 18-month follow-up refuted the hypothesis of bottle-fed obesity. Most students of this subject would question the population definitions. A study of adolescents retrospectively tested the question of whether breastfeeding and delayed introduction of solids protect against subsequent obesity. Yeung et al[113] concluded that breastfeeding does, but delayed solids alone do not protect against obesity.

Breastfed infants are rarely obese. The usual cause of obesity in these infants is the early addition of solids. Solids often provide excessive kilocalories. The obese breastfed infant should have the diet and feeding pattern scrutinized. If necessary, some restriction of prolonged feeding should be suggested. In the normal course of a breastfeeding, the fat content of the milk increases over the duration of the feeding and satisfies the infant after 10 to 15 minutes of nursing.

Because of general agreement that, once established, childhood obesity often becomes chronic and resistant to treatment,[74] it is appropriate to focus attention on prevention and early intervention. The physician can counsel a family whose breastfed infant meets the criteria for obesity (above the 85th percentile for weight for length).

The routine use of skinfold measurements as part of well-baby care will increase the ability to diagnose obesity because it distinguishes the constitutionally larger body frame from the fat infant.

Recommendations that will help taper unusual weight gain include the following:

1. Limit excessive feedings that are being provided on the mistaken belief that all the infant's needs are nutritional.
2. Encourage nonnutritive cuddling. If feeding is a response to all distress signals, the infant may expect feeding inappropriately, causing disassociation between appetite and energy need.
3. Use exclusive breastfeeding, that is, no solids for 4 to 6 months.
4. Increase activity and energy utilization by encouraging movement rather than containing or restricting the infant in carriers or swaddlings. For the older infant, encourage play activity and crawling and minimize sitting.
5. If there is persistent growth excess, it is appropriate to obtain a sample of maternal milk to rule out the rare case of hyperlipidemia with a "creamatocrit" (see Chapter 20).

REFERENCES

1. Ahn CH, MacLean WC: Growth of the exclusively breast-fed infant, *Am J Clin Nutr* 33:183, 1980.
2. Anand SK, Sandborg C, Robinson RG et al: Neonatal hypernatremia associated with elevated sodium concentration of breast milk, *J Pediatr* 96:66, 1980.
3. Asnes RS, Wisotsky DH, Migel PF et al: The dietary chloride deficiency syndrome occurring in a breastfed infant, *J Pediatr* 100:923, 1982.
4. Axelsson I, Borulf S, Righard L et al: Protein and energy intake during weaning. I. Effects on growth, *Acta Paediatr Scand* 76:321, 1987.
5. Barker DJP: Symposium on "Impact of diet on critical events in development": the effect of nutrition of the fetus and neonate on cardiovascular disease in adult life, *Proc Nutr Soc* 51:135, 1992.
6. Barness LA: Nutrition for healthy neonates. In Gracy M, Falkner F, editors: *Nutritional needs and assessment of normal growth,* New York, 1985, Vevey/Raven.
7. Behrman RE, Driscoll JM Jr, Seeds AE, editors: *Neonatal-perinatal medicine: diseases of the fetus and infant,* ed 2, St . Louis, 1977, Mosby.

8. Birch E, Birch D, Hoffman D et al: Breastfeeding and optimal visual development, *J Pediatr Ophthalmol Strabismus* 30:33, 1993.
9. Blass EM, Teicher MH: Suckling, *Science* 210:15, 1980.
10. Brown KH, Robertson AD, Akhtar NA: Lactational capacity of marginally nourished mothers: infants' milk nutrient consumption and patterns of growth, *Pediatrics* 78:920, 1986.
11. Budd SC, Erdman SH, Long DM et al: Improved lactation with metoclopramide, *Clin Pediatr* 32:53, 1993.
12. Butte NF, Garza C, Smith EO et al: Human milk intake and growth in exclusively breastfed infants, *J Pediatr* 104:187, 1984.
13. Castillo-Duran C, Rodriguez A, Venegas G et al: Zinc supplementation and growth of infants born small for gestational age, *J Pediatr* 127:206, 1995.
14. Caufield LE, Bentley ME, Ahmed S: Is prolonged breastfeeding associated with malnutrition? Evidence from nineteen demographic and health surveys, *Int J Epidemiol* 25:693, 1996.

15. Clarke TA, Markarian M, Griswold W et al: Hyper-natremic dehydration resulting from inadequate breast-feeding, *Pediatrics* 63:931, 1979.

16. Cohen RJ, Brown KH, Canahuah J et al: Effects of age of introduction of complementary foods on infant breast milk intake, total energy intake, and growth: a randomised intervention study in Honduras, *Lancet* 343:288, 1994.

17. Committee on Dietary Allowances, Food and Nutrition Board, National Research Council: *Recommended dietary allowances,* Washington, DC, 1989, National Academy of Sciences.

18. Cowie AT, Forsyth IA, Hart IC: Hormonal control of lactation. In *Monographs on endocrinology,* Heidelberg–New York, 1980, Springer Verlag.

19. Czajka-Narins DM, Jung E: Physical growth of breastfed and formula-fed infants from birth to age two years, *Nutr Res* 6:753, 1986.

20. De Andraca I, Uauy R: Breastfeeding for optimal mental development. In Simopoulos AP, Dutra DC, Olivena JE et al, editors: *Behavioral and metabolic aspects of breast-feeding,* Basel, 1995, Karger.

21. Dewey KG, Cohen RJ, Rivera LL et al: Do exclusively breast-fed infants require extra protein? *Pediatr Res* 39:303, 1996.

22. Dewey KG, Heinig MJ, Nommsen LA et al: Growth of breastfed and formula-fed infants from 0 to 18 months: the DARLING study, *Pediatrics* 89:1035, 1992.

23. Dewey KG, Heinig MJ, Nommsen LA et al: Breastfed infants are leaner than formula-fed infants at one year of age: the DARLING study, *Am J Clin Nutr* 57:140, 1993.

24. Dewey KG, Heinig MJ, Nommsen LA et al: Adequacy of energy intake among breastfed infants in the DARLING study: relationships to growth velocity, morbidity, and activity levels, *J Pediatr* 119:538, 1991.

25. Dewey KG, Lönnerdal B: Infant self-regulation of breast milk intake, *Acta Paediatr Scand* 75:893, 1986.

26. Dewey KG, Peerson JM, Brown KH et al: Growth of breast-fed infants deviates from current reference data: a pooled analysis of US, Canadian, and European data sets, *Pediatrics* 96:495, 1995.

27. Dewey KG, Peerson JM, Heinig MJ et al: Growth patterns of breastfed infants in affluent (US) and poor (Peru) communities: implications for timing of complementary feeding, *Am J Clin Nutr* 56:1012, 1992.

28. Duncan B, Schafer C, Sibley B et al: Reduced growth velocity in exclusively breast-fed infants, *Am J Dis Child* 138:309, 1984.

29. Ereman RR, Lönnerdal B, Dewey KG: Maternal sodium intake does not affect postprandial sodium concentrations in human milk, *J Nutr* 117:1154, 1987.

30. Fall C: Nutrition in early life and later outcome, *Eur J Clin Nutr* 46(suppl 4):57, 1992.

31. Fawzi WW, Forman MR, Levy A et al: Maternal anthropometry and infant feeding practices in Israel in relation to growth in infancy: the North African Infant Feeding Study, *Am J Clin Nutr* 65:1731, 1997.

32. Fergusson DM, Beautrais AL, Silva PA: Breastfeeding and cognitive development in the first seven years of life, *Soc Sci Med* 16:1705, 1982.

33. Fergusson DM, Horwood LJ, Shannon FT: Breastfeeding and subsequent social adjustment in six- to eight-year-old children, *J Child Psychol Psychiatry* 28:379, 1987.

34. Finberg L, Kiley J, Luttrell CN: Mass accidental salt poisoning in infancy: a study of a hospital disaster, *JAMA* 184:187, 1963.

35. Fomon SJ: *Infant nutrition,* ed 2, Philadelphia, 1974, Saunders.

36. Fomon SJ, Filer LJ Jr, Thomas LN et al: Growth and serum chemical values of normal breast fed infants, *Acta Paediatr Scand Suppl* 273:1, 1978.

37. Fomon SJ, Rogers RR, Ziegler EE et al: Indices of fatness and serum cholesterol at age eight years in relation to feeding and growth during early infancy, *Pediatr Res* 18:1233, 1984.

38. Forman MR, Lewando-Hundt G, Graubard BI et al: Factors influencing milk insufficiency and its long term health effects: the Bedouin Infant Feeding Study, *Int J Epidemiol* 21:53, 1992.

39. Frank DA, Silva M, Needlman R: Failure to thrive: mystery, myth and method, *Contemp Pediatr* 10:114, 1993.

40. Garza C, Frongillo E, Dewey KG: Implications of growth patterns of breastfed infants for growth references, *Acta Paediatr Suppl* 402:4, 1994.

41. Gilmore HE, Rowland TW: Critical malnutrition in breast-fed infants, *Am J Dis Child* 132:885, 1978.

42. Ghishan FK, Roloff JS: Malnutrition and hypernatremic dehydration in two breast-fed infants, *Clin Pediatr* 22:592, 1983.

43. Grummer-Strawn LM: Does prolonged breastfeeding impair child growth? A critical review, *Pediatrics* 91:766, 1993.

44. Gupta AP, Gupta PK: Metoclopramide as a lactagogue, *Clin Pediatr* 24:269, 1985.

45. Habbick BF, Gerrard JW: Failure to thrive in the contented breastfed baby, *Can Med Assoc J* 131:765, 1984.

46. Hall DMB, Kay G: Effect of thyrotrophin-releasing factor on lactation, *Br Med J* 1:777, 1977.

47. Hamill PVV, Drizd TA, Johnson CL et al: *Growth curves for children: birth to 18 years, United States,* National Center for Health Statistics, Series 11, No 165, Hyatts-ville, Md, 1977, US Department of Health, Education and Welfare.

48. Hamosh M: Does infant nutrition affect adiposity and cholesterol levels in the adult? *J Pediatr Gastroenterol Nutr* 7:10, 1988.

49. Heinig MJ, Nommsen LA, Peerson JM et al: Energy and protein intakes of breastfed and formula-fed infants during the first year of life and their association with growth velocity: the DARLING study, *Am J Clin Nutr* 58:152, 1993.

50. Hill ID, Bowie MD: Chloride deficiency syndrome due to chloride-deficient breast milk, *Arch Dis Child* 58:224, 1983.
51. Hilson JA, Rasmussen KM, Kjolhede CL: Maternal obesity and breast-feeding success in a rural population of white women, *Am J Clin Nutr* 66(6):1371, 1997.
52. Hitchcock NE, Gracey M, Owles EN: Growth of the healthy breast-fed infants in the first six months, *Lancet* 2:64, 1981.
53. Hoefer C, Hardy MC: Later development of breast-fed and artificially fed infants, *JAMA* 92:615, 1929.
54. Hopkinson JM, Schanler RJ, Fraley JK et al: Milk production by mothers of premature infants: influence of cigarette smoking, *Pediatrics* 90:934, 1992.
55. Horwood LJ, Fergusson DM: Breastfeeding and later cognitive and academic outcomes, *Pediatrics* 101:e9, 1998 (electronic article).
56. Jacobson SW, Jacobson JL: Breastfeeding and intelligence, *Lancet* 339:926, 1992.
57. Jakobsen MS, Sodemann M, Molbak K et al: Reason for termination of breastfeeding and the length of breastfeeding, *Int J Epidemiol* 25:115, 1996.
58. Jelliffe DB, Jelliffe EFP: *Human milk in the modern world,* Oxford, 1978, Oxford University Press.
59. Juez G, Diaz S, Casado ME et al: Growth pattern of selected urban Chilean infants during exclusive breastfeeding, *Am J Clin Nutr* 38:462, 1983.
60. Kramer MS: Do breast-feeding and delayed introduction of solid foods protect against subsequent obesity? *J Pediatr* 98:883, 1981.
61. Kramer MS, Barr RG, Leduc DG et al: Determinants of weight and adiposity in the first year of life, *J Pediatr* 106:10, 1985.
62. Lampl M, Veldhuis JD, Johnson ML. Saltation and stasis: a model of human growth, *Science* 258:801, 1992.
63. Lawrence RA: Successful breastfeeding, *Am J Dis Child* 135:595, 1981.
64. Lawrence RA: Infant nutrition, *Pediatr Rev* 5:133, 1983.
65. Lawrence R: Maternal factors in lactation failure. In Hamosh M, Goldman AS, editors: *Human lactation.* II. *Maternal and environmental factors,* New York, 1986, Plenum.
66. Lawton ME: Alcohol in breast milk, *Aust NZ J Obstet Gynaecol* 25:71, 1985.
67. Lewis DS, Bertrand HA, McMahan CA et al: Preweaning food intake influences the adiposity of young adult baboons, *J Clin Invest* 78:899, 1986.
68. Li JR, Bale LK, Kottke BA: Effect of neonatal modulation of cholesterol homeostasis on subsequent response to cholesterol challenge in adult guinea pig, *J Clin Invest* 65:1060, 1980.
69. Little RE, Anderson KW, Ervin CH et al: Maternal alcohol use during breastfeeding and infant mental and motor development at one year, *N Engl J Med* 321:425, 1989.
70. Lucas A, Fewtrell MS, Davies PSW et al: Breastfeeding and catch-up growth in infants born small for gestational age, *Acta Paediatr* 86:564, 1997.
71. Lucas A, Morley R, Cole TJ et al: Early diet in premature babies and developmental status at 18 months, *Lancet* 335:1477, 1990.
72. Lucas A, Morley R, Cole TJ et al: Breast milk and subsequent intelligence quotient in children born premature, *Lancet* 339:261, 1992.
73. Lukefahr JL: Underlying illness associated with failure to thrive in breastfed infants, *Clin Pediatr* 29:468, 1990.
74. Marmot MG, Page CM, Atkins E et al: Effect of breastfeeding on plasma cholesterol and weight in young adults, *J Epidemiol Community Health* 34:164, 1980.
75. McGill HC Jr:; The relationship of dietary cholesterol to serum cholesterol concentration and to atherosclerosis in man, *Am J Clin Nutr* 32:2664, 1979.
76. Mennella JA, Beauchamp GK: The transfer of alcohol to human milk, *N Engl J Med* 325:981, 1991.
77. Michaelson KF: Nutrition and growth during infancy: the Copenhagen Cohort Study, *Acta Paediatr* 86(suppl 420):1, 1997.
78. Michaelson KF, Larsen PS, Thomsen BL et al: The Copenhagen Cohort Study on Infant Nutrition and Growth: breast-milk intake, human milk macro nutrient content, and influencing factors, *Am J Clin Nutr* 59:600, 1994.
79. Moore BJ, Brasel JA: One cycle of reproduction consisting of pregnancy, lactation or no lactation, and recovery: effects on fat pad cellularity in ad libitum–fed and food-restricted rats, *J Nutr* 114:1560, 1984.
80. Morley R, Cole TJ, Powell R et al: Mother's choice to provide breast milk and developmental outcome, *Arch Dis Child* 63:1382, 1988.
81. Motil KJ, Sheng H-P, Montandon CM et al: Case report: failure to thrive in a breast-fed infant is associated with maternal dietary protein and energy restriction, *J Am Coll Nutr* 13:203, 1994.
82. Motil KJ, Sheng H-P, Montandon CM et al: Human milk protein does not limit growth of breast-fed infants, *J Pediatr Gastrenterol Nutr* 24:10, 1997.
83. Mott GE: Deferred effects of breastfeeding versus formula feeding on serum lipoprotein concentration and cholesterol metabolism in baboons. In Report of the 91st Ross Conference on Pediatric Research: *The breastfed infant: a model performance,* Columbus, Ohio, 1986, Ross Laboratories.
84. Mott GE, Jackson EM, McMahan CA et al: Cholesterol metabolism in juvenile baboons: influences of infant and juvenile diets, *Arteriosclerosis* 5:347, 1985.
85. National Center for Health Statistics: *Trends in breastfeeding: advance data from vital and health statistics,* DHHS Pub No 59, Washington, DC, 1980, US Department of Health, Education and Welfare.

86. Neifert MR, Seacat JM: Mammary gland anomalies and lactation failure. In Hamosh M, Goldman AS, editors: *Human lactation.* II. *Maternal and environmental factors,* New York, 1986, Plenum.

87. Neifert MR, Seacat JM, Jobe WE: Lactation failure due to insufficient glandular development of the breast, *Pediatrics* 76:823, 1985.

88. Nelson SE, Rogers RR, Ziegler EE et al: Gain in weight and length during early infancy, *Early Hum Dev* 19:223, 1989.

89. O'Connor ME, Szekely LJ: Failure to thrive in breastfed 8-11 month olds: a manifestation of the "vulnerable child syndrome," *ABM News Views* 2(2):9, 1996.

90. Oliva-Rasbach J, Neville MC: Longitudinal growth patterns of a reference population of breastfed infants, *Fed Proc* 45:362, 1986.

91. Palmer MM, Crawley K, Blanco IA: Neonatal oral-motor assessment scale: a reliability study, *J Perinatol* 13:28, 1993.

92. Paneth N: Hypernatremic dehydration of infancy, *Am J Dis Child* 134:785, 1980.

93. Podratz RO, Broughton DD, Gustafson DH et al: Weight loss and body temperature changes in breastfed and bottle-fed neonates, *Clin Pediatr* 25:73, 1986.

94. Pomerance HH: Growth in breastfed children, *Hum Biol* 59:687, 1987.

95. Pugliese MT, Weyman-Daum M, Moses N et al: Parental health beliefs as a cause of nonorganic failure to thrive, *Pediatrics* 80:175, 1987.

96. Ramsay M, Gisel EG, Boutry M: Non-organic failure to thrive: growth failure secondary to feeding skills disorder, *Dev Med Child Neurol* 35:285, 1993.

97. Roddey OF, Martin ES, Swetenburg RL: Critical weight loss and malnutrition in breastfed infants, *Am J Dis Child* 135:597, 1981.

98. Rogan WJ, Gladen BC: Breastfeeding and cognitive development, *Early Hum Dev* 31:181, 1993.

99. Rowland TW, Zori RT, Lafleur WR et al: Malnutrition and hypernatremic dehydration in breastfed infants, *JAMA* 247:1016, 1982.

100. Smith MM, Lifshitz F: Excess fruit juice consumption as a contributing factor in nonorganic failure to thrive, *Pediatrics* 93:436, 1994.

101. Štrbák V, Škultétyová M, Randušková A et al: Late effects of breastfeeding and early weaning: seven-year prospective study in children, *Endocr Regul* 25:53, 1991.

102. Subcommittee on Nutrition during Lactation, Committee on Nutritional Status during Pregnancy and Lactation, Food and Nutrition Board, Institute of Medicine, National Academy of Sciences: *Nutrition during lactation,* Washington, DC, 1991, National Academy Press.

103. Taylor B, Wadsworth J: Breastfeeding and child development at five years, *Dev Med Child Neurol* 26:73, 1984.

104. Volz VR, Book LS, Churella HR: Growth and plasma amino acid concentrations in term infants fed either whey-predominant formula or human milk, *J Pediatr* 102:27, 1983.

105. Weichert CE: Lactational reflex recovery in breastfeeding failure, *Pediatrics* 63:799, 1979.

106. Weston JA, Stage AF, Hathaway P et al: Prolonged breast-feeding and nonorganic failure to thrive, *Am J Dis Child* 141:242, 1987.

107. Whitehead RG, Paul AA: Growth charts and the assessment of infant feeding practices in the Western world and in developing countries, *Early Hum Dev* 9:187, 1984.

108. Whitehead RG, Paul AA, Ahmed EA: Weaning practices in the United Kingdom and variations in anthropometric development, *Acta Paediatr Scand* 323(suppl):14, 1986.

109. Wissler RW, McGill HC Jr, chairmen: Conference on blood lipids in children: optimal levels for early prevention of coronary artery disease, *Prev Med* 12:868, 1983.

110. Woolridge MW, Ingram JC, Baum JD: Do changes in pattern of breast usage alter the baby's nutrient intake? *Lancet* 336:395, 1990.

111. World Health Organization/Centers for Disease Control: *Measuring change in nutritional status: guidelines for assessing the nutritional impact of supplementary feeding programmes for vulnerable groups,* Geneva, 1983, WHO.

112. World Health Organization Working Group on Infant Growth: An evaluation of infant growth: the use and interpretation of anthropometry in infants, *Bull WHO* 73:165, 1995.

113. Yeung DL, Pennell MD, Leung M et al: Infant fatness and feeding practices: a longitudinal assessment, *J Am Diet Assoc* 79:531, 1981.

114. Young HB, Buckley AE, Hamza B et al: Milk and lactation: some social and developmental correlates among 1000 infants, *Pediatrics* 69:169, 1982.

115. Zive MM, McKay H, Frank-Spohrer GC et al: Infant feeding practices and adiposity in year old Anglo- and Mexican-Americans, *Am J Clin Nutr* 55:1104, 1992.

$\mathcal{M}$aternal employment

Maternal employment has been cited by many authors as the major reason for the decline in breastfeeding worldwide.[8,48] The international data do not actually support this contention. Year after year the Ross Laboratories Mothers Survey[52] confirms that the highest percentage of women initiating breastfeeding in the hospital is among women who plan to return to full-time employment, the next highest among women who plan to return to part-time employment, and the lowest among those who plan to remain at home.[53,54] The duration, however, is affected by employment, with 23.4% of those employed part-time still breastfeeding at 5 to 6 months, 25.0% of non-employed women still breastfeeding, and only 14.3% of those employed full-time still breastfeeding at 5 to 6 months (Table 13-1).[44,52] The individual mother who chooses to return to work and breastfeed confronts significant constraints, regardless of the statistical data. The physician should be knowledgeable about the principles and practice of this dual role when counseling about maternal employment.[62]

Although economic, cultural, and political pressures often confound decisions about infant feeding, the American Academy of Pediatrics (AAP) firmly adheres to the position that breastfeeding ensures the best possible health and the best developmental and psychosocial outcomes for the infant. Enthusiastic support and involvement of pediatricians in the promotion and practice of breastfeeding are essential to the achievement of optimal infant and child health, growth, and development.[4]

HISTORICAL PERSPECTIVE

In modern cultures a stigma has been attached to a mother's earning money while her children are young, but no such stigma is associated with leaving her children for social interaction, personal reasons, or a volunteer job. All women work when work is defined as expending energy for a purpose, but not all women are employed when it is defined as earning money for labor. Before industrialization, the working mother was the rule and not the exception. Home and work were separated by industrialization, making parenting a separate role for women.

Sanday[55] has described women's work as domestic or productive, public or private, traditional or modern. Domestic work, when performed for the family, is unpaid and thus is undervalued and not counted as productive work. Domestic work is performed in the private domain, and "productive" work is associated with the public domain. Women had previously worked in agriculture and cottage industries as well as in small-scale marketing, whereas today they participate in formal work (i.e., they are *employees*), including clerical, factory, and professional jobs predominantly in urban settings.

More women are employed outside the home today than previously in the twentieth century.[57,58] In 1900, 20% of the labor force was female; in 1950, 29%; and in 1997, 56.6%. Women with children under 6 years old are the fastest-growing segment of the female work force, reaching 59% in

TABLE 13-1 **Breastfeeding in hospital and at 6 months of age by selected demographic characteristics, 1989 through 1995**

Characteristic	In hospital (%)			At 6 months (%)		
	1989	1995	Change*	1989	1995	Change*
All infants	52.2	59.7	14.4	18.1	21.6	19.3
White	58.5	64.3	9.9	21.0	24.1	14.8
Black	23.0	37.0	60.9	6.4	11.2	75.0
Hispanic	48.4	61.0	26.0	13.9	19.6	41.0
Maternal age						
<20	30.2	42.8	41.7	5.6	9.1	62.5
20-24	45.2	52.6	16.4	11.5	14.6	27.0
25-29	58.8	63.1	7.3	21.1	22.9	8.5
30-34	65.5	68.1	4.0	29.3	29.0	(1.0)‡
35+	66.5	70.0	5.3	34.0	33.8	(0.6)‡
Total family income						
<$10,000	31.8	41.8	31.4	8.2	11.4	39.0
$10,000-$14,999	47.1	51.7	9.8	13.9	15.4	10.8
$15,000-$24,999	54.7	58.8	7.5	18.9	19.8	4.8
≥$25,000	66.3	70.7	6.6	25.5	28.5	11.8
Maternal education						
Grade school	31.7	43.8	38.2	11.5	17.1	48.7
High school	42.5	49.7	16.9	12.4	15.0	21.0
College	70.7	74.4	5.2	28.8	31.2	8.3
Maternal employment						
Employed full time	50.8	60.7	19.5	8.9	14.3	60.7
Employed part time	59.4	63.5	6.9	21.1	23.4	10.9
Not employed	51.0	58.0	13.7	21.6	25.0	15.7
Birthweight						
Low (≤2500 g)	36.2	47.7	31.8	9.8	12.6	28.6
Normal	53.5	60.5	13.1	18.8	22.3	18.6
Parity						
Primiparous	52.6	61.6	17.1	15.1	19.5	29.1
Multiparous	51.7	57.8	11.8	21.1	23.6	11.8
WIC participation†						
Participant	34.2	46.6	36.3	8.4	12.7	51.2
Nonparticipant	62.9	71.0	12.9	23.8	29.2	22.7
US census region						
New England	52.2	61.2	17.2	18.6	22.2	19.4
Middle Atlantic	47.4	53.8	13.5	16.8	19.6	16.7
East North Central	47.6	54.6	14.7	16.7	18.9	13.2
West North Central	55.9	61.9	10.7	18.4	21.4	16.3
South Atlantic	43.8	54.8	25.1	13.7	18.6	35.8
East South Central	37.9	44.1	16.4	11.5	13.0	13.0
West South Central	46.0	54.4	18.3	13.6	17.0	25.0
Mountain	70.2	75.1	7.0	28.3	30.3	7.1
Pacific	70.3	75.1	6.8	26.6	30.9	16.2

From Ross Products Division, Abbott Laboratories: *Mothers survey: updated breast-feeding trend through 1996,* Columbus, Ohio, 1998, Abbott.
*Percent change was calculated using following formula: % breastfed in 1984 − % breastfed in 1989/% breastfed in 1984.
†Women, Infants, and Children supplemental food program.
‡Figures in parentheses indicate a decrease in rate of breastfeeding from 1989 to 1995.

1992 and more than 65% in 1996. Even more critical is that the number of employed mothers with infants under age 1 year escalated to 48% of all women in 1985 and has continued to climb. Many more women facing the decision about infant-feeding methods must include the early return to work. In 1998 at least 50% of women employed in the United States when they become pregnant return to the labor force by the time their children are 3 months old. U.S. Department of Labor[56] statistics show that 54.3% of mothers with children under age 1 year were in the work force in 1996. This figure rises to 63.3% for women with children under 2 years of age.

Generations ago, the woman who worked violated the Victorian norms of role definition. Even when forced to work by sheer necessity, she was accused of neglecting her primary responsibility to her children. The new ethic proclaims work a cardinal virtue for the liberated woman, so that the woman who can and does stay home may begin to feel inadequate.

Why women enter the work force is important to understanding the trend.[33] Before 1970, the need to earn money motivated 3 million women either because the mother was a single parent or because husband-fathers were unable to earn an adequate income. For women whose husbands earned "enough," there was the need to provide a higher standard of living or provide the father with greater freedom of career choice.[63] Few women sought careers for careers' sake because need for income was the only socially acceptable, defensible reason for a mother to work outside the home.

Since that time many women have found that the full-time care of a home leads only to higher standards of cleanliness with no greater sense of achievement or completion.[25] Some believed that the exclusive investment of energy and emotion in the rearing of one to three children would involve a considerable hazard not only to a mother, but also to her children's ultimate achievement and ability to form a variety of responsive and satisfying personal relationships.[33,43] Women are responding to the pressures of an inflationary economy, to the costs of higher education, to the opportunities for personal fulfillment, and to the growing market for service occupations.[8,11] Married women continue to carry at least 70% to 80% of the child care and household duties when both parents work.

ATTITUDES OF PROFESSIONALS TOWARD WORKING MOTHERS

Professional[9] and lay[39] books alike on child rearing have viewed working negatively except for economic necessity, thus enhancing the working mother's guilt and providing little substantial advice about how to balance or how to continue breastfeeding.

The AAP Committee on Psychosocial Aspects of Child and Family Health[3] wrote: "Many mothers work outside the home and most have concerns about substitute child care. In addition to providing advice to individual parents, pediatricians can make an important contribution by supporting subsidized parental leaves after birth of a newborn infant, by encouraging the active participation of fathers in child and household care, and by having the knowledge to aid parents in access to high quality substitute child care."[3] The AAP strongly stated in 1997 that pediatricians should "encourage employers to provide appropriate facilities and adequate time in the workplace for breast-pumping."[4]

The American College of Obstetricians and Gynecologists (ACOG)[5] has acknowledged the current trend to work throughout pregnancy and to return to work promptly after delivery by preparing a physician's guide to patient assessment and counseling, which has not been updated since 1987. ACOG also provides for a patient occupational questionnaire for the practitioner. This forms a basis of discussion with the patient and provides an opportunity to counsel the patient and her husband about plans to maintain a healthy environment and any special needs for child care. With few exceptions, "the normal woman with an uncomplicated pregnancy and a normal fetus, in a job that presents no greater potential hazards than those encountered in normal daily life in the community, may continue to work without interruption until the onset of labor and may resume

TABLE 13-2 **Responses for reasons to recommend work**	Frequency	
Reason	No.	%
Economic	1709	25
Never recommend mother work	1566	22
Mother's emotional needs	1220	18
Mother's fulfillment	1059	15
Child is better off without mother	644	9
Reassure mother	270	4
Adequacy of child care	266	4
Child's age	170	2
Mother does important work	64	1
TOTAL	6968	

From Heins M, Stillman P, Sabers D et al: *Pediatrics* 72:283, 1983.
Copyright American Academy of Pediatrics 1983.

TABLE 13-3 **Responses for reasons to recommend against working**	Frequency	
Reason	No.	%
Child's physical health	1724	24
Child's mental health	1445	20
Never recommend against work	1318	18
Inadequate child care	701	10
Child's age	591	8
Mother feels guilty	540	7
No economic need	459	6
Usually say, "Do not work"	72	1
Other	402	6
TOTAL	7252	

From Heins M, Stillman P, Sabers D et al: *Pediatrics* 72:286, 1983.
Copyright American Academy of Pediatrics 1983.

working several weeks after an uncomplicated delivery."[5] Frederick and Auerbach[21] put it in more practical terms when they suggest that the obstetrician has a role in facilitating continued breastfeeding after the return to work or school. This includes counseling regarding pumping and storing milk and avoiding exhaustion.

Attitudes of pediatricians toward mothers working outside the home have been measured by mail survey, because attitudes seem to determine advice given.[28] The majority of pediatricians responding thought that the children of working and nonworking women were similar, that the mother could return to work at any age of the child, and that it did not make any difference. Many respondents said they did not give advice about working (Tables 13-2 and 13-3). Only half the respondents provided special considerations, such as evening hours for employed mothers.

Some respondents, however, did express bias against employed mothers. Bias was related to the respondent's age and gender and to whether the respondent's spouse worked. Those whose spouses did not work outside the home, those in older age groups, and male pediatricians in general held more negative attitudes toward maternal employ-

ment. The researchers thought that a substantial number might give advice or cues that maternal employment might be detrimental to children, producing maternal conflict and guilt.

The physician plays an important role in guiding parents with information about quality and availability of child care facilities, as well as with advice about coping strategies.[20] As family counselor, the physician can help support mothers and fathers seeking to fulfill parental, occupational, and personal needs in a rapidly changing society. With the firm recommendation of the AAP to breastfeed throughout the first year and beyond, support from pediatricians will be critical.[4]

OUTCOME FOR CHILDREN OF EMPLOYED MOTHERS

Numerous studies since the early 1930s have looked at the effects of maternal employment. Assessment of infant behavior, school achievement and adjustment, children's attitudes, adolescence, and delinquency have all been used as outcome measures.[18] Annotated bibliographies covering the range of research in areas of medicine, psychology, sociology, and education are available.* The four major considerations are the variables that facilitate or impede maternal employment, the effect of maternal employment on children during the four developmental stages, the effects on the family, and the effects on society in general. Society is far more accepting of the working mother now.

It has been emphasized that the presence of the mother in the home does not guarantee high-quality mothering.[25] It has also been shown that well-educated (college) mothers, including those who are employed, spend time with their children at the expense of their own personal needs.[34] Because employed mothers encompass a large group of women with different educations, different reasons for working, and different opportunities for employment, it is difficult to generalize about effects. Literature reviews have emphasized critical factors that are more important than maternal employment, such as good substitute care, maternal role satisfaction, family stability, paternal attitude toward maternal employment, and the quality of the time spent with the children.[31] Despite the abundance of research on school-age children, there is still little reported about preschoolers because no school records or test results are available to use in large-population analysis.

To date, there is no direct effect of nonexclusive mothering per se. Studies of infants of adolescent mothers have shown that the children do better socially and academically if there are multiple caregivers instead of the adolescent alone.[40] No uniformly harmful effects on family life or on the growth and development of children have been demonstrated. Maternal employment may jeopardize family life when the conditions of the mother's employment are demeaning to self-esteem, when others are strongly disapproving of her work away from the home, or when arrangements for child care are not adequate.[55]

Questions have been raised about the impact of separation of mother and infant and the timing of this separation.[11] Resumption of full-time employment when the child is under 1 year has sparked

studies. Using the Ainsworth "Strange Situation" validated techniques, no relationship between maternal work status and the quality of the infants' attachment to their mothers is reported.[1,2] Early resumption of employment may not impede development of a secure infant-mother attachment.[13] A significantly higher proportion of insecure attachments to fathers in employed-mother families is reported for boys but not for girls. Boys are more insecurely attached than girls in most studies. It is believed that an infant's attachment relationship to mother emerges at about 7 months.[22] Other studies suggest that maternal employment can have a positive effect on girls but not boys. Whether breastfeeding accounts for some of the variability in these studies is not stated.[30-32,60] One of the strategies suggested is to advocate for infant care centers that provide breastfeeding facilities in the workplace, schools, and other locations serving working women.

BREASTFEEDING AND EMPLOYMENT

An important distinction must be made between work that separates the mother and infant for blocks of time and work that does not. In rural settings, women's work is usually compatible with all aspects of child care, including breastfeeding. Work in or around the home is usually flexible. If there are provisions for infants at the workplace, even formal urban work is compatible with child care and breastfeeding. The higher the education of the mother and the more advanced the job, the more opportunity exists for flexible arrangements that permit breastfeeding. Among the strategies available is pumping and saving milk while on the job to be fed to the baby by the babysitter the next day.

Dismissal from employment (i.e., losing one's job) of nursing mothers demonstrates the unique problems for working women in certain jobs. Overall, the breastfeeding rates for working women do not show that breastfeeding and employment are mutually exclusive.[63] In Finland the

*References 8, 19, 25, 32, 57, 58.

TABLE 13-4 **Frequency of breastfeeding in hospital by maternal ethnicity and employment status, 1992**

Ethnicity	Employment status			Total
	Full time	Part time	Not employed	
Hispanic				
Formula	2084	767	5695	8546
Breast alone	2074	946	4118	7138
Breast and supplement	815	358	1932	3105
Total breastfed	2889 (58%)	1304 (63%)	6050 (52%)	10,243 (55%)
Native American				
Formula	269	151	860	1280
Breast alone	293	154	763	1210
Breast and supplement	74	43	244	361
Total breastfed	367 (58%)	197 (57%)	1007 (54%)	1571 (55%)
Asian/Pacific islands				
Formula	866	212	987	2065
Breast alone	1234	432	1621	3287
Breast and supplement	597	157	611	1365
Total breastfed	1831 (68%)	589 (74%)	2232 (69%)	4652 (69%)
Black				
Formula	5075	1963	11,492	18,530
Breast alone	2554	817	2993	6364
Breast and supplement	1057	367	1578	3002
Total breastfed	3611 (42%)	1184 (38%)	4571 (28%)	9366 (34%)
White				
Formula	23,914	11,192	39,300	74,406
Breast alone	33,967	21,916	58,140	114,023
Breast and supplement	5515	3510	9489	18,514
Total breastfed	39,482 (62%)	25,426 (69%)	67,629 (63%)	132,537 (64%)
Total, all ethnic groups				
Formula	32,208	14,285	58,334	104,827
Breast alone	40,122	24,265	67,635	132,022
Breast and supplement	8058	4435	13,854	26,347
Total breastfed	48,180 (60%)	28,700 (67%)	81,489 (58%)	158,369 (60%)

From Ross Laboratories Mothers Survey data, 1992, compiled by Molly A. Anthony, PhD, Perinatal and Women's Health Branch, Department of Mothers', Infants', Children's, and Adolescents' Health (DMICAH).

incidence of mothers breastfeeding at 1 month is 78% among nonworking and 80% among working mothers. The duration is also unaffected; 29% of nonworking and 32% of working mothers are breastfeeding at 3 months and 8% and 7% at 6 months.[59] Similar statistics are reported from Nigeria, the Philippines, and Chile.

In 1987, Ryan and Martinez[54] conducted a study of the impact of employment on breastfeeding as part of the annual Ross Laboratories Mothers Survey exploring infant-feeding practices. Those mothers at 6 months who were employed full time numbered 22,316 (26.6%), part time 12,186 (14.5%), and not working 49,483 (58.9%). The same proportion of employed mothers (55%) as not employed were breastfeeding when they left the hospital. On the other hand, only 10% of full-time employed mothers were breastfeeding at 6 months compared to 24% of those who were not employed. The highest incidence of breastfeeding

TABLE 13-5   Frequency of breastfeeding at 6 months by maternal ethnicity and employment status, 1992

Ethnicity	Employment status			Total
	Full time	Part time	Not employed	
Hispanic				
Formula	4095	1559	8912	14,566
Breast alone	171	138	1117	1426
Breast and supplement	383	220	904	1507
Total breastfed	554 (12%)	358 (19%)	2021 (18%)	2933 (17%)
Native American				
Formula	497	252	1394	2143
Breast alone	23	32	207	262
Breast and supplement	70	38	157	265
Total breastfed	93 (16%)	70 (22%)	364 (21%)	527 (20%)
Asian/Pacific islands				
Formula	2154	519	2032	4705
Breast alone	119	102	538	759
Breast and supplement	257	130	443	830
Total breastfed	376 (15%)	232 (31%)	981 (33%)	1589 (25%)
Black				
Formula	7411	2622	13,479	23,512
Breast alone	224	132	824	1180
Breast and supplement	518	193	694	1405
Total breastfed	742 (9%)	325 (11%)	1518 (10%)	2585 (10%)
White				
Formula	50,927	24,455	69,448	144,830
Breast alone	3110	4923	20,733	28,766
Breast and supplement	5018	4646	9170	18,834
Total breastfed	8128 (14%)	9569 (28%)	29,903 (30%)	47,600 (25%)
Total, all ethnic groups				
Formula	65,084	29,407	95,265	189,756
Breast alone	3647	5327	23,419	32,393
Breast and supplement	6246	5227	11,368	22,841
Total breastfed	9893 (13%)	10,554 (26%)	34,787 (27%)	55,234 (23%)

From Ross Laboratories Mothers Survey data, 1992, compiled by Molly A. Anthony, PhD, Perinatal and Women's Health Branch, Department of Mothers', Infants', Children's, and Adolescents' Health (DMICAH).

at birth and at 6 months was among the over-30-year-old mothers who are well educated and in a higher socioeconomic group. The continuance rate* for all mothers was 18% breastfeeding among those employed and 44% among those not employed. Not surprisingly, working mothers also used more supplementary bottles. These trends are confirmed by more recent surveys.[37] Using data from the Ross Mothers Survey in 1992, Molly Anthony of the Perinatal and Women's Health Branch compared the percentage of breastfed infants by maternal employment status and ethnicity, as shown in Tables 13-4 and 13-5.

Although there was no association between planning to be employed within the first 6 months

*Continuance rate =
$$\frac{1.0 - \% \text{ breastfed in hospital} - \% \text{ breastfed at 6 months}}{\% \text{ breastfed in hospital}}$$

and initiation of breastfeeding, Gielen et al[24] found that there was a significant association with cessation of breastfeeding as early as 2 to 3 months postpartum, even with adjustment for demographics. Among employed mothers, working 20 hours a week or less was protective for continuation of breastfeeding. When the factors influencing the duration of breastfeeding were examined by West[61] by postal questionnaire at 6 months in Edinburgh, only 5 of 116 mothers listed "return to work" as a reason for discontinuing.

A comparison by Martinez and Stahle[42] of low-income mothers who were receiving assistance from Women, Infants, and Children (WIC) Program showed that of the 38% who planned to work full time and left the hospital breastfeeding, only 8.8% were breastfeeding at 6 months, whereas of the 42.4% who had no plans for employment on leaving the hospital, 17.1% were still breastfeeding at 6 months.

Employment among black women around Johannesburg, South Africa, following the birth of a baby strongly influenced duration of breastfeeding.[12] Although 97% had initiated breastfeeding, only 30% continued for 20 weeks; there was a direct association with return to work, because these women did not consider it feasible to do both. Similar findings were reported in Washington, DC, where 80% of black women worked during pregnancy and those who planned to return to work only part time were more likely to breastfeed.[38] In this study, those who returned to a professional occupation had a longer duration of breastfeeding than those who returned to sales or technical jobs, regardless of whether the individual was black or white.

Although work has been listed as the primary cause of early weaning, women seldom give employment as a reason for terminating breastfeeding. A review of the world literature documenting reasons for weaning, starting bottle feeding, or not initiating breastfeeding rarely mentioned employment.[59] In studies of the effect of mother's employment on the nutritional status of her children, poverty, not mother's work, was associated with poor nutrition.

The effect of employment on the duration of breastfeeding may be influenced by the fact that breastfeeding can be carried out while the mother performs other tasks around the house so that it is easier to breastfeed when she is home.[29] Many studies have found that employment has little or no effect on the duration of breastfeeding, especially where cottage industry was prevalent. The greatest problems are the difficulties encountered finding a place to pump and store the milk on the job. Those women who work outside the home must schedule and plan carefully and are motivated to continue once the complex schedule is established. They also are more able to accommodate themselves to the stresses.

A national study among women who responded to an advertisement in popular parenting magazines about working and breastfeeding found a relationship between work and breastfeeding success.[7] The timing of the return to work and the number of hours worked, not the type of work, influenced the duration of breastfeeding. Most of the respondents, however, were well educated and were motivated to respond to the advertisement and to fill out retrospectively a lengthy questionnaire. Results showed that mothers who pumped or hand-expressed milk (86% of the respondents) while at work continued to breastfeed longer than the small percentage who did not pump at work.

In times of economic downturn, work patterns are influenced by money. More women feel forced to return to work for economic reasons. Thus more women with less flexible jobs find it impossible to handle the job, the home, the baby, and breastfeeding. As a result, returning to work or inability to combine work and breastfeeding appears as a reason for early weaning. In a study by Morse et al[47] in Canada, monthly semistructured interviews were conducted with 61 mothers who intended to continue breastfeeding after returning to work.

Maternity leaves in Canada vary from 17 to 37 weeks. Mothers were hesitant to commit themselves to continuing to breastfeed because they believed too many factors were beyond their control despite elaborate plans and backup plans. The authors[46,47] concluded that financial constraints, increased education, and professional preparation were forcing women back to work in greater numbers, but few could manage to continue to breastfeed because there were no accommodations in the workplace. When the final results were reported, 36 mothers (of the 61) successfully combined breastfeeding and work for a mean of 18 weeks. Five different strategies for modifying feeding facilitated the transition from home to the workplace in this study: (1) breastfeeding on demand, (2) early introduction of a routine bottle, (3) transition to minimal breastfeeding, (4) transition to partial breastfeeding, and (5) transition to flexible breastfeeding (total breastfeeding weekends, partial during week). Only one mother expressed her milk at work; five expressed their milk at home to be given to the infant at day care.[46,47]

The introduction of a bottle at 2 weeks of age for 4 weeks before returning to work was studied by Cronenwett et al.[16] In a prospective study of 121 women who were committed to at least 6 weeks of breastfeeding, the mothers were randomly assigned to the "add-a-bottle" group or to the exclusive breastfeeding group. Some of the mothers pumped and gave their own milk by bottle. The mean breastfeeding duration for both groups exceeded 6 months, although there was a slight difference in rates between the two groups at 12 weeks. The most important predictor of duration of breastfeeding was the mother's goal. The authors[16] saw no evidence that a single daily bottle in the early weeks was incompatible with prolonged breastfeeding in women committed to breastfeeding. Mothers who returned to work in the early postpartum period were likely to wean earlier. The conclusion in this study was that no evidence supports the "nipple confusion" hypothesis, because the infants went back and forth between breast and bottle without difficulty.

Impact of stress on milk supply

The stability of a milk supply is an individual matter. Some women can cope with extreme pressures and maintain an abundant milk supply, whereas other women find milk production to be very volatile. In the early weeks of lactation, the effect of external factors is much greater, but fatigue is consistently the most detrimental factor to milk production. In a study of the influence of commonplace stresses represented by academic stress and season of the year, 24-hour concentrations of growth hormone and prolactin were measured in 37 male first-year medical students during examination week.[41] Although measurements of perceived stress (Perceived Stress Scale, PSS) rose sharply, there was no significant change in growth hormone or prolactin. This would suggest stress does not affect prolactin levels.

The workplace

Although working mothers are commonplace, companies who make working mothers comfortable are still rare. Efforts to increase parental leave, even unpaid leave, have not been widely established, although laws requiring minimal parental leave have been passed.

Some major companies, however, have been recognized by *Working Mother* magazine's annual survey as making some efforts to support mothers in the workplace.[48] The yardstick includes everything from the number of female vice presidents to fair advancement and equal pay for equal work. No company has been nominated for its support of breastfeeding, although maternity leave policies are considered important. The 1997 report of the 12th annual survey named Bayfront Medical Center, Beth Israel Deaconess, Rex Health Care, Inc., and the University of Pittsburgh Medical Center in the top 100 companies, but none was in the top 10, even though hospitals should be the model workplace.[48] Three health-related companies, however, were in the top 10: Glaxo Wellcome, Johnson and Johnson, and Merck. Hospitals employ a number of professional women in their childbearing years as physicians, nurses, therapists, psychologists, laboratory technicians, and child life specialists.

A very significant contribution could be made by allocating space and providing staff for day-care centers. This would allow mothers to interact with their infants and breastfeed them during the work day. Small experiments providing day care have shown a decrease in tardiness and absenteeism and a general increase in job satisfaction among employees who are mothers. For hospitals, where highly skilled and trained staff require as much as 6 months of costly on-the-job training, day care has been shown to be very cost effective in eliminating excessive turnover.

Moore and Jansa[45] sent surveys to 12 institutions known to support breastfeeding and to 100 of the Fortune 500 companies; only 29 were turned. Only two workplaces had breast pumps, and no documentable support of breastfeeding existed. Only an additional 14% of the 29 respondents even permitted breastfeeding in the workplace.

The Fortune 500 top companies so named in 1994 were contacted by Dusdieker et al,[17] who received 242 (48%) responses to their four-item questionnaire. Five corporations (2.0%) had written policies regarding infant feeding or breastfeeding in the workplace; the policy was company wide for only two (0.8%). Less than 70% of the 242 responding companies followed any infant-feeding policy. A room or facility (other than a rest room) was provided to express milk in private by 64%, and the other 36% stated that no space was provided. Only 12% provided breast pumps, but 83% provided refrigerators for storage of breast milk. Most (76%) allowed flexible time schedules to allow for pumping; 7% had on-site day-care facilities. This represents a vast improvement in the 7 years since the previous survey.

Almost half the companies in Auerbach's study were unaware that an employee was breastfeeding.[6] The *Working Mother* survey considers compassion for the mother's regular day-to-day activities the "acid test."[48] Physicians who serve as consultants to large and small industries, unions, not-for-profit agencies, and day-care centers are in very important positions to influence corporate trends, which are changing very slowly. Companies that have been recognized by *Working Mother* for their corporate efforts to support breastfeeding include but are not limited to Amoco Corporation,

Chicago; Dow Chemical Company, Midland, Mich; General Motors, Detroit; Kodak, Rochester, NY; and the Los Angeles Department of Water and Power.[48]

A comparison of maternal absenteeism and infant illness rates among breastfeeding and formula-feeding women showed breastfeeding reduced absenteeism.[14,15] In two corporations with on-site lactation programs, one had 100 births among 2400 and the second 30 births among 1200 female employees. Of the 101 mother-infant dyads studied, 59 were breastfed and 42 formula-fed. The company provided lactation counseling as well as pumping and storing facilities. Of the 28% of the infants who had no illnesses, 86% were breastfed and 14% formula-fed. Among mothers who were absent because of infant illness, 75% were formula feeding and only 25% were breastfeeding (Fig. 13-1).

Most of the studies concerning employment and breastfeeding were retrospective, relied on voluntary responses, and did not clearly define breastfeeding in terms of exclusivity or working in terms of part time or full time.[16,36] A prospective study reported by Kurinij et al[38] involving over 1000 women confirmed the reports of others that women with professional occupations breastfeed longer than nonprofessionals and that part-time work is more conducive to longer duration than full-time jobs. Both groups of women found equal satisfaction from breastfeeding. The duration of breastfeeding was evaluated in a separate study in the same two corporations mentioned previously. Cohen et al[14,15] reported that of the 187 participants, 75% who returned to work breastfed for 6 months or longer. The average duration for breastfeeding was 8.1 months. These rates were equal to the statistical norms for the region among women not employed outside the home.

In a provocative commentary, Furman[23] points out "the dilemma every woman faces, whether breastfeeding or bottle feeding, is leaving one's child." She further comments that mother's milk in a bottle given by any of several staff members at day care is not equal to nursing at the breast. Her solution was part-time work, which is not a new

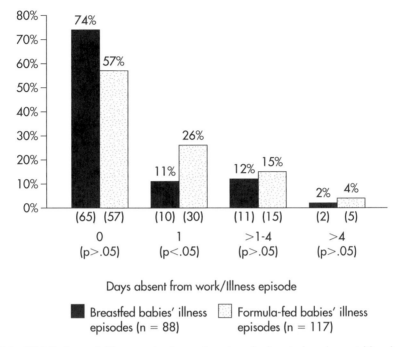

Fig. 13-1. Distribution of illness episodes and maternal absenteeism by nutritional groups. (Modified from Cohen R, Mrtek MB, Mrtek RG: *Am J Health Promotion* 10:148, 1995.)

idea but does depend on the nature of the mother's employment. The decision to work or not work is a very personal one and does not separate women into good and bad mothers. The role of the health professional is to discuss the mother's plans nonjudgmentally and then assist her in adjusting her infant and herself to the process.

Counseling breastfeeding mothers who choose to work

Part of the physician's counseling session before the birth of a baby should include inquiry about mother's plan to work postpartum. Open discussion about work, breastfeeding, child care arrangements, and general stress will be helpful. Most well-educated women who plan to return to a career have thought out the entire process carefully but may want some reassurance or alternative suggestions. The physician should know what services are available locally. It may be helpful to

have a list of other working mothers who are willing to share experiences and knowledge of resources. It is often helpful for a woman to know a real person who has experienced similar career choices.

Some women have no experience with newborns and are totally unrealistic about the new responsibility and what it entails. Even pediatricians in training may be unrealistic. The pediatrician may have to recommend a more realistic view of parenting and urge the parents to plan carefully and practically for working and parenting. The new mother needs to appreciate that events occur around children that cannot be totally controlled. Even when a woman has been an efficient career woman in total control of her destiny, an infant with normal needs may be overwhelming. Women who have jobs that are rigid from the standpoint of work hours and workplace will not find a few glib remarks in a pamphlet very helpful when they want to maintain their milk supply.

The physician may need to discuss specific issues of child care while the mother is working, as follows:

1. Child care arrangements should be sought that permit sufficient time for feeding an infant inexperienced with a bottle and sufficient time for extra cuddling of an infant who is used to a closer relationship with the "feeder." The child care specialist should be familiar with breastfeeding and sympathetic to the philosophy.

2. The advantages and disadvantages of child care in the infant's home, in the sitter's home, with or without the sitter's children, and with or without other children should be discussed. Is day care a good arrangement for this family, and what centers take young infants and will work with breastfeeding mothers? Despite low cost, nursery "warehousing" should be avoided.

3. Are there child care facilities available close to the workplace so that mother could leave work on her breaks to breastfeed?

Plans for feeding the infant while the mother is working depend on the infant's age and feeding pattern. If the infant is totally breastfed and under 6 months of age, the mother can breastfeed if she can leave work and go to the infant or if the infant can be brought to the workplace. If the mother cannot leave work to nurse, she may choose to pump her milk at work and save it for the following day. This necessitates having (1) a reasonably sanitary place to pump, such as a lounge or clean locker room, and (2) a means of storing the milk until she gets home, either in a refrigerator at work or in a portable refrigerator system. Mothers have used insulated containers with ice or dry ice. If no such arrangement for chilling can be made, the milk can be stored in a sterile container for 8 hours without refrigeration if collected under clean conditions.

A woman who is away from her breastfeeding infant past feeding time may need to pump to maintain her milk supply. A mother may also anticipate the infant's needs before she returns to work. She can practice pumping and storing a small amount of her milk daily for several weeks in her home freezer so that a stockpile is available while she is at work (see Chapter 20).

The mother should be instructed to introduce the baby to the bottle and an alternate caregiver before the first day of work. Developing a plan of organization and practicing it before the first day of work may avoid initial disaster. Also, returning to work part time at first may help minimize the adjustment.

No evidence indicates that it is necessary to introduce a bottle sooner than 10 days before returning to work. Unless a mother is returning to work immediately after delivery, a bottle should not be introduced before lactation is well established (at least 4 weeks for most primiparas) because it interferes with the mother's milk-making rhythm. Furthermore, it may confuse the infant. Although some infants readily go back and forth between breast and bottle, no way exists to identify the infant who will develop sucking difficulties and "nipple confusion," resulting ultimately in preference for the bottle if it is introduced too early. Babies given a bottle well before 3 months may easily reject it after 3 months. For the infant who does not accept the bottle gracefully, the following techniques may facilitate the process:

1. Someone other than the mother should give the feeding.

2. The mother should be out of sight and hearing range, preferably out of the building, so the infant does not await her arrival.

3. The infant should be held in the same position as for breastfeeding, that is, slightly elevated and close to the chest wall at about breast level. The bottle can be slipped down against the caregiver's chest wall.

4. Use a soft nipple and a small bottle at first for easy handling. A Volufeed, the clear plastic cylinder used for premature infants, allows a better view of the infant.

5. Create a soothing atmosphere; use a rocking chair, quiet music, and muted light.

6. The initial bottle feedings, if not all of them, should contain warm mother's milk to reduce the elements of change being introduced.

If the bottle feedings do not go well and alternate feedings are needed, milk can be provided by medicine cup feeding (see Chapter 14).

If the infant is over 6 months of age, the physician may consider introduction of other foods. The feeding given by the caregiver can be solids by spoon and liquids from a cup so that no breastfeeding is actually missed. The professional can anticipate these issues and tailor feeding counseling accordingly. Some infants quickly learn the mother's schedule and may adjust their sleep pattern to allow a long stretch while mother is away. This may result in feedings during the night instead, but if the mother is informed of this phenomenon, she may be less anxious if it occurs.

Bottle-fed infants have more infections and illnesses, which is another reason to encourage a mother to continue breastfeeding. This is especially important during the first weeks of adjustment to the transient, recurrent separation of mother and infant associated with the mother's return to work.

Maternal considerations

Counseling the breastfeeding family when the mother returns to work should also include attention to mothering the mother.[49] Fatigue is a significant problem for all postpartum women and many nursing mothers and can easily become a major stress when the mother adds outside employment to her schedule. Several days or more of adjustment are necessary for a major change in one's schedule. If the mother can focus on a few essential concerns (infant, job, own well-being) as opposed to housework, fancy meals, or a social schedule, she will weather this transition without despair. The first casualty of fatigue may be breastfeeding unless some anticipatory action is taken.

Once the schedule has been adjusted and a routine established, breastfeeding may offer tremendous satisfaction for both mother and infant in terms of a sustained relationship as well as a reaffirmation for the mother of the quality of her parenting. One of the most difficult adjustments to

motherhood is the need to set priorities and eliminate some chores of lesser urgency. The physician needs to reinforce this when the mother returns to work. Whether or not a mother continues to breastfeed, holding and cuddling her baby cannot become a lower priority. The mother's nourishment is also important and can be consumed during the time spent pumping. A mother should plan to have a beverage available every time she sits down to nurse or pump.

Day care

Infants in day care have created a special concern for parents, pediatricians, social scientists, and policymakers. The early published information did not discuss the impact of breastfeeding before or during the infant's involvement with day care. Haskins and Kotch[27] first reviewed the literature (172 articles) and concluded, "Children in day care, especially those under three years old and sometimes their teachers and household contacts, have higher rates of diarrhea, hepatitis A, meningitis and possibly also otitis media than children not in day care." The data are less clear for respiratory illnesses and cytomegalovirus. Extremely valuable but unavailable data would be the relationship between breastfeeding and illness in and out of day care. Revisions of state regulatory policy regarding health practices in day care are necessary. Parents choosing day-care facilities for their children need to select them with consideration for health and safety. More than 60% of the children under 6 years of age of women who work are in out-of-home care, approximately 8 million U.S. children in 1995. In some situations, day care may actually improve the infant's potential, especially when the mother is young, immature, depressed, overwhelmed, or without family support.

Concern about infant illness should result in pediatricians' involvement in ensuring quality day care in the local community. For the infant age appropriate for breastfeeding, one possible preventive measure would be to encourage a continuation of breastfeeding where possible. Furthermore, day-care policy and procedure should encourage and facilitate breastfeeding. Mothers should inquire about day-care centers' policies toward breastfeeding. Physicians who consult for day-care centers should be well informed as well. Breast milk can safely stand at room temperature for 6 to 8 hours and need not be discarded if the first feeding attempt is incomplete. In contrast, formula must be refrigerated and discarded after the first feeding attempt because it contains no antibodies or infection protection factors. No infant feeding of any kind should be warmed in a microwave oven. Protective gloves are not necessary to feed breast milk. The accidental feeding of a different mother's milk is not cause for alarm, although it should be reported to the parents for public health reasons. One feeding of milk produced by a mother who is positive for human immunodeficiency virus (HIV) will probably not transmit the disease. Women who are HIV positive in developed countries, however, are discouraged from breastfeeding.

Resources for parents

The popular press has been inundated with books on child care and child rearing, with a significant number on breastfeeding, specifically breastfeeding and employment. These volumes can be extremely helpful to young parents, providing detailed information about how to manage. Many recognize that mothers, fathers, infants, jobs, child care arrangements, and support resources are all different. A disturbing number, however, are dogmatic and single-minded, giving the impression that the author's method is the only recipe for successful lactation. The pediatrician should become familiar with a few of these guide books and certainly not recommend any without reading them first. A few of these books have instilled guilt in the working woman about leaving her infant.

The brochure *Working and Breastfeeding: Can You Do It?* was prepared by the National Healthy Mothers, Healthy Babies Coalition and is available free by calling the coalition in Washington, DC, at 202-863-2458. It is also available through local WIC nutritional programs. It is simple and direct, providing directions for managing a job and

breastfeeding as well as collecting and storing breast milk.

Women in health care head the list of authors, because many women physicians (especially residents), nurses, and hospital employees return to work while breastfeeding and then share their experiences in print.[26] Even the worst setup in a hospital may surpass the resources available to the women working in industry. Certainly hospitals and health care centers should provide models for other workplaces in supporting optimal day-care sources and making it possible for a mother-employee to return to work and maintain her milk supply.[35] Independent lactation practitioners provide an additional resource. Women should contact the International Lactation Consultants Association (ILCA) for referrals (see Chapter 21). Some industries have hired certified lactation consultants to provide assistance to their employees in maintaining their milk supply. The company also usually provides "a pumping room" and equipment. As pointed out by Cohen et al,[14,15] this also reduces absenteeism because the infant who is provided the mother's milk has fewer illnesses.

Responding to parental needs, Brazelton captured the quintessential challenge to parents in the title and the text *Working and Caring*.[10] It is possible for parents to both work and care! Freud and Dann[22] pointed out that the two most powerful requirements for human existence are "love" and "work." Our culture had suggested that men work and women love in relation to family obligations. Today it is possible not only for a mother to love her children and work, but also for a father to work and love his children. Although Brazelton's book was written for parents in his usual style of live reports of representative families, it also contains valuable guidance for the health care professional who counsels working parents.[10]

Surgeon General's Workshop

The *Report of the Surgeon General's Workshop on Breastfeeding and Human Lactation*[50] clearly enunciates that strategies need to be developed to reduce the barriers to breastfeeding while employed. All six categories address the issue in some capacity. Category 1, The World of Work, states that a national breastfeeding promotion initiative directed to all those who influence breastfeeding decisions and opportunities of women involved in school, job training, professional education, and employment is needed. Along with data collection, education, and change in institutional policy, the report suggests that legislation related to federal, state, and local tax incentives might be provided for institutions that successfully implement breastfeeding programs at work or at school. It also recommends the development of appropriate support services in the world of work, such as prenatal care, social and nutritional services, paid maternity leave, child care, and alternative types of work arrangements such as flextime and job sharing.

The workshop report also states that successful initiation and continuation of breastfeeding will require a broad spectrum of support services involving families, peers, care providers, employers, and community agencies and organizations.[50] Little has been accomplished toward these goals.

Maternal benefits

In 1919 the International Labor Organization established the Maternity Protection Convention for working women.[51] This document provided for two half-hour nursing breaks per day. It also recommended that employers provide crèches (day nurseries, especially European) or day care when more than a given number of women are employed, but few countries hold to its tenets today. Maternity benefits vary from country to country and may include maternity leave with or without pay, nursing breaks, provision of day-care facilities, and prohibition of dismissal. Physicians who care for mothers and infants should take a leadership role in ensuring that mothers can continue breastfeeding even when the mother is employed.

Many women, especially when faced with coping with a second or third child, reexamine the working issue in light of the needs of their children, even though they may have previously managed to breastfeed and work at one time. No

one else can or should decide for a woman how she will handle parenting, especially in the early years of a child's life. Furman[23] poignantly addresses some of the issues. No woman should be embarrassed to stay home or should apologize for working part time or not at all. Breast milk is not a substitute for good parenting, any more than quantity parenting is synonymous with quality parenting. It is possible to work and to care, however.

Physician's role

The primary role of the physician is as an advocate for children. Physicians can help support fathers and mothers alike who are faced with fulfilling the roles of parent, employee, and citizen in a rapidly changing society. Physicians should be able to provide understandable information concerning the child's growth and development combined with a realistic view of the issues in parenting and family life. They should show an openness and willingness to discuss nonjudgmentally with the parents their specific situation, options, and choices for caring for their child.

If the physician is the medical consultant to the day-care program, the role can be to assure mothers who want to provide their milk that they will be supported by the staff. The physician should develop policies and procedures for the storage and use of the breast milk provided. In addition, space and facilities (at least a rocking chair and a screen) should be available for the mother to nurse the infant before leaving the child and on her return later before going home. If the physician is in the medical department of a large company or the pediatrician for a working breastfeeding mother, he or she can advocate for time and resources for pumping while at work as part of good preventive care.

The success of breastfeeding depends to a degree on ever-widening circles of support for the breastfeeding infant-mother dyad. Support should come first from the husband/father, then from other family members, other caregivers in the home, day-care facilities, employers and other employees, and community members to help the mother and family comfortably and safely breastfeed, work, and care for their child as they choose. Breastfeeding is not just a woman's issue. It is a family issue and a public health issue as well.

The physician's role in achieving a successful return to work for the breastfeeding mother include the following steps:

1. Discuss the mother's plans for returning to work in advance.
2. Recommend appropriate local child care facilities that are "breastfeeding friendly."
3. Suggest that the mother discuss breastfeeding with her employer or supervisor.
4. Have a lactation consultant available in the practice or office, or if not, know where one can be contacted.
5. Provide recommendations for collecting and storing breast milk, which can be included in an office handout.
6. When medical problems arise, seek adequate information so that an appropriate solution can be recommended that supports continued breastfeeding.

REFERENCES

1. Ainsworth MDS: The development of infant-mother attachment. In Caldwell BM, Ricciuti HN, editors: *Review of child development research,* Chicago, 1973, University of Chicago Press.
2. Ainsworth MDS, Blehar MC, Waters E et al: *Patterns of attachment,* Hillsdale, NJ, 1978, Erlbaum.
3. American Academy of Pediatrics, Committee on Psychosocial Aspects of Child and Family Health: The mother working outside the home, *Pediatrics* 73:874, 1984.
4. American Academy of Pediatrics, Workgroup on Breastfeeding: Breast feeding and the use of human milk, *Pediatrics* 100:1035, 1997.
5. American College of Obstetricians and Gynecologists: *Guidelines on pregnancy and work,* Chicago, 1987, ACOG Publications.
6. Auerbach KG: Assisting the employed breastfeeding mother, *J Nurse Midwifery* 35:26, 1990.
7. Auerbach KG, Guss E: Maternal employment and breast feeding: a study of 567 women's experiences, *Am J Dis Child* 138:958, 1984.
8. Baden C: *Work and family: an annotated bibliography 1978-1980,* Boston, 1981, Wheelock College Center for Parenting Studies.
9. Brazelton TB: *Toddlers and parents,* New York, 1974, Delta.
10. Brazelton TB: *Working and caring,* Reading, Mass, 1985, Addison-Wesley.
11. Bronfenbrenner U, Crouter AC: Work and family through time and space. In Kamerman SB, Hayes CD, editors: *Families that work: children in a changing world,* Washington, DC, 1982, National Academy Press.
12. Chalmers B, Ransome OH, Herman A: Working while breastfeeding among coloured women, *Psychol Rep* 67: 1123, 1990.
13. Chase-Lansdale PL, Owen MT: Maternal employment in a family context: effects on infant-mother and infant-father attachments, *Child Dev* 58:1505, 1987.
14. Cohen R, Mrtek MB: The impact of two corporate lactation programs on the incidence and duration of breast-feeding by employed mothers, *Am J Health Promotion* 6:436, 1994.
15. Cohen R, Mrtek MB, Mrtek RG: Comparison of maternal absenteeism and infant illness rates among breast-feeding and formula-feeding women in two corporations, *Am J Health Promotion* 10:148, 1995.
16. Cronenwett L, Stukel T, Kearney M et al: Single daily bottle use in the early weeks post partum and breastfeeding outcomes, *Pediatrics* 90:760, 1992.
17. Dusdieker LB, Losch ME, Dungy CI: Breastfeeding and the workplace: a survey of Fortune 500 industrial corporations, *Pediatr Res* 37:136A, 1994.
18. Easterbrooks MA, Goldberg WA: Effects of early maternal employment on toddlers, mothers and fathers, *Dev Psychol* 21:774, 1985.
19. Eiger MS, Olds SW: *The complete book of breastfeeding,* ed 2, New York, 1987, Workman.
20. Eisenberg L: Caring for children and working dilemmas of contemporary womanhood, *Pediatrics* 56:24, 1975.
21. Frederick IB, Auerbach KG: Maternal-infant separation and breastfeeding: the return to work or school, *J Reprod Med* 30:323, 1985.
22. Freud A, Dann S: An experiment in group upbringing, *Psychoanal Study Child* 6:127, 1961.
23. Furman L: A second look at breastfeeding and full time maternal employment, *Am J Dis Child* 146:540, 1992.
24. Gielen AC, Faden RR, O'Campo P et al: Maternal employment during the early postpartum period: effects on initiation and continuation of breastfeeding, *Pediatrics* 87:298, 1991.

25. Ginzberg E: The changing pattern of women's work, *Am J Orthopsychiatry* 28:313, 1958.

26. Grams M: *Breastfeeding success for working mothers,* Carson City, Nev, 1985, National Capitol Resources.

27. Haskins R, Kotch J: Day care and illness: evidence, costs, and public policy, *Pediatrics* 77(suppl):951, 1986.

28. Heins M, Stillman P, Sabers D et al: Attitudes of pediatricians toward maternal employment, *Pediatrics* 72:283, 1983.

29. Hirschman C, Sweet JA: Social background and breast-feeding among American mothers, *Soc Biol* 21:39, 1974.

30. Hock E: Working and nonworking mothers and their infants: a comparative study of maternal caregiving characteristics and infant's social behavior, *Merrill-Palmer Q* 46:79, 1980.

31. Hoffman LW: Effects of maternal employment on the child: a review of the research, *Dev Psychol* 10:204, 1974.

32. Hoffman LW: Increased fathering: effects on mother. In Lamb M, Sagi A, editors: *Fatherhood and family policy,* Hillsdale, NJ, 1983, Erlbaum.

33. Howell MC: Employed mothers and their families, *Pediatrics* 52:252, 1973.

34. Hurst M, Zambrana RE: *Determinants and consequences of maternal employment,* Washington, DC, 1981, Business and Professional Women's Foundation.

35. Katcher AL, Lanese MG: Breastfeeding by employed mothers: a reasonable accommodation in the work place, *Pediatrics* 75:644, 1985.

36. Kearney MH, Cronenwett L: Breastfeeding and employment, *J Obstet Gynecol Neonatal Nurs* 20:471, 1991.

37. Krieger F: Ross Laboratories Mothers Survey: a marketing research tool. Presented at the Editors Conference, Sept 22, 1992, New York.

38. Kurinij N, Shiono PH, Ezrine SF et al: Does maternal employment affect breastfeeding? *Am J Public Health* 79:1247, 1989.

39. La Leche League: *The womanly art of breastfeeding,* ed 6, Schaumburg, Ill, 1997, La Leche League.

40. Lawrence RA: Early mothering by adolescents. In McAnarney ER, editor: *Premature adolescent pregnancy and parenthood,* New York, 1983, Grune & Stratton.

41. Malarkey WB, Hall JC, Pearl DK et al: The influence of academic stress and season on 24-hour concentrations of growth hormone and prolactin, *J Clin Endocrinol Metab* 73:1089, 1991.

42. Martinez GA, Stahle DA: The recent trend in milk feeding among WIC infants, *Am J Public Health* 72:68, 1982.

43. Mead M: A cultural anthropologist's approach to maternal deprivation. In *Deprivation of maternal care,* Public Health Papers No 14, Geneva, 1962, World Health Organization.

44. Mizera J: Personal communication, Ross Laboratories Mothers Survey, 1997.

45. Moore JF, Jansa N: A survey of policies and practices in support of breastfeeding mothers in the work place, *Birth* 14:191, 1987.

46. Morse JM, Bottorff JL: Intending to breastfeed and work, *J Obstet Gynecol Nurs* 18:493, 1989.

47. Morse JM, Bottorff JL, Boman J: Patterns of breastfeeding and work: the Canadian experience, *Can J Public Health* 80:182, 1989.

48. Moskowitz M: 100 best companies for working mothers, *Working Mother,* October, 1997, p 18.

49. Popkin BM: Time allocation of the mother and child nutrition, *Ecol Food Nutr* 9:1, 1980.

50. *Report of the Surgeon General's Workshop on Breastfeeding and Human Lactation,* Lawrence RA, chair, DHHS Pub No HRS-D-MC 84-2, Washington, DC, 1984, US Department of Health and Human Services.

51. Richardson JL: Review of the international legislation establishing nursing breaks, *J Trop Pediatr Environ Child Hlth* 21:249, 1975.

52. Ross Products Division, Abbott Laboratories: *Mothers survey: updated breastfeeding trend through 1996,* Columbus, Ohio, 1998, Abbott.

53. Ryan AS: The resurgence of breastfeeding in the United States, *Pediatrics* 99(4):e12, 1997(4): (electronic article).

54. Ryan AS, Martinez GA: Breastfeeding and the working mother: a profile, *Pediatrics* 83:524, 1989.

55. Sanday P: Female status in the public domain. In Rosaldo M, Lamphere L, editors: *Woman, culture and society,* Stanford, 1974, Stanford University Press.

56. US Department of Labor: *Facts on women workers,* Washington, DC, 1997, US Government Printing Office Web Page, www.gpo.gov.

57. US Department of Labor: *Manpower report of the president,* Washington, DC, 1974, US Government Printing Office.

58. US Department of Labor, Office of the Secretary: *Facts on women workers,* Washington, DC, 1980, Women's Bureau.

59. Van Esterik P, Greiner T: Breastfeeding and women's work: constraints and opportunities, *Stud Fam Plan* 12:184, 1981.

60. Vaugh BE, Gove FL, Egeland B: The relationship between out-of-home care and the quality of infant-mother attachment in an economically disadvantaged population, *Child Dev* 51:1203, 1980.

61. West CP: Factors influencing the duration of breast feeding, *J Biosoc Sci* 12:325, 1980.

62. Winikoff B, Baer EC: The obstetrician's opportunity: translating "breast is best" from theory to practice, *Am J Obstet Gynecol* 138:105, 1980.

63. Zambrana RE, Hurst M, Hite RL: The working mother in contemporary perspective: a review of the literature, *Pediatrics* 64:862, 1979.

*B*reastfeeding the infant with a problem

PREMATURE INFANTS

Research in the science of nutrition for the low-birthweight infant and the micropremature infant has advanced tremendously as the technology to study the important questions has improved. Neonatologists meanwhile have spent the last decades studying the physiology of respiration. Their advances have contributed to the survival of smaller and smaller infants. The edge of viability is 24 weeks and a weight of 500 g; however, there are examples of survivors under these values. One of the key points learned retrospectively about survival, generation after generation, has been the critical impact of fluid and nutrition. Although human milk has gained prominence in these studies, the early use of unsupplemented drip milk and some donor milks produced poor growth patterns. Drip milk is very low in fat and therefore low in calories. The protein levels in donor milk from women late in lactation (i.e., beyond 6 to 8 months, when the levels have dropped) parallel the biologic child's decreased needs with the addition of solid foods. These factors contributed to the abandonment of human milk until supplements were developed and studies of the milk of women who had delivered prematurely sparked new investigations.

This discussion highlights only the important issues; the reader is referred to reviews such as the exhaustive summary of human milk for the premature infant and the extensive bibliography by Steichen, Krug-Wispe, and Tsang.[215] *Nutritional Needs of the Preterm Infant,* the text by Tsang, Lucas, Uauy et al,[229] is an international collaboration that involved many major premature infant centers in discussions to create unity out of a tremendous disparity of practice and various recipes for nutritional support. This collaboration also produced a consensus on individual nutrient requirements for infants under 1000-g birthweight, for 1000-g to 1750-g infants, and for postdischarge management. Neonatologists, however, have not reached a consensus on the feeding of premature infants.[136] The absolute standard for evaluating the nutritional outcome of preterm infants remains undefined. A strategy to minimize mobilization of endogenous nutrient stores is moving away from a focus on intrauterine-based, short-term growth and nutrient retention rates to a system that considers long-term growth achievement.[199] The optimal time to initiate oral feedings in the smallest and sickest preterm infants is under revision.[198] Prolonged exclusive parenteral nutrition is being replaced with minimal amounts of oral feedings with parenteral nutrition to preserve and maintain intestinal function.[3,196] As nutritional markers shift, the preterm infant's own mother's milk may well be recognized, even by the most skeptical clinicians, as the "gold standard" to prevent short-term morbidities and enhance long-term outcome.[197] With this change may come the recognition that fortified donor milk is superior to artificial feeds.

No goal is universal, according to Gross and Slagle,[91] who define the task as (1) achieving well-defined, standard short-term growth, such as intrauterine growth curves or mimicking reference fetus composition; (2) preventing feeding-related morbidities, such as nosocomial infection and necrotizing enterocolitis; and (3) optimizing long-term neurodevelopmental and physical growth. This discussion addresses these goals. As the technology of ultrasound continues to advance, serial observations of fetuses that result in normal full-term infants are being assessed.[23] Intrauterine growth patterns so determined may come closer to a normal model than previous assessments done on infants delivered prematurely, which in itself is not normal.

A normal full-term infant can usually be breast-fed with only minor adjustment, even without the support of medical expertise. The infant with a medical or surgical problem presents special concerns that cannot be conquered simply by a strong-willed mother who is determined to overcome all obstacles to breastfeed.[128] An understanding of the infant's medical problem and special nutritional needs and the mechanical obstacles to feeding and nutritional absorption is necessary before a rational judgment can be made about breastfeeding. When the infant cannot nurse directly at the breast, is providing mother's milk appropriate? What is the overall prognosis for ever feeding at the breast or, perhaps, for survival itself? Parents are so awed by the medical staff of special and intensive care nurseries that they are often afraid to bring up the subject of breastfeeding. In addition, the nursery staff may be so busy balancing electrolytes and adjusting ventilators and monitors that they have not thought to ask what plans the mother might have had for feeding before the infant developed a problem.

Absolute contraindications exist to breastfeeding infants with certain conditions, but these problems are few and rare. This chapter discusses each medical problem separately. Chapter 18 provides general information on establishing a milk supply without the stimulus of the infant's suckling.

Initiation of enteral feeds

In the words of Lucas[137]: "It is fundamentally unphysiological to deprive an infant of any gestation of enteral feeding since the deprivation would never normally occur at any stage." This is based on the fact that the fetus normally makes sucking motions and swallows amniotic fluid from early gestation. This may even have a trophic effect on the gut. By the third trimester, the infant is swallowing up to 500 ml per day, which actually provides as much as 3 g of protein per day. The secretion of gastrointestinal hormones is believed to occur in response to the first postdelivery feedings.[229] In animals, after only a few days of deprivation of enteral feeds, atrophic changes take place in the gut.[139] In human infants who have never received enteral feedings, there are no gut peptide surges, not even those of the trophic hormones enteroglucagon, gastrin, and gastric inhibitory polypeptide.[108] These hormones are believed to be key to the activation of the enteroinsular axis.[139]

Although early enteral feedings are by no means universally accepted, a number of randomized controlled studies support the concept.[55,91] Berseth[23] reports that the response of the preterm infant's intestine to entire feedings at different postnatal ages showed significantly more mature motor patterns of the gut as well as higher plasma concentrations of gastrin and gastric inhibitory peptide. From a management standpoint, early-fed infants were able to tolerate full oral feeds sooner, had fewer days of feeding intolerance, and shorter hospital stays.[160] Studies varied from infants who were fed under 24 hours of age at 1 ml/hr to infants who were fed full feeds starting at days 2 to 7 compared to infants on usual delayed protocols. All showed an advantage to early feeds.[139]

Gross and Slagle[91] pointed out that human milk is better than formula in early feeds, in establishing enteral tolerance and discontinuation of parenteral nutrition, in long-term improved neurodevelopmental outcome, and in the psychologic benefit to the mother. They found human milk fell short after 4 to 6 weeks in the amount of protein, calcium, and phosphorus, a problem solvable with use of human milk fortifier. No substitute has been developed that replaces the many and varied advantages of human milk, however.

Many investigators have concluded that minimal enteral feedings with human milk can optimize growth, development, and progress for small prematures, even in ventilator-dependent infants.[3,108,139,212] In most studies the incidence of necrotizing enterocolitis (NEC) has been similar with and without early feeds.[137] The presence of an umbilical catheter has long been a contraindication to feeding because of the risk of NEC. When Davey et al[47] investigated this question, the incidence of NEC was comparable in infants with and without catheters.

Other advantages of early feeds include lower serum direct and indirect bilirubin and less phototherapy. Benefits from early feeds were measurable with raw maternal milk, pasteurized premature milk, and even infant formula.[139,212]

Low-birthweight infants

All premature infants are not the same. Infants who are born weighing less than 2500 g are referred to as being *low birthweight* (LBW). If the infants are less than 37 weeks of gestation, they are *premature;* if they are full term and LBW, they are *small for gestational age* (SGA).

Very low birthweight (VLBW) refers to an infant weighing less than 1500 g. The probability of survival has changed dramatically in all weight ranges. With the availability of surfactant for respiratory distress, infants between 500 and 1000 g are surviving in great numbers. The problems of nutrition, however, pose new challenges to the neonatologist. The feedings appropriate for a 2000-g premature infant vary only in volume and frequency from the full-term infant in most cases. Feedings for a VLBW infant must address the advantages

and disadvantages of human milk at this point in their growth curve. The composition of mother's milk varies in some constituents with the degree of prematurity[105] (Box 14-1).

The advantages of human milk for the LBW infant include the physiologic amino acid and fat profile,[28] the digestibility and absorption of these proteins and fats,[220] and the low renal solute load.[215] The presence of active enzymes enhances the maturation and supplements the enzyme activity of this underdeveloped gut. The antiinfective properties and living cells protect the immature infant from infection and may even protect against NEC. The psychologic benefit to the mother who can participate in her infant's care by providing her milk is a less tangible but no less important advantage.

The disadvantages are the gap in certain nutrients required for adequate growth, which include the volume of total protein and macrominerals, especially calcium and phosphorus.[65,76] Much of the attention to the shortcomings has been based on work done using pooled milk samples collected from women whose infants are full term and many months old. The source of the human milk and processing—freezing or pasteurizing—are signifi-

---

BOX 14-1 Milk of mothers who deliver preterm

Level increased in preterm	Level unchanged in preterm
Total nitrogen	Volume
Protein nitrogen	Calories
Long-chain fatty acids	Lactose (? less)
Medium-chain fatty acids	Fat (?) by
Short-chain fatty acids	"creamatocrit"
Sodium	Linolenic acid
Chloride	Potassium
Magnesium (?)	Calcium
Iron	Phosphorus
	Copper
	Zinc
	Osmolality
	Vitamin B_{1-12}

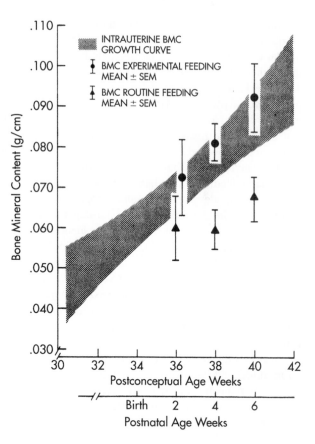

Fig. 14-1. Postnatal bone mineral content (BMC) in 33- to 35-week-old appropriate-for-gestational-age/preterm infants compared with intrauterine bone mineralization curve (IUBMC). Regression curve and 95th-percentile confidence limits for regression for BMC of infants born at different gestational ages (30 to 42 weeks' gestational age) represent IUBMC. Infants fed routine cow's milk formula *(closed triangles)* had significantly lower BMC than infants fed standard formula supplemented with calcium and phosphorus *(closed circles)*. In these infants, BMC was not different from IUBMC at 4 and 6 weeks' postnatal age. (From Steichen JJ, Gratton TL, Tsang RC: *J Pediatr* 96:528, 1980.)

cant to the question of nutritional adequacies. In the last decade, many laboratory and clinical scientists have studied the questions posed here and provided hundreds of reports regarding the nutrition and nurturance of the LBW and VLBW infant. Only a fraction of the resources can be referenced here.*

Optimal growth for premature infants

Optimal growth for infants born prematurely is considered to be the growth curve they would have followed had they remained in utero[67] (Fig. 14-1 and Tables 14-1 and 14-2). Achieving this goal utilizing the immature intestinal tract requires that the nutrients be digestible and absorbable and not

impose a significant metabolic stress on the other immature organs, especially the kidney. Although human milk provides the ideal nutrients, it would require an inordinate nonphysiologic volume to achieve adequate amounts of some nutrients without calculated supplementation. To fill these growth needs, one can use an artificial or chemical formula or use human milk as a base, with all its advantages, and add the deficit nutrients to it.

Special properties of preterm milk

The identification of special quantitative differences in nutrients in the milk of mothers who delivered prematurely brought new interest in the use of human milk for premature infants (Box 14-1). Many investigators have contributed to the pool of knowledge after the initial revelations by Atkinson et al in 1980, who reported the

---

*References 28, 84, 89, 137, 139, 141, 153-155, 184, 187, 188, 196.

TABLE 14-1   **Estimated requirements and advisable intakes for protein by infant's weight as derived by factorial approach**

Birthweight range	Tissue increment (per day)	Dermal loss (per day)	Urine loss (per day)	Intestinal absorption (% intake)	Estimated requirement (per day)	Advisable intake		
						Per day	Per kg*	Per 100 kcal†
800-1200 g	2.32 g	0.17 g	0.68 g	87 g†	3.64 g	4.0 g	4.0 g	3.1 g
1200-1800 g	3.01 g	0.25 g	0.90 g	87 g	4.78 g	5.2 g	3.5 g	2.7 g

From Ziegler EE, Biga RL, Fomon SJ: Nutritional requirements of the premature infant. In Suskind RM: *Textbook of pediatric nutrition*, New York, 1981, Raven.
*Assuming body weight of 1000 g and 1500 g for 800-g to 1200-g infant and 1200-g to 1800-g infant, respectively.
†Assuming calorie intake of 120 kcal/day.

TABLE 14-2   **Accumulation of various components during last trimester of pregnancy**

Component	Accumulation during various stages of gestation				
	26-31 wk	31-33 wk	33-35 wk	35-38 wk	38-40 wk
Body weight (g)*	500	500	500	500	
Water (g)	410	350	320	240	220
Fat (g)	25	65	85	175	200
Nitrogen (g)	11	12	12	6	7
Calcium (g)	4	5	5	5	5
Phosphorus (g)	2.2	2.6	2.8	3.0	3.0
Magnesium (mg)	130	110	120	120	80
Sodium (mEq)	35	25	40	40	40
Potassium (mEq)	19	24	26	20	20
Chloride (mEq)	30	24	10	20	10
Iron (mg)	36	60	60	40	20
Copper (mg)	2.1	2.4	2.0	2.0	2.0
Zinc (mg)	9.0	10.0	8.0	7.0	3.0

Modified from data of Widdowson, from Heird WC, Anderson TL: Nutritional requirements and methods of feeding low birth weight infants. In Gluck L et al, editors: *Current problems in pediatrics,* vol 7, no 8, Chicago, 1977, Year Book.
*Body weight of 26-week fetus is 1000 g and of 40-week fetus, 3500 g.

nitrogen concentrations of milk from mothers of premature infants to be greater than that of milk from mothers delivering at term.[12,13,25,105,177]

Preterm milk is higher in protein content during the first months of lactation, containing between 1.8 and 2.4 g/dl. Preterm milk contains similar fat in quality and quantity,[93] although Anderson et al[8] reported increased values for preterm milk over term milk. Lactose in preterm milk averages 5.96 g/dl and up to 6.95 g/dl at 28 days, whereas the values in term milk are 6.16 and 7.26 g/dl, respectively. Preterm milk has higher energy than term milk, 58 to 70 kcal/dl, compared with 48 to 64 over the first month postpartum.

The macronutrients calcium and phosphorus are slightly higher in preterm milk (14 to 16 mEq/L vs. 13 to 16 mEq/L calcium and 4.7 to 5.5 mM/L vs. 4.0 to 5.1 mM/L phosphorus). Neither term nor preterm milk has adequate calcium and phosphorus for the VLBW infant. Magnesium levels in preterm milk are 28 to 31 mg/L, dropping to 25 mg/L at

28 days, and term milk are 25 to 29 mg/L. Zinc levels are higher in preterm milk, beginning at 5.3 mg/L and dropping to 3.9, whereas term milk begins at 5.4 and drops to 2.6 mg/L. Sodium levels in preterm milk are higher (26.6 mEq/L, dropping to 12.6 mEq/L) whereas term milk is 22.3 mEq/L, decreasing to 8.5 mEq/L at 28 days.[201] Chloride has a similar average (preterm 31.6 decreasing to 16.8 mEq/L and term 26.9 decreasing to 13.1 mEq/L).

Requirements for growth in premature infants

The *whey protein* in human milk is an advantage for all infants but especially the premature infant. It includes the nine amino acids known to be essential to all humans, as well as taurine,[220] glycine, leucine, and cystine, which are considered essential for the premature infant.[198] The premature infant lacks the necessary enzymes for metabolism and has been noted to accumulate nonphysiologic levels of methionine, tyrosine, phenylalanine, blood urea, and ammonia.[92] The protein requirement for the LBW infant based on intrauterine accretion rates is 2.5 g/100 kcal or 325 mg/kg of body weight/day.[215] Metabolizable energy requirement is 109 kcal/kg/day.

The requirement for fat is based on the *essential fatty acid* proportion as 3% of total caloric intake. Human milk has high levels of linoleic acid (9% of lipids) and adequately meets this requirement. Human milk fat is more readily absorbed in the presence of milk lipase and other enzymes in milk. It is reported that infants under 1500 g absorb 90% of human milk fat and 68% of cow's milk–based formula fats.[200]

Fat digestion is very efficient in LBW infants who receive their own mother's milk fresh and untreated. Fat absorption is decreased by calcium supplementation, however, and by sterilizing the milk. If human milk is supplemented with lipids, it will change the vitamin E/polyunsaturated fatty acid (PUFA) ratio. Vitamin E may need to be added to keep the E/PUFA ratio greater than 0.6 (human milk E/PUFA is 0.9 normally).[101]

Special attributes of human milk for VLBW infants have been confirmed as investigators inspect the value of adding nutrients to formulas specifically for these infants.[232] In a study of omega-3 (ω-3) fatty acids on retinal function, using electroretinograms, human milk was associated with the best function, followed by formula supplemented with ω-3 fatty acids. This supports that ω-3 fatty acids are essential to retinal development.[26]

Preterm and term milk do not contain sufficient calcium and phosphorus for bone accretion. *Rickets* has developed in LBW infants who are not supplemented, because the requirement for bone growth at this point in the growth curve is high. *Calcium* and *phosphorus* fetal accretion increases steadily over the last trimester. *Magnesium* accretion is unchanged in that period.[155]

Mineral accretion is a complex phenomenon dependent on a number of variables beyond simple levels of calcium, phosphorus, magnesium, and vitamin D.[2] Absorption and retention are altered by the quantities of other minerals as well as other nutrients, including fat, protein, and carbohydrate. Although the calcium/phosphorus ratio in human milk is more physiologic than that of cow's milk, the low levels of phosphorus lead to loss of calcium in the urine.[208]

Even with optimal vitamin D and magnesium, the amount of calcium absorbed from preterm milk is not enough to meet intrauterine accretion rates without supplementation.[215] Because human milk phosphorus levels are low even with high intestinal absorption and high renal tubular reabsorption compared with the needs of the premature infant, supplementation is necessary to avoid depletion or deficiency.[34] Intrauterine accretion rates for calcium phosphorus were achieved when Schanler and Abrams[198] fed human milk supplemented with calcium gluconate and glycerophosphate to VLBW infants. In their study, supplementation with magnesium was not indicated. The authors concluded that greater intakes of calcium and phosphorus and not improved bioavailability were responsible for the improved net retention.

Vitamin D requirements in this period of high

skeletal development depend on maternal vitamin D status, because significant correlation exists between maternal serum and preterm infant cord serum 25-hydroxyvitamin D (25-OHD) values. LBW infants quickly become dependent on exogenous vitamin D because fetal storage is minimal. The recommended daily allowance (RDA) of 400 units of vitamin D appears to be appropriate for all LBW infants, regardless of feedings, as well as for term infants. Although unresolved questions surround its absorption and excretion, vitamin D has a toxic level, so more may not be better.

Other vitamin needs of LBW infants depend on body stores, intestinal absorption, bioavailability of the vitamin, and rates of utilization and excretion.[68] Little information suggests that major differences exist in absorption between term and LBW infants, although fat-soluble vitamins depend on bile acids for absorption. (See Chapter 9 and Appendix P for vitamin requirements.) It is recommended that LBW infants receive daily vitamin supplements especially to address the increased need and borderline levels provided in the volume of human milk they can reasonably consume (Box 14-2).

The mineral supplementation required for LBW infants fed human milk is based on intrauterine accretion rates, which may not actually be achieved (Table 14-3). Not all premature infants fed human milk develop rickets, which occurs infrequently in infants greater than 1500 g. The VLBW infant does need supplementation, and cases of rickets are well documented in the literature for this group.[201] Supplements are usually not necessary when the infant reaches 40 weeks' postconceptual age. *Hypophosphatemia* is a sensitive biochemical indicator of low bone mineralization in VLBW infants fed human milk. Weekly measurements of serum phosphorus for the first month and biweekly until 2000 g or 40 weeks' gestation are recommended by Steichen et al.[215] A level below 4 mg/dl should be followed by x-ray films of the wrists for osteopenia and rickets. Supplementation should be based on the infant's needs. Calcium levels should also be obtained

---

BOX 14-2   Vitamin supplements for low-birthweight (LBW) infants fed human milk (HM)

Vitamin B_{12}: only if mother's diet deficient
Folic acid: HM usually adequate
Thiamin (B_1): borderline
Riboflavin (B_2): borderline
Vitamin B_6: HM usually adequate
Niacin: HM usually adequate
Vitamin A: 1000-1500 IU/day
Vitamin C: if infant receives supplementary protein up to 60 mg/day
Vitamin D: 400 IU/day
Vitamin K: all infants should receive 0.5-1.0 mg at birth; recommended 5 µg/kg/day; HM borderline
Vitamin E: 25 IU/day for first month; 5 IU/day after first month; HM adequate

Data from multiple sources.

---

weekly to evaluate levels above 11 mg/dl for too much calcium or too little phosphorus.[201] Supplements of calcium and phosphorus are incorporated in available human milk supplements (Tables 14-4 to 14-6).

Trace minerals in general appear in physiologic amounts in human milk and are more bioavailable from human milk than artificial feedings. The minimum daily requirements for LBW infants are based on daily accretion rates as calculated from third-trimester data and calculated obligatory losses.

Zinc is known to be readily available in human milk, although zinc deficiency syndromes from hyperalimentation are well known in the literature and in neonatal intensive care units (NICUs). Zinc requirements are probably met by the mother's own milk, but pooled milk levels are lower because zinc levels drop from term birth through 6 months, and this milk will need supplementation.

TABLE 14-3 **Required calcium (Ca), phosphorus (P), and magnesium (Mg) intake to meet fetal accretion rate of 27 and 30 weeks***

	27 weeks			30 weeks		
	Ca	P	Mg	Ca	P	Mg
Accretion (mg/kg/day)	121	72	3.37	123	72	3.17
Retention (% intake)	50	89	59	50	89	59
Intake (mg/kg/day)	242	81	5.70	246	81	5.37

From Steichen JJ, Krug-Wispe SK, Tsang RC: *Clin Perinatol* 14:131, 1987.
*Assuming a weight of 1000 g and 1250 g, respectively, in an infant fed human milk.

Copper accretion requires 59 μg/kg/day, and absorption is thought to be 50% to 70%. Copper levels also decline in milk from term to 6 months postpartum. It is recommended that VLBW infants receive an additional 30 to 40 μg/day of copper for the first 3 months.[215]

Manganese represents an apparent deficiency because the minimum daily requirement is calculated to be 7 μg/kg/day. The provision in human milk is 0.35 ng/ml or 0.5 μg/k/day, but no information is available recommending supplementation.

The *selenium* suggested requirement is 1.5 to 2.5 μg/kg/day (1 μg minimum). Human milk provides 1 to 2 μg/dl and is stable throughout lactation so that no supplementation has been recommended.[87]

Iodine levels in human milk are sufficient to meet daily requirements in the LBW infant.

Chromium requirements are calculated to 1.0 to 2.0 μg/kg/day based on an accretion rate of 0.1 to 0.2 μg/kg/day and only 10% absorption. Levels in human milk are reported to be 0.03 μg/dl, which with 150 ml/kg/day intake would supply 0.045 μg/kg/day. Supplementation is not usually provided, and absorption in human milk is probably greater than 10%.

Molybdenum levels in human milk are believed sufficient to meet LBW accretion rates (1 μg/kg/day).[215]

Iron requirements are a complex issue, and intrauterine accretion rates are not appropriate values on which to base requirements.[115,178] Iron stores partially enlarged by hemoglobin break-

down in early life will eventually be used up if no iron is provided. Providing iron, however, interferes with the immunologic properties of human milk, especially the bacteriostatic properties of lactoferrin in the gut.

The recommendations for iron supplementation for infants receiving human milk (either own mother's or donor milk, which are similar in iron) are based on age and weight of the infant. Supplementation should begin at 2 to 3 months or when birthweight has doubled. For birthweight under 1000 g, the infant should receive 4 mg elemental iron/kg/day; infants weighing 1000 to 1500 g should receive 3 mg/kg/day.[115,178] It is necessary also to ensure adequate vitamin C and vitamin E supplementation (4 to 5 mg/day), even though human milk normally contains 5 mg/dl vitamin C and 0.25 mg/dl vitamin E.

Brain growth and subsequent intelligence

Although physical growth and plasma levels of nutrients have been closely scrutinized by investigators following nutrition in LBW infants,[113] adequate measurement of brain growth is not currently possible except indirectly in long-range studies of neurodevelopment and intelligence. A carefully controlled, long-range study of preterm infants by Lucas et al[143,144] over a 10-year period has produced some remarkable results. Mothers who provide their milk have a special desire to be good parents and embrace positive health behav-

TABLE 14–4   Composition of infant feeding using human milk with and without various supplements

	Preterm human milk*		Similac Natural Care*	50:50 Mix Similac Natural Care and preterm human milk*		Enfamil human milk fortifier (4 packets)	Enfamil human milk fortifier (4 packets) added to preterm human milk*	
Weeks postpartum	1	4		1	4	14	1	4
Kilocalories	67	70	81	72	76	14	81	84
Protein (g)	2.44	1.81	2.1	2.27	1.96	0.7	3.14	2.5
Carbohydrate (g)	6.05	6.95	8.6	7.3	7.8	2.7	8.75	9.65
Fat (g)	3.81	4.00	3.6	3.7	3.8	0.04	3.85	4.04
Vitamin A (IU)†	330	230	550	440	390	780	1110	1010
Vitamin E (mg)†	0.9	0.25	3	2.0	1.61	3.4	4.3	3.65
Vitamin K (µg)†	NA	1.5	10	NA	5.8	9.1	NA	10.6
Vitamin D (IU)†	NA	2.5	120	NA	61	260	NA	262
Thiamin (µg)	5.4	8.9	200	103	104	187	192	196
Riboflavin (µg)	36.0	26.6	500	268	263	250	286	277
Niacin (mg)	0.11	0.21	4.0	2.1	2.1	3.1	3.2	3.3
Pyridoxine (µg)	2.6	6.2	200	101	103	193	196	199
Folate (µg)	2.1	3.1	30	16.1	16.6	23	25	26
Vitamin B$_{12}$ (µg)†	0.1		0.45		0.27	0.21		0.3
Vitamin C (mg)†	7	5	30	19	18	24	31	29
Calcium (mg)	25	22	170	98	96	60	85	82
Phosphorus (mg)	14	14	85	50	50	33	47	47
Magnesium (mg)	3	2.5	10	6.5	6.3	4	7	6.5
Iron (mg)	0.1	0.1	0.3	0.2	0.2	0	0.1	0.1
Sodium (mEq)	2.2	1.3	1.7	2.0	1.5	0.3	2.5	1.6
Potassium (mEq)	1.8	1.7	2.9	2.4	2.3	0.4	2.2	2.1
Chloride (mEq)	2.5	1.6	2.0	2.3	1.8	0.5	3.0	2.1
Zinc (mg)	0.48	0.39	1.2	0.84	0.80	0.31	0.79	0.70
Copper (mg)	0.08	0.06	0.2	0.14	0.13	0.08	0.16	0.14
Manganese (µg)†	NA	0.4	NA	NA	NA	9	NA	9.4
Biotin (µg)	0.15	0.54	NA	NA	NA	0.8	0.95	1.34
Pantothenic acid (mg)	0.16	0.23	1.5	0.83	0.87	0.79	0.95	1.02
Osmolality (mOsm/kg H$_2$O)†	302	305	300	301	303	+60	362	365

NA, Not available.

*Volume 100 ml (1 dl).

†Listed values for 1 and 4 weeks reflect reported values for full-term transitional and mature human milk, respectively.

TABLE 14-5   Protein, calcium, and sodium requirements by growing premature infants and composition of banked human milk

	Protein (g/100 kcal)	Calcium (mg/100 kcal)	Sodium (mEq/100 kcal)
Estimated requirements for hypothetic, growing premature infants*	2.54	132†	2.3
Composition of banked human milk	1.50	43	0.8

From Fomon SJ, Ziegler EE, Vazquez HD: *Am J Dis Child* 131:463, 1977.
*Assumed body weight is 1200 g; weight gain, 20 g/day, energy intake, 120 kcal/kg/day. The basis for estimating requirements is described in the text.
†This estimate does not apply to infants fed formulas from which calcium absorption is less than 65% of intake.

TABLE 14-6   Weight gain (g/day) supported by intake of 180 ml human milk/kg at selected body weights

	Weight gain (g/day)			
	800 g	1000 g	1500 g	2000 g
Calcium	4	5	6.7	8.4
Phosphorus	4	5	6.8	8.7
Nitrogen	10	12	16	21
Sodium	5	7	11	15
Magnesium	12	15	22	28
Chloride	22	30	48	68
Potassium	21	33	49	66

Data from Forbes GB: Nutritional adequacy of human breast milk for premature infants. In Lebenthal E, editor: *Textbook of gastroenterology and nutrition,* New York, 1981, Raven.

iors, which has been suggested as the real cause of this study's measured differences. Several points deserve attention, however. LBW infants are born at a time of rapid brain growth. In fact, term infants have considerable brain growth ahead in the first year of life, doubling the size of the brain by 1 year of age. Several nutrients in human milk have been associated with brain tissue growth, including taurine, cholesterol, ω-3 fatty acids, and amino sugars in the free and bound forms.[101] Amino sugars such as *N*-acetylneuraminic acid are important constituents of brain glycoproteins and gangliosides.

The Lucas study[143,144] included infants weigh-

ing less than 1850 g at birth, delivered at multiple centers, who were entered in four parallel trials of preterm feedings from 1982 to 1985. Mothers decided whether to provide their milk; the remaining infants were assigned to receive preterm formula. All feedings were by feeding tube the first 4 weeks. At both age 18 months and age 7½ to 8 years, when the children were tested by an examiner blinded to their feeding method, the children who had received their mother's milk scored better. At 18 months, they were more advanced on the Bayley Developmental Scales.[143] In a subset of the larger study, comparison groups of infants who received preterm formula were more advanced than infants who received regular formula. At the second point, 7½ to 8 years of age, using the Weschler Intelligence Scale for Children, the children who received their mother's milk had an 8.3 point advantage, even after adjustments for mother's education and social class ($p < 0.0001$).[144]

A subset of this large study was also reported in 1990 on infants who had been randomly assigned for 30 days to receive preterm formula, unfortified donor milk, or their mother's milk (with donor milk supplements as necessary).[143] The infants fed donor milk or those whose mothers produced less than 50% of the diet and were supplemented with donor milk were disadvantaged by 0.25 standard deviation (SD) on the developmental scales. This was not pronounced in infants with mental growth retardation. The method of collection of milk from the donors was by drip; that is, the mother fed her baby at the breast and collected milk by drip from the other breast.[143] Drip milk is low in fat and fat-soluble nutrients. Donor milk actively pumped has a higher fat and calorie content. An important feature of these studies was that they focused on the first month of life, a critical time to protect the brain and facilitate its growth.[142-144] The infants were all tube fed, thus removing the physical interaction of the breastfeeding mother. Impact of early diet on long-term neurodevelopment demands continued review and assessment. Unfortified human milk has been shown to have measurable impact on neurodevelopment, but investigation of these same parameters comparing fortification of human milk has not shown improvement over unfortified milk. Neurodevelopmental outcomes at 18 months were not affected by fortification.[141,142]

Visual function is improved in premature infants fed human milk. This is believed to be a result of the long-chain polyenic fatty acids and the antioxidant activity of human milk in β-carotene, taurine, and vitamin E.[141] The diagnosis of retinopathy of prematurity was 2.3 times greater in formula-fed infants than in those fed human milk in a report by Hylander et al.[110] Few infants fed human milk advanced to severe retinopathy, and none required cryotherapy. Results were similar in fortified and unfortified human milk feeds.

Mother's own milk has clear advantages. Donor milk is now regulated and requires pasteurization, which may destroy some valuable properties, but is still advantageous.

Gastrointestinal characteristics of premature infants

The anatomic differentiation of the intestinal tract begins at 20 weeks' gestation, but the functional development is very limited before 26 weeks.[129] Different parts of the fetal gut develop at different times so that some nutrients are better tolerated than others (Tables 14-7 and 14-8). The present concentration of digestive enzymes determines the rate of digestion and absorption, along with the maturity of membrane carriers. (See Chapter 3 for impact of human milk on gut maturation.) The

presence of active enzymes in the gut improves the digestion and absorption of human milk. The gastric emptying time in preterm infants when given human milk is biphasic, with an initial fast phase in which 50% has left the stomach in the first 25 minutes.[35] After an hour, 25 ml of human milk has left the stomach. The formula feeding, on the other hand, follows a linear pattern, with half emptying in 51 minutes and a total of 19 ml in 1 hour.

Use of human milk for premature infants

A clear distinction must be made between an infant's own mother's milk and pooled human milk for the feeding of LBW infants. The mother's milk has some higher level of nutrients but never lower levels than term milk. Mothers who donate to milk banks are also feeding their own infants, who may be any age from birth to 6 months (but no donor should be more than 6 months postpartum). Donor milk must also be prepared by sterilization, and in only a few milk banks is fresh or fresh-frozen donor milk ever available. An infant's own mother's milk may be fed fresh or fresh frozen and is rarely heat treated. Chapter 20 discusses milk storage and milk banking.

When the volume of milk produced by the mother is not sufficient to meet the infant's needs each day, there is a clear need to provide additional nourishment by formula or donor milk.[86]

A 2001-g to 2500-g infant without complications may be weaned from the incubator to an open crib within 24 hours. Although the suck reflex may be poor, the infant can usually be nipple fed. The infant vigorous enough to nipple feed can be nursed at the breast. If the infant can stimulate the breast briefly and obtain the rich, antibody-containing, cell-filled colostrum, it will protect against infection while providing nutrition. Adequate stimulation of the breast also will require mechanical pumping after the feeding. If the infant cannot suck and must be tube fed, any colostrum the mother can manually express or pump from the breast can be given by gavage tube along with donor milk or the prescribed formula necessary for

TABLE 14-7   **Gastrointestinal tract in human fetus: first appearance of developmental markers**

Anatomic part	Developmental marker	Weeks of gestation
Esophagus	Superficial glands develop	20
	Squamous cells appear	28
Stomach	Gastric glands form	14
	Pylorus and fundus defined	14
Pancreas	Differentiation of endocrine and exocrine tissue	14
Liver	Lobules form	11
Small intestine	Crypt and villi develop	14
	Lymph nodes appear	14
Colon	Diameter increases	20
	Villi disappear	20
Functional ability		
Suckling	Mouthing only	24
Swallowing	Immature suck-swallow	26
Stomach	Gastric motility and secretion	20
Pancreas	Zymogen (proenzyme) granules	20
Liver	Bile metabolism	11
	Bile secretion	22
Small intestine	Active transport of amino acids	14
	Glucose transport	18
	Fatty acid absorption	24
Enzymes	α-Glucosidases	10
	Dipeptidases	10
	Lactase	10
	Enterokinase	26

Modified from Lebenthal E, Leung Y-K: *Pediatr Ann* 16:215, 1987.

nourishment. Chapter 5 reviews the protective value of colostrum to the infant.

A study in Guatemala that was repeated in the special care nursery of the Rainbow Children's Hospital in Cleveland showed that the infection rate among sick and premature newborns was greatly diminished by providing 15 ml of human colostrum contributed by random donors daily.[48] These findings were especially dramatic in Guatemala, where the mortality from infection in the nursery is extremely high. It has been suggested that mixed feedings of an infant's own mother's milk and formula to necessary volume be calculated over a 24-hour period so that the infant receives some mother's milk at each feeding and a supplement of formula, in contrast to alternating feedings or using all mother's milk until it runs out and finishing the day with formula. The reasoning is based on the concept of "inoculating" every feeding with human milk to provide the enzymes and immunologic properties with each feeding. Generous levels of active enzymes in the milk will also assist in the digestion and absorption of the formula. The immunologic properties are less measurable, but the only known interference with function is the addition of iron, which blocks the effectiveness of lactoferrin. Therefore the nutritional and infection-protective properties are also spread throughout each feeding around the clock.

The quantities of direct-acting antimicrobial factors in human milk vary according to the method of collection, processing, and storage.

	First detectable (week gestation)	Term neonate (% of adult)
TABLE 14-8 Digestion and absorption in human fetus and neonate		
Factors	First detectable (week gestation)	Term neonate (% of adult)
Protein		
H⁺ (hydrogen ion)	At birth	<30
Pepsin	16	<10
Trypsinogen	20	10-60
Chymotrypsinogen	20	10-60
Procarboxypeptidase	20	10-60
Enterokinase	26	10
Peptidases (brush border and cytosol)	<15	>100
Amino acid transport	?	>100
Macromolecular absorption	?	>100
Fat		
Lingual lipase	30	>100
Pancreatic lipase	20	5-10
Pancreatic co-lipase	?	?
Bile acids	22	50
Medium-chain triglyceride uptake	?	100
Long-chain triglyceride uptake	?	10-90
Carbohydrate		
α-Amylases		
Pancreatic	22	0
Salivary	16	10
Lactase	10	>100
Sucrase-isomaltase	10	100
Glucoamylase	10	50-100
Monosaccharide absorption	11-19	>100 (?)

From Lebenthal E, Leung Y-K: *Pediatr Ann* 16:215, 1987.

Donor milk's ability to protect against infection in the premature infant has not been tested in clinical studies.[77]

Supplementation of mother's own milk or pooled milk

Although some banks can provide single-donor milk for a specific baby and resources are usually more than enough for the newborn recipient, no supplement to human milk is usually needed if the infant is over 1500 g at birth.

The options for supplementing an infant's own mother's milk depend on need for additional volume or for specific nutrients, especially protein, calcium, and phosphorus, based on birthweight and growth rates.[117,118,225]

The ideal supplementation is one using human milk nutrients and is referred to as *lactoengineering,* in which nutrient concentration is increased by adding specific nutrients derived from human milk.[76] Techniques involve separating the cream and protein fractions, reducing the lactose content, and heat-treating the product by high-temperature short-time (HTST) process of pasteurization. This completely human milk product provides higher protein and energy needs so that weight gains and nitrogen retention are similar to intrauterine rates.

Using a feeding prepared from human milk protein and medium-chain triglyceride supplementation of human milk for VLBW infants was reported by Rönnholm et al.[187] Forty-four infants averaging 30 weeks' gestation with birthweights ranging from 710 to 1510 g were nourished by one of four protocols: plain human milk, human milk and protein, human milk and triglycerides, or human milk and protein and triglycerides. The triglycerides did not influence weight and length, but the two groups receiving added protein gained along a curve comparable with the intrauterine growth for their birthweight, gaining faster from 4 to 6 weeks than the unsupplemented infants. The protein-supplemented groups also grew more in length; however, head circumference growth was similar in all groups.[184]

Fortified mother's milk containing an infant's own mother's milk plus skim and cream components derived from mature donor milk was fed *fresh* during the first two postnatal months to 18 VLBW infants (birthweight of 1180 ± 35 g, gestation of 29 ± 0.2 weeks).[37] A comparison group of 16 VLBW infants (birthweight of 1195 g $\pm$ 30 g, gestation of 29 ± 0.1 weeks) were fed commercial formula with comparable nitrogen and energy distribution. Balance studies were performed on both groups. Growth measurements were similar in the two groups. Metabolizable energy was similar (109 kcal/kg/day) in both groups, as was fat absorption. The only recorded difference was a high serum calcium but lower serum phosphorus in the mother's milk group.

Total protein is usually calculated by determining the total nitrogen content (Kjeldahl method) and multiplying the number by the protein factor (6.25). Total protein corrected for nonprotein nitrogen (NPN), which is high in human milk, is true protein.[18] *True protein* is a heterogeneous mixture of casein and whey proteins. All caseins but not all whey proteins have nutritional value. Whey proteins include lactoferrin, immunoglobulins, and lysozyme. True protein minus those more or less indigestible proteins is called *digestible protein.* Analysis of preterm milk by Beijers et al[18] demonstrated that NPN was dependent on the degree of prematurity and averaged 20% to 25%,

increasing over the time of lactation. Only 30% to 60% of total protein is available for synthesis. However, in absolute amounts over lactation time, it remains stable.

Schanler and Garza[199] compared plasma amino acid levels in VLBW infants (mean age 16 days, mean birthweight 1180 g, mean gestation 29 weeks) fed either human milk fortified with human milk or whey-dominant cow's milk–based formula. The infants received continuous enteral infusions of isonitrogenous, isocaloric preparations. Taurine and cystine were significantly higher in the human milk–fed infants, and threonine, valine, methionine, and lysine were significantly higher in the formula-fed infants.[188]

The authors[199] suggest that synthesis of specific functional proteins in the cow's milk protein–based formula fed to VLBW infants requires further review. Human milk supplements for human milk are not commercially available although ideal from most standards.[199-201]

Supplementing an infant's own mother's milk with specially prepared formula supplements is an alternative that still provides the riches of human milk.[231] Available commercial preparations for such supplementation are intended to complement human milk and not to be used as an exclusive formula. They are different and are used differently (Table 14-4). The powdered supplement is intended to add special nutrients to an adequate volume of mother's own milk (Enfamil human milk fortifier), or it can be used to enhance pooled donor human milk. The osmolality is increased by 60 mOsm/kg H_2O. The liquid supplement (Similac Natural Care) is intended to provide 50% of the volume of the daily feeding for an infant whose mother's own milk supply has diminished below daily needs. This extends the mother's milk and provides additional nitrogen, calcium, phosphorus, and vitamins for an LBW infant.[30] If an infant is fed the mother's milk, pooled donor milk, and a fortifier, the sum total should meet the infant's daily requirements (Table 14-5).

Studies comparing fortified mother's milk with premature infant formulas have shown comparable growth in weight, length, and head circumference, making it possible to retain the many advantages of mother's milk while providing the additional nutrients for appropriate accretion rates.[216]

Trials have been conducted to assess both the Similac Natural Care liquid (81 kcal/dl) mixed 1:1 with human milk and the human milk–fortified powder protein-mineral supplement with 14 kcal/3.8 g, used by adding 3.8 g to each 100 ml (deciliter) of human milk.[91] Neither fortifier contains fat. When liquid fortifier in which unsupplemented and supplemented milks were kept isocaloric was used, fortification did not alter growth.[121] When powdered fortifier was added to mother's milk, the supplemented infants had significantly greater weight gain, linear growth, and head growth than those not supplemented.[82] The supplemented infants also had higher blood urea nitrogen levels.[87]

When a preterm infant's own mother's milk was fortified with protein (0.85 g/dl), calcium (90 mg/dl), and phosphorus (45 mg/dl), the rate of weight gain was greater than that of the unfortified group and comparable with that of the Similac Natural Care formula group.[82-84] Bone mineralization improved over the 6 weeks of the study but did not reach the intrauterine accretion rate of 150 mg/kg/day. A relative phosphorus deficiency occurred in the human milk groups both with and without supplementation. Greer and McCormick[82] conclude that fortifying preterm mother's milk permits biochemically adequate growth comparable with that provided by special care formula. Similar results using fortified human milk have been obtained by other investigators.[97]

The effect of calcium supplementation on fatty acid balance studies in LBW infants fed human milk or formula has been shown to be significant by Chappell et al.[37] They showed a decrease in total fatty acid absorption both in LBW infants fed their own mother's milk and in formula-fed (SMA 20) infants when calcium was added. Fecal output of fat and fatty acid excretion were higher in the formula-fed infants. Mother's milk–fed infants' total fat absorption and coefficient of absorption were higher.

Preterm milk with routine multivitamin supplementation (providing 4.1 mg of tocopherol) uniformly resulted in vitamin sufficiency in VLBW infants when they received iron as well as when they were not iron supplemented in a control study by Gross and Gabriel.[90] VLBW infants were fed preterm milk, bank milk, or formula, utilizing 2 mg/day of iron. Vitamin E content of preterm milk does not differ significantly from that of term human milk from days 3 to 36.[101]

Jocson et al[119] studied the effects of nutrient fortification and varying storage conditions on host-defense properties of human milk. Total bacterial colony counts and immunoglobulin A (IgA) were not affected by the addition of fortifier.

A novel fortification scheme for human milk was compared with the traditional system of fortification and a group of infants receiving human milk fortifier. To achieve a better match between individual infant needs and actual intakes, Moro et al[167] designed a regimen in which the amount of fortifier is based on the infant's metabolic response, which is monitored by frequent determinations of serum urea nitrogen (SUN). Twelve infants were studied with each of the three regimens—traditional, adjusted, and human milk protein fortification—for 3 weeks. Protein intake was generally higher and weight gain somewhat higher in the adjusted-fortification group. SUN was also higher in this group, as were calcium, phosphorus, and potassium. Plasma amino acid levels were also increased but not out of range. The authors conclude that adjustable fortification is feasible and safe but needs further work. In general the adjusted fortifier was equivalent to human milk fortifier.[167]

Long-term follow-up of growth parameters in very-low-birthweight infants

Weight gain and growth in length and head circumference are similar in VLBW infants breastfed or given standard formula postdischarge.[230] *Bone mineral content* (BMC) was also followed at 10, 16, and 25 postnatal weeks in those NICU graduates who had formerly received fortified human milk. At 16 and 25 weeks the breastfed infants had lower BMC and BMC/bone width ratio and serum phosphorus concentration and higher alkaline phosphatase activity than the formula-fed group. These data suggest a need to monitor this select group of VLBW infants very carefully for suboptimal bone accretion while receiving their mother's milk.[103]

Reduced bone mineralization is common in preterm infants and has been associated with growth stunting at 18 months of age and dietary insufficiency of calcium and phosphorus. Bishop et al[27] evaluated 54 children at a mean age of 5 years who were born prematurely and had been part of a longitudinal dietary growth study. The diets included were banked donor milk or preterm formula as a supplement to mother's own milk. Increasing human milk intake was strongly associated with better BMC. Those children who had the greater proportion of human milk had greater BMC than children born at term; that is, supplementing with donor milk produced a better outcome at age 5 years than supplementing with infant formula, even though the nutrient content of formula was greater. The authors suggest that the early nutritional environment of the preterm infant could play an important role in determining later skeletal growth and mineralization.

Iron status has also been studied in LBW infants at 6 months' chronologic age. The incidence of iron deficiency was 86% in the breastfed group of LBW and only 33% in those receiving iron-fortified formula.[2] The breastfed group had significantly lower serum ferritin and hemoglobin values at 4 months of age. The authors recommend that these special breastfed infants should receive iron from 2 months of age, because they have a risk of developing iron deficiency not seen in term infants.

Late *hypertriglyceridemia* was detected in a group of VLBW infants fully breastfed at home after premature births (30 weeks) and with a mean birthweight of 1140 g.[83] Blood samples were collected at 31, 33, and 35 days postconceptual age and 6 weeks after hospital discharge. During hospitalization triglycerides averaged 153 to 166 mg/dl. The mean fat content of the mother's milk was 3.2 to 3.4 g/dl and mean fat intake 5.0 to 5.5 g/kg/day. At home they received ad lib feedings at the breast, and the formula-fed infants received standard 20 cal/oz formula with 3.6 g/dl fat. Six of the 13 LBW infants fed human milk had serum triglyceride concentrations greater than 300 mg/dl, none of the formula fed infants had levels over 300, and only three were less than 200. Only 2 of 25 term breastfed infants had levels greater than 300 mg/dl. Three LBW infants had levels over 700 mg/dl and demonstrated hyperchlomicronemia. The meaning of these findings is unclear but deserves watching.[83] The role of lipase and postheparin plasma lipolytic activity is undetermined.

The feedings of these special VLBW infants after discharge and for the next 6 to 9 months is an important consideration. Although no data yet exist on breastfeeding with added supplementation, there are some important results from a randomized double-blind trial of the effect of supplementary standard formula feedings.[138] Growth and clinical status of infants receiving nutrient-enriched "postdischarge" formula were significantly affected, without vomiting, gas, or stool problems. The group receiving the enriched formula ingested volumes similar to those receiving regular formula. The neurodevelopmental status of these infants is being studied.[138] Box 14-3 lists recommendations modified from the work of Steichen et al[215] and Schanler and Hurst.[202]

Antimicrobial properties of preterm breast milk

The infection-protective properties of human milk have been considered a key reason to provide human milk to high-risk infants who are prone to devastating infections such as NEC, sepsis, meningitis, and viral infections such as respiratory syncytial virus (RSV) and rotavirus. The antimicrobial properties of milk produced by mothers who deliver preterm have been studied by several investigators.

The antiinfective factors in preterm human colostrum were studied by Mathur et al,[156] who compared the colostrum values of a comparable group of postpartum mothers. The mean concentrations of IgA, lysozyme, and lactoferrin were significantly higher than in full-term colostrum. IgG and IgM were similar in both groups. The absolute counts of total cells, macrophages, lymphocytes, and neutrophils were significantly higher in preterm colostrum. The mean percentage of IgA in the premature colostrum was also significantly higher. The degree of prematurity had no effect, although the study group ranged in gestation from 28 to 36 weeks (mean 33 ± 2.1) compared with the controls, who were at 38 to 40 weeks (mean 39.1 ± 0.8). Colostrum of preterm mothers had even greater potential for preventing infection than term colostrum and is an additional reason to begin early enteral feeds with human colostrum.[156] Table 14-9 lists the specific antiinfective components.

BOX 14-3   Feeding schedule for human milk in low-birthweight (LBW) infants

1. Use *refrigerated milk* from the preterm infant's mother when it is available and has been collected within 48 hours of feeding.
2. When fresh milk is not available, use *frozen human milk* from the infant's mother. This milk should be provided in the sequence that it was collected to provide the greatest nutritional benefit.
3. When the preterm infant is tolerating human milk at greater than 100 ml/kg/day, supplementation using a human milk *fortifier* is started.
    a. If it requires more than 1 week to reach 100 ml/kg/day intake, fortifier is added even though volume tolerance has not been achieved.
    b. Milk volumes should increase to 150 but not exceed 200 ml/kg/day. Weight gain is optimally 15 g/kg/day and length increment 1.0 cm/wk. Urinary excretion of calcium should be less than 6 mg/kg/day and phosphorus greater than 4 mg/kg/day.
    c. If weight gain is less than 15 g/kg/day, hindmilk is used if mother's milk production exceeds the infant's requirements by 30%.
4. If the mother's milk supply is inadequate to meet her infant's feeding needs, an *infant formula* designed for preterm feeding is used as described.
5. *Fortification of human milk* is recommended until the infant is taking all feedings from the breast directly or weighs 1800 g to 2000 g, depending on nursery policy on infant discharge weight. During the transition from feeding human milk by gavage or bottle and nipple to feeding at the breast, only those feedings given by gavage or bottle require fortification.
6. *Multivitamin supplementation* is started once feeding tolerance has been established. This supplementation varies depending on the composition of human milk fortifier.
7. *Iron supplementation* providing 2 mg/kg/day is started by the time the infant has doubled birthweight.

TABLE 14-9   Comparison of antiinfective properties in colostrum of preterm vs. term mothers

	Preterm colostrum	Term colostrum
Total protein (g/L)	0.43 ± 1.3	0.31 ± 0.05
IgA (mg/g protein)	310.5 ± 70	168.2 ± 21
IgG (mg/g protein)	7.6 ± 3.9	8.4 ± 1
IgM (mg/g protein)	39.6 ± 23	36.1 ± 16
Lysozyme (mg/g protein)	1.5 ± 0.5	1.1 ± 0.3
Lactoferrin (mg/g protein)	165 ± 37	102 ± 25
Total cells/ml^3	6794 ± 1946	3064 ± 424
Macrophages	4041 ± 1420	1597 ± 303
Lymphocytes	1850 ± 543	954 ± 143
Neutrophils	842 ± 404	512 ± 178

Modified from Mathur NB, Dwarkadas AM, Sharma VK et al: *Acta Paediatr Scand* 79:1039, 1990.

The cells of preterm milk were compared with those of term milk and found to be similar in number and in capacity to phagocytose and kill staphylococci.[168] The ability of the preterm cells to produce interferon on stimulation with mitogens was marginally better than that of term cells. The cells survived 24 hours refrigerated at $4°$ C ($39.2°$ F); at 48 hours, cell number, but not function, was reduced. Passing the milk through a feeding tube did not diminish the number or function of the cells. The levels of lactoferrin and lysozyme were greater in preterm milk than in term milk from the second to the twelfth week postpartum.[78]

Secretory IgA (sIgA) was the predominant form of IgA, and values increased from the sixth to the twelfth week in preterm milk. The increase in IgA was not dependent on method of collection, rate of flow, or time of day, but the concentration varied inversely with the milk volume; thus total production of IgA in 24 hours is thought by some investigators to be comparable for the two groups.[36,88] When preterm (31 to 36 weeks' gestation) infants were fed human milk and compared with a matched group of premature infants fed infant formula, the serum levels of IgA at 9 to 13 weeks were higher in the formula-fed infants.[193] Those infants who received at least 60% of their own mother's milk had higher IgA levels at 3 weeks of age than those receiving less than 30% of the feedings from their mother's milk.

Serum IgG levels were higher in the breast milk group, and serum IgM levels were similar in the two feeding groups. Samples of precolostrum collected from undelivered mothers were assayed and found to contain equal or greater amounts of IgA, IgG, IgM, lactoferrin, and lysozyme as mature colostrum.[132]

When the impact on actual prevention of infection among premature infants is reviewed, significantly less infection is found in infants receiving human milk as compared with those receiving formula (9 of 32 breast milk; 24 of 38 formula).[171] In a planned prospective evaluation of the antiinfective property of varying quantities of expressed human milk for high-risk LBW infants, infections were found to be significantly less in the groups that received human milk.[219]

NEC is a major cause of morbidity and mortality in preterm and other high-risk infants. The absolute cause has eluded neonatologists, although many theories have been put forth and associations suggested.[140] When researchers investigate its prevention, the role of human milk is prominent. In a large prospective multicentered study of 926 infants, 51 (5.5%) infants developed NEC. Mortality was 26%. In exclusively formula-fed infants, the incidence was 6 to 10 times more common than in those who received human milk exclusively. In those who received human milk and formula, it was three times more common than in the exclusively breastfed group. Pasteurization did not diminish the effect of human milk. The comparison was more dramatic above 30 weeks' gestation, when formula-fed infants were 20 times more apt to develop NEC than human milk–fed infants. Early enteral feeding did not change the risk in those receiving breast milk, whereas delaying feedings of formula did lower the rate of NEC.[125] In a study of the prevention of NEC in LBW infants with feedings higher in IgA and IgG, none of the infants in the study group or the breastfeeding comparison group developed NEC, whereas six cases developed among the 91 infants in the untreated group.[58]

The intestinal flora in the second week of life in hospitalized preterm infants who had been treated previously with antibiotics and were fed stored frozen human milk was compared with the flora of those fed formula.[171,172] The flora was very different from term infants, and both groups contained Enterobacteriaceae predominantly. Human milk did not alter the flora in these antibiotic-treated infants. Studies have shown that the acidic pH in the stomach of the human milk–fed LBW infants protects against the bacteria in the unpasteurized milk.[234] Although cultures of the milk (feeding sample) had grown both pathogens and nonpathogens, the 2-hour postfeeding cultures of the gastric contents had no growth and a pH less than 3.5.

In South Africa, where mothers remain with and help care for their premature babies, a study compared feeding an infant its own mother's milk with feeding pooled pasteurized breast milk. Birthweights were between 1000 and 1500 g. Nonventilator babies were begun on feedings by 96 hours of age. There was significantly greater weight gain using untreated mother's milk, both for regaining birthweight and reaching 1800 g sooner. The SGA and appropriate-for-gestational-age (AGA) infants both did better on their own mother's milk. This decreased hospital stays and decreased hospital-acquired infection. The authors attribute the advantages to milk being fed fresh with early initiation of feeding at the breast compared to pasteurization of the bank milk.[216]

The Committee on Nutrition, American Academy of Pediatrics (AAP),[41] has published the "Nutritional needs of low-birth-weight infants," in which they suggest that mother's own milk and new special formulas for those babies needing breast milk substitutes are promising alternatives. *Nutrition and Feeding of Preterm Infants* is published as a report of the Committee on Nutrition of the Preterm Infant, European Society of Paediatric Gastroenterology and Nutrition.[42] The report enthusiastically supports mother's own milk as the preferred nourishment, recognizing the need to supplement certain nutrients for the VLBW infant. It recommends 180 to 200 ml/kg/day mother's milk as soon as possible, adding sodium, phosphate, and, in some cases, protein and calcium. The committee recommends heat treatment for donor milk.[42]

A joint effort of the AAP Committee on the Fetus and Newborn and the American College of Obstetricians and Gynecologists (ACOG) Committee on Obstetric Practice states that "human milk has a number of special features that make its use desirable in feeding preterm babies."[43]

Milk production by mothers of premature infants

The production of milk by a mother who is not actively nursing her infant, as is frequently the case in LBW infants and other neonates in ICUs, is a challenge to the resources of the NICU and the postpartum staff.[159] Insufficient milk production is a common problem that becomes more critical as time passes, as production continues to drop, and as the infant's needs increase. Evaluation of various protocols has been undertaken by investigators who looked at times of onset of pumping postpartum, frequency of pumping, and duration in total minutes per day and length of time when no pumping occurred.

Thirty-two healthy mothers, 19 of whom had no previous breastfeeding experience, were entered into a study protocol by Hopkinson et al.[107] Their infants were 28 to 30 weeks' gestation. All the mothers initiated pumping between days 2 and 6, and the day of initiation was correlated with the volume of milk at 2 weeks but not at 4 weeks with mothers who had nursed previously and initiated pumping sooner. Parity, gravidity, age, and prior nursing experience were not correlated with volumes at 2 weeks. Parity and prior nursing experience were associated with milk volume at 4 weeks, with multiparas producing 60% greater volumes. These investigators found no significant relationship between 24-hour milk volume and frequency, duration, or maximal night interval. The change in milk volume from 2 weeks to 4 weeks was correlated with frequency and duration of pumping but not to maximal night intervals. The range in number of pumpings per day was four to nine. The authors[107] concluded that optimal milk production occurs with at least five expressions per day and pumping durations that exceed 100 minutes/day.

The frequency of milk expression was evaluated by de Carvalho et al[48] in a crossover design study of 25 mothers who delivered between 28 and 37 weeks' gestation. Frequent expression of milk was significantly associated with greater milk production (342 ± 229 ml) than with infrequent expression (221 ± 141 ml). They compared three or less pumpings a day to four or more times. The mean number was 2.4 versus 5.7, neither number being the frequency with which a mother would usually feed her infant in the first few weeks.

Although minimum frequency and duration figures have been provided, it is advisable to increase the frequency of pumping as the need to raise production increases and as it comes closer to time for discharge and feeding the infant exclusively at the breast. Consideration for increasing nighttime pumpings is also important as discharge approaches. Some mothers experience a dread of the pump when demands are increased for "more milk production." The management of the mother producing milk for her hospitalized infant should be coordinated by the neonatologist and primary care physician with the assistance of the primary care nurse and the unit's lactation coordinator to maximize support and minimize stress.

When the physiology of lactation is applied to the practical management of inducing a milk supply without benefit of the infant's participation, it is apparent that mimicking natural breastfeeding is more effective. Although some women succeed with manual expression, it is rare, and a good pump should be recommended. None of the hand pumps can truly duplicate the milking action of the infant, and all are essentially vacuum extractors. They should only be used as a stopgap measure when the electric pump is unavailable (see Chapter 20). A pump that is provided for pumping both breasts simultaneously saves time but may generate higher levels of prolactin and greater total milk volume compared with pumping each breast separately for the same length of time.[173] Subsequent studies have not confirmed this observation. Groh-Wargo et al[85] studied 32 women randomly assigned to single or double pumping for 6 weeks. No difference was found in prolactin levels or total volume of milk produced, although the time-saving effect was considered important.

Pumping should be initiated as soon as the mother's condition permits, and offering this opportunity to the mother should be part of the supportive care offered by the postpartum staff. All the points of preparation for pumping should be included: comfortable position, tranquil atmosphere, preparation of the breast with gentle stroking and warmth, confidence, and reassurance. The obstetrician is in an important position to initiate the offer to pump by knowing during the mother's prenatal care that she wants to breastfeed. She may not know it is appropriate to ask about it.

Providing knowledgeable, accurate, consistent, and sensitive support should be the rule in every perinatal center, especially for mothers of high-risk infants who choose to breastfeed.[173,236]

Providing an appropriate room for pumping after the mother has been discharged is critical to individual success and is an expression of commitment to breastfeeding. This room should be clean, bright, and cheery and accommodate more than one mother and companion at a time unless several rooms are available. It should have a sink for washing hands and storing equipment and supplies. A nurse call button or other alarm system is also essential. Additional conducive features are soft music, a telephone, and reading material. The hospital should have a supply of approved electric pumps and individual disposable attachment packets for each mother. A place should be available to store her properly labeled and dated milk in a freezer or refrigerator. Sterile storage containers should be readily available.

A mother should be encouraged to rent a pump for home use and around-the-clock pumping. These are available from medical supply stores, pharmacies, home care services, hospitals, and some lactation consultants. Insurance companies reimburse for the cost of rental when the milk is prescribed for a high-risk infant. The neonatologist can provide an appropriate letter of support. The hospital support staff who are coordinating the mother's care or the NICU staff should be sure that the mother understands how to use the equipment effectively. Ideally, NICUs have at least one staff member experienced in lactation counseling who will coordinate this effort under the direction of the obstetrician, pediatrician, and neonatologist. As more equipment and technology become available, the physician should be alert to avoid subjecting the mother to pressures of pump equipment entrepreneurs and unsolicited advice. The best remedy is for the NICU to provide on-staff, up-to-date experience and support to the mother in her efforts to provide milk and breastfeed her high-risk infant. Box 14-4 outlines key strategies for successful pumping when the infant is unable to suckle the breast.

1. Begin as soon after delivery as maternal condition permits.
2. Initiate use of electric pump while in hospital.
3. Begin slowly, increasing time over first week.
4. Pump on more regular basis as soon as engorgement is evident.
5. Pump at least five times in 24 hours.
6. Allow a rest period for uninterrupted sleep of at least 6 hours.
7. Pump a total of at least 100 minutes/day.
8. Use "double" pump to pump both breasts simultaneously; can cut total time proportionately.
9. Prepare breast with warm soaks, gentle stroking, and light massage to maximize production of milk.
10. Encourage skin-to-skin care (kangaroo care).

Milk production for low-birthweight or small-for-gestational-age infants

Maternal choice to breastfeed or provide milk for an LBW infant is influenced by many factors beyond those that interplay in most feeding decisions of normal full-term infants.[159] Lucas et al[142,143] sought to answer two major questions in a study of 925 mother/infant pairs in five hospitals from 1982 to 1985: Do health care professionals in neonatal units exert a major influence on a mother's feeding preference and availability of her milk for her infant, and are there population differences between mothers who do and do not provide their milk?

Mothers had delivered at a mean of 31 weeks' gestation infants weighing less than 1850 g with a mean of 1370 g. More educated mothers provided their milk (98%) than uneducated (40%). Higher socioeconomic class, lower parity or fewer living children, being married, and being over 20 years of age were associated with providing milk. Boys were more apt to receive mother's milk, as shown in other studies. Birthweight and extreme immaturity were not a determinant, nor was transfer of the infant to another center. In this study a mother who had cesarean delivery was more likely to breastfeed than one who had delivered vaginally.[236] In this study among five centers, the demographic characteristics of the mother were important, not the staff. This study did not look at success rates, however. Another study of breastfeeding LBW infants showed an inverse relationship between maturity and size; the smaller and less mature infants were not breastfed, nor were those with respiratory distress syndrome (RDS).

Feeding premature infants at the breast

Large premature infants of 36 weeks' gestation or older may be nursed at the breast if otherwise stable. Particular care should be given to assist the mother in getting the infant to suckle, especially if the breast and nipples are large or engorged.[173] Weight should be followed closely to prevent excessive weight loss. In our experience, infants who receive sugar water and formula supplements lose more weight than those who are nursed frequently at the breast without supplementation. If breastfeeding is going well, the infant could be discharged with the mother from the hospital as soon as the infant begins to gain substantially, with close follow-up at home.

Feeding at the breast when the infant is under 1500 g is considered too strenuous by many neonatologists. When the feeding of infants of less than 1500 g was examined, however, the growth of those fed at the breast was comparable with that of matched control infants fed expressed human milk by bottle. Breastfeeding was started when sucking movements were observed. Initially, they all received supplementary human milk by tube plus 800 units vitamin D and 60 mg vitamin C daily. Unrestricted visiting of parents to the neonatal unit, an optimistic and knowledgeable attitude of the nursing staff toward breastfeeding, and the avoidance of a bottle for the infants are important to success. They also encourage the expression of milk by the mothers early in the postpartum period.

The main deterrent to successful breastfeeding was lack of maternal interest and commitment.

Bier et al[24] undertook a clinical study of breastfeeding and bottle feedings in *extremely low-birthweight* (ELBW) *infants* (birthweight 800 g or less) when they were considered ready to bottle-feed. This was at a mean age since conception of 35 weeks. One breastfeeding and one bottle feeding were monitored each day for 10 days. Prefeeding and postfeeding weights, oxygen saturation, respiratory and heart rates, and axillary temperature were recorded. Higher oxygen saturation and higher temperatures during breastfeeding and less likelihood of desaturation below 90% were noted. The weights reflecting intake were higher in the bottle-fed infants. The authors concluded that it was physiologically safe and less stressful to breastfeed. The lower intake requires monitoring, however.

The ontogenic and temporal organization of nonnutritive sucking during active sleep were studied by Hack et al[96] in preterm infants. One infant of the six studied had recognizable rhythmic sucking bursts at 28 weeks, and all had bursts by 31 to 32 weeks. The number of bursts increased and the interval between bursts decreased as the infants matured, with the earliest indications of intrinsic rhythm beginning at 30 weeks.

Nonnutritive sucking has become a subject of controversy in NICUs. Allowing premature infants to suck on a pacifier during gavage feedings was initially reported to be associated with increased weight gain and shorter hospitalizations.[91] When nutrient intake and other parameters were controlled, however, there were no advantages to nonnutritive sucking in somatic growth, serum proteins, energy absorption, or feeding tolerance, nor was there any increase in tropic hormones or growth promoters.[51,62] Infants have been observed to have transcutaneous oxygen measurements increase by 3 to 4 mm during nonnutritive sucking.[51] Nonnutritive sucking does not appear to carry risk for infants destined for further bottle feeding but should be avoided for infants destined to breastfeed in order to avoid interference with normal sucking.

Of greater significance is the value of having

these infants placed at the "emptied" breast during gavage tube feedings. When Narayanan et al[170] studied this practice, they found no change in weight gain or length of hospital stay. It did, however, result in more successful and longer duration of breastfeeding after discharge. This technique was originally designed in our nursery to improve mother's milk production and encourage mothers who were becoming discouraged. As the infant matures and begins swallowing with sucking, it becomes unnecessary to pump the breast "empty" before presenting to the infant because any milk provided could be suckled and swallowed. Suckling at the breast initiates a peristaltic action that also triggers swallowing, and the physiologic response of the entire gastrointestinal tract (see Chapter 8).

Kangaroo care

Kangaroo care is the term applied to skin-to-skin contact first introduced in 1979 in a hospital in Bogota, Columbia, because of a shortage of incubators, high death rate from infection, and abandonment of premature infants by their mothers. Since that time, many investigators have carefully evaluated kangaroo care and found it to be beneficial to mother and infant.

Dressed only in a diaper, the infant is held skin to skin against the mother's chest between her breasts, snug inside the mother's clothing, often for hours. The father can do the same. Many advantages have been noted, including more stable respirations, heart rates, and temperatures. The infants spend less time crying and more time in a quiet, alert state and deep sleep. Some studies suggest better weight gain and earlier discharge. Hurst et al[109] also reported an increase in milk volume.

Mothers who give kangaroo care breastfeed longer and more frequently. They also report greater confidence in caring for their fragile infant than those who experience traditional care.[9]

Small-for-gestational-age infants

Infants who are below the tenth percentile (or 2 SD) in weight for their gestational age are termed *small for gestational age* (SGA). These infants may also be shorter in length and have smaller heads, depending on when in gestational life the insult to their growth occurred. The more general the growth failure, the earlier the intrauterine effect appears. For example, rubella in the first trimester causes total growth retardation, whereas hypertension in the mother in the third trimester predominantly affects weight. The more profound the growth retardation, the more difficult are the nutritional problems.

SGA infants are prone to be hypocalcemic; however, if they can be provided with adequate breast milk early, this complication may be avoided because the calcium/phosphorus ratio is more physiologic than formula. Other problems, including hypothermia and hypoglycemia, which lead to a vicious circle of acidosis and associated problems, can be triggered by unmonitored exposure of the infant to thermal stress in the first hours of life and failure to identify the hypoglycemia early. Hypoglycemia in an SGA infant cannot be ignored because the potential exists for significant stress to the nervous system, which can result in seizures requiring aggressive therapy and a detailed diagnostic workup.

Using human α-lactalbumin as a marker protein, Boehm et al[30] demonstrated that SGA infants with intrauterine growth retardation have delayed postnatal decrease in macromolecular absorption and delayed intestinal maturation, even compared with premature infants of the same weight. Their management demands special care. The enzymes in human milk can facilitate catch-up maturation of the intestinal tract.

Thus the perinatal nursery staff may appear to be obstructive to breastfeeding when they hover over this infant or even insist on transfer to the nursery. Initial breastfeeding at delivery is permissible, however, if adequate external heat is provided. Testing the blood sugar should be performed in the delivery room recovery area and the infant sent to the nursery if hypoglycemia or hypothermia cannot be controlled. Frequent breastfeeding can be initiated unless the blood sugar level is too low (below 30 mg/dl) or unresponsive to oral treatment. It may not be possible for even an actively lactating multipara to sustain an SGA infant

initially, but the infant should be put to breast at least every 3 hours and given intravenous (IV) glucose as well.

SGA infants often have a poor suck and poor coordination with the swallow reflex. There may be considerable mucus with gagging and spitting. A simple lavage of the stomach with a no. 8 feeding tube (or no. 5, if the infant weighs less than 2600 g) and warmed glucose water usually relieves the gagging. Once this SGA infant begins to eat, he will do well and will require sufficient kilocalories to meet the needs of an AGA infant. The mother may need to use a breast pump to stimulate lactation initially.

Concluding recommendations

Infants who are less than 1800 g at birth and have to be gavage-fed, or infants of any weight who are acutely ill present a complex problem. The mother should be instructed to express her milk initially and contribute any colostrum she produces. This can be given by gastric tube. An electric pump is effective in helping a mother increase the volume produced. When the infant is born at 1000 g, requires ventilator support for days, and is not discharged for 8 weeks, it is difficult to maintain a large volume of milk by pumping, but it can be done with supportive counseling by staff. Milk volumes usually increase when the infant begins actually to breastfeed, not unlike relactation (see Chapter 18).

When nipple feeding is possible, the infant can be put to the breast. It requires less energy to suckle at the breast than to feed from a bottle. The peristaltic motion of the tongue, which is the normal innate suckling mode, initiates the peristaltic motion of the gastrointestinal tract and triggers the swallow. If no pacifiers or rubber nipples have been given, the infant may be able to suckle at the breast before he reaches 1500 g. Figure 18-3 illustrates an infant who first nursed at 1100 g. If little or no breastfeeding has been done in the hospital and the mother has been unable to pump enough to sustain the daily needs, the infant may be frustrated at the breast when sent home from the hospital (Fig. 14-6).

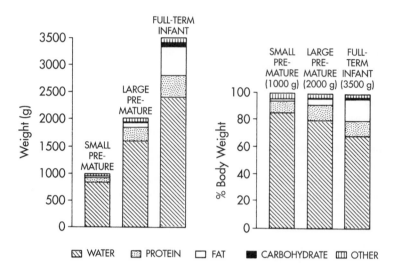

Fig. 14-2. Absolute and relative body composition of infants weighing 1000, 2000, and 3500 g at birth. (From Heird WC, Anderson TL: Nutritional requirements and methods of feeding low birth weight infants. In Gluck L et al, editors: *Current problems in pediatrics,* vol 7, no 8, Chicago, 1977, Year Book.)

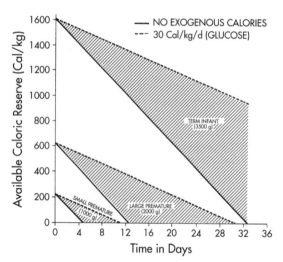

Fig. 14-3. Estimated survival of starved and semistarved infants weighing 1000, 2000, and 3500 g at birth. (From Heird WC, Anderson TL: Nutritional requirements and methods of feeding low birth weight infants. In Gluck L et al, editors: *Current problems in pediatrics,* vol 7, no 8, Chicago, 1977, Year Book.)

One can see that the reserves of the premature infant are limited if one studies the absolute and relative body compositions of infants at birth (Fig. 14-2). If one considers how little time it takes to starve a premature compared with a full-term infant, the risks of starving a premature infant while the infant adapts to nursing at the breast are

real (Fig. 14-3). The solution to the problem is to provide nourishment while the infant stimulates maternal milk production by suckling at the breast. Equipment called a *nursing supplementer* will provide this setup very effectively (see Fig. 18-4). It was developed to provide nourishment for the adopted infant who is being nursed by a mother who has not been pregnant or has never lactated and sustains the infant while the mother's milk supply develops (see Chapter 18). The same effect can be provided for the premature or sick infant who has not nursed at the breast since birth and needs nourishment while the mother's supply develops, even though she has been pumping.

Experience to date at the University of Rochester with mothers who have taken home infants 4 to 12 weeks of age to nurse has been good. The infant can continue to gain weight while stimulating the breast. The volume required from the nursing supplementer dropped continually in all but one case so that the infants were on the breast alone after a week. One infant required the supplementer for a month.

The nursing supplementer provides a simple means of ensuring adequate nourishment while adapting to the breast. It is preferable to using supplemental bottles because the infant is not confused by the rubber nipple, which requires a different mechanism of sucking than the human nipple. Furthermore, the suckling of the breast provides the continued stimulus necessary for increasing milk production. Cup feeding is an alternative to the bottle if the infant needs additional nourishment.

POSTMATURE INFANTS

Postmature infants are full-grown, mature infants who have stayed in utero beyond the full vigor of the placenta and have begun to lose weight in utero. They are usually "older looking" and look around wide eyed. Their skin is dry and peeling, and subcutaneous tissue is diminished; thus the skin appears too large. These infants have lost subcutaneous fat and lack glycogen stores. Initially, they may be hypoglycemic and require early feedings to maintain blood glucose levels of 40 mg/dl or higher. If breastfed, the infant should go to the breast early, taking special care to maintain body temperature, which is quite labile in postmature infants. Blood sugar levels should be followed. These infants may feed poorly initially and require considerable prodding to suckle. If the infant becomes hypoglycemic despite careful management, consideration should be given to a feeding of 10% glucose in water. In extreme cases of hypoglycemia, an IV infusion may be necessary, and management should follow guidelines for any infant who has hypoglycemia that is resistant to routine early feedings.

Calcium problems, on the other hand, although common in these infants, generally are rare if the infant is adequately breastfed early because of the physiologic calcium/phosphorus ratio in breast milk. Once postmature infants begin to feed well, they tend to catch up quickly and continue to adapt very well. Problems with hyperbilirubinemia seldom occur.

Fetal distress and hypoxia

Infants who have been compromised in utero or during delivery because of insufficient placental reserve, cord accidents, or other causes of intrauterine hypoxia have very low Apgar scores at birth and need special treatment. An asphyxiated infant cannot be fed for at least 48 hours, and depending on associated findings, it may be 96 hours or more before it is safe to put food in the gastrointestinal tract. The infant must be maintained on IV fluids. If the mother is to breastfeed, her colostrum will be valuable to the infant and will be better tolerated by the infant's intestinal tract, which has usually suffered hypotoxic damage in these circumstances. *Hypoxia* decreases the motility of the gut and decreases stimulating hormones.

The mother will need help initiating lactation and understanding the pathophysiology of the infant's disease. These infants often have a poor suck and do not coordinate with the swallow, making nursing at the breast difficult. The mother may need to hold her breast in place and hold the infant's chin as well. These infants are especially susceptible to "nipple confusion," so means of sustaining nourishment other than a bottle should be sought. Weaning slowly from the IV hyperalimentation fluids while introducing breastfeeding is helpful. Using a dropper and employing the nursing supplementer are options. These infants may continue to feed poorly for neurologic reasons. They do not do better with a bottle. If the mother is taught to cope with the problem, nursing should progress satisfactorily.

The infant can be held in positions that may help an individual baby adapt better. The "football hold" is a popular but poorly named position in which the infant is held to the mother's side with the infant's feet to her side. The head and face are squarely in front of the breast and steadied by the mother's arm and hand on that side. Cupping the breast and the jaw in one hand facilitates the infant's seal around the breast with the mouth (Fig. 14-5). This position has been called the "dancer hold" by Sarah Coulter Danner, who has prepared a pamphlet for mothers feeding the neurologically impaired infant.* It is well illustrated and is directed toward the mother and her specific problem. One of the most valuable suggestions is the use of a sling or pleat seat to hold

---

*Danner SC, Cerutti ER: *Nursing your neurologically impaired baby,* Childbirth Graphics, Ltd, Division of WRS Group, Inc, PO Box 21207, Waco, Texas 76702-1207.

the infant's body in a flexed position, thus giving the mother both hands free to hold the head and the breast in position for feeding (Fig. 14-4).

Pacing the feedings and pumping after feedings will increase mother's milk supply when the infant is unable to suck vigorously enough. Giving the pumped milk by lactation supplementer, small cup, or dropper ensures proper weight gain in the early weeks.[157] Holding the infant in a flexed position mimicking the fetal position relaxes an infant who is often hypertonic.

In a study of energetics and mechanics of nutritive sucking in preterm and term neonates, Jain et al[116] compared 38-week infants with 35-week infants and noted that preterm infants use less energy to suck the same volume of milk. The preterm infant took up to 0.5 ml per suck and generated lower pressures and a lower frequency.

Exploring the hypothesis that milk flow achieved during feeding contributes to ventilatory depression during rubber-nipple feeding, Mathew[154] compared nipples with different flow rates. Decreases in minute ventilation and breathing frequency were significantly greater with high-flow nipples, thus confirming that milk flow influences breathing in the premature infant who is unable to self-regulate the flow.

The work of feeding, and more important "the work" of feeding at the breast, has been the argument against allowing an immature infant in the Western world to breastfeed at under 1800 g. Survival of LBW infants in Third World countries has been dependent on early breastfeeding. Nonnutritive sucking using a pacifier was evaluated measuring transcutaneous oxygen tension, heart rate, and respiratory rate while sleeping. Infants were 32 to 35 weeks' postconceptual age.[22] The oxygen tension increased 2.3 mm Hg during suckling the pacifier at 32 to 33 weeks and 4.0 mm Hg at 34 to 35 weeks but not at 36 to 39 weeks. Respiratory rates remained stable, and heart rate rose slightly. Transcutaneous oxygen pressure (to Po_2) and body temperature were monitored during feedings in five VLBW infants during bottle feeding and breastfeeding.[161,162] Tracings were made from the first oral feeding to time of

discharge. Serial Po_2 values showed small undulations across baseline (above and below) while breastfeeding and substantial dips while bottle feeding with recovery, but not above baseline. The quality and quantity of variation were very different in the two modes, with large drops occurring during actual sucking of the bottle but only during burping or repositioning while breastfeeding. Meier[161] concludes that the findings do not support the widely held view that breastfeeding is more stressful. The comparative data suggest that both pacifier and bottle feeding are more stressful than suckling at the breast. If the infant has significant motor tone disabilities or lacks the usual oral reflexes in response to stimulus of the rooting and sucking reflexes, a neonatal neurologist should assess the infant before any routine exercises are initiated.

It has been suggested that perioral stimulation enhances an immature or neurologically impaired infant's ability to suck and to coordinate suck and swallow.[130] Perioral stimulation, consisting of stimulating the skin overlying the masseter and buccinator muscles by manually applying a quick-touch pressure stimulus lasting 1 second, was studied. This is accomplished by simultaneously squeezing (the buccal fat) both cheeks. Suck-monitoring equipment revealed that perioral stimulation increased the sucking rate, suggesting that this may facilitate sucking.[157] Exercising the mouths of infants who already have excessive mouth movements may not be appropriate.[130]

When the infant is ready for nonnutritive sucking in the NICU, it is possible to allow sucking at the empty breast (prepumped) instead of a pacifier. Although it is not clear that digestion and gastrointestinal motility are enhanced by sucking,[180] enteral tube feedings are usually given while using a pacifier in most NICUs. Mothers who have been using an electric pump to produce milk for their VLBW infant find "nonnutritive" suckling at the breast by their infant very helpful. Premature infants with a postconceptual age of 35 weeks can discriminate between sweet and nonsweet tastes.[223] They respond with greater sucking when given glucose water rather than plain water, so that the popular vanilla-flavored pacifiers may be significantly preferred over the human nipple. These pacifiers should not be used in infants who breastfeed. Studies of nonnutritive suckling at the breast have been associated with more successful breastfeeding of longer duration. Whitelaw et al[239] found skin-to-skin contact or kangaroo care to be associated with increased success and duration of breastfeeding. In a randomized trial of stable infants weighing 700 to 1500 g, half the mothers used skin-to-skin contact and half only fondled their infants. Skin-to-skin contact was deemed not only safe but enjoyable for the mother. We observed that the kangaroo care given in the NICU at the Providence Hospital in Anchorage, Alaska, which was surrounded by snow drifts and snow-covered mountains, was most successful in raising the body temperature and enhancing the maturation of their premature infants.

Medication-induced milk production

Stimulating milk production pharmacologically in mothers of LBW infants who are pumping to provide milk for their infants has been recommended by several authors, as reported by Ehrenkranz and Ackerman.[57] They used 10 mg metoclopramide orally every 8 hours for 7 days, tapering over 2 more days. Milk production increased within 2 days, but after therapy decreased, milk production decreased. Prolactin levels also increased during the treatment.

Improved lactation occurred in 67% of mothers with no breast milk at onset and in 100% of mothers with poor supply given metoclopramide (10 mg three times a day for 10 days) by Gupta and Gupta.[95] They reported that the improvement persisted when the drug was discontinued. None of the 32 women had any symptoms or side effects. This drug is a substituted benzamide, which has selective dopamine-antagonist activity.

Although growth hormone (GH) has been observed to enhance milk supply, no recommended protocol exists for its clinical use. A study of 20 healthy mothers with insufficient milk who

delivered between 26 and 34 weeks were given GH, 0.2 IU/kg/day subcutaneously for 7 days. A group of 10 received a placebo. Milk volume increased in the treated mothers. No change was noted in plasma GH levels, but an increase was seen in insulinlike growth factor. No other changes were noted during this short-term therapy.[94]

BREASTFEEDING TWINS AND TRIPLETS

Many case reports support that a mother can nurse twins and triplets. It has been documented for centuries that an individual mother can provide adequate nourishment for more than one infant. In seventeenth-century France, wet nurses were allowed to nurse up to six infants at one time. Foundling homes provided wet nurses for every three to six infants.

The key deterrent to nursing twins is not usually the milk supply but time. If the mother can nurse both infants simultaneously, the time factor is minimized. Many tricks have been suggested to achieve this feat. As the infants become larger and more active, it may be difficult to keep them simultaneously nursing with only two hands to cope. However, twins trained from birth to nurse simultaneously will often continue to nurse in a position that allows both to nurse when they are older, even if the other is not nursing at the moment. If the mother has help at home to assist with feedings, breastfeeding can be accomplished. The first year of life for the mother of a set of twins is an extremely busy one and really requires additional help, particularly if the mother is going to breastfeed. She will need time for adequate rest and nourishment. She often benefits from suggestions from other mothers of twins.

The challenge of breastfeeding twins was investigated by Addy,[4] who reviewed 173 questionnaires returned by mothers who were members of the Mothers of Twins Clubs of Southern California. This is a national organization that offers help and advice to mothers of twins. No other socioeconomic information was available. Forty-one mothers (23.7%) breastfed from birth, although 30% of the infants were premature. Of those who did not breastfeed, 9% were told not to do so by their physician, 11% did not think it was possible, and 11% did not think they would have enough milk for two. Of multiparas who had breastfed their first child, an equal number breastfed and bottle fed. Of those mothers who breastfed, 39 breastfed over 1 month and 12 over 6 months.

Eight healthy women breastfeeding twins and one breastfeeding triplets participated in a study by Saint et al[192] to determine the yield and nutrient content of their milk at 2, 3, 6, 9, and 12 months postpartum. At 6 months, they fed on the average 15 feeds per day. Fully breastfeeding women produced 0.84 to 2.16 kg of milk in 24 hours. Those partially breastfeeding produced 0.420 to 1.392 kg in 24 hours. The mother feeding triplets at 2½ months produced 3.08 kg/day, and the three infants were fed a total of 27 times per day. At 6 months the twins received 64% to 100% of total energy and at 12 months received 6% to 13%. This demonstrates that the breast is capable of responding to nutritional demands on it, contrary to previous suggestions that milk production had a finite limit that was much less than a liter.

FULL-TERM INFANTS WITH MEDICAL PROBLEMS

Infants who have self-limited acute illnesses, such as fever, upper respiratory infection, colds, diarrhea, or contagious diseases such as chickenpox, do best if breastfeeding is maintained. Because of breast milk's low solute load, an infant can be kept well hydrated despite fever or other increased fluid losses. If respiratory symptoms are significant, an infant seems to nurse well at the breast and poorly with a bottle. This observation has been documented many times when nursing mothers have roomed-in with their sick infants in the hospital. The studies of Johnson and Salisbury[120] on the synchrony of respirations in breastfeeding in contrast to the periodic breathing or gasping apnea

pattern of the normal bottle-fed infant may well provide the underlying explanation for the phenomenon of an acutely ill infant continuing to nurse at the breast.

In addition to the appropriateness of the human milk for a sick infant, there is the added comfort of nursing because of the closeness with the mother. If the infant is suddenly weaned, psychologic trauma is added to the stress of the illness.

It may become difficult to distinguish the effect of the trauma of acute weaning from the symptoms of the primary illness, such as poor feeding or lethargy, if the acutely weaned infant fails to respond to adequate treatment. Going back to breastfeeding may be the answer because the stress of acute weaning will be removed.

It is not appropriate to give the mother medicine intended to treat the infant, especially antibiotics. This has been tried, to the detriment of the child, because variable amounts of the drug reach the infant, depending on the dose, dosage schedule, and amount of milk consumed. Maternal drugs can produce symptoms in the infant in some cases,[114] and thus maternal history of ingestants is important in assessing symptoms in the breastfed infant (Appendix D).

Gastrointestinal disease

Bouts of diarrhea and intestinal tract disease are much less common in breastfed infants than in bottle-fed infants, but when they occur, the infant should be maintained on the breast if possible.[194] Human milk is a physiologic solution that normally causes neither dehydration nor hypernatremia. Occasionally, an infant will have diarrhea or an intestinal upset because of something in the mother's diet. It is usually self-limited, and the best treatment is to continue to nurse at the breast. If the mother has been taking a laxative that is absorbed or has been eating laxative foods such as fruits in excess, she should adjust her diet. Intractable diarrhea should be evaluated as it would be in any infant. Allergy to mother's milk is extremely rare and would require substantial evidence to support the diagnosis.

Colitis while breastfeeding

Severe colitis in a totally breastfed infant, usually with onset in the neonatal period, suggests an intrinsic metabolic disorder in the infant or an exquisite intolerance to something in mother's milk, such as cow's milk protein.[126] Six infants with protein-induced enterocolitis presenting in the first month of life with severe bloody diarrhea responded to weaning and use of hydrolyzed protein formula. Other cases have been reported requiring long periods of hyperalimentation and utilization of special formulas such as Nutramigen.

Induced colitis in infants is usually caused by some dietary insult, such as exposure to cow's milk.[126,209] It has been reported in breastfed infants, most of whom responded to removal of cow's milk from the maternal diet. Several had been given formula at birth. The symptoms included bloody diarrhea, and sigmoidoscopy revealed focal ulcerations, edema, and increased friability of the intestinal mucosa. On relief of symptoms by dietary change, the intestinal tract biopsy returns to normal.

A prospective study examined 35 consecutive infants who had fresh blood mixed with stools at approximately 4 weeks of age.[148] All infants were otherwise asymptomatic and had no infection, bleeding diathesis, or NEC. Thirty-one had histopathologic evidence of colitis characterized by marked eosinophilic infiltrate (more than 20/high-power field) compared with controls and low mean serum albumin. Ten of these 31 were exclusively breastfed, nine were fed cow's milk formula, nine soy formula, two mixed breast milk and formula, and one Nutramigen. The low serum albumin and high peripheral eosinophil count suggested the diagnosis of allergic colitis. All cases cleared with dietary change. The breastfed infants were weaned and not managed by dietary adjustment in the mother.

Protein-induced colitis can follow a benign course with proper treatment. Israel et al[112] studied 13 infants with blood from the rectum, negative stool cultures, and colonoscopic and histologic evidence of colitis. The infants were all less than $3\frac{1}{2}$ months of age, and six were breastfed and five

had been supplemented. All were gaining weight well. The mothers of the breastfed infants restricted cow's milk in their diet, and the infants were exclusively breastfed. All recovered.

Harmon et al[100] described a case of perforated pseudomembranous colitis in a breastfed infant. Other cases have been associated with giving antibiotics to the infant. The infant's stool was *Clostridium difficile* toxin positive, and the child required bowel resection for abscess and perforation. The mother had taken ciprofloxacin without consulting a physician for days before the infant's admission.

The Lactation Study Center has been notified of other cases of bloody diarrhea with a diagnosis of colitis that did appear to respond to maternal dietary restrictions. One infant showed brief improvement when all cow's milk products were removed from the mother's diet and then had a relapse. Removing all bovine (both meat and milk) products from the maternal diet resulted in recovery without relapse with exclusive breastfeeding. In retrospect the mother recalled switching from a vegetarian diet to high meat, especially beef, intake throughout pregnancy.

A case of fucose intolerance is reported in a breastfed infant who was not intolerant of lactose but of the byproduct of the oligosaccharides in human milk, passing large amounts of fucose in the stool.[17] The infant tolerated Pregestemil and then was weaned to SMA.

The management of protracted diarrhea in infants never breastfed is reported by many human milk banks on a case-by-case basis. Eleven of 24 children managed by MacFarlane and Miller[147] in a hyperalimentation referral unit recovered when fed banked human milk orally without protracted IV therapy. All the infants had been tried on all the available special formulas first. A study of oral rehydration in 26 children under the age of 2 years showed that the children who continued to breastfeed while receiving rehydration fluid had fewer stools and recovered more rapidly than those receiving only rehydration fluid.[123] The PIMA Infant Feeding Study clearly showed that in less developed and more disadvantaged communities in the United States, exclusive breastfeeding protected against severe diarrhea and other gastrointestinal disorders.[69]

Lactose intolerance

Suckling milk is the defining characteristic of mammals. *Lactose,* the major carbohydrate in milk, is hydrolyzed by lactase–phlorhizin hydrolase, an enzyme of the small intestine. *Lactase* plays a critical role in the nutrition of mammalian neonates. Congenital lactase deficiency, present from birth, is extremely rare and is inherited as an autosomal recessive gene.[166] Most humans (except Northern Europeans) and other adult mammals do not drink milk, which causes indigestion and mild to severe gastrointestinal symptoms because of an adult's inability to digest lactose. Low lactose levels result from injury or genetic expression of lactase. The enzyme hydrolyzes lactose, phlorhizin, and glycosyl ceramides. A decline in lactase-specific activity occurs at the time of weaning in most mammalian species. In humans it may occur as early as 3 to 5 years of age; in other species the elevated juvenile levels of lactase-specific activity persist. The developmental patterns of lactase expression are regulated at the level of gene transcription.[166]

Premature infants and those recovering from severe diarrhea have transient lactose intolerance. The only treatment is a temporarily lactose-free diet. Reports of lactose-hydrolyzed human milk suggest that banked human milk can be treated with lactase (Kerulac), which will hydrolyze the lactose (900 enzyme activity units to 200 ml breast milk degraded 82% of the lactose).[210] In one case the reason for using human milk was that the infant became infection prone when he was weaned from the breast at the time the initial diagnosis was made. He showed marked improvement with treated human milk. In the breastfed infant, lactase deficiency may be manifest by chronic diarrhea and marked failure to thrive.

An additional clinical syndrome related to slow gaining or failure to thrive is excessive lactose, resulting when the fat level in the milk is low and an excessive amount of milk is consumed because of the low calorie content. The first documented case was reported by Woolridge and Fisher.[242] Lactose production drives the milk-making capacity. When a feeding at one breast does not last long enough for the fat to let down, the result is low-calorie milk. The authors recommend in such cases that an entire feeding be taken at one breast. (For further discussion of this phenomenon, see Chapter 8.)

Celiac and Crohn's disease

Some chronic diseases are better controlled with the infant kept on breast milk, and symptoms become more severe with weaning. Should an infant be weaned and do poorly on formula, relactation of the mother might be considered. With the availability of the nursing supplementer, this possibility is no longer remote (see Chapter 18).

Childhood *celiac disease* is disappearing, according to Littlewood et al,[135] a trend they attribute to the increasing incidence of breastfeeding and the decreased use of straight cow's milk. They have seen a reduction in gastroenteritis. The delayed use of *gluten* in the diet may also be secondarily important. Infants who have been breastfed and had introduction of solids after 4 months have not been seen to have celiac disease.

In a retrospective study of 146 children with celiac disease, Greco et al[81] initially confirmed that children breastfed 3 months or more showed a marked delay in onset of the disease unrelated to when gluten was introduced. In a case control study of 216 children in Italy with celiac disease and their siblings, Auricchio et al[15] reported that infants formula fed from birth or infants breastfed less than 1 month have four times greater risk of celiac disease than infants breastfed over 1 month. The time of introduction of gluten into the diet was not a factor. The incidence in Ireland of celiac disease is also decreasing and was related by Stevens et al[217] to the protective effect of breastfeeding. Troncone et al[228] measured the passage of *gliadin* into breast milk after the ingestion of 20 g of wheat gluten. Fifty-four of 80 samples showed 5 to 95 ng/ml of gliadin, which peaked in the milk 2 to 4 hours after ingestion but did not appear in serum. The authors suggest that the transfer of gliadin from mother to infant might be critical for the development of an appropriate specific immune response. The epidemiologic data suggest that breastfeeding would be especially appropriate in celiac disease–positive families.

The development of *Crohn's disease* later in life has increased in recent decades. Because it has been suggested that breast milk is essential for the development of the normal immunologic competence of the intestinal mucosa, investigators have studied the association between breastfeeding and later Crohn's disease. Bergstrand and Hellers[20] studied 826 patients who developed Crohn's disease between 1955 and 1974 and their matched controls. Mean length of breastfeeding was 4.59 months among patients and 5.76 among controls ($p < 0.01$). Patients with Crohn's disease were overrepresented among those with no or very short periods of breastfeeding.

Respiratory illness and otitis media

Infants who develop respiratory illnesses should be maintained at the breast. The added advantages of antibodies and antiinfective properties are valuable to the infant. Sick infants can nurse more easily than they can cope with a bottle. Furthermore, the comfort of having the mother nearby is important whenever the infant has a crisis; weaning during illness may be devastating to the infant.

Otitis media in infants occurs less frequently in breastfed infants. Recurrent otitis media is associated with bottle feeding in a study of 237 children, in contrast to prolonged breastfeeding, which had a long-term protective effect up to 3 years of age.[190]

A regional birth cohort of 5356 children was followed prospectively regarding the occurrence of infectious disease in the first year of life.[122] One-third developed otitis media. Median age of onset was 8 months, and 10% had had three episodes by 1 year of age. Breastfeeding for 9 months or longer had a significant impact on otitis, as did the number of siblings and day care. Otitis media in Greenland in 3- to 8-year-old children was studied as a national concern for the incidence and associated deafness. Children who were breastfed were spared, especially if nursed a long time.[181]

Young infants who have older siblings may well be exposed to some virulent viruses and bacteria. Developing croup or chickenpox, for instance, may make the infant seriously ill. Hydration can be maintained by frequent, short breastfeedings. Studies have shown that respirations are maintained more easily when feeding on human milk than on cow's milk from a bottle. Nursing at the breast permits regular respirations, whereas bottle feeding is associated with a more grasping pattern. Thus, breastfed infants should continue to nurse when they are ill. If the infant is hospitalized, every effort should be made to maintain the breastfeeding to provide expressed breast milk if the infant can be fed at all. Staff should provide rooming-in for the mother if a care-by-parent ward is not available.

Colostrum and milk contain large amounts of IgA antibody, some of which is respiratory syncytial virus (RSV) specific. Breastfed but not bottle-fed infants have IgA in their nasal secretions. Neutralizing inhibitors to RSV have been demonstrated in the whey of most samples of human milk tested.[227] IgG anti-RSV antibodies are present in milk and in reactive T-lymphocytes. Breastfeeding-induced resistance to RSV was associated with the presence of interferon as well as virus-specific lymphocyte transformation activity, suggesting that breastfeeding has unique mechanisms for modulating the immune response of infants to RSV infection.[38] Clinical studies indicating a relative protection from RSV in breastfed infants were clouded by other factors.[226] The populations were unequal because of socioeconomic factors and smoking (i.e., bottle-feeding mothers were in lower socioeconomic groups and smoked more). In general, if breastfed infants become ill, they have less severe illness.[226,227] Although breastfeeding protects, parental smoking and day care are important negative factors as well in the incidence of respiratory infection.

Galactosemia

Galactosemia, caused by deficiency of galactose-1-phosphate uridyltransferase, is a rare circumstance in which the infant is unable to metabolize galactose and must be placed on a galactose-free diet. The disease can be rapidly fatal in the severe form. The infant may have severe and persistent jaundice, vomiting, diarrhea, electrolyte imbalances, cerebral signs, and weight loss. This does necessitate weaning from the breast to a special formula because human milk contains high levels of lactose, which is a disaccharide that splits into glucose and galactose. The diagnosis is suspected when reducing substances are found in the urine and it is confirmed by measuring the enzyme uridyltransferase in the red and white blood cells.

Inborn errors of metabolism

Other metabolic deficiency syndromes are usually only apparent as mild failure-to-thrive syndrome until the infant is weaned from the breast and the symptoms become severe. This particularly applies to inborn errors of metabolism caused by an inability to handle one or more of the essential amino acids. Infection is often a complication early in the lives of these infants with inborn errors. While the acute infection is being treated, the infant may be weaned, and the metabolic disorder then becomes apparent precipitously.

As shown in Table 4-13, certain amino acids have significantly lower levels in human milk than in cow's milk, including phenylalanine, methionine, leucine, isoleucine, and others associated with metabolic disorders. Management of an amino acid metabolic disorder while breastfeeding depends on careful monitoring of blood and urine levels of the specific amino acids involved. Because these are essential amino acids, a certain amount is necessary in the diet of all infants, including those with disease. An appropriate combination of breastfeeding and a milk free of the offending amino acid should be developed. The care of such infants should be in consultation with a pediatric endocrinologist. Transient neonatal *tyrosinemia,* which has been reported to occur in a high percentage (up to 80%) of neonates fed cow's milk, is associated with blood tyrosine levels 10 times those of adults. Wong et al[241] have associated severe cases with learning disabilities in later years.

Phenylketonuria

The most common of the amino acid metabolic disorders is phenylketonuria (PKU), in which the amino acid accumulates for lack of an enzyme. The treatment has been phenylalanine-free formula, available from Abbott Laboratories and Bristol-Myers, combined with added formula or breast milk to provide a little phenylalanine because every infant needs a small amount. If the infant is breastfed, the mother is usually willing to continue on an adjusted schedule. An infant may supplement the Lofenalac or Analog XP with breast milk. With careful monitoring of the blood levels and control of the amount of breastfeeding, a balance can be struck that permits optimal phenylalanine levels and breastfeeding. The infant will require some phenylalanine-free formula to provide enough calories and nutrients. A detailed outline of management called *Guide to Breast Feeding the Infant with PKU,* prepared by Ernest et al,[61] is available from the Superintendent of Documents, U.S. Government Printing Office, Washington, DC 20402.

Literature values for phenylalanine range from 29 to 64 mg/dl in human milk. The amount for Lofenalac or Analog XP and human milk for a given baby are calculated by weight, age, blood levels, and needs for growth. As an example, a 3-week-old weighing 3.7 kg whose blood level was 52.5 mg/dl when he was ingesting an estimated 570 ml of breast milk would receive 240 ml Lofenalac and 360 ml breast milk (four breastfeedings a day with before and after weighing). The details of every step of management are available in the guide to assist the physician in planning treatment.[61]

A simpler approach is described by Clark,[39] who suggests that as soon as the diagnosis is made, the infant be placed on the low-phenylalanine formula to reduce the levels in the plasma promptly. The mother should pump her breasts to maintain her milk supply. Human milk has less phenylalanine than formula, but it exceeds the tolerance of most infants with PKU. The breastfed infant is offered a small volume of special formula (10 to 30 ml) first and then completes the feeding at the breast. As long as the blood phenylalanine levels can be maintained between 120 and 300 μmol/L, exact intake need not be measured. Initially, weight checks to ensure adequate growth are essential because poor intake leading to a catabolic state will interfere with control. Because human milk is low in phenylalanine, the offending amino acid, more than half the diet can be breast milk.

The weaning of this special infant should be similar to that of other infants. Adding solid foods can be initiated at 6 months.[39] The liquid part of the diet continues as before, that is, two feeding components of low-phenylalanine formula and breastfeeding plus solids with little or no phenylalanine (fruits, vegetables, low-protein foods). Rice and wheat contain too much phenylalanine. When the decision is made to wean from the breast, solid foods can be used to replace the phenylalanine in the breast milk as needed. Growth should be followed closely. When weaning is complete, the infant should be given other less bulky sources of protein free of phenylalanine. This stage will be carefully orchestrated by the endocrinologist and nutritionist. Because infants with PKU are more prone to thrush infection, the mother should be alerted to watch for symptoms in the infant and the onset of sore nipples that could be caused by *Candida albicans*. Treatment is nystatin for mother and baby.

The other benefits of human milk make the effort to breastfeed valuable for the infant and for the mother, who usually wants to continue to contribute to her infant's nurturing and nourishment. The prognosis for intellectual development is excellent if treatment is initiated early and the blood levels maintained at less than 10 mg/dl phenylalanine (120 to 300 μmol/L).

A retrospective study of 26 school-age children who had been breastfed or formula fed for 20 to 40 days before dietary intervention was conducted by Riva et al.[185] The children who had been breastfed had a 14-point IQ advantage, which persisted at 12.9 points when corrected for maternal social and educational status. The age of treatment onset for PKU was not related to IQ scores. This study strongly supports the belief that breastfeeding in the prediagnostic stage has an impact on the long-range neurodevelopmental performance of PKU patients.

Nutrition management of infants with *organic acidemias* involves limiting the intake of the offending amino acid(s) to the minimum necessary for normal growth and development and suppressing amino acid degradation during catabolic periods by providing alternative fuels such as glucose. In some disorders, including isovaleric acidemia, specific treatment is included to increase the excretion of toxic metabolites by enhancing the body's capacity to make isovalerylglycine, a diisovalerylcarnitine. As more specific amino acid–free formulas are made available, a recipe for combining breastfeeding with the special formula can be engineered to specific infants' needs. The endocrinologist and nutritionist can provide such a recipe.

Cystic fibrosis

The first symptom in infants with cystic fibrosis (CF) is often failure to thrive. If the infant is breastfed, the mother may be forced to wean, yet the infant feeds even less well and has no weight gain. Infants do better if placed back on the breast. In a study of CF centers, 77% recommended breastfeeding either alone or with pancreatic enzyme supplements.[145] The recommended breastfeeding duration was 3 to 6 months by 43% of the centers (Tables 14-10 to 14-12). If supplementation is required, hydrolyzed formula is recommended. Generic and name-brand enzymes are not biologically equal, and some formulas were more frequently associated with greasy stools and abdominal cramping. Use of enzymes may be a way to improve tolerance and weight gain in these special breastfed infants rather than weaning to formula.[33]

α₁-Antitrypsin deficiency

α_1-Antitrypsin (α_1AT) is a serum protease inhibitor that inactivates a number of proteases. More than 24 genetic variants of this disease are designated B through Z, with the M variant being most common. Children with α_1AT deficiency are at

TABLE 14-10   **Recommendations about breastfeeding by cystic fibrosis (CF) center directors for CFIM***

Recommendations	Response, no. (%)	
Breastfeeding		
Only	3	(2.6)
Plus pancreatic enzymes	39	(34.2)
Plus hydrolyzed formula	7	(6.1)
Plus pancreatic enzymes and hydrolyzed formula	39	(34.2)
Hydrolyzed formula with pancreatic enzymes	18	(15.8)
Hydrolyzed formula only	2	(1.8)
Not applicable and/or others category	6	(5.3)
TOTAL	114	(100)

Modified from Luder E, Kattan M, Tanzer-Torres G et al: *Am J Dis Child* 144:1153, 1990.
**CFIM,* Mothers of infants with CF. Many centers chose more than one answer; therefore response rate for each answer is calculated as a percent of total responses.

TABLE 14-11   **Factors for discontinuation of breastfeeding according to CF center directors for CFIM***

Factors for discontinuation	Response, no. (%)	
Protein-energy malnutrition	69	(51.1)
Marked steatorrhea	29	(21.5)
Meconium ileus	16	(11.9)
Chronic bacterial pathogen(s) carrier	8	(5.9)
Not applicable and/or others category	13	(9.6)
TOTAL	135	(100)

Modified from Luder E, Kattan M, Tanzer-Torres G et al: *Am J Dis Child* 144:1153, 1990.
**CFIM,* Mothers of infants with CF. Many centers chose more than one answer; therefore response rate for each answer is calculated as a percent of total responses.

increased risk for liver disease, which occurs most often during infancy and often progresses to cirrhosis and death. Udall et al[233] investigated the relationship between early feedings and the onset of liver disease. Severe liver disease was present in eight (40%) of the bottle-fed and one (8%) of the

TABLE 14-12   **Duration of breastfeeding as reported by CF center directors for CFIM***

Duration (months)	Centers, no. (%)	
<3	34	(40)
3-6	37	(43)
>6	5	(5.8)
Not applicable and/or others category	10	(12)
TOTAL	86	(100)

Modified from Luder E, Kattan M, Tanzer-Torres G et al: *Am J Dis Child* 144:1153, 1990.
**CFIM,* Mothers of infants with CF. Many centers chose more than one answer; therefore response rate for each answer is calculated as a percent of total responses.

breastfed infants (breastfed for only 5 weeks). Of the 32 infants, 24 were still alive at the end of the study; 12 had been breastfed and 12 bottle fed during their first month of life. All eight of the deceased children had been bottle fed; SGA and preterm infants had been excluded from the study so that all infants were equally stable at birth and capable of breastfeeding. A bottle-fed infant was seven times more likely to develop liver disease.

With the increasing early diagnosis of $\alpha_1 AT$ deficiency, encouraging a mother to breastfeed if her infant is affected would appear to have a significant impact on long-range liver disease in her infant.

Acrodermatitis enteropathica (Danbolt-Closs syndrome)

Acrodermatitis enteropathica is a rare but unique disease in which feeding the infant with human milk may be lifesaving. It is inherited as an autosomal recessive trait and is characterized by a symmetric rash around the mouth, genitalia, and periphery of the extremities. The rash is an acute vesicobullous and eczematous eruption often secondarily infected with *C. albicans*. It may be seen by the third week of life or not until late in infancy and has been associated with weaning from the breast. Failure to thrive, hair loss, irritability, and chronic severe intractable diarrhea are often life threatening. The disease has been associated with extremely low plasma zinc levels. Oral zinc sulfate has produced remission of the syndrome.

Human milk contains less zinc than does bovine milk, with zinc concentrations of both decreasing throughout lactation. Eckert et al[56] studied the zinc binding in human and cow's milk and noted that the low-molecular-weight (LMW) binding ligand isolated from human milk may enhance absorption of zinc in these patients. Gel chromatography indicated that most of the zinc in cow's milk was associated with high-molecular-weight fractions, whereas zinc in human milk was associated with LMW fractions. The copper/zinc ratio may also be of significance, because the ratio is lower in cow's milk.

The zinc-binding ligand from human milk was further identified as prostaglandin E by chromatography, ultrafiltration, and infrared spectroscopy by Evans and Johnson.[63] Patients also have low arachidonic acid levels. Arachidonic acid is a precursor of prostaglandin. The efficacy of human milk in the treatment of acrodermatitis enteropathica results from the presence of the zinc-prostaglandin complex.

The clinical significance of the relationship of human milk to onset of the disease and its treatment is in developing lactation in the mother of such an infant, rare as the disease may be. Delayed lactation or relactation is possible and should be offered as an option to the mother of such an infant (see Chapter 18).

Several reports of isolated cases of zinc deficiency during breastfeeding have appeared in the literature.[5,6,11,163] In some cases, zinc levels in the milk were low; in others, they were not measured.[243] One child had a classic "zinc-deficient" rash that responded to oral zinc therapy. One should keep in mind that any deficiency is possible and consider intake deficiency when symptoms occur in the breastfed infant. The basic defect is presumed to be related to gastrointestinal malabsorption of zinc.

The treatment of choice is oral administration of zinc in the sulfate or gluconate form. It is usually well tolerated, safe, inexpensive, effective, and expedient. When zinc deficiency occurs in a breastfed infant, the possibility of zinc deficiency in the milk, although a rare disorder, should be considered.[205]

Down syndrome

Infants with Down syndrome or other trisomies may be difficult to feed. When they are breastfed, the mother needs patience to teach the infant to suck with sufficient vigor to initiate the let-down reflex and to stimulate adequate production of milk. Using manual expression to start flow and holding the breast firmly for the infant so that the nipple does not drop out of the mouth when the infant stops suckling will assist the process.

Initially, an infant with Down syndrome may have surprisingly good tone and may even suck well at the breast, only to develop problems once the mother and infant have been discharged home. Providing support for the head, the jaw, and the general body hypotonia will require considerable coordination by the mother. Propping the baby firmly with a pillow in mother's lap or supporting the infant in a sling frees up a much-needed hand for steadying the jaw and breast (Fig. 14-4).[157]

A nurse clinician knowledgeable and experienced in dealing with neurologically impaired infants should be available to the parents. The initial goals for the mother-infant pair are developing confidence in handling the infant, adjusting to the infant's problem, and dealing with the parental grief and sense of loss, loss of the normal infant that was expected. If the mother has breastfed other children, the emphasis on breastfeeding modifications are more successful, and milk supply usually responds to manual expression and pumping. Initiating sufficient stimulus to the breast to increase milk production is critical in the first few days to induce good prolactin response, especially in a primipara. Renting an electric breast pump is a good investment, justifiable for reimbursement from health insurance by physician prescription.

In developing a discharge plan for this infant,

Fig. 14-4. Pleat-seat or sling baby carrier holds infant in a flexed position that facilitates infant suckling, leaving mother's hands free to support her breast and the infant. (Redrawn from McBride MC, Danner SC: *Clin Perinatol* 14:109, 1987.)

the pediatrician will need to coordinate the team to avoid the fragmented care that develops with a multiproblem situation, which may require the consultation of a geneticist, genetic counselor, cardiologist, and other medical experts to deal with the problems. Ideally, the pediatrician and the office nurse practitioner can provide the additional support and counsel necessary. Many families prefer to leave the hospital early to retreat to the comfort and privacy of their home and the health care provider they selected. Home visits by the pediatrician's staff can provide the necessary monitoring of weight gain and nutrition, as well as counseling by someone capable of handling all the problems that arise, including the breastfeeding. No referrals should be made without the pediatrician's knowledge and agreement. The pediatrician has the advantage of knowing both the family and the child.

In a study of 59 breastfed infants with Down syndrome, Aumonier and Cunningham[14] reported that 31 had no sucking difficulty, 12 were successfully nursing within a week, and 16 required tube feeding initially, which was associated with other medical problems, including LBW, cardiac lesions, and jaundice. Hyperbilirubinemia is common in trisomy and was seen in 49% of these study infants. Eighteen babies had multiple medical conditions, and 11 of them sucked poorly. The authors point out that the initial sucking ability of the infants did not appear to be a major cause for nonmaintenance of breastfeeding. Ten of the 13 mothers who discontinued breastfeeding cited insufficient milk as a contributing cause, which might have been prevented by early pumping of the breasts between feedings.

The birth of an infant with a major genetic abnormality is a shock, even to the strongest parents. If the mother wants to breastfeed, she should be offered all the encouragement and support necessary. Usually she needs to talk with someone just to express her anguish about the infant, not the feeding per se. A sympathetic nurse practitioner can be invaluable in providing the support as well as the expertise necessary to help with the various management problems. If the mother chooses not to breastfeed, appropriate support can also be provided without disrupting treatment continuity.

It is especially important that these infants be breastfed if possible because they are particularly prone to infection. Before the advent of antibiotics, they often died of overwhelming infection and rarely survived past 20 years of age. These infants and most other infants with developmental disorders do better with stimulation and affection, so the body contact and communication while at the breast are especially important. Those who have associated cardiac lesions not only can suckle, swallow, and breathe with less effort at the breast, but also can receive a fluid more physiologic for their needs. Breastfed or bottle fed, these infants gain poorly; thus, switching to a bottle does not solve the problem. The recommendation that the Down syndrome child receive extra vitamins was tested in a controlled study in children 5 to 13 years of age, and there was no sustained improvement in the children's appearance, growth, behavior, or development with added vitamins.[19]

Hypothyroidism

Bode et al[29] reported that an infant with congenital cretinism was spared the severe effects of the disease because he was breastfed. This was attributed to significant quantities of thyroid hormone in the milk. In a prospective study of 12 cases of hypothyroidism in breastfed infants, Letarte et al[131] found no protective effect against the disease, nor was the onset of the disease delayed. Anthropometric measurements, biochemical values, and psychologic testing at 1 year of age did not differ from those in the 33 bottle-fed hypothyroid infants. Abbassi and Steinour[1] also reported successful diagnosis of congenital hypothyroidism in four breastfed neonates.

Sack et al[191] measured thyroxine (T_4) concentrations in human milk and found it to be present in significant amounts. Varma et al[235] studied T_4, triiodothyronine (T_3), and reverse T_3 (rT_3) concentrations in human milk in 77 healthy euthyroid mothers from the day of delivery to 148 days postpartum. They calculated from their data that if infants received 900 to 1200 ml of milk/day, they would receive 2.1 to 2.6 µg of T_4/day, based on 238.1 ng/dl of milk after the first week. This amount of T_4 is much less than the recommended dose for the treatment of hypothyroidism (18.8 to 25 µg/day of levo-T_3). T_4 was essentially unmeasurable in the milk sampled. In another study, however, comparing 22 breastfed and 25 formula-fed infants who were 2 to 3 weeks old, the levels of T_3 and T_4 were significantly higher in the breastfed infants.[98] No definite relationship between the levels of T_3 and rT_3 could be found.

A 6-week-old female was diagnosed to have congenital hypothyroidism by routine neonatal screening when T_4 was reported at 3 µg/dl (normal above 7 µg/dl).[45] The mother gave a history of multiple applications of povidone-iodine during pregnancy and continuing during lactation. Further testing revealed thyroid-stimulating hormone levels of 0.9 µU/ml (normal 0.8 to 5 µU/ml). Iodine

treatment was stopped and breastfeeding continued while treatment of thyroid replacement was begun. At 1 year, growth and development were normal. It is therefore suggested that neonatal screening for thyroid disease may be even more urgent if the clinical symptoms are apt to be masked in a breastfed infant. No contraindication exists to breastfeeding when the infant is hypothyroid, and it would be beneficial. Appropriate therapy should also be instituted promptly.

Adrenal hyperplasia

In an analysis of 32 infants with salt-losing congenital adrenal hyperplasia who were in adrenal crisis, 8 had been breastfed, 5 had been breastfed with formula supplements, and 19 had been formula fed.[44] Infants who were breastfed were admitted to the hospital later than the formula-fed infants, although the breastfed infants had lower serum sodium levels on admission. The breastfed infants did not vomit and remained stable longer, although they all had severe failure to thrive. Weaning initiated vomiting and precipitated crises in the breastfed infants. The authors suggest that congenital adrenal hyperplasia should be considered in a breastfed infant with failure to thrive. Electrolytes should be obtained before weaning to make the diagnosis and avoid precipitating a crisis by weaning.

Neonatal breasts and nipple discharge

The newborn may have swelling of the breasts for the first few days of life, whether male or female; this is unrelated to being breastfed. If the breast is squeezed, milk can be obtained. This has been called *witch's milk*. The constituents of neonatal milk were studied in the milks of 18 normal newborns and infants with sepsis, adrenal hyperplasia, CF, and meconium ileus.[21] Electrolyte values were similar to those in adult women in all the infants except one with a mastitis, in whom the sodium level was elevated and the potassium decreased. Total protein and lactose were also similar to those in adult women. The fat was different, increasing with postnatal age and being higher in short-chain fatty acids. It was indeed true milk.

Two infants, one female and one male, were reported to have bilateral bloody discharge from the nipples at 6 weeks of age. Cultures and smears were unrevealing.[21] No biopsy was done. The female infant's swelling and discharge cleared up after 5 months; the male's was still present at 10 weeks, when he was lost to follow-up. Galactorrhea or persistent neonatal milk has been reported in association with neonatal hyperthyroidism. In another report, a 21-day-old infant female was seen because of a goiter and galactorrhea. The infant had 50% 24-hour iodine-131 uptake and elevated prolactin levels, which slowly responded to Lugol's solution treatment for hyperthyroidism.[146]

Hyperbilirubinemia and jaundice

Jaundice in the newborn has become a source of considerable misinformation, confusion, and anxiety in recent years. There is a higher incidence of jaundice in full-term infants than a decade ago. More physicians are paying attention to the development of hyperbilirubinemia in newborns. These two factors serve to increase the frequency of the question of the role of breastfeeding in the development of hyperbilirubinemia. Some of the confusion and inconsistencies associated with the management can be attributed to the indecisive terminology. This discussion clarifies the issues and outlines the causes and effects of hyperbilirubinemia.

Why the concern about jaundice?

Bilirubin is a cell toxin, as can be demonstrated dramatically by adding a little bilirubin to a tissue culture, which will be quickly destroyed. Excessive bilirubin causes concern because when there is free, unbound, unconjugated bilirubin in the system, it can be deposited in various tissues, ultimately causing necrosis of the cells. The brain and brain cells, if destroyed by bilirubin deposits, do not regenerate.[99] The full-blown end result is bilirubin encephalopathy, or *kernicterus,* which is

essentially a pathologic diagnosis that depends on identifying the yellow pigmentation and necrosis in the brain, especially in the basal ganglion, hippocampal cortex, and subthalamic nuclei. About 50% of the infants with kernicterus at autopsy also have other lesions caused by bilirubin toxicity. There may be necrosis of the renal tubular cells, intestinal mucosa, or pancreatic cells or associated gastrointestinal (GI) hemorrhage.

The classic clinical manifestations of bilirubin encephalopathy are characterized by progressive lethargy, rigidity, opisthotonos, high-pitched cry, fever, and convulsions. The mortality rate is 50%. Survivors usually have choreoathetoid cerebral palsy, asymmetric spasticity, paresis of upward gaze, high-frequency deafness, and mental retardation.[52] Premature infants are particularly susceptible to bilirubin-related brain damage and may have kernicterus at autopsy without the typical clinical syndrome. A significant correlation exists between level of bilirubin and hearing impairment in newborns when other risk factors are present. Classic full-blown kernicterus rarely occurs today, but mild effects on the brain may be manifested clinically in later life as incoordination, hypertonicity, and mental retardation or perhaps learning disabilities, symptoms sometimes collectively called *minimal brain damage.*[99] *Bilirubin encephalopathy* is the appropriate term for conditions in which bilirubin is thought to be the cause of brain toxicity.

In response to the continued concern about hyperbilirubinemia, several collaborative long-range studies have been done.[92,149,150,203] Each one confirms the observation that in normal full-term infants who do not have an incompatibility, the neurodevelopmental outcome is normal, as is hearing acuity.[158,203] In a study of 60 breastfed infants in whom the maximum bilirubin was 18.3 mg% and the duration was 12 weeks or more, there were no late neurodevelopmental or hearing defects. The authors describe a peak level at 4 to 5 days and a second peak at the fourteenth to fifteenth day. All 60 infants had blood typing, direct and indirect Coombs' (antiglobulin) tests, blood count, glucose-6-phosphate dehydrogenase

(G6PD) activity, urinalysis, urine culture, T_4 and TSH, total reducing substances in the urine, and spot tests for galactose and aminotransferase to rule out other causes of hyperbilirubinemia. The authors also reported a 14% incidence of familial jaundice, that is, a previous infant with jaundice (6 of 43 breastfeeders who had siblings).[240]

Mechanism of bilirubin production in the neonate

The normal full-term infant has a hematocrit in utero of 50% to 65%. Because of the low oxygen tension delivered to the fetus via the placenta, the fetus requires more hemoglobin (Hb) to carry the oxygen. As soon as the infant is born and begins to breathe room air, the need is gone. The infant bone marrow does not make more cells, and excess cells are destroyed and not replaced. The life span of a fetal red blood cell (RBC) is 70 to 90 days instead of the adult's 120 days. Normally when RBCs are destroyed, the released Hb is broken down to heme in the reticuloendothelial system (RES). The RES cells contain a microsomal enzyme, heme oxygenase, which is capable of oxidizing the α-methene bridge carbon of the heme molecule after the loss of the iron and the globin to form biliverdin, a green pigment.[71,75] *Biliverdin* is water soluble and is rapidly degraded to bilirubin. A gram of hemoglobulin will produce 34 mg of bilirubin.

The reticuloendothelial cell releases the bilirubin into the circulation, where it is rapidly bound to albumin. Bilirubin is essentially insoluble (less than 0.01 mg/dl soluble). Adult albumin can bind two molecules of bilirubin, the first more tightly than the second. Newborn albumin had reduced molar binding capacities that vary with maturity and other factors.[189]

Unconjugated bilirubin is removed from the circulation by the hepatocyte, which converts it by conjugation of each molecule of bilirubin with two molecules of glucuronic acid into direct bilirubin. *Direct bilirubin* is water soluble and is excreted via the bile to the stools. The balance between hepatic cell uptake of bilirubin and the rate of bilirubin production determines the serum unconjugated bilirubin concentration.

Evaluation and management

Normal full-term newborns have serial bilirubin tests to determine the range of values. The cord bilirubin level may be as high as 2 mg/dl and rise over the first 72 hours to 5 to 6 mg/dl, which is barely in the visible range, and gradually taper off, assuming adult levels of 1 mg/dl after 10 days. Fewer than 50% of normal infants are visibly jaundiced in the first week of life. Why any normal infant is visibly jaundiced is not known, although Gartner and Lee[75] suggest the results from insufficient enzyme synthesis, inhibition of enzymatic activity by naturally occurring substances, deficient synthesis of the glucuronide donor uridine diphosphoglucoronic acid (UDPGA), or a combination of factors. This would suggest the jaundice is *idiopathic,* not physiologic. The acceptance level of bilirubin depends on a number of factors. In some premature infants, even bilirubin levels under 10 mg/dl may be of concern.

Factors that influence significance. For a given level of bilirubin, several associated factors may need to be considered. If the infant has acidosis, anoxia, asphyxia, hypothermia, hypoglycemia, or infection, even lower levels of bilirubin may have a significant risk of causing deposition of bilirubin in the brain cells. The most important factor is prematurity, which affects both liver and brain metabolism. An increased incidence of elevated bilirubin levels occurs in certain races and populations. Asian populations, including Chinese, Japanese, and Korean, and Native Americans may have bilirubin levels averaging 10 to 14 mg/dl. A higher incidence of autopsy-identified kernicterus also is seen in these populations. It does not seem to be related to G6PD deficiency, however, which is also common in these groups.

Determination of cause of jaundice. Following the chain of events from the RBC and its destruction in the newborn through the final excretion of conjugated bilirubin in the stools simplifies understanding the cause of a specific case of jaundice.[133] Causes include (1) increased destruction of RBCs, (2) decreased conjugation in the glucuronidase system, (3) decreased albumin binding, and (4) increased reabsorption from the GI tract.

When albumin binding is altered, the visibility of the jaundice is not affected. The bilirubin level may not be very high, but the substance is not bound to albumin and is available at lower levels to pass into the brain cells.[186] Premature infants have much lower albumin levels and thus have fewer binding sites. Drugs that also bind to albumin (e.g., aspirin, sulfadiazine) compete for binding sites. A lower level of bilirubin puts infants who have these medications in their system at risk because the bilirubin is unbound and available to enter tissue cells, including brain cells.

Reabsorption of bilirubin from stool in the GI tract can increase the bilirubin level. This occurs when the conjugated bilirubin that was excreted into the colon is unconjugated by the action of intestinal bacteria and reabsorbed, which happens when stools are decreased or slowed in passage. Poor feedings, pyloric stenosis, and other forms of intestinal obstruction are common causes of this type of jaundice. Some bacteria are more likely than others to unconjugate conjugated bilirubin.

Sepsis, on the other hand, was not found in more than 300 infants readmitted for hyperbilirubinemia while healthy and breastfeeding. Lower total bilirubin and direct bilirubin levels greater than 2.0 mg% in a sick baby have a high correlation with sepsis.[79]

Safe levels of bilirubin. Safe levels of bilirubin depend on a number of factors, including acidosis, hypoxia or anoxia, and sepsis. A handy rule of thumb is the correlation of birthweight in the premature infant and the indirect bilirubin level, using a value 2 to 3 mg lower when the infant has multiple problems. The risk of elevated bilirubin is related to the availability of albumin to bind the indirect bilirubin and prevent it from entering the brain cells. The amount of albumin is related to the degree of prematurity, and thus the rule of thumb is based on birthweight. When the infant is sick, fewer albumin-binding sites are available, and the bilirubin level of concern is even lower.

In a well infant weighing under 2000 g, the peak tolerated bilirubin level, above which an exchange transfusion might be done, corresponds roughly as follows: 1800 g/18 mg%, 1500 g/15 mg%,

1200 g/12 mg%, and 1000 g/10 mg%. Photo-therapy is usually initiated when the bilirubin is about 5 mg% lower than the exchange level. Because of stripping of bilirubin from the binding sites in the brain capillaries in some situations, such as prematurity, or presence of a competing drug in the serum, more bilirubin is available to be deposited than is measured to be "free" in the plasma.[189]

Any value of 20 mg% or greater warrants consideration of treatment. Jaundice visible under 24 hours of age is of special concern because it is usually associated with an incompatibility or infection. Rapidly rising bilirubin levels are also of concern, and a 0.5 mg% rise/hr is an indication for treatment.

The AAP has published a practice parameter for the management of hyperbilirubinemia in the healthy term newborn[182] (Table 14-13). Term infants who are visibly jaundiced at or before 24 hours of life are not considered healthy and require a diagnostic workup regardless of feeding method. The AAP also addresses jaundice associated with breastfeeding in a healthy term infant as follows:

> The AAP discourages the interruption of breast-feeding in healthy term newborns and encourages continued and frequent breastfeeding (at least eight to ten times every 24 hours). Supplementing nursing with water or dextrose water does not lower the bilirubin level in jaundiced, healthy, breastfeeding infants. Depending on the mother's preference and the physician's judgment, how-ever, a variety of options are presented in Table 14-13 for possible implementation beyond obser-vation, including supplementation of breast-feeding with formula or the temporary interrup-tion of breastfeeding and substitution with formula, either which can be accompanied by phototherapy.[182]

Hyperbilirubinemia and breastfeeding. Two major clinical conditions exist (one common, one rare) that associate the breastfed infant with hyperbilirubinemia. Table 14-14 outlines the major clinical features of these two conditions. The more common condition has been called *early breast milk jaundice* by Gartner[71] et al[73-75] but might be

TABLE 14-13   **Management of hyperbilirubinemia in healthy term newborns**

Age (hours)	Total serum bilirubin (TSB) level (mg/dl, µmol/L)			
	Consider phototherapy*	Phototherapy	Exchange transfusion if intensive phototherapy fails†	Exchange transfusion and intensive phototherapy
≤24‡	—	—	—	—
25-48	≥12 (170)	≥15 (260)	≥20 (340)	≥25 (430)
49-72	≥15 (260)	≥18 (310)	≥25 (430)	≥30 (510)
>72	≥17 (290)	≥20 (340)	≥25 (430)	≥30 (510)

From Provisional Committee for Quality Improvement, Subcommittee on Hyperbilirubinemia, American Academy of Pediatrics: *Pediatrics* 94:558, 1994.
*Phototherapy at these TSB levels is a clinical option, meaning that the intervention is available and may be used *on the basis of individual clinical judgment.*
†Intensive phototherapy should produce a decline of TSB of 1 to 2 mg/dl within 4 to 6 hours, and the TSB level should continue to fall and remain below the threshold level for exchange transfusion. If this does not occur, it is considered a failure of phototherapy.
‡Term infants who are clinically jaundiced at ≤24 hours old are not considered healthy and require further evaluation.

called *jaundice while breastfeeding,* because the failure to produce stool and the decreased intake of calories, probably not the breastfeeding, are at fault. Some bottle-fed infants also are jaundiced, so the appropriate term would be *bottle-feeding jaundice* for this group.

Early jaundice while breastfeeding. Many studies of bilirubin levels in normal newborn nurseries have been conducted looking at method of feeding. Unfortunately, very few have detailed frequency of feeds, supplementation, and stool pattern.[49,149,211] A review summarizing results in 13 studies covering more than 20,000 infants was reported by Schneider[204] to show a relationship between breastfeeding and jaundice. A pooled analysis of 12 studies showed 514 of 3997 breast-fed infants to have total serum bilirubin levels of 12 mg/dl or higher versus 172 of 4255 bottle-fed infants. In a smaller group of studies, 54 of 2655 breastfed infants had bilirubin levels of 15 mg/dl or greater versus 10 of 3002 bottle-fed infants. Eleven of 13 studies reported that breastfed infants had higher mean bilirubin levels. In a series of more than 12,000 infants, the risk of a breastfed infant becoming jaundiced was 1:8. The risk of becoming jaundiced for a premature was 3:6; for an Asian race, 3:56; and with prolonged rupture of membranes, 1:91. Jaundice is more common in normal newborns now compared with those in the

TABLE 14-14   **Comparison of early and late jaundice associated with hyperbilirubinemia while breastfeeding**

Early jaundice	Late jaundice
Occurs 2-5 days of age	Occurs 5-10 days of age
Transient: 10 days	Persists >1 month
More common in primiparas	All children of a given mother
Infrequent feeds	Milk volume not a problem
	May have abundant milk
Stools delayed and infrequent	Normal stooling
Receiving water or dextrose water	No supplements
Bilirubin peaks ≤15 mg/dl	Bilirubin may be >20 mg/dl
Treatment: none or phototherapy	Treatment: phototherapy
	Discontinue breastfeeding temporarily
	Rarely, exchange transfusion
Associations: low Apgar scores, water or dextrose water supplement, prematurity	Associations: none identified

1950s, when bilirubin was rarely measured in normal babies, although hospital stays averaged 5 to 7 days.

Rates of significant jaundice in Australia rose from 0.9% to 3.5% from 1975 to 1987. The associated factors most likely to be present in jaundiced infants were infrequent breastfeeding, less frequent stooling, and excessive weight loss.[230] It is clear from many studies that more breastfed than bottle-fed infants are jaundiced, and the cause requires further study.[204]

Relationship of bilirubin level to passage of stools. There are 450 mg of bilirubin in the intestinal tract meconium of the average newborn infant. Passing this meconium is critical to avoid the deconjugation and reabsorption of bilirubin from the gut into the serum. Failure to pass meconium is correlated with elevated serum bilirubin. Time of first stool is also correlated with level of serum bilirubin. Bottle-fed infants were reported by de Carvalho et al[50] to excrete more stool (82 g) and more bilirubin (23.8 mg) in the first 3 days than breastfed infants, who excreted 58 g of stool and 15.7 mg bilirubin. The serum bilirubin levels were 6.8 mg/dl in bottle-fed and 9.5 mg/dl in breastfed infants. Furthermore, when the breastfed infants excreted more stools and more bilirubin, they had lower bilirubin levels. This relationship has been confirmed in other studies from days 3 to 21.[79]

Feeding practices and early hyperbilirubinemia. A retrospective study of over 200 infants in our nursery looked at weight loss, number of feedings, amount of supplementation with water or dextrose water, body temperature, number of stools, and third-day serum bilirubin. The infants who received water or dextrose water passed fewer stools, had higher bilirubins, and had more problems nursing beyond 4 days of life. Full-term breastfed infants who were receiving water or dextrose supplements had higher serum bilirubin levels on the sixth day of life than bottle-fed babies in a study by Nicoll et al.[176] Supplementation with water or dextrose did not reduce hyperbilirubinemia that had already developed. This is not surprising because bilirubin is excreted in the stool

rather than the urine, and these jaundiced infants usually show no signs of dehydration.

When the number of feedings at the breast in the first 3 days of life was related to bilirubin levels, de Carvalho et al[50] were able to display a significant relationship. The greater the number of breastfeedings, the lower was the bilirubin. Those infants with more than eight feedings per day were not significantly jaundiced. These authors also found that water and dextrose supplements were associated with higher bilirubin levels. When they studied feeding practices in breastfed infants, Kuhr and Paneth[124] noted that sugar-water intake in the first 3 days negatively affected the volume of breast milk available on the fourth day. The infants with high glucose intake had higher bilirubin levels. These studies do not appear to show a correlation between weight loss and bilirubin level, although breastfed infants may lose more weight than bottle-fed infants.

When Stevenson[218] measured bilirubin production by calculating pulmonary carbon monoxide excretion in both breastfed and bottle-fed infants, he found no difference in the amount of bilirubin produced in the two groups.

Caloric deprivation and starvation. Elevated bilirubin did not impede sucking ability in a study by Alexander and Roberts.[7] Reduced caloric intake or starvation has been associated with hyperbilirubinemia in adult humans and in many animals. Gartner[71] has described the association between starvation and early neonatal jaundice. Gartner and Lee[75] have postulated that starvation may increase bilirubin production, shift bilirubin pools, reduce hepatic bilirubin uptake, diminish hepatic bilirubin conjugation, or increase enteric bilirubin reabsorption. Adequate caloric intake may simply diminish intestinal bilirubin absorption. Infants with intestinal obstruction (pyloric stenosis) at birth or in the early weeks of life are often jaundiced.

Treatment of early hyperbilirubinemia. When Maisels and Gifford[149] measured serum bilirubin levels in the newborn and the relationship to breastfeeding, they reported 8 of 10 infants with serum bilirubin greater than 12.9 mg/dl were breastfed. They suggested that rather than use phototherapy to treat the jaundice, the cause (i.e., breastfeeding) should be treated by temporary cessation of breastfeeding. This approach implies a substance in the milk causes the problem, whereas it is the process of altered nourishment. The amount of stress for the mother generated by separation from her infant for phototherapy was measured by urine cortisol levels and compared with levels in mothers who roomed-in with their jaundiced infants during phototherapy. The separated mothers were more stressed and were more likely to discontinue breastfeeding than those who remained with their infant.[60]

In a controlled trial of four interventions,[174] 125 of the 1685 infants in the birth cohort whose bilirubin levels reached 17 mg/dl (291 μmol/L) were randomly assigned to treatment. The four interventions were (1) continue breastfeeding and observe; (2) discontinue breastfeeding and substitute formula; (3) discontinue breastfeeding, substitute formula, and use phototherapy; and (4) continue breastfeeding and use phototherapy. The bilirubin reached 20 mg/dl (342 μmol/L) in 24% of group 1, 19% of group 2, 3% of group 3, and 14% of group 4. Phototherapy clearly adds to the decline in bilirubin, and the authors suggest that the parents can be offered the management of their choice. Newman and Maisels[175] recommend that because jaundiced infants are rarely sick, the only laboratory work necessary is a blood type and Coombs test; only when jaundice is excessive should bilirubin levels be followed closely. Infants with incompatibilities should be treated aggressively. In an attempt to apply logic to a very conflicting picture, a provocative report by Newman and Maisels[175] recommended a kinder, gentler approach to the evaluation and treatment of jaundice in the healthy term infant, with less interference with feeding.

The cumulative evidence from various studies published over the last 10 years, according to Gartner,[72] is that breastfeeding jaundice is the exaggeration of the first phase of physiologic jaundice of the newborn in the breastfed infant. It results from unphysiologic management of breastfeeding, expressed largely through insufficient frequency of breastfeeding. To treat the actual cause, that is, failed breastfeeding or inadequate stooling or underfeeding, the breastfeeding should be reviewed for frequency, length of suckling, and apparent supply of milk, adjusting the breastfeeding to improve any deficits. If stooling is the problem, the infant should be stimulated to stool. If starvation is the problem, the infant should receive additional calories (formula) while the milk supply is being increased by better breastfeeding techniques. The same would apply to bottle-feeding jaundice (i.e., any infant with *idiopathic* jaundice who is being bottle fed and has a bilirubin over 12.9 mg/dl). Stooling, frequency of feeds, and kilocalories would be improved. Box 14-5 provides a management schema for preventing or treating jaundice in the breastfed infant. All infants must have the appropriate laboratory studies performed.

BOX 14-5   Management outline for early jaundice while breastfeeding

1. Monitor all infants for initial stooling. Stimulate stool if no stool in 24 hours.
2. Initiate breastfeeding early and frequently. Frequent, short feeding is more effective than infrequent, prolonged feeding, although total time may be the same.
3. Discourage water, dextrose water, or formula supplements.
4. Monitor weight, voidings, and stooling in association with breastfeeding pattern.
5. When bilirubin level approaches 15 mg/dl, stimulate stooling, augment feeds, stimulate breast milk production with pumping, and use phototherapy if this aggressive approach fails and bilirubin exceeds 20 mg/dl.
6. Be aware that no evidence suggests early jaundice is associated with "an abnormality" of the breast milk, so withdrawing breast milk as a trial is only indicated if jaundice persists longer than 6 days or rises above 20 mg/dl or the mother has a history of a previously affected infant.

Breast milk jaundice, late-onset jaundice, or breast milk jaundice syndrome. Apart from the frequent but low-level (usually under 12 mg/dl) hyperbilirubinemia, breastfeeding rarely is associated with delayed but prolonged hyperbilirubinemia, which, if unchecked, may exceed 20 mg/dl. This has been called variously *breast milk jaundice, late-onset jaundice,* or *breast milk jaundice syndrome.*[73] It occurs in less than 1 in 200 births; the numbers are imprecise because not all mothers breastfeed. This is a syndrome associated with the milk of a particular mother and will occur with each pregnancy in varying degrees, depending on each infant's ability to conjugate bilirubin (i.e., a premature sibling might be more severely affected).[73] Early-onset jaundice is related to the process of breastfeeding, not the milk itself. It is essential to rule out other causes of prolonged or excessive jaundice, especially hemolytic disease, hypothyroidism, G6PD deficiency, inherited hepatic glucuronyl transferase deficiency (Gilbert syndrome, etc.), and intestinal obstruction.

The pattern of this jaundice is distinctly different. Normally, idiopathic jaundice peaks on the third day and then begins to drop. Breast milk jaundice, however, becomes apparent or continues to rise after the third day, and bilirubin levels may peak any time from the seventh to the tenth day, with untreated cases being reported to peak as late as the fifteenth day. Values have ranged from 10 to 27 mg/dl during this time. No correlation exists with weight loss or gain, and stools are normal.

The syndrome of breast milk jaundice was attributed by Arias et al[10] to a substance in the milk of some mothers that inhibits the hepatic enzyme glucuronyl transferase, preventing the conjugation of bilirubin. The substance has been identified as 5β-pregnane-3α,20α-diol, a breakdown product of progesterone and an isomer of pregnanediol that is not usually found in milk but occurs normally in about 10% of the lactating population. Although this substance had also been isolated from the milk and serum of mothers whose infants were not jaundiced, this work has not been duplicated.

In a definitive study of breast milk β-glucuronidase, Wilson et al[240] examined 55 mother-infant pairs. No correlation was found between serum bilirubin levels and breast milk β-glucuronidase between days 3 and 6 postpartum.

The role of lipoprotein lipase and bile salt–stimulated lipase in breast milk jaundice continues under investigation. The role of free fatty acids and the possibility of abnormal lipases are unresolved. The undisputed cause of breast milk jaundice continues to elude investigators.

As in early jaundice associated with breastfeeding, jaundiced infants at 3 weeks do not produce more bilirubin than their unjaundiced breastfed peers or bottle-fed infants.

Gartner and Auerbach[74] have suggested that bilirubin reabsorption from the gut may be enhanced by the milk of mothers whose infants are jaundiced. The studies relate 60% reabsorption of bilirubin in the presence of this milk when reabsorption is usually close to zero. This abnormal milk also inhibited hepatic glucuronyl transferase and contained 10 times the free fatty acids in normal milk. The authors speculate that these three abnormal properties may enhance enterohepatic circulation of bilirubin, with this increased load of bilirubin exceeding the capacity of the liver.[71]

Diagnosis depends on circumstantial evidence, because no easy, rapid laboratory test exists. All other causes, including infection, should be ruled out in the usual manner and a thorough history taken, including medications and family history. If the mother has nursed other infants, were they jaundiced? Usually 70% of the previous children of a given mother whose infant has breast milk jaundice have been jaundiced. The difference may be related to the greater maturity of the liver of a given infant who then is able to handle the increased demands on the glucuronyl transferase system. To establish the diagnosis firmly, and this is necessary when the bilirubin level is above 16 mg/dl for more than 24 hours, a bilirubin reading should be obtained 2 hours after a breastfeeding and then breastfeeding discontinued for at least 12 hours.[175] The infant must be fed fluids and calories. The infant's mother should be assisted in pumping her breasts to maintain her supply. Even more urgent is providing the mother with a sympathetic explanation of the problem and the process. After at least 12 hours without mother's milk, the bilirubin level should be measured. If a significant drop of more than 2 mg/dl occurs, it is diagnostic. When the level is below 15 mg/dl, the infant can be put to the breast. Bilirubin levels should be obtained to determine if the bilirubin rises again and, if so, how much. In most cases, in the time not breastfeeding the infant's body equilibrates the levels sufficiently, so there is only a slight increase in bilirubin on return to breastfeeding followed by a slow but steady drop. If that is the case, breastfeeding can continue. The bilirubin level should be checked at 10 to 14 days to be certain the bilirubin is truly clearing.

If the bilirubin has not dropped significantly after 12 hours off the breast, the time off the breast should be extended to 18 to 24 hours, measuring bilirubin levels every 6 hours. If the bilirubin rises while the infant is off the breast, the cause of jaundice is clearly not the breast milk; breastfeeding should be resumed and other causes for the jaundice reevaluated.

Phototherapy and breast milk jaundice. If the bilirubin is substantially over 20 mg/dl in a full-term infant (or proportionately lower in a preterm infant), it is important to lower the bilirubin promptly; thus phototherapy should be initiated as soon as the blood work is drawn. The relationship to breastfeeding can be established later. Often, IV fluids are also necessary.

If one is attempting to establish the diagnosis of breast milk jaundice, phototherapy should not be used while breast milk is being discontinued. If establishing the diagnosis is not necessary (perhaps because of the same diagnosis in older siblings), phototherapy can be used to bring the values to a more acceptable range (i.e., under 12 mg/dl). When phototherapy is discontinued, it is most important to establish that no rebound hyperbilirubinemia occurs. In addition, it is important to follow the infant at home after discharge through at least 14 days of life or longer if the values are not below 12 mg/dl. It should not be assumed that the diagnosis is breast milk jaundice when breastfeeding has been stopped and phototherapy initiated simultaneously.

Late diagnosis of breast milk jaundice. With the frequency of early discharge from the hospital, especially for families enjoying the birthing center concept, breastfed infants are often discharged before jaundice for any reason has developed. Because breast milk jaundice is likely to be delayed to the fourth or fifth day, peaking at 10 to 14 days of age, most normal infants are already home. Occasionally, an infant is observed in the pediatrician's office at 10 days of age or older with a bilirubin level over 20 mg/dl, often 23 to 25 mg/dl. This necessitates the admission of the infant to the hospital for a complete bilirubin workup. It is important to recognize that other causes of hyperbilirubinemia must be ruled out, including blood-type incompatibilities. At this age it is also necessary to rule out biliary obstruction and hepatitis, which might have a high direct or conjugated bilirubin level.

Phototherapy is used for 4 to 6 hours to establish whether this therapy will be effective in dropping the level sufficiently. It is necessary to stop breastfeeding temporarily and start phototherapy immediately on admission while the diagnostic workup is being performed when the bilirubin is substantially over 20 mg/dl if a possible association with breast milk exists. Otherwise, breastfeeding may continue even though IV fluids may also be necessary.

Suckling problems related to anatomy and neural disorders

Most problems with latch-on during breastfeeding can be solved with adjustment of position and approach, but a few cannot because the infant has an anatomic variation of the mouth or a neurodevelopmental problem. A thorough examination is required to evaluate the mouth and check for potential associated lesions and syndromes. Premature infants are more often identified with suckling problems because they not only are immature but also have been suctioned, intubated, and perhaps ventilated. Much has been put in their mouths. They may also have a high arched or grooved palate from the endotracheal tube.

When the mouth is carefully examined, an infant may have cysts on the dental ridge or under the tongue, the tongue may have limited range of motion, or the palate may be abnormal. A number of new observations are being reported in the literature, such as "bubble palate" or variation in infant palatal structure (VIPS). Snyder[213] recommends alternative positioning and repatterning oral behavior to increase the transfer of milk and reduce the trauma to the maternal nipple. Breastfeeding in the supine position with the infant prone encourages the infant's tongue to fall down and forward and keeps the nipple from being abraded by "the bubble." Marmet and Shell[151] describe a bubble palate as a concavity in the hard palate, usually about ⅜ to ¾ inch (1 to 2 cm) in diameter and ¼ inch (0.5 cm) deep. Similar adjustments to positioning would be appropriate for high arched palates.

Macroglossia presents a problem of too much tongue for the oral cavity. These infants do better at the breast than with a bottle. The main problem is to have the infant bring the tongue forward to avoid gagging.

Abnormal oral motor patterns are more common in premature infants and those who have been asphyxiated at birth. These include exaggerated tongue thrust (often from bottle feeding and nipple confusion), tonic bite, jaw thrust, jaw clenching, and lip pursing. Some of these behaviors are associated with postural muscle tone abnormalities.[237] Normal muscle tone and strength throughout breastfeeding, especially alignment of the head and neck, are required to form a stable base to anchor the oral and pharyngeal musculature.[179] Hypertonic and hypotonic infants may pose problems. Hypertonic infants are usually overflexed or overextended and have hypertonic mouths with tonic bite, jaw thrusting, and clenching. Inducing relaxation, minimizing handling, and using gentle strokes to calm the infant can be effective. If infant is extended, flexion may be achieved with a pleat-seat carrier (Fig. 14-4) or pillows.

Oral tactile hypersensitivity is often seen in infants who have had oral tubes, especially feeding tubes. Touching around the mouth causes feeding rejection. Decreased oral awareness may result in drooling and poor suckling. These infants may respond to stroking the oral area gently. Most

infants have a very strong arching reflex, which is elicited by touching or applying pressure on the back of the head, causing the infant to arch back away from the breast. Positions that require the mother to hold the head (e.g., "football hold") may trigger this reflex. Infants prefer to be swaddled but always respond better to a firm supportive hold of the body, slightly flexing the arms, legs, and trunk.

The development of an infant's oral motor and feeding skills parallels general physical development, especially gross and fine motor skills. When an infant is having persistent feeding problems, the infant needs total neuromotor assessment.[179] Minor problems may be solved by the firm supportive hold of a swaddled infant who is gently handled and encouraged.

Illingworth and Lister[111] first put forth the concept of a critical or sensitive period for the development of a skill. *Conditioned dysphagia* is a learned disorder, acquired and maintained through a behavioral conditioning process that occurs when a noxious stimulus is paired with the act of swallowing.[54] This is noted with suctioning of the mouth or nasopharynx and nasogastric feeding tubes in the NICU.

An infant with a true feeding disorder requires an assessment with a neonatal oral-motor review by a trained physical therapist.[179]

INFANTS WITH PROBLEMS REQUIRING SURGERY

Immediate neonatal period
First-arch disorders

Feeding of any sort may be greatly hindered by abnormalities of the jaw, nose, and mouth. A receding chin may be a minor problem and require only positioning the jaw forward. It is essential to establish that the jaw is not dislocated. A mother can hook the angle of the jaw with her finger and draw it forward. If the tongue is too large for the jaw, the infant will actually nurse better at the breast than at the bottle because the human nipple fits into the mouth with less bulk. Infants with first-arch abnormalities usually require considerable help in feeding. A cleft palate may also be present. If choanal atresia is present, it may be necessary to insert semipermanent nasal tubes so that the infant can be fed orally until older; definitive surgery may be necessary later. Once the nasal tubes are in place, the infant can manage at the breast. Feeding by any technique, however, is never easy.

Cleft lip

A solitary cleft lip is usually repaired in the first few weeks of life. Before surgery the infant will need some help, but the infant can nurse at the breast if a seal around the areola can be developed. Actually the breast may fill the defect, and suckling will go well. The mother may be able to put her thumb in the cleft to create a seal as she holds the breast to the infant's mouth. It is important to encourage the infant to suck to strengthen the tongue and jaw muscles. If all else fails, a breast shield can be tried, affixing a special cleft lip nipple to the shield.

The mother may have to express or pump milk and offer it by dropper or other means if sucking is ineffective. The pediatrician, plastic surgeon, and parents should work together as a team from the time of birth to determine a coordinated plan of treatment. Some surgeons have special protocols before and after surgery to ensure optimal healing. It is important to make all plans for feeding around the surgical plan. The literature reports individual mothers' experiences nursing infants with lip defects. The major caution in sharing these experiences is to consider that the supportive surgical approach may differ from those reported in the literature.[104]

Cleft palate

The prognosis for successful feeding of an infant with a cleft palate depends on the size and position of the defect (soft palate, hard palate) as well as the associated lesions. Lubit[136] recommends the application of an orthopedic appliance to the neonatal maxilla to close the gap, thus aiding nursing,

stimulating orofacial development, developing the palatal shelves, preventing tongue distortions, preventing nasal septum irritation, and decreasing the number of ear infections. This will aid the plastic surgeon and help the mother psychologically as well. Lubit further relates that a cleft involving the secondary palate can interfere with normal nursing. For the infant to suckle, the nose must be sealed off from the mouth, creating a negative pressure in the oral cavity. The milk may also run out the nose. The absence of palatal tissue can prevent expulsion of milk from the nipple. The orthopedic appliance prosthetically restores the anatomy of the palate, permitting normal suckling.

Because the purpose of the negative pressure in the mouth is to hold the nipple and areola in place and not to extract milk from the breast, a seal is needed to keep the pressure. A mother may be able to perform the positioning task by holding the breast to her infant's mouth firmly between two fingers, as shown in Figs. 8-13, 14-4, 14-5, and 14-6. The infant is then able to milk the areola and nipple with the tongue pressing it against the roof of the mouth, even with the cleft. The breast must be held in position just as a bottle must be held throughout the feeding.[80]

In assessing 143 infants with cleft lip and palate over a 5-year period, Clarren et al[40] found that by assessing the infant's ability to generate negative intraoral pressure and to move the tongue against the nipple, they could identify effective feeding techniques. They summarized these findings in relation to the possibility of breastfeeding (Table 14-15). They point out that normal children with a cleft can swallow normally. A defect in the bony structure of the palate, however, creates a hole that is difficult to plug; thus these children are more difficult to feed.

The authors[40] point out that problems with intraoral muscular movements are associated with bilateral cleft lip, which causes severe anterior projection of the premaxilla that precludes stabilizing the nipple, and with wide palatal clefts, which offer no back guard for tongue movements and retroplaced tongues that cannot compress the nipple effectively. When there are neurologic problems

Fig. 14-5.   Dancer hold. **A,** Hand position of mother. **B,** Infant in position at breast with support. (From McBride MC, Danner SC: *Clin Perinatol* 14:109, 1987.)

Fig. 14-6.   **A,** Infant with cleft lip and palate opening wide to latch on for a feeding. **B,** Same infant suckling at breast. Defect in lip and palate is comfortably filled by breast tissue. (Photos obtained with assistance of Marie Biancuzzo, RN, MSN.)

causing dysrhythmic tongue movements or a weak tongue or grinding of the gum on the nipple, it is more than a simple anatomic problem and is usually part of a syndrome (e.g., first-arch syndrome). These children usually have swallowing problems as well (e.g., Pierre Robin syndrome).

Feeding procedures for each infant vary. Early assessment of the infant and the mother can usually lead to successful feeding within 1 to 2 days. The infant should not go hungry, and the mother should not spend hours struggling with a system that is not successful for her child. The Lact-Aid or the lactation supplementer can be very helpful, because the mother can control the flow by squeezing

TABLE 14-15   Assessment of sucking and feeding techniques for infants with clefts of lip and palate

Condition	Assessment* Generation of negative pressure	Assessment* Ability to make mechanical movements	Feeding techniques
Cleft lip and palate	–	+/–	Breastfeeding is unlikely. Deliver milk into infant's mouth.
Cleft palate only	+/–	+	Breastfeeding sometimes succeeds. Soft artificial nipples with large openings are effective. Infant may need delivery of milk into the mouth.
Cleft of soft palate	+/–	+	Breastfeeding or normal bottle feeding usually works well.
Pierre Robin malformation sequence	+/–	–	Breastfeeding is unlikely. Nipple position is critical. Many infants need delivery of milk into mouth.
Cleft lip only	+/–	+	Breastfeeding works well. Artificial nipple with large base works well.

From Clarren SK, Anderson B, Wolf LS: *Cleft Palate J* 24:244, 1987.
*+, Present; –, absent; +/–, partial.

the reservoir, and the infant can have some suckling experience, which will strengthen the oral structure and avoid the trauma of invasive devices. The mother may need to pump to increase her milk supply.

Weatherley-White et al[238] report a program of early repair in breastfeeding infants with cleft lip. Repair has been initiated earlier and earlier, but these authors present 100 consecutive repairs: 51 infants were older than 3 weeks, and 49 were younger, of whom 26 underwent surgery at age 1 week or less. There was no increase in complication rate and no increase in need for revision of repair. Sixty mothers were offered the opportunity to breastfeed immediately postoperatively; 38 began within hours. Of these, 16 infants breastfed more than 6 weeks, 22 converted by 6 weeks, and 22 were fed by cup or syringe. Breastfed infants gained more weight, and hospital stay was a day shorter. A prospective randomized trial of 40 infants showed that early postoperative breastfeeding after cleft lip repair is safe and results in

more weight gain by 6 weeks after surgery when compared with infants randomized to be spoon-fed postoperatively.[46]

Similar experience with early surgery and breastfeeding is confirmed by Fisher,[64] who reports performing reconstructive surgery in the Third World, where breastfeeding is undisputed and is very successful. He also reports greater success rate with breastfeeding but notes it requires the conviction not only of the surgeon and pediatrician but also of the nurse, nutritionist, mother, and grandmother. It takes all these for success but only one for failure.

As noted earlier, breastfed infants have fewer bouts with otitis media, which has been attributed to the position of the infant while feeding at the breast as well as the antiinfective properties of the milk. This is an important consideration in infants with cleft palates, who have been identified as having more ear infections in general than other infants.[54]

Children with cleft palates may also fail to

thrive, not only as a function of their feeding difficulty but also because they may have an underlying increased metabolic need. In a study of 37 children with cleft palates and no other anomalies, the median birthweight was at the thirtieth percentile.[16] By 1 to 2 months, weights had dropped to the twentieth percentile and did not recover to the thirtieth until 6 months of age.

It is important to have the plastic surgeon involved promptly after birth so management plans can be developed with the family immediately. This also avoids conflicting information from others.

Oral defects: feeding recommendations

Feeding infants with oral defects requires extra effort. Each infant is slightly different. Usually mothers learn to feed their own infants more effectively, even when bottle feeding, than the skilled professional can advise them. This amplifies that it requires a special patience and knack. Breastfeeding can be successful. Infants with cleft lip or palate should be managed as normal infants. Cupping of the infant's jaw and filling the defect with the mother's thumb while supporting the breast in place for suckling will allow effective breastfeeding in the infant with cleft lip. This has been referred to as the "dance hold"[157] (Fig. 14-5). The infant should be brought to the mother to feed and for rooming-in, as with any infant. Reinforcing that the infant is normal and merely needs some reconstructive surgery is important in helping the parents adjust. Parent-to-parent programs are most helpful. The primary care physician coordinates care with the specialist and the rest of the health care team.

Pediatric reconstructive surgeons usually have a team of professionals, including otolaryngologists, audiologists and affiliated therapists, social workers and nurses, familiar and experienced with these first-arch problems. Parent support groups have often been developed through these sources. Most reconstructive surgeons will see the infant in the first 24 to 48 hours and reassure the parents while designing the plan of action. Usually a member of the nursing staff of the surgeon's

practice will also visit and provide the practical advice about feeding, especially if the mother chooses to breastfeed.[54]

Other syndromes may be associated with feeding difficulties because of an anatomic variation that interferes. *High arched palate* is seen in trisomies, in Turner syndrome, and in small premature infants who have been intubated, which causes a characteristic groove in the palate. In one study, 10 infants under 29 months of age with Turner syndrome had difficulty feeding from birth when compared with normal children.[155] Breastfeeding was less successful and terminated early. The infants were noted to have marked hypertonia of the cheeks and lips, dysfunctional tongue movements, and poor chewing skills later. The infants had difficulty latching on and had a slow, weak suck. The study infants did not demand food and had not developed a diurnal cycle of hunger and satiety. No efforts were reported to remedy these problems.

Intestinal tract disorders

Infants with anomalies of the GI tract that cause obstruction develop symptoms that depend on the location of the problem in the GI tract.

Tracheoesophageal fistula. Tracheoesophageal (TE) fistula is apparent early and, depending on the exact anatomy of the lesions, results in respiratory symptoms and signs of obstruction. This is a surgical emergency. If no feedings have been given or no milk has been aspirated, surgery can be done as soon as possible. If pneumonia develops, the course is protracted and the infant may have to be maintained on peripheral venous alimentation until healing takes place and surgery can be done.

A mother who wants to breastfeed an infant with a TE fistula can manually express milk or pump, saving all samples in the freezer until the infant can take oral milk feedings. If the infant has a gastrostomy tube in place, small feedings may be started fairly early postoperatively, and human milk is ideal if available because of its easy digestibility and antiinfective properties. If there is initially a need to supplement the milk partially with IV fluids, the fluids can be calculated to make up the difference between needs and nutrients supplied by breast milk taken by tube. As nutrition progresses, if supply does not keep up with requirements, feedings can be supplemented with other nutrients. When ready for oral feedings, a full-term or large premature infant can nurse at the breast. Unless the mother is able to spend most of the day and night at the hospital, the infant will have to receive bottle or cup feedings as well (Fig. 14-7). If the mother has been able to store up enough milk, the infant may be able to fulfill needs from breast milk. Once the infant is discharged and begins to nurse at the breast every feeding for a few days, the supply will increase immediately. If concern exists about nutritional lag between needs and production, the Lact-Aid or lactation supplementer device can be used briefly to stimulate the breast without starving and exhausting the infant (see Chapter 18).

Gastroesophageal reflux. Gastroesophageal (GE) reflux, persistent nonprojectile, postprandial vomiting or regurgitation, is being diagnosed with

Fig. 14-7. When infant must be fed but cannot be breastfed (e.g., when mother is ill), infant can be fed using a small, soft medicine cup. Infant is swaddled and held semiupright, and liquid is given inside lower lip.

increasing frequency. Part of this increase is occurring in graduates of NICUs who have been tube fed or perhaps intubated. Previously compromised infants are more frequently bottle fed, thus the increase in bottle feeding associated with this diagnosis is to be expected. Little is written about GE reflux in breastfed infants because it is usually asymptomatic. The position for feeding is more upright than for bottle feeding, and the suckling motion of the tongue, which triggers peristaltic waves from tongue to GI tract, provides some protection for breastfed infants.

The effect of milk type on physiologic GE reflux was evaluated in 37 breastfed and 37 bottle-fed healthy term infants at 2 to 8 days of life by Heacock et al.[102] The GE reflux episodes in breastfed infants were less frequent (83) and shorter than those in bottle-fed infants (144). Breastfed infants had more quiet sleep than active sleep. There was no apparent difference in volume consumed. The pH of breast milk was initially slightly higher than formula; a significantly lower pH was found for refluxes in the breastfed infants. The researchers did not test whether the differences were caused by the variations in human milk and formula or the differences in suckling at the breast, a physiologic process, or sucking a bottle.

Pyloric stenosis. Pyloric stenosis occurs in about 2 to 5 of 1000 live births. A family tendency exists, but the disease is more common in first-born males. Usually it occurs between the second and sixth weeks of life, although it can occur any time after birth. Vomiting is characteristic, is intermittent at first and progresses to include every feeding, and is often projectile. These infants are eager feeders and go back for more milk until the weight loss and dehydration make them anxious and irritable.

Large epidemiologic studies have failed to show a relationship between pyloric stenosis and breastfeeding. Although pyloric stenosis and breastfeeding have both increased in the last decades, a relationship does not appear to exist. The study in western Australia links LBW, short gestational age, and paternal family history.[106] In Atlanta the rates were unchanged, but the infants were white male, had greater birthweight, were from upper-class families, and were most likely to be breastfed in this generation but not in 1970.[127]

In an analysis of 91 infants with pyloric stenosis born in Saskatchewan from 1970 to 1985, matched with control infants who did not have the disease and were born at the same time and place, the ratio of males to females was 4:1, and 39 of the 91 were firstborns. Bottle feeding was more prevalent in the disease group than in the controls.

In the investigation of vomiting, it is important to keep in mind that overfeeding can cause spitting and vomiting, even projectile vomiting, but it is not associated with weight loss, decreased urine and stools, and dehydration. Therapy consists of pyloromyotomy following correction of the dehydration and associated electrolyte abnormalities. If the procedure is uncomplicated (i.e., intestinal lumen was not entered), the infant can go back to the breast in 6 to 8 hours after a trial of water at 4 hours shows the infant is alert and sucking well. The breastfed infant may be discharged in 24 hours if nursing has gone well. If the duodenum is entered at the time of surgery, gastric decompression and IV fluids will be necessary and oral feeding delayed several days until signs of healing occur. A breastfed infant may resume nursing earlier than a bottle-fed infant returns to formula because of the rapid emptying time of the stomach and the zero curd tension of the breast milk.

Disorders of the small intestine. Disorders such as duodenal obstruction, malrotation, jejunal obstruction, and duplications require surgery. Depending on the extent of the lesion, whether the bowel wall is opened, whether bowel segments are removed, and whether there are associated lesions such as annular pancreas, the infant will need postoperative maintenance on IV fluids and possibly alimentation. The mother who chooses to breastfeed may or may not have ever nursed the infant, depending on the time of onset of symptoms and their severity. The mother should be counseled about the prognosis and encouraged to express milk manually and pump if it appears feasible for her to breastfeed eventually. The decision should be made among the parents, surgeon, neonatolo-

gist, and pediatrician. Frequently, infants with atresias are also small or premature and have protracted recovery periods.

Disorders of the colon. Disorders of the colon occur more often in full-term infants. *Hirschsprung's disease,* or *congenital aganglionic megacolon,* is the most common lesion. Passage of meconium is usually delayed; however, only 10% to 15% of all children with delayed passage of meconium have Hirschsprung's disease. Constipation and abdominal distention are the most frequent initial symptoms. They may begin during the first few days of life and gradually progress to include bilious vomiting. The clinical picture may be indistinguishable from meconium ileus, ileal atresia, or large bowel obstruction. In any infant with perforation of the colon, ileum, or appendix, Hirschsprung's disease should be considered. The breastfed infant may have milder symptoms and delayed onset of real stress because the breast milk stools are normally loose and seedy and easily passed. The pH and flora of the intestinal tract are also different, leading to less distention. Enterocolitis may occur at any age and is the major cause of death.

No data have been found to distinguish the incidence of this complication in breastfed and bottle-fed infants, although an argument could be mounted regarding the projected value of sIgA and intestinal flora of the breastfed infant. The treatment depends on the symptoms, x-ray findings, and biopsy results for the identification of the aganglionic segment. Colostomy is usually done at the time of diagnosis, with definitive surgery later in the first year of life. Feedings can be resumed as soon as the infant is stable, after the colostomy has healed sufficiently to permit bowel activity. Human milk has the same advantages for early postoperative feeding in this disease as well because of its antiinfective properties and easy digestibility.

Meconium plug syndrome and meconium ileus. Meconium plug syndrome and meconium ileus are less common and less severe in breastfed infants who have received a full measure of colostrum, which has a cathartic effect and stimulates the passage of meconium. If either disorder is diagnosed, the infant should continue to nurse in addition to any other treatment, which should include an assessment for cystic fibrosis (CF).

Necrotizing enterocolitis. Although NEC has been known for 100 years, only since 1960 has it been identified with any frequency, which suggests an iatrogenic component. It is most common in premature infants and infants compromised by asphyxia. It has been associated with umbilical catheters, exchange transfusions, polycythemia, hyperosmolar feedings, and infection. Its cause is not clear. Work with animals has suggested that human breast milk, specifically colostrum, provides protection against the disease. A good control study to evaluate this in human infants has not been reported. A "dose or two" of human milk may not be enough. Reported cases of NEC have occurred so early in life that no feedings had been given. Present regimens of treatment call for cessation of all oral feedings and use of oral and systemic antibiotics, gastric decompression, plasma or blood transfusions, and rigorous monitoring for progression or perforation with serial x-ray studies as well as a septic workup. Further study is necessary to determine cause and possible prevention and the role colostrum or breast milk might play, as discussed earlier.

The organisms generally associated with NEC are gram-negative organisms such as *Bacteroides, Escherichia coli,* and especially *Klebsiella.* Brown et al[32] reported that 89% of the infants with NEC had received cow's milk formulas and that gram-negative bacteria and endotoxins were present in the stool. Colonization of breastfed infants with *Klebsiella* does not occur, and *Lactobacillus bifidus* predominates, according to Mata and Urrutia.[152] The unusual occurrence of NEC in Helsinki, at the University of Helsinki Children's Hospital intensive care nursery, is remarkable. All the premature infants are routinely fed colostrum and breast milk in Helsinki.

Imperforate anus. Defects in the rectum and anal sphincter are usually diagnosed in the first few hours on physical examination or because a rectal thermometer cannot be passed. When the blind pouch is more generous, diagnosis may depend on the evaluation of failure to pass stool. Depending on associated lesions and fistulas to bladder or vagina, surgical decompression can be performed. Until this time, oral feedings are withheld. High lesions require an immediate colostomy with later final repair, whereas low lesions may be repaired at the primary procedure through a perineal approach. Infants may be breastfed as soon as any bowel activity can be permitted, often 2 to 3 days postoperatively.

Gastrointestinal bleeding. The most common cause of vomiting blood or passing blood via the rectum in a breastfed infant is a bleeding nipple in the mother, which may or may not be painful. Any time fresh blood is found in the vomitus or stool of any newborn, the blood should be tested for adult or fetal hemoglobin (Hb). If adult Hb, it indicates the source is maternal. This is done by a qualitative test, the Apt test. (Mix blood with 2 to 3 ml normal saline solution, add this to 3 ml of 10% NaOH [0.25 M]. Mix gently. Observe for color change. Fetal Hb is stable in alkali and will remain pink, whereas adult Hb turns brown. Use a known adult sample as a color control.) If the blood is adult Hb in a breastfed infant, the possibility of a cracked and bleeding nipple should be ruled out by inspection of the maternal breast (see Chapter 8).

If the blood is fetal Hb, the differential diagnosis for bleeding in any neonate should be followed. Breastfeeding can be maintained, unless a lesion requiring surgery is identified. More than 50% of cases of GI bleeding in the neonate go undiagnosed. Anorectal fissure is an uncommon cause in breastfed infants. Allergy to human milk has not been reported as a cause of intestinal bleeding. The distribution of causes of intestinal bleeding in the neonate, without selection for type of feeding, follows: idiopathic, 50%; hemorrhagic disorders, 20%; swallowed maternal blood, 10%; anorectal fissures, 10%; intestinal ischemia, 5%; and colitis, 5%. When the bleeding occurs beyond the newborn period, colitis (see earlier discussion) becomes a more frequent cause as does Meckel diverticulum. Sullivan[221] has reviewed the subject of cow's milk–induced intestinal bleeding in infancy.[221]

Otitis media

Acute otitis media is a very common affliction among young children that has increased in incidence paralleling the increasing attendance at day care. Population density and air pollution have also been identified as factors. In a Finnish study of 471 2- to 3-year-old children, 188 had three or more attacks of otitis media, 76 had one to two attacks, and 207 had none.[183] Incidence was increased in those who attended day care or had several siblings. Prolonged breastfeeding (longer than 6 months) was associated with a decreased risk. A prospective study of 1011 children in Boston evaluated the duration of middle ear effusion, and it was significantly diminished by breastfeeding.[224]

Breastfeeding is protective against otitis media. With day-care exposure and other environmental risk factors, it does have a measurable minimizing effect. Breastfeeding is also more comfortable for the infant with a painful otitis when suckling at the breast than bottle feeding because of the physiologic suck/swallow mechanism. If the infant is having difficulty feeding, providing a dose of acetaminophen or ibuprofen before the feeding can be helpful.

Congenital dislocation of hip

When procedures or treatments need to be initiated for an infant previously thought to be normal, breastfeeding may not go smoothly. Using congenital dislocation of the hip as a prototype, Elander[59] looked at overall breastfeeding success. Compared with a randomly chosen control group of 113 infants, the 30 study infants who required the von Rosen splint were less successfully fed. However, a higher incidence of cesarean birth was seen in the study group (30% vs. 4%). There were equal numbers of primiparas (50% vs. 48%). Once breastfeeding was established, the long-range success rate was no different. Mothers were pleased to be able to do something special for their splinted children (i.e., breastfeed). This would suggest that special support and guidance regarding breastfeeding issues may be needed along with details on how to apply the splint and how to cope with the splint while positioning for breastfeeding.

Malformations of central nervous system

Malformations of the central nervous system (CNS) diagnosed at birth include the clinical spectrum from anencephaly and complete craniorachischisis to dermal sinuses. Defects of the spinal column range from complete spinal rachischisis to spina bifida occulta. Those that are incompatible with life or are inoperable present the additional problem to the mother who had planned to breastfeed of coping with her desire to nurse her infant. If the infant is to be given normal newborn care and the mother desires to nurse this infant, breastfeeding should be discussed by the pediatrician and parents together. It has been well demonstrated that parents grieve more physiologically if they have contact with their abnormal infants, but their imaginations are more vicious than some abnormalities of development. The professional's personal bias as to how to deal with this infant should not overshadow the discussion with the parents. If the mother chooses to nurse the infant who has no life expectancy and the infant is to be fed at all by mouth, she should have that choice.

Infants with CNS abnormalities requiring surgery can be breastfed until the procedure and postoperatively as soon as oral intake is permitted. In these cases, when the GI tract is not involved, breastfeeding can be initiated 6 to 8 hours postoperatively, at the surgeon's discretion. The risk of lung irritation from breast milk is minimal. The rapid emptying time of the stomach and presence of antiinfective factors serve as advantages in the postoperative course.

Surgery or rehospitalization beyond neonatal period

Anesthesia is a main concern when any patient is scheduled for surgery. Traditionally, the patient has been ordered "nothing by mouth" after midnight or 6 to 8 hours preoperatively. Young infants used to feeding every 4 hours are frantic when ready for the operating room.

Recommendations for fasting intervals preoperatively have changed with the belief that clear liquids are safe up to within 2 hours of anesthesia, with similar gastric volumes and pH at 2 hours or 8 hours.[206,214] Children under 1 year had not been studied until the report by Litman et al,[134] who evaluated 77 infants between 2 weeks and 1 year of age. Bottle-fed infants had no solids within 6 hours and only clear liquids up to 8 ounces within 2 hours of surgery. Breastfed infants had no solids but were permitted to breastfeed up to within 2 hours of surgery. After 0.02 mg/kg oral atropine 30 to 45 minutes before surgery, induction anesthesia, and tracheal intubation, gastric fluid was aspirated by a blinded researcher who measured volume and pH. The study was discontinued when an unacceptable number of infants in the breastfed group had gastric volumes greater than 1 ml/kg (7 of 24 breastfed and 2 of 46 bottle fed). The pH of the gastric contents of bottle-fed infants was less than 2.5 in 9 of 10 (90%) infants with measurable fluid, whereas pH greater than 2.5 in breastfed infants was 3 of 8 (38%). Low pH is probably a greater risk than volume, but the residual in breastfed infants is much greater than with clear fluids.[134] Instructions to breastfeeding mothers should limit the amount of breastfeeding after 4 hours and permit feeding on a prepumped breast, predominantly for comfort.

The infant who requires surgery or rehospitalization can and should be breastfed postoperatively in most cases. The gravity of the surgery and the length of the recovery phase will determine the time necessary for the mother to pump and manually express her milk to keep her supply available. The infant who is hospitalized is already traumatized by the separation, the strange surroundings and people, and the underlying discomfort of the disease process itself. If the infant is to be fed orally, feeding should be at the breast as often as possible. If the mother can room-in or the hospital has a care-by-parent ward, this works well. If obligations to other family members make it impossible for the mother to stay, she can pump her milk and bring it in fresh day by day or frozen if the time interval between visits is longer than a day. Freezing will destroy the cellular content, but this is not a major problem beyond the immediate neonatal period. The infant should not be subjected to the added trauma of being weaned from the breast when the infant needs the security and intimacy of nursing most, unless weaning is absolutely unavoidable.

The medical profession needs to be aware of this infant and mother and their special needs for support. An opportunity to discuss the breastfeeding aspect of the infant's management should be offered by the physician. The pediatrician should assume the advocacy role. The parents should not have to fight for the right to maintain breastfeeding. Plans for pumping and saving milk should be discussed and provided for. If the infant is recovering in an open ward or even a room with other infants and their parents without adequate privacy, a separate room should be provided for the mother to nurse or pump her milk. This room should be clean, neat, adequately illuminated, and equipped with a sink for washing hands. Storerooms, broom closets, and staff dressing rooms are inappropriate. If a mechanical pump is to be used, it should be kept clean and operable with disposable tubing and attachments that come in contact with the milk or the breast.

Arrangements for providing sterile containers for collecting milk and storing it are discussed (see Chapter 20). Occasionally a mother may become so concerned about the adequacy of her milk for her infant that she may nurse much too frequently. Actually her child will need much more nonnutritive cuddling and holding than usual. The physician may need to reassure the mother when pointing this out. The father should also be encouraged to understand all the tubes, bandages, and appliances the infant may have attached. He is an important member of the parenting team and should provide some of the soothing and especially the nonnutritive cuddling.

Congenital heart disease

When an infant who is diagnosed with congenital heart disease is already feeding at the breast, this is usually not a medical indication to interrupt the process unless surgery is imminent. Even infants with cyanotic heart disease, if they can be fed orally, can be breastfed. The "work" required to breastfeed is less than the "work" required to bottle-feed. Heart and respiratory rates remain stable during feeding at the breast. If the infant is unable to generate enough sucking stimulus to the breast to increase the milk supply, an electric pump can be used between feedings to increase the mother's supply.

Cardiac surgeons frequently plan surgery for a certain weight and/or age. The mother can be assisted in helping the infant reach the goal. Human milk is low in sodium and easily digested, thus permitting frequent feedings. The nurse practitioner or lactation consultant should assist the mother in increasing her production and increasing fat content at each feeding. Feeding at one breast usually increases fat. In the case of a cardiac-compromised infant, using one breast also diminishes the stress of switching to the other side. The mother may need extra support and encouragement. Providing one's milk for one's sick infant may be extremely important. The breastfeeding relationship may be important for the infant as well. Research has shown that infants have important cardiovascular responses to nutrient intake.[169] These responses are regulated by changes in autonomic activity to the heart and vasculature. These early life-shaping interactions that occur when the offspring is fed by the mother have been demonstrated in the animal model. Interactions between mothers and their young serve as hidden regulators of physiologic function.

If oral intake must be restricted preoperatively or immediately postoperatively, "nonnutritive" suckling at the previously pumped breast can be very calming and comforting for the infant.

SUDDEN INFANT DEATH SYNDROME

Sudden infant death syndrome (SIDS) is the leading cause of death in infants after 1 month of age, accounting for one third of all deaths in the first year. Healthy, full-term infants account for 85% of the deaths.[70]

In a 3-year, multicenter, controlled study of SIDS in New Zealand reported in 1993,[207] The

National COT Death Prevention Programme[164] sought to reduce the rising incidence of infant death by determining associated factors. Sleeping prone, maternal smoking, lack of breastfeeding, and the infant sharing a bed were the four modifiable risk factors. New Zealand launched a major prevention program to educate the public about these risk factors.[165] The American Academy of Pediatrics has launched a similar program focusing only on sleeping prone. Although breastfeeding offers protection, there are cases of SIDS among breastfed infants; the incidence is much lower, however, than with bottle feeding. A case-control study in the United States by Frederickson et al[70] analyzed births of infants weighing more than 2000 g between 1988 and 1989. There were 7102 controls and 499 SIDS and 584 non-SIDS deaths. Breastfeeding offered dose-response protection against SIDS across races and socioeconomic levels. For white infants, the risk of SIDS increased 19% for every month of not breastfeeding and 100% for every month of nonexclusive breastfeeding. For black infants, the risk was 19% and 113%, respectively.

Numerous studies have been conducted to define further the associations with SIDS. Prone sleeping position continues to be the most important correlation, and the AAP continues the "back to sleep" campaign. The protective influence of breastfeeding is actually strongest among infants of smoking mothers. SIDS rates are higher among infants of mothers who smoke, but breastfeeding by a smoking mother lowers that to a rate equal to that of bottle-fed infants. An association has also been suggested with pacifier use in bottle-fed infants. Pacifiers are not known to lower SIDS rates among breastfed infants beyond normal breastfeeding rates. Although some studies show a protective effect of bed sharing, the AAP has not endorsed bed sharing because of the reported risk of roll-over deaths and the need for additional studies.[222] Frederickson et al[70] suggest that breastfeeding promotion, especially among low-income women where rates of breastfeeding are lowest and SIDS are higher, would reduce the national SIDS rates.

NURSING BOTTLE CARIES IN BREASTFED INFANTS

The development of rampant dental caries can occur in breastfed infants.[31] Usually the children have been nursed for 2 or 3 years, spending long stretches at the breast. One infant had early signs at 9 months, and by 18 months she required full mouth reconstruction.

The physician should be alert to the potential for dental decay when infants nurse frequently, especially through the night. Family history of dental enamel problems is worth investigating. Certainly these children are candidates for fluoride treatment.

The levels of mutant streptococci in saliva and plaque are higher in children with rampant cavities than in controls.[153] All breastfed infants have mutant streptococci and lactobacilli on their teeth. Tooth susceptibility is genetically programmed. Children with a strong family history of caries may need fluoride supplements while breastfeeding.[53] They are at special risk if they suckle all night after age 1 year.

REFERENCES

1. Abbassi V, Steinour TA: Successful diagnosis of congenital hypothyroidism in four breast-fed neonates, *J Pediatr* 97:259, 1980.
2. Abrams SA, Schanler RJ, Garza C: Bone mineralization in former very low birth weight infants fed either human milk or commercial formula, *J Pediatr* 112:956, 1988.
3. Adamkin DH: Enteral and total parenteral nutrition in the very low birth weight infant. I. Enteral nutrition, *Neonatal Intensive Care* 10:19, 1997.
4. Addy HA: The breastfeeding of twins, *J Trop Pediatr Environ Child Health* 21:231, 1975.
5. Aggett PJ, Atherton DJ, More J et al: Symptomatic zinc deficiency in a breast-fed preterm infant, *Arch Dis Child* 55:547, 1980.
6. Ahmed S, Blair AW: Symptomatic zinc deficiency in a breast-fed infant, *Arch Dis Child* 56:315, 1981.
7. Alexander GS, Roberts SA: Sucking behavior and milk intake in jaundiced neonates, *Early Hum Dev* 16:73, 1988.
8. Anderson DM, Williams FH, Merkatz RB et al: Length of gestation and nutritional composition of human milk, *Am J Clin Nutr* 37:810, 1983.
9. Anderson GC: Touch and the kangaroo care method. In Field TM, editor: *Touch in early development,* Mahwah, NJ, 1995, Erlbaum Associates.
10. Arias IM, Gartner LM, Seifter S et al: Prolonged neonatal unconjugated hyperbilirubinemia associated with breast feeding and steroid pregnane-3α,20β-diol in maternal milk that inhibits glucuronide formation in vitro, *J Clin Invest* 43:2037, 1964.
11. Atinmo T, Omololu A: Trace element content of breast milk from mothers of preterm infants in Nigeria, *Early Hum Dev* 6:309, 1982.
12. Atkinson SA, Anderson GH, Bryan MH: Human milk: comparison of the nitrogen composition in milk from mothers of premature and full-term infants, *Am J Clin Nutr* 33:811, 1980.
13. Atkinson SA, Radde IC, Chance GW et al: Macromineral content of milk obtained during early lactation from mothers of premature infants, *Early Hum Dev* 4:5, 1980.
14. Aumonier ME, Cunningham CC: Breastfeeding in infants with Down's syndrome, *Child Care Health Dev* 9:247, 1983.
15. Auricchio S, Follo D, de Ritis G et al: Does breast feeding protect against the development of clinical symptoms of celiac disease in children? *J Pediatr Gastroenterol Nutr* 2:428, 1983.
16. Avedian LV, Ruberg RL: Impaired weight gain in cleft palate infants, *Cleft Palate J* 17:24, 1980.
17. Barfoot RA, McEnery G, Ersser RS et al: Diarrhoea due to breast milk: a case of fucose intolerance? *Arch Dis Child* 63:311, 1988.
18. Beijers RJW, Graaf FVD, Schaafsma A et al: Composition of premature breastmilk during lactation: constant digestible protein content (as in full term milk), *Early Hum Dev* 29:351, 1992.
19. Bennett FC, McClelland S, Kriegsmann EA et al: Vitamin and mineral supplementation in Down's syndrome, *Pediatrics* 72:707, 1983.
20. Bergstrand O, Hellers G: Breastfeeding during infancy in patients who later develop Crohn's disease, *Scand J Gastroenterol* 18:903, 1983.
21. Berkowitz CD, Inkelis SH: Bloody nipple discharge in infancy, *J Pediatr* 103:755, 1983.

22. Bernbaum JC, Pereira GR, Watkins JB et al: Nonnutritive sucking during gavage feeding enhances growth and maturation in premature infants, *Pediatrics* 71:41, 1983.

23. Berseth CL: Effect of early feeding on maturation of the preterm infant's small intestine, *J Pediatr* 120:947, 1992.

24. Bier JAB, Ferguson AE, Morales Y et al: Breastfeeding infants who were extremely low birth weight, *Pediatrics* 100:e3, 1997.

25. Billeaud C, Senterre J, Rigo J: Osmolality of the gastric and duodenal contents in low birth weight infants fed human milk or various formulae, *Acta Paediatr Scand* 71:799, 1982.

26. Birch DG, Birch EE, Hoffman DR et al: Retinal development in very-low-birth-weight infants fed diets differing in omega-3 fatty acids, *Invest Ophthalmol Vis Sci* 33:2365, 1992.

27. Bishop NJ, Dahlenburg SL, Fewtrell MS et al: Early diet of preterm infants and bone mineralization at age five years, *Acta Paediatr* 85:230, 1996.

28. Bitman J, Wood L, Hamosh M et al: Comparison of the lipid composition of breast milk from mothers of term and preterm infants, *Am J Clin Nutr* 38:300, 1983.

29. Bode HH, Vanjonack WJ, Crawford JD: Mitigation of cretinism by breastfeeding, *Pediatrics* 62:13, 1978.

30. Boehm G, Jakobsson I, Mansson M et al: Macromolecular absorption in small-for-gestational age infants, *Acta Paediatr* 81:864, 1992.

31. Brams M, Maloney J: "Nursing bottle caries" in breastfed children, *J Pediatr* 103:415, 1983.

32. Brown EG, Ainbender E, Sweet AY: Effect of feeding stool endotoxins: possible relationship to necrotizing enterocolitis, *Pediatr Res* 10:352, 1976.

33. Cannella PC, Bowser EK, Guyer LK et al: Feeding practices and nutrition recommendations for infants with cystic fibrosis, *J Am Diet Assoc* 93:297, 1993.

34. Carey DE, Rowe JC, Goetz CA et al: Growth and phosphorus metabolism in premature infants fed human milk, fortified human milk, or special premature formula, *Am J Dis Child* 141:511, 1987.

35. Cavell B: Gastric emptying in preterm infants, *Acta Paediatr Scand* 68:725, 1979.

36. Chandra RK: Immunoglobulin and protein levels in breast milk produced by mothers of preterm infants, *Nutr Res* 2:27, 1982.

37. Chappell JE, Clandinin MT, Kerney-Volpe C et al: Fatty acid balance studies in premature infants fed human milk or formula: effect of calcium supplementation, *J Pediatr* 108:439, 1986.

38. Chiba Y, Minagawa T, Mito K et al: Effect of breastfeeding on responses of systemic interferon and virus-specific lymphocyte transformation in infants with respiratory syncytial virus infection, *J Med Virol* 21:7, 1987.

39. Clark BJ: After a positive Guthrie—what next? Dietary management for the child with phenylketonuria, *Eur J Clin Nutr* 46(suppl I):S33, 1992.

40. Clarren SK, Anderson B, Wolf LS: Feeding infants with cleft lip, cleft palate, or cleft lip and palate, *Cleft Palate J* 24:244, 1987.

41. Committee on Nutrition, American Academy of Pediatrics: Nutritional needs of low-birth-weight infants, *Pediatrics* 75:976, 1985.

42. Committee on Nutrition of the Preterm Infant, European Society of Paediatric Gastroenterology and Nutrition: Nutrition and feeding of preterm infants, *Acta Paediatr Scand Suppl* 336:3, 1987.

43. Committee on Obstetric Practice, American College of Obstetricians and Gynecologists; Committee on the Fetus and Newborn, American Academy of Pediatrics: *Guidelines for perinatal care*, ed 4, Elk Grove, Ill, 1997, American Academy of Pediatrics.

44. Curtis JA, Bailey JD: Influence of breastfeeding on the clinical features of salt-losing congenital adrenal hyperplasia, *Arch Dis Child* 58:71, 1983.

45. Danziger Y, Pertzelan A, Mimouni M: Transient congenital hypothyroidism after topical iodine in pregnancy and lactation, *Arch Dis Child* 62:295, 1987.

46. Darzi MA, Chowdri NA, Bhat AN: Breast feeding or spoon feeding after cleft lip repair: a prospective, randomised study, *Br J Plast Surg* 49:24, 1996.

47. Davey AM, Wagner CL, Phelps DL et al: Do premature infants with umbilical artery catheters tolerate oral feeds? *Pediatr Res* 31:199A, 1992.

48. de Carvalho M, Anderson DM, Giangreco A et al: Frequency of milk expression and milk production by mothers of non-nursing premature neonates, *Am J Dis Child* 139:483, 1985.

49. de Carvalho M, Klaus M, Merkatz RB: Frequency of breast-feeding and serum bilirubin concentration, *Am J Dis Child* 136:737, 1982.

50. de Carvalho M, Robertson S, Klaus M: Fecal bilirubin excretion and serum bilirubin concentrations in breastfed and bottle-fed infants, *J Pediatr* 107:786, 1985.

51. DeCurtis M, McIntosh N, Ventura V et al: Effect of nonnutritive sucking on nutrient retention in preterm infants, *J Pediatr* 109:888, 1986.

52. DeVries LS, Lary S, Whitelaw AG et al: Relationship of serum bilirubin levels and hearing impairment in newborn infants, *Early Hum Dev* 15:269, 1987.

53. Deyano MP, Degana RA: Breastfeeding and oral health, *NY State Dent J* 59:30, 1993.

54. DiScippio W, Kaslon KR: Conditioned dysphagia in cleft palate children after pharyngeal flap surgery, *Psychol Med* 44:247, 1982.

55. Dunn L, Hulman S, Weiner J et al: Beneficial effects of early hypocaloric enteral feeding on neonatal gastrointestinal function: preliminary report of a randomized trial, *J Pediatr* 112:622, 1988.

56. Eckert CD, Sloan MV, Duncan JR et al: Zinc binding: a difference between human and bovine milk, *Science* 195:789, 1977.

57. Ehrenkranz RA, Ackerman BA: Metoclopramide effect on faltering milk production by mothers of premature infants, *Pediatrics* 78:614, 1986.
58. Eibl MM, Wolf HM, Furnkranz H et al: Prevention of necrotizing enterocolitis in low-birth-weight infants by IgA-IgG feeding, *N Engl J Med* 319:1, 1988.
59. Elander G: Breastfeeding of infants diagnosed as having congenital hip joint dislocation and treated in the von Rosen splint, *Midwifery* 2:147, 1986.
60. Elander G, Lindberg T: Hospital routines in infants with hyperbilirubinemia influence the duration of breastfeeding, *Acta Paediatr Scand* 75:708, 1986.
61. Ernest AE, McCabe ERB, Neifert MR et al: *Guide to breast feeding the infant with PKU,* Washington, DC, 1980, US Government Printing Office.
62. Ernst JA, Rickard KA, Neal PR et al: Lack of improved growth outcome related to non-nutritive sucking in very low birth weight premature infants fed a controlled nutrient, *Pediatrics* 83:706, 1989.
63. Evans GW, Johnson PE: Defective prostaglandin synthesis in acrodermatitis enteropathica, *Lancet* 1:52, 1977.
64. Fisher JC: Early repair and breastfeeding for infants with cleft lip, *Plast Reconstr Surg* 79:886, 1987.
65. Forbes GB: Nutritional adequacy of human breast milk for premature infants. In Lebenthal E, editor: *Textbook of gastroenterology and nutrition,* New York, 1981, Raven.
66. Forbes GB: Human milk and the small baby, *Am J Dis Child* 136:577, 1982.
67. Forbes GB: Fetal growth and body composition: implications for the premature infant, *J Pediatr Gastroenterol Nutr* 2(suppl):552, 1983.
68. Ford JE, Zechalko A, Murphy J et al: Comparison of the B vitamin composition of milk from mothers of preterm and term babies, *Arch Dis Child* 58:367, 1983.
69. Forman MR, Graubard BI, Hoffman HJ et al: The PIMA infant study: breastfeeding and gastroenteritis in the first year of life, *Am J Epidemiol* 119:335, 1984.
70. Frederickson DD, Sorenson JR, Biddle AK et al: Relationship of sudden infant death syndrome to breastfeeding duration and intensity, *Am J Dis Child* 147:460, 1993.
71. Gartner LM: Disorders of bilirubin metabolism. In Nathan DG, Oski FA, editors: *Hematology of infancy and childhood,* ed 3, Philadelphia, 1987, Saunders.
72. Gartner LM: On the question of the relationship between breastfeeding and jaundice in the first 5 days of life, *Semin Perinatol* 18:502, 1994.
73. Gartner LM, Arias IM: Temporary discontinuation of breast feeding in infants with jaundice, *JAMA* 225:532, 1973.
74. Gartner LM, Auerbach KG: Breast milk and breastfeeding jaundice, *Acta Pediatr* 34:249, 1987.
75. Gartner LM, Lee KS: Effect of starvation and milk feeding on intestinal bilirubin absorption, *Pediatr Res* 14:498, 1980.
76. Garza C, Hopkinson J, Schanler RJ: Human milk banking. In Howell RR, Morriss FH, Pickering LK, editors: *Human milk in infant nutrition and health,* Springfield, Ill, 1986, Thomas.
77. Goldman AS, Chheda S, Keeney SE et al: Immunologic protection of the premature newborn by human milk, *Semin Perinatol* 18:495, 1994.
78. Goldman AS, Garza C, Nichols B et al: Effects of prematurity on the immunologic system in human milk, *J Pediatr* 101:901, 1982.
79. Gourley GR, Kreamer B, Arend R: The effect of diet on feces and jaundice during the first three weeks of life, *Gastroenterology* 103:660, 1992.
80. Grady E: Breastfeeding the baby with a cleft of the soft palate: success and its benefits, *Clin Pediatr* 16:978, 1977.
81. Greco L, Mayer M, Grimaldi M et al: The effect of early feeding on the onset of symptoms in celiac disease, *J Pediatr Gastroenterol Nutr* 4:52, 1985.
82. Greer FR, McCormick A: Improved bone mineralization and growth in premature infants fed fortified own mother's milk, *J Pediatr* 112:961, 1988.
83. Greer FR, McCormick A, Kashyap ML et al: Late hypertriglyceridemia in very low birth weight infants fed human milk exclusively, *J Pediatr* 111:466, 1987.
84. Greer FR, Tsang RC: Calcium, phosphorus, magnesium, and vitamin D requirements for preterm infants. In Tsang RC, editor: *Vitamin and mineral requirements for preterm infants,* New York, 1985, Marcel Dekker.
85. Groh-Wargo S, Toth A, Mahoney K: The utility of a bilateral breast pumping system for mothers of premature infants, *Neonatal Network* 14:31, 1995.
86. Gross SJ: Growth and biochemical response of preterm infants fed human milk or modified infant formula, *N Engl J Med* 308:237, 1983.
87. Gross SJ: Bone mineralization in preterm infants fed human milk with and without mineral supplementation, *J Pediatr* 111:450, 1987.
88. Gross SJ, Buckley RH, Wakil SS et al: Elevated IgA concentration in milk produced by mothers delivered of preterm infants, *J Pediatr* 99:389, 1981.
89. Gross SJ, David RJ, Bauman L et al: Nutritional composition of milk produced by mothers delivering preterm, *J Pediatr* 96:641, 1980.
90. Gross SJ, Gabriel E: Vitamin E status in preterm infants fed human milk or infant formula, *J Pediatr* 106:635, 1985.
91. Gross SJ, Slagle TA: Feeding the low birth weight infant, *Clin Perinatol* 20:193, 1993.
92. Grunebaum E, Amir J, Merlop P et al: Breast milk jaundice: natural history, familial incidence and late neurodevelopmental outcome of the infant, *Eur J Pediatr* 150:267, 1991.

93. Guerrini P, Bosi G, Chierici R et al: Human milk: relationship of fat content with gestational age, *Early Hum Dev* 5:187, 1981.

94. Gunn AJ, Gunn TR, Rabone DL et al: Growth hormone increases breast milk volumes in mothers of preterm infants, *Pediatrics* 98:279, 1996.

95. Gupta AP, Gupta PK: Metoclopramide as a lactagogue, *Clin Pediatr* 24:269, 1985.

96. Hack M, Estabrook MM, Robertson SS: Development of sucking rhythm in preterm infants, *Early Hum Dev* 11:133, 1985.

97. Hagelberg S, Lindblad BS, Lundsjo A et al: The protein tolerance of very low birth weight infants fed human milk protein enriched mother's milk, *Acta Paediatr Scand* 71:597, 1982.

98. Hahn HB, Spiekerman AM, Otto WR et al: Thyroid function tests in neonates fed human milk, *Am J Dis Child* 137:220, 1983.

99. Hansen TWR, Bratlid D: Bilirubin and brain toxicity, *Acta Paediatr Scand* 75:513, 1986.

100. Harmon T, Burkhart G, Applebaum H: Perforated pseudomembranous colitis in the breastfed infant, *J Pediatr Surg* 27:744, 1992.

101. Haug M, Laubach C, Burke M et al: Vitamin E in human milk from mothers of preterm and term infants, *J Pediatr Gastroenterol Nutr* 6:605, 1987.

102. Heacock HJ, Jeffery HE, Baker JL et al: Influence of breast versus formula milk on physiological gastroesophageal reflux in healthy, newborn infants, *J Pediatr Gastroenterol Nutr* 14:41, 1992.

103. Heine W: Is mother's milk the most suitable food for low birth weight infants? *Early Hum Dev* 29:345, 1992.

104. Hemingway L: Breastfeeding a cleft-palate baby, *Med J Aust* 2:626, 1972.

105. Hibberd CM, Brooke OG, Carter ND et al: Variations in the composition of breast milk during the first 5 weeks of lactation: implications for the feeding of preterm infants, *Arch Dis Child* 57:658, 1982.

106. Hitchcock NE, Gilmour AI, Gracey M et al: Pyloric stenosis in western Australia, 1971-1984, *Arch Dis Child* 62:512, 1987.

107. Hopkinson JM, Schanler RJ, Garza C: Milk production by mothers of premature infants, *Pediatrics* 81:815, 1988.

108. Hughes CA, Dowling RH: Speed of onset of adaptive mucosal hypoplasia and hypofunction in the intestine of parenterally fed rats, *Clin Sci* 59:317, 1980.

109. Hurst NM, Valentine CJ, Renfro L et al: Skin-to-skin holding in the neonatal intensive care unit influences maternal milk volume, *J Perinatol* 17:213, 1997.

110. Hylander MA, Strobino DM, Dhanireddy R: Association of race, Apgar score at five minutes and formula feeding with retinopathy of prematurity (ROP) among very low birth weight (VLBW) infants, *Pediatr Res* 41:199A, 1997.

111. Illingworth RS, Lister J: The critical or sensitive period, with special reference to certain feeding problems in infants and children, *J Pediatr* 65:839, 1964.

112. Israel D, Levine J, Pettel M et al: Protein induced allergic colitis (PAC) in infants, *Pediatr Res* 25:116A, 1989.

113. Itabashi K, Hayashi T, Tsugoshi T et al: Fortified preterm human milk for very low birth weight infants, *Early Hum Dev* 29:339, 1992.

114. Ito S, Blajchman A, Stephenson M et al: Prospective follow-up of adverse reactions in breast-fed infants exposed to maternal medication, *Am J Obstet Gynecol* 168:1393, 1993.

115. Iwai Y, Takanashi T, Nakao Y et al: Iron status in low birth weight infants on breast and formula feeding, *Eur J Pediatr* 145:63, 1986.

116. Jain L, Sivieri E, Abbasi S et al: Energetics and mechanics of nutritive sucking in the preterm and term neonate, *J Pediatr* 111:894, 1987.

117. Järvenpää AL: Feeding the low-birth-weight infant. IV. Fat absorption as a function of diet and duodenal bile acids, *Pediatrics* 72:684, 1983.

118. Järvenpää AL, Raiha NCR, Rassin DK et al: Preterm infants fed human milk attain intrauterine weight gain, *Acta Paediatr Scand* 72:239, 1983.

119. Jocson MAL, Mason EO, Schanler RJ: The effects of nutrient fortification and varying storage conditions on host defense properties of human milk, *Pediatrics* 100:240, 1997.

120. Johnson P, Salisbury DM: Breathing and sucking during feeding in the newborn. In Hofer MA, editor: *Ciba Foundation Symposium no 33: Parent-infant interaction,* Amsterdam, 1975, Elsevier Scientific.

121. Kashyap S, Schulze KF, Forsyth M et al: Growth, nutrient retention, and metabolic response of low-birth-weight infants fed supplemented and unsupplemented preterm human milk, *Am J Clin Nutr* 52:254, 1990.

122. Kero P, Piekkala P: Factors affecting the occurrence of acute otitis media during the first year of life, *Acta Paediatr Scand* 76:618, 1987.

123. Khin-Maung-U, Nyant-Nyant-Wai, Myo-Khin et al: Effect on clinical outcome of breastfeeding during acute diarrhoea, *Br Med J* 290:587, 1985.

124. Kuhr M, Paneth N: Feeding practices and early neonatal jaundice, *J Pediatr Gastroenterol Nutr* 1:485, 1982.

125. LaGamma EF, Ostertag SG, Birenbaum H: Failure of delayed oral feedings to prevent necrotizing enterocolitis: results of studying very low birthweight neonates, *Am J Dis Child* 139:385, 1985.

126. Lake AM, Whitington PF, Hamilton SR: Dietary protein-induced colitis in breast-fed infants, *J Pediatr* 101:906, 1982.

127. Lammer EJ, Edmonds LD: Trends in pyloric stenosis incidence, Atlanta, 1968 to 1982, *J Med Genet* 24:482, 1987.

128. Lawrence RA: Infant nutrition, *Pediatr Rev* 5:133, 1983.

129. Lebenthal E, Leung Y-K: The impact of development of the gut on infant nutrition, *Pediatr Ann* 16:211, 1987.

130. Leonard EL, Trykowski LE, Kirkpatrick BV: Nutritive sucking in high-risk neonates after perioral stimulation, *Phys Ther* 60:299, 1980.

131. Letarte J, Guyda H, Dussault JH et al: Lack of protective effect of breastfeeding in congenital hypothyroidism: report of 12 cases, *Pediatrics* 65:703, 1980.

132. Lewis-Jones DI, Reynolds GJ: A suggested role for precolostrum in preterm and sick newborn infants, *Acta Paediatr Scand* 72:13, 1983.

133. Linn S, Schoenbaum SC, Monson RP et al: Epidemiology of neonatal hyperbilirubinemia, *Pediatrics* 75:770, 1985.

134. Litman RS, Wu CL, Quinlivan JK: Gastric volume and pH in infants fed clear liquids and breast milk prior to surgery. Abstract for presentation to The American Society of Anesthesiology, Washington, DC, October, 1993.

135. Littlewood JM, Crollick AJ, Richards IDG: Childhood coeliac disease is disappearing, *Lancet* 2:1359, 1980.

136. Lubit EC: Cleft palate orthodontics: why, when, how, *Am J Orthod* 69:562, 1976.

137. Lucas A: Enteral nutrition. In Tsang RC, Lucas A, Uauy R et al, editors: *Nutritional needs of the preterm infant,* Baltimore, 1993, Williams & Wilkins.

138. Lucas A, Bishop NJ, King FL et al: Randomized trial of nutrition for preterm infants after discharge, *Arch Dis Child* 67:324, 1992.

139. Lucas A, Bloom SR, Aynsley-Green A: Gut hormones and "minimal enteral feeding," *Acta Paediatr Scand* 75:719, 1986.

140. Lucas A, Cole TJ: Breast milk and neonatal necrotising enterocolitis, *Lancet* 336:1519, 1990.

141. Lucas A, Fewtrell MS, Morley R et al: Randomized outcome trial of human milk fortification and developmental outcome in preterm infants, *Am J Clin Nutr* 64:142, 1996.

142. Lucas A, Morley R, Cole TJ et al: Early diet in preterm babies and developmental status in infancy, *Arch Dis Child* 64:1570, 1989.

143. Lucas A, Morley R, Cole TJ et al: Early diet in preterm babies and developmental status at 18 months, *Lancet* 335:1477, 1990.

144. Lucas A, Morley R, Cole TJ et al: Breast milk and subsequent intelligence quotient in children born premature, *Lancet* 339:261, 1992.

145. Luder E, Kattan M, Tanzer-Torres G et al: Current recommendations for breastfeeding in cystic fibrosis centers, *Am J Dis Child* 144:1153, 1990.

146. Macaron C: Galactorrhea and neonatal hypothyroidism, *J Pediatr* 101:576, 1982.

147. MacFarlane PI, Miller V: Human milk in the management of protracted diarrhea of infancy, *Arch Dis Child* 59:260, 1984.

148. Machida HM, Smith AGC, Gall DG et al: Allergic colitis in infancy: clinical and pathologic aspects, *J Pediatr Gastroenterol Nutr* 19:22, 1994.

149. Maisels MJ, Gifford K: Normal serum bilirubin levels in the newborn and the effect of breastfeeding, *Pediatrics* 78:837, 1986.

150. Maisels MJ, Kring E: Risk of sepsis in newborns with severe hyperbilirubinemia, *Pediatrics* 90:741, 1992.

151. Marmet C, Shell E: *Lactation forms: a guide to lactation consultant charting,* Encino, Calif, 1993, Lactation Institute and Breastfeeding Clinic.

152. Mata LJ, Urrutia JJ: Intestinal colonization of breast fed children in a rural area of low socioeconomic level, *Ann NY Acad Sci* 176:93, 1971.

153. Matee MIN, Mikx FHM, Maselle SYM et al: Mutant streptococci and lactobacilli in breastfed children with rampant caries, *Caries Res* 26:183, 1992.

154. Mathew OP: Breathing patterns of preterm infants during bottle feeding: role of milk flow, *J Pediatr* 119:960, 1991.

155. Mathisen B, Reilly S, Skuse D: Oral-motor dysfunction and feeding disorders of infants with Turner syndrome, *Dev Med Child Neurol* 34:141, 1992.

156. Mathur NB, Dwarkadas AM, Sharma VK et al: Anti-infective factors in preterm human colostrum, *Acta Paediatr Scand* 79:1039, 1990.

157. McBride MC, Danner SC: Sucking disorders in neurologically impaired infants: assessment and facilitation of breastfeeding, *Clin Perinatol* 14:109, 1987.

158. McDonagh AF: Is bilirubin good for you? *Clin Perinatol* 17:359, 1990.

159. Meberg A, Willgraff S, Sande HA: High potential for breastfeeding among mothers giving birth to pre-term infants, *Acta Paediatr Scand* 71:661, 1982.

160. Meetze WH, Valentine C, McGuigan JE et al: Gastrointestinal priming prior to full enteral nutrition in very low birth weight infants, *J Pediatr Gastroenterol Nutr* 15:163, 1992.

161. Meier P: Bottle- and breast-feeding: effects on transcutaneous oxygen pressure and temperature in preterm infants, *Nurs Res* 37:36, 1988.

162. Meier P, Anderson GC: Responses of small preterm infants to bottle- and breast-feeding, *Matern Child Nurs J* 12:97, 1987.

163. Mendelson RA, Anderson GH, Bryan MH: Zinc, copper and iron content of milk from mothers of preterm and full-term infants, *Early Hum Dev* 6:145, 1982.

164. Mitchell EA, Aley P, Eastwood J: The National COT Death Prevention Programme in New Zealand, *Aust J Public Health* 16:158, 1992.

165. Mitchell EA, Taylor BJ, Ford RPK et al: Four modifiable and other major risk factors for cot death: the New Zealand study, *J Paediatr Child Health* 28(suppl 1):53, 1992.

166. Montgomery RK, Buller HA, Rings EHHM et al: Lactose intolerance and the genetic regulation of intestinal lactase-phlorizin hydrolase, *FASEB J* 5:2824, 1991.

167. Moro GE, Minoli I, Ostrom M et al: Fortification of human milk: evaluation of a novel fortification scheme and of a new fortifier, *J Pediatr Gastroenterol Nutr* 20:162, 1995.

168. Murphy JF, Neale ML, Mathews N: Antimicrobial properties of preterm breast milk cells, *Arch Dis Child* 58:198, 1983.

169. Myers MM, Shair HN, Hofer MA: Feeding in infancy: short- and long-term effects on cardiovascular function, *Experientia* 48:322, 1992.

170. Narayanan I, Mehta R, Choudhury DK et al: Sucking on the "emptied" breast: non-nutritive sucking with a difference, *Arch Dis Child* 66:241, 1991.

171. Narayanan I, Prakash K, Bala S et al: Partial supplementation with expressed breast-milk for prevention of infection in low-birth-weight infants, *Lancet* 2:561, 1980.

172. Narayanan I, Prakash K, Prabhakar AK et al: A planned prospective evaluation of the anti-infective property of varying quantities of expressed human milk, *Acta Paediatr Scand* 71:441, 1982.

173. Neifert MR, Seacat JM: Practical aspects of breastfeeding the premature infant, *Perinatol Neonatol* 12:24, 1988.

174. Newman TB, Maisels MJ: Does hyperbilirubinemia damage the brain of healthy full-term infants? *Clin Perinatol* 17:331, 1990.

175. Newman TB, Maisels MJ: Evaluation and treatment of jaundice in the term newborn: a kinder, gentler approach, *Pediatrics* 89:809, 1992.

176. Nicoll A, Ginsburg R, Tripp JH: Supplementary feeding and jaundiced newborns, *Acta Paediatr Scand* 71:759, 1982.

177. Oberkotter LV, Pereira GR, Paul MH et al: Effect of breastfeeding vs formula-feeding on circulating thyroxine levels in premature infants, *J Pediatr* 106:822, 1985.

178. Oski FA: Iron requirements of the premature infant. In Tsang RC, editor: *Vitamin and mineral requirements in preterm infants,* New York, 1985, Marcel Dekker.

179. Palmer MM, Crawley K, Blanco IA: Neonatal oral-motor assessment scale: a reliability study, *J Perinatol* 13:28, 1993.

180. Paludetto R, Robertson SS, Hack M et al: Transcutaneous oxygen tension during nonnutritive sucking in preterm infants, *Pediatrics* 74:539, 1984.

181. Pedersen CB, Zachau-Christiansen B: Otitis media in Greenland children: acute, chronic and secretory otitis media in three to eight year olds, *J Otolaryngol* 15:332, 1986.

182. Provisional Committee for Quality Improvement, Subcommittee on Hyperbilirubinemia, American Academy of Pediatrics: Practice parameters: management of hyperbilirubinemia in the healthy term newborn, *Pediatrics* 94:558, 1994.

183. Pukander J, Luotonen J, Timonen M: Risk factors affecting the occurrence of acute otitis media among 2-3-year-old urban children, *Acta Otolaryngol Stockh* 100:260, 1985.

184. Putet G, Rigo J, Salle B et al: Supplementation of pooled human milk with casein hydrolysate: energy and nitrogen balance and weight gain composition in very low birth weight infants, *Pediatr Res* 21:458, 1987.

185. Riva E, Agostoni C, Biasucci G et al: Early breastfeeding is linked to higher intelligence quotient scores in dietary treated phenylketonuric children, *Acta Paediatr* 85:56, 1996.

186. Robinson PJ, Rapoport SI: Binding effect of albumin on uptake of bilirubin by brain, *Pediatrics* 79:553, 1987.

187. Rönnholm KAR, Perheentupa J, Siimes MA: Supplementation with human milk protein improves growth of small premature infants fed human milk, *Pediatrics* 77:649, 1986.

188. Rönnholm KAR, Sipilä I, Siimes MA: Human milk protein supplementation for the prevention of hypoproteinemia without metabolic imbalance in breast milk-fed, very low-birth-weight infants, *J Pediatr* 101:243, 1982.

189. Rowe JC, Wood DH, Rowe DW et al: Nutritional hypophosphatemic rickets in a premature infant fed breast milk, *N Engl J Med* 300:293, 1979.

190. Saarinen UM: Prolonged breast feeding as prophylaxis for recurrent otitis media, *Acta Paediatr Scand* 71:567, 1982.

191. Sack J, Amado O, Lunenfeld B: Thyroxine concentration in human milk, *J Clin Endocrinol Metab* 45:171, 1977.

192. Saint L, Maggiore P, Hartman PE: Yield and nutrient content of milk in eight women breastfeeding twins and one woman breastfeeding triplets, *Br J Nutr* 56:49, 1986.

193. Savilahti E, Järvenpää A-L, Räihä NCR: Serum immunoglobulins in preterm infants: comparison of human milk and formula feeding, *Pediatrics* 72:312, 1983.

194. Sazawal S, Bhan MK, Bhandari N: Type of milk feeding during acute diarrhoea and the risk of persistent diarrhea: a case control study, *Acta Paediatr Suppl* 381:93, 1992.

195. Schanler RJ: Human milk fortification for premature infants, *Am J Clin Nutr* 64:249, 1996.

196. Schanler RJ: Quality of growth in preterm infants: use of fortified human milk. In Battaglia FC, Pedraz C, Sawatzki G et al, editors: *Maternal and extrauterine nutritional factors: their influence on fetal and infant growth,* Madrid, 1996, Ediciones Ergon.

197. Schanler RJ: Suitability of human milk for the low birthweight infant, *Clin Perinatol* 22:207, 1995.

198. Schanler RJ, Abrams SA: Postnatal attainment of intrauterine macromineral accretion rates in low birth weight infants fed fortified human milk, *J Pediatr* 126:441, 1995.

199. Schanler RJ, Garza C: Plasma amino acid differences in very low birth weight infants fed either human milk or whey-dominant cow milk formula, *Pediatr Res* 21:301, 1987.

200. Schanler RJ, Garza C, Nichols BL: Fortified mother's milk for very-low-birth-weight infants: results of growth and nutrient balance studies, *J Pediatr* 107:437, 1985.

201. Schanler RJ, Garza C, Smith EO: Fortified mother's milk for very-low-birth-weight infants: results of macro mineral balance studies, *J Pediatr* 107:767, 1985.

202. Schanler RJ, Hurst NM: Human milk for the hospitalized preterm infant, *Semin Perinatol* 18:476, 1994.

203. Scheidt PC, Graubard BI, Nelson KB et al: Intelligence at six years in relation to neonatal bilirubin level: follow-up of the National Institute of Child Health and Human Development clinical trial of phototherapy, *Pediatrics* 87:797, 1991.

204. Schneider AP: Breast milk jaundice in the newborn, *JAMA* 255:3270, 1986.

205. Schneider JR, Fischer H, Feingold M: Acrodermatitis enteropathica, *Am J Dis Child* 145:212, 1991.

206. Schreiner MS, Triebwasser A, Keon TP: Ingestion of liquids compared with preoperative fasting in pediatric outpatients, *Anesthesiology* 75:593, 1990.

207. Scragg LK, Mitchell EA, Tonkin SL et al: Evaluation of the cot death prevention programme in South Auckland, *NZ Med J* 106:8, 1993.

208. Senterre J, Patel G, Salle B et al: Effects of vitamin D and phosphorus supplementation on calcium retention in preterm infants fed banked human milk, *J Pediatr* 103:305, 1983.

209. Shmerling DH: Dietary protein-induced colitis in breastfed infants, *J Pediatr* 103:500, 1983.

210. Similä S, Kokkonen J, Kouvalainen K: Use of lactose-hydrolyzed human milk in congenital lactase deficiency, *J Pediatr* 101:584, 1982.

211. Sirota L, Nussinovirtch M, Landman J et al: Breast milk jaundice in preterm infants, *Clin Pediatr* 27:195, 1988.

212. Slagle TA, Gross SJ: Effect of early low-volume enteral substrate on subsequent feeding tolerance in very low birth weight infants, *J Pediatr* 113:526, 1988.

213. Snyder JB: Bubble palate and failure to thrive: a case report, *J Hum Lact* 13:139, 1997.

214. Splinter WM, Stewart JA, Muir JG: Large volumes of apple juice preoperatively do not affect gastric PH and volume in children, *Can J Anaesth* 37:36, 1990.

215. Steichen JJ, Krug-Wispe SK, Tsang RC: Breastfeeding the low birth weight preterm infant, *Clin Perinatol* 14:131, 1987.

216. Stein H, Cohen D, Herman AAB et al: Pooled pasteurized breast milk and untreated own mother's milk in the feeding of very low birth weight babies: a randomized controlled trial, *J Pediatr Gastroenterol Nutr* 5:242, 1986.

217. Stevens FM, Egan-Mitchell B, Cryan E et al: Decreasing incidence of coeliac disease, *Arch Dis Child* 62:465, 1987.

218. Stevenson DK: Pulmonary excretion of carbon monoxide in human infants as an index of bilirubin production. In Maisels MJ, editor: *Hyperbilirubinemia in the newborn: report of the 85th Ross Conference on Pediatric Research*, Columbus, Ohio, 1983, Ross Laboratories.

219. Stevenson DK, Yang C, Kerner JA et al: Intestinal flora in the second week of life in hospitalized preterm infants fed stored frozen breast milk or a proprietary formula, *Clin Pediatr* 24:338, 1985.

220. Sturman JA, Rassin DK, Gaull GE: A mini review: taurine in development, *Life Sci* 21:1, 1977.

221. Sullivan PB: Cows' milk induced intestinal bleeding in infancy, *Arch Dis Child* 68:240, 1993.

222. Task Force on Infant Positioning and SIDS, American Academy of Pediatrics: Positioning and sudden infant death syndrome (SIDS): update, *Pediatrics* 98:1216, 1996.

223. Tatzer E, Schubert MT, Timischl W et al: Discrimination of taste and preference for sweet in premature babies, *Early Hum Dev* 12:23, 1985.

224. Teele DW, Klein JO, Rosner B et al: Beneficial effects of breastfeeding on duration of middle ear effusion (MEE) after first episode of acute otitis media (AOM), *Pediatric Res* 14:494, 1980.

225. Tikanoja T, Simell O, Järvenpää AL et al: Plasma amino acids in preterm infants after a feed of human milk or formula, *J Pediatr* 101:248, 1982.

226. Toms GL, Gardner PS, Pullan CR et al: Secretion of respiratory syncytial virus inhibitors and antibody in human milk through lactation, *J Med Virol* 5:351, 1980.

227. Toms GL, Scott R: Respiratory syncytial virus and the infant immune response, *Arch Dis Child* 62:544, 1987.

228. Troncone R, Scarcella A, Donatiello A et al: Passage of gliadin into human breast milk, *Acta Paediatr Scand* 76:453, 1987.

229. Tsang RC, Lucas A, Uauy R et al: *Nutritional needs of the preterm infant*, Baltimore, 1993, Williams & Wilkins.

230. Tudehope D, Bayley G, Townsend M et al: Breastfeeding practices and severe hyperbilirubinemia, *J Pediatr Child Health* 27:240, 1991.

231. Tyson JE, Lasky RE, Mize CE et al: Growth, metabolic response, and development in very-low-birth-weight infants fed banked human milk or enriched formula. I. Neonatal findings, *J Pediatr* 103:95, 1983.

232. Uauy RD, Birch DG, Birch EE: Effect of dietary omega-3 fatty acids on retinal function of very low birth weight neonates, *Pediatr Res* 28:245, 1990.

233. Udall JN, Dixon M, Newman AP et al: Liver disease in α-1-antitrypsin deficiency, *JAMA* 253:2679, 1985.

234. Usowicz AG, Dab SB, Emery JR et al: Does gastric acid protect the preterm infant from bacteria in unheated human milk? *Early Hum Dev* 16:27, 1988.

235. Varma SK, Collins M, Row A et al: Thyroxine, tri-iodothyronine, and reverse tri-iodothyronine concentrations in human milk, *J Pediatr* 93:803, 1978.

236. Verronen P: Breastfeeding of low birth weight infants, *Acta Paediatr Scand* 74:495, 1985.

237. Walter RS: Issues surrounding the development of feeding and swallowing. In Tuchman DN, Walter RS, editors: *Disorders of feeding and swallowing in infants and children: pathophysiology, diagnosis, and treatment,* San Diego, 1994, Singular.

238. Weatherley-White RCA, Kuehn DP, Kuehn DP, Mirrett P et al: Early repair and breastfeeding for infants with cleft lip, *Plast Reconstr Surg* 79:879, 1987.

239. Whitelaw A, Heisterkamp G, Sleath K et al: Skin-to-skin contact for very low birth weight infants and their mothers, *Arch Dis Child* 63:1377, 1988.

240. Wilson DC, Afrasiabi M, Reid M McC: Breast milk beta-glucuronidase and exaggerated jaundice in the early neonatal period, *Biol Neonate* 61:232, 1992.

241. Wong PWK, Lambert AM, Komrowe GM: Tyrosinaemia and tyrosinuria in infancy, *Dev Med Child Neurol* 9:551, 1967.

242. Woolridge MW, Fisher C: Colic, "overfeeding" and symptoms of lactose malabsorption in the breastfed baby: a possible artifact of feed management, *Lancet* 2:382, 1988.

243. Zimmerman AW, Hambridge KM, Lepow ML et al: Acrodermatitis in breastfed premature infants: evidence for a defect of mammary gland zinc secretion, *Pediatrics* 69:176, 1982.

15

$\mathscr{M}$edical complications of the mother

OBSTETRIC COMPLICATIONS

Cesarean delivery

When birth takes place by cesarean delivery, the mother becomes a surgical patient with all the inherent risks and problems. If the procedure is anticipated because of a previous cesarean birth, cephalopelvic disproportion, or some other identifiable reason, a mother can prepare herself psychologically for the event and usually tolerates the process better. When the procedure is unplanned and done during the process of labor, it is psychologically more traumatic, and the mother tends to feel as if she has failed in her female role. In addition to this unexpected disappointment, medical emergencies may also have an impact on the mother's well-being, such as a long, difficult labor; abruptio placentae; blood loss; toxemia; or infection.

The mother who plans to breastfeed after a cesarean birth should be able to do so if the infant is well enough. The method of delivery makes no significant difference to the timing of the milk coming in or the changes in the concentration of the major milk constituents in the first 7 days postpartum.[115] Depending on the type of anesthesia and the associated circumstances, the mother may feel alert enough to put the infant to breast

within the first 12 hours. Mothers frequently nurse in the first hour after surgery.

Bupivacaine is being used as an epidural block for cesarean or vaginal delivery because it does not result in the decrease in muscle tone and strength reported in neonates whose mothers have received lidocaine or mepivacaine.[132,174] Bupivacaine and tetracaine are highly protein bound and appear in milk in very low concentrations, in contrast to lidocaine and mepivacaine, which are nonionized and unbound in serum. Because most local or regional anesthetics are used with epinephrine, which causes local vasoconstriction, thus slowing the rate of absorption, the anesthetic effects are prolonged and the amount secreted into the milk is minimal.

Epidural morphine is used for more prolonged analgesia and is used in cesarean delivery because it can then be continued postpartum for the relief of postoperative pain. Bernstein et al[15] showed that epidurally administered morphine enters the breast milk in very low levels compared with the levels in maternal urine, which were several thousand times higher. Most of the morphine in colostrum is in the conjugated form and thus pharmacologically inactive. Other studies report a milk/plasma ratio of 2:45; the amount received via the milk is calculated to be less than 50 µg/dl of milk, causing no untoward symptoms in any of the cases reported.

At birth infants may have morphine in their system from transplacental transfer of intrapartum maternal dosing. Transplacental medication has depressed some infants and may interfere with early attempts to suckle.

In a cesarean delivery under controlled circumstances, the procedure is initiated using local anesthesia to the skin and fascial layers. Systemic anesthesia is given as soon as the cord is clamped, sparing the transfer of anesthetics to the newborn.

Regional anesthesia permits the mother to remain awake, and she may be ready to nurse as soon as the intravenous (IV) lines and urinary catheter are stabilized. The mother will need considerable help from the nursing staff. She should remain flat if she has had a spinal anesthetic to prevent developing a spinal headache. She can turn to one side and offer the breast by placing the infant on its side and stroking the infant's perioral area with the nipple. The normal full-term infant who has not been depressed by maternal medication should do well. If the mother can be turned to the other side, the infant may nurse on both sides. In this first encounter, the emphasis is on some suckling, not switching. The bedside rails will help the mother turn as well as provide safety for her.

Maternal fluids and medications in the first 48 hours postoperatively should not affect the infant adversely. Pain medication is required usually for about 72 hours. It is best given immediately after breastfeeding to permit the level to peak before the next feeding. The medication used should be limited to short-acting drugs that the adult eliminates quickly (i.e., within 4 hours) and that the newborn is able to excrete. Ibuprofen and acetaminophen are in that category; codeine is also acceptable (see Chapter 11). Low-grade fever may occur and should not interrupt lactation.

Some very positive factors are associated with breastfeeding for the mother who has had a cesarean delivery. Lactation is advantageous to the postoperative uterus in that the oxytocin production stimulated by suckling will assist in its involution. In addition, the traumatized psyche of a mother whose delivery did not occur naturally as planned is more quickly healed when she can demonstrate her maternal capabilities by breastfeeding.

Whether breastfeeding can be introduced early or must await stabilization of medical problems in the mother or infant, it is a reasonable goal for the mother to seek in most cases. Supportive nursing care is critical to establishing successful lactation. None of this can take place, however, unless the physician has carefully assessed the condition of the mother and the infant in light of the advantages and disadvantages of breastfeeding to both.

The management should include the following:

1. A postoperative care plan must include sufficient rest. Most postpartum wards are not scheduled to include adequate rest for postoperative patients.
2. The family must be instructed on the needs for rest at home and assistance with the household chores. With shorter hospital stays, this is critical.
3. The infant should be considered, when possible, in writing medication orders.
4. If the infant cannot be put to breast, arrangements should be made to pump the mother's breasts on a regular basis with a quality electric pump at least every 3 hours during waking hours, even if separation will last only a day or two.

Toxemia

Toxemia presents a problem in management any time it occurs. The clinical onset is insidious and may be accompanied by a variety of subtle symptoms, but the diagnosis depends on the presence of hypertension and proteinuria.[29] Toxemia usually begins after the thirty-second week of gestation but has been observed to occur 24 to 48 hours or later postpartum. Convulsions, renal disease, and cerebral hemorrhage in the mother are complications that can be prevented by careful management. Because serious toxicity in the mother may necessitate delivery of a premature infant or an infant compromised by a poorly perfused placenta or maternal medications, a number of contraindications to breastfeeding exist in the immediate postpartum period.

Initial treatment of the preeclamptic patient includes bed rest, preferably lying on her side in a quiet room that is darkened to prevent photic and auditory stimuli. Blood pressure and proteinuria should be carefully watched. Sedation with phenobarbital or diazepam (Valium), salt restriction, and possibly diuretics such as thiazide or furosemide are used. Hydralazine (Apresoline) and methyldopa (Aldomet) may be indicated as well to bring down the blood pressure. Magnesium sulfate may also be used and is safest for the breastfeeding infant. Many patients recover quickly once the infant and placenta are delivered, requiring only 24 to 48 hours of postpartum sedation.

Often the infant is small for gestational age or premature and may require special or intensive care; therefore the decision when to initiate breastfeeding depends on the infant's condition. If the infant is full term and well, breastfeeding is initiated when toxemia precautions are discontinued and when the mother's phenobarbital intake has been tapered off to about 180 mg/day or less, calculating that initially the amount of milk obtained is not so great as to provide a large dose of drug to the infant. Careful observation should ensure the infant is not depressed by the accumulation of phenobarbital. Phenobarbital is given to newborns for several indications and therefore is low risk. It is preferable to wait until the other medications can be discontinued, especially the diuretics, hydralazine, and methyldopa.

Once the risk of convulsions is past, some attention can be given to manual expression or pumping even if the infant cannot be nursed yet. If medications are a problem temporarily, the milk may have to be discarded, but the expression of milk will serve to stimulate the breast and initiate lactation.

Diminution of stress is a critical factor in toxemia therapy, so maternal anxiety about being able to nurse must be managed with open discussion of the overall plan and nursing's role. On the other hand, the stress of early feedings that do not go

well because the infant has been confused by initial bottle feedings may also present a hazard in the course of toxemia management. This can be minimized by cup feedings. The most important element in every case is *communication* with the patient about her expectations or needs regarding breastfeeding. The physician's therapeutic management design can put this in appropriate perspective. Because of the effects of oxytocin and prolactin, it may be therapeutic to breastfeed.

Retention of placenta and lactation failure

Three cases of failed onset of lactation were reported by Neifert et al.[150] Although the original association of the placenta with delayed lactation was made a century ago, most reports of retained placenta merely discuss persistent hemorrhage as a recognized symptom. In each of three cases the failure of breast engorgement and leakage of milk was evident from delivery, but the hemorrhage and emergency curettage occurred at 1 week, 3 weeks, and 4 weeks postpartum, respectively. In each case, spontaneous milk flow began immediately postoperatively, after the removal of placental fragments. The authors suggest that failure of lactogenesis may be an early sign of retained placenta that should not be ignored.[150]

Venous thrombosis and pulmonary embolism

Venous thrombosis and pulmonary embolism are the most common serious vascular diseases associated with pregnancy and the postpartum period.[29] Pulmonary embolism has assumed relatively greater importance because of the decline in morbidity and mortality from sepsis and eclampsia. *Varicose veins* also present more problems during pregnancy than at any other time. These diseases all represent common features in vein physiology as associated with the perinatal period.

The major concerns during lactation, in addition to the well-being of the mother, include the procedures that might be necessary to establish the diagnosis and the systemic medications necessary for treatment that could have an impact on the nursing infant via the milk. Accurate diagnosis is urgent and is far more complex than therapy. Besides the health of the mother in this life-threatening state, any program of contraception after childbirth is fundamentally affected by the established diagnosis of thromboembolism. Thus the diagnosis must be accurate.

Diagnosis

Laboratory procedures such as evaluation of arterial blood gases, liver function studies, and fibrin/fibrinogen derivatives are not a problem to breastfeeding. The absence of fibrin split products in plasma and serum virtually excludes the diagnosis of embolism, although their presence does not confirm it. The most definitive diagnosis is made with radioactive scanning procedures and angiography.

Contrast venography is the most definitive method available for diagnosing deep vein thrombosis. The perfusion lung scan is the pivotal test for the investigation of patients with suspected pulmonary embolism. The radiopharmaceuticals used are technetium-99m–microaggregated albumin or microspheres (usual dose 3 mCi), which clear the milk promptly, thus requiring pumping and discarding the milk for 8 hours.[63] Pulmonary angiography, the most definitive test for pulmonary embolism, requires fluoroscopy, which is not a risk to the breastfeeding infant. The total dose is approximately 400 mrad and thus should not interfere with lactation. In deep vein thrombosis of the leg, fibrinogen leg scanning uses iodine-125 (^{125}I) fibrinogen, which requires 2 weeks of pumping and discarding the milk. Radioactive materials vary in their half-lives and disappearance time from breast milk. They all appear in breast milk (see Chapter 11).

Another technique is duplex ultrasonography. It consistently visualizes the iliac veins. Impedance plethysmography is noninvasive but not reliable for calf thromboses.[63] At present, computed tomography (CT) and ultrasound are effective in major arterial aneurysms only.

Treatment

Anticoagulant therapy is the treatment of choice for established venous thrombosis with or without embolism. *Heparin* can be given parenterally, because this large molecule does not cross the placenta or appear in breast milk. This therapy is adequate for the hospitalized patient, in whom constant monitoring of coagulation is possible. *Warfarin* has been considered the best replacement for heparin, but it is secreted in the breast milk (see Chapter 11 and Appendix D). The amount transmitted is minuscule, and it is considered safe to breastfeed while taking warfarin. In long-term therapy the prothrombin time should be monitored at least monthly in the infant and vitamin K given if necessary.

MEDICAL PROBLEMS

Pituitary and prolactinemic disorders

Galactorrhea

After an infant stops breastfeeding, it is not unusual for the mother to be able to express milk from the breasts for many weeks, although spontaneous flow ceases in 14 to 21 days. Postlactation milk is partially a function of the length of established lactation. When spontaneous lactation persists for more than 3 months after the infant has stopped nursing, the cause should be sought. The physician should evaluate the mother to make a specific diagnosis.

Galactorrhea is characterized by spontaneous milky, multiduct, bilateral nipple discharge. It is thought to result from increased prolactin production, either by the pituitary or by removal of hypothalamic inhibition.[197] Pituitary adenomas may be the cause. Galactorrhea can occur with normal ovulatory function for 1 or more years postpartum if everything else appears normal. Galactorrhea has been reported to occur in thyrotoxicosis with such frequency (80%) that it should be part of the differential for galactorrhea. Amenorrhea and galactorrhea are also associated with hypothyroidism, which is not surprising because thyrotropin-releasing hormone (TRH) is known to be a prolactin-stimulating hormone. More complex disorders are rare and are usually named for the physician who first described them.

During pregnancy a risk of pituitary tumor expansion exists, especially with large tumors. In a series of cases of microprolactinomas, Ikegami et al[81] noted no symptom of tumor enlargement in pregnancy. The serum prolactin levels were at or below pregnancy levels postpartum. The authors thought these breastfeeding patients diagnosed as having Chiari-Frommel syndrome may actually have occult microadenomas that may become radiologically evident later.[59]

Prolactin levels are elevated in about half the patients with galactorrhea, and the prolactin levels show little correlation with the copiousness of milk flow in the patients. Prolactin levels in milk and plasma in women with inappropriate lactation were compared with those of normally lactating women by Adamopoulos and Kapolla.[1] Women with galactorrhea had milk prolactin concentrations similar to nursing mothers, but plasma levels were significantly lower than in lactating women except for pituitary adenoma–related galactorrheas. Levels in milk remain relatively constant, whereas plasma levels vary by time of day and various stimuli.

Some drugs can cause galactorrhea, including phenothiazines, tricyclic antidepressants, rauwolfia alkaloids, theophylline, amphetamines, methyldopa, and even some contraceptives. A copper intrauterine device (IUD) was associated with normoprolactinemic galactorrhea in a fertile woman. When the IUD was removed, the secretion stopped, and when it was reinserted, the flow began again.[61]

The major causes of galactorrhea associated with amenorrhea are (1) medications (e.g., tranquilizers, antidepressants, reserpine, methyldopa, narcotics, oral contraceptives), (2) local stimulation of the nipples and breast, (3) hypothalamic dysfunction, (4) Forbes-Albright syndrome, (5) hypothyroidism, (6) chest lesion, (7) renal disease, and (8) a nonpituitary prolactin-producing tumor

(lungs or kidney). A patient has *idiopathic galactorrhea* if prolactin levels, menses, and fertility are normal. Idiopathic galactorrhea has five possible explanations[13]:

1. The abnormality may be in the breast itself, which is unusually sensitive to circulating prolactin.
2. The breast may have an increased number of prolactin receptors.
3. Prolactin levels may be intermittently high.
4. Excessive sleep-induced increases may occur in prolactin, which normally rises during sleep.
5. Biologically active prolactin may be elevated and is not immunoreactive (i.e., is not detected by immunoassay).

Prolactin exists in three sizes: small (molecular weight 25,000 daltons), large (50,000 daltons), and very large (100,000 daltons). Most of the biologic activity occurs in the small form. The large forms are immunoreactive but weakly biologically active. Thus, in patients with persistent galactorrhea with normal prolactin levels by immunoassay, magnetic resonance imaging (MRI) is necessary to rule out a tumor producing the large prolactin molecules.[13]

Hyperprolactinemia

Hyperprolactinemia with and without galactorrhea has been identified in patients with multiple sclerosis,[106] especially in relapse, suggesting hypothalamic dysfunction and not a pituitary prolactinoma.[73] Hyperprolactinemia is also seen in some connective tissue disorders[99] (see later discussion).

Since 1971, when human prolactin was identified as a distinct lactogenic hormone and was isolated and measurable by a specific radioimmunoassay, previously unrecognized clinical entities associated with hyperprolactinemia have been identified. *Physiologic hyperprolactinemia* occurs with excessive breast manipulation and is the reason induced lactation and relactation are physiologically possible. In susceptible women, a visit to the doctor, stress, a pelvic examination, venipuncture, or surgical procedures can produce elevated serum prolactin. The half-life of prolactin in these circumstances is 50 to 60 minutes.

Table 15-1 lists causes of hyperprolactinemia. Pathologic conditions associated with hyperprolactinemia include hypothyroid and hyperthyroid disease, chronic renal failure, and chest wall lesions such as thoracotomy scars and herpeszoster. Galactorrhea, or the secretion of a lactose/ fat-containing fluid independent of pregnancy, can occur in any of these hyperprolactinemic states. In general, pharmacologic hyperprolactinemia does not exceed 100 ng/ml. If a woman has achieved pregnancy with hyperprolactinemia, postpartum lactation is possible.

TABLE 15-1	Causes of chronic hyperprolactinemia in the female
Type	**Causes**
Physiologic	Excessive breast manipulation
	Stress, surgery, venipuncture, etc.
Pharmacologic	Depletion of tuberoinfundibular dopamine stores (by extrusion from intracellular granule to cytosol)
	Reserpine
	Blockade of dopamine receptor binding
	Phenothiazines (chlorpromazine, thioridazine, prochlorperazine, perphenazine, trifluoperazine)
	Thioxanthenes (chlorprothixene)
	Butyrophenones (haloperidol)
	Benzamines (metoclopramide, sulpiride)
	Dibenzoxapine antidepressants (amoxapine)
	Inhibition of dopamine release
	Chronic opiate use (methadone, morphine)
	Blockade of histamine (H_2) receptor binding
	Cimetidine
	Estrogen-containing oral contraceptives
	Interference with dopamine synthesis
	α-Methyldopa
	Calcium channel blockers
	Verapamil
	Mechanism unknown
	Tricyclic antidepressants (imipramine, amitriptyline)
	Papaverine derivatives
Pathologic	Primary hypothyroidism
	Hypothalamic disorders
	Neoplastic, infectious, vascular, degenerative, or granulomatous hypothalamic lesions
	Pituitary stalk section
	Pituitary disorders
	Prolactin-secreting adenoma
	Acromegaly, Cushing's disease, Nelson syndrome
	Ectopic production of prolactin
	Bronchogenic carcinoma, hypernephroma
	Chronic renal failure
	Chest wall lesions
	Surgical scars, herpes zoster
Functional	Idiopathic (no demonstrable tumor)

Modified from Katz E, Adashi EY: *Clin Obstet Gynecol* 33:623, 1990.

Chiari-Frommel syndrome

Patients with persistent postpartum or postlactation lactation extending over months or years should be evaluated for Chiari-Frommel syndrome, especially if abnormal menses exist.[59] Often, irregular menses will have occurred before the pregnancy as well. The galactorrhea will occur whether the mother breastfeeds or does not breastfeed. The clinical manifestations of Chiari-Frommel syndrome are not only persistent lactation with possible breast engorgement, but also oligomenorrhea or amenorrhea, obesity, uterine and ovarian failure, and in some cases hypothyroidism (Table 15-2). Spontaneous remission within 5 years occurs in 40% of patients.

Other possible causes of the galactorrhea include other hypothalamoadenohypophyseal disorders, including infection and trauma, ectopic production or lactogenic hormone as in hypernephroma, or end-organ hypersensitivity to prolactin.

Hyperprolactinemic women do not respond to breast stimulation with a rise in prolactin as breastfeeding women do. The hyperprolactinemic patient has no acute response to suckling in her growth hormone levels either, indicating that the central dopaminergic tonus was not altered but shows regulatory dysfunction.[59]

Del Castillo's syndrome

Del Castillo's syndrome was first described in 1932.[65] All patients have had galactorrhea and amenorrhea without evidence of pituitary tumor and with negative urinary gonadotropins and a small uterus but normal secondary sex characteristics and normal breasts, nipples, and areolae. Re-

mission is rare, as is pregnancy. Clomiphene citrate (Clomid) has been reported to be useful in decreasing the galactorrhea and achieving pregnancy (Table 15-2).

Forbes-Albright syndrome

Forbes-Albright syndrome was first described in 1954 by Forbes, who reported 15 cases of nonacromegalic women who had persistent lactation and amenorrhea or irregular menses, low urinary follicle-stimulating hormone (FSH), and pituitary tumor on x-ray films.[57] Both medical and surgical treatments have been used. Pregnancy may cause a recurrence of the galactorrhea (Table 15-2).

Sheehan's syndrome and hypopituitarism

Sheehan's syndrome is caused by postpartum hemorrhage of such severe degree that it leads to pituitary thrombotic infarction and necrosis or other vascular injury to the pituitary, including hypoperfusion. It is the only commonly recognized endocrine disorder associated with lactation failure.[1] It occurs in 0.01% to 0.02% of postpartum women. A highly vascular organ, the pituitary gland is particularly vulnerable to decreased blood flow at the end of gestation because of its increased size. It is thus more sensitive to hypoperfusion and necrosis. The degree of hypopituitarism is variable; hypoprolactinemia generally results following necrosis of the pituitary stalk, causing mammary involution and failure of lactation.[59]

Other signs of pituitary failure are diabetes insipidus, amenorrhea, hypothyroidism, loss of axillary hair, or sparse regrowth of pubic hair postpar-

TABLE 15-2 **Comparison of characteristics of various hyperprolactinemic disorders**

Syndrome	Amenorrhea	Galactorrhea	Postpartum	Pituitary tumor
Del Castillo	+	+	0	0
Chiari-Frommel	+	+	+	0
Forbes-Albright	+	+	±	+

From Gould BK, Randall RV, Kempers RD et al: *Galactorrhea,* Springfield, Ill, 1974, Thomas.

tum. Spontaneous recovery can occur, depending on the degree of infarction and regeneration.

Secretion of pituitary hormones including prolactin is usually deficient, and thus the patient may fail to lactate postpartum; this is considered a key clinical sign of the syndrome. Studies have reported women with Sheehan's syndrome who do lactate; the diagnosis had to be established by other means. This is believed to result from the pituitary *lactotropes,* which have compensatory activity of hypothalamoadenohypophyseal function.[196] Patients usually manifest hyposecretion of all pituitary hormones, with decreased thyroid and adrenal function. They may experience oligomenorrhea or amenorrhea and uteroovarian atrophy. Often the obstetric crisis that caused the hemorrhage has also required hysterectomy, however, and these findings are obscured.

Prolactin-stimulating drugs such as sulpiride to augment milk yields require investigation, although they have been successful in women delivering prematurely and unable to breastfeed immediately.[8] In a case of presumed Sheehan's syndrome in our service, use of nasal oxytocin spray (see Chapter 8) with each feeding for about 2 weeks resulted in a gradual increase in milk production. The mother weaned herself from the drug and the infant from the lactation supplementer over the next 2 weeks, achieving full lactation for 6 months.

Diabetes insipidus in a patient with Sheehan's syndrome requiring vasopressin injection therapy was described by Isbister.[82] The woman had been diagnosed and treated for 2 years before becoming pregnant and experiencing a normal labor and delivery. For 10 days postpartum, she required no replacement therapy. She breastfed without difficulty for 2 months until she was hospitalized with pneumonia. Lactation was temporarily interrupted until the infant was brought to the hospital. Lactation was reestablished by suckling at the breast and supplementing the infant with formula. The vasopressin injection did not cause a let-down or influence the feeding patterns. It was concluded that the patient produced adequate oxytocin but lacked antidiuretic hormone (ADH).

Treatment

In a review of normal lactation and galactorrhea, Benjamin[13] outlines four treatments for pituitary adenomas: (1) identify nonpituitary causes and eliminate (e.g., medications), (2) do nothing, (3) perform surgery, or (4) administer bromocriptine. Also, a significant cause of galactorrhea or hyperprolactinemia can be breast stimulation. Stimulation of breast and nipple can cause prolactin to rise 60 to 120 ng/ml (normal levels 15 to 25 ng/ml).

Acute lactation failure

Acute lactation failure (when women abruptly lose their milk) has been noted historically in times of great crises, fright, or accident. Two such cases have been reported in the literature by Ruvalcaba[171] after the Mexico City earthquake in 1985. Stress-induced lactation failure is described in a gravida 3 woman, 24 years old, who had been exclusively breastfeeding for 3 months and had fed two previous children for 14 and 18 months. The day of the quake, the building she was in collapsed. She ran home to her children past demolished buildings and could not produce a drop of milk when her infant suckled then or subsequently. Multiple attempts over the next weeks failed to produce a drop. The second woman was 39 weeks pregnant and had been dripping colostrum for several weeks as she had with her previous three pregnancies. The day of the quake, her house collapsed, her husband and two children were missing for several hours, and her sister was killed. She never leaked another drop of colostrum and was never able to breastfeed.[171]

Alactogenesis

Familial puerperal alactogenesis is described as probably a genetically transmitted, isolated prolactin deficiency. It is a rare disorder with only a few cases reported. Zargar et al[207] describe a mother and her daughter with eight pregnancies between them with no evidence of lactation at any time. Their only abnormal laboratory value was their prolactin levels, which were undetectable.

Hypergalactia

Hypergalactia is excessive milk production. It is often heralded by the initiation of milk production beginning in pregnancy, often as early as 25 weeks' gestation, and is characterized by persistent leaking that soaks the clothing and is independent of breast stimulation. Some women will note a drop or two on stimulation or while showering during pregnancy. This is considered to be within normal limits. Hypergalactia then persists after delivery with constant leaking between feedings. Mothers can pump or express several ounces after each feeding with no effort. This does not appear to minimize the leaking. Many women find early in lactation that they have a strong let-down reflex with a soaking spray of milk initially. This is not hypergalactia and usually diminishes over 1 or 2 weeks.

If this phenomenon persists for more than 1 or 2 weeks, an evaluation for prolactinoma is in order. A baseline level and a stimulus-associated level of prolactin after 10 minutes of suckling or pumping with a breast pump should be obtained. If the patient has associated symptoms of headache or visual disturbances, further workup for pituitary adenoma would be appropriate. The phenomenon, however, may not be associated with any identifiable pathology. Idiopathic hypergalactia may diminish over months of breastfeeding. It occurs more often with first pregnancies and may not recur with subsequent pregnancies.

Treatment is palliative, including a tight, well-fitting brassiere that is well padded between feedings. A trial of low-dose estrogen, as available in oral contraceptives, may be effective. A careful history to identify any medications or herbs that are galactagogues or any form of stimulus other than breastfeeding is essential to management. Although bromocriptine would theoretically be effective, it would only be indicated in patients with hyperprolactinemia associated with pituitary adenoma. In such a patient the diagnosis should be established first. Bromocriptine has potentially serious side effects and should not be used casually.

Excessive milk production has also been associated with hyperthyroidism and postpartum thyroiditis.

Hyperactive let-down reflex

Hyperactive let-down reflex may occur especially among primiparas. It is characterized by a spray of milk on initiation of a feeding. If the other breast is checked, it also is flowing. The infant is often overwhelmed by the rate of flow and begins to choke or is gulping frantically to keep up. Milk runs out the corners of the mouth. When the milk is high volume but low fat, it may be accompanied by increased gas formation and colic.[205]

Treatment involves controlling the flow. Initially, expressing a little milk (and saving it in the freezer) until the flow slows and then putting the infant to the breast usually solves the problem. If the fat of hindmilk is slow to come, additional milk can be expressed until the fat begins to be secreted. The high-fat milk or hindmilk will decrease the relative volume of lactose and the relative amount of gas produced, reducing the colic, thrashing at feedings, and green stools.

Diabetes mellitus

Interest in lactation among diabetic women is high, and clinical research on the topic is gradually increasing.[10,27,31,86] The laboratory has been the site of considerable study of the disease in the animal model and of the role of insulin.[10] The breast is known to be a target organ for insulin, and there are insulin receptors in the mammary gland acini. The mammary gland is an insulin-sensitive tissue where acute changes in insulin concentration result in a rapid alteration in the rate of lipogenesis and the utilization of glucose. Cultures of mammalian breast tissue serve as ideal models for the exploration of insulin activity.[128]

Pregnancy has become a more common event in the well-controlled diabetic woman, and fertility rates compare with those of nondiabetic women. Much has been said about labor and delivery in the diabetic mother and almost nothing about lactation in these mothers. Textbooks on diabetes often do not mention lactation, except those written before

1960, perhaps reflecting the national trends away from breastfeeding. A mother, although diabetic, should be offered the same opportunity to breastfeed that is offered to all patients unless her disease has so incapacitated her that any stress is contraindicated. When the progress of the infant of a diabetic mother is uneventful and the infant can be treated normally, no contraindication exists to breastfeeding. Lactation may be more difficult in diabetic mothers, perhaps as a result of cesarean delivery or the need to keep the infant in a special care unit for the first few days of life.[153]

In a retrospective study of 25 mothers who were insulin dependent before pregnancy, there were both successful (13) and unsuccessful (12) breastfeeders.[55] The successful ones were slightly older and better educated and had had diabetes longer (13.7 versus 8.2 years). The infants were half a week more mature and spent less time in the intensive care nursery (ICN) (1.8 versus 7.2 days). Delay to first breastfeeding and introduction of a bottle in the ICN were no different, and both groups of mothers experienced an adjustment period. Observations about diet, insulin, and control of diabetes were similar in the two groups and parallel the observations made in the study by Ferris et al.[55]

During the last stages of pregnancy in normal women, a more or less constant excretion of lactose occurs in the urine, with the peak reached on the day of delivery. After delivery the lactose excretion immediately drops to a low level, where it remains for from 2 to 5 days, followed by a sudden large excretion of lactose.[179] *Lactosuria* in the diabetic mother may lead to diagnostic confusion. It normally occurs late in pregnancy and in the postpartum period before the infant takes much milk, if the mother does not nurse, or if the supply of milk exceeds the infant's requirement. Lactose reabsorbed from the breasts is excreted in the urine. Urine sugar tests are not reliable during lactation.

The sparing effect of lactation on the insulin requirement has been observed by many, beginning with Joselin et al.[90] The depression of the level of the blood sugar in normal nursing diabetic women may lead to hypoglycemic symptoms. The simultaneous lactosuria may be misdiagnosed as glucosuria and excessive insulin taken. The improved tolerance has been explained by the transference of sugar from the blood to the breast for conversion to galactose and lactose. Joselin et al[90] reported that the majority of patients at the Joselin Clinic, as well as those at Johns Hopkins Hospital, breastfed in whole or in part. They recommended the increased administration of the B vitamins for the diabetic mother during lactation.

Milk composition in diabetes has been studied by Butte et al[30] in a group of moderately well-controlled insulin-dependent women (classes B, C, and D) at 3 months postpartum. Diabetic women in pregnancy and postpartum have been observed to have low levels of prolactin, placental lactogen, and parathyroid hormone. Whether the observed decreased placental blood flow is associated with diminished mammary blood flow in lactation has not been established.

In this small sample size, no significant difference was seen in the values for total nitrogen, lactose, fat, and calories given the normally wide variations found among control subjects as well. Mineral content was not different except for sodium, which averaged 140 µg/g compared with reference milk's 100 µg/g. The glucose concentrations were significantly higher in the milk of diabetic women, and this varied greatly without any pattern throughout the 24-hour collections, although lactose fluctuated little. The mean glucose value was 0.70 ± 0.11 mg/g in diabetic women and 0.32 ± 0.08 mg/g in the reference women. During the collections the diabetic women were noted to have periods of hyperglycemia. Total milk volumes were not measured in Butte's study, but the infants were noted to gain weight appropriately.[30] Measurements of glycosylated hemoglobin within a month of the milk collections were noted to be $8.1\% \pm 0.6\%$, that is, above the normal range of 4.0% to 7.6%. It is appropriate for the clinician to be aware of the slightly elevated sodium levels, especially if mastitis develops. The glucose elevations probably have little clinical significance to the infant because glucose makes up only about 0.4% of the total energy content.

When milk volume and composition were measured serially on days 3 to 7 postpartum in a diabetic woman by Bitman et al,[17] sodium, potassium, chloride, lactose, protein, calcium, magnesium, and citrate were within the limits of a nondiabetic reference population. Unlike Butte et al,[30] Bitman et al[17] found that fat content was lower, with free fatty acids 2% of total lipid on day 3 but 23% on days 4 through 7. Lipoprotein lipase was increased on days 4 and 5. Other changes suggested impaired fatty acid synthesis and high concentrations of polyunsaturated fatty acids. Jensen et al[87] studied serum levels at 3, 14, and 42 days postpartum from a large group of women. Serum cholesterol levels decreased significantly from days 3 and 14 to day 42 in both diabetic women and controls. Because lipids are a major source of calories, the lipid content of milks of diabetic women will require further study.

Diet for lactating diabetic mothers

Although it is clearly demonstrated that all lactating mothers have an increased energy requirement, it is critical to the diabetic woman to identify this need and provide for it in dietary adjustments (Fig. 15-1). The 300 kcal required by the infant initially means at least 500 to 800 additional kcal in the mother's diet. Because the milk is synthesized from maternal stores and substrates, the plasma glucose levels in the lactating diabetic mother will be lower. The daily maternal insulin requirement is usually much less. The balance is significant between the needs of the infant and the energy and nutrition production in the mother. Most postpartum women, including the diabetic mother, have fat stores developed during pregnancy in preparation by the body for lactation. The diabetic woman, when balancing diet and insulin, needs to consider that the course of lactation mobilizes these fat stores as substrate for the mammary gland. It has been recommended that the diet include no less than 100 g of carbohydrate and 20 g of protein. This will permit the continued mobilization of fat stores to produce the glucose needed for mother and milk. When a diabetic mother increases fat metabolism, there is always the risk of ketonemia and ketonuria. This indicates a need for increased kilocalories in both the diabetic and the nondiabetic mother. With some careful observations of blood and urine sugar levels and anticipatory guidance, lactation can be managed without hypoglycemia or hyperglycemia.

A critical analysis of dietary intake and outcome of lactation in a group of women with insulin-dependent diabetes mellitus (IDDM) was undertaken by Ferris et al[55] in three major obstetric services in Connecticut. Sixteen of the 30 women

DIET   (↑ caloric intake with ↑ carbohydrates and ↑ protein primarily)

AVAILABLE FOR METABOLISM

(Diet and Stores)

→ Maintenance requirements for daily activities

during lactation → Energy for milk synthesis

→ Substrate for lactose production

BODY STORES

Fig. 15-1. Glucose utilization in lactation. (From Asselin BL, Lawrence RA: *Clin Perinatol* 14:71, 1987.)

with IDDM chose to breastfeed and 14 to bottle feed (53%), compared with the 57% of the general maternity population at that time. The authors found that the women with IDDM who sustained lactation received average diet prescriptions of 31 kcal/kg/day (based on maternal weight at 3 days postpartum) or 35 kcal/kg/day (based on preconceptual weight). The mothers who stopped nursing had received only 25 kcal/kg/day (based on maternal weight at 3 days postpartum) or 31 kcal/kg/day (based on preconceptual weight), which was the same as that for bottle-feeding diabetic women. When compared with general recommendations, the recommended dietary allowance (RDA) for lactation is 2000 kcal plus 500 kcal extra. Only one mother who continued to nurse and none who had stopped nursing met this requirement. Mothers who lactated successfully actually consumed more than they thought, and those who "failed" consumed less than they thought when it was calculated, which supports the recommendation that breastfeeding mothers with IDDM need a knowledgeable dietary counselor as well as other support systems. The weight loss patterns of these women reinforced this observation. Those women who stopped lactating lost considerably more weight than the successful breastfeeders, the bottle feeders, or the normal controls. Fasting blood sugar levels were lower (60 mg/dl) in the successful lactators without an increased insulin dosage.

Adjustments to lactation for diabetic mothers

The mildly, or class A, diabetic woman whose condition can be controlled by diet alone must modify her diet to include the increased caloric needs, especially ensuring adequate protein intake. Class A diabetic women who have been taught to control the problem in pregnancy by diet often continue this dietary awareness postdelivery, and thus appropriate counseling for lactation should continue. The IDDM mother usually is able to increase her diet and maintain her insulin level, although some may find insulin requirements are also reduced. Monitoring blood sugar levels and

acetone is necessary at first to achieve the correct balance.

Although hypoglycemia does not cause a reduction in lactose in the milk, the phenomenon of hypoglycemia itself causes increased secretion of epinephrine in insulin shock. The epinephrine inhibits milk production and the ejection reflex. Acetone signals a need for increased calories and carbohydrate. In addition, elevated acetone can cause increased acetone in the milk itself, which is a stress to the newborn liver. If one merely increases insulin to clear the acetone, it may predispose the patient to hypoglycemia. Each mother will identify the point below which she cannot reduce her insulin dosage without producing acetonuria. While the infant is nursing exclusively at the breast, adjustment is usually smooth. Weaning may present some need for day-to-day adjustment, because the amount of milk taken by the infant varies. Many infants take more one day and less the next, and it is less predictable. If blood sugar levels cannot be controlled by diet during this time, insulin must be decreased. If the weaning is gradual and continuous, the adjustment is similar.

Social support, including help and encouragement with baby care and family responsibilities, was a significant difference between successful and unsuccessful breastfeeding among diabetic women in the report by Gagne et al.[60] The management problems, on the other hand, were not related to breastfeeding per se but to management of the diabetes. Physicians managing the maternal diabetes and the infant must work in concert to help the mother adjust her diabetes management to lactation and must understand the issues of diet and insulin.

Problems among mothers with IDDM in first days after delivery

Fewer infants of mothers with diabetes are put to the breast in the first few days, as noted by Ferris et al.[55] Most infants of diabetic mothers are admitted to the neonatal intensive care unit (NICU) for 8 hours or more of observation. Not only does this delay breastfeeding, but it also increases the amount of formula and number of bottle feedings.

The breastfeeding women with IDDM breastfed for the first time at 35 ± 5 hours, whereas the bottle-feeding mothers did so for the first time in 43 ± 24 hours! In this study, only two diabetic mothers and no control mothers were offered a pump. All the mothers who stopped breastfeeding had infants who received a total of 9 oz or more of formula while in the NICU.

Weaning was precipitated in these mothers by problems they saw with the baby, such as crying, fussing, and problems suckling, not because of insufficient milk. No woman with IDDM was told by her physician to stop. Control mothers all cited insufficient milk as the cause of weaning. Severity of the disease correlated with the decision to bottle feed and to wean early.

Hospital management is critical to successful lactation in diabetic mothers as well.[10] When 42 mothers with IDDM who breastfed were followed by Whichelow and Doddridge,[202] they found the most important factor in success was the lapsed time to the first breastfeeding. This is usually a function of the infant's medical stability. They were able to initiate a change in hospital policy that minimized separation of infant and mother. Duration of lactation was inversely related to the delay in the first suckling.[10]

The insulin requirement at 3 months in Whichelow and Doddridge's study[202] was an average 43 U daily, compared with 50 U prepregnancy in bottle feeders, and 40 U at 3 months, compared with 45 U prepregnancy in the breastfeeders. Ferris et al[55] reported that insulin dosages were no different among breastfeeders and bottle feeders, but the numbers were not provided. The subjects in Butte et al's study[30] received less insulin while lactating (35 ± 10 U/day compared with 63 ± 14 U/day during pregnancy).

Special features of lactation for diabetic mothers

Some diabetic mothers enjoy a postpartum remission of their diabetes that may be minimal or complete. The remission may last through lactation, or for several years. This remission has been attributed to the hormone interactions that affect the hypothalamus and pituitary gland during pregnancy, labor, delivery, and lactation. Many diabetic women report a feeling of well-being during lactation.

Diabetic women are prone to infection,[27] and therefore *mastitis* presents a particular problem. With careful anticipatory care, avoidance of fatigue, and antibiotics for at least 10 days when indicated, mastitis should not pose a threat. Candidal infections are more common because of the glucose-rich vaginal secretions, and most diabetic women are alert to the early signs of a fungal vaginitis. Infection of the nipples can also occur from *Candida albicans,* even though the infant does not have obvious thrush. Early specific treatment with nystatin ointment to the breast and nystatin suspension for the infant whenever sore nipples do not respond to the usual nonspecific treatment is recommended. Treatment of both mother and infant simultaneously is necessary or they will reseed each other.

Infants of diabetic women present a special problem in breastfeeding, because they are often premature, frequently have respiratory distress syndrome and hyperbilirubinemia, and may be poor feeders at first. Hypoglycemia is the immediate problem, and its management may initially preclude dependency on breast milk as the sole source of nourishment. Because less than half do develop problems, many need not be separated from their mothers. For those requiring special or intensive care, lactation may have to be postponed briefly, depending on the infant's status.

Providing an electric breast pump and assistance in pumping is essential if the infant is too ill to be fed. Attention to this detail is important regardless of the reason for separation of the mother and infant.[10]

The hypoglycemia of the infant of a diabetic woman occurs early and is proportional to the level of hyperglycemia in the mother at delivery. Cord blood sugar and microsugar levels at $\frac{1}{2}$ and 1 hour of age provide the curve of glucose disappearance and potential for hypoglycemia. If lactation can be established, the glucose can be managed by breastfeeding, but it must be closely monitored so that intervention can be initiated when necessary. There is also a high incidence of hypocalcemia in infants of diabetic mothers, which is believed to result from functional hypoparathyroidism because phosphorus and calcitonin levels are normal.[138] The role of magnesium in this balance has not been clearly defined.

Hyperbilirubinemia occurs more frequently in infants of diabetic mothers. β-Glucuronidase and bilirubin measurements were made on 10 breastfed infants of diabetic women and 10 normal breastfed controls by Sirota et al.[182] The concentrations of β-glucuronidase were higher in the serum of the milk of diabetic mothers, and the bilirubin levels were higher in their infants. None of the control infants required phototherapy, whereas 50% of the infants of the women with IDDM did. Other investigators compared β-glucuronidase and bilirubin levels in a group of normal breastfed infants on the third and fifth days of life and found no correlation between the values. Although infants of diabetic women clearly are more prone to hyperbilirubinemia, the central cause remains elusive.

Breastfeeding and onset of diabetes

Epidemiologic reports[21,58] continue to accumulate suggesting that breastfeeding has a protective effect on the onset of diabetes in childhood. Children to the age of 14 years who were studied in western Australia revealed an incidence of 0.59 diabetic children per 1000.[64] No significant trends or associations with illness were made, except that breastfeeding beyond 1 week of age was less frequent in diabetic than nondiabetic cohorts. In a study of 95 children of women with diabetes and their nondiabetic siblings and peers, the incidence of breastfeeding was only 18% but was comparable in all three groups. Twice as many diabetic children had received soy formula as the other children. In a study of IDDM in Scandinavian populations, fewer children with childhood-onset diabetes were breastfed, and those who were breastfed were breastfed for shorter periods.[21] The authors suggest that insufficient breastfeeding of genetically susceptible newborn infants may lead to β-cell infection and IDDM in later life. The

prevalence of diabetes in black populations throughout Africa, where breastfeeding is common, is usually considerably lower than in Western countries among those of African descent.[114]

The Colorado IDDM Registry was studied retrospectively to determine the possible relationship between breastfeeding and development of childhood diabetes in comparison with randomly selected controls.[136] There was less IDDM among breastfed infants, and the longer the breastfeeding, the greater the effect. The population percentage attributable risk ranged from 2% to 26%. Because of the increasing incidence of childhood diabetes throughout Scandinavia, a prospective study was conducted following children for 7 years. Results demonstrate a clear relationship between lack of breastfeeding and IDDM in the first 7 years of life, or conversely a protective effect of breastfeeding, which is strongest with at least 4 months of exclusive breastfeeding.[21]

Other investigators have been exploring the possible relationship of early exposure to cow's milk and the onset of diabetes. It is suggested there is both a genetic and an environmental component to the etiology of the disease. Karjalainen et al[98] report the identification of a bovine albumin peptide as a possible trigger of IDDM. The antibodies to this peptide are said to react with P69, a β-cell surface protein that may represent the target antigen for milk-induced β-cell-specific immunity. The antibodies decline over 1 to 2 years to normal values. Much lower values were found in all the control children.

Utilizing the Colorado IDDM Registry, Kostraba et al[113] compared children with high and low genetic risk for IDDM by an HLA-DQB1 molecular marker and a group of matched normal controls. Early exposure to cow's milk and solid foods was strongly associated with IDDM in genetically high-risk individuals. The authors suggest that the inclusion of the HLA-encoded risk in the analyses demonstrates the combined effect of genetic and environmental factors.

The association of serum immunoglobulin A (IgA) antibodies with milk antigens in patients with severe arteriosclerosis is under review. The presence of antibodies against dietary antigens is well documented. Its relevance is under study by Muscari et al[146] and others.

Rennie[167] showed a relationship between the consumption of cow's milk and the incidence of diabetes between the ages of 0 to 14 years in countries around the world (Fig. 15-2). The association between IDDM and early exposure to cow's milk may be explained by the generation of a specific immune response to β-casein. A cellular and humoral anti-β-casein immune response is triggered by exposure to cow's milk and may cross-react with β-cell antigen. Sequential homologies exist between β-casein and several β-cell molecules.[33] Much work remains to be done. In the meantime, this may be one more reason for mothers to consider breastfeeding, especially in families at high risk for diabetes.

Thyroid disease

The thyroid gland is intimately involved with hormone activity of pregnancy. The metabolic and hormonal demands of pregnancy alter the thyroid gland. Conversely, the outcome of pregnancy may be altered by changes in the thyroid gland.

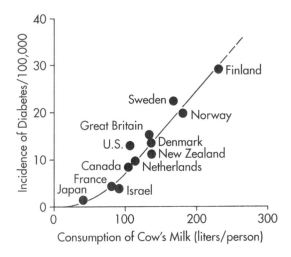

Fig. 15-2. Annual consumption of cow's milk and incidence of diabetes (ages 0-14). (Modified from Rennie J: *Sci Am* 267:24, 1992.)

Thyroxine-binding globulin increases secondary to the increased estrogens. The normal pregnant woman may be euthyroid, but changes occur in the basal metabolic rate, radioactive iodine uptake, and thyroid size.

Thyroid disease is four times more common in women than men, and thyroid abnormality is common in pregnancy. The diagnosis is more difficult to make during pregnancy because of problems with the interpretation of thyroid function tests. Treatment must take into account the presence of the fetus once the management decision is made.

Maternal hypothyroidism

It has long been held that hypothyroidism is associated with infertility. There is a low incidence of hypothyroidism during pregnancy. Because of the difficulty in maintaining pregnancy in hypothyroid individuals, the number of women who are truly hypothyroid at delivery is also low. Some women who are maintained on thyroid treatment for one reason or another do bear children. If hypothyroidism is diagnosed, it should be treated with full replacement therapy equivalent to 3 grains of desiccated thyroid daily. The medication should be continued after delivery. The mother should be permitted to breastfeed without question. Data from Bode et al[20] indicate there is measurable thyroid hormone in the milk of normal women. Breastfeeding is not contraindicated.

In experimental animals when the thyroid is removed before onset of lactation, lactation cannot be initiated. In hypothyroid states in the animal model, there may be associated hypoprolactinemia. This would suggest that a woman with hypothyroidism should be well controlled by thyroid replacement therapy to ensure full lactation. If the mother is truly hypothyroid, particular care should be used to rule out hypothyroidism in the infant, using neonatal screening with thyroxine (T_4) and thyroid-stimulating hormone (TSH) if necessary. Diagnosis can be performed by evaluating blood values and is not a hazard to the nursling.[195] Because of the small amount of thyroid hormone in breast milk, a breastfed hypothyroid child may be undiagnosed unless laboratory values are carefully reviewed.

An increase in hypothyroidism is being identified postpartum, especially when normal women have prolonged "baby blues" and fatigue or appear to have new-onset depression. Screening for thyroid disease is appropriate before prescribing antidepressants. Self-medication has led women to initiate treatment with St. John's wort, thus masking the thyroid disease. A thorough history is always important, including self-medication with other drugs and herbs.

Maternal hyperthyroidism

The diagnostic procedures and therapeutic management of the mother with possible hyperthyroidism present some hazards to the breastfed infant. The diagnosis can be made without radioactive material. The combination of an elevated serum T_4 level and a normal resin triiodothyronine (T_3) uptake is helpful. These two determinations can be combined to obtain a free-T_4 index, which reflects these determinations in a single value. Whether the patient eventually has a thyroidectomy or not, her thyrotoxicosis must first be medically stabilized.

In the experimental hyperthyroid model, rats given chronic doses of thyroid hormone, beginning before mating, were able to carry the pregnancy and delivery without difficulty but were unable to lactate. The mammary gland made milk, but the dams were unable to allow suckling and could not let down.[168]

Postpartum thyroiditis has also increased in frequency to about 1 in 20 women. It is characterized by symptoms of hyperthyroidism with pounding tachycardia, rapid weight loss, insatiable appetite, and excessive milk production.[97] One case reported to the lactation center was notable for the stimulating reaction to prenatal vitamins (possible iodine effect), caffeine, and high-protein beverages.

The treatment for hyperthyroidism includes antithyroid medication with thiourea compounds, which inhibit the synthesis of thyroid hormone by blocking iodination of the tyrosine molecule.

Propylthiouracil (PTU) and methimazole (Tapazole) are the drugs of choice for the mother. The major difficulty in their use in pregnancy is that PTU may cause fetal goiter and possibly hypothyroidism. The goiter is thought to be the result of inhibition of fetal thyroid hormone production by PTU with resulting increase in fetal TSH and thyroid gland enlargement. In 41 pregnancies in 30 patients receiving antithyroid medication, five infants developed goiters. Goiter development was not dose related. It has been recommended that the maternal therapy also include desiccated thyroid on the basis that the various components of thyroid metabolism cross the placenta at different rates.[29]

The lactating mother presents a somewhat similar problem. Thiouracil appears in the milk in significant levels and is contraindicated. Methimazole appears in the milk with a milk/plasma (M/P) ratio of 1. A 40-mg dose of methimazole would yield 70 µg for the infant. Lamberg et al[119] treated 12 lactating women with a methimazole derivative, carbimazole, in doses ranging from 5 to 15 mg daily, which is comparable with 3.3 to 10 mg methimazole. All the infants maintained normal thyroid function studies at 4, 14, and 21 days. Two infants were followed to 3 and 4 months and remained normal.

Levels of PTU in milk were reported by Kampmann et al,[95] who calculated that minimal amounts reach the milk because the drug is ionized and protein bound. They found no evidence of effect in the infants with careful follow-up with T_4 and TSH measurements. It has been suggested that the infant can be breastfed and monitored biochemically. Microtechniques are available for determining T_3, T_4, and TSH levels, and monitoring should not be a technical problem.[194] Physical examination would reveal bradycardia or other signs of hypothyroidism and goiter. It has also been suggested that the infant may be given 0.125 and 0.25 grain of thyroid daily.

This situation requires close medical surveillance and continual monitoring by microanalysis. The clinical judgment rests with the physician as to whether sufficient medication is reaching the infant. The older infant (over 6 months of age) who is receiving other dietary intake such as solids would be at less risk than the newborn, who depends solely on breast milk. Lamberg et al[119] recommend PTU doses of up to 150 mg/day.

When PTU is not an effective drug for the mother, Cooper[37] suggests methimazole or carbimazole in doses up to 10 mg with close monitoring of the breastfeeding infant and thyroid function tests biweekly. Lamberg et al[119] recommend methimazole doses up to 15 mg/day.

Because iodine appears in milk and the M/P ratio is greater than 1.0, a lactating mother with thyroid disease should not be given iodine for any reason.

Cystic fibrosis

Patients with cystic fibrosis (CF) are living longer and enjoying more stable lives as diagnostic and therapeutic advances in the disease continue. Reports have appeared indicating that a number of women with CF have become pregnant and have delivered normal infants. A case was reported of such a mother who had high sodium levels (132 and 280 mEq/L) in her milk. This mother had not been breastfeeding and expressed her milk for the studies only. As pointed out by Alpert and Cormier,[2] milk from involuting breasts is different, and sodium may be closer to serum levels. Since that time, Welch et al[201] reported one case and Alpert and Cormier[2] reported two cases of successful breastfeeding with maternal CF. Sodium and chloride levels in the milks were normal.

Hamosh et al[69] have investigated the fat content of the milk of mothers with CF and report lowered levels of fatty acids.

Another case of successful breastfeeding by a woman with CF is reported by Smith et al.[183] The infant grew along the 50th percentile for height, weight, and head circumference. Milk samples (fore and hind) at 11 weeks postpartum had sodium levels of 11 mmol/L (normal 2 to 19 mmol/L).

Michael and Mueller[139] reviewed five women with CF and their infants. Evaluations indicating

their need for enzyme therapy and their pulmonary disease status classified these women as mild cases. The infants averaged 37.4 ± 1.5 weeks' gestation with birthweights of 3.0 ± 0.5 kg. Sweat tests were negative for all the infants. Duration of breastfeeding ranged from 3 to 30 weeks. Four of the five infants maintained good growth during breastfeeding. Four of the five mothers were at or above their standard body weight throughout lactation. The authors conclude that women with mild CF can not only sustain a pregnancy but also support the growth of a healthy infant through breastfeeding while maintaining their own weight.[139]

Current recommendations for breastfeeding by mothers with CF have been published by Luder et al[130] following a survey of CF centers (Tables 15-3 to 15-5). For mothers with CF, 11% of centers recommend breastfeeding, 8% do not recommend it, 42% tailor their recommendations to the mother's health, and 32% make recommendations on the basis of mother's wishes. Of the centers, 41% report a breastfeeding duration of less than 3 months. Table 15-4 lists factors that preclude breastfeeding and factors contributing to discontinuation, as reported by directors of CF centers.

TABLE 15-3 Recommendations about breastfeeding by cystic fibrosis (CF) center directors for mothers with CF*

Recommendation	Response, no. (%)
Recommend breastfeeding	14 (11.2)
Do not recommend breastfeeding	10 (8.0)
Recommendation made according to each patient's health status	52 (41.6)
Recommendation made according to each patient's personal wishes	40 (32.0)
No applicable and/or others category	9 (7.2)
TOTAL	125 (100)

Modified from Luder E, Kaltan M, Tanzer-Torres G et al: *Am J Dis Child* 144:1153, 1990.
*Many centers chose more than one answer; therefore the response rate for each answer is calculated as a percent of total responses.

TABLE 15-4   **Factors for preclusion or discontinuation of breastfeeding according to cystic fibrosis (CF) center directors for mothers with CF**

Factor	Response, no. (%)
Preclusion	
Inadequate prepregnancy weight	54 (25.5)
Inadequate weight gain during pregnancy	57 (26.9)
Marked pulmonary disease	45 (21.2)
Marked pancreatic insufficiency	15 (7.1)
Diabetes	13 (6.1)
Chronic bacterial pathogen(s) carrier	10 (4.7)
Not applicable and/or others category	18 (8.5)
TOTAL	212 (100)
Discontinuation	
Mother's excessive weight loss	68 (32.7)
Infant's inadequate weight gain	64 (30.8)
Exacerbation of mother's respiratory disorder(s)	52 (25.0)
Passage of bacterial pathogen(s) from mother to infant	16 (7.7)
Not applicable and/or others category	8 (3.8)
TOTAL	208 (100)

Modified from Luder E, Kaltan M, Tanzer-Torres G et al: *Am J Dis Child* 144:1153, 1990.

Eighty-one centers (94%) have support services available throughout the course of lactation.

As the survival of patients with CF continues to improve and more women reach the childbearing years, an increasing number will choose to breast-feed.[130] Additional research is necessary to help mothers with CF maintain their health while lactating and to monitor growth in infants with CF and their general health status while breastfeeding. Breastfeeding usually enhances the health of an infant with CF because it helps to protect against infection and provide active enzymes (see Chapter 14).

Studies demonstrate that mothers with pulmonary and pancreatic disease of CF can breastfeed

TABLE 15-5   **Duration of breastfeeding as reported by cystic fibrosis (CF) center directors for mothers with CF**

Duration (months)	Centers, no. (%)
<3	35 (41)
3-6	9 (10)
>6	1 (1.2)
Not applicable and/or others category	41 (48)
TOTAL	86 (100)

Modified from Luder E, Kaltan M, Tanzer-Torres G et al: *Am J Dis Child* 144:1153, 1990.

and that their infants do well. It is appropriate, however, to test milk samples occasionally for sodium, chloride, and total fat and to follow the infant's growth pattern.

Hyperlipoproteinemia

The study of a mother with type I hyperlipoproteinemia nursing her second child is reported by Steiner et al.[187] The milk and plasma were carefully analyzed, and it appeared that the deficit of lipoprotein lipase extended to the mammary gland. The milk had low total lipids and a bizarre composition of fatty acids. Her milk differed greatly from her plasma triglycerides in comparison to normal mothers, whose fatty acid profile in the milk matches the plasma. Low concentrations of essential linoleic ($C_{18:2, 20:4}$) and arachidonic ($C_{20:4}$) acids in her milk made it inadequate for her infant. Other women in the literature have been reported to develop pancreatitis during pregnancy.

Galactosemia

The case of a 25-year-old woman, who had been diagnosed herself at the age of 3 weeks to have galactosemia, was reported by Forbes et al[57] at the time of her first baby, whom she breastfed. The woman had blood transferase activity that hovered from zero to 1.9 U (normal 18 to 25 U/g hemoglobin). Despite irregular menses, she conceived and delivered a normal female who thrived on breastfeeding exclusively. Solid foods were added at 5 months. The analysis of her milk at 4½ weeks postpartum revealed protein 1.42 g/dl, lactose 7.5 g/dl, fat 4.25 g/dl, and calculated energy content 74 kcal/dl. Fatty acid profile was normal except for 18:3, which was low. Macrominerals were all within normal range. Glucose was 26 mg/dl and galactose less than 15 mg/dl. The authors point out that because "lactose can be found from uridine diphosphogalactose (by means of epimerase) and glucose (a reaction stimulated by lactalbumin) in the absence of transferase enzyme, one could have predicted that lactose would be present in her milk."[57]

Phenylketonuria

The success of newborn screening and early treatment has resulted in a population of adolescents with phenylketonuria (PKU) moving into the childbearing years with normal intelligence. Matalon et al[134] reported a pregnancy and lactation experience in a woman who had stopped her diet and did not seek medical care until 16 weeks' gestation. They also reported their experience with 32 young adults who had discontinued their diets. The authors make the following recommendations:

1. Diet restrictions for PKU should not be discontinued at any age, especially in women.
2. Strict control should begin before conception to bring blood phenylalanine levels to 4 mg% or lower.
3. Breastfeeding is permitted.

Matalon et al[134] report that the milk of mothers with PKU controlled by diet is normal (Table 15-6).

Radiation exposure

The diagnosis and treatment of a lactating woman with malignancy may well necessitate the use of radioactive compounds or antimetabolites. Because the breast is a minor route of excretion for most of these compounds, it is probably inappropriate to continue nursing during such exposure. Although the dose of the material in a single

TABLE 15-6   Amino acid levels (n mol/dl) in milk of mothers with phenylketonuria (PKU)

Amino acid	PKU milk	Reference values
Phenylalanine	0.5	0.62
Tyrosine	0.5	1-2
Taurine	36.7	41-45

Iron, zinc, copper, magnesium, and selenium were also within normal range.

aliquot of milk may be small, the effects are cumulative (see Appendix D). No long-range studies indicate the outcome of offspring exposed in utero. In addition, a mother with malignancy should be encouraged to spare all her resources to overcome the disease. Lactation is as draining in such a situation as pregnancy.

Diagnostic or therapeutic measures using radioactive materials are contraindicated in pregnancy and lactation, because they tend to accumulate in the fetal and neonatal thyroid gland and the maternal breast. If radioactive testing is deemed essential before treatment can be carried out, a test dose of iodine-131 (^{131}I) can be given and breastfeeding discontinued for 48 hours. The validity of the test during lactation has been questioned because the mammary gland may divert a disproportionate amount of ^{131}I to the milk. The milk should be expressed during the 48-hour period and discarded.[24]

Breast cancer

In the young cancer patient, another concern is what risk lactation adds to the mother's long-range prognosis.[169] The automatic response tends to be not to become pregnant and, in any event, not to breastfeed. This question was examined by Hornstein et al,[79] who indicate that "the current data suggest that pregnant women with early breast carcinoma may be treated in the same way as nonpregnant women without affecting the pregnancy." Disease that is detected toward the end of pregnancy may be treated with surgery immediately, and then the patient may receive adjuvant therapy if indicated after delivery. Advanced disease should be treated aggressively, and the infant delivered and not breastfed. During lactation, the diagnosis of breast carcinoma requires the immediate suppression of lactation by medications other than estrogens. The carcinoma is then treated by standard methods. When a woman has already had a radical mastectomy for breast cancer, she can have subsequent pregnancies, but they should be delayed until the period of greatest risk is over (i.e., at least 3 to 5 years). She may also breastfeed.

Kalache et al[92] report that 7% of fertile women have one or more pregnancies after mastectomy. Seventy percent of these pregnancies have occurred within 5 years after treatment. Women who have pregnancies after potentially curative mastectomy have survival rates of 5 to 10 years—as good or better than those who do not become pregnant. The patients with the best prognosis, however, may be a function of selection because they are healthier and thus able to become pregnant. Uneventful pregnancy does not guarantee cure, although the highest rate of recurrence is in the first 3 years and gradually declines. It is never zero. Metastases to the axilla increase the risk. Recurrence in the chest wall during pregnancy can be treated with local shielded radiation, but anything more extensive requires aggressive intervention.

The importance of careful monitoring during pregnancy is obvious. One of the major contributors to a more grave prognosis of the original disease that appears during pregnancy and lactation is not the underlying disease, but the difficulty detecting the lesion during pregnancy and lactation and the reluctance of patient and physician to make a diagnosis and initiate treatment. The greatest risk of neoplastic growth occurs in the first 20 weeks of pregnancy, when the immune system is suppressed and growth of the mammary tissues is at its peak under the stimulus from estrogen, progesterone, and prolactin levels.[125,170] No data were provided on the influence of postmastectomy lactation on long-range survival. Some women have wanted to nurse on the remaining breast. The decision would necessitate consideration of the individual situa-

tion. It represents a different risk/benefit ratio than pregnancy itself. Extensive epidemiologic studies of large populations of women do not indicate that breastfeeding has any relationship to the overall risk of breast cancer. Epidemiologic data about breastfeeding on the remaining breast are not available.[125]

The incidence of cancer in the remaining breast has fueled the question of prophylactic contralateral mastectomy. The women who are at greatest risk for cancer in the second breast are those who have a family history of breast cancer in their mother or sister, who have had onset in childbearing years, or whose original cancer involved multiple lesions in the primary breast. In their discussion of the other breast, Leis and Urban[125] state that if a postmastectomy patient were to become pregnant and deliver, "it would be rare indeed that the patient would allow or the attending physician would condone the use of the remaining breast for nursing." Although some women cherish the remaining breast, most in the experience of Leis and Urban,[125] are ashamed of it and keep it hidden.

Lactation after primary radiation therapy for carcinoma of the breast was reported in a major literature search by Burns[28] to have occurred successfully in one patient whose primary lesion was in the tail of Spence. One year after radiation, she became pregnant and successfully breastfed. She had less milk on the treated side. Her malignancy had not recurred. Another patient received radiotherapy after biopsy for an invasive duct carcinoma known to be present for a year. She had a week of boost therapy 8 weeks later. She became pregnant a year later, delivering a full-term infant 22 months after the original radiation. She successfully established lactation on the uninvolved side but was unable to obtain any response from the irradiated breast. No comment was made about the radiated breast's response to pregnancy. She weaned her infant at 6 weeks.[44] Two years after treatment the patient had no evidence of recurrence.

The incidence of breast cancer diagnosed during pregnancy in a large series was 3 per 10,000 pregnancies, or 1% to 2% of breast cancer cases. Delay in diagnosis is the primary reason for the seemingly worse prognosis overall for breast cancer diagnosed during pregnancy and lactation, with the duration of symptoms averaging 5 to 15 months. The incidence of spread to the axilla is 70% to 80% in the perinatal period compared with a 40% to 50% node-positive rate in nonpregnant women.[77]

Any dominant mass during pregnancy or lactation should be evaluated promptly. Mammography may be difficult to interpret, however, because of the increased water density of the breast. Radiation exposure is minimal if the abdomen is properly shielded. A fine-needle biopsy will distinguish cystic from solid lesions. A solid mass can be biopsied during pregnancy or lactation.[173] The risk of milk fistulas is very low. Suppression of lactation is not necessary. Once the diagnosis of cancer is made, staging is essential before treatment is begun. Staging during pregnancy is more difficult because of the need for ionizing radiation.[77]

Further surgery, including mastectomy, can be done during pregnancy and lactation. Because radiation and chemotherapy will also be necessary, breastfeeding is not recommended. When breast cancer is diagnosed during lactation, treatment should be initiated promptly and the infant weaned when chemotherapy is begun.

When young patients are treated with breast-conserving therapy and radiation for early-stage breast cancer, they may experience full-term pregnancies subsequently. Successful breastfeeding on the untreated breast as well as the treated breast is possible after conservative lumpectomy and radiation in some patients. The volume and the duration of lactation are less on the treated side. When the incision is circumareolar, successful lactation is less likely. Usually the function of the untreated breast is unaffected.[74]

Autoimmune thrombocytopenic purpura

Reports are conflicting regarding the passage of antibodies to platelets via the breast milk in mothers with autoimmune thrombocytopenic purpura.[70,100,137] Laboratory efforts to demonstrate absorption of these antibodies from the breast milk failed. One case report detailed the successful breastfeeding of a severely affected premature infant who had required exchange transfusion and multiple platelet transfusions at birth.[133] No relapses occurred with introduction of maternal milk at 5 days of age. Steroids were discontinued at 2 weeks, and the infant thrived at the breast.

Rheumatoid arthritis and other connective tissue disorders

The influence of lactation on the development and progression of rheumatoid arthritis (RA) has been the subject of several epidemiologic studies. Previous observations noted an increased risk of RA developing postpartum, particularly after the first pregnancy. A national cohort of 187 women developed RA within 12 months of pregnancy. Of the 88 women who developed the disease after their first pregnancy, 71 breastfed (81%) compared with only half of control mothers. A smaller risk was noted after the second pregnancy. No added risk with the third pregnancy was associated with breastfeeding. The increase in risk was highest in those women whose disease was erosive and rheumatoid factor positive. The authors suggest that this may be a hormonal influence, especially by the proinflammatory hormone prolactin.[23]

Other investigators reviewed a cohort of 176 women with RA who had at least one child and a mean age of 46 years at diagnosis.[88] They concluded that parity and to a lesser degree breastfeeding before RA onset worsened the prognosis for severe disease. Oral contraceptive use had a protective effect.[89]

The evidence regarding reproductive events as risk factors for RA is conflicting. A population-based study of 63,090 women followed from 1961 to 1989 examined reproductive factors and mortality ratios. The role of parity, age at first and last birth, or age at menarche and menopause showed no relationship to RA. A protective effect of lactation was noted, however, with total time of lactation associated with decreased mortality from RA with a dose-response relationship.[26]

Rheumatic disease may necessitate treatment

of pregnant and lactating patients with disease-modifying active rheumatic disease (D-MARD) drugs or immunosuppressive drugs. For lack of information, breastfeeding is not recommended by Ostensen[158] in patients requiring antimalarials, penicillamine, cyclosporine, or cytotactic drugs. On the other hand, intramuscular gold and sulfasalazine impose no risk to the breastfed infant. Information about milk levels and general recommendations appear in Appendix D. Levels in milk of aurothioglucose, aurothiomalate, chloroquine, hydroxychloroquine, and sulfasalazine have less than 10% of maternal dose in milk, and in the few cases studied, the infants had no side effects.[158] Cyclosporine is not recommended as a therapy during breastfeeding.

Prolactin levels are greatly elevated during pregnancy in women with systemic lupus erythematosus (SLE).[85] Most patients with SLE have elevated prolactin levels, as do patients with RA, osteoarthritis, fibromyalgia, and polymyalgia. A dysregulation of pituitary response has been suggested as the etiology in RA. The role of prolactin in other autoimmune disorders is not understood but supports the concept that a close relationship exists between neuroendocrine and immune systems.

Primary *Sjögren's syndrome* is known to be associated with hyperprolactinemia, but because of the characteristic abnormalities of secreting glands, lactation may not be successful.[7] Sjögren's syndrome has also been seen in association with Raynaud's phenomenon[83] (see later discussion). Breastfeeding is not contraindicated.

Hypertension

The published literature on the excretion of antihypertensive agents into human milk has been reviewed by White[203] because successful management of hypertension is pharmacologic. Before one considers the drugs involved, it is appropriate to consider that lactation may present some therapeutic advantages. The high levels of prolactin may be physiologically soothing to the mother, and it has been shown in animals that females given high levels of prolactin respond with nesting and mothering behavior. The breast is also an organ of secretion, and a liter or so of fluid is produced a day. In dehydrated women, lactation continues while urine production diminishes. The appropriate use of low-dose diuretics may control hypertension, whereas high-dose thiazides can cause suppression of lactation. Chlorothiazide, hydrochlorothiazides, and chlorthalidone are minimally excreted in milk (see Chapter 11 and Appendix E), as are spironolactone and its metabolite canrenone, according to single-dose kinetics.

Propranolol has been widely studied and is probably the safest of the beta blockers during lactation because of its low level in milk compared with other beta blockers, which are weak bases with an average pKa of 9.2 to 9.5, predisposing them to appear in slightly acidic human milk. *Methyldopa* appears in low amounts in milk, but its direct action on the pituitary to suppress prolactin release presents a theoretic risk of suppressing milk production. The obstetrician should be aware of this potential if lactation is going poorly. *Reserpine* poses a recognized risk to the infant during delivery and postpartum. Other drugs appropriate to hypertension management are discussed in Chapter 11.

Cardiac, liver, and renal transplantation

The number and survival times of patients receiving heart transplants are increasing, as is their quality of life. In young recipients, childbearing becomes important. Teratogenicity has not been reported with traditional immunosuppressive agents such as prednisone and azathioprine or with cyclosporine. Osteoporosis prophylaxis is important in pregnancy and lactation associated with chronic use of prednisone. A successful pregnancy after cardiac transplantation is reported with the birth of a normal infant who had normal growth and development for the 3 years of follow-up. The infant was not breastfed.[104]

Successful pregnancy after liver transplant has been reported in at least six patients.[181] Immunosuppression was maintained throughout pregnancy, and the infants were normal. Breastfeeding was not recommended because of the cyclosporine therapy.

Of infants born to mothers with renal transplants, 60% to 70% have uncomplicated neonatal courses. Thymic atrophy, leukopenia, anemia, thrombocytopenia, chromosome aberrations in lymphocytes, and certain abnormalities of the immune system have been seen.[104]

Breastfed infants of mothers with renal transplants have normal blood counts and show no increase in infection and above-average growth rates.[112] The immunosuppressants azathioprine, 6-mercaptopurine, and 6-methylprednisolone have been found in milk in very low levels. Cyclosporine, however, has been detected in breast milk at levels approximating maternal concentrations. The advice when cyclosporine is the drug has been not to breastfeed, with varying decisions about 6-mercaptopurine and azathioprine.

Pregnancy following renal transplant is relatively safe when renal function is adequate before conception and when maintenance immunosuppressive therapy is instituted. Most patients receive azathioprine and prednisone or methylprednisolone. When the actual levels of these compounds were studied in two patients, one of whom breastfed her infant,[39] measurements of IgA were also done because of the concept that immunosuppressed women might produce immunoincompetent milk.

The levels of 6-mercaptopurine in the milk averaged 3.4 ng/ml in one patient and 18 ng/ml in the other. The therapeutic level is 50 ng/ml with the use of the normal daily dose. The levels of methylprednisolone in the milk (daily dose 6 mg) were at or below the levels measured in normal drug-free controls. The IgA determination in the milk was similar in both transplant and control mothers. The breastfed infant whose mother had a transplant had normal blood cell counts, no increase in infections, and an above-average growth rate.[39]

Breastfeeding and maternal donor renal allografts

With the advent of renal transplants, a new mode of investigation with the role of human milk in the host-graft relationship has developed.[10] Large numbers of living maternal lymphocytes are present in human milk. Campbell et al[32] investigated the question of whether exposure of an infant to maternal lymphocytes during breastfeeding would affect the subsequent reactivity of a patient to a maternal donor–related renal transplant. They studied the posttransplant course of 55 patients with a primary maternal donor transplant, 27 of whom were breastfed and 28 of whom were not. The 1-year graft function rate was 82% for those breastfed and 57% for the bottle-fed ($p \le 0.05$) infants. Five-year follow-up did not sustain the statistically significant difference. Paternal donor relationship in a small group of patients did not reveal significant difference.

The same group of investigators (Kois et al[111]) reported that a history of breastfeeding was associated with improved results in a different patient population (HLA-semiidentical sibling donors). Breastfed patients in whom both donor and recipient were breastfed by the same mother showed dramatic improvements in graft-function rates compared with nonbreastfed counterparts at all intervals studied up to 9 years ($p \le 0.001$). The authors[111] concluded that the breastfeeding effect is not entirely specific for maternal antigens, because both sibling donor and maternal donor transplantation was improved. They consider a history of being breastfed an important variable in clinically related renal transplantation.

Because these studies used retrospective questionnaires, they did not take into account the length of time breastfeeding took place, which included all cases "ever breastfed." Although this is potentially important, studies of graft recipients' donors are another means of understanding more about the role of breast milk for the human species.

In a study of renal transplants, 45 breastfed subjects with maternal donor transplants were compared with 43 bottle-fed subjects with maternal donor transplants and 62 subjects with paternal donor transplants.[56] No statistically significant differences were seen in graft survival between the groups. Length of breastfeeding was not stated.

Glomerular disease and lactation

A high percentage of pregnant patients show their first evidence of renal disease probably not because

TABLE 15-7	Calcium content of foods (mg per serving)		
100±	150±	200±	250±
10 Brazil nuts	1 cup ice cream	1 cup beet greens	1 cup almonds
1 med stalk broccoli	1 cup oysters	1 oz cheddar or	1 oz Swiss or Parmesan
1 cup instant Farina	1 cup cooked rhubarb	Muenster cheese	cheese
3 oz canned herring	3 oz canned salmon with		1 cup cooked collard
1 cup cooked kale	bones		greens
1 T blackstrap molasses	1 cup cooked spinach		1 cup cooked dandelion
3 T light (reg) molasses	1 oz feta or mozzarella		greens
1 cup cooked navy beans	cheese		4 oz self-rising flour
3.5 oz soybean curd	½ cup cooked chopped		1 cup milk
(tofu)	collard greens		3 oz sardines
3.5 oz sunflower seeds			½ cup cooked ricotta
5 T maple syrup			cheese
1 cup cottage cheese,			
regular or lowfat			

From Committee on Nutrition, American Academy of Pediatrics. In Barness LA, editor: *Pediatric nutrition handbook,* ed 3, Elk Grove Village, Ill, 1993, The Academy.

pregnancy precipitates the disease but because it is the first time these young women have had urinalysis and blood pressure studies. The series of glomerular disease in pregnancy published by Surian et al[189] reported that in most cases the disease is not made worse by pregnancy. A disease with a poor prognosis such as membranoproliferative glomerulonephritis is neither worsened nor bettered by pregnancy. When the nonpregnant serum creatine and urea nitrogen levels exceed 3 mg/dl and 300 mg/dl, respectively, normal pregnancy is uncommon. Lupus nephropathy, however, has a very poor prognosis in pregnancy with considerable fetal loss and morbidity.[45]

Hypertension as a complication influences the obstetric complication rate and the fetal outcome. The infant may be premature, small for gestational age (SGA), or both. The option to breastfeed is a matter of the risk/benefit ratio.[10] It involves not only the medical status of the mother but also that of the infant and the drugs that must be used to keep the mother stable. The obstetrician, nephrologist, and neonatologist must determine the appropriateness of breastfeeding on a case-by-case basis.

Osteoporosis

Tremendous attention has been focused on osteoporosis in women, particularly following childbirth and lactation. Clearly the demands for calcium and phosphorus during the perinatal period are great, but they can be met by diet with any degree of attention. In addition to dairy products, there are other sources of calcium (Table 15-7). Modern advertising in the wave of the calcium hysteria has suggested women take various medicinal forms of calcium. The incidence of calcium-containing renal calculi has increased as a result.

A syndrome of severe osteoporosis is associated with pregnancy and lactation. Three cases are reported by Gruber et al.[67] These young women had vertebral fractures and skeletal complications, but most of their studies were normal except for their bony structure. They had no osteomalacia, however. They apparently recovered after lactation ceased and had no residual high-turnover osteoporosis. The authors suggest an association with low calcium in the diet.[67]

Bone density changes during pregnancy and lactation in active women were followed in a longitudinal study by Drinkwater and Chesnut.[48]

The variations at the femoral neck, radial shaft, tibia, and lumbar spine were attributed to mechanical stress of weight gain and changes in posture in pregnancy and lactation. Further studies have confirmed that lactation-associated bone-mineral mobilization does not require parathyroid hormone (PTH) or parathyroid tissue.[75]

Extended lactation (≥ 70% of infant energy intake provided for ≥ 6 months) is associated with bone loss; however, there is evidence of return to baseline by 12 months.[185] Those who breastfed a month or less lost no bone mass. Age, diet, body size, and physical activity were not correlated in these healthy white women.

Hypomagnesemia caused by lactational losses

A case of hypomagnesemic tetany caused by excessive lactation was reported in 1963 by Greenwald et al.[66] The 20-year-old patient had been fully nursing her own 3-month-old infant and contributing 50 ounces a day to the local milk bank. She was hospitalized with painful muscle spasms of her hands and feet that improved slightly but did not clear with calcium (serum level 9.6 mg/dl). Serum magnesium levels were low (0.4 mEq/L).

Kamble and Ookalka[93] reported on a 24-year-old woman who was breastfeeding a 15-day-old full-term infant. She presented with the sudden onset of rapidly progressive weakness of all her limbs. She had successfully breastfed two previous children. Her electrocardiogram (ECG) showed "hypokalemia" and multiple ventricular premature beats. Serum magnesium was 0.5 mmol/L (normal 0.8 to 1.7); milk magnesium was 4.9 mmol/L (normal 1.6). Serum calcium was 2.8 mmol/L, phosphate 1.1 mmol/L, and PTH normal. Urinary potassium was 36 mmol/L. After treatment with potassium and magnesium, the ECG and muscle tone returned to normal. This woman continued to breastfeed. She had three times the normal level of magnesium in her milk.

Lactational hypomagnesia is well described in the bovine model.

Crohn's disease and ulcerative colitis

Ulcerative colitis and Crohn's disease (and recently RA) are treated with salazosulfapyridine (SASP). Because of the concern about exposing the fetus to sulfisoxazole at the end of pregnancy or during lactation because of the suggestion that sulfas, even at low levels, predispose to kernicterus, this therapy has been discontinued in the third trimester. Recently, it was noted that sulfapyridine (SP), the main split product of SASP, has a low affinity for albumin-binding sites.

Esbjorner et al[52] studied the binding capacities in both mothers and babies and found them low. They measured cord blood levels in the mothers of 11.5 µmol/L and in the infants of 20 µmol/L. Follow-up infant blood levels showed a clearance in 70 to 90 hours. Infants who were being breastfed did not increase their levels of SASP or SP. The milk/serum levels for SP were 0.4 to 0.6, and those for SASP were undetectable. Infant serum samples were 10% of maternal SP levels, and only one infant had detectable SASP. No children had complications of hyperbilirubinemia or kernicterus. All the infants were term infants without major complications. The authors[52] concluded that it is safe to continue the SASP throughout pregnancy and lactation in full-term infants. The effect on premature infants is under study.

Epilepsy

A history of epilepsy in a mother is of concern for the obstetrician during pregnancy, and much has been written on the topic. Seizures in pregnancy are more dangerous to the fetus than is the medication. Antiepileptic drugs (AEDs) include phenobarbital, primidone, phenytoin, carbamazepine, ethosuximide, valproic acid, and diazepam. The concern regarding lactation includes the effect of the disease on the fetus in terms of major and minor malformations, the level of drugs in the infant's serum at birth, and the state of the mother postpartum. Breastfeeding may provide a means of gradually withdrawing the infant from maternal medication and avoiding the syndrome of withdrawal[22] (i.e., hyperirritability, tremor, vomiting, poor sucking, hyperventilation, sleep disturbances). A good mother-infant relationship is important for a mother with epilepsy. Brodie[25] recommends alternating the breast with an occasional bottle (once a day or more) if the infant is sedated by maternal medication to reduce the effect.

Table 15-8 lists the half-lives of various AEDs. These compounds have a sedating effect and may prevent the infant from suckling adequately in the first few days. Attention must be paid to the infant's behavior to avoid not only undernutrition but also failure to provide sufficient stimulus to the breast. The infant may need some supplementation and the mother some stimulus with an electric pump, carefully coordinated with support.

Whether the infant is breastfed or bottle fed, it is necessary to establish that the mother will remain seizure free and be able to care for the infant. Forty-two infants of 32 epileptic mothers were studied by Kaneko et al[96] for harmful side affects of AEDs while breastfeeding. The duration of poor sucking was correlated with the drug and the levels. The poor weight gain of the mixed-fed infants (breast/bottle) was associated with vomiting and infant drowsiness during feeding. These authors recommend mixing feedings (breastfeeding and formula) early postpartum to reduce the medication to the infant until levels in infant serum taper a little and the infant's metabolism increases to promote drug clearance. Full breastfeeding can then proceed if care has been taken to establish a good milk supply with supplementary pumping.

Neuropathies associated with breastfeeding

A number of neurologic symptoms have been described in association with lactation.

During periods of engorgement, pressure on nerves in the axilla, especially from an engorged tail of Spence (see Chapter 2), has caused numbness and tingling down the arms on the flexor surface to the ulnar distribution of the hands similar to crutch palsy. The numbness and tingling usually abate as soon as the infant nurses and then gradually return as the breast fills again. Symptoms gradually disappear after several weeks as engorgement disappears.

Symptoms similar to those associated with tennis elbow—pain and tingling with flexion of the forearm—have developed in nursing women who are pumping milk with a Kaneson-style hand pump.[204] Similar symptoms have been experienced by mothers just holding a newborn over time, especially primiparas.

Carpal tunnel syndrome has been described in pregnancy, causing paresthesia of the hands. Two cases were reported by Yagnik[206] in which symptoms developed 1 month postpartum in breastfeeding women. The diagnosis was confirmed by electromyography (EMG) and nerve conduction studies. The second case was bilateral. Symptoms disappeared after the infants were weaned. Five other cases are described in the literature: all the women were breastfeeding, all showed improvement with temporary suspension of breastfeeding,

TABLE 15-8 Pharmacokinetic data on antiepileptic drugs (AEDs) in newborns

AED	Free fraction (% unbound)	Volume distribution (1/kg)	Half-life (hr)
Phenobarbital	57-72	0.6-1.5	40-500
Primidone	?	?	7-60
Phenytoin	15-30	0.7-2.0	15-105
Carbamazepine	?	1.1-2.6	8-28
Ethosuximide	?	?	40
Valproic acid	~15	0.2-0.4	14-88
Diazepam	~14	1.8-2.1	40-400

and all recovered completely within a month of complete weaning.[184]

In a retrospective study by mail[199,200] of 27 women who had developed carpal tunnel syndrome postpartum, the women affected were older, mean age 31.5 years, were primiparous, and 24 of 27 were breastfeeding. The three bottle feeders had less severe symptoms that cleared in less than 1 month. Symptoms (predominantly paresthesias, clumsiness, and pain) began at a mean of 3.5 weeks postpartum and lasted 6.5 months. Resolution began after 2 weeks of beginning to wean. Two women required surgical intervention. All were symptom free within a year.[199] The recommended treatment for carpal tunnel syndrome is conservative, with rest, diuretics, hand splint, and local corticosteroid injection, because it is usually reversible. No women had residual signs or symptoms, so perseverance with lactation and symptomatic treatment is appropriate.

Raynaud's phenomenon

Raynaud's phenomenon was first described by Maurice Raynaud in 1862 as episodic digital ischemia provoked by cold and emotion. The true cause remains obscure despite elaborate efforts to identify it.[50] It is widely thought to be a cutaneous manifestation of a generalized vascular disorder often associated in complex cases with scleroderma and vasoconstriction of the kidneys, heart, and lungs. Patients with Raynaud's phenomenon have significantly more migraine headaches.[91] The basic research on the subject does not mention vasospasm of the nipples.[50] The digital vessels of patients are more sensitive to the cold. All vasospasm is not Raynaud's phenomenon.

Five cases of Raynaud's phenomenon of the nipple are described in the literature as severe blanching and debilitating pain.[121] Several women had white, blue, and red color changes but only of the nipple. All were treated with nifedipine (10 mg three times a day or 30 mg by slow-release tablet). Nifedipine (Adalat, Procardia) is an antihypertensive calcium channel blocker. It does pass into the milk and is estimated to provide about 7.0 μg/kg/ day (5%) of the pediatric dose. The American Academy of Pediatrics (AAP) rates nifedipine a 6. All the women responded with a decrease or obliteration of the painful blanching.

The clinical parameters used to diagnose this disease are not universal.[49] Some history or other evidence of Raynaud's phenomenon is essential when associating it with nipple blanching.[18] Before prescribing a medication, the other therapeutic first options should be initiated.[120] Discontinuing smoking or secondhand smoke is imperative. Steady ambient temperature and warm clothing are important. Adding fish oil to the diet has helped some victims, as has evening primrose oil, which is a rich source of essential polyunsaturated fatty acid, especially γ-linoleic acid. Evening primrose oil has been used effectively in patients with mastalgia of unknown origin.

Peripheral tissue ischemia in neonates has been treated with topical nitroglycerin ointment, which is well absorbed through intact skin. Effects are usually seen within 30 to 60 minutes and last 6 to 8 hours.[18] Because of the risk of hypotension, constant observation is necessary. Although this is theoretically an effective therapy for blanched nipples, no studies report on its safety, and no data are available on its secondary effect on the infant, who would receive it through the milk or directly from the nipple. Other medications that have been used for Raynaud's phenomenon include angiotensin-converting enzyme (ACE) inhibitors (e.g., captopril, enalapril) and prostaglandins for severe prolonged attacks.

Smoking

The number of women who breastfeed and smoke varies from 5% to 20% of breastfeeding women.

Mothers who smoke choose bottle feeding more frequently than women who do not smoke. Of those smokers who are breastfeeding on discharge from the hospital, more have discontinued breastfeeding by 6 weeks than those who do not smoke.[131]

Smoking behavior patterns prenatally, during pregnancy, and postpartum, as studied by

O'Campo et al,[155] show that 41% of women quit during pregnancy, with the highest rate of quitters being older, better educated, and white. Among black women, only the intention to breastfeed affected behavior. Early postpartum relapse rates differed by ethnicity, with formula feeding being the strongest predictor. Clinicians may be able to assist women in their resolve to quit as well as to breastfeed by providing strong support at the critical time in the early postpartum period.

The pharmacologic effects of nicotine have been studied in the fetuses of experimental animals. The active components of cigarette smoke, nicotine and carbon monoxide, have been implicated in the birthweight reduction seen in infants of mothers who are heavy smokers. Nicotine has acetylcholine-like actions on the central nervous system (CNS), skeletal muscle, and upper sympathetic and parasympathetic ganglia. Nicotine initially stimulates and then depresses. Nicotine has been shown to interfere with the let-down reflex, but it does not appear to disrupt lactation once it has been initiated. Smoking has been associated with a poor milk supply. It has been reported that women who smoke 10 to 20 cigarettes a day have 0.4 to 0.5 mg of nicotine/L in their milk. Calculations indicate this is equivalent to a dose of 6 to 7.5 mg of nicotine in an adult. In an adult, 4 mg of nicotine has produced symptoms, and the lethal dosage is in the range of 40 to 60 mg for adults. On the basis of gradual intake over a day's time, the neonate would metabolize it in the liver and excrete the chemical through the kidney.

Multiple studies of nicotine and cotinine concentrations in the nursing mother and her infant have confirmed that although bottle-fed infants born to smoking mothers and raised in a smoking environment have significant levels of nicotine and metabolites in their urine, breastfed infants have higher levels.[43,117,129] A direct correlation exists between the mother's plasma level and the amount in the milk, but not with the amount in the infant's urine in a study of smokers.[117,176] When the infant was removed from the environment and second-hand smoke, the correlation between milk and infant urine levels was high. The half-life of nicotine in the milk of smokers was reported by Steldinger

and Luck[188] to be 95 minutes. Nicotine levels were higher in milk than in maternal serum because maternal serum is basic and milk is acidic. The total amount of nicotine and metabolites depends on the number of cigarettes per day and the time between the last cigarette and breastfeeding.[129]

When lactating women who smoked more than 15 cigarettes a day were compared with lactating women who did not smoke at all, the basal prolactin levels were significantly lower in smokers, but suckling-induced acute increments in serum prolactin and oxytocin-linked neurophysin were not influenced.[4] These experiments showed no influence on oxytocin when two cigarettes were smoked before a feeding. Serum nicotine and plasma epinephrine, but not dopamine or norepinephrine, were significantly increased in the mothers during smoking.

Somatostatin levels in plasma in smoking breastfeeding women were significantly higher at onset of lactation on day 4 postpartum and throughout lactation. *Somatostatin* is a widely distributed peptide with multiple hormonal and neurogenic actions. It inhibits the release of prolactin; it inhibits gastrointestinal functions; and its presence in milk suggests it may be produced by the mammary gland. That milk yield is significantly decreased in smoking women was demonstrated by deuterium-dilution methods by Vio et al.[195] Similar results were reported in the mothers of premature infants initiating lactation by pump in a carefully controlled study by Hopkinson et al.[78] The smokers weaned their babies more quickly than nonsmokers.[131] The heavy smokers had the lowest prolactin levels and weaned earliest.

Newborn infants nursed by smoking mothers and kept in the newborn nursery to avoid passive smoke showed serum concentration of nicotine 0.2 ng/ml and cotinine, the main metabolite, 5 to 30 ng/ml.[40] Newborns excrete measurable amounts in their urine as well. Infants exposed to passive smoking but not breastfed also had nicotine in their urine. Thus breastfeeding by smoking women contributes to the nicotine in infants.

The effect of maternal smoking on the infant includes decreased growth (Fig. 15-3). Weight increase of infants of smokers was 340 ± 170 g compared with 550 g ± 130 g in controls over 14 days, as reported by Vio et al.[195] In another comparison group of breastfeeders, Schulte-Hobein et al[176] reported no significant weight difference when the infants were 1 year old. Gross motor and mental development also were no different. A group of infants followed from the sixth month of pregnancy through 1 year of age included breastfed infants of 74 smokers, breastfed infants of 195 nonsmokers, and bottle-fed infants of 64 smokers. Every 10 cigarettes smoked while breastfeeding was related to an additional 3% infant body mass at 1 year of age. This group of infants whose mothers smoked paradoxically had significantly higher body mass and were heavier than those of nonsmokers.[127]

Children of smokers had more respiratory illnesses in the first year and had been weaned sooner.[68] In a matched-pair group of 28 smokers and 28 nonsmokers, the smokers weaned at 4.5 months and the nonsmokers at 6.7 months. The infants of smokers required treatment for respiratory infection with antibiotics 38 times and the infants of nonsmokers 19 times. The relationship to colic in infants breastfed by a smoker is significant.[172] Forty percent of infants breastfed by smokers (≥5 cigarettes/day) had infantile colic,

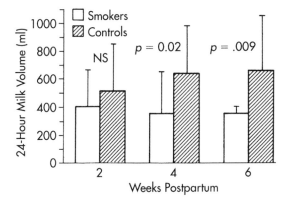

Fig. 15-3. Milk production of smokers. (From Hopkinson JM, Schanler RJ, Fraley JK et al: *Pediatrics* 90: 934, 1992.)

defined as 2 to 3 hours a day of excessive crying, compared with 26% of those breastfed by non-smokers, according to Matheson and Rivrud[135] ($p < 0.005$). This observation has been made for bottle-fed infants with one or more smokers in the home. A case of presumed nicotine poisoning was reported by Bisdom[16] in 1937 in a 6-week-old nursling whose mother smoked 20 cigarettes a day. The infant was restless and insomniac, with "spastic vomiting," diarrhea, rapid pulse, and "circulatory disturbances." The milk contained nicotine, and discontinuing breastfeeding caused "withdrawal," which was treated symptomatically. In a report of hair analysis as a marker for fetal exposure to nicotine and cotinine from maternal smoking by Klein et al,[107] there was a direct correlation of hair levels to maternal levels. Measurable levels were found in mothers and infants exposed to passive smoke. Hair analysis may be an estimate of long-term systemic exposure.

Sudden infant death syndrome (SIDS) is more common in infants of smokers. Breastfed infants of smokers have a SIDS rate equal to that of bottle-fed infants of nonsmokers. Infants of smokers have more respiratory disease, as do infants exposed to passive smoke. This effect is improved if the infant is breastfed.

Many women who want to stop smoking have tried *nicotine gum.*[126] Its safety in lactation has not been determined. Levels of nicotine in mothers and the physiologic effect on their fetuses have been measured by Doppler effect in Sweden. Nicotine gum exposes the child only to nicotine and its metabolites and not to the other effects of smoking, including thiocyanate and carbon monoxide. The Swedish Nicorette chewing gum containing 4-mg nicotine was compared with one cigarette (high dose provides 1.6 mg). The gum did not appear to affect the fetus. Maternal plasma levels after a high-dose cigarette are double the levels after the gum or a low-dose cigarette. Nicorette gum in the United States contains 2-mg nicotine, which produces a plasma level of 11.8 ng/ml (Table 15-9).

The *nicotine patch* provides nicotine transdermally continuously while worn (it is recommended that it be removed while sleeping). The estimated rate of release of nicotine depends on the total dose

TABLE 15-9	Available nicotine in tobacco products and nicotine therapies
Tobacco products	**Nicotine treatments**

Tobacco products	Nicotine treatments
Smoking tobacco 1-g cigarette contains about 1.5% nicotine, or 13-19 mg/cigarette Cigar 15-40 mg Cigarette butt 5-7 mg/butt *Snuff* 1.5% nicotine Snuff containers about 30 g, of which 1.5% is nicotine, or total of 45 mg Dry snuff inhaled Wet snuff more alkaline and absorbed more readily, reaching plasma levels of cigarette smoking in 10 minutes *Chewing tobacco* 2.5%-8% nicotine Sweeter in taste than smoking tobacco "Chaw" 7.8 mg nicotine/g of tobacco 8-10 "chaws" equivalent to smoking 30-40 cigarettes	*Nicotine gum* Nicotine polyacrolex, Nicorette Contains 2 mg nicotine/piece in United States or 4 mg/piece in Canada and Europe Buffered to pH of 8.5 for enhanced absorption Nicotine rapidly and completely absorbed through oral mucosa About 30 minutes of chewing releases 90% of nicotine 1 hour of chewing 2-mg piece produces 11.8 ng/ml and 4-mg piece 23.2 ng/ml nicotine plasma concentrations Gum must be chewed to release nicotine *Nicotine transdermal systems* Usually in three doses Provide 21, 14, and 7 mg of nicotine over 16-24 hours Provide average plasma nicotine concentrations of 17, 12, and 6 ng/ml, respectively (smoking provides 20-50 ng/ml) 21 mg/24 hr equivalent to smoking for 15 hours Elimination half-life of transdermally absorbed nicotine 3-6 hours

in the patch, the number of layers, and the size of the patch (skin contact area). Up to 114-mg nicotine may be in a patch with a delivery rate of 21 to 22 mg/hr. Lower doses (7 mg/24 hr) can be prescribed. The serum level will vary accordingly.

In counseling the nursing mother who smokes, consideration should be given to the data, which suggest that mothers should not smoke while nursing or in the infant's presence. If it is not possible to stop, they should cut down and also consider low-nicotine cigarettes. Feedings should be delayed as long as possible after smoking.

Because some vegetables contain measurable amounts of nicotine (but not cotinine), they should be avoided as well. Highest levels are found in eggplant, green and pureed tomatoes, and cauliflower. Ten grams of eggplant provides 1 μg of nicotine, the same amount obtained in 3 hours in a room with minimal tobacco smoke.[47]

Clove cigarettes

Clove cigarettes contain 60% to 70% tobacco and 30% to 40% clove. Exposure to tar, nicotine, and carbon monoxide is twice that from regular cigarettes. *Eugenol,* the major active ingredient, is used as a topical dental anesthetic. It is more toxic in smoke than by ingestion.

Marihuana

If the mother smokes marihuana (marijuana), an entirely different risk is created. Animal studies have shown that structural changes occur in the brain cells of newborn animals nursed by mothers whose milk contained cannabis. Nahas et al[147,148] describe impairment of deoxyribonucleic acid (DNA) and ribonucleic acid (RNA) formation and of proteins essential for proper growth and development. Results seen in some humans suggest that serious and long-lasting effects can occur. Impairment of judgment and behavioral changes may interfere with an individual's ability to care for the infant or adequately breastfeed. If the mother smokes while nursing, the infant not only ingests the drug in her milk but also inhales the effect of the smoke from the environment. Because brain cell development is still taking place in the first months of life, any remote chance that DNA and RNA metabolism is altered should be viewed with concern.

The mother who requires hospitalization

Emergency admission

The mother who suddenly develops an emergency condition that requires hospitalization presents a unique problem in management. The emergency condition must be dealt with appropriately, whether medically, surgically, or psychiatrically. It is equally important in all three situations to deal with the patient as a lactating mother. Failure to do so may have an impact on the successful outcome of the primary condition.

Medical admission. Medical problems such as acute infection or metabolic disturbances should be analyzed in relationship to lactation, to the infant, and to any other children at home. Is it contagious? In the case of lactation, will the drugs pass into the breast milk? If so, are there alternative treatments? What is the prognosis for recovery? Is the recovery phase more or less than 2 weeks, and is maintaining lactation realistic? This decision should not be made without an understanding of the mother's commitment to further breastfeeding. If the prognosis is poor for recovery or the drugs involved are contraindicated for the infant but necessary for the mother, provision should be made for the mother's adjustment. Abrupt cessation of lactation can cause a flulike syndrome, which will confuse the management picture. It may be advisable to include the

mother's obstetrician or pediatrician in the discussion to provide the mother with the necessary support to accept alternatives (see Chapter 11).

For instance, the management of asthma during pregnancy or lactation must consider the risk of drugs to the infant. Inhaled β_2-agonist medication (metaproterenol, terbutaline, albuterol) by metered dose delivers the least drug to the infant. Steroid therapy may be dramatic in the acute disease, and the breast milk levels are minimal and will drop slowly, providing a weaning mechanism from the drug. Theophylline, as with caffeine, can cause irritability and wakefulness in the infant and is no longer considered the primary treatment. The approach is initially focused to decrease the inflammation and not the spasm.

Surgical admission. As with any surgical procedure, communication must occur among the surgeon(s), anesthesiologist, other consultants, and the primary care physician to establish the process for breastfeeding when a lactating woman is the patient. Surgical emergencies such as trauma, appendicitis, or chylocystitis[12] require immediate attention, including anesthesia and surgery.

Breast biopsy during pregnancy and lactation represents special challenges to the surgeon and pathologist. The risk of milk fistula and infection is increased, although no published data are available. The risk is low in peripheral biopsies and high in central biopsies involving the areola. In 105 benign biopsies, 71% of patients had conditions similar to nonpregnant, nonlactating women. Those lesions peculiar to pregnancy and lactation in decreasing order of frequency are fibroadenoma, lipoma, papilloma, fibrocystic disease, galactocele, and inflammation. Localized breast infarcts also occur either from overgrowth of preexisting fibroadenoma or spontaneously. The risk of cancer diagnosis in one series was 22% of breastfeeding women compared with 19% of nonpregnant, nonlactating women overall. Most lumps were preexisting, but growth rate was accelerated by pregnancy.[162]

Thiopental sodium (thiopentone) as an induction agent was studied in lactating women, a group who had cesarean births and a group who had been fully lactating for at least 2 weeks and were to have elective surgery.[6] The dosage was 5.0 mg/kg for the first group and 5.4 mg/kg for the second. The maximum concentrations in colostrum were 1.3 ± 0.5 μmol/L and 3.4 ± 0.68 μmol/L in the mature milk, which were lower levels than those in the maternal serum (2.21 ± 0.31 and 7.09 ± 1.4, respectively). The maximum dose of drug in 100-ml mature milk was calculated to be 0.090 mg and in colostrum 0.034 mg. No effect was anticipated or seen in the fully breastfeeding infants.

Alfentanil has been measured in colostrum of nonlactating women having tubal ligations postpartum. When the women were in the operating room before medication, both breasts were pumped with an electric pump for 10 minutes.[6] The women received diazepam, D-turbocurarine, succinylcholine, and thiopental sodium. Mothers were maintained on mechanical ventilation for the procedure. Then 50-μg/kg alfentanil was given intravenously with additional 10-μg/kg doses as needed for control. Four hours after the last injection of alfentanil, colostrum was collected from the right breast and at 28 hours from the left breast. The mean level at 4 hours was 0.88 ng/ml and 0.05 ng/ml at 28 hours. The drug cleared the colostrum rapidly.[62]

In the immediate postpartum period, tubal ligation may be performed on a multiparous woman. This type of procedure requires anesthesia and a brief interruption of mother-infant contact. The choice of anesthetic is important. Specific information is slowly accumulating regarding actual milk levels and infant responses. The highest morphine levels were reached about 30 minutes after the intravenous, intramuscular, or epidural doses and were slightly higher than the maternal plasma levels at all points. Some specimens were pumped from lactating patients having tubal ligations in the immediate postpartum period.[53] The peak dose was estimated at 500 ng/ml in the milk. Because of the low oral bioavailability of morphine in the breastfed infant, the drug is of minimal risk.[15,53]

Interpleural bupivacaine in the seventh right interspace 10 cm from the spinous process was given for operative and postoperative pain to a woman for biliary surgery who was breastfeeding a 10-month-old infant four times a day.[11] The dosage of bupivacaine was 0.13 ml/kg/hr. Peak maternal serum level was 1.6 μg/ml at 47 hours. The drug was undetectable in the infant's blood; maximum milk levels occurred immediately postoperatively. Despite numbness of the right nipple, breastfeeding continued uninterrupted except for time in the operating room. The numbness would suggest that the pain fibers are from the thoracic spinal nerves and the suckling sensory nerve fibers from the median branches of the intracostal nerves.

Major surgical trauma has a rapid, profound, and long-lasting effect on gonadal activity and less effect on adrenal activity. Prolactin levels rise significantly and return to baseline slowly. Initiating lactation postoperatively may be influenced by hormonal changes and the effects of pain.

With self-limited trauma or disease with a short postoperative course, as in appendicitis, the mother can go back to breastfeeding on her return home. If the hospitalization will be more prolonged, as in trauma with immobilizing fractures, different considerations are important. The infant can be brought to the hospital several times a day for nursing. Unless the mother is mobile enough to provide some of the infant's bedside care, rooming-in is too taxing to the recovering patient. It is also stressful to other patients and staff who are not equipped for neonates. The mother would require a single room. If she has provision for her own nursing care or if the nursing staff is agreeable, an arrangement could be worked out. The only contraindication would be whether it would interfere with recovery.

When bone healing is important, attention should be given to the dietary demands of bone healing and lactation, especially in calcium, phosphorus, and vitamin intakes. If the mother is to be cared for but immobilized at home, nursing is easier, but provision for ample assistance is mandatory. The need for assistance does not differ for the breastfed or bottle-fed infant of the same age. Home care services are available in most communities.

Psychiatric admission. The onset of a psychiatric crisis in a lactating mother rarely occurs unless the mother has already been identified as having a psychiatric problem. Childbirth has an established etiologic role in postpartum psychosis. A report in the literature, however, details a case of mania precipitated in a mother each time she weaned her children from the breast but at no other time. We had treated a patient with a known psychiatric disorder who decompensated during pregnancy, did well during lactation, and had difficulty after weaning. With her fourth child, she weaned abruptly at 3 months and committed suicide 2 weeks later.

Breastfeeding of itself does not cause psychosis. Women with a postpartum psychosis have acutely decompensated when they wean abruptly. Thus the management of weaning is a very important part of the mother's treatment, and the process should be orchestrated by the psychiatrist and not the pediatrician or obstetrician.

As the number of women who breastfeed increases, there will be increased understanding of the relationship of these physiologic events to psychiatric disease.[122] The role of the mother in lactation will be a part of her psychiatric care, and the decision to breastfeed or not should be worked out with her psychiatrist. Most psychiatric wards can accommodate young infants whether they are breastfed or bottle fed, so it is less of a novelty than on medical or surgical wards. The management of postpartum psychosis includes the concerns of the mother caring for the infant as part of recovery. The drugs used when the mother is nursing should be appropriate for both mother and nursing infant.

Elective admission

At times a lactating mother may have to plan for hospitalization. The urgency will be determined by the underlying disease. If the admission date can be made for over a month away, there is time for gradual weaning of the infant, if necessary. If weaning is appropriate and/or necessary, the impact will largely be determined by the age of the infant. A very young infant who would profit greatly by continued breastfeeding is one type of problem. If the infant is a year old, it may be less traumatic for the child to be weaned when the separation is going to be greater than 48 to 72 hours. A child who is also receiving solids and some other liquids from a cup can be sustained during the separation without much more than sadness. If the caregiver and the surroundings are familiar, the support of this infant is easier. For the mother of the older child, the impact of forced separation during hospitalization is also easier and less likely to produce "milk fever."

The young infant can be sustained by cup feedings, bottle feedings, or "cross-nursing" by another lactating mother until the infant can be breastfed by the mother again. The mother in the first few months of lactation will have more problems with engorgement, discomfort, and even malaise. Provision should be made to express or pump milk to maintain the supply if the mother will be nursing again or pumping minimally for comfort if lactation is to be discontinued. Milk can be collected in sterile bottles and sent home for the infant. When the admission is elective, plans can be made in advance to have a pump available, renting one if the hospital is not equipped. Methods for collecting, refrigerating, and transporting milk home to the infant can be planned along with her other needs, such as a babysitter.

During an elective admission for a self-limited disease, rooming-in for the infant may be possible if the circumstances of the illness permit. The prime purpose of the hospitalization is to treat an illness. If surgery is involved, rooming-in should not be a stress to the mother when she is in the operating room, in the recovery room, or heavily medicated. Day-of-surgery, same-day surgery, and ambulatory surgery units have minimized hospital stays and the need for alternative nourishment for the infant.

The purpose of this section is to point out that it is possible to maintain lactation when hospitalization is necessary for the mother. It is also possible to have the infant accompany the mother, or vice versa, in a rooming-in arrangement. The theoretic threat of infection in the hospital setting is outweighed by the advantages of human milk in most cases. On the other hand, the decision rests with the physician in charge of the case, who will have the responsibility of looking at the total picture, including the medical problem in question, the necessary treatment, and the short-range prognosis for resuming normal breastfeeding. The expertise of the mother's obstetrician and the infant's pediatrician may be invaluable. They can also assist in coping with family and friends who have confused the mother with their experiences or opinions.

Evaluation of nipple discharge

Reports of nipple discharge usually exclude problems during lactation. In a consecutive series of 8703 breast surgeries, Leis and Urban[125] noted that 7.4% of patients had a discharge. To be significant, they point out, a discharge should be true, spontaneous, persistent, and nonlactational. Discharges can be milky, multicolored and sticky, purulent, clear (watery), yellow (serous), pink (serosanguineous), and bloody (sanguineous). The latter four are the surgically significant ones except in lactation.

Most nipple discharges are caused by benign lesions, and many do not require surgical intervention.[124] They could, however, represent a malignant condition and deserve careful investigation. Nipple discharges associated with lactation have a different etiologic incidence profile, but they are no less significant. In general, discharge is more common in older women. Most texts discussing discharge from the nipple are written by surgeons, and the distinction regarding the relationship to breastfeeding is not made.

A *discharge* from the nipple is defined as fluid that escapes spontaneously. A *secretion,* on the other hand, is fluid present in the ducts that must be collected by nipple aspiration or by other means, such as a conventional breast pump or gentle massage and expression from the ducts (*nonspontaneous secretion*).[105]

Nipple secretion is usually not observed in nonlactating women because the lactiferous sinuses are plugged with dense keratotic material. The secretions are seen on histologic sections. If the keratotic plugs are removed, fluid can be aspirated by use of a simple device in most women.[105] Various solutions have been injected into the duct system, and their absorption into tissue, lymphatics, and blood have been traced. The presence of fluid among nonlactating women depends on age, race, and menstrual, menopausal, and breast disease status.[3] The latter being the most important, lactation is still the ultimate secretory product.

Needle aspiration *biopsy* and aspiration biopsy cytology have made it possible to achieve a diagnosis without open biopsy and are standard clinical procedures for the evaluation of many palpable breast masses.[108] They are also used for nonpalpable lesions and can be used for multiple nodules, in mastitis, for evaluating vague masses and painful areas, and for assay of hormonal receptors. Biopsy is a prompt, cost-effective, safe procedure and can be done without interrupting lactation, often in the office setting.

Breast cytology is an important part of an evaluation during pregnancy and lactation and any other time. During pregnancy the ductal lobular system undergoes marked hyperplasia with rapid proliferation of the epithelial linings as they form new ductules.[157] Lymphocytes, plasma cells, and eosinophils infiltrate during the proliferation process. After 16 weeks, colostrum-like fluid is present in the ducts. Cytology of the breast during pregnancy is very cellular; the cell types are the same as in the resting breast, although the proportions differ.[76] Epithelial cells are numerous and suggest a papillary structure. Neutrophils are abundant as well. The most common cell types are foam cells, leukocytes, histocytes, and gland epithelial cells consisting of single cells and cell clusters.[76] The foam cells in pregnant patients exhibit nuclear enlargement, binucleation, multinucleation, and increased cytoplasmic vacuolization compared with those of nonpregnant women. Unexpectedly large numbers of ductal epithelial cells are present in pregnancy and lactation. Groups of cells are papillary in structure and similar to the papillary fronds of an intraductal papilloma. In the immediate postpartum period, the lactating woman's secretions are virtually acellular at the end of the first week; nonlactators exhibited cellularity characteristics of pregnancy, according to work by Holmquist and Papanicolaou.[76]

Biopsies during the third trimester of pregnancy, as described by Kline and Lash,[109] had "tufts of cells forming spurs or invaginations into duct and alveolar lumens and similar structures that were desquamated into lumens and groups of cells found in the breast secretions." The investigators also commented that the "spurs" were closely associated with the formation of new alveoli, suggesting their origin. Delicate capillary networks within these tufts of cells might easily be traumatized and result in the bloody secretion described in pregnancy and early lactation. Kline and Lash[110] reported the persistence of the antepartum cellular findings in 31 of 72 postpartum women. The correlation to lactation or its suppression was not made. Biopsies, however, demonstrated findings similar to those in pregnancy; these changes lasted up to 2 months.

Conclusions drawn from multiple studies by King and Goodson[105] are that breast-fluid cytology during pregnancy and lactation reveals the following:

1. Increased cellularity is seen and is most marked in late pregnancy.
2. Cellularity is variable postpartum.
3. Increased numbers of duct epithelial cells in groups are similar to intraductal papilloma or papillary hyperplasia.
4. Blood may be found in pregnancy and lactation in the absence of clinical lesion.
5. Interpretation of secretions in pregnancy and lactation justifies caution.

Cytologic findings referred to as "hyperplasia" in lactation have no apparent association with increased risk of breast cancer.[46] Lesions usually not associated with increased risk of cancer are apocrine metaplasia, cyst, duct ectasia, fibroadenoma, fibrosis, mastitis, periductal mastitis, squamous metaplasia, and milk hyperplasmia. According to a consensus meeting, "Is 'fibrocystic disease' of the breast precancerous?"[36]

Milky discharge

Persistent bilateral lactation is the presentation following breastfeeding and, as noted, may represent pituitary disease. If no surgical disease (e.g., adenoma) exists, medical treatment to suppress prolactin (e.g., estrogens, bromocriptine) is usually employed. In the nonlactating woman, this finding is called *galactorrhea* and is a spontaneous, milky, multiduct, bilateral discharge[164] (see earlier discussion).

Multicolored and sticky discharge

Multicolored, sticky, spontaneous bilateral discharges from multiple ducts usually show only normal skin flora when cultured.[125] It is usually green but may be yellow, brown, red brown, or gray; it is Hemostix or guaiac negative. The discharge can occur from puberty to the postmenopausal years and is most common in parous women. It is often associated with nipple manipulation, especially when seen in the third trimester or early lactation. Simple cases can be treated with good hygiene and discontinuing nipple manipulation. If it occurs at delivery, lactation can be initiated after cleansing and removal and discarding of early secretion. Normal colostrum usually follows.

Duct ectasia, or *comedomastitis,* is the most common cause of multicolored sticky discharge.[164] It begins as a dilatation of the terminal ducts and may occur during pregnancy, although it is most common between the ages of 35 and 40. It is rare in virgins and most common in women who have lactated. An irritating lipid forms in the ducts, producing an inflammatory reaction and nipple discharge. Cytology shows debris and epithelial cells. Duct ectasia may be associated with burning pain, itching, and swelling of the nipple and areola. Palpation reveals a wormlike tube once called *varicocele tumor of the breast.* As the disease progresses, a mass may develop that mimics cancer, and chronic inflammation leads to fibrosis. Surgery is not indicated unless the discharge becomes bloody. The disease is usually treated with thorough cleansing with pHisoHex or povidone-iodine (Betadine) daily and avoidance of nipple manipulation. Lactation would aggravate preexisting diseases but would not be an absolute contraindication.

Purulent discharge

Purulent discharge is caused by acute puerperal mastitis, chronic lactation mastitis, central breast abscess, or plasma cell mastitis. It is usually unilateral, involving one or two ducts. Once diagnosed, the treatment is antibiotics. When an abscess does not clear after cessation of lactation and adequate treatment, a biopsy should be done to rule out secondary necrosis and infection of an underlying lesion. Ultrasound or other imaging may assist in the diagnosis.

Watery, serous, serosanguineous, and bloody discharges

A volunteer survey among members of the Nursing Mothers Association of Australia resulted in a report of 37 cases in 32 women who had bloody or serosanguineous secretion in either pregnancy or lactation. The condition usually occurred in the first pregnancy (27 of 37) or was a recurrence in a second pregnancy (5 cases), with one case occurring in the third pregnancy. It was usually bilateral, although onset might be unilateral. The earliest case started in the fourth month of pregnancy, although most began at birth and in early lactation. More than 50% of the women had practiced prenatal nipple "exercising." Most cases cleared within 3 to 7 days of onset of lactation. These cases were distinct from trauma, cracked nipple, or mastitis.

Nipple discharges with blood visible or detected by cytologic examination are common during pregnancy and lactation. Lafreniere[118] estimated that 15% of asymptomatic lactating women have blood in their early secretions when they are examined cytologically.

The Lactation Study Center frequently receives calls regarding pink (guaiac positive) or frankly bloody milk, referred to by some as "rusty-pipe syndrome." It is painless and may go unnoticed unless the mother is pumping her milk or her infant vomits blood that is positive for adult hemoglobin (Apt test), eliminating cases of bleeding of the newborn gastrointestinal tract, which is positive for fetal blood by Apt test. If the infant tolerates the milk, breastfeeding can continue and the blood usually disappears in 3 to 7 days.

The explanation for this phenomenon is probably the increased vascularization of the breast coupled with the rapid development of the alveolae.[110] If the blood persists or is recurrent, the breast should be evaluated by mammography.

The cytology of breast secretions obtained during the third trimester from 50 pregnant women aged 16 to 39 years was reported by Kline and Lash.[110] There was increased cellularity with epithelial cell clusters and capillary groupings forming "spurs" or invaginations into duct and alveolar lumina. The authors noted that the spurs were closely associated with the formation of new alveoli; the delicate capillary networks within these tufts could be easily traumatized and result in blood escaping into the breast secretions.

The other cells found in secretions during pregnancy and lactation when breast secretions were aspirated were foam cells, leukocytes, histocytes, and gland epithelial cells.[51] Foam cells are also referred to as *colostrum bodies* and have large nucleae or are binuclear or multinucleated. When lactation is suppressed postpartum, the secretion is almost acellular by the seventh day.[110]

Nipple discharges are primarily of surgical significance. They are the second most common indication for breast surgery. Watery or colorless, serous or yellow, serosanguineous or pink and sanguineous discharges are more common over the age of 50, but younger women do not escape them.[164] Bloody discharge in pregnancy and lactation is most often caused by vascular engorgement or breast trauma. The next most common causes in pregnancy and lactation are intraductal papilloma (50%) and fibrocystic disease (31%). Because the type of discharge does not identify the malignant or nonmalignant nature of the problem, all patients with unusual discharge should be seen by an appropriate surgeon for diagnosis.

In intraductal papilloma the discharge is usually spontaneous, unilateral, and from a single duct. It is occasionally associated with a nontender lump in the subareolar area. Symptoms may include bleeding, which is usually painless during pregnancy. It is possible to excise the involved duct and wedge of tissue, leaving the rest intact to preserve mammary function, when surgery is required for intraductal papilloma. Painless bleeding during pregnancy may be bilateral or unilateral and may cease after delivery. After serious disease has been ruled out by physical examination and cytology, lactation is possible.[118]

To be significant, a discharge should be true, persistent, spontaneous, and nonlactational. Single-duct unilateral discharges are more apt to be surgically significant. A true discharge comes from a duct to the surface of the nipple. Pseudodischarges occur on the surface and may be associated with inverted nipples, eczematoid lesions, trauma, herpes simplex, infections of the Montgomery glands, and mammary duct fistulas. Discharges are more common in women taking oral contraceptives, tranquilizers, or rauwolfia alkaloids and in those who are postmenopausal and menopausal. Cytologic examination should be part of any examination for an abnormal discharge from the breast, although a high percentage of false-negative tests occur as well as some false-positive results. Absence of a mass is reassuring but should not dissuade one from further diagnostic studies.

Lumps in the breast

The lactating breast is lumpy to palpation, and the lumps shift day by day. The most common cause of a persistent lump is a plugged duct (see Chapter 8); the second most common cause is a mass associated with mastitis. Lumps that persist beyond a few days and do not respond to palliative treatment deserve investigation.[160,161]

Adenomas of the breast and ectopic breast under lactational influences were reviewed by O'Hara and Page.[156] They reported five ectopic lactating adenomas located in the axilla, chest wall, and vulva. Tubular adenomas have been associated with lactation and show lactational changes in a fibroadenoma, thus making diagnosis difficult by fine-needle aspiration. Fine-needle aspiration of the breast has been recommended as a safe, simple diagnostic tool to use in an ambulatory setting without interrupting lactation.[123]

Once a breast mass is palpated, prompt evaluation is indicated to rule out breast cancer. A palpable lump in pregnancy has been noted by investigators to delay the time to treatment as long as 8 months.[14]

Three percent of women diagnosed with breast cancer are pregnant or lactating.[162] Data suggest that pregnant or lactating women with breast cancer, stage for stage, have similar survival rates as nonpregnant women. Average delay during the perinatal period is 2.2 months compared with 0.59 month in the total population of breast cancer patients; thus a higher proportion of pregnant women are in advanced stages when first seen.[177]

Fibrocystic disease

Fibrocystic disease is a diffuse parenchymal process in the breasts that has many synonyms, none of which is satisfactory. The process involves hormonally produced benign proliferations of the alveolar system of varying degrees that occur in response to the normal menstrual cycle. A patient with full-blown disease has pain, tenderness, palpable thickenings, and nodules of varying sizes that are most symptomatic with menses. Fibrocystic disease is prominent in the childbearing years and regresses during pregnancy. It is not a contraindication to breastfeeding. Some women have achieved relief by totally eliminating caffeine and related products from their diet.

Diagnostic procedures include mammography and aspiration biopsy. When no fluid is obtained and a smooth, freely movable mass is present, lumpectomy can be performed. Microscopic examination will clarify the diagnosis and the need for further treatment.

Galactography

Galactography is radiography of the mammary ducts after the injection of radiopaque contrast material. It is done to identify the cause of abnormal nipple discharge, especially when there is no palpable or radiologically detectable lesion.

Cytology examination of the discharge material should always be done first. Positive cytology is helpful, but false-negative results do occur. The procedure involves cannulation of the duct with a blunt needle under sterile precautions with the slow injection of 2.0 ml of sterile, water-soluble contrast material. Preexisting mastitis or abscess is a contraindication to the procedure.

The nipple discharge may be caused by ductal ectasia, fibrocystic changes, papilloma, papillomatosis, or intraductal carcinoma. Galactography is performed to localize the abnormality and not to make a histologic diagnosis, because the appearance of some benign and malignant lesions overlaps significantly.

Breast cysts

Benign cysts of the breast are being identified in younger and younger women, probably because of the more careful self-examination of the breast now recommended. They should be removed and biopsied but do not interfere with lactation. Fibroadenomas that result from a disturbance in the normal menstrual cycle usually proliferate and regress before age 30. Pregnancy and lactation stimulate their growth. They are firm, smooth, lobulated masses and are freely movable without fixation. They can be diagnosed radiologically. They can be removed with the patient under local anesthesia if necessary without stopping breastfeeding.

Lipomas

Lipomas are very common in the breast, which has considerable fat in its stroma. They are usually solitary, asymptomatic, slowly growing, freely movable, soft, and well delineated. They can be easily identified radiologically or with ultrasound imagery in the lactating breast, which has less fat present.

Fat necrosis

Fat necrosis is usually associated with trauma and is caused by local destruction of fat cells with release of free lipid and variable hemorrhage. Organization with fibrosis may lead to fixation. Fat necrosis can be identified radiologically and appears as a fat density or oil cyst with a capsule.

Hematomas

Hematomas of the lactating breast may occur from trauma or in women receiving anticoagulant therapy. They generally regress without treatment. When they occur with minimal trauma, the presence of a tumor should be considered.

Breast hypertrophy with pregnancy (gigantomastia)

Massive hypertrophy of the breast with pregnancy is a rare condition of unknown etiology referred to as *gigantomastia of pregnancy*.[142] It is reported in all races during the childbearing years but is less common than juvenile or virginal hypertrophy,[19] which usually has its onset between ages 11 and 19. When associated with pregnancy, hypertrophy usually begins during the first trimester and progresses until delivery and may even lead to necrosis and incapacity. The first report was in 1948, and a total of 55 cases have been reported in the world literature.[142]

The typical case involves a previously healthy pregnant woman who observes excessive enlargement bilaterally early in pregnancy. The breasts may double or triple in size, becoming not only grotesque but incapacitating. They are firm, edematous, and tense, with a prominent venous pattern. The rapidity of the changes predisposes to necrosis, infection, and hemorrhage. After delivery, in the immediate postpartum period, the breasts recede to almost their previous size. With subsequent pregnancies, they almost always enlarge again and even more extensively.

A patient reported to our center who had moderate breast hypertrophy during pregnancy and massive enlargement during the immediate postpartum period. She had planned to breastfeed but was completely incapacitated. Her caregivers described her breasts as the size of basketballs. Some pain relief was achieved with a Velcro abdominal binder applied to support the breasts and provide some counterpressure. Pillows for support under the arms were also used. Ice packs did little for relief, and analgesics were mildly palliative. The mother was hospitalized for weeks, unable to get out of bed. Gentle pumping helped establish milk flow, and breastfeeding was initiated. Breast size diminished sufficiently to allow discharge home. At about 3 months postpartum, the excessive enlargement recurred, weaning was unpreventable, and surgical intervention was planned.

The cause of gigantomastia is unknown, but most authors agree it is hormonal in nature,[142] whether it is an overproduction or an overreaction of the target organ to the stimulus. Various hormonal therapies, including estrogen, testosterone, and hydrocortisone, have not been effective. Diuretics have been mildly helpful for some. Liver dysfunction has been postulated but essentially discarded.

Pseudohyperparathyroidism has been associated with this condition, with improvement after therapy for the underlying disease. A case of gigantic mammary hypertrophy during pregnancy was associated with severe nonparathyroid hypercalcemia. Vigorous diuresis reduced the calcium level to 11.1 mg/dl. No galactorrhea was present, and the prolactin level was 26 ng/ml. No enlargement of parathyroids was detected. An emergency partial bilateral mastectomy was performed because of necrosis and bleeding. Intraoperatively, 16 U of blood were required. The breast tissue removed weighed 12.5 kg (left) and 11.3 kg (right). Pathology showed virginal hypertrophy with no duct formation. Postoperatively, the serum calcium level returned to normal.[193]

If delivery is not imminent, surgical intervention to relieve severe pain, massive infections, ulceration, hemorrhage, or necrosis is an alternative. After delivery the patient should be counseled about the risk of recurrence and the option of reduction mammoplasty, preserving the nipple and duct system.[177]

Lactation after delivery has not been described in these patients.[142]

Surgical procedures

Surgical manipulation of the breast may result in residual loss of sensation for several months but only rarely permanently. The nerve involved is the anterior cutaneous branch of the fourth lateral cutaneous nerve, which passes deep into the breast tissue unaccompanied by arteries. Preoperative and postoperative evaluation of breast sensation was reported by Courtiss and Goldwyn.[41] Preoperatively, they found the areola to be the most sensitive. For 2 weeks following augmentation mammoplasty, sensation was decreased to the areola and nipple. Erectility did return in all patients. The return of significant sensitivity, however, usually took 6 months or longer, even 2 years, with the larger implants being associated with the greatest loss. Hyperesthesia and paresthesia were also reported.

Immediately after reduction mammoplasty (see next section), breasts were insensitive to testing, and it took about 6 months for sensation to return. The greater the resection, the greater was the loss of sensation. Nipple erectility returned before complete sensation in the skin in about 2 months, but complete recovery took about 1 year. With mastopexy for sagging breasts, normal sensation in the skin returned in about 2 months, but complete recovery could take up to a year.[41]

Augmentation mammoplasty

Augmentation mammoplasty has become a more acceptable procedure, and techniques have improved tremendously.[190] The implantation of inert material is the approach. Young women may request it and then choose to lactate. There should be no destruction of breast tissue or interruption of ducts, nerve supply, or blood supply to the gland or nipple so that breastfeeding is possible and successful (Fig. 15-4). Injections of silicone are no longer used. The silicone caused fibrosis and duct destruction.[190]

Implants for augmentation present different problems and different risk/benefit ratios than implants done after mastectomy as prostheses. An

Fig. 15-5. Asymmetric breasts, with right breast significantly smaller.

Fig. 15-4. Placement of implant in augmentation mammoplasty, with no interruption of vital ducts, nerve supply, or blood supply.

indication that still remains is the unilateral use when one breast is significantly underdeveloped (Fig. 15-5). The underdeveloped breast may present a problem of underproduction during lactation. The flood of reports of rupture of the implants and the leakage of silicone into the breast tissue caused considerable alarm. The U.S. Food and Drug Administration (FDA) concluded after extensive study that it is not necessary to remove intact implants or to check milk for silicone when the prosthesis is intact and the woman chooses to breastfeed. Measurements of levels of silicone and degradation products in urine and milk are not readily available. Silicone and simethicone were present in many medications and toiletries, and silicon is the second most common element on the earth's surface. Nonaugmented cadavers have measurable amounts of silicone.

The FDA's position is that breast implants filled with silicone gel will be available only through controlled clinical trials.[103] Women needing reconstruction will be assured of access. This is based on the lack of knowledge about the safety of silicone implants 35 years after their introduction. It has not been recommended that these implants be removed, except on a case-by-case basis for medical reasons.[103]

Silicon analysis of breast and periprosthetic capsular tissue from patients with saline or silicone gel breast implants demonstrated that silicon levels of breast tissue specimens from saline prostheses were in the same range as those of controls. The levels in the periprosthetic tissue with intact saline implants were significantly higher than those of controls but not as high as those of ruptured silicone gel implants.[175]

Polyurethane implants are no longer available. They had been associated with long-lasting complications, the most common being contractions. Polyurethane is a polymer formed by reaction of diisocyanates and polyols. The polymer sponge breaks down into its reactive monomers, toluene-2,4- and -2,6-diisocyanate. Diamine metabolites have been identified in the urine of patients implanted with the material.[34] The disfigurement of the breast from fibrosis and contractions has led to their removal from the market.

More than 700 articles are found in the literature relating to illness and silicone gel implants, many of them single-case reports. After a thorough study of the literature the Practice Committee of the American Academy of Neurology reports that studies to date (1) show no clear relationship between silicone breast implants and connective tissue disease and (2) do not support a casual relationship between silicone breast implants and neurologic disorders at present.[54]

Breasts requiring augmentation mammoplasty may lack adequate functional breast tissue. A woman may want to have this evaluated by real-time ultrasound before the insertion of an implant if she chooses to breastfeed later.

Postlactation involution

Postlactation involution of a severe degree occasionally occurs. After multiple pregnancies and lactation, some women note considerable regression and seeming atrophy after weaning, which alarms them. The fat deposition has not recurred when the ducts regress. In most of these women the breasts return to their normal contour in about 3 years if no further pregnancy or lactation has occurred. Loss of tissue turgor and fat padding occurs without pregnancy or lactation as well (Fig. 15-6). Augmentation is possible, if desired, once childbearing is completed. If subsequent pregnancy occurs, the breast regenerates and lactates well.

Reduction mammoplasty

Some women have breasts so large that they cause shoulder and back pain, deep grooves in the shoulders from brassiere straps, and negative self-image. These women sometimes want surgical correction. Reduction mammoplasty is more destructive than augmentation because of the necessity of replacing the nipple symmetrically, which requires interrupting the ducts.[190,191] Although reconstructive surgeons report that these women do not want to breastfeed, it is our experience that many of them do choose to breastfeed later when they bear a child and are suddenly aware of their maternal role. At surgery they are consumed with their perceived affliction. The surgeon should clearly discuss the options with the patient or provide a procedure that leaves the ducts intact. If the ducts are intact, breastfeeding can be successful

Fig. 15-6. Extreme postlactation involution.

postoperatively. The nerve must also be intact for tactile sensations to trigger let-down.

In general, surgery of the breast for nonmalignant lesions does not preclude breastfeeding unless the ductal structure has been interrupted. Surgeons need to consider mammary function in counseling young women about breast surgery.

A follow-up study by Harris et al[72] of 73 patients, all in the childbearing years, was done by mailed questionnaire. In the series of 68 patients with reduction mammoplasty procedures who responded, 20 patients became pregnant. All 20 lactated; 7 (35%) breastfed successfully; and 13

(65%) decided not to breastfeed or discontinued for a variety of personal reasons. These patients had all undergone an inferiorly based pedicle reduction mammoplasty, which retains the ability to lactate.[72]

A prospective study of 319 normal healthy women by Neifert et al[149] identified 22 women with previous breast surgery, including 11 excisional biopsies, 5 augmentations, 4 reductions, and 2 chest surgeries involving breast tissue. Ten of the 22 had periareolar incisions (4 reductions, 1 augmentation, 5 excisional biopsies). In this series, previous breast surgery was significantly correlated with the final outcome of lactation, that is, a threefold risk of insufficiency compared to women without surgery. Those women with a periareolar incision had a fivefold risk of lactation insufficiency. Breast reduction was the condition most highly correlated with insufficiency.

Dermatitis that involves the breast

Bacterial dermatitis

Infections of the skin can also involve the breast. Impetigo is extremely contagious and spreads by contact. If it affects the breast, it should be vigorously treated locally and systemically. Breastfeeding should be interrupted until lesions are clear. Milk should be pumped and discarded until systemic treatment has been under way for at least 24 hours. The infant should be inspected daily for possible lesions and treated vigorously if under 3 months of age. Local treatment may be adequate early in older children.

Viral dermatitis

Herpes simplex lesions on the breast are a contraindication for breastfeeding (see Chapter 16). Chickenpox lesions similarly are a contraindication for breastfeeding, unless the infant has already contracted the disease, until the lesions clear.

Contact dermatitis

Lesions from contact with irritating material usually do not affect the infant, so breastfeeding is not contraindicated unless the process interferes with maternal healing or puts the mother at risk for infection. Latex allergic dermatitis can usually be treated with cortisone ointment (by prescription to achieve adequate dosing), and breastfeeding can continue. The offending material should be eliminated. Latex may be in moisture-proof padding for nursing brassieres. Nipple shields are latex and have no purpose in lactation management.

Poison ivy (*Rhus* infection) anywhere on the body except the breast poses no problem to the suckling infant. The toxin from the plant is dissipated from the involved skin within 6 hours after contact. Toxic oils may remain on shoes or clothing until they are washed. The contents of the vesicles do not cause disease in others. The risk involved with continuing to breastfeed if the lesions are on the nipple or areola results from the possibility of secondary infection from infant to mother, which will cause skin breakdown and delayed healing. Treatment with hydrocortisone ointment 1% will hasten healing. Milk should be pumped and may be fed to the infant. Breastfeeding can resume as soon as lesions have healed, usually 4 to 5 days, and the risk of secondary infection is gone.

Anaphylaxis and breastfeeding

Anaphylaxis can be associated with breastfeeding. Urticaria and angioedema can be triggered by a number of factors, including physical stimuli, bites, stings, hormones, collagen vascular disease, and cyclooxygenase inhibitors.

The patient reported by Mullins et al[143] had symptoms when achieving a let-down with breastfeeding. The first episode occurred at first feeding with the first infant. The events were restricted to the early postpartum period. The role of progesterone is not clear, although in other cases unrelated to lactation, suppressing ovulation cleared the symptoms. Although the patient did not react to a skin test with oxytocin, manual expression of the breast precipitated laryngeal edema and hypotension, as did every attempt to breastfeed. Lactation was suppressed by bromocriptine and there were no recurrences. The patient remained symptom free for 5 years until the birth of her fourth child. At 48 hours postpartum, urticaria, upper airway angioedema, and hypotension occurred within minutes of each breastfeeding. She was again given bromocriptine, lactation ceased, and she was symptom free.

Less dramatic urticaria reported during lactation usually occurs at onset of let-down. The itching may be intense. Some relief has been achieved by medicating the mother about 15 minutes before breastfeeding with antihistamines. An alternative is a low-dose, sustained-release antihistamine preparation such as loratadine (Claritin), which does pass into milk but at levels less than 0.03% of the maternal dose. Because it dries mucous membranes and decreases secretions, such a preparation could decrease milk supply over time.

Cephalgia and lactational headache

The association of headache with lactation has been described in the literature and reported to our Lactation Study Center. Migraine headaches differ from lactational headaches.[180] *Migraine* is a hormonally sensitive, episodic headache disorder that may worsen during pregnancy and lactation.[198] Women are reported to have frequent headaches between the third and the sixth day postpartum. Research on periparietal migraines fail to mention the mode of infant feeding. The relationship to prolactin is of interest to neurogenic theorists because prolactin levels are high during migraine headaches. Hyperprolactinemic infertility is associated with increased headaches. The theory is that although hyperprolactinemia does not cause headaches per se, headaches and hyperprolactinemia reflect a derangement of neurotransmission.[94,186]

A detailed description of the onset of headache is provided by Askmark and Lundberg[9] in a 26-year-old woman who was gravida 4, para 2, Ab 2. At her previous term pregnancy, she had intense headaches the weeks before delivery. These increased in intensity, necessitating a complete diagnostic workup by 32 weeks. Because of the headache and facial edema, a cesarean delivery was done at 32⅚ weeks. The headache and edema

cleared in 2 days and recurred at 1 month about 2 minutes into breastfeeding. Each event lasted for 2 to 7 minutes. On occasion the headache would briefly clear while the infant interrupted feeding to burp or change breasts. There was no change in blood pressure and no exertion. Measurements of serum vasopressin, which is a vasoconstrictor, did not show a rise, and oral propranolol given 1 hour before nursing did not prevent the headache. Prolactin levels rose gradually and persisted long after the headache stopped. Oxytocin was not measured. The patient weaned the infant, and the headaches stopped. Wall[198] reported five milder but similar cases.

Headaches are reported to occur during sexual intercourse, which is also associated with oxytocin, which is a vasoconstrictor. This condition is called *benign orgasmic cephalgia.*

Medical evaluation of such a complaint requires the usual evaluation for headache. When associated with lactation and after assessment of pulse and blood pressure, a trial of oxytocin can be given by nasal spray to test the association with oxytocin. A prolactin level at baseline and after 10 minutes of breast stimulation might provide some information. With a negative workup for causes of headache, lactational headache can be considered. It appears to be self-limited.

Multiple sclerosis

Studies historically have reported an increased risk of exacerbation in multiple sclerosis (MS) during the postpartum period but have not considered the impact of breastfeeding. In a study of 435 women regarding their pregnancy and breastfeeding experience, Nelson et al[151] report that 191 pregnancies occurred in a nonprogressive phase of MS. During the 9 months of pregnancy, the exacerbation risk was 10%. During the first 9 months postpartum, the risk was more than three times higher, or 34%. The rate of exacerbation was highest in the first 3 months (44 of 65 women, or 68%) and tapered through 6 months postpartum. In 96 of 191 pregnancies, breastfeeding was initiated, and the average duration was 6.3 months. The exacerbation rate was 37.5% for breastfeeders compared with 31.5% for nonbreastfeeders. The average time of onset was similar—3.0 and 3.1 months, respectively. The exacerbation pattern was similar in breastfeeding and bottle-feeding women and was not correlated with duration of breastfeeding.

The relationship between the mode of feeding in infancy and MS development in later life was examined by Pisacane et al.[165] Patients with MS were less likely than healthy controls to have been breastfed for a prolonged period. Of the 93 MS patients and 93 controls, 76% of controls and 55% of MS patients breastfed for 7 months or longer (odds ratio 0.38).

Counseling a woman with MS regarding pregnancy should include discussion of the postpartum statistics. Breastfeeding is not contraindicated but unfortunately does not appear to protect against exacerbations. It does allow a mother the opportunity to provide her infant with a special gift.

PSYCHOLOGIC PROBLEMS WHILE BREASTFEEDING

Early works, including those of Hippocrates in the Third Book of Epidemics from the fourth century BC, described the "mental derangements" of women who recently delivered and were breastfeeding.[178] These disorders were considered to be etiologically linked to childbirth and lactation as a discrete disease entity. The women were described as febrile and toxic. With the introduction and liberal use of antibiotics, these symptoms disappeared. An extensive review by Seager[178] notes that after the middle of the twentieth century, the incidence of infection and delirious reactions dropped precipitously. Some investigators now believe that no unique pattern of illness exists in puerperal compared with nonpuerperal women. Whereas childbearing might render certain predisposed women more vulnerable to an acute psychiatric episode, the pattern of mental illness in women in the perinatal period does not differ from that seen in other women or in men. The terms *puerperal disorders* and *postpartum psychoses* have been removed from the nomenclature.

Interest in the temporal relationship of the postpartum period to psychiatric disorders continues, however, especially because the incidence of mental illness is lower in pregnant women than in matched nonpregnant women for age, race, and socioeconomic status. The highest incidence of hospitalization for mental problems in women 15 to 44 years of age is 1 to 2 months postpartum.[178] Although the risk of mental illness increases 15-fold postpartum, most reviews never consider the distinction between mothers who breastfeed and those who do not. Elaborate discussions of the influence of fluctuating hormone levels ignore lactation and the possible protective nature of the high levels of prolactin and oxytocin during lactation.

The major clinical issue when significant mental illness occurs during breastfeeding is the question of medications. The use of *lithium* for bipolar disorders during lactation has been of concern because lithium does enter the milk, and lithium in any dosage is considered a risk in an infant under 1 year of age. Infants have been reported to be hypotonic, flaccid, and "depressed" when the nursing mother is taking lithium, whereas others have remained asymptomatic.

In a study of 147 postpartum women 6 to 8 weeks after delivery of a normal, healthy infant, the Edinburgh, Montgomery-Asberg, and Raskin psychologic scales were completed. Fifteen percent were depressed on all three scales.[71] Significant correlations were seen between depression ratings and salivary progesterone and prolactin. Progesterone was positively associated with depression in bottle-feeding women and negatively associated in breastfeeding women. Prolactin levels were inappropriately low in depressed breastfeeders. The authors suggest management should be different for breastfeeding and bottle-feeding women.[71]

Chlorpromazine or phenothiazine used in psychotic disorders appears in the milk in small amounts. Even at doses of 1200 mg, it does not appear to accumulate. Doses of 100 mg/day do not appear to cause symptoms in the infants. *Fluoxetine* (Prozac) appears in breast milk at one-fourth to one-fifth the levels in maternal plasma.[84] (See Chapter 11.)

Clinical experience with significantly depressed patients has shown that abrupt weaning from the breast may precipitate severe depression or even suicidal behavior. Whenever weaning is initiated in a woman with a psychiatric disorder, it should be initiated gradually and take place over 2 to 4 weeks or longer.

The impact of mental illness on the lactation process has been evaluated. Depressed mothers had more difficulties during breastfeeding than other women, and their attitudes were more negative. Depressed mothers complained more of too little milk or too much, of too much crying, of too little sleep, and of not getting enough support and help. Tamminen and Salmelin[192] noted frequent difficulties when they studied psychosomatic interaction between mother and infant during breastfeeding. They found that "depressed mothers in particular did not seem to understand that problems in nursing may be due to somatic rather than psychic reasons. Depressed mothers lacked satisfaction in the mother-infant relationship, failing to create reciprocity with their infant."

In assessing the relationship between infant-feeding method and maternal role adjustment at 1 month, studies find that women who breastfeed their infants have less anxiety and more mutuality, the adaptation of appropriate maternal behavior to the infant's state and behavioral cues and the ability to adjust mothering activities to the infant's needs.[192]

It is not possible from present knowledge to state definitely the impact of breastfeeding on the potential for mental illness in the mother, but breastfeeding clearly enhances mothering and mother-infant interaction and mutuality.[152] Under most circumstances, it is better to continue breastfeeding than to terminate it unnecessarily or prematurely.

Postpartum depression

Much has been written in the lay press about the "baby blues," and many mothers, predominantly primiparas, will admit to a few hours or a day of incredible emotional seesawing some time in the first week after delivery. Episodes in which a mother dissolves in tears when she has "so much to be thankful for" is the usual description. This is a transient state that has been attributed to the tremendous change in hormonal levels after the delivery of the placenta, although no studies confirm this belief. It is usually successfully treated with reassurance and rest. True postpartum depression does occur, however, and contrary to popular fantasy, it occurs in women who are breastfeeding but usually only in women with a problem before pregnancy.

The incidence of psychiatric disorders during pregnancy is remarkably lower than age-adjusted rates in the general population. Rates in the postpartum period, however, increase dramatically to 1 to 2 per 1000, with 50% to 75% involving affective disorders, 10% to 20% schizophrenic illness, 2% to 12% organic psychiatric disorders, and 12% anxiety disorders.[35] Studies of clinically depressed postpartum women reveal that two out of three have a major depression. In an extensive review of postpartum mental illness, Seager[178] noted that with the introduction and use of antibiotics in the mid-1950s, many symptoms, described as puerperal fever or milk fever, resulting in toxic-confusional or delirious behavior no longer are reported.

A growing number of investigators have been unable to demonstrate significant evidence for a unique pattern of mental illness in puerperal compared with nonpuerperal psychiatric disorders. Although childbearing might make a woman more vulnerable to psychiatric stress, the patterns of illness symptomatology, course, and outcome are no different from those of nonpuerperal women or males. The relative risk of serious psychiatric illness when it is immediately preceded by the event of childbirth is 15-fold.[101] Causal mechanisms, however, remain uncertain. Prevailing views support a concept of multifactorial causes or the summation of stresses. Factors of ambivalence or negative attitude toward pregnancy, primary role conflict, lack of emotional and practical support, and increased numbers of life events are all part of the picture.

The relationship between breastfeeding and depression was studied by Kumar and Robson[116] in mothers who totally breastfed and in those who totally bottle fed. No relationship was found between depression and feeding method. A prospective study following 103 women postpartum recorded a 13% incidence of marked postnatal depressive illness and an additional 16% of minor depressive illness of at least 4 weeks' duration. No correlation was made with method of feeding until the mothers were asked about their feeding methods and oral contraceptive use in an attempt to determine the influence of hormones on depression. The authors speculated that the prolactin, estrogen, and progesterone levels would vary with the amount of breastfeeding, amount of other foods consumed by the baby, and amount of hormones taken in the form of contraceptives.[116] In this study the bottle feeders received estrogen and progesterone as contraceptives, but breastfeeders received only progesterone. Total breastfeeders who were not taking contraceptives were somewhat more likely to report depressive symptoms. Feelings of fatigue may have influenced this. The mothers least likely to be depressed were those who were likely to have normal hormonal levels, that is, partial breastfeeders not taking contraceptives. Clearly, breastfeeding women are not immune to postpartum depression.[42]

The impact of the mother's depression on her breastfeeding and nursing attitudes was reported by Tamminen and Salmeun[192] in a study of 119 healthy primparous women using the Beck Depression Inventory (BDI) attitude scales and other questionnaires. Eight percent of the participants were clinically depressed, but 25% did not return the questionnaire, which is possibly more common in depressed subjects. Depressed mothers had more difficulty with breastfeeding.

In a continuing study as part of a larger study, qualitative analysis of mother-infant interactions during breastfeeding showed depressed mothers to be less able to sense the infant's needs, cues, and problems.[154] Furthermore, they saw the problems in psychologic terms; that is, the infant did not want their milk or did not like it.[192] They did not understand that difficulties in breastfeeding could be somatic in nature. Depressed mothers

achieved less satisfaction and mutual pleasure in breastfeeding.

The impact of postpartum depression on the emotional and cognitive development of infants was found to be adverse in several studies, because depressed mothers are typically unresponsive to infant cues, which are manifest with flat affect or withdrawal.[144] Postnatally depressed mothers are likely to be socially isolated and emotionally unsupported. The relationship among family life events, maternal depression, and teacher and maternal ratings of child behavior up to age 6 was reported. Both maternal depression and family life events made significant contributions to negative child behavior.[141]

The prevalence of postpartum depression varied between 7% and 14% over 34 weeks of postpartum monitoring of a cohort of 293 women studied by Pop et al.[166] Peak incidence (14%) was at 10 weeks postpartum; in other studies the peak incidence has been as high as 40%. The symptoms of postpartum and other depressions are similar; however, the puerperium is a time of unique stress.[163] Table 15-10 lists major findings related to the "baby blues," postpartum depression, and psychosis.[102] The cause is uncertain, with hormonal change being a continuing theme. Other perinatal events have been noted to trigger true depression, especially negative birth experiences. At-risk infants, including premature infants, sick infants, and those with disabilities, are often triggers for maternal depressive episodes.[166]

Breastfeeding can be a source of distress for many new mothers who do not have a good support system at home, especially when no one knowledgeable about breastfeeding is available. The LaLeche League International has made an enormous difference with their mother-to-mother program. Isolation often contributes to the depression, and having telephone contact with a league mother or resources such as a lactation consultant to assess the breastfeeding progress may be therapeutic.

The physician and other health care team members should be sensitive to the subtle signs and vague symptoms. When a woman says, "I am

TABLE 15-10   Timing of onset, symptoms, and incidence of maternal psychologic problems

Problem	Onset	Duration	Symptoms	Incidence
The "blues" ("baby blues")	3-5 days postpartum typically	A few days	Lability of mood; tearfulness; cognitive confusion; forgetfulness; headaches; depersonalization; negative feelings toward baby; restlessness; irritability; nightmares	30%-84%; mean incidence across studies 55.75%
Postpartum depression	Within first postpartum year	At least 2 weeks, but usually longer	Tearfulness; despondency; feelings of inadequacy; numbness; suicidal ideation; sadness; reduced appetite and interest; insomnia; oversensitivity; feelings of helplessness and hopelessness; excessive dependency; anxiety and despair; irrational fears about infant or mother's health	27% had depressive symptoms at 3-5 months postpartum; 20% mild and 8% severe depression at 6 weeks postpartum; 40% mild and 17% severe depression at 12 months postpartum; 12% major and minor depression combined at 9 weeks postpartum; 10%-14% experienced depression of clinical severity at 3 days postpartum; 6.1% with major depression and 10.4% with minor depression at 8 weeks postpartum
Postpartum psychosis	Typically within 2-4 weeks or as late as 8 weeks postpartum	Depends on diagnosis and treatment prescribed	Heightened or reduced motor activity; hallucinations; marked deviation in mood; severe depression, mania, or both; confusion; delirium	1-2 per 1000 postpartum women

Modified from Kendall-Tackett KA, Kantor GK: *Postpartum depression, Sage series in clinical nursing research*, Newbury Park, Calif, 1993, Sage.

BOX 15-1   Edinburgh Postnatal Depression Scale (EPDS)

The Edinburgh Postnatal Depression Scale (EPDS) has been developed to assist primary care health professionals to detect mothers suffering from postnatal depression, a distressing disorder more prolonged than the "blues" (which occur in the first week after delivery) but less severe than puerperal psychosis.

Previous studies have shown that postnatal depression affects at least 10% of women and that many depressed mothers remain untreated. These mothers may cope with their baby and with household tasks, but their enjoyment of life is seriously affected, and it is possible that there are long-term effects on the family.

The EPDS was developed at health centers in Livingston and Edinburgh. It consists of 10 short statements. The mother underlines which of the four possible responses is closest to how she has been feeling during the past week. Most mothers complete the scale without difficulty in less than 5 minutes.

The validation study showed that mothers who scored above a threshold 12/13 were likely to be suffering from a depressive illness of varying severity. Nevertheless, the EPDS score should *not* override clinical judgment. A careful clinical assessment should be carried out to confirm the diagnosis. The scale indicates how the mother has felt *during the previous week,* and in doubtful cases it may be usefully repeated after 2 weeks. The scale will not detect mothers with anxiety neuroses, phobias, or personality disorders.

Instruction for users

1. The mother is asked to underline the response which comes closest to how she has been feeling in the previous 7 days.
2. All 10 items must be completed.
3. Care should be taken to avoid the possibility of the mother discussing her answers with others.

4. The mother should complete the scale herself, unless she has limited English or has difficulty with reading.
5. The EPDS may be used at 6-8 weeks to screen postnatal women. The child health clinic, postnatal check-up, or a home visit may provide suitable opportunities for its completion.

EDINBURGH POSTNATAL DEPRESSION SCALE (EPDS)
J.L. Cox, J.M. Holden, R. Sagovsky
Department of Psychiatry, University of Edinburgh
Name:

Address:

Baby's age:

As you have recently had a baby, we would like to know how you are feeling. Please **UNDERLINE** the answer which comes closest to how you have felt **IN THE PAST 7 DAYS,** not just how you feel today.

Here is an example, already completed.
I have felt happy:
    Yes, all the time
    Yes, most of the time
    No, not very often
    No, not at all
This would mean: "I have felt happy most of the time" during the past week. Please complete the other questions in the same way.

In the past 7 days:

1. I have been able to laugh and see the funny side of things
    As much as I always could
    Not quite so much now
    Definitely not so much now
    Not at all

J.L. Cox, MA, DM, FRCP(Edin), FRCPsych, *Professor of Psychiatry, Department of Postgraduate Medicine, University of Keele. Consultant Psychiatrist, City General Hospital, Stoke-on-Trent, formerly Senior Lecturer, Department of Psychiatry, University of Edinburgh* (Correspondence to: *University of Keele, Thornburrow Drive, Hartshill, Stoke-on-Trent, Staffs S17 7QB); J.M. Holden, BSc, SRN, HVCert, Research Psychologist; R. Sagovsky, MB, ChB, MRCPsych, Research Psychiatrist, Department of Psychiatry, University of Edinburgh.*

BOX 15-1   Edinburgh Postnatal Depression Scale (EPDS)—cont'd

2. I have looked forward with enjoyment to things
     As much as I ever did
     Rather less than I used to
     Definitely less than I used to
     Hardly at all
* 3. I have blamed myself unnecessarily when things went wrong
     Yes, most of the time
     Yes, some of the time
     Not very often
     No, never
4. I have been anxious or worried for no good reason
     No, not at all
     Hardly ever
     Yes, sometimes
     Yes, very often
* 5. I have felt scared or panicky for no very good reason
     Yes, quite a lot
     Yes, sometimes
     No, not much
     No, not at all
* 6. Things have been getting on top of me
     Yes, most of the time I haven't been able to cope at all

     Yes, sometimes I haven't been coping as well as usual
     No, most of the time I have coped quite well
     No, I have been coping as well as ever
* 7. I have been so unhappy that I have had difficulty sleeping
     Yes, most of the time
     Yes, sometimes
     Not very often
     No, not at all
* 8. I have felt sad or miserable
     Yes, most of the time
     Yes, quite often
     Not very often
     No, not at all
* 9. I have been so unhappy that I have been crying
     Yes, most of the time
     Yes, quite often
     Only occasionally
     No, never
*10. The thought of harming myself has occurred to me
     Yes, quite often
     Sometimes
     Hardly ever
     Never

*Response categories are scored 0, 1, 2, and 3 according to increased severity of the symptom.
Items marked with an asterisk are reverse-scored (i.e., 3, 2, 1, and 0). The total score is calculated by adding together the scores for each of the 10 items. Users may reproduce the scale without further permission, providing they respect copyright (which remains with the *British Journal of Psychiatry*) by quoting the names of the authors, the title, and the source of the paper in all reproduced copies (*Br J Psychiatry* 150:782, 1987).

overwhelmed," "Nothing will ever be the same," or "I feel hopeless or out of control," the other person must listen to her. When she is anxious or nervous or has insomnia, especially waking in the early morning when she is exhausted, the person must consider depression.[102] Use of a depression scale may be helpful when the mother answers general questions such as "How are things going?" with "Fine." A referral for professional psychiatric help or to a support program or hotline is the minimal response.

Studies support the recommendation that the primary care physician should identify the mother with depression using a simple inventory such as the 10-item Edinburgh Postnatal Depression Scale (Box 15-1). The EPDS has been validated and specifically designed for use by the primary health care team during routine health care visits and it relies on self-reporting.[144]

The role of infant factors in postnatal depression and mother-infant interactions was evaluated in a large group of infants born to 188 primiparous women at risk for postnatal depression and a smaller group born to 43 mothers at low risk. By 8 weeks postpartum, poor motor scores and high irritability in the infant were strongly predictive of maternal depression. These factors also predicted less optimal infant behavior in face-to-face interactions with the mother at 8 weeks.[145]

When the crying behaviors of 3- and 6-month-old infants were compared, infants of depressed mothers cried significantly more per day than infants of nondepressed mothers at 3 months but not at 6 months of age.[140]

A significant association exists with depressive disorder preceding the early cessation of breastfeeding, according to the results of two large, independent samples of puerperal women.[38] Other factors associated with early weaning were low social class, low education, and young age of the mother. Depression is more common in winter in the Northern Hemisphere, when days are short and darkness is prolonged. The relationship of lower prolactin levels in the winter is not understood.[159]

REFERENCES

1. Adamopoulos DA, Kapolla N: Prolactin concentration in milk and plasma of puerperal women and patients with galactorrhea, *J Endocrinol Invest* 7:273, 1984.
2. Alpert SE, Cormier AD: Normal electrolyte and protein content in milk from mothers with cystic fibrosis: an explanation for the initial report of elevated milk sodium concentration, *J Pediatr* 102:77, 1983.
3. Anbazhagan R, Bartek J, Monaghan P et al: Growth and development of the human infant breast, *Am J Anat* 192:407, 1991.
4. Andersen AN, Lund-Andersen C, Larsen JF et al: Suppressed prolactin but normal neurophysin levels in cigarette smoking breast-feeding women, *Clin Endocrinol* 17:363, 1982.
5. Andersen AN, Tabor A: Prl, TSH, GH and LH responses to metoclopramide and breast-feeding in normal and hyperprolactinaemic women, *Acta Endocrinol* 100:177, 1982.
6. Andersen LW, Qvist T, Hertz J et al: Concentrations of thiopentone in mature breast milk and colostrum following an induction dose, *Acta Anaesthesiol Scand* 31:30, 1987.
7. Angya JM, Gutierrez MA, Scopelitis E et al: Hyperprolactinemia in primary Sjögren's syndrome, *Arthritis Rheum* 37:10, 1994.
8. Aono T, Aki T, Koike K et al: Effect of sulpiride on poor puerperal lactation, *Am J Obstet Gynecol* 143:927, 1982.
9. Askmark H, Lundberg PO: Lactation headache—a new form of headache? *Cephalalgia* 9:119, 1989.
10. Asselin BL, Lawrence RA: Maternal disease as a consideration in lactation management, *Clin Perinatol* 14:71, 1987.
11. Baker PA, Schroeder D: Interpleural bupivacaine for postoperative pain during lactation, *Anesth Analg* 69:400, 1989.
12. Basso L, McCollum PT, Darling MRN et al: A study of cholelithiasis during pregnancy and its relationship with age, parity, menarche, breastfeeding, dysmenorrhea, oral contraception and a maternal history of cholelithiasis, *Surg Gynecol Obstet* 175:41, 1992.
13. Benjamin F: Normal lactation and galactorrhea, *Clin Obstet Gynecol* 37:887, 1994.
14. Berens P, Newton ER: Breast masses during lactation and the role of the obstetrician in breastfeeding, *ABM News Views* 3(2):4, 1997.
15. Bernstein J, Patel N, Moszczynski Z et al: Colostrum morphine concentrations following epidural administration, *Anesth Analg* 68:S23, 1989.
16. Bisdom CJW: Alcohol and nicotine poisoning in nurslings, *Maandschrift Kindergenees Kunde Leyden* 6:332, 1937.
17. Bitman J, Hamosh M, Hamosh P et al: Milk composition and volume during the onset of lactation in a diabetic mother, *Am J Clin Nutr* 50:1364, 1989.
18. Black C: Update on Raynaud's phenomenon, *Br J Hosp Med* 52:555, 1994.
19. Bland KI, Romnell LJ: Congenital and acquired disturbances of breast development and growth. In Bland KI, Copeland EM III, editors: *The breast: comprehensive management of benign and malignant diseases,* Philadelphia, 1991, Saunders.
20. Bode HH, Vanjonack K, Crawford JD: Mitigation of cretinism by breast feeding, *Pediatrics* 62:13, 1978.
21. Borch-Johnsen K, Joner G, Mandrup-Poulsen T et al: Relation between breastfeeding and incidence rates of insulin-dependent diabetes mellitus, *Lancet* 2:1083, 1984.
22. Bossi L: Neonatal period including drug disposition in newborns: review of the literature. In Janz D, Dam M, Richens A et al, editors: *Epilepsy, pregnancy, and the child,* New York, 1982, Raven.
23. Brennan P, Silman A: Breast-feeding and the onset of rheumatoid arthritis, *Arthritis Rheum* 37:808, 1994.
24. Briggs GG, Freeman RK, Yaffe S: *Drugs in pregnancy and lactation,* ed 3, Baltimore, 1990, Williams & Wilkins.
25. Brodie MJ: Management of epilepsy during pregnancy and lactation, *Lancet* 336:426, 1990.
26. Brun JG, Nilssen S, Kvale G: Breastfeeding, other reproductive factors and rheumatoid arthritis: a prospective study, *Br J Rheumatol* 34:542, 1995.

27. Buchanon TA, Unterman TG, Metzger BE: Medical management of diabetes in pregnancy, *Clin Perinatol* 12:625, 1985.

28. Burns PE: Absence of lactation in a previously radiated breast, *Int J Radiat Oncol Biol Phys* 13:1603, 1987 (letter).

29. Burrow GN, Ferris TF: *Medical complications during pregnancy,* Philadelphia, 1975, Saunders.

30. Butte NF, Garza C, Burr R et al: Milk composition of insulin-dependent diabetic women, *J Pediatr Gastroenterol Nutr* 6:936, 1987.

31. Bybee DE, Metzger BE, Freinkel N et al: Amniotic fluid prolactin in the third trimester of pregnancies complicated by gestational or pregestational diabetes mellitus, *Metabolism* 39:714, 1990.

32. Campbell DA, Lorber MI, Sweeton JC et al: Breastfeeding and maternal-donor renal allografts, *Transplantation* 37:340, 1984.

33. Cavallo MG, Fava D, Monetini L et al: Cell-mediated immune response to β casein in recent-onset insulin-dependent diabetes: implications for disease pathogenesis, *Lancet* 348:926, 1996.

34. Chan SC, Birdsell DC, Gradeen CY: Detection of toluenediamines in the urine of a patient with polyurethane-covered breast implants, *Clin Chem* 37:756, 1991.

35. Coble PA, Day NL: The epidemiology of mental and emotional disorders during pregnancy and the postpartum period. In Cohen RL editor: *Psychiatric consultation in childbirth setting,* New York, 1988, Plenum.

36. Consensus Meeting: Is "fibrocystic disease" of the breast precancerous? *Arch Pathol Lab Med* 110:171, 1986.

37. Cooper DS: Antithyroid drugs: to breastfeed or not to breastfeed, *Am J Obstet Gynecol* 157:234, 1987.

38. Cooper PJ, Murray L, Stein A: Psychological factors associated with the early termination of breastfeeding, *J Psychosom Res* 37:171, 1993.

39. Coulam CB, Moyer TP, Jiang NS et al: Breastfeeding after renal transplantation, *Transplant Proc* 14:605, 1982.

40. Counsilman JJ, Mackay EV: Cigarette smoking by pregnant women with particular reference to their past and subsequent breastfeeding behaviour, *Aust NZ Obstet Gynecol* 25:101, 1985.

41. Courtiss EH, Goldwyn RM: Breast sensation before and after plastic surgery, *Plastic Reconstruct Surg* 58:1, 1976.

42. Cox JL, Connor Y, Kendall RE: Prospective study of the psychiatric disorders of childbirth, *Br J Psychiatry,* 140:111, 1982.

43. Dahlström A, Lundell B, Curvall M et al: Nicotine and cotinine concentrations in the nursing mother and her infant, *Acta Paediatr Scand* 79:142, 1990.

44. David FC: Lactation following primary radiation therapy for carcinoma of the breast, *Int J Radiat Oncol Biol Phys* 11:1425, 1985.

45. Davidson JM, Katz AI, Lindheimer MD: Kidney disease and pregnancy: obstetric outcome and long term renal prognosis, *Clin Perinatol* 12:497, 1985.

46. Dawson EK: A histological study of the normal mamma in relation to tumor growth. II. The mammary gland in pregnancy and lactation, *Edinburgh Med J* 42:569, 633, 1935.

47. Domino EF, Hornbach E, Demana T: The nicotine content of common vegetables, *N Engl J Med* 329:437, 1993.

48. Drinkwater BL, Chesnut CH: Bone density changes during pregnancy and lactation in active women: a longitudinal study, *Bone & Mineral* 14:153, 1991.

49. Eglash A: Vasospasm of the nipples, *ABM News Views* 2(1):1, 1996.

50. Engelhart M: Clinical and physiological studies of Raynaud's phenomenon, *Danish Med Bull* 38:458, 1991.

51. Engels S: An investigation of the origin of the colostrum cells, *J Anat* 87:362, 1953.

52. Esbjorner E, Jarnerot G, Wranne L: Sulphasalazine and sulphapyridine serum levels in children of mothers treated with sulphasalazine during pregnancy and lactation, *Acta Paediatr Scand* 76:137, 1987.

53. Feilberg VL, Rosenborg D, Christensen CB et al: Excretion of morphine in human breast milk, *Acta Anaesthesiol Scand* 33:426, 1989.

54. Ferguson JH: Silicone breast implants and neurologic disorders, *Neurology* 48:1504, 1997.

55. Ferris AM, Dalidowitz CK, Ingardia CM et al: Lactation outcome in insulin-dependent diabetic women, *J Am Diet Assoc* 88:317, 1988.

56. Flores HC, Cromwell JW, Leventhal JR et al: Does previous breastfeeding affect maternal donor renal allograft outcome? A single-institution experience, *Transplant Proc* 25:212, 1993.

57. Forbes GB, Barton LD, Nicholas DL et al: Composition of milk produced by a mother with galactosemia, *J Pediatr* 113:90, 1988.

58. Fort P, Lanes R, Dahlem S et al: Breastfeeding and insulin-dependent diabetes mellitus in children, *J Am Coll Nutr* 5:439, 1986.

59. Frantz AG, Wilson JD: Endocrine disorders of the breast. In Wilson JD, Foster DW, editors: *Textbook of endocrinology,* ed 7, Philadelphia, 1985, Saunders.

60. Gagne MP, Leff EW, Jefferis SC: The breastfeeding experience of women with type I diabetes, *Health Care Women Int* 13:249, 1992.

61. Giampietro O, Ramacciotti C, Moggi G: Normoprolactinemic galactorrhea in a fertile woman with a copper intra-uterine device (copper IUD), *Acta Obstet Gynecol Scand* 63:23, 1984.

62. Giesecke AH Jr, Rice LJ, Lipton JM: Alfentanil in colostrum, *Anesthesiology* 63:A284, 1985.

63. Ginsberg JS, Hirsh J: Thromboembolic disorders of pregnancy. In Reese EA, Hobbins JC, Mahoney MJ et al, editors: *Medicine of the fetus and mother,* Philadelphia, 1992, Lippincott.

64. Glatthaar D, Whittall DE, Welborn TA et al: Diabetes in western Australian children: descriptive epidemiology, *Med J Aust* 148:117, 1988.

65. Gould BK, Randall RV, Kempers RD et al: *Galactorrhea,* Springfield, Ill, 1974, Thomas.

66. Greenwald JH, Dubin A, Cardon L: Hypomagnesemic tetany due to excessive lactation, *Am J Med* 35:854, 1963.

67. Gruber HE, Gutteridge DH, Baylink DJ: Osteoporosis associated with pregnancy and lactation: bone biopsy and skeletal features in three patients, *Metab Bone Dis Rel Res* 5:159, 1984.

68. Häkansson A, Cars H: Maternal cigarette smoking, breastfeeding and respiratory tract infections in infancy, *Scand J Prim Health Care* 9:115, 1991.

69. Hamosh M, Bitman J, Wood DL et al: Human milk in cystic fibrosis: composition and enzyme content, *Pediatr Res* 16:164A, 1982.

70. Hanson LA: The mammary gland as an immunological organ, *Immunol Today* 3:168, 1982.

71. Harris B, Johns S, Fung H et al: The hormonal environment of postnatal depression, *Br J Psychol* 154:660, 1989.

72. Harris L, Morris SF, Freiberg A: Is breastfeeding possible after reduction mammoplasty? *Plast Reconstr Surg* 89:836, 1992.

73. Hattori N, Ishihara T, Ikekubo K et al: Autoantibody to human prolactin in patients with idiopathic hyperprolactinemia, *J Clin Endocrinol Metab* 75:1226, 1992.

74. Higgins S, Haffty BG: Pregnancy and lactation after breast-conserving therapy for early stage breast cancer, *Cancer* 73:2175, 1994.

75. Hodnett DW, DeLuca HF, Jorgensen NA: Bone mineral loss during lactation occurs in absence of parathyroid tissue, *Am J Physiol* 262:E230, 1992.

76. Holmquist DG, Papanicolaou GN: The exfoliative cytology of the mammary gland during pregnancy and lactation, *Ann NY Acad Sci* 63:1422, 1956.

77. Hoover HC: Breast cancer during pregnancy and lactation, *Surg Clin North Am* 70:1151, 1990.

78. Hopkinson JM, Schanler RJ, Fraley JK et al: Milk production by mothers of premature infants: influence of cigarette smoking, *Pediatrics* 90:934, 1992.

79. Hornstein E, Skornick Y, Rozin R: The management of breast carcinoma in pregnancy and lactation, *J Surg Oncol* 21:179, 1982.

80. Humenick SS, Hill PD, Anderson MA: Breast engorgement: patterns and selected outcomes, *J Hum Lact* 10:87, 1994.

81. Ikegami H, Aono T, Koizumi K et al: Relationship between the methods of treatment for prolactinomas and the puerperal lactation, *Fertil Steril* 47:867, 1987.

82. Isbister C: Diabetes insipidus with a normal draught reflex, *Med J Aust,* Feb 11, 1956, p 234.

83. Isenberg DA, Black C: Raynaud's phenomenon, scleroderma, and overlap syndromes, *Br Med J* 310:795, 1995.

84. Isenberg KE: Excretion of fluoxetine in human breast milk, *J Clin Psychiatry* 51:169, 1990.

85. Jara LJ, Lavalle C, Espinoza LR: Does prolactin have a role in the pathogenesis of systemic lupus erythematosus? *J Rheumatol* 19:1333, 1992.

86. Jarrett RJ: Breastfeeding and diabetes, *Lancet* 2:1283, 1984 (letter).

87. Jensen RG, Ferris AM, Lammi-Keefe CJ: Cholesterol levels and the breastfeeding mom, *JAMA* 262:2092, 1989.

88. Jorgensen C, Maziad H, Bologna C et al: Kinetics of prolactin release in rheumatoid arthritis, *Clin Exp Rheumatol* 13:705, 1995.

89. Jorgensen C, Picot MC, Bologna C et al: Oral contraception, parity, breastfeeding, and severity of rheumatoid arthritis, *Ann Rheum Dis* 55:94, 1996.

90. Joselin EP, Root HF, White P et al: *The treatment of diabetes mellitus,* Philadelphia, 1959, Lea & Febiger.

91. Kahaleh B, Matucci-Cerinic M: Raynaud's phenomenon and scleroderma, *Arthritis Rheum* 38:1, 1995.

92. Kalache A, Vessey MP, McPherson K: Lactation and breast cancer, *Br Med J* 280:223, 1980.

93. Kamble TK, Ookalka DS: Lactation hypomagnesemia, *Lancet* 2:155, 1989.

94. Kamman E, Jones J: Hyperprolactinemia and headache, *Am J Obstet Gynecol* 145:668, 1983.

95. Kampmann J, Johansen K, Hansen JN et al: Propylthiouracil in human milk, *Lancet* 1:736, 1980.

96. Kaneko S, Suzuki K, Sato T et al: The problems of antiepileptic medication in the neonatal period: is breastfeeding advisable? In Janz D, Dam M, Richens A et al, editors: *Epilepsy, pregnancy, and the child,* New York, 1982, Raven.

97. Kapcala LP: Galactorrhea and thyrotoxicosis, *Arch Intern Med* 144:2349, 1984.

98. Karjalainen J, Martin JM, Knip M et al: A bovine albumin peptide as a possible trigger of insulin-dependent diabetes mellitus, *N Engl J Med* 327:302, 1992.

99. Katz E, Adashi EY: Hyperprolactinemic disorders, *Clin Obstet Gynecol* 33:622, 1990.

100. Kelemen E, Szalay F, Peterfy M: Autoimmune (idiopathic) thrombocytopenic purpura in pregnancy and the newborn, *Br J Obstet Gynecol* 85:239, 1978 (letter).

101. Kendall RE, Wainwright S, Hailey A et al: The influence of childbirth on psychiatric morbidity, *Psychol Med* 6:297, 1976.

102. Kendall-Tackett KA, Kantor GK: Postpartum depression, *Sage series in clinical nursing research,* Newbury Park, Calif, 1993, Sage.

103. Kessler DA: The basis of the FDA's decision on breast implants, *N Engl J Med* 326:1713, 1992.

104. Key TC, Resnik R, Dittrich HC et al: Successful pregnancy after cardiac transplantation, *Am J Obstet Gynecol* 160:367, 1989.

105. King EB, Goodson WH III: Discharges and secretions of the nipple. In Bland KI, Copeland EM III, editors: *The breast: comprehensive management of benign and malignant diseases,* Philadelphia, 1991, Saunders.

106. Kira J-i, Harada M, Yamaguchi Y et al: Hyperprolactinemia in multiple sclerosis, *J Neurol Sci* 102:61, 1991.

107. Klein J, Chitayat D, Koren G: Hair analysis as a market for fetal exposure to maternal smoking, *N Engl J Med* 328:66, 1993.

108. Kline TS, Kline IK: *Breast: guides to clinical aspiration biopsy,* New York/Tokyo, 1989, Igaku-Shoin Medical Publishers.

109. Kline TS, Lash SR: Nipple secretion in pregnancy: a cytologic and histologic study, *Am J Clin Pathol* 37:626, 1962.

110. Kline TS, Lash SR: The bleeding nipple of pregnancy and postpartum period: a cytologic and histologic study, *Acta Cytol* 8:336, 1964.

111. Kois WE, Campbell DA, Lorber MI et al: Influence of breastfeeding on subsequent reactivity to a related renal allograft, *J Surg Res* 37:89, 1984.

112. Kossoy LR, Herbert CM, Wentz AC: Management of heart transplant recipients: guidelines for the obstetrician-gynecologist, *Am J Obstet Gynecol* 159:490, 1988.

113. Kostraba JN, Cruickshanks KJ, Lawler-Heavner J et al: Early exposure to cow's milk and solid foods in infancy, genetic predisposition, and risk of IDDM, *Diabetes* 42:288, 1993.

114. Kostraba JN, Steenkiste AR, Dorman JS et al: Early infant diet and risk of IDDM in blacks and whites, *Diabetes Care* 15:626, 1992.

115. Kulski JK, Smith M, Hartmann PE: Normal and caesarean section delivery and the initiation of lactation in women, *Aust J Exp Biol Med Sci* 59:405, 1981.

116. Kumar R, Robson K: Neurotic disorders during pregnancy and the puerperium: preliminary report of a prospective study of 119 primigravidae. In Sandler MJ, editor: *Mental illness in pregnancy and the puerperium,* London, 1978, Oxford University Press.

117. Labrecque M, Marcoux S, Weber J-P et al: Feeding and urine cotinine values in babies whose mothers smoke, *Pediatrics* 83:93, 1989.

118. Lafreniere R: Bloody nipple discharge during pregnancy: a rationale for conservative treatment, *J Surg Oncol* 43:228, 1990.

119. Lamberg BA, Ikonen E, Osterlund K et al: Antithyroid treatment of maternal hyperthyroidism during lactation, *Clin Endocrinol* 21:81, 1984.

120. Lawlor-Smith LS, Lawlor-Smith CL: Raynaud's phenomenon of the nipple: a preventable cause of breastfeeding failure, *Med J Aust* 166:448, 1996.

121. Lawlor-Smith LS, Lawlor-Smith CL: Vasospasm of the nipple: a manifestation of Raynaud's phenomenon; case reports, *Br Med J* 314:644, 1997.

122. Lawrence R: Lactation, breastfeeding, infant care and mental illness. In Kuczmerczy AR, Reading AE, editors: *Handbook of behavioral obstetrics and gynecology,* New York, 1994, Plenum.

123. Lee GF: Fine-needle aspiration of the breast: the outpatient management of breast lesions, *Am J Obstet Gynecol* 156:1532, 1987.

124. Leis HP: Management of nipple discharge, *World J Surg* 13:736, 1989.

125. Leis HP, Urban JA: The other breast. In Gallager HS, editor: *The breast,* St Louis, 1978, Mosby.

126. Lindblad A, Maršál K: Influence of nicotine chewing gum on fetal blood flow, *J Perinat Med* 15:13, 1987.

127. Little RE, Lambert MD III, Worthington RB et al: Maternal smoking during lactation: relation to infant size at one year of age, *Am J Epidemiol* 140:544, 1994.

128. Lobato MF, Careche M, Ros M et al: Effect of prolactin and glucocorticoids on P-enolpyruvate carboxykinase activity in liver and mammary gland from diabetic and lactating rats, *Mol Cell Biochem* 67:19, 1985.

129. Luck W, Nau H: Nicotine and cotinine concentrations in serum and urine of infants exposed via passive smoking or milk from smoking mothers, *J Pediatr* 107:816, 1985.

130. Luder E, Kaltan M, Tanzer-Torres G et al: Current recommendations for breastfeeding in cystic fibrosis centers, *Am J Dis Child* 144:1153, 1990.

131. Lyon AJ: Effects of smoking on breast feeding, *Arch Dis Child* 58:378, 1983.

132. Magno R, Berlin A, Karlsson K et al: Anesthesia for cesarean section. IV. Placental transfer and neonatal elimination of bupivacaine following epidural analgesia for elective cesarean section, *Acta Anaesthesiol Scand* 20:141, 1976.

133. Martin JN, Morrison JC, Files YC: Autoimmune thrombocytopenic purpura: current concepts and recommended practices, *Am J Obstet Gynecol* 150:86, 1984.

134. Matalon R, Michals K, Gleason L: Maternal PKU: strategies for dietary treatment and monitoring compliance, *Ann NY Acad Sci* 477:223, 1986.

135. Matheson I, Rivrud GN: The effect of smoking on lactation and infantile colic, *JAMA* 261:42, 1989.

136. Mayer EJ, Hamman RF, Gay EC et al: Reduced risk of IDDM among breastfed children: the Colorado IDDM Registry, *Diabetes* 37:1625, 1988.

137. Meschengieser S, Lazzari MA: Breastfeeding in thrombocytopenic neonates secondary to maternal autoimmune thrombocytopenic purpura, *Am J Obstet Gynecol* 154:1166, 1986.

138. Metcalfe MA, Baum JD: Family characteristics and insulin dependent diabetes, *Arch Dis Child* 67:731, 1992.

139. Michael SH, Mueller DH: Impact of lactation on women with cystic fibrosis and their infants: a review of five cases, *J Am Diet Assoc* 94:159, 1994.

140. Milgrom J, Westley DJ, McCloud PI: Do infants of depressed mothers cry more than other infants? *J Paediatr Child Health* 31:218, 1995.

141. Morrow-Tlucak M, Haude RH, Ernhart CB: Breastfeeding and cognitive development in the first two years of life, *Soc Sci Med* 26:635, 1988.

142. Moss TW: Gigantomastia with pregnancy, *Arch Surg* 96:27, 1968.

143. Mullins RJ, Russell A, McGrath GJ et al: Breastfeeding anaphylaxis, *Lancet* 338:1279, 1991.

144. Murray L, Cooper PJ, Stein A: Postnatal depression and infant development: emotional and cognitive development of infants may be adversely affected, *Br Med J* 302:978, 1991.

145. Murray L, Stanley C, Hooper R: The role of infant factors in postnatal depression and mother-infant interactions, *Dev Med Child Neurol* 38:109, 1996.

146. Muscari A, Volta U, Bonazzi C et al: Association of serum IgA antibodies to milk antigens with severe atherosclerosis, *Atherosclerosis* 77:251, 1989.

147. Nahas GG: Marijuana, *JAMA* 233:79, 1975.

148. Nahas GG, Suciu-Foca N, Armand J-P et al: Inhibition of cellular mediated immunity in marijuana smokers, *Science* 183:419, 1974.

149. Neifert M, DeMarzo S, Seacat J et al: The influence of breast surgery, breast appearance and pregnancy-induced breast changes on lactation sufficiency as measured by infant weight gain, *Birth* 17:31, 1990.

150. Neifert MR, McDonough SL, Neville MC: Failure of lactogenesis associated with placental retention, *Am J Obstet Gynecol* 140:477, 1981.

151. Nelson LM, Franklin GM, Jones MC et al: Risk of multiple sclerosis exacerbation during pregnancy and breastfeeding, *JAMA* 259:3441, 1988.

152. Newton N, Newton M: Psychologic aspects of lactation, *N Engl J Med* 277:1179, 1967.

153. Nigro G, Campea L, DeNovellis A et al: Breastfeeding and insulin-dependent diabetes mellitus, *Lancet* 1:467, 1985.

154. Nordstrom UL, Dallas JH, Morton HG et al: Mothering problems and child morbidity amongst "mothers with emotional disturbances," *Acta Obstet Gynecol Scand* 67:155, 1988.

155. O'Campo P, Brown H, Faden RR et al: The impact of pregnancy on women's prenatal and postpartum smoking behavior, *Am J Prev Med* 8:8, 1992.

156. O'Hara MF, Page DL: Adenomas of the breast and ectopic breast under lactational influences, *Hum Pathol* 16:707, 1985.

157. Osborne MP: Breast development and anatomy. In Harris JR, Hellman S, Henderson IC et al, editors: *Breast diseases,* Philadelphia, 1987, Lippincott.

158. Ostensen M: Treatment with immunosuppressive and disease modifying drugs during pregnancy and lactation, *Am J Reprod Immunol* 28:148, 1992.

159. Partonen T: Prolactin in winter depression, *Med Hypotheses* 43:163, 1994.

160. Paulus DD: Benign diseases of the breast, *Radiol Clin North Am* 21:27, 1983.

161. Pellegrinc JR, Wagner RF Jr: Polythelia and associated conditions, *Am Fam Physician* 28:129, 1983.

162. Petrek JA: Abnormalities of the breast in pregnancy and lactation. In Harris JR, Lippman ME, Morrow M et al, editors: *Diseases of the breast,* Philadelphia, 1996, Lippincott-Raven.

163. Picazo O, Fernandez-Guasti A: Changes in experimental anxiety during pregnancy and lactation, *Physiol Behav* 54:295, 1993.

164. Pilnik S, Leis HP: Nipple discharge. In Gallager HS, editor: *The breast,* St Louis, 1978, Mosby.

165. Pisacane A, Impagliazzo N, Russo M et al: Breastfeeding and multiple sclerosis, *Br Med J* 308:1411, 1994.

166. Pop VJM, Essed GGM, deGeus CA et al: Prevalence of postpartum depression, *Acta Obstet Gynecol Scand* 72:354, 1993.

167. Rennie J: Formula for diabetes? *Sci Am* 267:24, 1992.

168. Rosato RR, Gimenez MS, Jahn GA: Effect of chronic thyroid hormone administration on pregnancy, lactogenesis and lactation in the rat, *Acta Endocrinol (Copenh)* 127:547, 1992.

169. Rudland PS: Histochemical organization and cellular composition of ductal buds in developing human breast: evidence of cytochemical intermediate between epithelial and myoepithelial cells, *J Histochem Cytochem* 39:1471, 1991.

170. Russo IH, Russo J: Progestagens and mammary gland development: differentiation versus carcinogenesis, *Acta Endocrinol (Copenh)* 125:7, 1991.

171. Ruvalcaba RHA: Stress-induced cessation of lactation, *West J Med* 146:228, 1987.

172. Said G, Patois E, Lellouch J: Infantile colic and parenteral smoking, *Br Med J* 289:660, 1984.

173. Sakakura T: New aspects of stroma-parenchyma relations in mammary gland differentiation, *Int Rev Cytol* 125:165, 1991.

174. Scanlon JW, Ostheimer GW, Lurie AO et al: Neurobehavioral responses and drug concentrations in newborns after maternal epidural anesthesia with bupivacaine, *Anesthesiology* 45:400, 1976.

175. Schnur PL, Weinzweig J, Harris JB et al: Silicon analysis of breast and periprosthetic capsular tissue from patients with saline or silicone gel breast implants, *Plast Reconstr Surg* 98:798, 1996.

176. Schulte-Hobein B, Schwartz-Bickenbach D, Abt S et al: Cigarette smoke exposure and development of infants throughout the first year of life: influence of passive smoking and nursing on cotinine levels in breastmilk and infant's urine, *Acta Paediatr Scand* 81:550, 1992.

177. Scott-Conner CEH, Schorr SJ: The diagnosis and management of breast problems during pregnancy and lactation, *Am J Surg* 170:401, 1995.

178. Seager CP: A controlled survey of postpartum mental illness, *J Ment Sci* 106:214, 1960.

179. Siemiatycki J, Colle E, Campbell S et al: Case-control study of IDDM, *Diabetes Care* 12:209, 1989.
180. Silberstein SD: Headaches and women: treatment of the pregnant and lactating migraineur, *Headache* 33:533, 1993.
181. Sims CJ, Porter KB, Knuppel RA: Successful pregnancy after a liver transplant, *Am J Obstet Gynecol* 161:532, 1989.
182. Sirota L, Ferrera M, Lerer N et al: Beta glucuronidase and hyperbilirubinemia in breastfed infants of diabetic mothers, *Arch Dis Child* 67:120, 1992.
183. Smith PK, Tamlin N, Robertson E: Breastmilk and cystic fibrosis, *Med J Aust* 157:283, 1992.
184. Snell NJC, Coysh HL, Snell BJ: Carpal tunnel syndrome presenting in the puerperium, *Practitioner* 224:191, 1980.
185. Sowers MF, Corton G, Shapiro B et al: Changes in bone density with lactation, *JAMA* 269:3130, 1993.
186. Stein G: Headaches in the first postpartum week and their relationship to migraine, *Headache* 21:201, 1981.
187. Steiner G, Myher JJ, Kuksis A: Milk and plasma lipid composition in a lactating patient with type I hyperlipoproteinemia, *Am J Clin Nutr* 41:121, 1985.
188. Steldinger R, Luck W: Half lives of nicotine in milk of smoking mothers: implications for nursing, *J Perinat Med* 16:261, 1988.
189. Surian M, Imbasciati E, Cosci P et al: Glomerular disease and pregnancy, *Nephron* 36:101, 1984.
190. Synderman RK: Augmentation mammoplasty. In Gallager HS, editor: *The breast,* St Louis, 1978, Mosby.
191. Synderman RK: Reduction mammoplasty. In Gallager HS, editor: *The breast,* St Louis, 1978, Mosby.
192. Tamminen TM, Salmelin RK: Psychosomatic interaction between mother and infant during breastfeeding, *Psychother Psychosom* 56:78, 1991.
193. VanHeerden JA, Gharib H, Jackson IT: Pseudohyperparathyroidism secondary to gigantic mammary hypertrophy, *Arch Surg* 123:80, 1988.
194. Varma SK, Collins M, Row A et al: Thyroxine, triiodothyronine, and reverse tri-iodothyronine concentrations in human milk, *J Pediatr* 93:803, 1978.
195. Vio F, Salazar G, Infante C: Smoking during pregnancy and lactation and its effects on breastmilk volume, *Am J Clin Nutr* 54:1011, 1991.
196. Voegeli DR: Galactography. In Peters ME, Voegeli DR, Scanlon KA, editors: *Breast imaging,* New York, 1989, Churchill Livingstone.
197. Vorherr H: *The breast: morphology, physiology, and lactation,* New York, 1974, Academic Press.
198. Wall VR: Breastfeeding and migraine headaches, *J Hum Lact* 8:209, 1992.
199. Wand JS: The natural history of carpal tunnel syndrome in lactation, *J R Soc Med* 82:349, 1989.
200. Wand JS: Carpal tunnel syndrome in pregnancy and lactation, *J Hand Surg* 15B:93, 1990.
201. Welch MJ, Phelps DL, Osher AB: Breastfeeding by a mother with cystic fibrosis, *Pediatrics* 67:664, 1981.
202. Whichelow MJ, Doddridge MC: Lactation in diabetic women, *Br Med J* 287:649, 1983.
203. White WB: Management of hypertension during lactation, *Hypertension* 6:297, 1984.
204. Williams JM, Auerbach KG, Jacobi A: Lateral epicondylitis (tennis elbow) in breastfeeding mothers, *Clin Pediatr* 28:42, 1989.
205. Woolridge MW: The "anatomy" of infant sucking, *Midwifery* 2:164, 1986.
206. Yagnik PM: Carpal tunnel syndrome in nursing mothers, *South Med J* 80:1468, 1987.
207. Zargar AH, Masoodi SR, Laway BA et al: Familial puerperal alactogenesis: possibility of a genetically transmitted isolated prolactin deficiency, *Br J Obstet Gynecol* 104:629, 1997.

Transmission of infectious diseases through breast milk and breastfeeding

ROBERT M. LAWRENCE

A large body of evidence clearly demonstrates the protective effects of breastfeeding and documents the transmission of specific infections to the infant through breast milk. The fear and anxiety that arise with the occurrence of any infectious disease are even greater in the situation of the breastfeeding mother-infant dyad. Uncertainty and lack of knowledge often lead to proscribing against breastfeeding out of fear, which then deprives the infant of the potential protective, nutritional, and emotional benefits of breastfeeding exactly at the time when they are most needed. Decisions concerning breastfeeding in the mother with an infectious illness should balance the potential benefits of breastfeeding versus the known or estimated risk of the infant acquiring a clinically significant infection via breastfeeding and the potential severity of the infection.

Documenting transmission of infection from mother to infant by breastfeeding requires not only the exclusion of other possible mechanisms of transmission but also the demonstration of the infectious agent in the breast milk and a subsequent clinically significant infection in the infant caused by a plausible infectious process. The first step is to establish the occurrence of a specific infection (clinically or immunologically evident) in the mother and demonstrate the persistence of the infectious agent in the mother such that it could still be transmitted to the infant. Isolation or identification of the infectious agent from the colostrum, breast milk, or an infectious lesion of the breast is important but not necessarily proof of transmission to the infant. Epidemiologic evidence of transmission must be considered, including identifying characteristics of the organism that relate an isolate from the infant to the maternal isolate. Infectious organisms can reach the breast milk either by secretion in the fluid or cellular components of breast milk or by contamination of the milk at the time of or after expression. A reasonable mechanism of infection via breast milk should be evident and proved through either animal or human studies. Demonstration of a subclinical or clinically evident infection in the infant should follow the just outlined steps.

Exclusion of other possible mechanisms of transmission (exposure to the mother or other persons/animals via airborne, droplet, arthropod, or vector modes of transmission or through direct contact with other infectious fluids) would complete the confirmation of transmission of infection via breastfeeding. It is essential to exclude prenatal or perinatal transmission of infection to the fetus/infant, but doing this can often be difficult.

Clinical case reports or studies confirming the isolation of an infectious agent from the milk are important. To determine a reasonable estimate of the risk of infection via breast milk, larger epidemiologic studies are needed comparing infection rates in breastfed infants versus formula-fed infants, addressing the issues just identified. Timing of breastfeeding is important relative to the timing of maternal infection and to the presence of a pathogen in colostrum or breast milk. The duration of breastfeeding is another important variable to consider in the estimate of risk, because shedding of a pathogen in breast milk may be intermittent.

These considerations are just some of the variables to be taken into account, in general, to assess the risk of transmission of an infectious agent from mother to infant via breast milk or breastfeeding. Efforts to prove transmission of infection in a particular maternal-infant dyad can be just as difficult and must consider many of the same factors.

This chapter focuses on a discussion of specific, clinically relevant, infectious agents and diseases, with reasonable estimates of the risk of infection to the infant from breastfeeding. The basic tenet concerning breastfeeding and infection is that *breastfeeding is rarely contraindicated in maternal infection.* The few exceptions relate to specific infectious agents with strong evidence of transmission and to the association of the infant's illness with significant morbidity and mortality.

The risk or benefit of breastfeeding relative to immunization of the mother or infant is discussed for certain microorganisms. Chapter 11 addresses use of antimicrobial agents in the breastfeeding mother, and Chapter 5 reviews how breastfeeding may protect against infection. Chapter 20 addresses specific concerns relating to banked breast milk and includes standards developed by the Human Milk Banking Association of North America to guide the appropriate handling of banked human milk relative to possible infectious agents.

INFECTION CONTROL CONSIDERATIONS

Isolation precautions have undergone some revisions in terminology and conceptualization in recent years.[68] Understanding that the transmission of microorganisms can occur with a known infection and with unrecognized sources of infection, recommendations have been made for standard precautions to be applied to all patients to protect health care workers from potentially infectious body fluids. Additionally, precautions based on the predominant modes of transmission have been recommended to protect against infection through the airborne route, direct contact, or contact with droplets. Although these precautions are intended to be used in clinical situations to protect health care workers, they may be applied in certain situations to the mother-infant dyad to prevent transmission of infectious agents from one to the other or to other hospitalized mothers and infants. These precautions are useful most often when the mother and infant are still hospitalized.

Standard precautions include preventing contact with blood, all body fluids, secretions and excretions, nonintact skin, and mucous membranes by (1) careful handwashing before and after every patient contact; (2) use of gloves when touching body fluids, nonintact skin, or mucous membranes or any items contaminated with body fluids (linens, equipment, devices, etc.); (3) use of nonsterile gowns to prevent contact of clothing with body fluids; (4) use of masks, eye protection, or face shields when splashing with body fluids is possible; and (5) appropriate disposal of these materials. Standard precautions should be applied to all patients regardless of actual or perceived risks.

In considering the breastfeeding infant-mother dyad and standard precautions, body fluids other than breast milk should be avoided, and only in specified situations should breast milk also be avoided. In general, clothing or a gown for the mother and bandages, if necessary, should prevent direct contact with nonintact skin or secretions. Avoiding infant contact with maternal mucous membranes requires mothers to be aware of and understand the risks and to make a conscious effort to avoid this type of contact. The use of gloves, gowns, and masks by the infant for protection is neither practical nor appropriate. The recommendations concerning the appropriateness of breastfeeding and breast milk are addressed for specific infectious agents throughout this chapter. Human immunodeficiency virus (HIV) infection is an example of one infection that can be prevented by the use of standard precautions, including avoiding breast milk and breastfeeding. The recommendations concerning breastfeeding and HIV and the various variables and considerations involved are discussed later.

Airborne precautions are intended to prevent transmission via droplet nuclei (dried respiratory particles less than 5 μm in size that contain microorganisms and can remain suspended in the air for long periods) or dust particles containing microorganisms. Airborne precautions include the use of a private room with a negative-air-pressure ventilation and masks at all times. In the case of pulmonary tuberculosis (TB), respiratory protective devices (requiring personal fitting and seal testing before use) should be worn. Airborne precautions are recommended with measles, varicella or disseminated zoster, and TB. Breastfeeding in the situation of these maternal infections is prohibited for the infectious period. This is to protect against airborne contact with the mother and to allow the infant to be fed the mother's expressed breast milk by another individual. The exception to allowing breast milk would be local involvement of the breast by varicella-zoster lesions or *Mycobacterium tuberculosis,* such that the milk becomes contaminated by the infectious agent.

Transmission via droplets occurs when an individual produces droplets that travel only a short distance in the air and then contact a new host's eyes, nose, mouth, or skin. The common mechanisms for producing droplets include coughing, sneezing, talking (singing or yelling), suction-ing, intubation, nasogastric tube placement, or bronchoscopy. Droplet precautions include the use of a private room (preferred) and a mask if within 3 feet (0.9 m) of the patient, in addition to standard precautions applied to all patients. Droplet precautions are recommended for adenovirus, diphtheria, respiratory infections, *Haemophilus influenzae, Neisseria meningitidis* or invasive infection, influenza, mumps, mycoplasma, parvovirus, pertussis, plague (pneumonic), rubella, and streptococcal pharyngitis, pneumonia, or scarlet fever. The institution of droplet precautions with a breastfeeding mother who has these infections should be specified for each particular infection. This may require some period of separation for the infant and mother (for duration of the illness, for short-term or complete treatment of the mother, for the infectious period) with use of expressed breast milk for nutrition in the interim. Prophylactic treatment of the infant, maternal use of a mask during breastfeeding or close contact combined with meticulous handwashing, and the mother's avoidance of touching her mucous membranes may be adequate and reasonable with regard to certain infections.

Contact precautions are meant to prevent transmission of infection via direct contact (contact between the body surfaces of one individual with another) and indirect contact (contact of a susceptible host with an object contaminated with microorganisms from another individual). Contact precautions include cohorting or a private room, gloves and gowns at all times, and handwashing after removal of gown and gloves. Contact precautions are recommended for a long list of infections, such as diarrhea in diapered or incontinent patients with *Clostridium difficile* infection, *Escherichia coli* O157:H7, shigella, rotavirus, hepatitis A, respiratory illness with parainfluenzae virus or respiratory syncytial virus, multidrug-resistant bacteria (e.g., enterococci, staphylococci, gram-negative organisms), enteroviral infections, cutaneous diphtheria, impetigo, herpes simplex virus infection, herpes zoster (disseminated or in immunocompromised individuals), pediculosis, scabies, *Staphylococcus aureus* skin infection, viral hemorrhagic fevers (e.g., Ebola, Lassa), conjunctivitis and abscesses, cellulitis, or decubiti that cannot be contained by dressings.[38] With regard to the breastfeeding infant-mother dyad, implementation of precautions for each of these infections in the mother requires meticulous attention to gowning and handwashing by the mother, as well as a specialized plan for each situation.

Each of these transmission-based precautions can be used together for organisms or illnesses that can be transmitted by more than one route. They should always be used in conjunction with standard precautions, which are recommended for all patients. The *Red Book: Report of the Committee on Infectious Diseases* by the American Academy of Pediatrics (AAP)[38] remains an excellent resource for infection control guidelines and recommendations to prevent transmission in specific situations and infections.

CLINICAL SYNDROMES AND CONDITIONS

Microorganisms produce a whole spectrum of clinical illnesses affecting the mother and infant. Many situations carry the risk of transmission of the involved organism from the mother to the infant, or vice versa; in general, however, the infant is at greater risk because of such factors as inoculum size and immature immune response. As always, the infection must be accurately diagnosed in a timely manner. Empiric therapy and initial infection control precautions should begin promptly, based on the clinical syndrome and the most likely etiologic agents. When dealing with a maternal infection, clarifying the possible modes of transmission and estimating the relative risk of transmission to the infant are essential first steps to decision making concerning the issues of isolating the mother from the infant and the appropriateness of continuing breastfeeding or providing expressed breast milk. Breastfeeding infrequently is contraindicated in specific maternal infections. Often the question of isolation and interruption of breastfeeding arises when symptoms of fever, pain, inflammation, or other manifestations of illness

first develop in the mother and the diagnosis is still in doubt. A clinical judgment must be made as to the site of infection, probable organisms involved, possible or actual mechanisms of transmission of these organisms to the infant, estimated virulence of the organism, and likely susceptibility of the infant. Many situations associated with maternal fever do not require separation of the mother and infant, such as engorgement of the breasts, atelectasis, localized nonsuppurative phlebitis, or urinary tract infection (UTI).

Appendix E lists a number of clinical syndromes, conditions, and organisms that require infection control precautions while in the hospital. This appendix also includes short lists of possible etiologic agents for these conditions and appropriate precautions and recommendations concerning breastfeeding for different scenarios or organisms. This chapter considers specific infectious agents that are very common, clinically significant, or of particular interest.

BACTERIAL INFECTIONS

Brucellosis

Brucella melitensis has been isolated in the milk of animals. Foods and animals represent the primary sources of infection in humans. Brucellosis demonstrates a broad spectrum of illness in humans, from subclinical to subacute to chronic illness with nonspecific signs of weakness, fever, malaise, body aches, fatigue, sweats, arthralgia, and lymphadenitis. In areas where the disease is enzootic, childhood illness has been described more frequently. The clinical manifestations in children are similar to those in adults.[111] Infection can occur during pregnancy, leading to abortion (infrequently), and can produce transplacental spread, causing neonatal infection (rarely). The transmission of *B. melitensis* through breast milk has been implicated in neonatal infection, although not proved.[111,112] Interruption of breastfeeding with breast pumping and discarding the milk to continue stimulation of milk production is appropriate;

breastfeeding should then continue after an initial period of 48 to 72 hours of therapy in the mother. Acceptable medications for treating the mother while continuing breastfeeding include streptomycin, tetracycline, trimethoprim-sulfamethoxazole (TMP-SMX), and rifampin (see Appendix E).

Botulism

Considerable justifiable concern has been expressed because of the reports of sudden infant death from botulism. Infant botulism is distinguished from food-borne botulism from improperly preserved food containing the toxin and from wound botulism from spores entering the wound. Infant botulism occurs when the spores of *Clostridium botulinum* germinate and multiply in the gut and produce the botulinal toxin in the gastrointestinal tract.[8] The toxin binds presynaptically at the neuromuscular junction, preventing acetylcholine release. The clinical picture is descending, symmetric flaccid paralysis. The gut of only some infants is susceptible, as many infants and adults are exposed. When a previously healthy infant under 6 months of age develops constipation, then weakness and difficulty sucking, swallowing, crying, or breathing, botulism is a likely diagnosis. The organisms should be looked for in the stools; electromyography (EMG) may or may not be helpful.

In a group reviewed by Arnon et al,[10] 33 of 50 patients hospitalized in California were still being nursed at onset of the illness. A beneficial effect of human milk was observed in the difference in the mean age at onset, with breastfed infants being twice as old as formula-fed infants with the disease, and the breastfed infants' symptoms were milder. Breastfed infants receiving iron supplements developed the disease earlier than those who were breastfed but unsupplemented. Of the cases of sudden infant death from botulism, no infants were breastfed within 10 weeks of death. All were receiving iron-fortified formulas. The only known food exposure that has been implicated is *honey*, in not more than 35% of the world cases. (Honey may contain botulism spores, which

can germinate in the infant gut. However, botulin toxin has not been identified in honey.) It has been recommended that honey not be given to infants under 12 months of age. This includes putting honey on a mother's nipples to initiate an infant's interest in suckling.

Arnon[9] reviewed the first 10 years of infant botulism monitoring worldwide. The disease has been reported from 41 of the 50 states and from eight countries on four continents. The relationship to breastfeeding and human milk is unclear. In general, the acid stools (pH 5.1 to 5.4) of human milk–fed infants encourage *Bifidobacterium* species but very few facultatively anaerobic bacteria, and clostridia as spores are virtually absent. In contrast, formula-fed infants have stool pHs ranging from 5.9 to 8.0, with few *bifidobacteria*, clostridia, anaerobic streptococci, and facultative anaerobic bacteria. *C. botulinum* and toxin production declines with pH and usually stops below 4.6. Breast milk also contains the protective immunologic components.

The relationship between the introduction of solid foods or weaning in both formula-fed and breastfed infants and the onset of botulism remains unclear. For the breastfed infant, the introduction of solid food may cause a major change in the gut with a rapid rise in the growth of enterobacteria and enterococci followed by progressive colonization by Bacteroides species, clostridia, and anaerobic streptococci. Feeding solids to formula-fed infants changes nothing. Although more hospitalized infants have been breastfed, sudden-death victims are younger and have been formula-fed, which supports the concept of immunologic protection in the gut of the breastfed infant.

Much work remains to understand the disease. Clinically, constipation, weakness, and hypotonicity in a previously healthy child constitute botulism until ruled out, especially with recent dietary changes. At this time, no reason exists to suspect breastfeeding as a risk for infant botulism, and some evidence suggests a possible protective effect from breastfeeding. Breastfeeding should continue if botulism is suspected in the mother or infant.

Chlamydial infections

Chlamydial infection is the most frequent sexually transmitted disease (STD) in the United States and is a frequent cause of conjunctivitis and pneumonitis in the infant from perinatal infection. The major determinant of whether chlamydial infection occurs in the newborn is the prevalence rate of chlamydial infection of the cervix.[153] Specific chlamydial immunoglobulin A (IgA) has been found in colostrum and breast milk in a small number of postpartum women who were seropositive for *Chlamydia*. No information is available on the role of milk antibodies in protection against infection in the infant.[161] It is not believed that *Chlamydia* is transmitted via breast milk. Use of erythromycin or tetracycline to treat the mother and oral erythromycin and ophthalmic preparations of tetracyclines, erythromycin, or sulfonamides to treat suspected infection in the infant are appropriate during continued breastfeeding. Separating the infant from a mother with chlamydial infection or stopping breastfeeding is not indicated.

Diphtheria

Corynebacterium diphtheriae causes several forms of clinical disease, including membranous nasopharyngitis, obstructive laryngotracheitis, and cutaneous infection. Complications can include airway obstruction from membrane formation and toxin-mediated central nervous system (CNS) disease or myocarditis. The overall incidence of diphtheria has declined even though immunization does not prevent infection but does prevent severe disease from toxin production. Less than five cases are reported annually in the United States.

Transmission occurs via droplets or direct contact with contaminated secretions from the nose, throat, eye, or skin. Infection occurs in individuals whether they have been immunized or not, but infection in those not immunized is more severe and prolonged. As long as the skin of the breast is not involved, no risk of transmission exists via breast milk. No toxin-mediated disease has been reported in a infant from toxin transmitted through breast milk.

Breastfeeding, along with chemoprophylaxis and immunization of the infant, is appropriate in the absence of cutaneous breast involvement (see Appendix E).

Haemophilus influenzae

Haemophilus influenzae type B can cause severe invasive disease such as meningitis, sinusitis, pneumonia, epiglottitis, septic arthritis, pericarditis, and bacteremia. Shock can also occur. Since the increased utilization of the *H. influenzae* type B conjugate vaccines, invasive disease caused by *Haemophilus* has decreased dramatically, more than 95%, in the United States. Most invasive disease occurs in children 3 months to 3 years of age. Older children and adults rarely experience severe disease but do serve as sources of infection for young children. Children less than 3 months of age seem to be protected because of passively acquired antibodies from the mother, and some additional benefit may be received from breast milk.

Transmission occurs through contact with respiratory secretions, and droplet precautions are protective. No evidence suggests transmission through breast milk or breastfeeding.

In the rare case of maternal infection, an inadequately immunized infant in the household is an indication to provide rifampin prophylaxis and close observation for all household contacts, including the breastfeeding infant. Expressed breast milk can be given to the infant during the 24-hour separation, or if the mother's illness prevents breastfeeding, it can be reinitiated when the mother is able (see Appendix E).

Leprosy

Although uncommon in the United States, leprosy occurs throughout the world. This chronic disease presents with a spectrum of symptoms depending on the tissues involved (typically the skin, peripheral nerves, and mucous membranes of the upper respiratory tract) and the cellular immune response to the causative organism, *Mycobacterium leprae*. Transmission occurs through long-term contact with individuals with untreated or multibacillary (large numbers of organisms in the tissues) disease.

Leprosy is not a contraindication to breastfeeding, according to Jeliffe and Jeliffe.[92] The importance of breastfeeding and urgency of treatment are recognized by experts who treat the infant and mother early and simultaneously. No mother-infant contact is permitted except to breastfeed. Dapsone, rifampin, and clofazimine are typically and safely used for the infant and mother regardless of the method of feeding (see Appendix E).

Listeriosis

Listeriosis is a relatively uncommon infection that can have a broad range of manifestations. In immunocompetent individuals, including pregnant women, the infection can vary from being asymptomatic to presenting as an influenza-like illness, occasionally with gastrointestinal (GI) symptoms or back pain. Severe disease occurs more frequently in immunodeficient individuals or infants infected in the perinatal period (pneumonia, sepsis, meningitis, granulomatosis infantisepticum).

Although listeriosis during pregnancy may manifest as mild disease in the mother and is often difficult to recognize and diagnose, it is typically associated with stillbirth, abortion, and premature delivery. It is believed that transmission occurs through the transplacental hematogenous route, infecting the amniotic fluid, although ascending infection from the genital tract may occur.[57] Early and effective treatment of the mother can prevent fetal infection and sequelae.[94,110] Neonatal infection occurs as either early or late-onset infection from transplacental spread late in pregnancy, ascending infection during labor and delivery, infection during passage through the birth canal, or, rarely, during postnatal exposure.

No evidence in the literature suggests transmission of *Listeria* through breast milk. Treatment of the mother with ampicillin, penicillin, or TMP-SMX is not a contraindication to breastfeeding as long as the mother is well enough. Expressed colostrum or breast milk also can be given as long

as the infant is able to feed orally. The management of lactation and feeding in neonatal listeriosis is conducted supportively, as it is in any situation in which the infant is extremely ill, beginning feeding with expressed milk or directly breastfeeding as soon as is reasonable.

Meningococcal infections

Neisseria meningitidis most often causes severe invasive infections, including meningococcemia or meningitis often associated with fever and a rash and progressing to purpura, disseminated intravascular coagulation (DIC), shock, coma, and death.

Transmission occurs via respiratory droplets. Spread can occur from an infected, ill individual or from an asymptomatic carrier. Droplet precautions are recommended until 24 hours after initiation of effective therapy. Despite the frequent occurrence of bacteremia, no evidence indicates breast involvement or transmission through breast milk.

The risk of maternal infection to the infant after birth is from droplet exposure and exists whether the infant is breastfeeding or bottle feeding. In either case the exposed infant should receive chemoprophylaxis with rifampin, 10 mg/kg/dose every 12 hours for 2 days (5 mg/kg/dose for infants less than 1 month of age), or ceftriaxone, 125 mg intramuscularly (IM) once, for children less than 12 years of age. Close observation of the infant should continue for 7 days, and breastfeeding during and after prophylaxis is appropriate. The severity of maternal illness may prevent breastfeeding, but it can continue if the mother is able once the mother and infant have begun receiving antibiotics for 24 hours. A period of separation from the index case for the first 24 hours of effective therapy is recommended; expressed breast milk can be given during this period.

Pertussis

Respiratory illness caused by *Bordetella pertussis* evolves in three stages: *catarrhal* (nasal discharge, congestion, increasing cough), *paroxysmal* (severe paroxysms of cough sometimes ending in an inspiratory whoop, i.e., whooping cough), and *convalescent* (gradual improvement in symptoms).

Transmission is via respiratory droplets. The greatest risk of transmission occurs in the catarrhal phase, often before the diagnosis of pertussis. The nasopharyngeal culture usually becomes negative after 5 days of antibiotic therapy. Chemoprophylaxis for all household contacts is routinely recommended. No evidence indicates transmission through breast milk, with similar risk to breastfed and bottle-fed infants.

In the case of maternal infection with pertussis, chemoprophylaxis for all household contacts, regardless of age or immunization status, is indicated. In addition to chemoprophylaxis of the infant, close observation and subsequent immunization (in infants greater than 6 weeks of age) are appropriate. Despite chemoprophylaxis, droplet precautions and separation of the mother and infant during the first 5 days of effective maternal antibiotic therapy are recommended. Expressed breast milk can be provided to the infant during this period.

Tuberculosis

The face of TB is changing throughout the world. In the United States the incidence of TB rose during 1986 through 1993 and has been declining since then.[26] Increased rates of TB were noted in adults between 25 and 45 years of age, and because these are the primary childbearing years, the risk of transmission to children increased.

Tuberculosis during pregnancy has always been a significant concern for patient and physician alike.[144] It is now clear that the course and prognosis of TB in pregnancy are less affected by the pregnancy and more determined by the location and extent of disease, as defined primarily by the chest radiograph, and by the susceptibility of the individual patient. Untreated TB in pregnancy is associated with maternal and infant mortality rates of 30% to 40%.[154] Effective therapy is crucial to the clinical outcome in both pregnant and nonpregnant women. TB during pregnancy rarely results in congenital TB.

Any individual in a high-risk group for TB should be screened with a tuberculin skin test (TST). No contraindication or altered responsiveness to the TST exists during pregnancy or breastfeeding. Interpretation of the TST should follow the most recent guidelines, using different sizes of induration in different-risk populations as cutoffs for a positive test, as proposed by the Centers for Disease Control and Prevention (CDC).[29] Figure 16-1 outlines the evaluation and treatment of a pregnant woman with a positive TST.[167]

Treatment of active TB should begin as soon as the diagnosis is made, regardless of the fetus' gestational age, because the risk of disease to the mother and fetus clearly outweighs the risks of treatment. Isoniazid, rifampin, and ethambutol have been used safely in all three trimesters. Isoniazid and pyridoxine therapy during breastfeeding is safe, although the risk of hepatotoxicity in the mother may be a concern during the first 2 months postpartum.[163]

Congenital TB is extremely rare if one considers that 7 to 8 million cases of TB disease occur each year worldwide and that less than 300 cases of congenital TB have been reported in the literature, although a case occurred in Rochester, NY in 1997. As with other infectious diseases presenting in the perinatal period, distinguishing congenital infection from perinatal or postnatal TB in the infant can be difficult.

Postnatal TB infection in infancy typically presents with severe disease and extrapulmonary extension (meningitis, lymphadenopathy, and bone, liver, spleen involvement). Airborne transmission of TB to infants is the major mode of postnatal infection because of close and prolonged exposure in enclosed spaces, especially in their own household, to any adult with infectious pulmonary TB. Potential infectious sources could be the mother or any adult caregiver, such as babysitters, day-care workers, relatives, friends, neighbors, and even health care workers.

The suspicion of TB infection or disease in a household with possible exposure of an infant is a highly anxiety-provoking situation (Fig. 16-2). Although protection of the infant from infection is

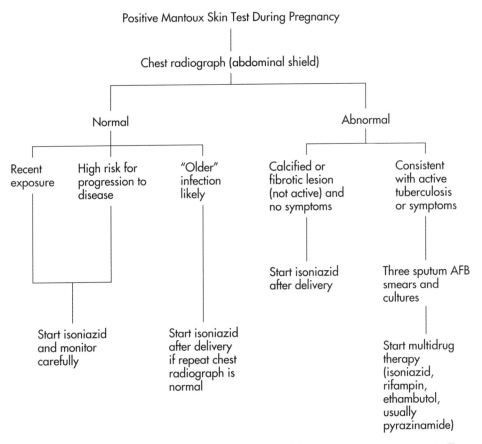

Positive Mantoux Skin Test During Pregnancy

Chest radiograph (abdominal shield)

Normal — Abnormal

Recent exposure

High risk for progression to disease

"Older" infection likely

Calcified or fibrotic lesion (not active) and no symptoms

Consistent with active tuberculosis or symptoms

Start isoniazid after delivery

Three sputum AFB smears and cultures

Start isoniazid and monitor carefully

Start isoniazid after delivery if repeat chest radiograph is normal

Start multidrug therapy (isoniazid, rifampin, ethambutol, usually pyrazinamide)

Fig. 16-1. Evaluation and treatment of pregnant woman with positive tuberculin skin test. (From Starke JR: *Clin Perinatol* 24:107, 1997.)

foremost in everyone's mind, separation of the infant from the mother should be avoided when reasonable. Every situation is unique, and the best approach will vary according to the specifics of the case and accepted principles of TB management. The first step in caring for the potentially exposed infant is to determine accurately the true TB status of the suspected case (mother or household contact). This prompt evaluation should include a complete history (previous TB infection or disease, previous or ongoing TB treatment, TST status, symptoms suggestive of active TB, results of most recent chest radiograph, sputum smears, or cultures), physical examination, a TST if indicated, a new chest radiograph, and mycobacterial cultures

and smears of any suspected sites of infection. All household contacts should be evaluated promptly, including history and TST with further evaluation as indicated. Continued risk to the infant can occur from infectious household contacts who have not been effectively evaluated and treated.

The infant should be separated temporarily from the suspected source if symptoms suggest active disease or a recent TST documents conversion, and separation should continue until the results of the chest radiograph. Because of considerable variability in the course of illness and the concomitant infectious period, debate continues without adequate data about the appropriate period of separation.[119] This should be individualized

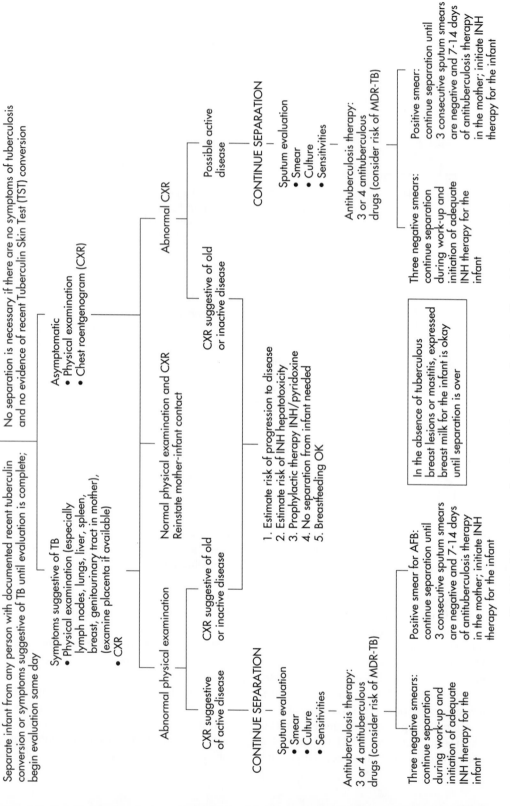

Positive Tuberculin Skin Test in the Postpartum Mother or a Household Contact of a Newborn Infant

Separate infant from any person with documented recent tuberculin conversion or symptoms suggestive of TB until evaluation is complete; begin evaluation same day

No separation is necessary if there are no symptoms of tuberculosis and no evidence of recent Tuberculin Skin Test (TST) conversion

Symptoms suggestive of TB
• Physical examination (especially lymph nodes, lungs, liver, spleen, breast, genitourinary tract in mother), (examine placenta if available)
• CXR

Asymptomatic
• Physical examination
• Chest roentgenogram (CXR)

Abnormal physical examination

Normal physical examination and CXR
Reinstate mother-infant contact

Abnormal CXR

CXR suggestive of active disease

CXR suggestive of old or inactive disease

1. Estimate risk of progression to disease
2. Estimate risk of INH hepatotoxicity
3. Prophylactic therapy INH/pyridoxine
4. No separation from infant needed
5. Breastfeeding OK

CXR suggestive of old or inactive disease

Possible active disease

CONTINUE SEPARATION

Sputum evaluation
• Smear
• Culture
• Sensitivities

Antituberculosis therapy:
3 or 4 antituberculous drugs (consider risk of MDR-TB)

In the absence of tuberculous breast lesions or mastitis, expressed breast milk for the infant is okay until separation is over

CONTINUE SEPARATION

Sputum evaluation
• Smear
• Culture
• Sensitivities

Antituberculosis therapy:
3 or 4 antituberculous drugs (consider risk of MDR-TB)

Positive smear for AFB: continue separation until 3 consecutive sputum smears are negative and 7-14 days of antituberculosis therapy in the mother; initiate INH therapy for the infant

Three negative smears: continue separation during work-up and initiation of adequate INH therapy for the infant

Positive smear: continue separation until 3 consecutive sputum smears are negative and 7-14 days of antituberculosis therapy in the mother; initiate INH therapy for the infant

Three negative smears: continue separation during work-up and initiation of adequate INH therapy for the infant

Fig. 16-2. Management of newborn infant exposed to tuberculin-positive household contact.

given the specific situation. HIV testing and assessment of the risk of multidrug-resistant TB (MDR-TB) should be done in every case of active TB. Sensitivity testing should be done on every *Mycobacterium tuberculosis* isolate. Table 16-1 summarizes the management of the newborn infant whose mother (or other household contact) has TB.

Initiation of prophylactic isoniazid therapy in the infant has been demonstrated to be effective in preventing TB infection and disease in the infant. Therefore continued separation of the infant and mother is unnecessary once therapy in both mother and child has begun.[49] The real risk to the infant requiring separation is from airborne transmission. Separation of the infant from a mother with active pulmonary TB is appropriate regardless of the method of feeding.

Tuberculous mastitis occurs very rarely in the United States but does occur occasionally in other parts of the world[75] and can lead to infection in the infant, frequently involving the tonsils. The mother usually has a single breast mass and associated axillary lymph node swelling and infrequently develops a draining sinus. TB of the breast can also present as a painless mass or edema. Involvement of the breast can occur with or without evidence of disease at other sites. Evaluation of extent of disease is appropriate, including lesion cultures by needle aspiration, biopsy, or wedge resection and milk cultures. Therapy should be with multiple antituberculous medications, but surgery should supplement this, as needed, to remove extensive necrotic tissue or a persistently draining sinus.[7] Neither breastfeeding nor breast-milk feeding should be done until the lesion is healed, usually 2 weeks or more. Continued antituberculous therapy for 6 months in the mother and isoniazid for the infant for 3 to 6 months is indicated.

In the absence of tuberculous breast infection in the mother, transmission of TB through breast milk has not been documented. Thus, even though temporary separation of the infant and mother may occur pending complete evaluation and initiation of adequate therapy in the mother and prophylactic isoniazid therapy (10 mg/kg/day as a single dose) in the infant, breast milk can be expressed

and given to the infant during the short separation. Breastfeeding can safely continue whether the mother, infant, or both are receiving antituberculous therapy. Antituberculous medications (isoniazid, rifampin, pyrazinamide, aminoglycosides, ethambutol, ethionamide, *p*-aminosalicylic acid) have been safely used in infancy, and therefore the presence of these medications in smaller amounts in breast milk is not a contraindication to breastfeeding.

Although conflicting, reports indicate that breastfeeding by TST-positive mothers does influence the infant's response to bacille Calmette-Guérin (BCG) vaccine, the TST, and perhaps the *M. tuberculosis* bacillus. Despite efforts to identify either a soluble substance or specific cell fractions (gamma/delta T cells) in colostrum and breast milk that affect the infant's immune responsiveness, no unified theory explains the various reported changes and no evidence has identified a consistent, clinically significant effect.[21,97,135,156]

Staphylococcal infections

Staphylococcal infection in the neonate can be caused by either *Staphylococcus aureus* or coagulase-negative staphylococci (most often *S. epidermidis*) and can manifest in a wide range of illnesses. Localized infection can be impetigo, cellulitis, or wound infection, and invasive or suppurative disease includes sepsis, pneumonia, osteomyelitis, arthritis, and endocarditis. *S. aureus* requires only a small inoculum (10 to 250 organisms) to produce colonization in the newborn, most often of the nasal mucosa and umbilicus.[89] By the fifth day of life, 40% to 90% of the infants in the nursery will be colonized with *S. aureus*.[59] The organism is easily transmitted to others from mother, infant, family, or health care personnel through direct contact. Outbreaks in the nursery were common in the past. Mothers, infants, health care workers, and even contaminated, unpasteurized, banked breast milk were sources of infection.[138] Careful use of antibiotics, changes in nursery layout and procedures, standard precautions, and cohorting as needed have decreased the spread

TABLE 16-1 Management of newborn whose mother (or other household contact) has tuberculosis (TB)

Mother/infant status	Additional workup recommended[1]	Therapy for mother/contact	Therapy for infant	Separation[2]	Breast milk[3]	Breast-feeding[3]
1. TB infection, no disease[4]	None for mother/contact	Prophylactic[5]	None	No	Yes	Yes
2. TB infection: abnormal CXR not suggestive of active disease		Decide active vs. inactive disease				
a. Symptoms or physical findings suggestive of active TB	Aerosolized sputums (culture, smears)[6]	Active disease: empiric[5] Inactive disease: prophylactic[5]	Isoniazid[7] None	Yes No	Yes Yes	No[8] Yes
b. No symptoms or physical findings suggestive of active TB	Aerosolized sputums in select cases	Prophylactic[5]	None	No	Yes	Yes
3. TB infection: abnormal CXR suggestive of active disease	Aerosolized sputums (culture, smears)[6]	Empiric therapy[5]	Isoniazid[7]	Yes	Yes	No[8]
4. Active pulmonary TB: suspected multi/drug-resistant (MDR) TB	Aerosolized sputums (culture, smears)[6]	Consult TB specialist for best regimen[9]	Consult pediatric TB specialist[9] Consider bacille Calmette-Guérin (BCG) vaccine	Yes	Yes	No
5. TB disease: suspected mastitis[10]	Aerosolized sputums (culture, smears)[6]	Empiric[5]	Isoniazid[7]	Yes	No[11]	No

	Perform/interpret CXR within 24 hours	Yes, until CXR interpreted (see a and b)	Yes	No
6. TB infection: status undetermined[12]		Yes, until CXR interpreted (see a and b)		
a. Abnormal CXR not suggestive of active disease	Proceed as in 2	As in 2	As in 2	
b. Abnormal CXR suggestive of active disease	Proceed as in 3	As in 3	As in 3	

Notes:

Data from Committee on Infectious Diseases, American Academy of Pediatrics: *Red book: report of the Committee on Infectious Diseases*, ed 24, Elk Grove Village, Ill, 1997, The Academy.

1. Further workup should always include evaluation of TB status of all other household (or close) contacts by tuberculin skin testing (TST), review of symptoms, physical examination, and chest x-ray film (CXR). Sputum smears and cultures should be done as indicated.

2. Separation should occur until interpretation of CXR confirms absence of active disease, or with active disease, separation should continue until individual is no longer considered infectious: three negative consecutive sputum smears, adequate ongoing empiric therapy, and decreased fever, cough, and sputum production. *Separation* means in a different house or location, not simply separate rooms in a household. Duration of separation should be individualized for each case in consultation with TB specialist.

3. This assumes no evidence of breast involvement, suspected TB mastitis, or lesion (except in status 5, when breast involvement is considered). Risk to infant is via aerosolized bacteria in sputum from the lung. Expressed breast milk can be given even if separation of mother and infant is advised.

4. TST positive, no symptoms or physical findings suggestive of TB, negative CXR.

5. *Prophylactic therapy:* isoniazid 10 mg/kg/day, maximum 300 mg for 6 months; pyridoxine 25 to 50 mg/day for 6 months. *Empiric therapy:* standard 3- or 4-drug regimens for 2 months, and treatment should continue for total of 6 months with isoniazid and rifampin when organism is shown to be sensitive. Suspected MDR-TB requires consultation with TB specialist to select optimum empiric regimen and for ongoing monitoring of therapy and clinical response.

6. Sensitivity testing should be done on any positive culture.

7. Isoniazid 10 mg/kg/day for 3 to 9 months depending on mother's or contact's status; repeat TST at 3 months. Before beginning therapy, workup of infant for congenital or active TB may be appropriate. This workup should be determined by clinical status of infant and suspected, potential risk. TST after 4 weeks of age, with CXR, complete blood count, and erythrocyte sedimentation rate. Liver function tests, cerebrospinal fluid analysis, gastric aspirates, sonography/computed tomography of liver/spleen, and chest if congenital TB is suspected.

8. Breastfeeding is proscribed when separation of mother and infant is indicated because of risk of aerosolized transmission of bacteria. Expressed breast milk given to infant via bottle is acceptable in absence of mastitis or breast lesions.

9. Consult with TB specialist about MDR-TB. Empiric therapy will be chosen based on the most recent culture sensitivities of index patient or perhaps suspected source case, if known, as well as medication toxicities and other factors.

10. TB mastitis usually involves a single nerve with associated axillary lymph node swelling and, infrequently, a draining sinus tract. It can also present as a painless mass or edema of breast.

11. With suspected mastitis or breast lesion caused by TB, even breast milk is contraindicated, until lesion or mastitis heals, usually 2 weeks or more.

12. Patient has a documented, recent TST conversion but has not been completely evaluated. Evaluation should begin and CXR done and evaluated in less than 24 hours to minimize separation of this person from infant. Further workup should proceed as indicated by symptoms, physical findings, and CXR results.

of *S. aureus* in nurseries. Now the occurrence of methicillin-resistant *S. aureus* (MRSA) is a more common problem, requiring cohorting and occasionally epidemiologic investigation and careful infection control intervention. Breastfeeding can continue during diagnosis and treatment of closed, minor staphylococcal infection in the mother along with standard precautions.

S. aureus is the most common cause of mastitis in lactating women. One case of *staphylococcal scalded skin syndrome* (SSS) was reported by Katzman and Wald[95] in an infant breastfed by a mother with a lesion on her areola that did not respond to ampicillin therapy for 14 days. Subsequently the infant developed conjunctivitis with *S. aureus,* which produced an exfoliative toxin, and a confluent erythematous rash without mucous membrane involvement or Nikolsky's sign. No attempt to identify the exfoliative toxin in the breast milk was made, and the breast milk was not cultured for *S. aureus.* The child responded to intravenous (IV) therapy with nafcillin. This emphasizes the importance of evaluating the mother and infant at the time of a suspected infection and the need for continued observation of the infant for evidence of a pyogenic infection or toxin-mediated disease, especially with breast lesions.

This case also raises the issue of when and how infants and mothers become colonized with *S. aureus* and what factors lead to illness and infection in each. Empiric therapy may be indicated depending on the infant's clinical status. For patients with major open lesions caused by *S. aureus* that cannot be fully contained, with MRSA, or with SSS, the CDC recommends contact precautions in addition to standard precautions for the duration of the illness. The concern is that staphylococci can be easily transmitted, colonization occurs, and potentially serious infection can occur later. With SSS the primary site of infection can be minimal (e.g., conjunctivitis, infection of a circumcision site), but a clinically significant amount of toxin can be produced and lead to severe disease in the infant. However, it seems reasonable that after initiating appropriate antistaphylococcal therapy for the mother for 24 hours, standard precautions

and breastfeeding can be continued whether or not mastitis is present. Some individuals recommend bathing the mother and infant once with hexachlorophene to change the skin flora, but this does not address nasal carriage of *S. aureus.* Evaluation of the infant's status at the time of decision making, continued close observation of the infant, and timely empiric therapy as needed in the infant are also appropriate. The mother and infant can room-in together, without contact with other mothers or infants until discharge.

Toxic shock syndrome (TSS) can result from *S. aureus* or *Streptococcus pyogenes* infection and probably from a variety of antigens produced by other organisms. TSS-1 has been identified as a "superantigen" affecting the T-lymphocytes and other components of the immune response, producing an unregulated and excessive immune response and resulting in an overwhelming systemic clinical response. TSS has been reported in association with vaginal delivery, cesarean birth, mastitis, and other local infections in the mother. Mortality in the mother may be as high as 5%.

The case definition of staphylococcal TSS includes meeting all four major criteria: fever greater than 38.9° C, rash (diffuse macular erythroderma), hypotension, and desquamation (associated with subepidermal separation seen on skin biopsy). The definition also includes involvement of three or more organ systems (GI, muscular, mucous membrane, renal, hepatic, hematologic, or CNS); negative titers for Rocky Mountain spotted fever, leptospirosis, and rubeola; and lack of isolation of *S. pyogenes* from any source or *S. aureus* from the cerebrospinal fluid (CSF).[157] A similar case definition has been proposed for streptococcal TSS.[187] Aggressive empiric antibiotic therapy against staphylococci and streptococci and careful supportive therapy are essential to decreasing morbidity and mortality. Oxacillin, nafcillin, first-generation cephalosporins, clindamycin, erythromycin, and vancomycin are all acceptable antibiotics, even for the breastfeeding mother. The severity of illness in the mother may preclude breastfeeding, but it can be reinitiated when the mother is improving and wants to restart.

Standard precautions, but allowing breastfeeding, are recommended.

Staphylococcal enterotoxin F (SEF) has been identified in breast milk specimens collected on days 5, 8, and 11 from a mother who developed TSS at 22 hours postpartum.[179] *S. aureus* that produced SEF was isolated from the mother's vagina but not from breast milk. The infant and mother lacked significant antibody against SEF in their sera. The infant remained healthy beyond 60 days of follow-up. SEF is pepsin inactivated at pH 4.5 and therefore is probably destroyed in the stomach environment and presents little or no risk to the breastfeeding infant.[20] Breastfeeding can continue if the mother is able.

Coagulase-negative staphylococcal infection (*S. epidermidis* is the predominant isolate) produces minimal disease in healthy, full-term infants but is a significant problem in hospitalized or premature infants. Factors associated with increased risk of this infection include prematurity, high colonization rates in specific nurseries, invasive therapies (e.g., IV lines, chest tubes, intubation), and antibiotic use. Illness produced by coagulase-negative staphylococci can be invasive and severe in high-risk neonates, but rarely in mothers. At 2 weeks of age, for infants still in the nursery, *S. epidermidis* is a frequent colonizing organism at multiple sites, with colonization rates as high as 75% to 100%. Serious infections with coagulase-negative staphylococci (e.g., abscesses, IV line bacteremia/sepsis, endocarditis, osteomyelitis) require IV therapy. Many strains are resistant to penicillin and the semisynthetic penicillins, so sensitivity testing is essential. Empiric or definitive therapy may require treatment with vancomycin, gentamicin, rifampin, teicoplanin, or combinations of these for synergistic activity. Transmission of infection in association with breastfeeding appears to be no more common than with bottle feeding. Infection control includes contact and standard precautions, as with *S. aureus*. Occasionally, during presumed outbreaks, careful epidemiologic surveillance may be required, including cohorting, limiting overcrowding and understaffing, surveillance cultures of infants and nursery personnel,

reemphasis of meticulous infection control techniques for all individuals entering the nursery, and rarely, removal of colonized personnel from direct infant contact.

Streptococcal infections
Group A

Streptococcus pyogenes (β-hemolytic group A *Streptococcus* [GAS]) is a common cause of skin and throat infections in children, producing pharyngitis, cellulitis, and impetigo. Illnesses produced by GAS can be classified in three categories: (1) impetigo, cellulitis, or pharyngitis without invasion or complication; (2) severe invasive infection with bacteremia, necrotizing fasciitis, myositis, or systemic illness (e.g., streptococcal TSS); and (3) autoimmune-mediated phenomena, including acute rheumatic fever and acute glomerulonephritis. GAS can also cause puerperal sepsis, endometritis, and neonatal omphalitis. Significant morbidity and mortality are associated with invasive GAS infection; mortality is approximately 20% to 50%, with almost half the survivors requiring extensive tissue débridement or amputation.[147] Infants are not at risk for the autoimmune sequelae of GAS (rheumatic fever or poststreptococcal glomerulonephritis). Transmission is through direct contact (rarely indirect contact) and droplet spread. Outbreaks of GAS in the nursery are rare, unlike with staphylococcal infections. Either mother or infant can be initially colonized with GAS and transmit it to the other.

In the situation of maternal illness (extensive cellulitis, necrotizing fasciitis, myositis, pneumonia, TSS, mastitis), it is appropriate to separate the mother and infant until effective therapy (penicillin, ampicillin, cephalosporins, erythromycin) has been given for 24 hours. Breastfeeding should also be suspended and may resume after 24 hours of therapy.

Group B

Group B *Streptococcus* (GBS, *S. agalactiae*) is a significant cause of perinatal bacterial infection. In parturient women, infection can lead to asymptomatic bacteriuria, UTI (often associated with premature birth), endometritis, or amnionitis. In infants, infection usually occurs between birth and 3 months of age (1 to 4 cases per 1000 live births). It is routinely classified by the time of onset of illness in the infant: early onset (0 to 7 days, majority less than 24 hours) and late onset (7 to 90 days, generally less than 4 weeks). Infants may develop sepsis, pneumonia, meningitis, osteomyelitis, arthritis, or cellulitis. Early-onset GBS disease is often fulminant, presenting as sepsis or pneumonia with respiratory failure. Almost three quarters of neonatal disease is early onset. Type III is the most common serotype causing disease.

Transmission is believed to occur in utero and during delivery. Colonization rates of mothers and infants have varied between 5% and 35%. Postpartum transmission is thought to be uncommon,

although it has been documented. Risk factors for early-onset GBS disease include delivery before 37 weeks' gestation, rupture of membranes for longer than 18 hours before delivery, intrapartum fever, heavy maternal colonization with GBS, or low concentrations of anti-GBS capsular antibody in maternal sera.[38,39] The common occurrence of severe GBS disease before 24 hours of age in the neonate has lead to prevention strategies. Revised guidelines developed by the AAP Committees on Infectious Diseases and on the Fetus and Newborn[39] have tried to combine various variables for increased risk of GBS infection (prenatal colonization with GBS, obstetric and neonatal risk factors for early-onset disease) and provide intrapartum prophylaxis to those at high risk (Fig. 16-3).

Late-onset GBS disease is thought to be the

* Includes CBC and differential, blood culture, and chest radiograph if respiratory symptoms. A lumbar puncture is performed at the discretion of the physician.
† Duration of therapy will vary depending on results of blood culture and CSF findings (if obtained), as well as on the clinical course of the infant. *If* laboratory results and clinical course are unremarkable, duration may be as short as 48 to 72 hours.
‡ Applies to penicillin or ampicillin chemoprophylaxis.
§ CBC and differential, blood culture.
‖ Does *not* allow early discharge.

Fig. 16-3. Empiric management of neonate born to mother who received intrapartum antimicrobial prophylaxis (IAP) for prevention of early-onset group B streptococcal (GBS) disease. (From Committee on Infectious Diseases and Committee on the Fetus and Newborn, American Academy of Pediatrics: *Pediatrics* 99:489, 1997.)

result of transmission during delivery or in the postnatal period from maternal, hospital, or community sources. Dillon et al[47] demonstrated that 10 of 21 infants with late-onset disease were colonized at birth, but the source of colonization was unidentified in the others. Gardner et al[66] showed that only 4.3% of 46 children who were culture negative for GBS at discharge from the hospital had acquired GBS by 2 months of age. Anthony et al[6] noted that many infants are colonized with GBS, but the actual attack rate for GBS disease is low and difficult to predict.

Acquisition of GBS through breast milk or breastfeeding is rare. Three cases of late-onset GBS disease associated with GBS in the maternal milk have been reported.[98,155] Two of the three mothers had bilateral mastitis, and the third was asymptomatic. It was not clear when colonization of the infants occurred or when infection or disease began. The authors discussed the possibility that the infants were originally colonized during delivery, subsequently colonized the mothers' breasts during breastfeeding, and then became reinfected at a later time. Butter and DeMoor[25] showed that infants initially colonized on their heads at birth had GBS cultured from their throat, nose, or umbilicus 8 days later. Whenever they cultured GBS from the nipples of mothers, the authors also found it in the nose or throat of the infants.

When a breastfed infant develops late-onset GBS disease, it is appropriate to culture the milk and treat the mother to prevent reinfection. Breastfeeding can continue depending on the infant's ability to feed during GBS disease. Routine culturing of infants or breast milk to detect colonization is not recommended or useful. (See Chapter 15 for management of mastitis in the mother.) A mother or infant colonized or infected with GBS should be managed with standard precautions[38] while in the hospital. GBS endometritis in the mother necessitates separation of mother and infant for the first 24 hours of the mother's therapy, but expressed breast milk can be given to the infant during the separation. Timely evaluation of the infant for infection or illness and empiric therapy for GBS in the infant are appropriate until the child has

remained well and cultures are subsequently negative at 72 hours. Occasionally, epidemiologic investigation in hospital will utilize culturing to detect a source of late-onset GBS disease in the nursery. This can be useful when more than one case of late-onset disease is detected with the same serotype. Cohorting in such a situation may be appropriate, but prophylactic therapy to eradicate colonization is impractical. Unlike GAS infection, GBS infection in nurseries has not been reported to cause outbreaks.

Gonococcal infections

Maternal infection with *Neisseria gonorrhoeae* can produce a large spectrum of illness ranging from uncomplicated vulvovaginitis, proctitis, pharyngitis, conjunctivitis, or more severe and invasive disease, including pelvic inflammatory disease (PID), meningitis, endocarditis, or disseminated gonococcal infection. The risk of transmission from the mother to the infant occurs mainly during delivery in the passage through the infected birth canal and occasionally from postpartum contact with the mother (or her partner). There is negligible risk of transmission from breast milk, and *N. gonorrhoeae* does not seem to cause local infection of the breast. Infection in the neonate is most often ophthalmia neonatorum and less often a scalp abscess or disseminated infection. Mothers with presumed or documented gonorrhea should be reevaluated for other STDs, especially *Chlamydia trachomatis* and syphilis, because some therapies for gonorrhea are not adequate for either of these infections.

With the definitive identification of gonorrhea in the mother, empiric therapy should begin immediately, and the mother should be separated from the infant until completion of 24 hours of adequate therapy. Treatment of the mother with ceftriaxone, cefixime, penicillin, or erythromycin is without significant risk to the infant. Single-dose treatment with spectinomycin, ciprofloxacin, ofloxacin, or azithromycin has not been adequately studied but would presumably be safe for the infant given the 24-hour separation and a delay in breastfeeding without giving the infant the expressed breast milk (pump and discard). Doxycycline use in the nursing mother is not recommended.

Careful preventive therapy for ophthalmia neonatorum should be provided, and close observation of the infant should continue for 2 to 7 days, the usual incubation period. Empiric or definitive therapy against *N. gonorrhoeae* may be necessary depending on the infant's clinical status and should be chosen on the basis of the maternal isolate's sensitivity pattern. The mother should not handle other infants until 24 hours of adequate therapy, and the infant should be separated from the rest of the nursery population, with or without breastfeeding.

VIRAL INFECTIONS

Arboviruses

Arboviruses were originally a large collection of viruses grouped together because of the common mode of transmission through arthropods. They have now been reclassified into several different families: Bunyaviridae, Togaviridae, Flaviviridae, Reoviridae, and others. They include more than 30 human pathogens.

These organisms primarily produce either CNS infections (encephalitis, meningoencephalitis) or undifferentiated illnesses associated with fever and rash, severe hemorrhagic manifestations, and involvement of other organs (hepatitis, myalgia, polyarthritis). Infection with this array of viruses may also be asymptomatic and subclinical, although how often this occurs is uncertain. Some of the notable human pathogens include Bunyaviridae (California serogroup viruses), Hantavirus, Hantaan virus, Phlebovirus (Rift Valley fever), Nairovirus (Crimean-Congo hemorrhagic fever [CCHF]), Alphavirus (western, eastern, and Venezuelan equine encephalomyelitis viruses), Flavivirus (St. Louis encephalitis virus, Japanese encephalitis virus, dengue viruses, yellow fever virus, tick-borne encephalitis viruses), and Orbivirus (Colorado tick fever). Other than for CCHF

and for reported cases of Colorado tick fever associated with transfusion, direct person-to-person spread does not seem to occur.

No evidence indicates that these organisms can be transmitted through breast milk. Standard precautions are sufficient. With any of these infections in a breastfeeding mother, the severity of the illness may determine the mother's ability to continue breastfeeding. Providing the infant with expressed breast milk is acceptable.

In general, treatment for these illnesses is supportive. However, ribavirin appears to decrease the severity of and mortality from Hantavirus pulmonary syndrome, hemorrhagic fever with renal failure, and CCHF. Ribavirin has been described as teratogenic in various animal species and is contraindicated in pregnant women. No information is available concerning ribavirin in breast milk, with little information on the use of IV or oral ribavirin in infants.

Arenaviruses

Arenaviruses are single-stranded ribonucleic acid (RNA) viruses that infect rodents and are acquired by humans through the rodents. The six major human pathogens in this group are (1) lymphocytic choriomeningitis virus (LCMV), (2) Lassa fever virus, (3) Junin virus (Argentine hemorrhagic fever), (4) Machupo virus (Bolivian hemorrhagic fever), (5) Guanarito virus (Venezuelan hemorrhagic fever), and (6) Sabia virus. The geographic distribution of these viruses and the illness they cause are determined by the living range of the host rodent (reservoir). The exact mechanism of transmission to humans is unknown and hotly debated.[13,31,64] Direct contact and aerosolization of rodent excretions and secretions are probable mechanisms.

LCMV is well recognized in Europe, the Americas, and other areas. Perinatal maternal infection can lead to severe disease in the newborn, but no evidence suggests transmission through breast milk.[15,100] Standard precautions with breastfeeding are appropriate.

Lassa fever (West Africa) and Argentine hemorrhagic fever (Argentine pampas) are usually more severe illnesses with dramatic bleeding and involvement of other organs, including the brain. These fevers more frequently lead to shock and death than do the forms of hemorrhagic fever caused by the other viruses in this group. Person-to-person spread of Lassa fever is believed to be common, and transmission within households does occur.[96] This may relate to prolonged viremia and excretion of the virus in the urine of humans for up to 30 days.[140] The possibility of persistent virus in human urine, semen, and blood after infection exists for each of the arenaviruses. The possibility of airborne transmission is undecided. Current recommendations by the CDC[31] are to use contact precautions for the duration of the illness in situations of suspected viral hemorrhagic fever. No substantial information describes the infectivity of various body fluids, including breast milk, for these different viral hemorrhagic fevers. Considering the severity of the illness in the mother and the risk to the infant, it is reasonable to avoid breastfeeding in these situations if alternative forms of infant nutrition can be provided.

As more information becomes available, reassessment of these recommendations is advisable. There is a vaccine in clinical trials in endemic areas for Junin virus and Argentine hemorrhagic fever. Preliminary studies suggest it is very effective, but data are still being accumulated concerning the vaccine's use in children and pregnant or breastfeeding women.

Cytomegalovirus

Cytomegalovirus (CMV) is one of the human herpesviruses. Congenital infection of infants, postnatal infection of premature infants, and infection of immunodeficient individuals represent the most serious forms of this infection in children. The time at which the virus infects the fetus or infant and the presence or absence of antibodies against CMV from the mother are important determinants of the severity of infection and the likelihood of significant sequelae (congenital infection syndrome, deafness, chorioretinitis, ab-

normal neurodevelopment, learning disabilities). About 1% of all infants are born excreting CMV at birth, and approximately 5% of these congenitally infected infants will demonstrate evidence of infection at birth (approximately five symptomatic cases per 10,000 live births). Approximately 15% of infants born after primary infection in the pregnant woman will manifest at least one sequela of prenatal infection.[38]

Various studies have detected that 3% to 28% of pregnant women have CMV in cervical cultures and that 4% to 5% of pregnant women have CMV in their urine.[55,78] Perinatal infection certainly occurs through contact with virus in these fluids but usually is not associated with clinical illness in full-term infants. The lack of illness is believed to result from transplacental passive transfer of protective antibodies from the mother.

Postnatal infection later in infancy occurs via breastfeeding or contact with infected fluids (e.g., saliva, urine) but, again, rarely causes clinical illness in full-term infants. Seroepidemiologic studies have documented transmission of infection in infancy, with higher rates of transmission occurring in day-care centers, especially when the prevalence of CMV in the urine and saliva is high. CMV has been identified in the milk of CMV-seropositive women at varying rates (10%-85%) using viral cultures or CMV deoxyribonucleic acid polymerase chain reaction (DNA-PCR).[78,129,166,181] CMV is more often identified in the breast milk of seropositive mothers than in vaginal fluids, urine, and saliva. The CMV isolation rate from colostrum is lower than that from mature milk.[78,165] The reason for the large degree of variability in identification of CMV in breast milk in these studies probably relates to the intermittent nature of reactivation and excretion of the virus, in addition to the variability, frequency, and duration of sampling of breast milk in the different studies. Some authors have hypothesized that the difference in isolation rates between breast milk and other fluids is caused by viral reactivation in cells (leukocytes or monocytes) in the breast leading to "selective" excretion in breast milk.[129] Vochem et al[181] reported that the rate of virolactia was greatest at 3 to 4 weeks postpartum, and Yeager et al[190] reported significant virolactia between 2 and 12 weeks postpartum. Antibodies (e.g., secretory IgA) to CMV are present in breast milk, along with various cytokines and other proteins (e.g., lactoferrin). These may influence virus binding to cells, but they do not prevent transmission of infection.*

Several studies have documented increased rates of postnatal CMV infection in breastfed infants (50% to 69%) compared with bottle-fed infants (12% to 27%) observed through the first year of life.[55,122,166,181] In these same studies, full-term infants who acquired CMV infection postnatally were only rarely mildly symptomatic at the time of seroconversion or documented viral excretion. Also, no evidence of late sequelae from CMV was found in these infants.

Postnatal exposure of susceptible infants to CMV, including premature infants without passively acquired maternal antibodies against CMV, infants born to CMV-seronegative mothers, and immunodeficient infants, can cause significant clinical illness (pneumonitis, hepatitis, thrombocytopenia). In one study of premature infants followed up to 12 months, Vochem et al[181] found CMV transmission in 17 of 29 infants (59%) exposed to CMV virolactia and breastfed compared with no infants infected of 27 exposed to breast milk without CMV. No infant was given CMV-seropositive donor milk or blood. Five of the 12 infants who developed CMV infection after 2 months of age had mild signs of illness, including transient neutropenia, and only one infant had a short increase in episodes of apnea and a period of thrombocytopenia. Five other premature infants with CMV infection before 2 months of age had acute illness, including sepsislike symptoms, apnea with bradycardia, hepatitis, leukopenia, and prolonged thrombocytopenia.[181] Exposure of CMV-seronegative or premature infants to CMV-positive milk (donor or natural mother's) should be avoided. Various methods of inactivating CMV in

breast milk have been reported, including Holder pasteurization, freezing ($-20°$ C for 3 days), and brief high temperature ($72°$ C for 10 seconds).[55,65,74,164,190] The efficacy of such treatments to prevent CMV infection in premature infants has not been studied prospectively.

However, CMV-seropositive mothers can safely breastfeed their full-term infants because, despite a higher rate of CMV infection than in formula-fed infants observed through the first year of life, infection in this situation is not associated with significant clinical illness or sequelae.

Epstein-Barr virus

Epstein-Barr Virus (EBV) is a common infection in children, adolescents, and young adults. It is usually asymptomatic but most notably causes infectious mononucleosis and has been associated with chronic fatigue syndrome (CFS), Burkitt's lymphoma, and nasopharyngeal carcinoma. Because EBV is one of the human herpesviruses, concern has been raised about lifelong latent infection and the potential risk of infection to the fetus and neonate from the mother. Primary EBV infection during pregnancy is unusual because few pregnant women are susceptible.[71,86] Although abortion, premature birth, and congenital infection from EBV are suspected, no distinct group of anomalies is linked to EBV infection in the fetus or neonate. Also, no virologic evidence of EBV as the cause of abnormalities has been found in association with suspected EBV infection.

Culturing of EBV from various fluids or sites is difficult. The virus is detected by its capacity to transform B lymphocytes into persistent lymphoblastoid cell lines. PCR and DNA hybridization studies have detected EBV in the cervix and in breast milk. One study, which identified EBV-DNA in breast milk cells in more than 40% of women donating milk to a breast milk bank, demonstrated that only 17% had antibody to EBV (only IgG, no IgM).[93]

The question of the timing of EBV infection and the subsequent immune response and clinical disease produced requires continued study. Differ-

*References 2, 3, 101, 122, 129, 139, 188.

ences exist among the clinical syndromes manifest at different ages. Infants and young children are asymptomatic, have illness not recognized as related to EBV, or have mild episodes of illness, including fever, lymphadenopathy, rhinitis and cough, hepatosplenomegaly, or rash. Adolescents or young adults who experience primary EBV infection more often demonstrate infectious mononucleosis syndrome or are asymptomatic. CFS is more common in young adults. Burkitt's lymphoma, observed primarily in Africa, and nasopharyngeal carcinoma, seen in southeast Asia, where primary EBV infection usually occurs in young children, are tumors associated with early EBV infection.[173] These tumors are related to "chronic" EBV infection and tend to occur in individuals with persistently high antibody titers to EBV viral capsid antigen and early antigen. The questions of why these tumors occur with much greater frequency in these geographic areas and what cofactors (including altered immune response to infection) may contribute to their development remain unanswered.[11]

It also remains unknown to what degree breast milk could be a source of early EBV infection compared with other sources of EBV infection in the infant's environment. Similar to the situation of postnatal transmission of CMV in immunocompetent infants, clinically significant illness rarely is associated with primary EBV infection in infants. More data concerning the pathogenesis of EBV-associated tumors should be obtained before proscribing against breastfeeding is warranted, especially in areas where these tumors are common but the protective benefits of breastfeeding are high. In areas where Burkitt's lymphoma and nasopharyngeal carcinoma are uncommon, EBV infection in the mother or infant is not a contraindication to breastfeeding.

Filoviridae

Marburg and Ebola viruses cause severe and highly fatal hemorrhagic fevers. The illness often presents with nonspecific symptoms (conjunctivitis, frontal headache, malaise, myalgia, bradycar-

dia) and progresses with worsening hemorrhage to shock and subsequent death in 50% to 90% of patients. Person-to-person transmission through direct contact, droplet spread, or airborne spread is the common mode of transmission. However, the reservoir or source of these viruses for humans has not been identified. Attack rates in families are 5% to 16%.[140] No postexposure interventions have proved useful in preventing spread, and no treatment other than supportive is currently available.

No information is available concerning these viruses in breast milk or additional risks or benefits from breastfeeding. Contact precautions are recommended for Marburg virus infections and contact and airborne precautions for Ebola virus infection. Given the high attack and mortality rates, these precautions should be carefully instituted and breastfeeding not allowed. If any other suitable source of nutrition can be found for the infant, expressed breast milk should also be proscribed for the infant of a mother with either of these infections.

Human herpesvirus 6

Human herpesvirus 6 (HHV-6) is a cause of exanthema subitum (roseola, roseola infantum) and is associated with febrile seizures. HHV-6 appears to be most similar to CMV based on genetic analysis. No obvious congenital syndrome of HHV-6 infection has been identified, although prenatal infection has been reported.[53] Seroepidemiologic studies show that most adults have already been infected by HHV-6. Therefore primary infection during pregnancy is unlikely, but reactivation of latent HHV-6 infection may be more common. No case of symptomatic HHV-6 prenatal infection has been reported. The significance of reactivation of HHV-6 in the pregnant woman and the production of infection and disease in the fetus and infant remains to be determined. Primary infection in children occurs most often between 6 and 12 months of age, when maternally acquired passive antibodies against HHV-6 are waning. Febrile illnesses in infants less than 3 months of age have been described with HHV-6 infection, but infection before 3 months or after 3 years is uncommon.

Various studies involving serology and restriction enzyme analysis of HHV-6 isolates from mother/infant pairs support the idea that postnatal transmission and perhaps perinatal transmission from the mother are common sources of infection. At least one study was unable to detect HHV-6 in breast milk by PCR analysis in 120 samples, although positive controls seeded with HHV-6-infected cells did test positive.[54]

Given the limited occurrence of clinically significant disease and the absence of sequelae of HHV-6 infection in infants and children, the almost universal acquisition of infection in early childhood (with or without breastfeeding) and the absence of evidence that breast milk is a source of HHV-6 infection, breastfeeding can continue in women known to be seropositive for HHV-6.

Herpes simplex virus

Herpes simplex virus types 1 and 2 (HSV-1, HSV-2) can cause prenatal, perinatal, and postnatal infection in the fetus and infant. Prenatal infection can lead to abortion, prematurity, or a recognized congenital syndrome. Perinatal infection is the most common (1 in 2000 to 5000 live births, 700 to 1500 cases/year in the United States) and is often fatal or severely debilitating. The factors that facilitate intrapartum infection and predict the severity of disease have been extensively investigated. Postnatal infection is uncommon but can occur from a variety of sources, including oral or genital lesions and secretions in mothers or fathers, hospital or home caregivers, and breast lesions in breastfeeding mothers. A number of case reports have documented severe HSV-1 or HSV-2 infections in infants in association with HSV-positive breast lesions in the mother.[51,143,172] Cases of infants inoculating the mother's breast have also been reported.

Breastfeeding, in the absence of breast lesions, in HSV-seropositive or culture-positive women is reasonable when accompanied by careful handwashing, covering other lesions, and avoiding fondling or kissing with oral lesions until all lesions are crusted. Breastfeeding during maternal therapy with oral or IV acyclovir can continue safely. Inadequate information exists concerning valacyclovir, famiciclovir, ganciclovir, and foscarnet in breast milk to make a recommendation at this time. Breastfeeding in women with active herpetic lesions on their breasts should be proscribed until the lesions are dried. Treatment of the mother's breast lesion with topical, oral, or even IV antiviral preparations may hasten recovery and decrease the length of viral shedding.

Rotaviruses

Rotavirus infections usually result in diarrhea accompanied by emesis and low-grade fever. In severe infections the clinical course can include dehydration, electrolyte abnormalities, and acidosis and can contribute to malnutrition in developing countries. In developed countries, rotavirus is often associated with diarrhea requiring hospitalization in children less than 2 years of age. Fecal-oral transmission is the most common route, but fomites and respiratory spread may also occur. Spread of infection occurs most often in homes with young children or in day-care centers and institutions. In hospitalized infants or mothers with rotavirus infection, contact precautions are indicated for the duration of the illness. No evidence indicates prenatal infection from rotavirus, but perinatal or postnatal infection from contact with the mother or others can occur.

There are no documented cases of transmission of rotavirus via breast milk. Breast milk does contain antibodies to rotavirus for up to 2 years. Although breastfeeding does not prevent infection with rotavirus, it seems to decrease the severity of rotavirus-induced illness in children less than 2 years old.[37,58,84] At least one study suggested that this may represent simply the postponement of severe rotavirus infection until an older age.[37] This delay in rotavirus infection until the child is older may be beneficial in that the older child may be able to tolerate the infection or illness with a lower likelihood of becoming dehydrated or malnourished. Continuing breastfeeding during an episode of rotavirus illness with or without vomiting is appropriate and often helpful.

Several types of rotavirus vaccines are undergoing study in a variety of situations. Evidence indicates that maternal immunization with rotavirus vaccine can increase both transplacental acquisition of antibodies and secretory IgA (sIgA) in breast milk.[141] Additionally, oral rotavirus vaccines have been able to stimulate a good serologic response in both formula-fed and breastfed infants, although the antigen titers may need to be modified to create an optimal response in all infants.[34] The actual protective effect of these vaccines in different situations and strategies will require measurement in prospective studies.

Rubella virus

Congenital rubella infection has been well described, and the contributing variables to infection and severe disease have been elucidated. The primary intervention to prevent congenital rubella has been to establish the existence of maternal immunity to rubella before conception, including immunization with rubella vaccine and reimmunization if indicated. Perinatal infection is not clinically significant. Postnatal infection occurs infrequently in children less than 1 year of age because of passively acquired maternal antibodies. The predominant age of infection is 5 to 14 years old, and more than half of those with infections are asymptomatic. Postnatal rubella is a self-limited, mild viral infection associated with an evanescent rash, shotty adenopathy, and low-grade transient fever. It most often occurs in the late winter and spring. Infants with congenital infection shed the virus for prolonged periods from various sites and may serve as a source of infection throughout the year. Contact isolation is appropriate for suspected and proven congenital infection for at least 1 year, including exclusion from day care and avoidance of pregnant women, whereas postnatal rubella infection requires droplet precautions for 7 days after the onset of rash.

Rubella virus has been isolated from breast milk after natural infection (congenital or postnatal) and after immunization with live attenuated vaccine virus. Both IgA antibodies and immunoreactive cells against rubella have been identified in breast milk. Breastfed infants can acquire vaccine virus infection via milk but are asymptomatic. Because postpartum infection with this virus (natural or vaccine) is not associated with clinically significant illness, no reason exists to prevent breastfeeding after congenital infection, postpartum infection, or maternal immunization with this virus.

Varicella–zoster virus

Varicella-zoster virus (VZV) infection (varicella/chickenpox, zoster/shingles) is one of the most communicable diseases of humans, in a class with measles and smallpox. Transmission is believed to occur via respiratory droplets and virus from vesicles. Varicella in pregnancy is a rare event, although disease can be more severe with varicella pneumonia, and can be fatal.

Congenital VZV infection occurs infrequently, causing abortion, prematurity, and congenital malformations. A syndrome of malformations has been carefully described with congenital VZV infection, typically involving limb deformity, skin scarring, and nerve damage, including to the eye and brain.[70]

Perinatal infection can lead to severe infection in the infant if maternal rash develops 5 days or less before delivery and within 2 days after delivery. Illness in the infant usually develops before 10 days of age and is believed to be more severe because of the lack of adequate transfer of antibody from the mother during this period and transplacental spread of virus to the fetus and infant during viremia in the mother. Varicella in the mother occurring prior to 5 days before delivery allows sufficient formation and transplacental transfer of antibodies to the infant to ameliorate disease even if the infant is infected with VZV. Mothers who develop varicella rash more than 2 days after delivery are less likely to transfer virus to the infant transplacentally; they pose a risk to the infant from postnatal exposure, which can be diminished by

TABLE 16-2 **Guidelines for preventive measures after exposure to chickenpox in the nursery or maternity ward**

Type of exposure or disease	Chickenpox lesions present		Disposition
	Mother	**Neonate**	
A. Siblings at home have active chickenpox when neonate and mother are ready for discharge from hospital.	No	No	1. Mother: if she has a history of chickenpox, she may return home. Without a history, she should be tested for varicella-zoster virus (VZV) antibody titer.* If test is positive, she may return home. If test is negative, varicella-zoster immune globulin (VZIG)† is administered and she is discharged home. 2. Neonate: may be discharged home with mother if mother has history of varicella or is VZV antibody positive. If mother is susceptible, administer VZIG to infant and discharge home or place in protective isolation.
B. Mother has no history of chickenpox; exposed during period 6-20 days antepartum.‡	No	No	1. Exposed mother and infant: send home at earliest date unless siblings at home have communicable chickenpox.§ If so, may administer VZIG and discharge home, as above. 2. Other mothers and infants: no special management indicated. 3. Hospital personnel: no precautions indicated if there is a history of previous chickenpox or zoster. In absence of history, immediate serologic testing is indicated to determine immune status.* Nonimmune personnel should be excluded from patient contact until 21 days after an exposure. 4. If mother develops varicella 1 to 2 days postpartum, infant should be given VZIG.

From Gershon AA: Chickenpox, measles and mumps. In Remington JS, Klein JO, editors: *Infectious diseases of the fetus and newborn infant,* ed 4, Philadelphia, 1995, Saunders.

*Send serum to virus diagnostic laboratory for determination of antibodies to VZV by a sensitive technique (e.g., FAMA, LA, ELISA). Personnel may continue to work for 8 days after exposure pending serologic results because they are not potentially infectious during this period. Antibodies to VZV >1:4 probably are indicative of immunity.

†VZIG is available through the American Red Cross. The dose for a newborn is 1.25 ml (1 vial). The dose for a pregnant woman is conventionally 6.25 ml (5 vials).

‡If exposure occurred less than 6 days antepartum, mother would not be potentially infectious until at least 72 hours postpartum.

§Considered noninfectious when no new vesicles have appeared for 72 hours and all lesions have crusted.

the administration of varicella-zoster immune globulin (VZIG) to the infant. Postnatal transmission is believed to occur through aerosolized virus from skin lesions or the respiratory tract entering the susceptible infant's respiratory tract. Airborne precautions are therefore appropriate in the hospital setting. Infants infected with VZV in utero or in the perinatal period (less than 1 month of age) are more likely to develop zoster (reactivation of latent VZV) during childhood or as young adults. Table 16-2 summarizes management of varicella in the hospitalized mother or infant.[70]

Postnatal varicella from nonmaternal exposure can occur but is generally mild when it develops after 3 weeks of age or when the mother has passed on antibodies against VZV via the placenta. Severe

TABLE 16-2   **Guidelines for preventive measures after exposure to chickenpox in the nursery or maternity ward—cont'd**

Type of exposure or disease	Chickenpox lesions present		Disposition
	Mother	**Neonate**	
C. Onset of maternal chickenpox occurs antepartum‡ or postpartum.	Yes	No	1. Infected mother: isolate until no longer clinically infectious. If seriously ill, treat with acyclovir.‖ 2. Infected mother's infant: administer VZIG† to neonates born to mothers with onset of chickenpox less than 5 days before delivery and isolate separately from mother. Send home with mother if no lesions develop by the time mother is noninfectious. 3. Other mothers and infants: send home at earliest date. VZIG may be given to exposed neonates. 4. Hospital personnel: same as B-3.
D. Onset of maternal chickenpox occurs antepartum.§			1. Mother: isolation unnecessary. 2. Infant: isolate from other infants but not from mother. 3. Other mothers and infants: same as C-3 (if exposed). 4. Hospital personnel: same as B-3 (if exposed).
E. Congenital chickenpox	No	Yes	1. Infected infant and mother: same as D-1 and D-2. 2. Other mothers and infants: same as C-3. 3. Hospital personnel: same as B-3.

‖Dosage of acyclovir for pregnant woman is 30 mg/kg/day; for seriously ill infant with varicella, 750 to 1500 mg/m²/day.

postnatal varicella does occur in premature infants or infants of varicella-susceptible mothers. When the mother's immune status relative to VZV is uncertain and measurement of antibodies to VZV in the mother or infant cannot be performed promptly (less than 72 hours), administration of VZIG to the infant exposed to varicella or zoster in the postnatal period is indicated. Ideally the mother's varicella status should be known before pregnancy, when varicella virus vaccine could be given if indicated.

VZV virus has not been cultured from milk, but VZV-DNA has been identified in breast milk.[192] Antibody against VZV has also been found in breast milk.[116] One case of suspected transfer of VZV to an infant via breastfeeding has been reported, but virus may have been transmitted by respiratory droplet or exposure to rash before the mother began antiviral therapy.[192] Isolation of the infant from the mother and interruption of breastfeeding should occur only while the mother remains clinically infectious, regardless of the method of feeding. Expressed breast milk can be given to the infant if no skin lesions involve the breasts, as soon as the infant has received VZIG. Persons with varicella rash are considered non-infectious when no new vesicles have appeared for 72 hours and all lesions have crusted, usually 6 to 10 days. Immunocompetent mothers who develop zoster can continue to breastfeed if the lesions do not involve the breast and can be covered, because antibodies against VZV are provided to the infant via the placenta and breast milk and will diminish the severity of disease even if not preventing it. Conservative management in this scenario would include giving the infant VZIG as well (Table 16-2).

Measles

Measles is another highly communicable childhood illness that can be more severe in neonates and adults. Measles is an exanthematous febrile illness following a prodrome of malaise, coryza, conjunctivitis, and cough and often Koplik's spots in the mouth. The rash usually appears 10 to 14 days after exposure. Complications can include pneumonitis, encephalitis, and bacterial superinfection. With the availability of vaccination, measles in pregnancy is rare (0.4 in 10,000 pregnancies),[70] although respiratory complications (primary viral pneumonitis, secondary bacterial pneumonia), hepatitis, or other secondary bacterial infections often lead to more severe disease in these situations.

Prenatal infection with measles may cause premature delivery without disrupting normal uterine development. No specific group of congenital malformations have been described in association with in utero measles infection, although teratogenic effects of measles infection in the pregnant woman may rarely manifest in the infant.

Perinatal measles includes transplacental infection when measles occurs in the infant in the first 10 days of life. Infection from extrauterine exposure usually develops after 14 days of life. The severity of illness after suspected transplacental spread of virus to the infant varies from mild to severe and does not seem to vary with the antepartum or postpartum onset of rash in the mother. It is uncertain what role maternal antibodies play in the severity of the infant's disease. More severe disease seems to be associated with severe respiratory illness and bacterial infection. Postnatal

exposure leading to measles after 14 days of life is generally mild, probably because of passively acquired antibodies from the mother. Severe measles in children less than 1 year of age may occur because of declining passively acquired antibodies and complications of respiratory illness and rare cases of encephalitis.

Measles virus has not been identified in breast milk, whereas measles-specific antibodies have been documented.[1] Infants exposed to mothers with documented measles while breastfeeding should be given immune globulin and isolated from the mother until 72 hours after the onset of rash, which is often only a very short period after diagnosis of measles in the mother. The breast milk can be pumped and given to the infant because sIgA begins to be secreted in breast milk within 48 hours of onset of the exanthem in the mother. Table 16-3 summarizes management of the hospitalized mother and infant with measles exposure or infection.[70]

Mumps

Mumps is an acute transient benign illness with inflammation of the parotid gland and other salivary glands and often involving the pancreas, testicles, and meninges. Mumps occurs infrequently in pregnant women (1 to 10 cases/10,000 pregnancies) and is generally benign. Mumps virus has been isolated from saliva, respiratory secretions, blood, testicular tissue, urine, CSF in cases of meningeal involvement, and breast milk. The period of infectivity is believed to be between 7 days before and 9 days after the onset of parotitis, with the usual incubation period being 14 to 18 days.

Prenatal infection with the mumps virus causes an increase in the number of abortions when infection occurs in the first trimester. A small increase in the number of premature births was noted in one prospective study of maternal mumps infection.[70] No conclusive evidence suggests congenital malformations associated with prenatal infection, not even with endocardial fibroelastosis, as originally reported in the 1960s.

Perinatal mumps (transplacentally or postna-

TABLE 16-3   Guidelines for preventive measures after exposure to measles in the nursery or maternity ward

Type of exposure or disease	Measles (prodrome or rash) present*		Disposition
	Mother	Neonate	
A. Siblings at home have measles* when neonate and mother are ready for discharge from hospital.	No	No	1. Neonate: protective isolation and immune globulin (IG) indicated unless mother has unequivocal history of previous measles or measles vaccination.† 2. Mother: with history of previous measles or measles vaccination, she may either remain with neonates or return to older children. Without previous history, she may remain with neonate until older siblings are no longer infectious, or she may receive IG prophylactically and return to older children.
B. Mother has no history of measles or measles vaccination exposure 6 to 15 days antepartum.‡	No	No	1. Exposed mother and infant: administer IG to each and send home at earliest date unless siblings at home have communicable measles. Test mothers for susceptibility if possible. If susceptible, administer live measles vaccine 8 weeks after IG. 2. Other mothers and infants: same unless clear history of previous measles or measles vaccination in the mother. 3. Hospital personnel: unless clear history of previous measles or measles vaccination, administer IG within 72 hours of exposure. Vaccinate 8 weeks or more later.
C. Onset of maternal measles occurs antepartum or postpartum.§	Yes	Yes	1. Infected mother and infant: isolate together until clinically stable, then send home. 2. Other mothers and infants: same as B-3 except infants should be vaccinated at 15 months of age. 3. Hospital personnel: same as B-3.
D. Onset of maternal measles occurs antepartum or postpartum.§	Yes	No	1. Infected mother: isolate until no longer infectious.§ 2. Infected mother's infant: isolate separately from mother. Administer IG immediately. Send home when mother is no longer infectious. Alternatively, observe in isolation for 18 days for modified measles,‖ especially if IG administration was delayed more than 4 days. 3. Other mothers and infants: same as C-2. 4. Hospital personnel: same as B-3.

From Gershon AA: Chickenpox, measles and mumps. In Remington JS, Klein JO, editors: *Infectious diseases of the fetus and newborn infant,* ed 4, Philadelphia, 1995, Saunders.
*Catarrhal stage or less than 72 hours after onset of exanthem.
†Vaccination with live attenuated measles virus.
‡With exposure less than 6 days antepartum, mother would not be potentially infectious until at least 72 hours postpartum.
§Considered infectious from onset of prodrome until 72 hours after onset of exanthem.
‖Incubation period for modified measles may be prolonged beyond the usual 10 to 14 days.

tally acquired) has rarely if ever been documented. Natural mumps virus has been demonstrated to infect the placenta and infect the fetus, and live attenuated vaccine virus has been isolated from the placenta but not from fetal tissue in women vaccinated 10 days before induced abortion. Antibodies to mumps do cross the placenta.

Postnatal mumps in the first year of life is typically very benign. No epidemiologic data suggest that mumps infection is more or less common or severe in breastfed infants compared with formula-fed infants. Although mumps virus has been identified in breast milk and mastitis is a rare complication of mumps in the mature female, no evidence indicates that breast involvement occurs more frequently in lactating women. If mumps occurs in the mother, breastfeeding can continue because exposure has already occurred throughout the 7 days before the development of the parotitis, and sIgA in the milk may help to mitigate the symptoms in the infant.

Polioviruses

Poliovirus infection (types 1, 2, and 3) cause a range of illness, with 90% to 95% subclinical, 4% to 8% abortive, and 1% to 2% manifest as paralytic poliomyelitis. A review by Bates[16] from 1955 of 58 cases of poliomyelitis in infants less than 1 month of age demonstrated paralysis or death in more than 70% and only one child without evidence of even transient paralysis. More than half the cases were ascribed to transmission from the mothers, although no mention was made of breastfeeding. Breastfeeding rates at the time were about 25%.

Prenatal infection with polioviruses does cause an increased incidence of abortion. Prematurity and stillbirth apparently occur more frequently in mothers who developed paralytic disease versus inapparent infection.[85] Although individual reports of congenital malformations in association with maternal poliomyelitis exist, no epidemiologic data suggest that polioviruses are teratogenic. Also, no evidence indicates that live attenuated vaccine poliovirus given during pregnancy is associated with congenital malformations.[35,77]

Perinatal infection has been noted in several case reports of infants infected in utero several days before birth who had severe disease manifesting with neurologic manifestations (paralysis) but without fever, irritability, or vomiting. Additional case reports of infection acquired postnatally demonstrate illness more consistent with poliomyelitis of childhood. These cases were more severe and involved paralysis, which may represent reporting bias.[35]

No data are available concerning the presence of poliovirus in breast milk, although antibodies to poliovirus types 1, 2, and 3 have been documented.[116] In this era of increasing worldwide poliovirus vaccination, the likelihood of prenatal or perinatal poliovirus infection is decreasing. Maternal susceptibility to poliovirus should be determined before conception and poliovirus vaccine offered to susceptible women. An analysis of the last great epidemic in Italy in 1958 was done using a population-based case-control study.[142] In 114,000 births, 942 infants were reported with paralytic poliomyelitis. A group of matched controls was selected from infants admitted to the hospital at the same time. Using the dichotomous variable of never breastfed and partially breastfed, 75 never-breastfed infants were among the cases and 88 among the controls. The authors determined an odds ratio of 4:2, with 95% confidence interval of 1.4 to 14, demonstrating that the risk of paralytic polio was higher in infants never breastfed and lowest among those exclusively breastfed. Because by the time the diagnosis of poliomyelitis is made in a breastfeeding mother, the exposure of the infant to poliovirus from maternal secretions has already occurred, and because the breast milk already contains antibodies that may be protective, no reason exists to interrupt breastfeeding. Breastfeeding also does not interfere with successful immunization against poliomyelitis with oral or inactivated poliovirus vaccine.[33]

Tumor virus in breast milk

No documented evidence indicates that women with breast cancer have RNA of tumor virus in their milk. No correlation between RNA-directed DNA polymerase activity has been found in women with a family history of breast cancer. RNA-directed DNA polymerase activity, a reserve transcriptase, is a normal feature of the lactating breast.[36,62,149]

Epidemiologic studies

Epidemiologic data conflict with the suggestion that the tumor agent is transmitted through the breast milk. The incidence of breast cancer is low among groups who had nursed their infants, including lower economic groups, foreign-born groups, and those in sparsely populated areas.[113] The frequency of breast cancer in mothers and sisters of a woman with breast cancer is two to three times that expected by chance. This could be genetic or environmental. Cancer actually is equally common on both sides of the family of an affected woman. If breast milk were the cause, it should be transmitted from mother to daughter. When mother-daughter incidence of cancer was studied, no relationship was found to breastfeeding.

Sarkar et al[152] reported that human milk, when incubated with mouse mammary tumor virus, caused degradation of the particular morphology and decreased infectivity and reverse transcriptase activity of the virions. They suggest that the significance of this destructive effect of human milk on mouse mammary tumor virus may account for the difficulty in isolating the putative human mammary tumor agent. Sanner[151] showed that the inhibitory enzymes in milk can be removed by special sedimentation technique. He ascribes the discrepancies in isolating virus particles in human milk to these factors, which inhibit RNA-directed DNA polymerase.

Current position

The fear of cancer in the breastfed female offspring of a women with breast cancer does not justify avoiding breastfeeding. Breastfed women have the same breast cancer experience as nonbreastfed women, and no increase is seen in benign tumors. Daughters of breast cancer patients have an increased risk of developing benign and malignant

tumors because of their heredity, not their breastfeeding history.[121,123]

Unilateral breastfeeding (limited to the right breast) is a custom of Tanka women of the fishing villages of Hong Kong. Ing et al[90] investigated the question, Does the unsuckled breast have an altered risk of cancer? They studied breast cancer data from 1958 to 1975. Breast cancer occurred equally in the left and the right breast. Comparison of patients who had nursed unilaterally with nulliparous patients and with patients who had borne children but not breastfed indicated a highly significantly increased risk of cancer in the unsuckled breast. The authors conclude that in postmenopausal women who have breastfed unilaterally, the risk of cancer is significantly higher in the unsuckled breast. They believed that breastfeeding may help protect the suckled breast against cancer.[90]

Others[117] have suggested that Tanka women are ethnically a separate people and that left-sided breast cancer may be related to their genetic pool and not to their breastfeeding habits. No mention has been made of other possible influences, such as the impact of their role as "fishermen" or any inherent trauma to the left breast.[137]

In 1926, Lane-Claypon[103] stated that the breast that had never lactated was more liable to become cancerous. Nulliparity and absence of breastfeeding had been considered important risk factors for breast cancer. MacMahon et al[113] reported in 1970 that age at first full-term pregnancy was the compelling factor, and the younger the mother, the less the risk.

Papaioannou,[137] in a collective review of the etiologic factors in cancer of the breast in humans, concludes, "Genetic factors, viruses, hormones, psychogenic stress, diet and other possible factors, probably in that order of importance, contribute to some extent to the development of cancer of the breast."

Wing[185] concluded in her 1977 review on human milk and health that "in view of the complete absence of any studies showing a relationship between breastfeeding and increased risk of breast cancer, the presence of virus-like particles in breast milk should not be a contraindication to breastfeeding." Henderson et al[79] made a similar statement in 1979, whereas Vorherr[182] concluded in 1979 that the roles of pregnancy and lactation in the development and prognosis of breast cancer had not been determined.

Gradually, studies have appeared challenging the dogma. Brinton et al,[24] McTiernan and Thomas,[118] and Layde et al[106] showed the clearly protective effects of breastfeeding. Another example is a study conducted to clarify whether lactation has a protective role against breast cancer in an Asian people, regardless of confounding effects of age at first pregnancy, parity, and closely related factors.[191] In a hospital-based case-control study of 521 women without breast cancer, statistical adjustment for potential confounders and a likelihood ratio test for linear trend were done by unconditional logistic regression. Total months of lactation regardless of parity was the discriminator. Regardless of age of first pregnancy and parity, lactation had an independent protective effect against breast cancer in Japanese women.[191] Although breast cancer incidence is influenced by genetics, stress, hormones, and pregnancy, breastfeeding clearly has a protective effect. "There is a reduction in the risk of breast cancer among premenopausal women who have lactated. No reduction in the risk of breast cancer occurred among postmenopausal women with a history of lactation," according to Newcombe et al,[128] reporting a multicenter study in 1993.

Hepatitis in the mother

The diagnosis of hepatitis in the pregnant woman or nursing mother causes significant anxiety. The first issue is determining the etiology of the hepatitis, which then allows an informed discussion of the risk to the fetus/infant. The differential diagnosis of acute hepatitis includes (1) common causes of hepatitis, such as hepatitis A, B, C, and D; (2) uncommon causes of hepatitis, such as hepatitis E and G, CMV, echoviruses, enteroviruses, EBV, HSV, rubella, VZV, yellow fever virus; (3) rare causes of hepatitis, such as Ebola virus, Junin virus and Machupo virus (cause hemorrhagic fever), Lassa virus, and Marburg virus; and

(4) nonviral causes, such as hepatotoxic drugs, alcoholic hepatitis, toxoplasmosis, autoimmune hepatitis, bile duct obstruction, ischemic liver damage, Wilson's disease, α_1-antitrypsin deficiency, and metastatic liver disease. The following sections focus on hepatitis viruses A to G. Other infectious agents that can cause hepatitis are considered individually in other sections. Box 16-1 provides hepatitis terminology.

Martin et al[115] outline a succinct diagnostic approach to the patient with acute viral hepatitis and chronic viral hepatitis (Figs. 16-4 and 16-5). The

---

BOX 16-1   Terminology for hepatitis

Hepatitis A Virus (HAV)

IgM anti-HAV	Immunoglobulin M antibody against HAV
HAV-RNA	HAV ribonucleic acid

Hepatitis B Virus

HBsAg	Hepatitis B surface antigen
HBeAg	Hepatitis Be antigen
HBcAg	Hepatitis B core antigen
Anti-HBe	Antibody against hepatitis Be antigen
IgM anti-HBcAg	IgM antibody against hepatitis B core antigen
HBV-DNA	HBV deoxyribonucleic acid
HBIG	Hepatitis B immune globulin

Hepatitis C Virus (HCV)

Anti-HCV	Antibody against HCV
HCV-RNA	HCV ribonucleic acid

Hepatitis D Virus (HDV)

Anti-HDV	Antibody against HDV

Hepatitis E Virus (HEV)

HEV-RNA	HEV ribonucleic acid

Hepatitis G Virus (HGV)

HGV-RNA	HGV ribonucleic acid

Other

NANBH	Non-A, non-B hepatitis
ISG	Immune serum globulin

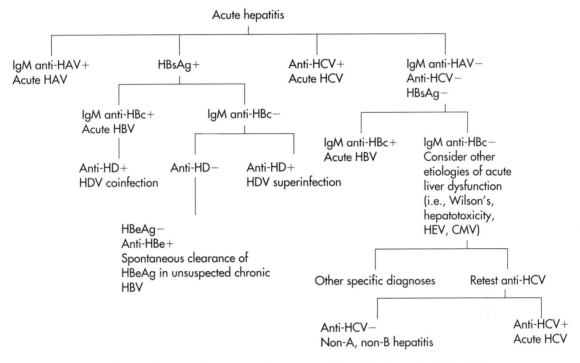

Fig. 16-4. Diagnostic approach to patient with acute viral hepatitis. (From Martin P, Friedman L, Dienstag J: Diagnostic approach. In Zuckerman A, Thomas H, editors: *Viral hepatitis: scientific basis and clinical management,* Edinburgh, 1993, Churchill Livingstone.)

Fig. 16-5. Diagnostic approach to patient with chronic viral hepatitis. (From Martin P, Friedman L, Dienstag J: Diagnostic approach. In Zuckerman A, Thomas H, editors: *Viral hepatitis: scientific basis and clinical management,* Edinburgh, 1993, Churchill Livingstone.)

approach involves using the four serologic markers (IgM anti-HAV, HBsAg, IgM anti-HBcAg, anti-HCV) as the initial diagnostic tests. Simultaneous consideration of other etiologies of acute liver dysfunction is appropriate depending on the patient's history. If the initial diagnostic tests are all negative, subsequent additional testing for anti-HDV, HCV-RNA, HGV-RNA, anti-HEV, or HEV-RNA may be necessary. If initial testing reveals positive HBsAg, testing for anti-HDV, HBeAg, and HBV-DNA is appropriate. These additional tests are useful in defining the prognosis for the mother and the risk of infection to the infant. During the diagnostic evaluation, it is appropriate to discuss with the mother or parents the theoretic risk of transmitting infectious agents that cause hepatitis via breastfeeding. The discussion should include an evaluation of the positive and negative effects of suspending or continuing breastfeeding until the exact etiologic diagnosis is determined. The relative risk of transmission of infection to the infant can be estimated and specific preventive measures provided for the infant (Table 16-4).

Hepatitis A

Hepatitis A virus (HAV) is usually an acute self-limited infection. The illness is typically mild, and generally subclinical in infants. Occasionally, HAV infection is prolonged or relapsing, extending over 3 to 6 months, rarely is fulminant, but does not lead to chronic infection. The incidence of prematurity after maternal HAV infection is increased, but no evidence to date indicates obvious birth defects or a congenital syndrome.[159,195] HAV infection in premature infants may lead to prolonged viral shedding.[148] Transmission is most often person to person (fecal-oral), and transmission in food-borne or water-borne epidemics has been described. Transmission via blood products and vertical transmission (mother to infant) are rare.[183] Transmission in day-care settings has been clearly described.

Infection with HAV in the newborn is uncommon and does not seem to be a significant problem. The usual period of viral shedding and presumed contagiousness lasts 1 to 3 weeks. Acute maternal HAV infection in the last trimester or in the postpartum period could lead to infection in the infant. Symptomatic infection can be prevented by immune globulin (IG) administration, and 80% to 90% of disease can be prevented by IG administration within 2 weeks of exposure. HAV vaccine can be administered simultaneously with IG without affecting the seroconversion rate to produce rapid and prolonged HAV serum antibody levels.

Transmission of HAV via breast milk has been implicated in one case report, but no data exist on the frequency of isolating HAV from breast milk.[183] Because HAV infection in infancy is rare and usually subclinical without chronic disease, and because exposure has already occurred by the time the etiologic diagnosis of hepatitis in the mother is made, no reason exists to interrupt breastfeeding with maternal HAV infection. The infant should receive IG and HAV vaccine, administered simultaneously.

Hepatitis B

Hepatitis B virus (HBV) infection leads to a broad spectrum of illness, including asymptomatic seroconversion, nonspecific symptoms (fever, malaise, fatigue), clinical hepatitis with or without jaundice, extrahepatic manifestations (arthritis, rash, renal involvement), fulminant hepatitis, and chronic HBV infection. Chronic HBV infection occurs in up to 90% of infants infected via perinatal and vertical transmission and in 30% of children infected between 1 to 5 years of age. Given the increased risk of significant sequelae from chronic infection (chronic active hepatitis, chronic persistent hepatitis, cirrhosis, primary hepatocellular carcinoma), prevention of HBV infection in infancy is crucial. Transmission of HBV is usually through blood or body fluids (stool, semen, saliva, urine, cervical secretions).[38]

Vertical transmission either transplacentally or perinatally during delivery has been well described throughout the world. Vertical transmission rates in areas where HBV is endemic (Taiwan and Japan) are very high, whereas transmission to infants from

TABLE 16–4 Viral hepatitis in association with breastfeeding*

Hepatitis	Virus	Identified in breast milk	Factors for peri/postnatal transmission	Prevention	Breastfeeding†
A	Picornaviridae (RNA)	?	Vertical transmission uncertain or rare HAV in pregnancy associated with premature birth	ISG HAV vaccine	Limited evidence of transmission via breastfeeding or of serious disease in infants Breastfeeding OK after ISG and vaccine
B	Hepadnaviridae (DNA)	HBsAg HBV-DNA	Increased risk of vertical transmission with HBeAg+, in countries where HBV is endemic or early in maternal infection, before Ab production	HBIG HBV vaccine	Low theoretic risk Virtually no risk after HBIG and HBV vaccine Breastfeeding OK after HBIG and vaccine
C	Flavivirus (RNA)	HCV-RNA detected	Increased risk when mother HIV+ and HCV+ or with increased HCV-RNA titers Vertical transmission uncommon	None	Positive theoretic risk Inadequate data on relative risk Breastfeeding OK after informed discussion with parents
D	Deltaviridae (RNA negative strand, circular)	?	Requires co-infection/superinfection with HBV Vertical transmission rare	None (except to prevent HBV infection, give HBIG/HBV vaccine)	Prevent HBV infection with HBIG and vaccine Breastfeeding OK after HBIG and vaccine
E	Caliciviridae (RNA)	?	Severe disease in pregnant women (20% mortality)	ISG and subunit vaccine being tested	Usually subclinical infection in children Breastfeeding OK
G	Related to calicivirus and flaviviruses (RNA)	?	?	None	Inadequate data

Data from Committee on Infectious Diseases, American Academy of Pediatrics: *Red book: report of the Committee on Infectious Diseases,* ed 24, Elk Grove, Ill, 1997, The Academy.

*See Box 16-1 for abbreviations. *Ab,* Antibody; *HIV,* human immunodeficiency virus.

†With any type of infectious hepatitis, discussion of what is known and not known concerning transmission should be related to the mother/parents, and together an informed decision can be made concerning breastfeeding.

HBV carrier mothers in other areas where HBV carrier rates are low is uncommon.[168] Transmission of HBV to infants occurs in up to 50% of infants when the mother is acutely infected immediately before, during, or soon after pregnancy.[194]

Hepatitis B surface antigen (HBsAg) is found in breast milk, but transmission by this route is not well documented. Beasley et al[17,18] demonstrated that although breast milk transmission is possible, seroconversion rates are no different between breastfed and nonbreastfed infants in a long-term follow-up study of 147 HBsAg-positive mothers. Transmission, when it does happen, probably occurs during labor and delivery. The AAP Committee on Infectious Diseases[38] stated in 1997 that "studies from Taiwan and England have indicated that breastfeeding by HBsAg-positive women does not increase significantly the risk of infection among their infants."

Screening of all pregnant women for HBV infection is an essential first step to preventing vertical transmission. Universal HBV vaccination at birth and during infancy, along with administration of hepatitis B immune globulin (HBIG) immediately after birth to infants of HBsAg-positive mothers, prevents HBV transmission in more than 95% of cases. Breastfeeding by HBsAg-positive women is not contraindicated, but immediate administration of HBIG and HBV vaccine should occur. Two subsequent doses of vaccine should be given at the appropriate intervals and dosages for the specific HBV vaccine product. This decreases the small theoretic risk of HBV transmission from breastfeeding to almost zero.

When acute peripartum or postpartum hepatitis occurs in the mother and HBV infection is a possibility, with its associated increased risk of transmission to the infant, a discussion with the mother or parents should identify the potential risks and benefits of continuing breastfeeding until the etiology of the hepatitis can be determined. If an appropriate alternative source of nutrition is available for the infant, breast milk should be withheld until the etiology of the hepatitis is identified. HBIG and HBV vaccine can be administered to the infant who has not already been immunized or has no documented immunity against HBV.[169] If acute HBV infection is documented in the mother, breastfeeding can continue once immunization has begun.

Hepatitis C

Acute infection with hepatitis C virus (HCV) can be indistinguishable from hepatitis A or B infection; however, it is typically asymptomatic or mild. HCV infection is the major cause of blood-borne non-A, non-B hepatitis (NANBH). Chronic HCV infection is reported to occur 70% to 85% of the time regardless of age at time of infection. Sequelae of chronic HCV infection are similar to those associated with chronic HBV infection. Bortolotti et al[23] described two groups of children with HCV infection whom they observed for 12 to 48 months. The first group of 14 children, who acquired HCV infection early in life, presumably from their mothers, all demonstrated biochemical evidence of liver disease in the first 12 months of life. Two of these children subsequently cleared the viremia and had normal liver function, an additional three children developed normal liver function despite persistent HCV viremia, and the remaining children had persistent viremia and abnormal liver function. The second group of 16 children, with chronic HCV infection, remained free of clinical symptoms of hepatitis, while 10 (62%) of them had mild alanine aminotransferase (ALT) elevations, and 7 (44%) of the 16 who had liver biopsies had histologic evidence of mild to moderate hepatitis.

The two commonly identified mechanisms of transmission of HCV are transfusions of blood or blood products and IV drug use. However, other routes of transmission exist, because HCV infection occurs even in the absence of obvious direct contact with significant amounts of blood. Other body fluids contaminated with blood probably serve as sources of infection. Transmission through sexual contact occurs infrequently and probably requires additional contributing factors, such as co-infection with other sexually transmitted agents or promiscuity. Studies of transmission in households without other risk factors has demonstrated either very low rates of transmission or no transmission.

The reported rates of vertical transmission vary widely. In mothers with unknown HIV status or known HIV infection, the rates of vertical transmission were 4% to 100%, whereas the rates varied between 0% and 42% in known HIV-negative mothers.[48] These same studies suggest that maternal co-infection with HIV, HCV genotype, active maternal liver disease, and the serum titer of maternal HCV-RNA may be associated with increased rates of vertical transmission.[114,131,193] The clinical significance and risk of liver disease after vertical transmission of HCV are still unknown. The timing of HCV infection in vertical transmission is also unknown. In utero transmission has been suggested by some studies, whereas intrapartum or postpartum transmission was proposed by Ohto et al[132] when they documented the absence of HCV-RNA in the cord blood of neonates who later became HCV-RNA positive at 1 to 2 months of age.

The risk of HCV transmission via breast milk is uncertain. Anti-HCV antibody and HCV-RNA has been demonstrated in colostrum and breast milk, although the levels of HCV-RNA in milk did not correlate with the titers of HCV-RNA in serum.[76,109] Nevertheless, transmission of HCV via breastfeeding (and not in utero, intrapartum, or from other postpartum sources) has not been proved in the small number infants studied. Transmission rates in breastfed and nonbreastfed infants appear to be similar, but various important factors have not been controlled, such as HCV-RNA titers in the mothers, examination of the milk for HCV-RNA, exclusive breastfeeding versus exclusive formula feeding versus partial breastfeeding, and duration of breastfeeding.[109,114,124,132,193] Zanetti et al[193] documented the absence of HCV transmission in 94 mother-infant pairs when the mother had only HCV (no HIV) infection and no transmission in 71 mother-infant pairs who breastfed, including 23 infants whose mothers were seropositive for HCV-RNA. Eight infants in that study were infected with HCV, their mothers had both HIV and HCV, and three of these eight infants were infected with both HIV and HCV. The

HCV-RNA levels were significantly higher in the mothers co-infected with HIV compared with those mothers with HCV alone.

Because (1) the risk of HCV infection via breastfeeding is very low, (2) the risk of HCV infection appears to be more frequent in association with HIV infection and higher levels of HCV-RNA in maternal serum, (3) no effective preventive therapies (IG or vaccine) exist, and (4) the risk of chronic HCV infection and subsequent sequelae with any infection is high, it is therefore appropriate to discuss the theoretic risk of breastfeeding in HCV-positive mothers with the mother or parents and to consider proscribing breast milk when appropriate alternative sources of nutrition are available for the infant. HIV infection is a separate contraindication to breastfeeding. Additional study is necessary to determine the exact role of breastfeeding in the transmission of HCV, including the quantitative measurement of HCV-RNA in colostrum and breast milk, the relative risk of HCV transmission in exclusively or partially breastfed infants versus the risk in formula-fed infants, and the effect of duration of breastfeeding on transmission.

The current position of the CDC is that no data indicate HCV virus is transmitted through breast milk. Therefore breastfeeding by a HIV-negative mother is not contraindicated.[14]

Hepatitis D

Hepatitis delta virus (HDV) is a defective RNA virus that causes hepatitis only in persons also infected with HBV. The infection occurs as either an acute co-infection of HBV and HDV or a superinfection of HBV carriers. This "double" infection results in more frequent fulminant hepatitis and chronic hepatitis, which can progress to cirrhosis. The virus uses its own HBV-RNA (circular, negative-strand RNA) with an antigen, HDAg, surrounded by the surface antigen of HBV, HBsAg. HDV is transmitted in the same way as HBV, especially through the exchange of blood and body fluids. HDV infection is uncommon where the prevalence of HBV is low. In areas where HBV is endemic, the prevalence of HDV is highly variable. HDV is very common in tropical Africa and South America as well as in Greece and Italy but is uncommon in the Far East and in Alaskan Eskimos, despite the endemic occurrence of HBV in these areas.[162]

Transmission of HDV has been reported to occur from household contacts and rarely through vertical transmission. No data are available on transmission of HDV by breastfeeding. HDV infection can be prevented by blocking infection with HBV; therefore HBIG and HBV vaccine are the best protection. In addition to HBIG and HBV vaccine administration to the infant of a mother infected with both HBV and HDV, discussion with the mother or parents should include the theoretic risk of HBV and HDV transmission through breastfeeding. As with HBV, once HBIG and HBV vaccine have been given to the infant, the risk of HBV or HDV infection from breastfeeding is negligible. Therefore breastfeeding after an informed discussion with the parents is acceptable.

Hepatitis E

Hepatitis E virus (HEV) is a cause of sporadic and epidemic, enterically transmitted NANBH, which is typically self-limited and without chronic sequelae. HEV is notable for causing high mortality in pregnant women. Although transmission is by the fecal-oral route, as with HAV, the highest infection rates occur in adolescents and young adults (ages 15 to 40 years) rather than in the first decade of life, as usually occurs with HAV in endemic areas. Epidemics are usually related to contamination of water. Person-to-person spread is minimal, even in households and day-care settings. Although IG may be protective, no controlled trials have been done. Animal studies suggest that a recombinant subunit vaccine may be feasible.[146]

HEV infection in infancy is rare, and no data exist on transmission of HEV by breastfeeding. With no evidence of clinically significant postnatal HEV infection in infants or of chronic sequelae in association with HEV infection and no documented HEV transmission through breast milk, currently no contraindication exists to breastfeed-

ing with maternal HEV infection. IG has not been shown to be effective in preventing infection, and no vaccine is available for HEV.

Hepatitis G

Hepatitis G virus (HGV) has recently been confirmed as a cause of NANBH distinct from hepatitis viruses A through E. Several closely related genomes of HGV, currently named GBV-A, -B, and -C, appear to be related to HCV, the pestiviruses, and the flaviviruses. Epidemiologically, HGV is most often associated with transfusion of blood, although studies have identified nontransfusion-related cases. Apparently both acute and chronic infection with HGV occurs but is not associated with significant liver disease. HGV-RNA has been detected in 1% to 3% of healthy blood donors in the United States.[4] Feucht et al[61] described maternal-to-infant transmission of HGV in three of nine children. Two of the three mothers were co-infected with HIV and the third with HCV. None of these infants developed signs of liver disease. Neither the timing nor the mode of transmission was clarified. Lin et al[108] reported no HGV transmission in three mother-infant pairs after cesarean delivery and discussed transplacental spread via blood as the most likely mode of HGV infection in vertical transmission.

Fischler et al[63] followed eight children born to HGV-positive mothers and found only one to be infected with HGV. That child remained clinically well, while his twin, also born by cesarean delivery and breastfed, remained HGV negative over 3 years of observation. Five of the other six children breastfed for variable periods without evidence of HGV infection. Insufficient data are available to make a recommendation concerning breastfeeding by the HGV-infected mother.

Human papillomavirus

Human papillomavirus (HPV) is a DNA virus with at least 70 different types. These viruses cause warts, genital dysplasia, cervical carcinoma (types 6 and 11), and laryngeal papillomatosis. Transmission occurs through direct contact and sexual contact. Laryngeal papillomas are believed to result from acquiring the virus in passage through the birth canal. Infection in pregnant women or during pregnancy does not lead to an increase in abortions or the risk of prematurity, and no evidence indicates intrauterine infection.

Diagnosis is usually by histologic examination or DNA detection. Spontaneous resolution does occur, but therapy for persistent lesions or growths in anatomically problematic locations is appropriate. Therapy can be with podophyllum preparations, trichloroacetic acid, cryotherapy, electrocautery, and laser surgery. Interferon is being tested in the treatment of laryngeal papillomas, with mixed results.[46] Prevention against transmission means limiting direct or sexual contact, but this may not be sufficient because lesions may not be evident, and transmission may still occur.

The breast is a rare site of involvement. Without breast lesions, there is no apparent risk from breast milk, and breastfeeding is acceptable.

Parvovirus

Human parvovirus B19 causes a broad range of clinical manifestations, including asymptomatic infection (most frequent manifestation in all ages), erythema infectiosum (fifth disease), arthralgia and arthritis, red blood cell (RBC) aplasia (less often decreased white blood cells or platelets), chronic infection in immunodeficient individuals, and rarely myocarditis, vasculitis, or hemophagocytic syndrome.

Vertical transmission can lead to severe anemia and immune-mediated hydrops fetalis, which can be treated, if accurately diagnosed, by intrauterine transfusion. Inflammation of the liver or CNS can be seen in the infant, along with vasculitis. If the child is clinically well at birth, hidden or persistent abnormalities are rarely identified. No evidence indicates that parvovirus B19 causes an identified pattern of birth defects.

Postnatal transmission usually occurs person to person via contact with respiratory secretions, saliva, and rarely blood or urine. Seroprevalence in children at 5 years of age is less than 5%, with the peak age of infection occurring during the school-

age years (5% to 40% of children infected). The majority of infections are asymptomatic or undiagnosed seroconversions.[176] Severe disease, such as prolonged aplastic anemia, occurs in individuals with hemoglobinopathies or abnormal RBC maturation. Attack rates have been estimated to be 17% to 30% in casual contacts but up to 50% among household contacts. In one study of 235 susceptible pregnant women, the annual seroconversion rate was 1.4%.[99]

There are no reports of transmission to an infant through breastfeeding. Excretion in breast milk has not been studied because of limitations in culturing techniques. Rat parvovirus has been demonstrated in rat milk. The very low seroconversion rate in young children and the absence of chronic or frequent severe disease suggest that the risk of parvovirus infection via breast milk is not significant. The possibility of antibodies against parvovirus or other protective constituents in breast milk has not been studied. Breastfeeding by a mother with parvovirus infection is acceptable.

Retroviruses
Human T-cell leukemia virus type I

The occurrence of human T-cell leukemia virus type I (HTLV-I) is endemic in parts of the West Indies, sub-Saharan Africa, Brazil, and southwestern Japan.[186] Seroprevalence increases throughout life in endemic areas. HTLV-I–associated illness covers a broad spectrum, including T-cell leukemia and lymphoma, myelopathy, dermatitis, arthritis, uveitis, and Sjögren's syndrome in adults and infective dermatitis and persistent lymphadenitis in children. HTLV-I is not a major disease in the United States.[170]

Transmission of HTLV-I occurs most often through sexual contact, contact with blood or blood products, and via breast milk and infrequently through transplacental transmission and casual or household contact. No infected cells were found in 115 cord blood samples from newborns of mothers infected in Japan.[126] Other studies have confirmed this observation.[45,184]

The evidence for horizontal transmission of the virus through breast milk is strong. HTLV-I-infected lymphocytes have been found in the milk of infected mothers, 10% of whose milk cells are T-lymphocytes, of which 1% are infected. It is estimated that 1 ml of milk harbors 1000 infected T cells, which equals half the infectious dose used in animal experiments in which rabbits and common marmosets were infected by human milk.[189] Hino[82] showed that the rate of mother-to-child transmission of HTLV-I was 30% among 47 breastfed infants, 10% among 40 mixed-fed infants, and 0% among nine formula-fed infants. These rates were confirmed in a study by Ando et al,[5] who showed a 46% transmission rate (11 of 24) in breastfed infants and a 9% rate (1 of 11) in formula-fed infants. Hino et al[83] demonstrated an approximately 80% decrease in infant HTLV-I infection in a Japanese population by refraining from breastfeeding. A more recent study by Takezaki et al[174] reported a decreased risk of transmission for short-term breastfeeders. The seroconversion rates were different for formula-fed infants (4 of 162, 2.5%) and short-term breastfeeders (less than 6 months, 2 of 51, 3.9%) compared with long-term breastfeeders (longer than 6 months, 13 of 64, 20.3%). The authors hypothesized that passively acquired maternal antibodies may have protected infants for the first 6 months of breastfeeding.

The percentage of individuals infected with HTLV-I during childhood is unknown because the majority of individuals do not manifest illness until much later in life. Despite that a greater risk of progression to disease has not been proved for HTLV-I infection through breast milk, early-life infections are associated with the greatest risk of adult T-cell leukemia.[171] It seems prudent to discuss the available information with the mother or parents and to proscribe against breastfeeding or at least to limit the duration of breastfeeding to 5 or 6 months if the risks from the lack of breast milk are not too great and formula is readily available.

Human T-cell leukemia virus type II

Human T-cell leukemia virus type II (HTLV-II) is endemic in IV drug users and their sexual partners, as well as in specific geographic groups, including the Guayami Indians in Panama, Native Americans

in New Mexico, and populations in equatorial Africa. Transmission seems to occur mainly through contact with blood or blood products and sexual transmission. Transplacental transmission and horizontal transmission via breast milk both probably occur, but the relative rates of transmission have not been documented. HTLV-II has been found in breast milk. A 1% to 2% prevalence rate is seen in preadolescent Guayami Indians, and seropositive children have seropositive mothers.[180] Less is known about the disease associated with HTLV-V-II, although glomerulonephritis has been described in children and adults, with myelopathy, arthritis, and T-hairy cell and large granulocytic leukemia possibly associated.

It is difficult to make definite recommendations concerning breastfeeding in the absence of evidence relative to HTLV-II. With the current understanding of the retroviruses, it is appropriate in cases of documented maternal infection to avoid breastfeeding, provide alternative nutrition, and test the breast milk and infant serially for evidence of the virus or infection. As additional information becomes available, discussion with the mother or parents about HTLV-II transmission is appropriate.

Human immunodeficiency virus I

The debate continues concerning the potential risks and benefits of breastfeeding for the infant of a mother with HIV-I infection. Although HIV-I clearly can be transmitted through breast milk, the relative risk is not well quantified. Recommendations from various agencies are based on perceived risks and benefits, data projected from various statistical models, and social, economic, and medical considerations specific to different geographic areas. The question of the role of breastfeeding in HIV-I transmission is not trivial when one considers that (1) heterosexual transmission is the most common mode of transmission worldwide; (2) the World Health Organization (WHO) projects that by the year 2000, 30 to 40 million people will be HIV-I infected; (3) 20% to 50% of infants born to HIV-I-infected women are HIV infected; (4) almost 90% of children less than 13 years of age are infected vertically (mother to infant); and (5) about

10% of all cases of acquired immunodeficiency syndrome (AIDS) are children born to HIV-I–infected women. Despite the advances in antiretroviral therapy with improved survival rates, prevention in any form is essential to halting or diminishing this epidemic.

HIV-I and antibodies against the virus have been described in the breast milk of HIV-I-positive women.[19,175,177] Transmission of HIV-I from mother to infant through breastfeeding when the primary HIV infection occurs postpartum (most frequently from contaminated blood) has been well publicized.[134] One study suggested that the risk of transmission to the infant was as high as 29% when primary maternal HIV infection occurs during lactation.[136] The more important questions concerning breastfeeding relate to the possible benefits versus the risk of transmission in women with established HIV infection, because this is the more common situation.

The major dilemma in estimating the risk from breastfeeding is the difficulty in determining when the HIV infection actually occurs in the infant: prenatal (in utero), perinatal (intrapartum), or postnatal. Estimates suggest that approximately one third of infants are infected prenatally (intrauterine transmission), almost two thirds are infected perinatally (contact with maternal blood and secretions during delivery), and a small number are infected postpartum (contact with maternal secretions or breast milk).[40]

Many studies trying to estimate the risk of HIV infection from breast milk have had difficulties because of retrospective analysis, determination of timing of HIV infection in the infant, and historic reporting of the amount and duration of breastfeeding.[43,91] A metaanalysis of five reports on infants of mothers infected before delivery demonstrated an additional 14% (confidence interval 7% to 22%) risk of transmission via breastfeeding. However, differences between the analyzed reports and the wide confidence interval make this estimate of risk questionable.[52] The duration of breastfeeding seems to relate to the risk of transmission via breast milk.[41,43,125] The analysis by de Martino et al[43] of mothers and infants in Italy suggested that

the risk of HIV infection increased with the longer that breastfeeding continued beyond the first 28 days of life. Nagelkerke et al[125] analyzed the duration of breastfeeding as an independent risk factor for HIV infection in less developed countries. They concluded that the risk of HIV infection from breastfeeding beyond 7 months of age is greater than the decreased-mortality benefit from continued breastfeeding.

Others have attempted to quantify the virus or specific antiviral properties against HIV-I in breast milk. Detection of HIV-I–P24 antigen by antigen capture method and HIV-I-DNA by PCR analysis was done in the milk of 47 seropositive women. HIV-I-DNA was identified in 70% of samples at 0 to 4 days postpartum and in 50% of samples collected 6 to 12 months postpartum. P24 antigen was identified in 24% of samples at 0 to 4 days postpartum but not in subsequent specimens.[150,177] The variable detection of HIV-I-DNA in breast milk over time suggests intermittent viral shedding.[150]

The detection of HIV-I in breast milk may relate to various maternal factors, such as stage of clinical illness, viral load, CD4-lymphocyte counts, and the presence of antiviral factors in the breast milk. HIV-I-specific antibodies have been detected in the breast milk of seropositive women. IgG, IgM, and sIgA were present to varying degrees in specimens collected at 15 days, 6 months, and 18 months.[43] A glycosaminoglycan that inhibits binding of HIV-I to CD4 molecules (which could possibly block infection of cells by HIV-I) was identified in breast milk of seropositive and seronegative women.[127]

Although HIV-I-DNA is readily identifiable in breast milk, isolation of the virus is not so easy. This could relate to the culture methods, the existence of inhibitory factors in milk, or factors relating to the quantity, tropism, or viability of the virus in breast milk. Pasteurization of breast milk, (heating at 62.5° C for 30 minutes) blocks the infectivity of breast milk inoculated with both cell-free HIV-I and HIV-I-infected cells.[133] Much is still to be learned about the relationship between breastfeeding and HIV transmission to the infant and about the associated factors, because all infants breastfed by HIV-positive mothers do not become infected with HIV.[105]

Advances in treatment and prevention may provide added protection for the infant even as they make it more difficult to assess the contribution of breastfeeding to HIV-I transmission. The Pediatric AIDS Clinical Trial Group Protocol 076 demonstrated a two-thirds reduction in transmission of HIV from mother to infant in a placebo-controlled trial of zidovudine (AZT) administered to the mother during pregnancy and delivery and to the infant for the first 6 weeks postpartum.[40] Other studies on prevention of perinatal transmission are investigating perinatal nevirapine, vaginal washes to inactivate the HIV in blood and secretions, and other therapies. The recent advances in antiretroviral therapy, protease inhibitors, and combination therapy, with their improved survival rates and decreases in viral load, may enhance the ability to diminish vertical transmission. The potential risks and benefits of combinations of these various agents in pregnant women will require careful study.

With the current proscription against breastfeeding in many countries where these new medical advances are available, it will be almost impossible to measure their effect on HIV-I transmission via breast milk. The challenges to creating an effective HIV-I vaccine remain substantial. Various engineered vaccines have produced immune responses, but generation of a measurable protective effect remains elusive. The role of vaccines relative to breastfeeding remains to be studied.

Major issues on the role of breastfeeding in HIV infection that require further study include the following[42]:
1. Reasonable estimates of the risk of vertical transmission of HIV through breastfeeding
2. Effect of breastfeeding on HIV-infected infants (possible beneficial effect)
3. Effect of breastfeeding on noninfected infants of HIV-infected mothers (e.g., risk of infection versus protective effects against HIV, other infectious agents, and malnutrition)
4. Effect of lactation on HIV-infected women
5. Effect of AZT or other antiretroviral agents used by women on the transmission of HIV through breastfeeding
6. Effect of various measures to prevent vertical transmission (e.g., AZT, vaginal washes, nevirapine perinatally)
7. How duration of breastfeeding influences the risk of transmission

A number of investigators have resorted to decision analysis models and computer models to estimate the impact of breastfeeding practices on the mortality of children under 5 years of age in developing countries.[44,81,88,107] Studies in Africa have suggested that breastfed infants with HIV do better than nonbreastfed infants with HIV.[134] Of HIV-positive infants in Africa, 15% die in the first year of life from HIV infection when they are breastfed, whereas 50% of all nonbreastfed infants (HIV infected, HIV exposed, or non-HIV exposed) die in the first year when deprived of the benefits of breast milk.[44,134,136,150] Del Fante et al[44] projected that stopping breastfeeding (in a hypothetic East African country) would lead to a 108% increase in mortality in children less than 5 years of age born to mothers who are HIV negative at delivery and to a 27% additional increase in mortality in infants born to HIV-positive mothers. Projected estimates for rural areas were even higher.[44]

The analysis for developed countries relies on several basic assumptions: (1) HIV education and testing with consent are routinely available to all individuals, especially pregnant women; (2) formula is available, easy to use, without stigma; and (3) the ready access to clean water, adequate nutrition, and medical care somewhat offsets the loss of breastfeeding benefits for the infant. In developed countries, therefore, the additional risk of HIV transmission through breast milk outweighs the potential benefits of breastfeeding.

The current recommendations by various health agencies on breastfeeding by HIV-positive women depend on the risk of infant mortality without breastfeeding. In the United States the CDC and the AA Pediatrics recommend against breastfeeding for all HIV-positive mothers[105,177,178] (Box 16-2). WHO advises that in areas where the risk of infant mortality is significant, breastfeeding of all

---

BOX 16-2   Recommendations on breastfeeding and transmission of human immunodeficiency virus (HIV)

- Women and their health care providers need to be aware of the potential risk of transmission of HIV infection to infants during pregnancy and in the peripartum period, as well as through breast milk.
- Documented, routine HIV education and routine testing with consent of all women seeking prenatal care are strongly recommended so that each woman knows her HIV status and the methods available both to prevent the acquisition and transmission of HIV and to determine whether breastfeeding is appropriate.
- At delivery, education about HIV and testing with consent of all women whose HIV status during pregnancy is unknown are strongly recommended. Knowledge of the woman's HIV status assists in counseling on breastfeeding and helps each woman understand the benefits to herself and her infant of knowing her serostatus and the behaviors that would decrease the likelihood of acquisition and transmission of HIV.
- Women who are known to be HIV infected must be counseled not to breastfeed or provide their milk for the nutrition of their own or other infants.
- In general, women who are known to be HIV seronegative should be encouraged to breastfeed. However, women who are HIV seronegative but at particularly high risk of seroconversion (e.g., injection drug users and sexual partners of known HIV-positive persons or active drug users) should be educated about HIV with an individualized recommendation concern-

ing the appropriateness of breastfeeding. In addition, during the perinatal period, information should be provided on the potential risk of transmitting HIV through breast milk and about methods to reduce the risk of acquiring HIV infection.
- Each woman whose HIV status is unknown should be informed of the potential for HIV-infected women to transmit HIV during the peripartum period and through breast milk and the potential benefits to her and her infant of knowing her HIV status and how HIV is acquired and transmitted. The health care provider needs to make an individualized recommendation to assist the woman in deciding whether to breastfeed.
- Neonatal intensive care units should develop policies that are consistent with these recommendations for the use of expressed breast milk for neonates. Current standards of the U.S. Occupational Safety and Health Administration (OSHA) do not require gloves for the routine handling of expressed human milk. However, health care workers should wear gloves in situations in which exposure to breast milk might be frequent or prolonged, such as in milk banking.
- Human milk banks should follow the guidelines developed by the U.S. Public Health Service, which include screening all donors for HIV infection and assessing risk factors that predispose to infection, as well as pasteurization of all milk specimens.

From Lawrence RA: A review of the medical benefits and contraindications to breastfeeding in the United States, *Maternal and child health technical information bulletin,* October, 1997, US Health Resources and Services Administration.

---

infants regardless of maternal HIV status should be encouraged. In areas where the risk of mortality from other infections is less, alternatives to breastfeeding are recommended. WHO is continually reviewing new information and data and reevaluating these recommendations.

As additional information on the potential benefits and risks of breastfeeding by HIV-positive women becomes available and new data on various

therapies and preventive strategies accumulate, these guidelines will have to be reassessed.

Human immunodeficiency virus type II

HIV-II is an RNA virus in the nononcogenic, cytopathic lentivirus genus of retroviruses and is genetically closer to *simian immunodeficiency virus* (SIV) than to HIV-I. The clinical disease associated with HIV-II is more benign than that with HIV-I, producing similar symptoms but a slower progression to AIDS. HIV-II is endemic in West Africa but is found infrequently throughout Caribbean countries, Europe, North America, and South America.[87] HIV-II is most common in prostitutes in West Africa, with increasing seropositivity with age. High-risk groups for HIV-II include sexual partners of those with known HIV-II infection, recipients of blood products in countries where HIV-II is endemic, individuals from areas where HIV-II is endemic, and children of women with HIV-II infection or at high risk for HIV-II infection.[130]

Routine testing for HIV-II is recommended in blood banks. HIV-I enzyme-linked immunosorbent essays (ELISAs) are only 50% to 90% sensitive for detecting HIV-II.[27] Specific HIV-II ELISA testing is appropriate whenever HIV infection is suspected but not proved by testing for HIV-I and when the individual is in a high-risk group for HIV-II.

Vertical transmission occurs infrequently and is more common when primary HIV-II infection occurs during pregnancy.[60] To date, little information exists on HIV-II transmission through breast milk. Ekpini et al[56] followed children born to 138 HIV-I-seropositive women, 132 HIV-II–seropositive women, 69 women seroreactive to both HIV-I and HIV-II, and 274 HIV-seronegative women. Although some perinatal HIV-II transmission occurred, no late postnatal transmission of HIV-II was seen in any of these children. Even with the likelihood that HIV-II transmission via breast milk is less common than with HIV-I, guidelines for breastfeeding by women who are HIV-II positive should follow those for HIV-I until additional information is available.

Rabies

Rabies virus produces a severe infection with progressive CNS symptoms (anxiety, seizures, altered mental status) that ultimately proceeds to death; few reports of survival exist. Rabies occurs worldwide except in Australia, Antarctica, and several island groups. In 1992 more than 36,000 cases of rabies were reported to WHO, which is probably a marked underestimate of the actual

cases.[28] In the United States, five or six cases per year have been reported over the last 6 to 7 years.[30,32] Postexposure prophylaxis is given to thousands of patients each year.

Rabies virus is endemic in various animal populations, including raccoons, skunks, foxes, and bats. Because of aggressive immunization programs, rabies in domesticated dogs and cats in the United States is uncommon. The virus is found in the saliva and nervous tissue of infected animals. Transmission occurs by bites, licking, or simply contact of oral secretions with mucous membranes or nonintact skin. Many cases of rabies in humans now lack a history of some obvious contact with a rabid animal. This may be a result of the long incubation period (generally 4 to 6 weeks, but can be up to 1 year, with reports of incubation periods of several years), a lack of symptoms early in an infectious animal, or airborne transmission from bats in enclosed environments (caves, laboratories, houses). Person-to-person transmission via bites has not been documented, although it has occurred in corneal transplants.[22] No evidence indicates transmission through breast milk.

In the case of maternal infection with rabies, many scenarios can occur before the onset of progressive, severe CNS symptoms. The progression and severity of maternal illness can preclude breastfeeding, but separation of the infant from the mother is appropriate regardless of the mother's status and method of infant feeding. Breastfeeding should not continue when the mother has symptoms of rabies, and the infant should receive postexposure immunization and close observation. Depending on the scenario, the nature of the mother's illness, the possible exposure of the infant to the same source as the mother, and the exposure of the child to the mother, postexposure immunization of the infant may be appropriate. A more common scenario is the mother's apparent exposure to rabies (without exposure for the infant) necessitating postexposure immunization of the mother with rabies vaccine. In the majority of cases, in the absence of maternal illness, breastfeeding can reasonably continue during the mother's five-dose immunization series over 28 days. In a rare situation in which apparent exposure of the mother and infant to rabies occurs together, postexposure treatment of both mother and infant should be instituted, and breastfeeding can continue.

Respiratory syncytial virus

Respiratory syncytial virus (RSV) is a common cause of respiratory illness in children and is relatively common in adults, usually producing milder upper respiratory tract infection in adults. No evidence indicates that RSV causes intrauterine infection, adversely affects the fetus, or causes abortion or prematurity. RSV does produce infection in neonates, causing asymptomatic infection, afebrile upper respiratory tract infection, bronchiolitis, pneumonia, and apnea. Mortality can be high in neonates, especially in premature infants and ill full-term infants, particularly those with preexisting respiratory disease (hyaline membrane disease, bronchopulmonary dysplasia) or cardiac disease associated with pulmonary hypertension.

RSV is believed to be transmitted via droplets or direct contact of the conjunctiva, nasal mucosa, or oropharynx with infected respiratory secretions. Documentation of RSV infection is rarely made in adults, and spread from the mother or other household contacts probably occurs before a diagnosis can be made. Therefore risk of RSV transmission from breast milk is probably insignificant compared with transmission via direct or droplet contact in families. In nurseries, however, it is appropriate to make a timely diagnosis of RSV infection in the neonate to gain the benefit of treatment with ribavirin and to isolate the infant from the others to prevent spread in the nursery. RSV infection should be suspected in any infant with rhinorrhea, nasal congestion, or unexplained apnea, especially in October through March in temperate climates. Prophylaxis against RSV with specific intravenous immune globulin (RSV-IGIV) during this season for infants at highest risk of severe disease may be appropriate.

Considerable debate surrounds the effect of passively acquired antibodies against RSV on the occurrence and severity of illness in the neonate and infant. It appears that a higher level of neutralizing antibody against RSV in the neonate decreases the risk of severe RSV disease.[73,102] However, some controversy remains concerning the measurable benefit of breastfeeding for preventing serious RSV disease.[50] Different studies have shown benefit and others no effect. Controlling for possible confounding factors (e.g., smoking, crowded living conditions) in these studies has been difficult. At this point, no reason exists to stop breastfeeding with maternal RSV infection, and infants with RSV infection should breastfeed unless their respiratory status precludes it.

SPIROCHETES

Lyme disease

Lyme disease, as with the other human illnesses caused by spirochetes, especially syphilis, is characterized by a protean course and distinct phases (stages) of disease. Lyme borreliosis was described in Europe in the early twentieth century. Since the 1970s, tremendous recognition, description, and investigation of Lyme disease have occurred in the United States and Europe. Public concern surrounding this illness is dramatic.

Lyme disease is a multisystem disease characterized by involvement of the skin, heart, joints, and nervous system (peripheral and central). Stages of disease are identified as *early localized* (erythema migrans [EM], often accompanied by arthralgia, neck stiffness, fever, malaise, and headache), *early disseminated* (multiple EM lesions, cranial nerve palsies, meningitis, conjunctivitis, arthralgia, myalgia, headache, fatigue, and, rarely, myocarditis), and *late disease* (recurrent arthritis, encephalopathy, and neuropathy). The varied manifestations of disease may relate to the degree of spirochetemia, the extent of dissemination to specific tissues, and the host's immunologic response.

The diagnosis of Lyme disease is often difficult in part because of the broad spectrum of presentations, inapparent exposure to the tick, and the lack of adequately standardized serologic tests. Culture of the spirochete, *Borrelia burgdorferi,* is not readily available. ELISA, immunofluorescent assay (IFA), and immunoblot assay are the usual tests. PCR detection of spirochetal DNA requires additional testing in clinical situations to clarify and standardize its utility.

Gardner[67] reviewed infection during pregnancy, summarizing a total of 46 adverse outcomes from 161 cases reported in the literature. The adverse outcomes included miscarriage and stillbirth (11% of cases), perinatal death (3%), congenital anomalies (15%), and both early- and late-onset progressive infection in the infant. Silver[160] reviewed 11 published reports and concluded that Lyme disease during pregnancy is uncommon, even in endemic areas. Although the spirochete can be transmitted transplacentally, a significant immune response in the fetus is often lacking, and the association of Lyme infection with congenital abnormalities is weak.

Little published information exists on whether *B. burgdorferi* can be transmitted via breast milk. One report showed the detection of *B. burgdorferi* DNA by PCR in the breast milk of two lactating women with untreated EM, but no evidence of Lyme disease or transmission of the spirochete in the one infant followed for 1 year.[158] No attempt to culture the spirochete was made, so it is not possible to determine if the detectable DNA was from viable spirochetes or noninfectious fragments. In that same study, of 56 women with untreated EM who had detectable *B. burgdorferi* DNA in the urine, 32 still had detectable DNA in the urine 15 to 30 days after starting treatment, but none had detectable DNA in urine 6 months after initiating therapy.

The lack of adequate information on transmission of *B. burgdorferi* via breast milk cannot be taken as proof that it is not occurring. If one extrapolates from data on syphilis and the *Treponema pallidum* spirochete, it would be prudent to discuss the lack of information on the transmission of *B. burgdorferi* via breast milk with the mother or parents and to consider withholding breast milk at least until therapy for Lyme disease has begun or been completed. If the infection occurred during pregnancy and treatment has already been completed, the infant can breastfeed. If infection occurs postpartum or the diagnosis is

made postpartum, infant exposure may have already occurred; again, discussion with the mother or parents about withholding versus continuing breastfeeding is appropriate.

After prenatal or postnatal exposure, the infant should be closely observed and empiric therapy considered if the infant develops a rash or symptoms suggestive of Lyme borreliosis. Treatment of the mother and infant with ceftriaxone, penicillin, or amoxicillin is acceptable during breastfeeding relative to the infant's exposure to these medications. Doxycycline should not be administered for more than 14 days while continuing breastfeeding because of possible dental staining in the neonate. Continued surveillance for viable organisms in breast milk and evidence of transmission through breastfeeding is recommended.

A large body of information is available on various "Lyme vaccines" used in dogs, which are only partially protective and must be repeated yearly. Preliminary information suggests that a vaccine for use in humans safely produces good serologic responses, but protective efficacy has not been demonstrated, and no information exists on its use during pregnancy or breastfeeding.

Syphilis

Syphilis is the classic example of a spirochetal infection that causes multisystem disease in various stages. Both acquired syphilis and congenital syphilis are well-described entities. *Acquired syphilis* is almost always transmitted through direct sexual contact with open lesions of the skin or mucous membranes of individuals infected with the spirochete, *Treponema pallidum*. *Congenital syphilis* occurs by infection across the placenta (placentitis) at any time during the pregnancy or by contact with the spirochete during passage through the birth canal. Any stage of disease (primary, secondary, tertiary) in the mother can lead to infection of the fetus, but transmission in association with secondary syphilis approaches 100%. Infection with primary syphilis during pregnancy, without treatment, leads to spontaneous abortion, stillbirth, or perinatal death in 40% of cases. Similar to acquired syphilis, congenital syphilis manifests with moist lesions or secretions from rhinitis (snuffles), condylomata lata, or bullous lesions. These lesions and secretions contain numerous spirochetes and are therefore highly infectious.

Postnatal infection of the infant can occur through contact with open, moist lesions of the skin or mucous membranes in the mother or other infected individuals. If the mother or infant has potentially infectious lesions, isolation from each other and from other infants and mothers is recommended. If lesions are on the breasts or nipples, breastfeeding or using expressed milk is contraindicated until treatment is complete and the lesions have cleared. Spirochetes are rarely identified in open lesions after more than 24 hours of appropriate treatment. Penicillin remains the best therapy.

Evaluation of the infant with suspected syphilis should be based on the mother's clinical and serologic status, history of adequate therapy in the mother, and the infant's clinical status. Histologic examination of the placenta and umbilical cord, serologic testing of the infant's blood and CSF, complete analysis of the CSF, long bone and chest radiographs, liver function tests, and a complete blood cell count are all appropriate given the specific clinical situation. Treatment of the infant should follow recommended protocols for suspected, probable, or proven syphilitic infection.[38]

No evidence indicates transmission of syphilis via breast milk in the absence of a breast or nipple lesion. When the mother has no suspicious breast lesions, breastfeeding is acceptable as long as appropriate therapy for suspected or proven syphilis is begun in the mother and infant.

PARASITES

Toxoplasmosis

Toxoplasmosis is one of the most common infections of humans throughout the world. The infective organism, *Toxoplasma gondii,* is ubiquitous in nature. The prevalence of positive serologic test titers increases with age, indicating past exposure and infection. The cat is the definitive host,

although infection occurs in most species of warm-blooded animals.

Postnatal infection with toxoplasmosis is usually asymptomatic. Symptomatic infection typically manifests with nonspecific symptoms, including fever, malaise, myalgia, sore throat, lymphadenopathy, rash, hepatosplenomegaly, and occasionally a mononucleosis-like illness. The illness usually resolves without treatment or significant complications.

Congenital infection or infection in an immunodeficient individual can be persistent and severe with significant morbidity and mortality. Although most infants with congenital infection are asymptomatic at birth, visual abnormalities, learning disabilities, and mental retardation can occur months or years later in many children. There is a clearly defined syndrome of *congenital toxoplasmosis,* with the most severe manifestations involving the CNS, including hydrocephalus, cerebral calcifications, microcephaly, chorioretinitis, seizures, or simply isolated ocular involvement. The risk of fetal infection is related to the timing of primary maternal infection, although transmission can occur with preexisting maternal toxoplasmosis. In the last months of pregnancy the protozoan is more readily transmitted to the fetus, but the infection is more likely to be subclinical. Early in pregnancy the transmission to the fetus occurs less frequently but does result in severe disease. Treatment of documented congenital infection is currently recommended, although the duration and optimal regimen have not been determined, and reversal of preexisting sequelae generally does not occur.[145]

Prevention of infection in susceptible pregnant women is possible by avoiding exposure to cat feces or the organism in the soil. Pregnant or lactating women should not change cat litter boxes, but if they must, it should be done daily and while wearing gloves. The oocyst is not infective for the first 24 to 48 hours after passage. Mothers can avoid ingestion of the organism by fully cooking meats and carefully washing fruits, vegetables, and food preparation surfaces.[38]

In various animal models, *T. gondii* has been transmitted through the milk to the suckling young.

The organism has been isolated from colostrum as well. The newborn animals became asymptomatically infected when nursed by an infected mother whose colostrum contained *T. gondii*. Only one report has identified *T. gondii* in human milk, and some question surrounds the reliability of that report.[104] Transmission during breastfeeding in humans has not been demonstrated. Breast milk may contain appropriate antibodies against *T. gondii*. Given the benign nature of postnatal infection, the absence of documented transmission in human breast milk, and the potential antibodies in breast milk, no reason exists to proscribe breastfeeding by a mother known to be infected with toxoplasmosis.

Giardia lamblia

Giardiasis is a localized infection limited to the intestinal tract and causing diarrhea and malabsorption. Immunocompetent individuals show no evidence of invasive infection, and no evidence indicates fetal infection from maternal infection during pregnancy. Giardiasis is rare in children under 6 months of age, although neonatal infection from fecal contamination at birth has been described.[12] Human milk has an in vivo protective effect against *G. lamblia* infection, as documented by work from central Africa, where the end of breastfeeding heralds the onset of *Giardia* infection.[69] This has been reaffirmed in undeveloped countries around the world.

The protective effect of breast milk has been identified in the milk of noninfected donors.[71] The antiparasitic effect does not result from specific antibodies but rather from lipase enzymatic activity. The lipase acts in the presence of bile salts to destroy the trophozoites as they emerge from their cysts in the GI tract. Hernell et al[80] demonstrated that free fatty acids have a marked giardiacidal effect, which supports the conclusion that lipase activity releasing fatty acids is responsible for killing *G. lamblia*.

G. lamblia have also been reported to appear in the mother's milk, and the parasite has been transmitted to newborns via that route. The exact relationship of breastfeeding to transmission of *G. lamblia* and the effect on the infant continue to be studied, even though symptomatic infection in the breastfed infant is rare.[72] Breastfeeding by mothers with giardiasis is mainly problematic because of the medications used for therapy. Metronidazole's safety in infants has not been established, and little information is available on quinacrine hydrochloride and furazolidone in breast milk. Paramomycin, a nonabsorbable aminoglycoside, is a reasonable alternative recommended for treatment of pregnant women. Breastfeeding by the mother with symptomatic giardiasis is acceptable when consideration is given to the presence of the therapeutic agents in the breast milk.

Trichomonas vaginalis

Trichomonas vaginalis is a flagellated protozoan that can produce vaginitis (see Chapter 15) but frequently causes asymptomatic infection in both males and females. The parasite is found in 10% to 25% of women in the childbearing years. It is transmitted predominantly by sexual intercourse, but it can be transmitted to the neonate by passage through the birth canal. This parasite often coexists with other STDs, especially gonorrhea.

Infection during pregnancy or while taking oral contraceptives is more difficult to treat. Some evidence suggests that infection with and growth of the parasite are enhanced by estrogens or their effect on the vaginal epithelium. No evidence indicates adverse effects on the fetus in association with maternal infection during pregnancy. Occasionally the female newborn has a vaginal discharge during the first weeks of life caused by *T. vaginalis*. This is thought to be influenced by the effect of maternal estrogen on the infant's vaginal epithelium and acquisition of the organism during passage through the birth canal. The organism does not seem to cause significant disease in the healthy infant. No documentation exists on transmission of *T. vaginalis* via breast milk.

The difficulty encountered with maternal infection during lactation stems from metronidazole (Flagyl), the drug of choice, being contraindicated for infants. Case reports describe treatment of neonates with metronidazole without adverse effect. Although topical agents containing povidone-iodine (Betadine) or sodium lauryl sulfate (Trichotine) can be effective when given as douches, creams, or suppositories, metronidazole remains the treatment of choice. The AAP advises using metronidazole only with the physician's discretion and considers its effect on the nursing infant unknown but possibly a concern. The potential concerns are metronidazole's disulfiram-like effect in association with alcohol, tumorigenecity in animal studies, and the leukopenia and neurologic side effects described in adults. On the other hand, metronidazole is given to children beyond the neonatal period to treat serious infections with various other parasites, such as *Entamoeba histolytica.*

The current recommendation for lactating women is to try local treatment first, and if these fail, then to try metronidazole. A 2-g single-dose treatment produces peak levels after 1 hour, and discarding expressed breast milk for the next 12 to 24 hours is recommended. If this treatment also fails, a 1-g twice-daily regimen for 7 days or a 2-g single daily dose for 3 to 5 days is recommended, with discarding of some breast milk close to the dose and timing of feedings distant from the dose. Infants who exclusively breastfeed are presumed at greater risk from exposure to metronidazole than those who are only partially breastfed.

Malaria

Malaria is recognized as a major health problem in many countries. The effect of malaria infection on pregnant and lactating women and thus on the developing fetus, neonate, and growing infant can be significant. The four species of malaria, *Plasmodium vivax, ovale, malariae,* and *falciparum,* vary in the specific aspects of the disease they produce. *P. vivax* exists throughout the world, but *P. falciparum* predominates in the tropics and is most problematic in its chloroquine-resistant form. Malaria in the United States is most often seen in individuals traveling from areas where malaria is endemic. The parasite can exist in the blood for weeks, and infection with *P. vivax* and *P. malariae* can lead to relapses years later. Transmission occurs through the bite of the anopheline mosquito and can occur via transfusion of blood products and transplacentally.

Congenital malaria is rare but seems to occur more often with *P. vivax* and *P. falciparum.* It usually presents in the first 7 days of life (range 1 day to 2 months). It may resemble neonatal sepsis, with fever, anemia, and splenomegaly occurring in the most neonates and hyperbilirubinemia and hepatomegaly in less than half.

Malaria in infants less than 3 months of age generally manifests with less severe disease and mortality than in older children. Possible explanations include the effect of less exposure to mosquitoes, passive antibody acquired from the mother, and the high level of fetal hemoglobin in the infant at this age.[11] The variations in the infection rates in children less than 3 months of age during the wet and dry seasons support the idea that postnatal infection is more common than congenital infection. No evidence indicates that malaria is transmitted through breast milk. The greatest risk to the infant is exposure to the anopheline mosquito infected with malaria.

The main issues relative to malaria and breastfeeding are how to protect both the mother and the infant effectively from mosquitoes and what drugs for treating malaria in the mother are appropriate during lactation. Protection from mosquito bites includes screened-in living areas, mosquito nets while sleeping, protective clothing with or without repellents on the clothes, and community efforts to eradicate the mosquitoes. Chloroquine, quinine, and tetracycline are acceptable during breastfeeding. Sulfonamides should be avoided in the first month of the infant's life, but pyrimethamine-sulfadoxine (Fansidar) can be used later.

Mefloquine is not approved for infants or pregnant women. However, the milk/plasma ratio for mefloquine is less than 0.25, there is a large volume of distribution of the drug, high protein binding of the drug limits its presence in breast milk, and the relative importance of breastfeeding in areas where malaria is prevalent shifts the risk/benefit ratio in favor of treatment with mefloquine. The single dose recommended for treatment or the once-weekly dose for prevention allows for continued breastfeeding with discarding of the milk for short periods after a dose (1 to 6 hours). Inadequate information exists to make a recommendation for primaquine.[38] Therefore breastfeeding during maternal malaria even with treatment is appropriate with specific medications.

CANDIDAL FUNGAL INFECTIONS

Candida consists of multiple species. The most common species affecting humans include *C. albicans* as the dominant agent and *C. tropicalis, C. krusei,* and *C. parapsilosis,* as well as many other uncommon species. In general, *Candida* exists as a commensal organism colonizing the oropharynx, GI tract, vagina, and skin without causing disease until some change disrupts the balance between the organism and the host. Mild mucocutaneous infection is the most common illness, often leading to vulvovaginitis and rarely to mastitis in the mother (see Chapter 15) and thrush (oral candidiasis) and candidal diaper rash in the infant.

Invasive candidal infection occurs infrequently, usually when the individual has other illness, impaired resistance to infection (HIV, diabetes mellitus, neutropenia; decreased cell-mediated immunity in premature infants), and disrupted normal mucosal and skin barriers and has received antibiotics or corticosteroids. Invasive disease can occur through local spread, as may occur more often in the genitourinary tract (urethra, bladder, ureters, kidneys), but usually develops in association with candidemia. The bladder, kidney, and meninges are more frequently involved, but when dissemination occurs via candidemia, a careful search for other sites of infection should be made (e.g., retina, liver, spleen).

Transmission usually occurs from healthy individuals colonized with *Candida* through direct contact with them or through their oral or vaginal secretions. Intrauterine infection can occur through ascending infection up through the birth canal but is rare. No distinct syndrome of congenital candidal infection exists. Most often the infant is infected in passing through the birth canal and remains colonized. Postnatal transmission can occur through direct contact with caregivers. Reports on how the mother and infant serve as an immediate source of recolonization after one or the other is treated for mucocutaneous candidiasis suggest that the infant and breastfeeding mother should be treated simultaneously when treating thrush, vulvovaginitis, diaper candidiasis, or mastitis. Because colonization with this organism usually occurs in the absence of any clinical evidence of infection, simultaneous treatment should occur regardless of any evidence of *Candida* in the apparently uninvolved individual in the dyad.

Treatment of mucocutaneous candidiasis should begin with a topical agent, such as nystatin, clotrimazole, miconazole, econazole, butaconazole, terconazole, or ciclopirox. Treatment should continue for at least 2 weeks, even with obvious improvement in 1 or 2 days. Failures most often result from inadequate therapy involving the frequency of application, careful washing and drying before application, or in the case of diaper candidiasis, decreasing moisture as well.

When careful instructions and retreatment with topical agents again fail, systemic therapy is appropriate. Fluconazole, ketoconazole, and IV amphotericin B with or without oral flucytosine are reasonable choices in different situations. Although fluconazole and ketoconazole have not been used extensively in infants less than 6 months of age, and their safety and efficacy is not well established by controlled studies, their use in chronic or invasive candidal infection is indicated in certain situations. Treatment of chronic mucocutaneous candidiasis or invasive disease with amphotericin B with or without oral flucytosine is appropriate. Use of itraconazole in infants has not been adequately studied to date. Using these agents in the breastfeeding mother is not contraindicated because they are used in infants in specific situations. Breastfeeding can continue. Whenever the mother is treated for candidal mastitis or vulvovaginitis, the infant should be treated simultaneously at least with nystatin oral suspension as the first choice of medication.

Any predisposing risk factors for candidal infection in the mother and infant should be reduced or eliminated to improve the chance of rapid, successful treatment and to decrease the likelihood of chronic or recurrent disease. For the mother, such interventions might include decreasing sugar consumption, stopping antibiotic use as soon as possible, and eating yogurt with active acidophilus, which can alter the normal colonizing bacterial flora, increasing the presence of acidophilus or lactobacillus. For the infant, breastfeeding can help enhance the growth of specific colonizing bacterial flora such as lactobacillus, which can successfully limit fungal growth. Standard precautions are appropriate even between the mother and infant, emphasizing careful handwashing, but breastfeeding can continue.

REFERENCES

1. Adu FD, Adeniji JA et al: Measles antibodies in the breast milk of nursing mothers, *Afr J Med Med Sci* 24:385, 1995.
2. Alford C: Breast milk transmission of cytomegalovirus (CMV) infection. In Mestecky J et al, editors: *Immunology of milk and the neonate,* New York, 1991, Plenum.
3. Alford CA, Stagno S, Pass RF et al: Congenital and perinatal cytomegalovirus infections, *Rev Infect Dis* 12: S745, 1990.
4. Alter HJ: The cloning and clinical implications of HGV and HGBV-C, *N Engl J Med* 334:1536, 1996.
5. Ando Y, Saito K, Nakano S et al: Bottle feeding can prevent transmission of HTLV-I from mothers to their babies, *J Infect* 19:25, 1989.
6. Anthony BF, Okada DM, Hobel CJ: Epidemiology of group B streptococcus: maternal and nosocomial sources for acquisition, *J Pediatr* 95:431, 1979.
7. Armstrong L, Garay SM: Tuberculosis and pregnancy and tuberculous mastitis. In Rom WN, Garay SM, editors: *Tuberculosis,* Boston, 1996, Little, Brown.
8. Arnon SS: Infant botulism, *Ann Rev Med* 31:541, 1980.
9. Arnon SS: Infant botulism: anticipating the second decade, *J Infect Dis* 154:201, 1986.
10. Arnon SS, Damus K, Thompson B et al: Protective role of human milk against sudden death from infant botulism, *J Pediatr* 100:568, 1982.
11. Arvin AM, Maldonado YA: Other viral infections of the fetus and newborn. In Remington JS, Klein JO, editors: *Infectious diseases of the fetus and newborn infant,* ed 4, Philadelphia, 1995, Saunders.
12. Arvin AM, Maldonado YA: Protozoan and helminth infections (including *Pneumocystis carinii*). In Remington JS, Klein JO, editors: *Infectious diseases of the fetus and newborn infant,* ed 4, Philadelphia, 1995, Saunders.
13. Bannister BA: Stringent precautions are advisable when caring for patients with viral hemorrhagic fevers, *Rev Med Virol* 3:3, 1993.
14. Barden LS: Personal communication, 1998.
15. Barton LL, Budd SC, Morfitt WS et al: Congenital lymphocytic choriomeningitis virus infection in twins, *Pediatr Infect Dis J* 12:942, 1993.
16. Bates T: Poliomyelitis in pregnancy, fetus and newborn, *Am J Dis Child* 90:189, 1955.
17. Beasley RP: Transmission of hepatitis by breastfeeding, *N Engl J Med* 292:1354, 1975 (letter).
18. Beasley RP, Stevens CE, Shiao I et al: Evidence against breast feeding as a mechanism for vertical transmission of hepatitis B, *Lancet* 2:740, 1975.
19. Belec L, Bouquety JC, Georges AJ et al: Antibodies to HIV in the breastmilk of healthy, seropositive women, *Pediatrics* 85:1022, 1990.
20. Bergdoll MS, Crass BA, Reisser et al: A new staphylococcal enterotoxin, enterotoxin F, associated with TSS *Staphylococcus aureus* isolate, *Lancet* 1:1017, 1981.
21. Bertotto A, Gerli R, Castellucci G et al: Mycobacteria-reactive T cells are present in human colostrum from tuberculin-positive, but not tuberculin-negative nursing mothers, *Am J Reprod Immunol* 29:131, 1993.
22. Bleck TP, Rupprecht CE: Rhabdoviruses. In Richman DD, Whitley RJ, Hayden FG, editors: *Clinical virology,* New York, 1997, Churchill Livingstone.
23. Bortolotti F, Resti M, Giacchino R et al: Hepatitis C virus infection and related liver disease in children of mothers with antibodies to the virus, *J Pediatr* 130:990, 1997.
24. Brinton LA, Hoover R, Fraumeni JF Jr.: Reproductive factors in the aetiology of breast cancer, *Br J Cancer* 47:757, 1983.
25. Butter MNW, DeMoor CE: *Streptococcus agalactiae* as a cause of meningitis in the newborn and bacteraemia in adults, *Antonie Van Leeuwenhoek* 33:439, 1967.
26. Cantwell M, Snider DE Jr, Cauthen G et al: Epidemiology of tuberculosis in the United States, 1985-1992, *JAMA* 272:535, 1994.

27. Centers for Disease Control and Prevention: *Testing for antibodies to HIV-2 in the United States, MMWR* 41:1, 1992.

28. Centers for Disease Control and Prevention: Compendium of animal rabies control, 1995, *MMWR* 44(RR-2): 1, 1995.

29. Centers for Disease Control and Prevention: Screening for tuberculosis and tuberculosis infection in high-risk populations, *MMWR* 44(RR-11):19, 1995.

30. Centers for Disease Control and Prevention: Human rabies—Alabama, Tennessee, and Texas, 1994, *MMWR* 44:269, 1995.

31. Centers for Disease Control and Prevention: Update: management of patients with suspected viral hemorrhagic fever—United States, *MMWR* 44:475, 1995.

32. Centers for Disease Control and Prevention: Human rabies—Washington, 1995, *MMWR* 44:625, 1995.

33. Centers for Disease Control and Prevention, Advisory Committee on Immunization Practices: Poliomyelitis prevention in the United States: introduction of a sequential vaccination schedule of inactivated poliovirus vaccine followed by oral poliovirus vaccine—United States, *MMWR* 46:1, 1997.

34. Ceyhan M, Kaura G, Secmeer G et al: Take of rhesus-human reassortment tetravalent rotavirus vaccine in breastfed infants, *Acta Pediatr* 82:223, 1993.

35. Cherry JD: Enteroviruses: polioviruses (poliomyelitis), coxsackieviruses, and enteroviruses. In Feigin RD, Cherry JD, editors: *Textbook of pediatric infectious diseases,* ed 3, Philadelphia, 1992, Saunders.

36. Chopra H, Ebert P, Woodside N et al: Electron microscopic detection of simian-type virus particles in human milk, *Nat Biol* 243:159, 1973.

37. Clemens J, Rao M, Eng M et al: Breastfeeding and the risk of life-threatening rotavirus diarrhea: prevention or postponement? *Pediatrics* 92:680, 1993.

38. Committee on Infectious Diseases, American Academy of Pediatrics: *Red book: report of the Committee on Infectious Disease,* ed 24, Elk Grove Village, Ill, 1997, The Academy.

39. Committee on Infectious Diseases and Committee on the Fetus and Newborn, American Academy of Pediatrics: Revised guidelines for prevention of early-onset group B streptococcal (GBS) infection, *Pediatrics* 99:489, 1997.

40. Connor EM, Mofenson LM: Zidovudine for the reduction of perinatal human immunodeficiency virus transmission: Pediatric AIDS Clinical Trials Group Protocol O76—results and treatment recommendations, *Pediatr Infect Dis J* 14:536, 1995.

41. Datta P, Embree JE, Kreiss JK et al: Resumption of breast-feeding in later childhood: a risk factor for mother to child human immunodeficiency virus type 1 transmission, *Pediatr Infect Dis J* 11:974, 1992.

42. Davis MK: Human milk and HIV infection: epidemiologic and laboratory data. In Mestecky J et al, editors: *Immunology of milk and the neonate,* New York, 1991, Plenum.

43. De Martino M, Tovo PA, Tozzi et al: HIV-1 transmission through breast-milk: appraisal of risk according to duration of feeding, *AIDS* 6:991, 1992.

44. Del Fante P, Jenniskens F, Lush L et al: HIV, breastfeeding and under 5 mortality: modelling the impact of policy decisions for or against breastfeeding, *J Trop Med Hyg* 96:203, 1994.

45. Del Mistro A, Chotard J, Hall AJ et al: HTLV-I/II seroprevalence in The Gambia: a study of mother-child pairs, *AIDS Res Hum Retroviruses* 10:617, 1994.

46. Derkay CS: Task Force on Recurrent Respiratory Papillomatosis, *Acta Otolaryngol Head/Neck Surg* 121:1386, 1995.

47. Dillon HC Jr, Khare S, Gray BM: Group B streptococcal carriage and disease: a 6 year prospective study, *J Pediatr* 110:31, 1987.

48. Dinsmoor MJ: Hepatitis in the obstetric patient, *Infect Obstet* 11:77, 1997.

49. Dormer BA, Swarit JA, Harrison I et al: Prophylactic isoniazid protection of infants in a tuberculosis hospital, *Lancet* ii:902, 1959.

50. Downham M, Scott R, Sims DG et al: Breast-feeding protects against respiratory syncytial virus infections, *Br Med J* 2:274, 1976.

51. Dunkle LM, Schmidt RR, O'Connor DM: Neonatal herpes simplex infection possibly acquired via maternal breast milk, *Pediatrics* 63:250, 1979.

52. Dunn DT, Newell ML, Ades AE et al: Risk of human immunodeficiency virus type 1 transmission through breastfeeding, *Lancet* 340:585, 1992.

53. Dunne WM, Demmler GJ: Serologic evidence for congenital transmission of human herpesvirus, 6, *Lancet* 340:121, 1992.

54. Dunne WM, Jevon M: Examination of human breastmilk for evidence of human herpesvirus 6 by PCR, *J Infect Dis* 168:250, 1993.

55. Dworsky M, Yow M, Stagno S et al: Cytomegalovirus infection of breast milk and transmission in infancy, *Pediatrics* 72:295, 1983.

56. Ekpini ER, Wiktor SZ, Satten GA et al: Late postnatal mother-to-child transmission of HIV-1 in Abidjan, Cote d'Ivoire, *Lancet* 349:1054, 1997.

57. Enocksson E, Wretlind B, Sterner G et al: Listeriosis during pregnancy and in neonates, *Scand J Infect Dis Suppl* 71:89, 1990.

58. Espinosa F, Paniagua M, Hallander H et al: Rotavirus infections in young Nicaraguan children, *Pediatr Infect Dis J* 16:564, 1997.

59. Fairchild JP, Graber CD, Vogel EH et al: Flora of the umbilical stump: 2479 cultures, *J Pediatr* 53:538, 1958.

60. Faye A, Burgard M, Crosnier H et al: Human immunodeficiency virus type 2 infection in children, *J Pediatr* 130:994, 1997.

61. Feucht HH, Zollner B, Polywka S et al: Vertical transmission of hepatitis G, *Lancet* 347:615, 1996.

62. Fieldsteel AH: Nonspecific antiviral substances in human milk against arbovirus and murine leukemia virus, *Cancer Res* 34:712, 1974.

63. Fischler B, Lara C, Chen M et al: Genetic evidence for mother-to-infant transmission of hepatitis G virus, *J Infect Dis* 176:281, 1997.

64. Fisher-Hoch SP: Stringent precautions are not advisable when caring for patients with viral hemorrhagic fevers, *Rev Med Virol* 3:7, 1993.

65. Friis H, Andersen HK: Rate of inactivation of cytomegalovirus in raw banked milk during storage at −20 degrees C and pasteurisation, *Br Med J Clin Res* 285:1604, 1982.

66. Gardner SE, Mason EO Jr, Yow MD: Community acquisition of group B streptococcus by infants of colonized mothers, *Pediatrics* 66:873, 1980.

67. Gardner T: Lyme disease. In Remington JS, Klein JO, editors: *Infectious disease of the fetus and newborn infant,* ed 4, Philadelphia, 1995, Saunders.

68. Garner JS: Hospital Infection Control Practices Advisory Committee: Guidelines for isolation precautions in hospitals, *Infect Control Hosp Epidemiol* 17:53, 1996.

69. Gendrel D, Richard-Lenoble D, Kombila M et al: Giardiasis and breastfeeding in urban Africa, *Pediatr Infect Dis J* 8:58, 1989.

70. Gershon AA: Chickenpox, measles and mumps. In Remington JS, Klein JO, editors: *Infectious diseases of the fetus and newborn infant,* ed 4, Philadelphia, 1995, Saunders.

71. Gervais F, Joncas JH: Seroepidemiology in various population groups of the greater Montreal area, *Comp Immunol Microbiol Infect Dis* 2:207, 1979.

72. Gillin FD, Reiner DS, Gault MJ: Cholate-dependent killing of *Giardia lamblia* by human milk, *Infect Immunol* 47:619, 1985.

73. Glezen WP, Paredes A, Allison JE et al: Risk of respiratory syncytial virus infection for infants from low-income families in relationship to age, sex, ethnic group, and maternal antibody level, *J Pediatr* 98:708, 1981.

74. Goldblum RM, Dill CW, Albrecht TB et al: Rapid high temperature treatment of human milk, *J Pediatr* 104:380, 1984.

75. Gupta R, Gupta AS, Duggal N: Tubercular mastitis, *Int Surg* 67:422, 1982.

76. Gurakan B, Oran O, Yigit S et al: Vertical transmission of hepatitis C virus, *N Engl J Med* 331:399, 1994 (letter).

77. Harjulhto T, Aro T, Hovi T et al: Congenital malformations and oral poliovirus vaccination during pregnancy, *Lancet* I:771, 1989.

78. Hayes K, Danks DM, Gibas H et al: Cytomegalovirus in human milk, *N Engl J Med* 287:177, 1972.

79. Henderson BE, Powell D, Rosario I et al: An epidemiologic study of breast cancer, *J Natl Cancer Inst* 53:609, 1974.

80. Hernell O, Ward H, Blackberg L: Killing of *Giardia lamblia* by human milk lipases: an effect mediated by lipolysis of milk lipids, *J Infect Dis* 153:715, 1986.

81. Heyman SJ: Modeling the impact of breastfeeding by HIV infected women on child survival, *Am J Public Health* 80:1305, 1990.

82. Hino S: Milk-borne transmission of HTLV-I as a major route in the endemic cycle, *Acta Pediatr Jpn* 31:428, 1989.

83. Hino S, Katamine S, Kawase K et al: Intervention of maternal transmission of HTLV-I in Nagasaki, Japan, *Leukemia* 94:S68, 1993.

84. Hjelt K, Granbella PC, Haagen O et al: Rotavirus antibodies in the mother and her breastfed infant, *J Pediatr Gastroenterol Nutr* 4:414, 1985.

85. Horn P: Poliomyelitis in pregnancy: a twenty-year report from Los Angeles County, California, *Obstet Gynecol* 6:121, 1955.

86. Horowitz CA, Henle W, Henle G et al: Long-term serologic follow-up of patients for Epstein-Barr virus after recovery from infectious mononucleosis, *J Infect Dis* 151:1150, 1985.

87. Horsburgh CR, Holmberg SC: The global distribution of human immunodeficiency virus type 2 (HIV-2) infection, *Transfusion* 28:192, 1988.

88. Hu DJ, Heyward WL, Byers RH et al: HIV infection and breastfeeding: policy implications through a decision analysis model, *AIDS* 6:1501, 1992.

89. Hurst V: *Staphylococcus aureus* in the infant upper respiratory tract. I. Observations on hospital-born babies, *J Hyg* 55:299, 1957.

90. Ing R, Ho JHC, Petrakis NL: Unilateral breast feeding and breast cancer, *Lancet* 2:124, 1977.

91. Italian Register for HIV Infection in Children: HIV-1 infection and breastmilk, *Acta Paediatr Suppl* 400: 51, 1994.

92. Jeliffe DB, Jeliffe EFP: *Human milk in the modern world,* Oxford, 1978, Oxford University Press.

93. Junker AK, Thomas EE, Radcliffe A et al: Epstein-Barr virus shedding in breast milk, *Am J Med Sci* 302:220, 1991.

94. Kalstone C: Successful antepartum treatment of listeriosis, *Am J Obstet Gynecol* 164:57, 1991.

95. Katzman DK, Wald ER: Staphylococcal scalded skin syndrome in a breastfed infant, *Pediatr Infect Dis J* 6:295, 1987.

96. Keelyside RA, McCormick JB, Webb PA et al: Case-control study of *Mastomys natalensis* and humans in Lassa virus–infected households in Sierra Leone, *Am J Trop Med Hyg* 32:829, 1983.

97. Keller MA, Rodriguez AI, Alvarez S et al: Transfer of tuberculin immunity from mother to infant, *Pediatr Res* 22:277, 1987.

98. Kenny JF, Zedd AJ: Recurrent group B streptococcal disease in an infant associated with the ingestion of infected mother's milk, *J Pediatr* 91:158, 1977.

99. Koch WC, Adler SP: Human parvovirus B19 infection in women of childbearing age and within families, *Pediatr Infect Dis J* 8:83, 1989.

100. Komrower GM, Williams BL, Stones PB: Lymphocytic choriomeningitis in the newborn, *Lancet* 1955, part 1:697.

101. Kumar ML, Nankervis GA, Jacobs IB et al: Congenital and postnatally acquired cytomegalovirus infections: long-term follow-up, *J Pediatr* 104:674, 1984.

102. Lamprecht CL, Krause HE, Mufson MA: Role of maternal antibody in pneumonia and bronchiolitis due to respiratory syncytial virus, *J Infect Dis* 134:211, 1976.

103. Lane-Claypon JE: A further report on cancer of the breast, with special reference to its associated antecedent conditions, Report No. 32, *Reports of the Ministry of Health,* London, 1926.

104. Langer H: Repeated congenital infection with *Toxoplasma gondii, Obstet Gynecol* 21:318, 1963.

105. Lawrence RA: A review of the medical benefits and contraindications to breastfeeding in the United States, *Maternal and Child Health Technical Information Bulletin,* October 1997, US Health Resources and Services Administration.

106. Layde PM, Webster LA, Braughman AL et al: The independent associations of parity, age at first full term pregnancy, and duration of breastfeeding with risk of breast cancer, *J Clin Epidemiol* 42:963, 1989.

107. Lederman SA: Estimating infant mortality from HIV and other causes in breastfeeding and bottle-feeding populations, *Pediatrics* 89:290, 1992.

108. Lin HH, Kao JH, Chen PJ et al: Mechanism of vertical transmission of hepatitis G, *Lancet* 347:1116, 1996.

109. Lin HH, Kao JH, Hsu HY et al: Absence of infection in breast-fed infants born to hepatitis C virus–infected mothers, *J Pediatr* 126:589, 1995.

110. Liner RI: Intrauterine listeria infection: prenatal diagnosis by biophysical assessment and amniocentesis, *Am J Obstet Gynecol* 163:1596, 1990.

111. Lubani MM, Dudin KI, Sharda DC et al: Neonatal brucellosis, *Eur J Pediatr* 147:520, 1988.

112. Lubani MM, Dudin KI, Sharda DC et al: A multicenter therapeutic study of 1100 children with brucellosis, *Pediatr Infect Dis J* 8:75, 1989.

113. MacMahon B, Lin TM, Lowe CR et al: Lactation and cancer of the breast: a summary of an international study, *Bull World Health Organ* 42:185, 1970.

114. Manzini P, Saracco G, Cerchier A et al: Human immunodeficiency virus infection as risk factor for mother-to-child hepatitis C virus transmission: persistence of anti–hepatitis C virus in children is associated with the mother's anti–hepatitis C virus immunoblotting pattern, *Hepatology* 21:328, 1995.

115. Martin P, Friedman L, Dienstag J: Diagnostic approach. In Zuckerman A, Thomas H, editors: *Viral hepatitis: scientific basis and clinical management,* Edinburgh, 1993, Churchill Livingstone.

116. May JT: Antimicrobial factors and microbial contaminants in human milk: recent studies, *J Pediatr Child Health* 30:470, 1994.

117. McManus IC: Predominance of left-sided breast tumors, *Lancet* 2:297, 1977.

118. McTiernan A, Thomas DB: Evidence for a protective effect of lactation on risk of breast cancer in young women: results from a case-control study, *Am J Epidemiol* 124:353, 1986.

119. Menzies D: Effect of treatment on the contagiousness of patients with active pulmonary tuberculosis, *Infect Control Hosp Epidemiol* 18:582, 1997.

120. Miller MJ: Fungal Infections. In Remington JS, Klein JO, editors: *Infectious diseases of the fetus and newborn infant,* ed 4, Philadelphia, 1995, Saunders.

121. Miller RN, Fraumeni JF: Does breast feeding increase the child's risk of breast cancer? *Pediatrics* 49:645, 1972.

122. Minamishima I, Ueda K, Minematsu T et al: Role of breast milk in acquisition of cytomegalovirus infection, *Microbiol Immunol* 38:549, 1994.

123. Morgan RW, Vakil DV, Chipman ML: Breastfeeding family history and breast disease, *Am J Epidemiol* 99:117, 1974.

124. Moriya T, Sasaki F, Mizui M et al: Transmission of hepatitis C virus from mothers to infants: its frequency and risk factors revisited, *Biomed Pharmacother* 49:59, 1995.

125. Nagelkerke NJ, Moses S, Embree JE et al: The duration of breastfeeding by HIV-1 infected mothers in developing countries: balancing benefits and risks, *J Acquir Immune Defic Syndr Hum Retrovirol* 8:176, 1995.

126. Nakano S, Ando Y, Ichijo M et al: Search for possible routes of vertical and horizontal transmission of adult T-cell leukemia virus, *Acta Obstetrica et Gynaecologica Japonica* 37(1):145, 1985.

127. Newburg DS, Linhardt RJ, Ampofo SA et al: Human milk glycosaminoglycans inhibit HIV glycoprotein gp 120 binding to its host cell CD4 receptor, *J Nutr* 125:419, 1995.

128. Newcombe PA, Storer BE, Longnecker MP: Lactation and a reduced risk of premenopausal breast cancer, *N Engl J Med* 330:81, 1994.

129. Numazaki K: Human cytomegalovirus infection of breast milk, *FEMS Immunol Med Micro* 18:91, 1997.

130. O'Brien TR, George JR, Holmberg SD: HIV-2 infection in the United States: epidemiology, diagnosis and public health implications, *JAMA* 267:2775, 1992.

131. Ohto H, Okamoto H, Mishiro S: Vertical transmission of hepatitis C virus, *N Engl J Med* 331:400, 1994 (letter).

132. Ohto H, Terazawa S, Sasaki N et al: Transmission of hepatitis C virus from mothers to infants, *N Engl J Med* 330:744, 1994.

133. Orloff SL, Wallingford JC, McDougal JS: Inactivation of human immunodeficiency virus type I in human milk: effects of intrinsic factors in human milk and of pasteurization, *J Hum Lact* 9:13, 1993.

134. Oxtoby MJ: Human immunodeficiency virus and other viruses in human milk: placing the issues in broader prospective, *Pediatr Infect Dis J* 7:825, 1988.

135. Pabst HF, Grace M, Godel J et al: Effect of breast-feeding on immune response to BCG vaccination, *Lancet* I:295, 1989.

136. Palasanthiran P, Ziegler JB, Stewart GJ et al: Breast-feeding during primary maternal human immunodeficiency virus infection and risk of transmission from mother to infant, *J Infect Dis* 167:441, 1993.

137. Papaioannou AN: Etiologic factors in cancer of the breast in humans: collective review, *Surg Gynecol Obstet* 138:257, 1974.

138. Parks YA, Nuy MF, Aukett MA et al: Methicillin-resistant *Staphylococcus aureus* in milk, *Arch Dis Child* 62:82, 1987.

139. Peckham CS, Johnson C, Ades A et al: Early acquisition of cytomegalovirus infection, *Arch Dis Child* 62:780, 1987.

140. Peters CJ: Arenaviruses. In Richman DD, Whitley RJ, Hayden FG, editors: *Clinical virology,* New York, 1997, Churchill Livingstone.

141. Pickering LK, Morrow AL, Herrera I et al: Effect of maternal rotavirus immunization on milk and serum antibody titers, *J Infect Dis* 172:723, 1995.

142. Pisacane A, Grillo G, Cafiero M et al: Role of breastfeeding in paralytic poliomyelitis, *Br Med J* 305:1367, 1992.

143. Quinn PT, Lofberg JV: Maternal herpetic breast infection: another hazard of neonatal herpes simplex, *Med J Aust* 2:411, 1978.

144. Raucher HS, Grimbetz I: Care of the pregnant woman with tuberculosis and her newborn infant: a pediatrician's perspective, *Mt Sinai J Med* 53:70, 1986.

145. Remington JS, McLeod R, Desmonts G: Toxoplasmosis. In Remington JS, Klein JO, editors: *Infectious diseases in the fetus and newborn infant,* ed 4, Philadelphia, 1995, Saunders.

146. Reyes GR: Hepatitis E virus. In Richman DD, Whitley RJ, Hayden FG, editors: *Clinical virology,* New York, 1997, Churchill Livingstone.

147. Roggiani M, Schlievert PM: Streptococcal toxic shock syndrome, including necrotizing fasciitis and myositis, *Curr Opin Infect Dis* 7:423, 1994.

148. Rosenblum LS, Villarino ME, Nainan OV et al: Hepatitis A outbreak in a neonatal intensive care unit: risk factors for transmission and evidence of prolonged viral excretion among preterm infants, *J Infect Dis* 164:476, 1991.

149. Roy-Burman P, Rongey RW, Henderson BE et al: Attempts to detect RNA tumour virus in human milk, *Nat Biol* 24 4:146, 1973.

150. Ruff AJ, Coberly J, Halsey NA et al: Prevalence of HIV-1 DNA and p24 antigen in breastmilk and correlation with maternal factors, *J AIDS* 7:68, 1994.

151. Sanner T: Removal of inhibitors against RNA-directed DNA polymerase activity in human milk, *Cancer Res* 36:405, 1976.

152. Sarkar NH, Charney J, Doion AS et al: Effect of human milk on mouse mammary tumor virus, *Cancer Res* 33:626, 1973.

153. Schachter J, Grossman M: Chlamydial infections, *Ann Rev Med* 32:45, 1981.

154. Schaefer G, Zervoudakis IA, Fuchs FF et al: Pregnancy and pulmonary tuberculosis, *Obstet Gynecol* 46:706, 1975.

155. Scheiner RL, Coates T, Shackelford PG et al: Possible breast milk transmission of group B streptococcal infection, *J Pediatr* 91:159, 1977.

156. Schlesinger JJ, Covelli HD: Evidence for transmission of lymphocyte responses to tuberculin by breast-feeding, *Lancet* I:529, 1977.

157. Schlievert PM: Toxic shock syndrome, *Postgrad Med* 94:108, 1993.

158. Schmidt B, Aberer E, Stockenhuber C et al: Detection of *Borrelia burgdorferi* DNA by PCR in the urine and breastmilk of patients with Lyme borreliosis, *Diagn Microbiol Infect Dis* 21:121, 1995.

159. Schwer M, Moosa A: Effects of hepatitis A and B in pregnancy on the mother and fetus, *S Afr Med J* 54:1092, 1978.

160. Silver HM: Lyme disease during pregnancy, *Infect Obstet* 11:93, 1997.

161. Skaug K, Otnaess Ab, Orstavik I et al: Chlamydial secretory IgA antibodies in human milk, *Acta Pathol Microbiol Immunol Scand* 90:21, 1982.

162. Smedile A, Niro G, Rizzetto M: Hepatitis D virus. In Richman DD, Whitley RJ, Hayden FG, editors: *Clinical virology,* New York, 1997, Churchill Livingstone.

163. Snider DE Jr, Powell KE: Should women taking antituberculous drugs breast feed? *Arch Int Med* 144:589, 1984.

164. Speer CHP, Gahr M, Pabst MJ: Phagocytosis-associated oxidative metabolism in human milk macrophages, *Acta Pediatr Scand* 75:444, 1986.

165. Stagno S, Cloud GA: Working parents: the impact of day care and breast-feeding on cytomegalovirus infection in offspring, *Proc Natl Acad Sci USA* 91:2384, 1994.

166. Stagno S, Reynolds DW, Pass RF et al: Breast milk and the risk of cytomegalovirus infection, *N Engl J Med* 302:1073, 1980.

167. Starke JR: Tuberculosis, an old disease but a new threat to mother, fetus, and neonate, *Clin Perinatol* 24:107, 1997.

168. Stevens CE, Beasley PR, Tsui J et al: Vertical transmission of hepatitis B antigen in Taiwan, *N Engl J Med* 292:771, 1975.

169. Stevens CE, Taylor PE, Tong MJ et al: Yeast-recombinant hepatitis B vaccine: efficacy with hepatitis B immune globulin in prevention of perinatal hepatitis B virus transmission, *JAMA* 257:2612, 1987.

170. Subcommittee on Nutrition During Lactation, Food and Nutrition Board, Institute of Medicine, National Academy of Sciences, *Nutrition during lactation,* Washington, DC, 1991, National Academy Press.

171. Sugiyama H, Doi H, Yamaguchi et al: Significance of postnatal mother-to-child transmission of HTLV-I on the development of adult T-cell leukemia/lymphoma, *J Med Virol* 20:253, 1986.

172. Sullivan-Bolyai JZ, Fife KH, Jacobs RF et al: Disseminated neonatal herpes simplex virus type I from a maternal breast lesion, *Pediatrics* 71:455, 1983.

173. Sumaya CV: Epstein-Barr virus. In Feigin RD, Cherry JD, editors: *Textbook of pediatric infectious diseases,* ed 3, Philadelphia, 1992, Saunders.

174. Takezaki T, Tajima K, Ito M et al: Short-term breastfeeding may reduce the risk of vertical transmission of HTLV-I, *Leukemia* 11(suppl 3):60, 1997.

175. Thiry L, Sprecher-Goldbrecker S, Jonckheer T et al: Isolation of the AIDS virus from cell-free breastmilk of three healthy virus carriers, *Lancet* 2:891, 1985.

176. Torok TJ: Human parvovirus B19. In Remington JS, Klein JO, editors: *Infectious diseases of the fetus and newborn infant,* ed 4, Philadelphia, 1995, Saunders.

177. Van de Perre P, Lepage P, Homsy J et al: Mother-to-infant transmission of human immunodeficiency virus by breastmilk: presumed innocent or presumed guilty? *Clin Infect Dis* 15:502, 1992.

178. Van de Perre P, Simonon A, Hitimana D et al: Infective and antiinfective properties of breastmilk from HIV-1 infected women, *Lancet* 341:914, 1993.

179. Vergeront JM, Everson ML, Crass BA et al: Recovery of staphylococcal enterotoxin F from the breast milk of a woman with toxic-shock syndrome, *J Infect Dis* 146:456, 1982.

180. Vitek CR, Gracia FI, Giusti RA et al: Evidence for sexual and mother-to-child transmission of human T lymphotrophic virus type II among Guaymi Indians, Panama, *J Infect Dis* 171:1022, 1995.

181. Vochem M, Hamprecht K, Jahn G et al: Transmission of cytomegalovirus to preterm infants through breast milk, *Pediatr Infect Dis J* 17:53, 1998.

182. Vorherr H: Pregnancy and lactation in relation to breast cancer risk, *Semin Perinatol* 3:299, 1979.

183. Watson JC, Fleming DW, Borella AJ et al: Vertical transmission of hepatitis A resulting in an outbreak in a neonatal intensive care unit, *J Infect Dis* 167:567, 1993.

184. Wiktor SZ, Pate EJ, Barnett M et al: Maternal-infant transmission of HTLV-I: frequency and time course of seroconversion, Abstract W-53. In *Proceedings of the Fifth International Conference of Human Retrovirology,* Tokyo, May 1992.

185. Wing JP: Human versus cow's milk in infant nutrition and health, *Curr Probl Pediatr* 8(1):entire issue, 1977.

186. Wong-Staal F, Gallo RC: Human T-lymphocyte retroviruses, *Nature* 312:395, 1985.

187. Working Group on Severe Streptococcal Infections: Defining GAS streptococcal toxic shock syndrome: rationale and consensus definition, *JAMA* 269:390, 1993.

188. Wu J, Tang ZY, Wu YX et al: Acquired cytomegalovirus infection of breast milk in infancy, *Chin Med J* 102:124, 1989.

189. Yamanouchi K, Kinochita K, Moriuchi R et al: Oral transmission of human T-cell leukemia virus type 1 into a common marmoset as an experimental model for milk-borne transmission, *Jpn J Cancer Res* 76:481, 1985.

190. Yeager AS, Palumbo PE, Malachowski N et al: Sequelae of maternally derived cytomegalovirus infections in premature infants, *J Pediatr* 102:918, 1983.

191. Yoo K-Y, Tajima K, Kuroishi T et al: Independent protective effect of lactation against breast cancer: a case-control study in Japan, *Am J Epidemiol* 135:726, 1992.

192. Yoshida M, Yamagami N, Tezuka T et al: Case report: detection of varicella-zoster virus DNA in maternal breast milk, *J Med Virol* 38:108, 1992.

193. Zanetti AR, Tanzi E, Paccagnini S et al: Mother-to-infant transmission of hepatitis C virus, *Lancet* 345:289, 1995.

194. Zeldis JB, Crumpacker CS: Hepatitis. In Remington JS, Klein JO, editors: *Infectious diseases of the fetus and newborn infant,* ed 4, Philadelphia, 1995, Saunders.

195. Zhang RJ, Zeng JS, Zhang HZ: Survey of 34 pregnant women with hepatitis A and their neonates, *Chin Med J* 103:552, 1990.

$\mathscr{H}$uman milk as a prophylaxis in allergy

THE NATURAL HISTORY OF ATOPIC DISEASE

The association of allergy with cow's milk has been documented in the literature for decades.[17,49,67] The incidence of this allergy in the general population has been noted to increase progressively since the original comments on the subject by Rowe[69] in 1931. The incidence has reportedly increased 10 times in 20 years and has been attributed to increased recognition, increased incidence of exposure to known allergens, and a gradual decrease in infection as a source of morbidity because use of antibiotics and immunization revealed an underlying allergic component to chronic symptoms. Glaser[22] attributed this rapid increase in the development of allergic diseases to the abandonment of breastfeeding when safe pasteurized milk became available. It was noted that 20% of all children were allergic by 20 years of age.

Studies of office pediatrics[82] have shown that one third of the visits are a result of allergy.[82] One third of all chronic conditions under age 17 result from allergy and one third of lost school days from asthma. In the evaluation of 2000 consecutive unselected newborns in pediatric practice, 50% had family histories of allergy. Grulee et al[28] observed as early as 1934 that eczema was seven times more common in infants fed cow's milk than in breast-fed infants. McCombs et al[62] reported in 1979 that asthma caused more than 2000 deaths and the loss of 94 million days of activity and initiated 183,000 hospital admissions and more than 1 million hospital days in 1 year in the United States alone.

Asthma is the most common chronic disease of childhood, affecting an estimated 4.8 million children, according to a Centers for Disease Control and Prevention (CDC) report in 1996.[66] These data indicate that now people with asthma collectively have more than 100 million days of restricted activity and 470,000 hospitalizations annually, with mortality increased more than 5000 people annually. Asthma hospitalization rates have been highest among blacks and children, with mortality death rates consistently highest among blacks ages 15 to 24 years. Asthma costs the American public billions of dollars annually.

The question of heredity

Heredity undoubtedly plays a part in the development of allergic disease, an observation first recorded by Maimonides in his *Treatise on Asthma* in the twelfth century. Most studies in the past 60 years have concurred with the concept of a recessive mode of inheritance.[39]

Kern[48] has noted that the outstanding etiologic

factor in human hypersensitivity is heredity. He states that few diseases exist in which heredity is so clearly identified and so common.

Hamburger[31] reported that children with two atopic parents had a 47% chance of developing atopic disease. One atopic parent meant a 29% chance of developing atopy, and only a 13% risk with no allergic parent.

Falliers et al,[14] in a study of asthmatic monozygotic twins, observed similar serum immunoglobulin E (IgE), blood eosinophil counts, and positive skin tests to allergens in both twins but dissimilar responses to infection and methacholine. This finding suggests there is also an acquired component to bronchial hyperactivity. Apparently several mechanisms are involved in antigen processing.

To identify infants at high risk for developing atopy, several approaches have been suggested. Cord serum total IgE levels of greater than 100 U/ml are associated with five to ten times greater risk than lower levels. Eosinophilia and lymphocytes may prove to be markers, but at present only the family allergy history and the cord blood IgE have been significantly reliable predictors.[1]

Glaser speculated in the 1930s that if a child was at high risk for developing allergy, prophylaxis should be able to change the outcome. The original work on prophylaxis was done by Glaser and Johnstone[25] and reported in 1953. Only 15% of a group of children whose mothers controlled their own diet in pregnancy and controlled the infant's diet and environment at birth did develop eczema, whereas 65% of the sibling controls and 52% of nonrelated controls receiving cow's milk developed similar allergic illnesses. Although as a retrospective study it was open to some criticism, it did begin to look at a very significant issue, that is, reducing the incidence of allergic manifestations in high-risk individuals by a new type of preventive measure.

A second study was designed in 1953 and carried out prospectively by Johnstone and Dutton[40] to investigate dietary prophylaxis of allergic disease. They observed a difference of more than 10 years in the incidence of asthma and perennial

allergic rhinitis in those fed soybean milk (18%) and those fed evaporated milk (50%). No infant in this study of 283 children was breastfed, however. Halpern et al[30] reported the study of 1753 children fed breast milk, soy milk, and cow's milk from birth to 6 months of age who were followed until they were 7 years or older. The children included those with high-risk, low-risk, and no-risk family histories for allergy. No difference in outcome was related to early diet, but a relationship to the family history was seen.

In a prospective study to identify the development of reaginic allergy, infants of allergic parents were placed in a study or control group. The study group followed an allergen-avoidance regimen, including breastfeeding. At 6 months and 1 year, the study infants had less eczema than the controls, as well as lower serum total IgE levels.[49]

PROPHYLAXIS OF ATOPIC DISEASE

Efforts to alter the incidence of atopic illness have continued to challenge investigators, who now have access to increased methodologic sophistication. Prevention of IgE-mediated disorders can be directed at interfering with any of the major forces responsible for the phenotypic expression of atopy. Practically, however, it is not yet possible to mask IgE genes or manipulate cellular components of the response organ. Clinicians are limited to manipulating the effect of the environment by reducing the allergenic load.

Review of the plethora of studies directed at measuring the impact of dietary manipulations on the incidence of atopic disease demonstrates that retrospective studies show little or no difference in the incidence of asthma and eczema. Prospective studies, however, tend to demonstrate a significant reduction in atopic disease in the treated group (Table 17-1). In looking at these data, it is important to recognize that some studies did not consider the risk of the population developing atopic disease on a hereditary basis. In other studies, breastfeeding may have been carried out

TABLE 17-1 Prevention of atopy: prospective studies

Study	Year published	No. of years followed	No. of subjects*	Type of milk/feeding	Impact on atopy†
Johnstone and Dutton[40]	1966	10	235	Soy, cow's	↓ Asthma, rhinitis
Matthew et al[60]	1977	1	53 (26)	Breast, soy	↓ Eczema
Chandra[7]	1979	>2	134	Breast	↓ Eczema, asthma
Saarinen et al[71]	1979	3	(256)	Breast	↓ Eczema, food allergy, asthma
Hamburger[32]	1981	1	(300)	Breast	↓ Eczema, asthma
Kaufman and Frick[46,47]	1976, 1981	2	(94)	Breast	↓ Asthma
Hide and Guyer[35]	1981	1	843 (266)	Breast <6 mo, soy, cow's (maternal diet not controlled)	↓ Eczema slight, rhinitis
Gruskay[29]	1982	15	908 (328)	Breast 4 mo, soy, cow's	↓ Breast symptoms; soy no effect
May et al[61]	1982	½	67 normal	Soy, cow's, modern formula	↑ Antibodies with no disease symptoms
Businco et al[4]	1983	2	(101)	Breast <6 mo; soy, cow's	↓ Asthma, eczema
Kajosaari and Saarinen[45]	1983	1	(135)	All breast milk <6 mo; half solid foods early	↑ Eczema/food intolerance in those fed solids
Moore et al[64]	1985	1	525	Study—breastfed 3 mo; control—SMA	Not clear: 74% failed to breastfeed or gave cow's milk in study group
Zeiger et al[90]	1989	4	288	Maternal avoidance diet last trimester Controls unrestricted; mothers diet; infants given Nutramigen	↓ Atopy 16% in restricted infants ↑ Atopy in control infants (to 27%) ↓ Urticaria/GI symptoms in restricted group
Sigurs et al[81]	1992	4	115	All breastfed; 65 mothers restricted diet for first 3 mo of lactation; 50 no restrictions	↓ Atopy/asthma among both groups ↓ Greater among restricted group

Modified from Busino L, Marchetti F, Pellegrini G et al: *Ann Allergy* 51:296, 1983.
*Number in study; parentheses indicate number at risk for atopy.
†Arrows indicate decrease or increase compared with control group.

for only a few weeks or months. The evidence is clear that 6 months or longer of exclusive breast-feeding makes a difference. No study controlled for smoking in the household, and no data were reported on incidence of respiratory syncytial virus. In addition, some studies did not control the breastfeeding mother's diet, the weaning foods, or use of cow's milk–based beverages.

Hamburger et al[33] carried out prospective pro-phylactic studies to include measuring IgE and skin radioallergosorbent test (RAST) on mother, father, and infant. They found a significant corre-lation between maternal IgE and infant IgE and potential allergy in the infant (Tables 17-2 and 17-3). This study was done by controlling the environment and the diet. The process was initiated in pregnancy to begin by protecting the fetus and then was continued at birth. Therefore, consider-able attention was directed toward breastfeeding in this and other studies.

Human milk consistently contains antibodies, especially secretory immunoglobulin A (sIgA) to major food proteins. The levels are influenced by the mother's own external antigen exposure.

In a study of 500 babies born to families at high risk for allergies, one group was deliberately not given cow's milk and was fed soy milk by random assignment.[63] No benefit resulted from withhold-ing cow's milk, but breastfeeding even for a short period was clearly associated with a lower inci-dence of wheezing, prolonged colds, diarrhea, and vomiting. Smoking and environmental molds were also associated with wheezing. Merrett et al[63] concluded from this that breastfeeding played a significant role in prophylaxis.

The effect of breastfeeding on allergic sensitiza-tion is both *direct* through the elimination of non-human milk protein as an exposure to antigen and *indirect* by affecting the absorption of antigen through the intestinal tract.[49] Maternal antibody is

---

TABLE 17-2   Relationship of maternal total serum IgE level to cord and 4-month serum IgE level in prophylaxis group infants

Maternal IgE (U/ml)	Cord IgE (U/ml)		4-month IgE (U/ml)	
	<0.5 Number (%)	≥0.5 Number (%)	<5.0 Number (%)	≥5.0 Number (%)
≤100	35 (71)	14 (29)	41 (87)	6 (13)
>100	14 (42)	19 (58)	24 (73)	9 (27)
TOTAL	49	33	65	15

From Hamburger RN, Heller S, Mellon MH et al: *Ann Allergy* 51:281, 1983.
$p < 0.01$ by chi square for maternal IgE <100 vs >100 U/ml for cord IgE with a trend ($p < 0.08$) at 4-month IgE measurement.

TABLE 17-3   Relationship of paternal total serum IgE level to cord and 4-month serum IgE level in prophylaxis group infants

Paternal IgE (U/ml)	Cord IgE (U/ml)		4-month IgE (U/ml)	
	<0.5 Number (%)	≥0.5 Number (%)	<5.0 Number (%)	≥5.0 Number (%)
≤100	29 (63)	17 (37)	40 (83)	8 (17)
>100	10 (56)	8 (44)	14 (82)	3 (18)
TOTAL	39	25	54	11

From Hamburger RN, Heller S, Mellon MH et al: *Ann Allergy* 51:281, 1983.

transferred to the breastfed infant as part of what has been called the *enteromammary immune system*[50] (Fig. 17-1). The secretory IgA (sIgA) antibody present in the milk is the result of the mother's enteric immune response to antigens in her gut. sIgA in her milk provides protection against bacterial, viral, and toxic exposures. Prospective studies have shown that infants at high risk for atopic illness from a hereditary standpoint had significantly less disease when breastfed, especially if reared in a protected environment with delayed use of solid foods, compared with children of similar risk fed cow's milk and regular solid foods. Serum IgE concentrations were also greatly reduced under 6 months and 12 months of age in the breastfed group.[84]

Infants with a low incidence of T-lymphocytes are at greater risk to develop allergies if fed cow's milk rather than breast milk, according to Juto[41] and Bjorksten.[42] Infants with reduced T cells fed cow's milk also demonstrated higher serum IgE levels and peripheral eosinophil counts. Juto and Strannegard[43] also reported that with careful prophylaxis, greater than 50% of infants who had both parents with IgE levels above 100 μg/ml showed elevated cord and 4-month IgE levels. More than 80% of those infants whose parents had IgE levels below 100 μg/ml, however, had both low cord blood and low 4-month IgE levels. Such data confirm the genetic effect of both maternal and paternal genes.

The predictive value of cord blood IgE in the development of atopic disease was tested by Chandra et al[10] in a study of 226 infants, 120 of whom had a positive family history of atopic disease in first-degree relatives (parents and siblings) and 106 whose family history was negative for atopy. Using 0.7 U/ml or less of IgE, these authors found the level of cord blood IgE correlated significantly with the subsequent development of atopic disease. These investigators further tested the effect of feeding.[11] In the group with IgE levels less than 0.7 mg/dl who were breastfed, none developed atopy, and only one on formula did by 2 years of age. Of the 39 breastfed infants with elevated IgE, 12 developed atopy (30.7%), whereas in the 31 with elevated IgE who were formula fed, 26 (83.3%) developed eczema and/or wheezing in the first 2 years, a highly significant finding ($p = 0.001$). Of the entire study group, 12%

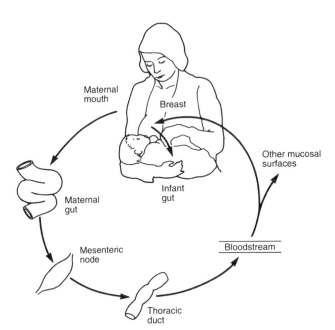

Fig. 17-1. Maternal serum antibodies affect passage of foreign antigens into milk and processing of antigen in infant's intestine. (Redrawn from Kleinman RE: *Ann Allergy* 51:222, 1983.)

of breastfed and 32% of formula-fed infants developed atopy. The authors[11] consider cord blood IgE antibody levels a significant marker for development of atopy when the level of 0.7 or less µg/ml is used. The history of family atopy was a significant indicator of high IgE levels.

Investigating the influence of maternal food antigen avoidance during pregnancy and lactation on the incidence of atopic eczema in infants, Chandra et al[11] reported the outcome of a randomly assigned prospective study of 120 women with a history of a previous child with atopic disease. The study group avoided all milk, dairy products, eggs, fish, beef, and peanuts throughout pregnancy and lactation. The control group had no restrictions. Maternal antigen avoidance was associated with less and milder eczema, particularly in those who were breastfed. Of 55 women who completed the avoidance regimen, 17 infants developed atopy, 5 from the 35 who were breastfed and 12 from the 20 who were formula fed. Of the 54 unrestricted mothers, 11 of 36 breastfed infants and 13 of 18 formula-fed infants developed atopy. The researchers thus concluded that avoidance of common dietary allergens during pregnancy and lactation enhances the preventive beneficial effect of exclusive breastfeeding on the incidence of atopic eczema among high-risk infants.[11] Diets eliminating dairy products and eggs are deficient in calcium, however, and require special efforts to correct this by diet or supplementation.

In one study, 162 women with respiratory allergies to animal danders or pollens were randomly allocated to two groups: one on a diet of limited eggs and cow's milk and the other on a diet of a daily egg and a liter of cow's milk the last 3 months of pregnancy. Genetic factors rather than maternal diet during pregnancy were thought to have a greater effect on the incidence of atopic diseases in the first 18 months of life.[54] Almost all the infants in both groups were breastfed, a few received soy milk, and 13 received some cow's-milk formula. Mothers had no diet restrictions during lactation. Thus, as an isolated effort, diet restriction for the last trimester of pregnancy does not influence neonatal allergy in the first 18 months when it is associated with environmental allergens and not with diet.

Long-term effects of allergy prophylaxis

In an 18-month study of atopic outcome, atopic mothers were randomly allocated to an intervention group or an unrestricted-diet group, and both were compared to nonatopic mothers on unrestricted diets.[56] The intervention was a milk/dairy product–free diet during late pregnancy and lactation. After 7 weeks of the diet, serum β-lactoglobulin and immunoglobulin G (IgG) levels in the mother were collated to the levels in the cord blood. The infants were examined at 12 and 18 months by a single-blind allergy assessment by a pediatrician. The infants born to nonatopic parents had significantly less allergy than those born to atopic mothers with the unrestricted diets.[55] The "restricted-diet group" of infants had comparable levels to the atopy-free group and had significantly less allergy than the unrestricted-diet group. The nature of the parents' disease also played a role in the type of illness in both groups.

A prospective longitudinal study of 988 healthy infants from birth to 6 years of age recorded feeding-history episodes of lower respiratory tract infection in the first 3 years of life and recurrent episodes of wheezing.[89] Being breastfed was associated with lower rates of recurrent wheeze (3.1% vs. 9.7%, $p < 0.01$) for nonatopic children. The authors concluded that recurrent wheeze at age 6 is less common among nonatopic children who were breastfed as infants. This effect was independent of whether or not the child had a wheezing lower respiratory tract illness in the first 6 months of life (Table 17-4). These authors recorded smoking history, but it did not alter the compelling influence of breastfeeding on the outcome.

Additional long-term studies have demonstrated that children who had ever been breastfed had a 50% lower incidence of wheezing than those who had not breastfed and that the effect persisted for

TABLE 17-4   Odds ratios and confidence intervals for recurrent wheeze at age 6 years by logistic regression

	Odds ratio (confidence interval)*		
Factor	Total group (n = 970)	Nonatopic children (n = 420)	Atopic children (n = 280)
Not breastfed	1.49 (0.80-2.77)	3.03† (1.05-8.69)	1.36 (0.49-3.73)
Maternal education ≤12 yr	1.48 (0.87-2.53)	1.58 (0.56-4.43)	0.92 (0.36-2.38)
Hispanic	2.48‡ (1.39-4.40)	2.45 (0.82-7.27)	2.50† (1.01-6.18)
Maternal hay fever	2.66§ (1.49-4.72)	2.64 (0.96-7.22)	2.35† (1.07-5.16)
Wheezing lower respiratory tract illness in first 6 mo	1.68 (0.88-3.19)	1.86 (0.55-6.25)	2.01 (0.74-5.48)

From Wright AL, Holberg CJ, Taussig LM et al: *Arch Pediatr Adolesc Med* 149:762, 1995.
*Excludes children who were missing information for one or more of these factors.
†*p* < 0.05.
‡*p* < 0.005.
§*p* < 0.0005.

the 7 years of the study in nonatopic children.[2] These authors attribute this in part to breastfeeding's protective effect against respiratory illness. They did not distinguish minimal from prolonged breastfeeding.

In a 17-year prospective study of 150 healthy children, researchers did consider length of breastfeeding.[70] The three groups had been breastfed less than 1 month or not at all, 1 to 6 months, or more than 6 months. Prolonged breastfeeding was associated with the least eczema at 1 to 3 years, as well as fewer food and respiratory allergies. At age 17 years the trends continued, leading the authors to conclude that breastfeeding is protective against atopic eczema, food allergy, and respiratory asthma throughout childhood and adolescence[70] (Figs. 17-2 and 17-3).

IMMUNOLOGIC ASPECTS OF ALLERGY

Interest in identifying the immunologic aspects of clinical allergy led to a number of additional studies on infant feeding.[32,33] Kletter et al[51] reported that hemagglutinating antibodies to cow's milk were present in the sera of some newborns but

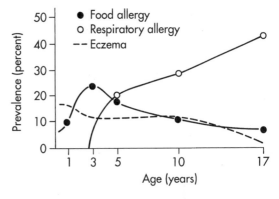

Fig. 17-2. Prevalence of atopic eczema, food allergy, and respiratory allergy in full cohort of initially 236 children during follow-up for 17 years. (Modified from Saarinen UM, Kajossari M: *Lancet* 346:1065, 1995.)

usually at levels lower than those of the mother. The earliest rise in titer was detected at 1 month, and a peak was seen at 3 months in infants given cow's milk from birth. Antibodies belonged mainly to the IgG group, with their rise and fall paralleling hemagglutinating antibodies. IgA antibodies were in low titer, and IgM antibodies were rarely detected. The delayed exposure to cow's milk in breastfed infants resulted in lower mean values of cow's milk antibodies, and peak values were attained more slowly. An inverse relationship exists between duration of breastfeeding and levels of titers of humoral antibodies.

Freed and Green[15] investigated antibody-facilitated digestion and its implications for infant nutrition. They suggest a model of digestion in which oligopeptides in the small bowel are bound to secretory antibodies, which hold them in contact with proteases. This facilitates the breakdown and utilization of the oligopeptides. They consider immunity and digestion to be closely related. Breastfeeding with colostrum and then mature human milk provides the immature gut of the infant with both immunity and "digestivity."

The presence of periods of transient IgA deficiency in saliva in the first 12 months of life has been identified as a possible risk factor for the development of asthma, bronchial hyperactivity and atopy.[26]

Eighteen patients with documented malabsorption of cow's milk who were studied by Savilahti[72] et al[74] improved by feeding them human milk after challenge with powdered milk. Eight patients had clinical reactions; the number of IgA- and IgM-

containing cells increased by almost 2.5 times in the intestinal mucosa. When breast milk resumed, the findings returned to normal. Serum antibodies of both hemagglutination and IgA increased. No change was seen in IgE antibodies or serum complement. Many other findings, including villous atrophy and round cell infiltration, were noted. After age 2 years, all the infants became tolerant of milk, which may indicate that immunologic immaturity is part of the pathogenesis. Walker[88] presented similar arguments and conclusions in a symposium discussion.

When studying problems related to infant feeding, it is difficult to randomize groups to breastfeed or not, and many women are particularly adamant about breastfeeding with a strong family history of allergy. This was a factor in a study of 69 preterm infants and subsequent allergic symptoms in childhood, as well as the premature infant's intestine being more permeable to proteins and the immune system more immature. The long-term incidence of atopy, however, was no different between the feeding groups at age 11, although those receiving breast milk had a strong family history of atopy.[74]

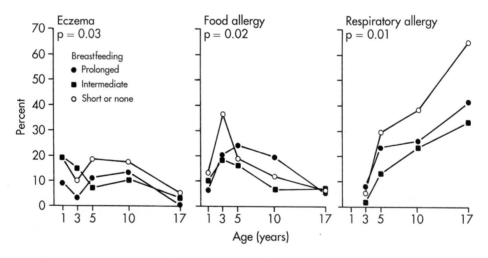

Fig. 17-3. Prevalence of atopic eczema, food allergy, and respiratory allergy in infant-feeding groups during follow-up for 17 years. Tests for differences during the appropriate age periods (eczema 1 to 3 years, food allergy 1 to 3 years, respiratory allergy at 5, 10, and 17 years) were done by analysis of variance and covariance with repeated measures. (Modified from Saarinsen UM, Kajossari M: *Lancet* 346:1065, 1995.)

Low IgA content of milk, especially low colostral IgA, has been correlated with cow's milk allergy in a group of 198 infants, seven of whom became allergic to cow's milk.[73] All other measurements (immunoglobulins G, A, M; cow's milk–specific antibodies; β-lactoglobulin) were similar among all 198 infants. The authors[55] suggest that an infant is more likely to develop cow's milk allergy if the mother has insufficient protective factors, namely, IgA.

Some discrepancies between studies may be explained by measuring the concentration of bovine IgG in human milk using different methods. When levels were tested on the same milk samples using competition radioimmunoassay (RIA), competition enzyme-linked immunosorbent assay (ELISA), and sandwich ELISA, IgG levels were significantly higher using RIA or ELISA.[58] Levels in the milk of mothers on a dairy product–free diet for a month still have measurable levels by RIA and ELISA but not by sandwich ELISA.

To resolve the question of the presence of specific IgE (sIgE) for cow's milk protein in the sera of breastfed infants who had never received cow's milk, Cantisani et al[6] measured sIgE in the sera of six breastfed infants with atopic dermatitis who were never in contact with cow's milk. The sIgE to bovine β-lactoglobulin was not detected in any of the sera examined.

Studying the role of heredity in allergy, Kaufman and Frick[46] described unilateral family history as allergy in one parent and bilateral as involving both parents. They followed 94 infants from birth for 24 months. Significantly more infants developed allergy if they were from a bilaterally allergic family. In the first 3 months there was less atopic dermatitis in the breastfed infants with unilateral history than with bilateral history. Businco et al[4] present similar relationships to family history in a study of breastfed infants.

These data are augmented by findings by Murray[65] examining nasal-secretion eosinophilia in relationship to respiratory allergy, associated with a screening procedure for hearing loss. In a group of children with a history of allergy in the immediate family, an association between early introduction of solid food and the presence of a nasal-secretion eosinophilia was significantly positive.

Further follow-up on the Isle of Wight Infant Feeding Survey was conducted by Hide and Guyer[35,36] when the children were 2 and 4 years old, producing data on 486 of the original 843 children. The authors reported not only on eczema and asthma but also on recurrent croup. Both asthma and recurrent croup showed strong predictability with a positive family history. More atopy was seen in the breastfed group; however, more mothers with a family history of eczema choose to breastfeed. Breastfeeding had a protective effect against asthma at 1 year but not at 4 years. Recurrent croup did not have a clear relationship to feeding method, but any breastfeeding at all was considered breastfeeding. The authors found a male preponderance and a close association with other signs of allergy in children with recurrent croup.

Although modern processing of cow's milk has diminished the problem, it has not eliminated it. Given high-risk factors or strong family history of allergy, an effort to avoid unnecessary exposure to known allergens is an easy way to avoid some medical problems (Table 17-5).

TABLE 17-5   Some diseases possibly preventable by protecting relatively immunodeficient infants from adverse antigen experience

Disease	Status
Eczema	Established
Asthma	Probable
Hay fever	Probable
Infantile gut and respiratory infection	Probable
Intestinal allergy	Probable
Septicemia and renal *E. coli* infection	Probable
Sudden death	Probable
Ulcerative colitis	Possible

From Soothill JF: *Proc R Soc Med* 69:439, 1976.

PATTERNS OF CLINICAL DISEASE ASSOCIATED WITH COW'S-MILK ALLERGY IN CHILDHOOD

Cow's-milk allergy affects 2% to 7% of infants. Many poorly defined illnesses and pathologic lesions have been associated with the ingestion of milk, making clear diagnosis difficult.[37] Definitions have been proposed by the American Academy of Allergy and Immunology and are described in a consensus paper,[37,87] as follows:

- *Food intolerance* is an adverse reaction to the ingestion of a food related to an enzyme deficiency.
- *Food adverse reaction with unknown mechanism* is an idiosyncrasy; there is no associated immunologic mechanism.
- *Food allergy* or *food hypersensitivity* is an adverse reaction to food caused by one or more immune hypersensitivity mechanisms and is not confined to IgE.
- *Food anaphylaxis–type reactions* are immediate hypersensitivity involving the immunologic activity of IgE homocytotropic antibody and release of chemical mediators.
- *Anaphylactoid reaction* to food is an anaphylaxis-like reaction to food as a result of nonimmune release of chemical mediators.

Symptoms associated with food allergy include asthma, eczema, urticaria, and rhinitis, as well as colic and failure to thrive with chronic respiratory and gastrointestinal disease.[87] Well-defined but uncommon syndromes, including pulmonary hemosiderosis, bronchitis, protein- and iron-losing enteropathy, neonatal thrombocytopenia, and colitis, have been reported to result from cow's-milk allergy in both breastfed and formula-fed infants.[8] Sleep disturbances have been reported in a series of children evaluated with a prospective double-blind crossover design.[44] Another symptom reported in two siblings was insatiability despite adequate weight gain.[13] This was confirmed by history and reproducible reaction to dietary elimination and subsequent oral challenges.

The *intestinal permeability test* is a noninvasive but rigorous technique for detecting the deleterious effect of food on the intestinal mucosa of allergic children. It requires overnight fasting of 6 hours, test feeding, and nothing but water for 5 additional hours to collect urine samples for analysis. A 1-month-old breastfed infant with a history of regurgitation, diarrhea, difficult feeding, and malaise did not respond clinically to the elimination of dairy products from the mother's diet.[12] When the intestinal permeability test was performed with the mother's milk before and after dietary elimination of milk, there was no change. When the mother eliminated pork and egg, however, clinical and test results improved.

ACUTE REACTIONS TO COW'S MILK IN BREASTFED INFANTS

Hippocrates and Gojen described classic cases of milk allergy.[69] External reaction to cow's milk was first described in the literature in the nineteenth century by Schloss[78] in 1920 and Tisdale and Erb[85] in 1925. At that time the reaction was noted to occur at the first feeding of cow's milk provided in an effort to wean from the breast at several months of age. The event included sudden crying as if in pain; swelling of the lips, tongue, and throat; stridor; and even generalized urticaria and wheezing lasting for up to an hour.

This type of cow's-milk allergy is the first of two types described by Gerrard and Shenassa[19] and others. The second type is the well-known reaction to large amounts of cow's milk in a cow's-milk–fed infant and is manifested by vomiting, diarrhea, or colic and is not associated with cow's milk–specific IgE antibodies. It usually subsides over time. The acute anaphylactic reactions, however, are associated with α-lactalbumin, β-lactoglobulin, and casein immunity.

Schwartz et al[77] studied 29 breastfed or soy formula–fed infants who had experienced acute urticarial reactions while being fed cow's milk for the first time. One infant had the reaction in the newborn nursery, suggesting in utero sensitization. When charts were carefully reviewed, 16 infants were identified as having been given formula, often without an order, in the newborn nursery. Twelve could have been sensitized in utero or through the breast milk. The authors identified elevated serum IgE levels; positive RASTs for α-lactalbumin, β-lactoglobulin, and casein; and recurrent wheezing in 55% of infants (16 of 29).

In a follow-up study challenging this group of children with whey and casein hydrolysate products, Schwartz[75] et al[76] found 69% with positive prick tests to whey hydrolysate and 38% positive to casein hydrolysate. Children with reactions to cow's milk and both hydrolysates had very severe reactions, including urticaria, angioedema, and wheezing. Hydrolysates of cow's milk protein are not therefore hypoallergic. Breastfeeding with occasional, small amounts of cow's milk can be a major risk factor in the development of IgE-mediated cow's milk allergy in the rare, susceptible infant. Early exposures may occur in utero, through the breast milk, or with inadvertent feeds. Schwartz suggests that isolated cow's milk not be given to exclusively breastfed infants in the newborn period.[75,76]

The study confirms the importance of heredity in this acute reaction by its occurrence in twins and human leukocyte antigen (HLA)–identical siblings as well as in children of 28 (89%) parent pairs also sensitive to cow's milk. Genetic homogeneity could not be demonstrated by HLA typing.

A case of anaphylactic shock from cow's-milk hypersensitivity in a breastfed infant has been reported by Lifschitz et al.[53] They describe three episodes of shock from two separate feedings of formula and one while breastfeeding. After a prolonged course and the diagnosis of colitis, associated with numerous eosinophils, the infant was able to breastfeed at 21 days of age without difficulty after his mother had been placed on a cow's milk–free diet. When challenged, however, with breast milk that had been pumped and stored while the mother was still consuming dairy products, the infant went into profound shock. The child was finally stabilized on breast milk and meat-based formula. At 6 months, cereal was added to the diet. At 12 months, soy and cow's milk were well tolerated.

Intrauterine sensitization and allergy in the newborn breastfed infant were described by Matsumura et al[59] in Japan. Glaser[23] also identified that under certain conditions an infant with a predisposition for allergy may become actively sensitized in utero because of the mother's overindulgence in certain foods in pregnancy. For example, Shannon[80] demonstrated in 1922 the presence of egg antigen in human breast milk. The infant then responded to reexposure with allergic symptoms on first contact with that same food.[18,52] Kuroume et al[52] showed that with intrauterine sensitization, hemagglutinating antibody titers against lactalbumin and soybean in the amniotic fluid are high. They suggest using measurement of amniotic fluid as an instrument to predict future allergy. Infant colic associated with maternal ingestion of cow's milk is discussed in Chapter 14.

Multiple studies continue to confirm the value of elimination diets in pregnancy for women at high risk for having an allergic infant.[5,16,34] These studies not only report a significantly reduced incidence of symptoms in the infants, but also a significant reduction in β-lactoglobulin–specific IgA and α-casein–specific IgA levels in maternal serum and milk. Similar observations have been made with the elimination of egg. Consistently breastfeeding was associated with reduced incidence of atopy in the infant with, and to a lesser degree without, dietary restrictions in mothers.

When Giovannini et al[20] studied growth and metabolic parameters of infants fed special formulas for atopy prevention, they noted differences compared with infants exclusively breastfed. Lower body mass index values and higher blood urea nitrogen levels were seen at 3 months.[21] Plasma aminoacidograms showed higher essential amino acids but lower branched-chain amino acids. Furthermore, the plasma taurine levels were lower in the formula-fed infants even though the formulas had added taurine. These observations have been confirmed by other investigators, who are most concerned about the elevated threonine levels.[68]

The allergens of specific foods ingested by the mother have now been identified in the milk.

β-Lactoglobulin was studied by Machtinger and Moss[57] and identified in milk. These same investigators measured IgA in milk and attempted to correlate these levels with symptoms in the infants. High IgA levels were seen in asymptomatic infants. Cant et al[5] found 49 eczematous infants who were solely breastfed to be sensitized to cow's milk and egg protein; these researchers also concluded that infants can be sensitized by foods eaten by the mother. They were able to demonstrate ovalbumin in the breast milk of 14 of 19 mothers tested 2 to 4 hours after eating raw egg, whether or not their infants had tested positive to egg albumin.

Trocone et al[86] collected samples of breast milk at various times after the mothers were fed 20 g of gluten, following a period of deliberate gluten avoidance. Gliadin was found in 54 of 80 samples; levels peaked at 2 to 4 hours. Gliadin could not be detected in maternal serum. The transfer of gliadin to the infant through the milk could be one of the factors producing a protective effect, because breastfeeding is known to decrease the risk of celiac disease.[27]

RECOMMENDATIONS FOR MANAGEMENT

It has been suggested that for the first 6 weeks or so of life, the intestinal tract is immature anatomically and immunologically. The early absorption of protein macromolecules in young animals is well recognized.[79] The subepithelial plasma cells of the lamina propria mucosae and lymph nodes do not make IgA initially. Gradually, the levels increase until they reach adult values at 2 years of age. Children with a strong family history of allergy have a more prolonged deficiency of IgA, lasting 3 months or longer. The early introduction of foods other than human milk has been associated with a rise in antibodies in the blood and eosinophilia, as noted earlier. Providing infants with breast milk so that they will not become sensitized to it is the most direct way of dealing with the problem.[24]

The total approach to the potentially allergic infant involves exclusion of known common food allergens from the pregnant mother's diet and avoidance of products known to cause problems in

TABLE 17-6 Idealized strategy and mechanisms for the prevention of allergic diseases in humans

Strategy	Mechanisms
Identify at-risk families	Document IgE reactivity in parents with history of allergic disorders or with existing atopic child
Prevent intrauterine sensitization	Reduce maternal dietary allergenic load during last trimester, when potential for sensitization increases
Prevent postnatal sensitization to:	
1. Food allergens	
a. Transmitted through breast milk	Continue maternal avoidance diet during lactation
b. Ingested by infant	Withhold *all* nonbreast-milk foods except casein hydrolysate formula for at least 6 months
2. Environmental allergens	Encourage, instruct, and document avoidance of animals, mites, dust, and molds, as well as unnecessary medications
Maximize immunologic competence	Encourage, instruct, and support breastfeeding for at least 6 months
Minimize nonspecific enhancing factors	Discourage parental smoking; encourage avoidance of viral illnesses (?); delay pertussis immunization (?)

From Hamburger RN, Heller S, Mellon MH et al: *Ann Allergy* 51:281, 1983.

members of that family[83] (Table 17-6). From birth until 6 months, the infant should receive no cow's-milk formula. In addition, the diet of the mother should be restricted as in pregnancy and the environment made as allergen free as possible. If not breastfed, the infant should receive cow's-milk–free formula. Even though this regimen will not totally prevent all the potentials for allergy, it will help to minimize the insults by foreign protein. Another compelling reason to consider prophylaxis is the costly medical care required for the affected individual (Fig. 17-4).[9]

The possible alleviation of atopic eczema in a

Fig. 17-4. Estimated cost of management of symptomatic children with atopy in Newfoundland. Costs include physician fees, laboratory tests, hospitalization, and medication. For those fed Similac, cost of management until age 5 is $740,000 per annum. Standard cow's milk formula (e.g., Similac) during first 6 months of life for all infants with parental history of allergy would cost $504,000. In those fed hydrolyzed formula (e.g., Food Start), cost is about the same as for standard formula, but with savings of about 50% on management. An almost similar magnitude of reduction in allergic disease by feeding extensively hydrolyzed casein formula (e.g., Nutramigen) would cost three times more than in the cow's milk group because of higher purchase value of such a formula. (Modified from Chandra RK: *J Pediatr Gastroenterol Nutr* 24:388, 1997.)

breastfed infant by maternal supplementation with a fish oil concentrate has been reported by Jensen et al.[38] A 6-week-old infant who had eczema from the first week of life despite treatment cleared when the mother, who was part of a study of effects of fish oil supplementation, began the supplementation. The eczema returned when the fish oil was stopped and cleared again when the mother added fish to her diet.

This clinical experience has been corroborated in the laboratory. Essential fatty acids are important in promoting the renewal of the protective hydrolipidic layer of the skin. Altered essential fatty acid metabolism has been associated with atopic dermatitis,[20] and reduced levels of γ-linolenic acid and dihomo-α-linolenic acid appear in the plasma of patients with atopic dermatitis. The ratio of linoleic acid to the sum of its metabolites was found to be the relevant feature related to atopy. Increased marine fat consumption by the breastfeeding mother appears to improve the ratio of polyunsaturated fatty acids,[3] although this treatment has not been incorporated into routine care.

Walker[88] summarizes his extensive research on the subject by stating that antigens have been shown to cross the intestinal barrier in physiologic and pathologic states. He further states that it is most important to prevent excessive penetration of antigens in patients who are susceptible to the disease by implementing the following steps:

1. Identify the population at risk.
2. Encourage breastfeeding in infancy.
3. Decrease antigen load with elemental formulas.
4. Continue to conduct direct research at identification and prevention.

SUMMARY

The role of prophylactic management in pregnancy and the initiation of breastfeeding at birth have a major impact on the long-term incidence of reactive airway disease. Beyond the medical risks, the high cost of medical management must be considered when an infant is not breastfed.

REFERENCES

1. Bousquet J, Menardo J, Viala J et al: Predictive value of cord serum IgE determination in the development of "early-onset" atopy, *Ann Allergy* 51:291, 1983.
2. Burr M, Limb ES, Maguire MJ et al: Infant feeding, wheezing, and allergy: a prospective study, *Arch Dis Child* 68:724, 1993.
3. Businco L, Ioppi M, Morse NL et al: Breast milk from mothers of children with newly developed atopic eczema has low levels of long chain polyunsaturated fatty acids, *J Allergy Clin Immunol* 91:1134, 1993.
4. Businco L, Marchetti F, Pellegrini G et al: Prevention of atopic disease in "at-risk newborns" by prolonged breast-feeding, *Ann Allergy* 51:296, 1983.
5. Cant AJ, Bailes JA, Marsden RA et al: Effect of maternal dietary exclusion on breast fed infants with eczema: two controlled studies, *Br Med J* 293:231, 1986.
6. Cantisani A, Giuffrida MG, Fabris C et al: Detection of specific IgE to human milk proteins in sera of atopic infants, *Fed Eur Biochem Soc* 412:515, 1997.
7. Chandra RK: Prospective studies on the effect of breast feeding on incidence of infection and allergy, *Acta Pediatr Scand* 68:691, 1979.
8. Chandra RK: Long-term health consequences of early infant feeding. In Atkinson SA, Hanson LA, Chandra RK, editors: *Breastfeeding, nutrition, infection, and infant growth in developed and emerging countries,* St Johns, Newfoundland, Canada, 1990, ARTS Biomedical.
9. Chandra RK: Five-year follow-up of high-risk infants with family history of allergy who were exclusively breast-fed or fed partial whey hydrolysate, soy, and conventional cow's milk formulas, *J Pediatr Gastroenterol Nutr* 24:380, 1997.
10. Chandra RK, Puri S, Cheema PS: Predictive value of cord blood IgE in the development of atopic disease and role of breastfeeding in its prevention, *Clin Allergy* 15:517, 1985.
11. Chandra RK, Puri S, Suraiya C et al: Influence of maternal food antigen avoidance during pregnancy and lactation on incidence of atopic eczema in infants, *Clin Allergy* 16:563, 1986.
12. de Boussieu D, Dupont C, Badoval J: Allergy to non-dairy proteins in mother's milk as assessed by intestinal permeability tests, *Allergy* 49:882, 1994.
13. Ducharme FM, Rousseau E, Seidman EG et al: Apparent insatiability: an unrecognized manifestation of food intolerance in breast-fed infants, *Pediatrics* 93:1006, 1994.
14. Falliers CJ, Cardoso RR de A, Bane HN et al: Discordant allergic manifestations in monozygotic twins: genetic identity vs. clinical, physiologic, and biochemical differences, *J Allergy* 47:207, 1971.
15. Freed DLJ, Green FHY: Hypothesis: antibody-facilitated digestion and its implications for infant nutrition, *Early Hum Dev* 1:107, 1977.
16. Fukushima Y, Kawata Y, Onda T et al: Consumption of cow milk and egg by lactating women and the presence of β-lactoglobulin and ovalbumin in breast milk, *Am J Clin Nutr* 65:30, 1997.
17. Gerrard JW: Allergy in infancy, *Pediatr Ann* 3:9, 1974.
18. Gerrard JW, Shenassa M: Sensitization to substances in breast milk: recognition, management and significance, *Ann Allergy* 51:300, 1983.
19. Gerrard JW, Shenassa M: Food allergy: two common types as seen in breast and formula fed babies, *Ann Allergy* 50:375, 1983.
20. Giovannini M, Agostoni C, Fiocchi A et al: Antigen-reduced infant formulas versus human milk: growth and metabolic parameters in the first 6 months of life, *J Am Coll Nutr* 13:357, 1994.
21. Giovannini M, Fiocchi A, Agostoni C et al: Nutrition in infancy and childhood. In Wüthrich B, Ortolani C, editors: *Highlights in food allergy,* Basel, 1996, Karges.
22. Glaser J: Prophylaxis of allergic disease in infancy and childhood. In Speer F, Dockhorn RJ, editors: *Allergy and immunology in children,* Springfield, Ill, 1973, Thomas.
23. Glaser J: Intrauterine sensitization and allergy in the newborn breast fed infant, *Ann Allergy* 35:256, 1975 (editorial).
24. Glaser J, Dreyfuss EM, Logan J: Dietary prophylaxis of atopic disease. In Kelley VC, editor: *Brennemann's practice of pediatrics,* vol 2, Hagerstown, Md, 1976, Harper & Row.
25. Glaser J, Johnstone DE: Prophylaxis of allergic disease in newborn, *JAMA* 153:620, 1953.
26. Gleeson M, Cripps AW, Clancy RL et al: The significance of transient mucosal IgA deficiency on the development of asthma and atopy in children, *Adv Exp Med Biol* 371B:861, 1995.
27. Greco L, Mayer M, Grimaldi M et al: The effect of early feeding on the onset of symptoms in celiac disease, *J Pediatr Gastroenterol Nutr* 4:52, 1985.
28. Grulee GG, Sanford HN, Herron PH: Breast and artificial feeding, *JAMA* 103:735, 1934.
29. Gruskay FL: Comparison of breast, cow, and soy feedings in the prevention of onset of allergic disease, *Clin Pediatr* 21:486, 1982.
30. Halpern SR, Sellars WA, Johnson RB et al: Development of childhood allergy in infants fed breast, soy, or cow milk, *J Allergy Clin Immunol* 51:139, 1973.
31. Hamburger RN: Allergy and the immune system, *Am Sci* 64:157, 1976.
32. Hamburger RN: Development of atopic allergy in children. In Johansson SGO, editor: *International symposium on diagnosis and treatment of IgE-mediated diseases,* Amsterdam, 1981, Excerpta Medica.

33. Hamburger RN, Heller S, Mellon MH et al: Current status of the clinical and immunologic consequences of a prototype allergic disease prevention program, *Ann Allergy* 51:281, 1983.

34. Herrmann ME, Danneman A, Grüters A et al: Prospective study on the atopy preventive effect of maternal avoidance of milk and eggs during pregnancy and lactation, *Eur J Pediatr* 155:770, 1996.

35. Hide DW, Guyer BM: Clinical manifestations of allergy related to breast and cow's milk feeding, *Arch Dis Child* 56:172, 1981.

36. Hide DW, Guyer BM: Clinical manifestations of allergy related to breastfeeding and cow's milk–feeding, *Pediatrics* 76:973, 1985.

37. Hill DJ, Hosking CS: Patterns of clinical disease associated with cow milk allergy in childhood, *Nutr Res* 12:109, 1992.

38. Jensen RG, Ferris AM, Lammi-Keefe CJ et al: Possible alleviation of atopic eczema in a breastfed infant by maternal supplementation with a fish oil concentrate, *J Pediatr Gastroenterol Nutr* 14:474, 1992 (letter).

39. Johnstone DE: The natural history of allergic disease in children. In *Proceedings of Advances in Pediatric Allergy Workshop,* Rome, 1982.

40. Johnstone DE, Dutton AM: Dietary prophylaxis of allergic disease in children, *N Engl J Med* 274:715, 1966.

41. Juto P: Elevated serum immunoglobulin E in T cell–deficient infants fed cow's milk, *J Allergy Clin Immunol* 66:402, 1980.

42. Juto P, Bjorksten B: Serum IgE in infants and influence of type of feeding, *Clin Allergy* 10:593, 1980.

43. Juto P, Strannegard O: T lymphocytes and blood eosinophils in early infancy in relation to heredity for allergy and type of feeding, *J Allergy Clin Immunol* 64:38, 1979.

44. Kahn A, Mozin MJ, Rebuffat E et al: Milk intolerance in children with persistent sleeplessness: a prospective double-blind crossover evaluation, *Pediatrics* 84:595, 1989.

45. Kajosaari M, Saarinen UM: Prophylaxis of atopic disease by six months' total solid food elimination, *Acta Paediatr Scand* 72:411, 1983.

46. Kaufman HS, Frick OL: The development of allergy in infants of allergic parents: a prospective study concerning the role of heredity, *Ann Allergy* 37:410, 1976.

47. Kaufman HS, Frick OL: Prevention of asthma, *Clin Allergy* 11:549, 1981.

48. Kern RA: Prophylaxis in allergy, *Ann Intern Med* 12:1175, 1939.

49. Kleinman RE: The role of developmental immune mechanisms in intestinal allergy, *Ann Allergy* 51:222, 1983.

50. Kleinman RE, Walker WA: The enteromammary immune system: an important new concept in breast milk host defense, *Dig Dis Sci* 24:876, 1979.

51. Kletter B, Gery I, Freier S et al: Immune response of normal infants to cow's milk. I. Antibody type and kinetics of production, *Int Arch Allergy* 40:656, 1971.

52. Kuroume T, Oguri M, Matsumura T et al: Milk sensitivity and soybean sensitivity in the production of eczematous manifestations in breast-fed infants with particular reference to intrauterine sensitization, *Ann Allergy* 37:41, 1976.

53. Lifschitz CH, Hawkins HK, Guerra C et al: Anaphylactic shock due to cow's milk protein hypersensitivity in a breastfed infant, *J Pediatr Gastroenterol Nutr* 7:141, 1988.

54. Lilja G, Dannaeus A, Foucard T et al: Effects of maternal diet during late pregnancy and lactation on the development of atopic diseases in infants up to 18 months of age—in vivo results, *Clin Exp Allergy* 18:473, 1989.

55. Lovegrove JA, Hampton SM, Morgan JB: The immunological and long-term outcome of infants born to women following a milk-free diet during late pregnancy and lactation: a pilot study, *Br J Nutr* 71:223, 1994.

56. Lovegrove JA, Morgan JB, Hampton SM: Dietary factors influencing levels of food antibodies and antigens in breast milk, *Acta Paediatr* 85:778, 1996.

57. Machtinger S, Moss R: Cow's milk allergy in breastfed infants: the role of allergen and maternal secretory IgA antibody, *J Allergy Clin Immunol* 77:341, 1986.

58. Maeda S, Morikawa A, Tokuyama K et al: The concentration of bovine IgG in human breast milk measured using different methods, *Acta Paediatr* 82:1012, 1993.

59. Matsumura T, Kurome T, Iwasaki I et al: Congenital sensitization to food in humans, *Jpn J Allergy* 16:858, 1967.

60. Matthew DJ, Taylor B, Norman AP et al: Prevention of eczema, *Lancet* 1:321, 1977.

61. May CD, Fomon SJ, Remigio L: Immunologic consequences of feeding infants with cow milk and soy products, *Acta Paediatr Scand* 71:43, 1982.

62. McCombs R, Lowell F, Ohman J: Myths, morbidity, and mortality in asthma, *JAMA* 242:1521, 1979.

63. Merrett TG, Burr ML, Butland BK et al: Infant feeding and allergy: 12-month prospective study of 500 babies born into allergic families, *Ann Allergy* 61:13, 1988.

64. Moore WJ, Midwinter RE, Morris AF et al: Infant feeding and subsequent risk of atopic eczema, *Arch Dis Child* 60:722, 1985.

65. Murray AB: Infant feeding and respiratory allergy, *Lancet* 1:497, 1971.

66. National Asthma Education Program: *Expert Panel Report II,* Atlanta, 1996, Centers for Disease Control and Prevention.

67. Ratner B: A possible causal factor of food allergy in certain infants, *Am J Dis Child* 36:277, 1928.

68. Rigo J, Salle BL, Cavero E et al: Plasma amino acid and protein concentrations in infants fed human milk or a whey protein hydrolysate formula during the first month of life, *Acta Paediatr* 83:127, 1994.

69. Rowe AH: *Food allergy,* Philadelphia, 1931, Lea & Febiger.

70. Saarinen UM, Kajossari M: Breastfeeding as prophylaxis against disease: prospective follow-up study until 17 years old, *Lancet* 346:1065, 1995.
71. Saarinen UM, Kajosaari M, Backman A et al: Prolonged breast-feeding as prophylaxis for atopic disease, *Lancet* 1:163, 1979.
72. Savilahti E: Intestinal immunoglobulins in children with coeliac disease, *Gut* 13:958, 1972.
73. Savilahti E, Tainio V-M, Salmenpera L et al: Low colostral IgA associated with cow's milk allergy, *Acta Paediatr Scand* 80:1207, 1991.
74. Savilahti E, Tuomikoski-Jaakkola P, Järvenpää A-L et al: Early feeding of preterm infants and allergic symptoms during childhood, *Acta Paediatr* 82:340, 1993.
75. Schwartz RH: IgE-mediated allergic reactions to cow's milk, *Immunol Allergy Clin North Am* 11:717, 1991.
76. Schwartz RH, Keefe MW, Harris N et al: The spectrum of IgE-mediated acute allergic reactions to cow's milk in children as determined by skin testing with cow's milk protein hydrolysate formulas, *Pediatr Asthma Allergy Immunol* 3:207, 1989.
77. Schwartz RH, Kubicka M, Dreyfuss EM et al: Acute urticarial reactions to cow's milk in infants previously fed breast milk or soy milk, *Pediatr Asthma Allergy Immunol* 1:81, 1987.
78. Schloss OM: Allergy in infants and children, *Am J Dis Child* 19:433, 1920.
79. Shannon WR: Demonstration of food proteins in human breast milk by anaphylactic experiments in guinea pigs, *Am J Dis Child* 22:223, 1921.
80. Shannon WR: Eczema in breast-fed infants as a result of sensitization to foods in the mother's diet, *Am J Dis Child* 23:392, 1922.
81. Sigurs N, Hattevig G, Kjellman B: Maternal avoidance of eggs, cow's milk, and fish during lactation: effect on allergic manifestations, skin-prick tests and specific IgE antibodies in children at age 4 years, *Pediatrics* 89:735, 1992.
82. Soothill JF: Some intrinsic and extrinsic factors predisposing to allergy, *Proc R Soc Med* 69:439, 1976.
83. Soothill JF: Prevention of atopic allergic disease, *Ann Allergy* 51:229, 1983.
84. Stevenson DD, Orgell HA, Hamburger RN et al: Development of IgE in newborn human infants, *J Allergy Clin Immunol* 48:61, 1971.
85. Tisdale FF, Erb IH: Extreme sensitization in infants to cow's milk protein, *J Can Med Assoc* 15:497, 1925.
86. Troncone R, Scarcella A, Donatiello A et al: Passage of gliadin into human breast milk, *Acta Paediatr Scand* 76:453, 1987.
87. Vandenplas Y, Bahna SL, Bousquet J et al: Extraintestinal manifestations of food allergy in infants and children, *Nutr Res* 12:161, 1992.
88. Walker WA: Antigen absorption from the small intestine and gastrointestinal disease, *Pediatr Clin North Am* 22:731, 1975.
89. Wright AL, Holberg CJ, Taussig LM et al: Relationship of infant feeding to recurrent wheezing at age 6 years, *Arch Pediatr Adolesc Med* 149:758, 1995.
90. Zeiger RS, Heller S, Mellon MH et al: Effect of combined maternal and infant food-allergen avoidance on development of atopy in early infancy: a randomized study, *J Allergy Clin Immunol* 84:72, 1989.

Induced lactation and relactation (including nursing the adopted baby) and cross-nursing

I nduced lactation is the process by which a nonpuerperal woman is stimulated to lactate, in other words, breastfeeding without pregnancy. Relactation is the process by which a woman who has given birth but did not initially breastfeed is stimulated to lactate. This may also apply to a mother who may have initially breastfed her infant, weaned the infant, and then chooses to reinstitute lactation.

HISTORIC PERSPECTIVE

Induced lactation and relactation are not new concepts but rather are well known to history and to other cultures. The motivation historically has been to provide nourishment for an infant whose mother has died in childbirth or is unable to nurse for some reason. A friend or relative would take on the care of the child and with it the responsibility to nourish the infant at the breast, because no other alternatives were available.

Relactation has been used in times of disaster or epidemics to provide safe nutrition to weaned or motherless infants. Numerous accounts of induced

lactation are recorded in medical literature and reviewed in the writings of Brown.[6] Mead[26] recorded the phenomenon in her writings about New Guinea in 1935. Other anthropologists have made similar observations in other preindustrialized societies of women who have not borne children and, after a few weeks of placing the suckling infant to the breast, produce milk adequate to nourish the infant.[33] Until recently, Western world literature reported the phenomenon as an anecdotal report as part of the discussion of aberrant lactation. Cohen[11] reported in 1971 a patient who had been nursing an adopted child very successfully for weeks when first seen in his pediatric office.

Today, the interest in induced lactation in the industrialized world stems from a desire on the part of some adopting mothers to nurture the adopted child at the breast even if she was unable to carry the infant in utero. The interest in relactation comes from mothers of sick or premature infants who want to breastfeed their infants after the days and weeks of neonatal intensive care are over. These mothers, although postpartum, have not been lactating.

INDUCED VERSUS INAPPROPRIATE LACTATION

The process of induced lactation is separate from *galactorrhea,* or inappropriate lactation, which has been described in the medical literature for over 100 years.[39] Abnormal lactation has been observed in a number of circumstances in nulliparous and parous women and even in males. There are many eponyms for these conditions, usually based on the name of the physician who first described the syndrome, such as Chiari-Frommel and Ahumada–del Castillo.

Normally in the absence of suckling, lactation ceases 14 to 21 days after delivery. Milk flow that continues beyond 3 to 6 months after abortion or any termination of pregnancy is termed *abnormal* or *inappropriate lactation,* or *galactorrhea. Galactorrhea* also refers to lactation in a woman 3 months after weaning or the secretion of milk in a nulliparous woman in association with hyperprolactinemia and amenorrhea. Although these cases are pathologic in nature and therefore different from the groups under discussion, it is noteworthy that some knowledge of the initiation and maintenance of lactation has been gained from the study of these syndromes.

ANIMAL STUDIES

Information on the incidence of nonoffspring nursing in 100 mammalian species has been assembled by Packer et al.[29] The incidence of nonoffspring nursing is increased by captivity. It is more common in species with large litters (polytocous taxa) and differs from that which occurs with single young species (monotocous taxa). In the latter, it is more common for females to continue nursing after they have lost their own young. Among nondomesticated animals, spontaneous lactation has been observed repeatedly only in the dwarf mongoose *(Helogale parvula).*

Lactation has been induced for scientific and commercial purposes in nonpregnant and nonparturient animals by the continual systematic application of a mechanical milking apparatus to the mammary gland of the animal.[23] The response is effected through the release of mammotropic hormone from the anterior pituitary gland. This effect is abolished if the pituitary stalk is transected. Ruminants respond to the addition of estrogen or estrogen-progesterone combinations, which facilitate mammary growth. Experiments in goats involved applying ointment containing estradiol benzoate to the udders of virgins, which resulted in development of the udder and milk yield almost comparable to normal postpartum animals.[12] It was subsequently shown, however, that a combination of estrogen-progesterone not only resulted in better milk yield, but histologically the lobuloalveolar growth was normal, whereas with estrogen alone growth was cystic and irregular. It was also demonstrated that ovariectomized goats could be stimulated to lactation with these two hormones, with resultant normal histology of the udder and good milk production. Initiation of regular milkings had a significant impact on production of milk.

Because lactation can be stimulated when the ovaries have been removed but not when the pituitary stalk has been severed, this has significance for understanding some of the postpartum lactation failures in women. Again in ruminants, growth hormone and thyroid hormone have been shown to increase milk yield, although prolactin does not. This suggests that prolactin is not deficient in ruminants. Selye and McKeown[32] showed in 1934 that suckling stimulus inhibits sexual cyclicity in rats. They further showed that when the main milk ducts to all the nipples are cut and the escape of milk has been rendered impossible, the mechanical stimulation of the nipples by nursing would also inhibit the sexual cyclicity of the normal estric, nonlactating adult rat. These studies demonstrate the significance of suckling in triggering the lactation cycle and suppressing ovulation.

• • •

Because the motivation, goals, and physiologic problems may be slightly different, induced lactation and relactation are discussed separately.

INDUCED LACTATION

When a mother chooses to nurse her adopted infant, the goal is usually to achieve a mother-infant relationship that may also have the benefit of some nutrition.[27] In that perspective, success can be evaluated on the basis of whether the infant will suckle the breast and achieve some comfort and security from this opportunity and close relationship with the new mother. As has been well described by Avery,[4] this is nurturing with the emphasis on *nurturing,* not on "breastfeeding" or nutrition. A mother who is interested in inducing lactation to nurse an adopted infant may need to understand that she may never be able to sustain the infant completely by her milk alone without supplementation. Neither the physician nor the mother should be disappointed. The nurturing goal is still achieved.

Preparation of the breast

Normally the breast is prepared by the proliferation of the ductal and alveolar system through pregnancy in anticipation of the time when lactation will begin.[26] Thus it is appropriate to assume that a period of similar preparation should take place in induced lactation. It has been suggested that the woman should begin systematically to express the breasts manually and stimulate the nipples for up to 2 months before the arrival of the infant, if time permits. A hand pump or other pumping devices can be used, but manual expression may work as well or better. Sometimes some secretion can be produced in this manner if it is carried out systematically on a uniform schedule throughout the day. The schedule should be practical, that is, include times when a mother could take a moment for this activity, such as morning and night plus any times she uses the bathroom or can conveniently handle her breasts.

In other cultures in which lactation is induced as a survival tactic for the infant, no period of preparation is available. The infant is put to the adoptive mother's breast and allowed to suckle. Emphasis has been placed on herbal teas as galactogogues

and good nourishment for the mother, while the infant is also given prechewed food, gruel, or animal milk. Mead[26] attributed much of the success of induced lactation to the ingestion of ample supplies of coconut milk by the new mother.

Adoption is not an easy process, and in fact, it can be quite stressful to become an instant parent. In assisting such a mother, consideration should be given to the infant's age, previous feeding experience, and any medical problems that may exist. Provision for additional nourishment during the process of establishing some milk secretion is most important. Onset of lactation varies from 1 to 6 weeks, averaging about 4 weeks after initiation of stimulation with the appearance of the first drops of milk. When the infant is actually nursing at the breast and being nourished by supplements, milk may appear as early as 1 to 2 weeks.

Some infants are easily confused by switching back and forth between breast and bottle because the sucking technique is slightly different. Other nourishment can be offered by dropper, by small medicine cup, or as solid foods. A unique system is available, however, for providing nourishment for the infant while suckling at the breast. It involves the use of a device to provide a source of nourishment while the infant suckles at the breast, thus stimulating production. It is further described later in this chapter and in Appendix F and is called *Supplemental Nursing System* (Medela's SNS) or *Lact-Aid Nursing Trainer System.*

Drugs to induce lactation

As described in Chapter 3, estrogen and progesterone stimulate the proliferation of the alveolar and ductal systems. These hormones work in association with an increase in prolactin production. Although the prolactin level is high during pregnancy, milk secretion is inhibited by the presence of the estrogen, progesterone, and placental lactogen, the prolactin-inhibiting hormone. After delivery has occurred and the placenta is removed, there is a marked fall in these hormones, and prolactin initiates milk production.[37] Efforts to stimulate this hormonal response have had variable success and are not usually recommended because of the possible effect on the infant through the milk. Women taking oral contraceptives have been noted in some cases to have breast enlargement. In addition, although estrogen and progesterone may enhance proliferation, they may inhibit lactation per se.

The dosage of conjugated estrogens recommended by Waletzky and Herman[41] is 2.5 mg twice a day for 14 days beginning on the fourth day of a regular menstrual cycle. Giving 0.35 mg norethindrone once daily for the morning dose of estrogen prevents breakthrough bleeding. Medication is given for 2 weeks and is comparable in dosage to 2 weeks of oral contraceptives. This may be accompanied by some side effects. The regimen should include direct efforts to stimulate lactation by pumping the breasts.

A report from Papua New Guinea, where inducing lactation is critical to adequate infant nutrition, recommends priming the breast tissue of nulliparous women or those who have not lactated with 50-µg ethinyl estradiol three times a day for a week.[20] An alternative would be medroxyprogesterone acetate (Depo-Provera), 100 mg as a single injection. When relactation is the goal in women who have previously lactated, pumping and massaging alone are initiated.

Growth hormone (GH) and prolactin have considerable genetic similarity, as reflected in some overlap of function.[10] High concentrations of GH can cause lobuloalveolar development and casein expression. GH may play a role in optimization of milk production during lactation and even an accessory role in the induction of lactogenesis. Both natural and recombinant human growth hormones (HGHs) are potent inductors of milk synthesis in pregnant and lactating rats. This effect is attributed to their effect on the prolactin receptor.[10]

Oxytocin is a critical component in the milk ejection reflex and may be helpful in the early initiation of ejection. Physiologically, stimulation of the nipple in the lactating woman results in the release of oxytocin by the hypothalamus, which then triggers the release of milk by stimulating the contraction of myoepithelial cells and the ejection of milk (see Chapter 8). The effect of intranasal administration of oxytocin on the let-down reflex

in lactating women was well described by Newton and Egli.[28] (Oral administration by tablet has not been as effective, because oxytocin is destroyed in the stomach.) Oxytocin nasal spray has been used in cases of nonpuerperal lactation with some success in enhancing let-down but not necessarily altering the volume produced. Continued use of oxytocin over weeks has been associated with diminished effect or even suppression of lactation. The chief benefit of oxytocin is often to break the cycle of failure and instill a feeling of confidence once it has been demonstrated that some secretion can be produced.

Chlorpromazine has been observed to act as a galactogogue as well as a tranquilizer when given to patients in large doses (up to 1000 mg or more). The effect has been observed in both male and female patients in mental institutions. The drug has been reported to increase pituitary prolactin secretion severalfold. It acts via the hypothalamus, probably by reducing levels of prolactin inhibitory factor. Using this information, women well motivated to lactate who have attempted induced lactation by suckling a normal infant have had the process enhanced by small doses of chlorpromazine.[8]

In a program to induce lactation in refugee camps in India and in Vietnam, nonlactating women were given 25 to 100 mg of chlorpromazine three times a day for a week to 10 days while infants were initially put to breast. Brown[7] reports apparent enhancement of lactation with this treatment. Chlorpromazine has the added pharmacologic effect of acting as a tranquilizer. The program of management in these women was supportive in other ways and also included the usual herbal medicines associated with lactation in these Eastern cultures. There was no control group. It is possible that the drug contributed to both the physiologic and the psychologic well-being of the women wanting to lactate. It has been suggested that the desire to lactate is a strong component of success, because women whose breasts are frequently stimulated sexually do not begin to lactate.

Theophylline can also increase pituitary prolactin secretions.[40] Therefore both tea and coffee should enhance prolactin secretion and thus lactation. Excessive amounts may inhibit milk let-down, however.

Because the role of prolactin is the initiation and maintenance of lactation, whereas oxytocin regulates the glandular emptying through the milk-ejection reflex, it is reasonable to speculate that enhancing prolactin release would be productive in inducing lactation. The exact activating mechanism of the neuronal reflex arc from breast to brain has not been deciphered. Secretion of prolactin appears to be influenced, if not controlled, by changes in hypothalamic dopamine turnover. Correspondingly, suckling has been observed to deplete dopamine stores.

Investigation of other drugs that are known to stimulate prolactin release has identified some possible therapeutic materials.[1] Kramer[20] and McNeilly et al[25] have reported that *metoclopramide* induces prolactin release regardless of the route of administration. Prolactin levels are increased three to eight times normal levels within 5 minutes when a 10-mg dose is given either intravenously or intramuscularly. The effect is achieved within an hour when metoclopramide is given orally. The effect persists for 8 hours. The suggested regimen is 10 mg of metoclopramide, four times a day for a week.[14] This is then gradually tapered.

Metoclopramide also is used in neonates with esophageal reflux. The side effects are irritability and diarrhea. Rarely, susceptible infants experience dystonic reactions. Metoclopramide has also been used in combination with chlorpromazine, 25 mg four times a day, in Papua New Guinea.[20] Metoclopramide has been used to enhance lactation as well, especially among mothers of premature infants.

The regulation of prolactin secretion in humans has been studied to further the understanding of abnormal lactation as well as to provide information on the regulation of pituitary function of the brain.[13] It has been shown experimentally that the hypothalamus secretes prolactin inhibitory factor (PIF), which acts on the mammotropin-releasing cells of the pituitary to inhibit release of the hormone prolactin. The hypothalamus can also regulate prolactin secretion by a stimulatory mechanism, the secretion of thyrotropin-releasing hormone (TRH). When human volunteers (nonpregnant, nonlactating) are given infusions of TRH, increases in thyrotropin and prolactin are observed within minutes of injection, with values peaking in 20 minutes. The level of thyroid hormone in the volunteers initially influences the results. Hypothyroid patients have been observed to secrete excessive amounts of prolactin, whereas hyperthyroid patients are relatively insensitive to TRH. This may explain some of the variable results obtained with prolactin-stimulating drugs used to enhance lactation. Studies of relactation have been done using TRH but not of newly induced lactation.

Table 18-1 summarizes the influence of drugs on prolactin secretion.

Any pharmacologic regimen to stimulate milk production is most effective if it is initiated after the breast tissue has responded to mechanical stimulation or after the hormones that act as the prolactin-stimulating compounds are ineffective in unprimed breast tissue. Jelliffe[18] points out that the most important factor for continued production of milk is not drugs or hormones but "mulging." He explains that *mulging* (stimulation) is a word created in 1975 by N.W. Pirie to mitigate the confusion between the words *sucking* and *suckling*. The word comes from the Latin *mulgere,* to milk. Suck, according to the dictionary,[16] means to draw into the mouth by means of a partial vacuum created by action of the lips and the tongue. Suckle, however, refers specifically to the breast and means "to give suck to," as at the breast, or to take nourishment from the breast.

Composition of milk

Concern has been expressed that the composition of the milk produced by stimulation of suckling rather than as a result of pregnancy might differ from "normal human milk."[35] Such induced milk is not different in other species that have been studied extensively, including bovine and rat. In developing countries, that the infants showed normal growth and weight gain was taken as evidence that induced milk is adequate.

Vorherr[39,40] reported the analysis of the galac-

TABLE 18-1	Influence of drugs on prolactin secretion	

Pharmacologic agents	Plasma prolactin concentration	Mechanism of drug action
L-Dopa	Decrease	Increase in hypothalamic dopamine-catecholamine levels, leading to enhanced activity of prolactin inhibitory factor (PIF)
Ergot alkaloids (ergocornine, ergocryptine)	Decrease	Direct inhibition of adenohypophyseal prolactin secretion; possible increase of hypothalamic PIF activity (continued PIF function)
Thyrotropin-releasing hormone (TRH; pyroglutamyl-histidyl-prolinamide)	Increase	Direct stimulation of adenohypophyseal lactotrophs for increased prolactin secretion
Theophylline		
Phenothiazines (chlorpromazine)	Increase	Decreases in hypothalamic dopamine-catecholamine levels, leading to diminution of PIF activity
Metoclopramide	Increase	Inhibition of hypothalamic PIF secretion through dopamine antagonism
Sulpiride	Increase	Increase in hypothalamic prolactin-releasing hormone
Growth hormone (GH)	Increase	Causes lobulo-alveolar development and casein expression
Recombinant human growth hormones (HGHs)	Increase	Affects prolactin receptors

Modified from Vorherr H: Human lactation and breast feeding. In Larson BL, editor: *Lactation,* New York, 1978, Academic Press.

TABLE 18-2	Composition of normal breast milk and "galactorrhea milk"		

Milk components and properties	Normal breast milk	"Galactorrhea milk"	Induced lactation
Components			
Fat (g/dl)	3.7	3-8	
Lactose (g/dl)	7.0	3-5	5.4
Total protein (g/dl)	1.2	2-7	1.6
Sodium (mg/dl)	15	70	22.0
Potassium (mg/dl)	50	5	19.8
Calcium (mg/dl)	35	38	
Chlorine (mg/dl)	45	50	18.4
Phosphorus (mg/dl)	15	2	
Ash (mg/dl)	20	40-70	
Properties			
Specific gravity	1030-1033	1031	
Milk pH	6.8-7.3	7.3	
Daily volume	400-800 ml	1-120 ml	

From Vorherr H: *The breast: morphology, physiology and lactation,* New York, 1974, Academic Press; and Kulski JK, Hartmann PE, Saint WJ et al: *Am Obstet Gynecol* 139:597, 1981. Reprinted with permission from the American College of Obstetricians and Gynecologists.

torrheal secretion produced by the breast after hyperstimulation; Table 18-2 shows the comparative analysis. The induced lactational milk did not differ from puerperal milk. Brown[6] reported higher values of fat, protein, and lactose in galactorrheal milk, but the volume of secretion was small in these subjects.

The composition of the breast secretion produced by two women who induced lactation artificially by breast hyperstimulation was close to the composition obtained for women with normal lactation, according to Kulski et al[22] (see Table 18-2). These investigators also examined the milk of a woman in whom lactation had occurred when medicated with a psychotropic drug (haloperidol). She had been pregnant 4 years previously. Her galactorrhea lasted 38 months. Her milk had composition like that of colostrum for a week but resembled mature milk at 1 month. A woman with hypothyroidism and elevated prolactin and TSH had colostrum-like milk for 53 days of sampling. Two women with galactorrhea and amenorrhea associated with pituitary tumor and hyperprolactinemia had transient colostrum-like secretion, which changed to mature milk.

Protein values of milk samples from five mothers without biologic pregnancies were measured by Kleinman et al.[19] Two of the mothers had nursed previous babies, and three had never been pregnant and had never breastfed. These authors did not distinguish between them. The mean total protein concentration of milk samples from the "nonbiologic" mothers differs from the "biologic" mothers (Figs. 18-1 and 18-2). If the goal of induced lactation is nurturing, these differences are clinically less important. However, the clinician needs to keep these values in mind when counseling a mother-infant dyad about induced-lactation nutrition, especially if the infant was premature or small for gestational age. A creamatocrit test for fat and energy content is an appropriate first step (see Chapter 20).

In tandem nursing, when a mother continues to nurse an older child and puts an adopted newborn on the breast simultaneously, the composition of milk will not return to colostrum as it does with a biologic pregnancy.

Management of the mother and infant

The collected experiences of counseling women in the Western world who want to induce lactation

Fig. 18-1. Total protein changes over time: biologic versus nonbiologic mother's milk, protein value ± standard deviation. (From Kleinman R, Jacobson L, Hormann E et al: *J Pediatr* 97:613, 1980.)

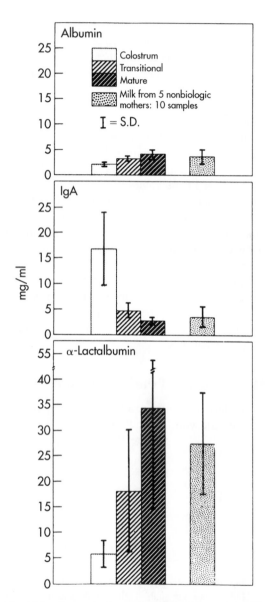

Fig. 18-2. Concentrations of albumin, immunoglobulin A (IgA), and α-lactalbumins: biologic versus nonbiologic mother's milk. *S.D.,* Standard deviation. (From Kleinman R, Jacobson L, Hormann E et al: *J Pediatr* 97:614, 1980.)

have reported on several thousand women. The request for information and advice is increasing and becoming widespread throughout the United States and other Western countries.[35]

Because there are simple means of supplement-

ing the nutritional needs of the infant, the counseling should center on the relationship and the nurturing aspects. When the process is undertaken in preindustrialized nations, the antiinfective properties become important even though total nourishment may not be possible. Success is measured by having the infant content to nurse at the breast.

The woman should be encouraged to come to the physician's office for a counseling visit before the arrival of the adoptive infant to discuss the process of induced lactation. Actually, parents who are planning to adopt an infant should have at least one visit with their pediatrician so that some understanding of parenting can be discussed, just as any couple should do before the birth of their first child. At this visit, while discussing lactation with the couple, it is helpful to explore their motives and general concepts of what is involved. All authors on the subject have pointed out that the husband's interest in and support of lactation is critical to success. His participation in the preparation of the breasts may be a means by which the father can share intimately and constructively in the process.

Instruction of the mother in preparation of the breast for suckling is critical in induced lactation, whereas with puerperal lactation it may not be necessary at all. Exercises to stimulate the nipple should be undertaken several times a day and will be most successful if they are scheduled for times when and situations in which it is easy, feasible, and readily remembered. A few minutes multiple times a day is more successful and less likely to *overemphasize* milk versus mothering than rigid excessive exercises once or twice a day. Manual manipulation with gentle traction or horizontal and vertical stretching can be suggested. Avery[4] suggests that the father be encouraged to assist in breast massage and other techniques. She notes that "many adoptive parents felt that this technique (fondling and suckling of the breasts by the husband) added to the mutual sharing in preparation for adoptive nursing similar to the closeness many couples experience in preparing for natural childbirth." Raphael[31] reports that among 40 adoptive nursing mothers, dozens of variations on the theme of preparation were used. A positive attitude seemed to be the only consistent factor.

The need for dietary counseling is obvious. Lip service in behalf of well-balanced nutritious meals is not enough. Discussion should center around the absolute needs in kilocalories, fluids, and nutrients to produce milk (see Chapter 9).

The physician should point out that stimulation of the nipples may well cause amenorrhea. Although the variation in menses is not uniform, decreased flow, irregular cycles, and total cessation of menstrual flow are possible. On the other hand, the menstrual cycle may be maintained and the flow of milk may seem to vary during menses. Changes in breast size, heaviness, and feeling of fullness may accompany the induced lactation. The woman may have an associated weight gain of 10 to 12 pounds (4.5 to 5.4 kg), on the average,[4] attributed to the response of the body to developing stores for lactation, just as in pregnancy (i.e., increased fluid retention and appetite increase). The weight gain may be a simple phenomenon of excessive intake. There is no need to gain excessive weight, however, during this experience. Mothers (who may be nutritionally depleted) in non-Western countries who induce lactation are given added diet, nourishment, and herbal teas but do not usually gain weight. Failure to experience change in breast size, menstrual regularity, or weight should not be construed as a failed response.

Auerbach and Avery[3] reported a retrospective questionnaire study of 240 women: 83 had never been pregnant or lactated, 55 had been pregnant but never lactated, and 102 had breastfed one or more biologic children before the adoptive nursing (lactation). Most respondents used more than one technique to stimulate their nipples. These mothers stated that the most effective method of nipple stimulation was nipple exercises combined with infant suckling. Hand-operated pumps caused soreness and irritation. The nipple exercises included nipple stroking, massaging the breast, and rolling the nipple between thumb and finger.

In this study the infant's willingness to suckle improved over time and was related to the age at which the infant was first put to breast. Infants who were under 8 weeks of age had over a 75% success rate; those over 8 weeks of age had only 50% success. No infants failed to thrive, but nearly all needed some type of supplementation. Mothers who had nursed a biologic baby before were able to wean from supplementation partially or completely. This group was also more disappointed if they had to supplement.[3]

The following simple guidelines, developed as a result of experiences reported by several authors and many mothers, may be helpful to the physician in counseling the mother to induce lactation:

1. Before arrival of the baby, initiate frequent, brief manual stimulation of nipples and breasts, increasing time gradually to about 10 minutes per session. Initiate mechanical pumping stimulus after 2 weeks or so of manual stimulus, if time permits. Hand pumps usually cause more soreness. Modern electric pumps with milking action and pressure cycling are most effective. Pumps that can be controlled in cycle frequency and strength are best. Double-sided pumps maximize stimulus and save time.
2. On arrival of the baby, depending on the infant's age, limit sucking to breastfeeding, using a lactation supplementer if necessary.
3. Breastfeed before any other nourishment is provided for a given feeding.
4. Avoid stressing baby with hunger.
5. When supplementing, use donor human milk or prepared formula, not cow's milk, with its long stomach-emptying time.
6. Avoid rubber nipples and pacifiers to encourage appropriate suckling at breast.
7. Provide other supplements by dropper, spoon, cup, or supplementer.
8. Create a positive atmosphere; "mother the mother."

A trial of oxytocin nasal spray once the infant is established at the breast may facilitate let-down and even encourage prolactin release (see instructions, p. 268).

Rigid conformity to a system of feeding may be a symptom of a more serious problem. Women who are rigid and compulsive may have trouble lactating because of the inability to have a good ejection reflex, which can be inhibited by stress and emotional conflict. Mothers who demonstrate an inordinate attention to volume of production of milk over and above the value of the relationship may feel as if they have failed.

Nutritional supplementation

The need to supplement the infant's intake while the milk supply is being developed should be discussed. The older infant who has already been receiving solid foods can be continued on solids by spoon with careful attention to nutritional content so that the diet includes a balance of protein and other nutrients. Supplements with milk or formula should be appropriate to the age of the infant. The infant under 6 months should receive infant formula rather than whole milk if donor breast milk is not available. The milk supplements should be full strength, 20 kcal/oz, and provided during the feeding by dropper or supplementer or after the nursing by dropper, spoon, or cup in preference to rubber nipple, which may confuse the infant during adaptation to nursing at the breast.

Support systems

The process of induced lactation requires considerable commitment and determination.[42] It is far more arduous a task than initiating postpartum lactation, but it is possible and worth the effort, according to the many mothers who have attempted it. The situation is better managed if a doula is available. It is appropriate for the physician to suggest that in addition to medical support, the mother seek counseling from a lactation consultant experienced in induced lactation. Day-by-day contact for verbal support may be helpful, and these needs may be beyond the scope of a busy office practice. The nurse practitioner may be invaluable in this situation, particularly if home visits are made.

Ensuring that the child grows appropriately is the responsibility of the pediatrician; however, this task is best carried out in a nonthreatening way so the mother can concentrate on nurturing and nourishing the infant.[15] Monitoring the usual growth parameters of weight and height as well as the patterns of voiding and stooling is essential.

RELACTATION

The need to relactate exists in a number of circumstances, including the following:
1. A sick or premature infant cannot be fed initially or at all until several weeks or months old (Fig. 18-3).
2. An infant is weaned prematurely because of illness in the infant or in the mother.
3. An infant who was not previously breastfed develops an allergy or food intolerance.
4. A mother who has lactated weeks, months, or years earlier wants to nurse an adopted infant.
5. A mother who is nursing a biologic child wants to nurse an adopted child (without benefit of pregnancy).

Historic reviews provide many examples of infants suckled in times of crisis by women who have not lactated for years. The process of reestablishing lactation under these circumstances is generally easier than that of nonpuerperal lactation. Investigations have shown that a breast that has been previously primed by pregnancy to respond to prolactin will produce milk more readily.

An early unpublished report of relactation describes a woman who had breastfed her first child, who was full term, for 9 months. Then the woman experienced two premature births and deaths and then breastfed two adopted infants. The first adoptee was 6 weeks old when the mother began breastfeeding. She had full milk supply within 3 months and nursed for 9 months. Nursing required supplementary formula for the infant at first, but the volume was gradually reduced. Three years later, she adopted a 2-week-old infant. She had to entice the infant with honey on the nipple, expressed milk, and spoon feedings. The mother used oxytocin nasal spray to obtain let-down the first few weeks. This infant was also fully breastfed for months.

Psychologic factors

Although the general process of nipple stimulation, having the infant suckle the breast, and setting the stage for lactation is similar, the woman who has

Fig. 18-3. Premature infant at breast: infant weighed 1300 g at time of photograph.

experienced successful lactation previously may have not only the physiologic but also the psychologic edge.

A prospective study of mothers whose infants were in the neonatal intensive care unit in Durham, NC, was reported by Bose et al.[5] The profile of the mothers is listed in Table 18-3. Mother and baby were admitted to the Clinical Research Unit, where they were assisted with relactating, including help using the Lact-Aid. The infant's nutritional intake was recorded. Mother and infant were discharged when the mother was comfortable with the Lact-Aid and feeding was established (about 3 days). Follow-up occurred every week or two. All but one infant were initially reluctant to suckle, but all received their entire nutritional intake at the breast, with or without Lact-Aid, within the first week of the study. Most of the mothers had trouble initiating suckling, with the most significant factor being the length of separation from their infant and not degree of prematurity, postnatal age, weight, or feeding regimen. Nipple tenderness occurred in all mothers transiently. All the mothers (except number seven, who was an adoptive mother), produced milk in 1 week, with maximum milk production

occurring from 8 to 58 days, proportional to the time since delivery.

Although it was done with a small population, this study established some important information. Given appropriate techniques and support, many women appear to be able to relactate, and premature infants can learn to breastfeed after initial bottle feeding.

A retrospective study of relactation was reported by Auerbach and Avery[2] in which 366 women responded with a completed questionnaire out of over 500 contacted from a list of names obtained from manufacturer's lists, magazine ads, and requests to breastfeeding support groups. The bias was in favor of well-educated, affluent women who had probably obtained their lactation goals. The population included those who had untimely weaning (n = 174), following delivery of low-birthweight infants (n = 117), and following hospitalization of mother or baby or both (n = 75).

The infant's willingness to nurse was related to previous suckling experience, but responses in the first week of effort were not directly correlated with ultimate successful suckling. Fifty percent of mothers were able to discontinue supplementing in

TABLE 18-3   Historic and clinical data of mothers in relactation study

Case no.	Gestational age	Time from delivery to entry into study (days)	Time from last lactation to entry into study (days)	Postpartum breast involution*	Time to first breast milk (days)	Time to half breast milk supply† (days)	Time to complete relactation (days)
1	Term	10	10	None	1	4	8
2	Term	120	120	Incomplete	4	20	28
3‡	Twins, 31 wk	49	49	Complete	7	28	Never
4	32 wk	70	42	Complete	7	39	Never
5	28 wk	150	135	Complete	9	Never	Never
6	32 wk	30	16	None	4	17	58
7	Term (adopted)	5 yr	5 yr	Complete	21	Never	Never

From Bose CL, D'Ercole J, Lester AG et al: *Pediatrics* 67:565, 1981.

*Mothers were asked if their brassiere size was different from that before this pregnancy.

†Estimated on the basis of a decrease in formula intake.

‡Ceased to suckle her infant after 28 days in the study to return to full-time employment.

1 month, and 24% were never able to eliminate supplements completely. Once established, the nursing patterns were similar to those of ordinary breastfeeding. The authors[2] point out that keeping the baby hungry in the mistaken notion that the infant will nurse more often and for longer periods does not help and may negatively influence outcome. For the professional, it is of interest that fewer than 10% of respondents received helpful advice from health care professionals.

Relactation in mothers of children over 12 months of age was reported.[30,36] Six Australian children 12 to 18 months of age had been weaned by the mother with no further stimulus to the breast, then were reinitiated to breastfeeding. The length of time without breastfeeding ranged from 1 week to 6 months (Table 18-4). All the children had been actively weaned and initiated the suckling, although the mothers did not forcibly resist. All the mothers reestablished milk supplies and nursed for 48 months to 5 years.[30,36]

Tandem nursing

Tandem nursing an adoptive child is a phenomenon in which the adoptive mother is still nursing a biologic child and puts an adopted infant to the breast and intends to nourish the newcomer totally. Usually the older child is a toddler and feeding only a few times a day or for comfort and receiving the major nourishment from other food and drink. In biologic tandem nursing, the milk returns to colostrum-like constituency with the birth of the new baby; in the absence of a pregnancy, however,

TABLE 18-4	Relactation in children over 12 months of age					
Case no.	Age of child	Length of time off breast	Methods	Evidence of presence of milk	How long from relactation to weaning	Age at final weaning
1	48 mo	4 mo	Child suckled from breast Mother relaxed, not anxious over outcome	Child verbally reported presence of milk Mother saw whitish milk	After milk appeared	48 mo
2	12 mo	1 wk	Child took four feeds daily	Milk had not quite dried up	1 yr	2 yr
3	20½ mo	2½ mo	Mother gave in to demands of child and suckled her	Mother noticed child's swallowing while breastfeeding	>10 mo	Some time after 2½ yr
4	2 yr	1 mo	Child suckled from both breasts avidly	Mother saw the milk Flow was enough to soak the bed next morning Mother heard swallowing	Approx. 1 yr	>3 yr
5	>3 yr	6 wk	Child suckled from both breasts	Mother saw the milk Mother noticed swallowing	Approx. 2 yr	5 yr
6	Approx. 2 yr	Approx. 6 mo	Mother attached child to breast to demonstrate	Mother began to feel let-down of milk	12 mo	Almost 3 yr

From Phillips N: *J Trop Pediatr* 39:45, 1993.

TABLE 18-5 Basal and stimulated serum prolactin concentrations (ng/ml)

Case no.	TRH stimulation		Suckling stimulation: presuckling/postsuckling					
	Basal	15 min/30 min	1st wk*	2nd wk	3rd wk	4th-5th wk	6th-7th wk	8th-9th wk
1	179.2	611.1/423.5	136.9/155.4	72.3/123.8	—	—	—	—
2	38.7	80.9/70.3	17.2/119.3	38.6/214.3	16.6/180.6	186.2/244.5	—	—
3	19.9	89.6/77.3	17.9/23.5	—	—	—	—	—
4	9.5	89.9/63.4	12.5/12.7	—	7.0/437.6	5.5/47.3	—	—
5	13.9	40.6/36.3	21.1/58.2	37.8/82.0	38.3/57.7	77.2/98.5	24.6/54.2	—
6	31.7	335.6/274.7	9.5/11.4	—	16.5/18.4	11.8/16.3	7.8/13.3	—
7	43.6†	78.8/69.9	8.8/59.6	17.0/77.7	—	—	34.4/147.1	19.2/60.5

From Bose CL, D'Ercole J, Lester AG et al: *Pediatrics* 67:565, 1981.

*Suckling test performed on day 1 or 2 of study.

†In this mother, suckling test was done first, followed 1 hour later by thyrotropin-releasing hormone (TRH) infusion; thus 8.8 is the true basal concentration.

the milk volume may increase with increased nipple stimulus while the constituents do not change. Data on milk constituents beyond a year postpartum or in the case of relactation have been noted earlier. In most cases reported anecdotally, the adopted infant is several weeks or months old, so the absence of colostrum is less of a problem. On the other hand, the active state of lactation in terms of immediate availability of milk is actually an advantage.

An additional concern, as in any situation of tandem nursing, is the development of the younger child. The physician will need to be alert to these issues in counseling the family and ensuring adequate total nutrition for the adopted child.

Eighteen respondents to the survey on adoptive nursing by Auerbach and Avery[3] reported tandem-nursing experiences. Eleven of these mothers were able to discontinue supplements totally (two within the first month). Most of the infants were started on solids by 4½ months, which may be the most effective method of supplementing if nutritional value is maintained. For the physician, it is important to be knowledgeable about tandem adoptive nursing and to support the family accordingly.

Drugs to induce relactation

Some medications that have been tried in relactation seem to work only when the breast has been primed by mammogenesis, that is, by pregnancy.

TRH (Thyroliberin) has been used by Tyson[38] and others to induce lactation (Table 18-1). Each woman in the study was primed with estrogens beforehand. TRH stimulates the pituitary to release both thyrotropin-stimulating hormone (TSH) and prolactin. Drugs that produce a decrease in hypothalamic catecholamines, such as phenothiazines, reserpine, meprobamate, amphetamines, and α-methyldopa, cause an increase in prolactin secretion by blocking hypothalamic PIF.

The feasibility of pharmacologically manipulating puerperal lactation was demonstrated by Canales et al[9] using bromocriptine and TRH sequentially. They suppressed lactation using bromocriptine orally for 8 days in four mothers whose infants were premature and/or ill and could not be nursed. These mothers did not lactate during this time. On the eighth day, they were given TRH intravenously and then orally daily for 4 days (eighth to twelfth postpartum day). On the fourteenth day, they initiated breastfeeding by putting the infant to the breast. Prolactin levels were measured from the day of birth. Levels were depressed by bromocriptine and rose when the TRH was given. The mothers subsequently nursed successfully.

Bose et al[5] also studied TRH and the basal and stimulated serum prolactin concentrations. Prolactin concentrations were measured followed by levels at 15 and 30 minutes after intravenous infusion of 200 µg of TRH. Prolactin levels were also measured before and after suckling at weekly intervals. Serum prolactin levels rose 15 minutes after infusion of TRH (Table 18-5). The absolute rise in prolactin concentrations did not appear to be related to establishment of milk production. The change over time in the basal prolactin levels was not predictably related to lactation progress.

Lactation can be reestablished with metoclopramide, according to Sousa et al.[34] Metoclopramide is a derivative of procainamide, as is sulpiride. Studies done by McNeilly et al[25] showed that metoclopramide and sulpiride are potent stimulators of prolactin release. These authors demonstrated marked increase in prolactin when metoclopramide is given, as noted earlier in this chapter. Sousa et al[34] used metoclopramide to reestablish lactation in women who had experienced diminished milk supply. All five mothers experienced increased production of milk when 10 mg was given orally every 8 hours for 7 to 10 days. No side effects were noted, although this drug is known to cause cardiac arrhythmias and extrapyramidal signs in some adults. No side effects were noted in the infants either, but the level of drug was not measured in the milk. The results were encouraging, but further study is needed to determine the minimum dosage necessary to produce the effect and the amount passed into the milk. The summation of the data on patients treated by Sousa et al[34] is recorded in Table 18-6.

Case no.	Age of mother (yr)	Age of infant (mo)	Daily dose (mg)	Length of treatment (days)	Side effects	Results	Education level of mother
						TABLE 18-6 **Data regarding mothers taking metoclopramide**	
1	27	2	30	6	None	Increase in milk volume; infant not weaned	University
2	25	10	30	10	None	Same as above	University
3	29	1	20	7	None	Same as above	High school
4	35	3	30	7	None	Same as above	University
5	20	2	20	7	None	Same as above	High school

From Sousa PLR, Barros FC, Pinheiro GNM et al: *J Trop Pediatr Environ Child Health* 21:214, 1975.

In a controlled double-blind study with a placebo, Lewis et al[24] found no difference in the success rate of induced lactation in 10 patients medicated with 10-mg metoclopramide orally three times daily for 7 days compared with 10 matched patients medicated with lactose capsules. Successful lactation was attributed to the special advice and support provided equally for these women by the nursery staff. Before conducting the study, these authors measured the amount of drug that appeared in the milk of 10 women after a single 10-mg dose of metoclopramide given orally at 7 to 10 days postpartum. The mean 2-hour postdose plasma level was 68.5 ± 29.6 ng/ml. The simultaneous mean concentration in the breast milk was 125.7 ± 41.7 ng/ml. If the infant consumed a liter of milk a day, the dose to the infant would be calculated at 130 mg or 45 mg/kg, a subtherapeutic dose. These data do not address possible accumulation in the infant, however, when multiple doses are given to the mother.

SPECIAL DEVICES

Although many mechanical devices have been developed since Roman times to augment lactation and give other feeding opportunities, lactation-supplementing devices provide a unique ability to adequately nourish an infant while it is suckling at the inadequately lactating breast (Fig. 18-4). The suckling stimulates the mother's own supply. On the other hand, the infant continues to suckle the breast because milk is available. The devices have been carefully engineered to provide a source of milk that is obtained by suckling, not by gravity. The capillary tube through which the milk flows can be placed along the human nipple without interfering with suckling. The plastic containers that serve as reservoirs for the supplemental milk are sterilizable or disposable. The milk is naturally warmed by hanging the bag beside the mother's breast, as shown in Fig. 18-4. See Appendix F for a full description.

Gradual weaning from the supplementer can be provided by putting less and less in the container each day. Thus the infant can obtain milk from the breast in increasing amounts because the nipple stimulation affects milk production.

An increasing number of mothers want to nurse their sick premature infants; however, it is often not possible for the infant to breastfeed for weeks. Meanwhile, the mother may pump but only obtain minimal volume. When the infant is finally ready for discharge from the hospital, it is mandatory that the baby continue to receive reliable nourishment every day. Starving the infant into submission is inappropriate and dangerous. A lactation supplementer is an excellent alternative.

For years, mothers of premature and sick infants have been assisted in breastfeeding their infants in preparation for discharge from the hospital and during the early weeks at home by using dropper feeding, complementary feeds by bottle after each breastfeeding, or solids. The success rate was low and the aggravation for the mother often insurmountable.

Weaning from the device is usually not a problem for most of the infants. It was a problem, however, for an occasional mother who could not nurse without the supplementer even though it contained less than an ounce of formula per feeding and the breast was supplying the rest. Because the mother may use this as a "crutch," careful anticipatory counseling should address this issue.

Special equipment should be started with a full understanding of its role in nourishment of the infant as well as with a plan for weaning from it that begins the first day. Weaning should be appropriate to the infant's age and nutritional needs. The nourishment provided should be donor human milk or regular-strength formula, 20 kcal/oz, and not just water, sugar water, or diluted formula. Starvation, even for a day or so, in a premature infant compromises growth, especially of the brain. An infant who has been in the intensive care nursery is in special jeopardy (see Fig. 14-3).

Several alternative devices have been suggested by professionals interested in the transient supplementation of lactation while a mother increased her milk supply for her full-term baby. Usually in these situations, lactation failure has been the result of inadequate initial advice. The devices are rigged from readily available feeding tubes and syringes but lack the special engineering and safety features of the supplementer. Special precautions are advised when employing such handmade equipment to avoid milk aspiration by the infant, which is the chief hazard. Because they will allow milk to flow without sucking, they do not stimulate the infant to suck. Other devices, such as hand pumps and a variety of electric pumps, which are useful in initiating relactation or induced lactation as well as in puerperal nursing, are illustrated in Chapter 20.

SUMMARY

Careful medical management of the adopted infant who is breastfed is important. Many times the

Fig. 18-4. A, Lact-Aid Nursing Trainer System (Lact-Aid International, Inc.). **B,** Supplemental Nursing System (SNS) by Medela, which provides additional nourishment to infant while suckling at underproducing breast.

prenatal care of this infant as a fetus in utero has not been optimal. Any failure in growth should be identified quickly so that appropriate supplementation can be provided. In cases of relactation to provide for sick or premature infants, close follow-up is mandatory. A child who does not have a powerful suck may well appear to be very content yet be underfed. This situation was clearly described by Gilmore and Rowland,[17] who reported three cases of malnutrition while breastfeeding, attributed to the failure of the mother to recognize signs of growth failure and dehydration.

Relactation and induced lactation are special events requiring the positive support of medical personnel.[42] The physician can serve as a well-informed stable resource in a process that will require considerable effort and commitment by the participants.

Mother-initiated preparation

1. Nipple stimulation: hand massage and nipple exercise, hand pump, electric "milkers"
2. Diet supplementation: fluids and calories, especially protein
3. Reading, learning, and communication with others with similar experience

Physician-initiated preparation

1. Knowledgeable, sympathetic support
2. Preparatory hormones and lactogogues to promote mammogenesis may be considered
3. Induction of let-down: oxytocin nasal drops to initiate or enhance let-down
4. Counseling about breast preparation and diet supplementation in the context of total care of the mother and the infant
5. Use of lactation-supplementing devices

WET NURSING OR CROSS-NURSING

Although feeding an infant by one who is not the mother is an established means of sustaining life, it has been uncommon in Western cultures since the 1930s. There were no medical contraindications provided the nursing woman was in good health, was infection free, and was taking no medications. The threat of human immunodeficiency virus (HIV) infection has altered the risk. In special cases, surrogate nursing would be acceptable by individual arrangement, with HIV testing in both mother and infant. The chief obstacle had been psychologic or social. Actually, women who are trying to develop a supply of milk when their own infant cannot nurse because of prematurity or illness would be greatly benefited by having a vigorous, normal suckling infant nurse at their breasts.

In contemporary society, the term *cross-nursing* has replaced *wet nursing* to disassociate the phenomenon from the negative historic connotations.[21] In cross-nursing the mother continues to breastfeed her own child in addition to the child she takes for a feeding or two per day. The circumstances described in the report by Krantz and Kupper[21] usually involve babysitting arrangements, which may be daily and formal or random and informal. They interviewed three women involved in a mutual agreement for babysitting purposes. The mothers were married and well educated. The babies were female and 4 months old. The mothers reported no physical effects on the babies. The behavioral reactions of the babies were "looking puzzled" and being disturbed if the surrogate mother spoke. Some difficulty was noticed in let-down, and all three mothers noted a difference in the way each baby suckled.

Another purpose of cross-nursing is for maternal benefit, wherein an experienced, vigorous infant is nursed by a woman whose own baby is unable to give proper stimulus to milk production. This has been done by private arrangement and has not caused any known problems. Usually the normal newborn is younger than 2 months. Cross-nursing has also been used to stimulate lactation in adoptive nursing. In this situation, the infants are exchanged to stimulate the adoptive mother's breasts and also to show the adopted infant that milk comes from breasts and how to suckle at the breast.

Cross-nursing had been used in neonatal intensive care units by mothers to encourage their own milk production. It was usually a private arrangement between mothers who had babies to nourish. A mother of an immature infant who cannot be put to the breast sought out a friend who was actively feeding a full-term infant and borrowed the infant to stimulate her production. An infant who needs to learn how to suckle correctly after weeks of bottle feeding or no feeding may benefit from being nursed by a fully lactating woman.

The hazards to cross-nursing are undocumented but worthy of consideration. The physical problems are the potential for infection, either of mother or of baby; interruption of milk supply for the mother's own baby; and the difference in composition of milk if babies are of different chronologic or conceptual ages. The psychologic hazards could include failure of mother to letdown, refusal of infant to nurse (which does occur when infants are introduced to the phenomenon beyond 4 months of age), and negative impact on siblings and the household environment. The long-range effects are not documented.

Reasonable caution is certainly appropriate, taking care to ensure that the cross-nursing mother is healthy and well nourished without any general or local infection, not taking any medications, and not smoking. The infants should probably be close in age to the mother's own baby and also free of infection, especially thrush. If this were a commercial venture in a public day-care setting, regulations of certification screening for tuberculosis, syphilis, hepatitis, cytomegalovirus, herpesvirus, HIV, and other infectious agents might be in order. Documents of liability might be required.

Perhaps as breastfeeding knowledge and understanding reach a greater number of professionals and women, such opportunities may be more common. At present, it is significant to recognize cross-nursing as a viable option, as long as appropriate infection precautions are taken. The hospital or physician cannot be the agent of arrangement.

REFERENCES

1. Arya DK, Taylor WS: Lactation associated with fluoxetine treatment, *Aust NZ J Psychiatry* 29:697, 1995.
2. Auerbach KG, Avery JL: Relactation: a study of 366 cases, *Pediatrics* 65:236, 1980.
3. Auerbach KG, Avery JL: Induced lactation: a study of adoptive nursing by 240 women, *Am J Dis Child* 135:340, 1981.
4. Avery JL: *Induced lactation: a guide for counseling and management,* Denver, 1979, Resources in Human Nurturing, International.
5. Bose CL, D'Ercole J, Lester AG et al: Relactation by mothers of sick and premature infants, *Pediatrics* 67:565, 1981.
6. Brown RE: Some nutritional considerations in times of major catastrophe, *Clin Pediatr* 11:334, 1972.
7. Brown RE: Breastfeeding in modern times, *Am J Clin Nutr* 26:556, 1973.
8. Brown RE: Relactation: an overview, *Pediatrics* 60:116, 1977.
9. Canales ES, Lasso P, Murrieta S et al: Feasibility of suppressing and reinitiating lactation in women with premature infants, *Am J Obstet Gynecol* 128:695, 1977.
10. Caron RW, Janh GA, Deis RP: Lactogenic actions of different growth hormone preparations in pregnant and lactating rats, *J Endocrinol* 142:535, 1994.
11. Cohen R: Breastfeeding without pregnancy, *Pediatrics* 48:996, 1971 (letter).
12. Cowie AT, Forsyth IA, Hart IC: Hormonal control of lactation, *Monogr on Endocrinol* 15, 1980.
13. Creel SR, Monfort SL, Wildt DE et al: Spontaneous lactation is an adaptive result of pseudopregnancy, *Nature* 351:660, 1991.
14. Ehernkranz RA, Ackerman BA: Metoclopramide effect on faltering milk production by mothers of premature infants, *Pediatrics* 78:614, 1986.
15. Evans TJ, Davies DP: Failure to thrive at the breast: an old problem revisited, *Arch Dis Child* 52:974, 1977.
16. *Funk and Wagnalls' standard dictionary,* international edition, vol II, New York, 1960, Funk and Wagnalls.
17. Gilmore HE, Rowland TW: Critical malnutrition in breast fed infants, *Am J Dis Child* 132:885, 1978.
18. Jelliffe DB: Hormonal control of lactation. In Schams D, editor: *Breast feeding and the mother,* Ciba Foundation Symposium no 45, Amsterdam, 1976, Elsevier.
19. Kleinman R, Jacobson L, Hormann E et al: Protein values of milk samples from mothers without biologic pregnancies, *J Pediatr* 97:612, 1980.
20. Kramer P: Breastfeeding of adopted infants, *Br Med J* 310:188, 1995 (letter).

21. Krantz JZ, Kupper NS: Cross-nursing: wet-nursing in a contemporary context, *Pediatrics* 67:715, 1981.

22. Kulski JK, Hartmann PE, Saint WJ et al: Changes in the milk composition of nonpuerperal women, *Am J Obstet Gynecol* 139:597, 1981.

23. Larson BL: *Lactation: a comprehensive treatise.* IV. The mammary gland/human lactation/milk synthesis, New York, 1978, Academic Press.

24. Lewis PJ, Devenish C, Kahn C: Controlled trial of metoclopramide in the initiation of breastfeeding, *Br J Clin Pharmacol* 9:217, 1980.

25. McNeilly AS, Thorner MO, Volans G et al: Metoclopramide and prolactin, *Br Med J* 2:729, 1974.

26. Mead M: *Sex and temperament in three primitive societies,* New York, 1963, Dell.

27. Mobbs GA, Babbage NF: Breastfeeding adopted children, *Med J Aust* 2:436, 1971.

28. Newton M, Egli GE: The effect of intranasal administration of oxytocin on the let-down of milk in lactating women, *Am J Obstet Gynecol* 76:103, 1958.

29. Packer C, Lewis S, Pusey A: A comparative analysis of non-offspring nursing, *Animal Behav* 43:265, 1992.

30. Phillips V: Relactation in mothers of children over 12 months, *J Trop Pediatr* 39:45, 1993.

31. Raphael D: Breast feeding the adopted baby. In Raphael D: *The tender gift: breast feeding,* New York, 1976, Schocken.

32. Selye H, McKeown T: The effect of mechanical stimulation of the nipples on the ovary and the sexual cycle, *Surg Gynecol Obstet* 59:886, 1934.

33. Slome C: Nonpuerperal lactation in grandmothers, *J Ped* 49:550-552, 1956.

34. Sousa PLR, Barros FC, Pinheiro GNM et al: Reestablishment of lactation with metoclopramide, *J Trop Pediatr Environ Child Health* 21:214, 1975.

35. Thearle MJ, Weissenberger R: Induced lactation in adoptive mothers, *Aust NZ J Obstet Gynecol* 24:283, 1984.

36. Thorley V: Relactation and induced lactation: what the exceptions can tell us, *Birth Issues* 6:24, 1997.

37. Turkington RW: Human prolactin, *Am J Med* 53:389, 1972.

38. Tyson JE: Mechanisms of puerperal lactation. In Symposium on pregnancy, *Med Clin North Am* 61:153, 1977.

39. Vorherr H: *The breast: morphology, physiology and lactation,* New York, 1974, Academic Press.

40. Vorherr H: Human lactation and breast feeding. In Larson BL, editor: *Lactation,* New York, 1978, Academic Press.

41. Waletzky LR, Herman EC: Relactation, *Am Fam Pract* 14:69, 1976.

42. Waterson T: Any questions? *Br Med J* 310:780, 1995.

$\mathscr{R}$eproductive function during lactation

FERTILITY

Although gonadotropic and ovarian function during lactation have been investigated, the major body of knowledge has been collected about the postpartum return of the menstrual cycle and ovulation in the woman who is lactating compared with the nonlactating woman.

Lactational amenorrhea

The amenorrhea of lactation has been attributed to an imperfect balance of hypothalamoanteropituitary function and gonadotropin secretion. However, the complex process by which lactation inhibits ovulation and the menstrual cycle is incompletely understood. Frequent suckling, which results in high prolactin levels, is closely associated with altered luteinizing hormone (LH) secretion and amenorrhea.[63]

Figure 19-1 illustrates the usual menstrual cycle and gonadotropic control. The key points include the following:
1. Follicular development is initiated by pituitary gonadotropin follicle-stimulating hormone (FSH).
2. Continued growth requires FSH and estradiol from the growing follicle in response to LH, which is released in a pulsatile fashion from the pituitary.

3. At midcycle, an increase in estradiol triggers the release of preovulatory surges of LH and FSH.
4. The follicle secretes predominantly progesterone (luteinization).
5. The oocyte is released 36 hours later.

Gonadotropin-releasing hormone (Gn-RH), through pulsatile release from the hypothalamus, stimulates the release of LH. Estrogen increases Gn-RH secretion, and the combination of progesterone and estrogen decreases it.[63]

In lactation the pulsatile secretion of Gn-RH is altered, suggesting that suckling affects ovarian activity at the hypothalamic Gn-RH generator.[63] The follicular development is suppressed because of suppression of estradiol. Ultrasound studies show the absence of medium- or large-size follicles during lactation.[62] The period of lactational amenorrhea depends on suckling (Figs. 19-2 to 19-4).

The levels of gonadotropin in all postpartum women for the first weeks of the postpartum period are decreased, which substantiates the theory of *postpartum ovarian refractoriness*. In the first 2 weeks postpartum, low levels of FSH are found in urine and plasma. Beling et al[5] report estrogen excretion to be low with a linear increase during the first 5 to 8 weeks. When lactating postpartum women are given intramuscular gonadotropins, urinary steroids do not increase, according to studies by Zarate et al.[95] The prolactin-cell pre-

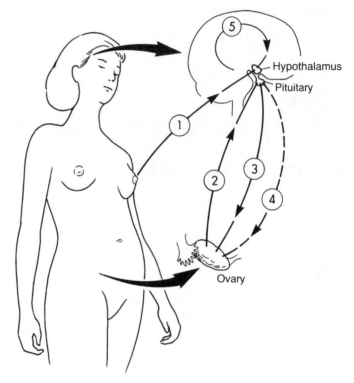

Fig. 19-1. Possible mechanisms of lactational amenorrhea: Nervous impulse from nipple produces not only a rise in prolactin *(1)* but also changes in hypothalamic sensitivity to ovarian steroid feedback *(2)* and changes in gonadotropin releasing hormone (Gn-RH) *(3)*, leading to changes in pituitary release of luteinizing hormone (LH) and follicle-stimulating hormone (FSH) *(4)*. Suckling may also stimulate release of β endorphin *(5)*, thus suppressing Gn-RH from hypothalamus. (Redrawn from Winikoff B, Semeraro P, Zimmerman M: *Contraception during breastfeeding: a clinician's source book,* New York, 1988, Population Council.)

Fig. 19-2. 17β-Estradiol levels in postpartum period in lactating *(open circles)* and nonlactating *(dots)* women. Levels in lactating women vary with intensity of suckling. (From Neville MC: Regulation of mammary development and lactation. In Neville MC, Neifert MR, editors: *Lactation: physiology, nutrition, and breastfeeding,* New York, 1983, Plenum.)

Fig. 19-3. Progesterone levels in postpartum period in lactating *(open circles)* and nonlactating *(dots)* women. (From Neville MC: Regulation of mammary development and lactation. In Neville MC, Neifert MR, editors: *Lactation: physiology, nutrition, and breastfeeding,* New York, 1983, Plenum.)

Fig. 19-4. Prolactin levels in postpartum period in lactating *(open circles)* and nonlactating *(dots)* women. Levels in lactating women vary with intensity of suckling. (From Neville MC: Regulation of mammary development and lactation. In Neville MC, Neifert MR, editors: *Lactation: physiology, nutrition, and breastfeeding,* New York, 1983, Plenum.)

dominance may be responsible for the decreased activity of the pituitary-ovarian axis postpartum.

Myometrial and endometrial involution are also considered to reduce fertility. Animal studies have shown that the release of FSH and LH is inhibited by intense suckling. In addition, animals in whom the nipple is stimulated while the milk ducts have been tied off still show a suppression of estrous and menstrual cycles. Selye and McKeown[79] concluded that interruption of sexual cyclicity during lactation is a result of the suckling and not

of the secretory activity of the mammary gland. The more the suckling stimulus in frequency and duration, the more consistent is the suppression of ovulation.[63]

In a longitudinal study of 48 women, endocrine profiles were assessed with morning blood samples from the first postpartum month until the recovery of ovulation.[22,23] Additional samples were drawn throughout 24 hours at the end of the third postpartum month in 10 of the exclusively nursing amenorrheic women. Prolactin, LH, FSH, estradiol

(E_2), progesterone, cortisol, and dehydroepiandrosterone sulfate were measured. In response to suckling, there was a smaller increase in prolactin and higher levels of E_2 in women who ovulated within 6 months postpartum compared with those who had not. Diaz et al[22-24] suggest that this may explain some of the variability in duration of lactational amenorrhea. The greater prolactin response to suckling associated with longer amenorrhea may result from higher sensitivity to the breast-hypothalamus-pituitary system.[24]

Prolactin and dopamine

The relationship between lactational infertility and physiologic hyperprolactinemia is not clear. In an extensive study of prolactin levels in lactating women, Tay et al[83] measured by the pattern of prolactin secretion in relation to suckling and the return of ovarian activity. Blood samples were drawn at 10-minute intervals for 24 hours at 4 and 8 weeks and when weaning was initiated and suckling reduced, at first menses and in the follicular phase of the first menstrual cycle after weaning. Mothers fed their infants on their usual pattern, with no restrictions or alterations, in an effort to replicate natural lactation.

These data confirmed that during frequent suckling, prolactin levels remain high with little decline between feeds. When suckling became less frequent, prolactin dropped to baseline levels between feeds but surged when suckling was initiated (see Chapter 3). The natural increase in prolactin at night was evident only after weaning. Prolactin response also declined greatly in association with suckling after the return of menses. This occurred about 33.6 weeks (± 3.5 weeks) postpartum. No relationship was seen between the duration of amenorrhea and plasma prolactin levels over a day, at night, or throughout lactation. The timing of the introduction of solids was strongly correlated with the duration of amenorrhea. The authors concluded that no exact link exists between release of prolactin during lactation and the duration of lactational infertility in breastfeeding women.[83]

The inhibition of dopamine secretion from the hypothalamus has been associated with the neural impulses from stimulation of the nipple during lactation. Normally, dopamine inhibits the secretion of prolactin, and conversely, when dopamine is inhibited, prolactin rises. Two pathways of ovulation inhibition are possible as a result of the rise in prolactin. One is a lack of responsiveness to ovarian steroids of the hypothalamic-pituitary axis of the lactating woman, leading to nonpulsatile release of pituitary gonadotropins, FSH, and LH, which in turn results in absent or reduced ovarian activity. FSH may actually be higher at some points; LH is nonpulsatile. The second possible pathway is through the impaired ovarian response to gonadotropins. It is possible that both pathways function as a result of prolactin[12] (Fig. 19-1).

Return of menses

Clinically, the perceptible measurement of the return of fertility is the onset of menstruation. Return of reproductive function varies, depending on the length and degree of lactation. Most studies do not, in fact, report the completeness of lactation, that is, whether the infant is totally breastfed or is also receiving solid foods or supplemental bottles.[38] By the end of the third month, only 33% of lactating women have had a menstrual period, whereas 91% of nonlactating women have had at least one period.[39]

In 72 fully breastfeeding women studied prospectively from 42 days postpartum, vaginal bleeding was recorded daily if it occurred. Almost half the women had some bleeding or spotting between 6 and 8 weeks postpartum. Those who experienced this bleeding eventually menstruated and ovulated earlier than those who did not, but differences were not significant. Seven women had ovarian follicular development before day 56, but neither bleeding nor follicular development was associated with ovulation in the first 8 weeks. The authors stated it was unlikely that vaginal bleeding in a fully breastfeeding woman indicates a return to fertility before 8 weeks.[87,88]

The period of lactational amenorrhea does offer a measure of conception protection for 3 months.

The nonlactating woman has a return of her period at 25 days at the earliest, a return of ovulation at 25 to 35 days, and a 5% chance of regaining fertility before 6 weeks postpartum. In a detailed study of 130 women in Chile, Diaz et al[25] found the cumulative probability of pregnancy at the end of 6 months postpartum in women who were exclusively nursing and amenorrheic to be 1.8%. For exclusively nursing women who had a return of menses, it was 27.2%, and for those partially nursing it was 40.5%.

Perez et al[72] diagnosed the first postpartum ovulation by endometrial biopsy, basal body temperature, vaginal cytology, and cervical mucus in a group of 200 women in a prospective study. The dates of first ovulation, first menses, and nursing status were analyzed. No woman ovulated before day 36, whether lactating or not. The intensity and length of nursing affected the date when ovulation occurred. About 78% of the women ovulated before the first menses, but only 12 pregnancies occurred with first ovulation. Of the 170 women who breastfed, 24 ovulated while completely nursing, 49 while partially nursing, and 97 after weaning.

Although many investigators continue to evaluate the impact of lactation on ovulation and menstruation, the fundamental observations remain the same[3,31,46] (Table 19-1). Available data on return of ovulation and menstruation can be summarized as follows[90]:

I. Nursing mothers
    A. Earliest possible menstruation is 4 to 6 weeks postpartum (pp).
    B. Ovulation before end of amenorrhea varies 14% to 75%.
    C. The longer the first menses is delayed, the more likely the first cycle will be ovulatory.
    D. Continued suckling and elevated prolactin levels produce inadequate luteal function in first cycles.
    E. Exclusive breastfeeding (day and night): return of menses
        1. 9% to 30% in 3 months
        2. 19% to 53% in 180 days

TABLE 19-1   Relative risk of ovulation in relation to breastfeeding frequency*

Average number of feeds per day	Relative risk
0	1.0
1	0.62
2	0.43
3	0.28
4	0.19
5	0.12
6	0.08
7	0.05
8	0.04
9	0.02
10	0.01

From Gray RH, Campbell O, Eslamic S et al: The return of ovarian function during lactation: results of studies from the United States and the Philippines. In *Biomedical and demographic determinants of reproduction*, Oxford, 1993, Clarendon.
*Breastfeeding episodes per day before ovulation:
$B_1 = -0.4207$
$p < 0.0001$
Average duration of suckling episodes per day:
$B_2 = -0.6566$ $\xi^2 = 36.05$
$p = 0.0071$ 2 d.f.

II. Nonnursing mothers
    A. Earliest possible menstruation is 4 weeks pp.
    B. Most women are menstruating by third month pp.
    C. Return of menstruation
        1. 6 weeks pp—40%
        2. 12 weeks pp—65%
        3. 24 weeks pp—90%
    D. Earliest possible ovulation is 3½ to 5 weeks pp.
    E. Ovular cycles occur in about 50% with first menstrual period pp.
    F. Early pp ovulation may occur late in menstrual cycle: shortening of secretory phase and greater tendency toward irregular menses.
    G. Return of ovulation
        1. 6 weeks pp—15%
        2. 12 weeks pp—40%
        3. 24 weeks pp—75%

III. Amenorrheic nonnursing mothers: return of ovulation
  A. 12 weeks pp—20%
  B. 16 weeks pp—40%

Breastfeeding and birth interval

Data collected where women practice more intensive breastfeeding show more prolonged lactational amenorrhea as a result of more prolonged total breastfeeding.[49] Nutritional status has virtually no effect on amenorrhea, except in the extremes. In a study of Guatemalan women, maternal energy supplements did not shorten length of lactational amenorrhea; however, supplementing their breastfed infant did shorten amenorrhea by reducing suckling. A difference exists between postpartum and nutritional amenorrhea: *true nutritional amenorrhea* is predictable on the basis of the height/weight ratio; lactational amenorrhea is hormonal, and when it occurs, nutrition has only a trivial role.[30,49]

Among !Kung hunter-gatherers, long intervals pass between births, which has puzzled investigators because the tribes are well nourished, have low fetal wastage, and do not employ contraceptives or prolonged abstinence. The !Kung eat only what they hunt and gather. They have no agriculture. They are lean, spare people. They have late menarche (about 16 years of age), first pregnancy at age 18, and early menopause at about 40, leaving 24 reproductive years during which they produce 4.4 children, which, with some perinatal mortality, exactly replaces their society. This compares with industrial society, where productive years begin at 11 and end at 51. Konner and Worthman[48] report that the !Kung have unusual temporal patterns of nursing characterized by highly frequent nursing bouts with short space between nursings. The !Kung nurse several times an hour with only 15 minutes at most between bouts, which last only 15 to 120 seconds each. Serum estradiol and progesterone levels are correspondingly low. Infants are always in the immediate proximity of their mothers until they are weaned, at about 3½ years, during a new sibling's gestation.

In Nigeria the effect of duration and frequency of breastfeeding on postpartum amenorrhea is comparable in that Nigerians breastfeed for 16.5 months with a frequency of 4.5 times a day. The mean length of amenorrhea is 12.5 months. Amenorrheic mothers who were lactating had lower levels of serum estradiol and lactic dehydrogenase (LDH). A significant association was seen between hyperprolactinemia with amenorrhea. The incidence of amenorrhea declined parallel to that of the hyperprolactinemia.[20]

When fertility postpartum during lactation was studied in Edinburgh, suckling was the most important factor inhibiting the return to ovulation.[69] Suckling duration was the first factor to discriminate the mothers who experienced early ovulation. Those mothers who ovulated while breastfeeding had all introduced two or more supplementary feeds per day and had reduced suckling to under six times a day, with 60 minutes or less suckling time per day. The basal prolactin levels were below 600 μU/L. The mothers who did not ovulate until after 40 weeks postpartum breastfed longest, suckled most intensely, maintained night feeds longest, and introduced supplementary feeds most slowly.[38] The prolactin levels remained substantially above 600 μU/L.

Another review of the effects of hormonal contraceptives on lactation by Hull[40] concludes that a significant number of reports indicate decrease in milk yield. The description of severe growth failure[30] in the nursling, even leading to "contraceptive marasmus," in Egypt and Tunisia is cause for concern.

Most large studies of birth interval and its relationship to method of feeding have been conducted in developing countries. However, Rosner and Schulman[75] reported on 112 metropolitan New York, Orthodox Jewish women with 266 birth experiences. The women strictly adhered to biblical and Rabbinic law prohibiting birth control. They were well-nourished, middle-class, educated women who breastfed on demand (210 infants) for a mean duration of 10.7 months, with 177 of the infants receiving formula less than once a week. Significant positive correlations were found with duration of lactational amenorrhea, which increased as duration of breastfeeding increased. Delay in starting solids, continuation of night feedings, and postponement of other liquid feeds all were associated with prolongation of birth interval. The investigators found a longer mean duration of lactational amenorrhea (8.6 months) and mean birth interval (22 months) than other studies because of the more intensive feeding patterns[75] (Table 19-2).

Lactational amenorrhea method

The Bellagio Consensus Conference[18] on breastfeeding as a family-planning method established that a mother who is fully or nearly fully breastfeeding her infant and remains amenorrheic will have more than 98% protection from pregnancy in the first 6 months postpartum.[16,43] In a large prospective study of duration of lactational anovulation and amenorrhea in well-nourished Australian women—members of the Nursing Mothers' Association of Australia who breastfed for a long time—Short et al[81] found that breastfeeding alone is not an effective form of contraception because all the women resumed ovulation while

still breastfeeding. They compared breastfeeding women who had unprotected sex with breastfeeding women who had unprotected sex only during lactational amenorrhea and adopted other contraceptive measures after resumption of menstruation. Only 1.7% became pregnant during the first 6 months of amenorrhea, only 7% after 12 months, and 13% after 24 months.[72] Only one woman in a study of 422 middle-class urban women in Chile became pregnant using the lactational amenorrhea method (LAM) as the only method of pregnancy avoidance in the first 6 months,[22,45] a protective rate of 99.5% (Figs. 19-5 and 19-6).

Although it has long been recognized that breastfeeding has an effect on fertility, the mechanism is only beginning to be explored. The use of LAM for child spacing is based on the natural infertility associated with lactation, especially during the early months postpartum, which are associated with frequent around-the-clock suckling.[47] Infertility is the result of hormonal suppression during lactation.[91]

Menses as an indicator of ovulation has been studied with data collected not only on onset of menses but on urinary hormone assays. Among women who menstruated before 6 months postpar-

TABLE 19-2   **Comparison of studies of breastfeeding and its relationship to birth interval when practiced in absence of birth control**

Study	Mean duration of breastfeeding (mo)	Mean lactational amenorrhea (mo)	Mean birth interval (mo)
Bonte and van Balen[9]	N/A	15.2	25.2
Berman et al[7]	7.0	7.1	21.6
Prema et al[73]	19.8	11.1	23.8
Perez[71]*	4.0	3.03†	N/A
Gioiosa[32]	10.27	N/A	21.92
Rosner and Schulman[75]	10.74	8.56	21.95
Adnan and Bakr[3]	36.0	12.0	N/A
Howie et al[38]	10.0	8.1	N/A
Ojofeitimi[69]	16.5	12.5	N/A

Modified from Rosner AE, Schulman SK: *Pediatrics* 86:747, 1990.
N/A, Not available.
*Women did introduce family planning after menses return or after supplementation after 6 months.
†First postpartum ovulation.

Fig. 19-5. Cumulative probability of pregnancy during breastfeeding. – – – –, Nonlactating women of normal fertility having unprotected intercourse; ━■━, study breastfeeding women having unprotected intercourse throughout 24 months of lactation; ━●━, study breastfeeding women having unprotected intercourse only during lactational amenorrhea and adopting effective contraceptive measures at resumption of menstruation. Percentage of women in lactational amenorrhea by month postpartum (▽) is also shown. (From Short RY, Lewis PR, Renfree MB et al: *Lancet* 337:715, 1991.)

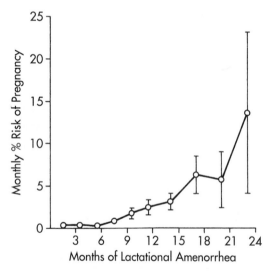

Fig. 19-6. Monthly percentage probability of pregnancy during lactational amenorrhea with estimated standard errors. With cumulative percentage probability of pregnancy by months postpartum for these three groups of women, 50% of nonlactating women would be pregnant in less than 3 months, and 85% would be pregnant by 6 months. (From Short RY, Lewis PR, Renfree MB et al: *Lancet* 337:715, 1991.)

tum, 67% of cycles were anovulatory, and the lag between anovular first menses and subsequent ovulation was 15.7 weeks.[27] On the other hand, after 6 months postpartum, the proportion of anovular first menses declined to 22%, and the lag

to ovulation declined to 7.3 weeks. Comparing all menstrual episodes, the mean interval between first observed menses and ovulation was 8.4 weeks the first 6 months and only 0.1 week after 6 months postpartum.

A significant distinction should be made between token breastfeeding with early solids and more rigid feeding schedules and the ad lib breastfeeding around the clock with no solids until the infant is 6 months old. The amount and frequency of sucking are closely related to the continued amenorrhea in most women. When a totally breastfed infant sleeps through the night at an early age, requiring no suckling for 6 hours or so at night, the suppressive effect on menses diminishes. It has also been shown that if the infant uses a pacifier rather than receiving nonnutritive sucking at the breast, the suppression of ovulation is diminished.[57]

The degree of fertility inhibition associated with breastfeeding has decreased remarkably since the time of hunter-gatherers, cautions Diaz.[23] She points out that fertility rates vary; population and socioeconomic factors, urbanization, and nutrition all influence not only breastfeeding patterns but associated ovarian quiescence. Lactational amenorrhea can provide protection against pregnancy for the first 6 months even in well-nourished women who are giving the infant some supplemental foods[50-55] (Fig. 19-7).

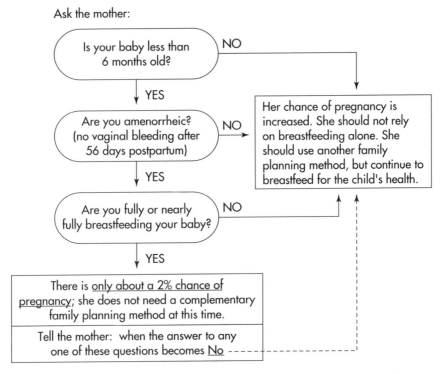

Ask the mother:

Fig. 19-7.   Use of lactational amenorrhea method (LAM) for child spacing during first 6 postpartum months.

TABLE 19-3	Life table analysis of lactational amenorrhea method (LAM) efficacy*

Month	No. of pregnancies	WM	WMAC	R × 100	P × 100
1	0	384	384	0.00	0.00
2	0	327	711	0.00	0.00
3	0	272	983	0.00	0.00
4	0	243	1226	0.00	0.00
5	0	224	1450	0.00	0.00
6	1	221	1671	0.45	0.45

From Perez A, Labbok MH, Queenan JT: *Lancet* 339:968, 1992.
WM, Number of women using LAM; *WMAC*, cumulative women-months of use; *R × 100*, monthly risk of conception; *P × 100*, cumulative risk of conception.
*Characteristics of women: Mean age (SEM, range) was 27.1 years (5.0, 18 to 39). Mean parity (SEM, range) was 2.0 (1.0, 1 to 5). 23.6% of the women had primary education, and only 5.4% had completed university studies.

For women who practice LAM, the efficacy is remarkably good (Table 19-3). Table 19-4 details the reestablishment of menses in breastfeeding women using LAM. *Bellagio and Beyond: Breastfeeding and LAM in Reproductive Health* was published as a final report in 1997 of the many years of work worldwide involving the use of LAM.[18] It was concluded that the efficacy of LAM is well established in prospective studies. Policy support is still needed to institute an additional

TABLE 19-4   Life table of reestablishment of menses among exclusively breastfeeding women using lactational amenorrhea method (LAM)*

Month	Bleeding	WM	WMAC	R × 100	P × 100
1	0	384	384	0.00	0.00
2	8	327	711	2.45	2.42
3	18	272	983	6.62	8.67
4	11	243	1226	4.55	12.72
5	10	224	1450	4.46	16.53
6	6	221	1671	2.73	18.78

From Perez A, Labbok MH, Queenan JT: *Lancet* 339:968, 1992.
WM, Number of women using LAM; *WMAC,* cumulative women-months of use; *R × 100,* monthly bleeding risk; *P × 100,* cumulative risk of bleeding.
*Characteristics of women: mean age (SEM, range) was 27.1 years (5.0, 18 to 39); mean parity (SEM, range) was 2.0 (1.0, 1 to 5); 23.6% of women had primary education, and only 5.4% had completed university studies.

method that increases the family-planning choices of postpartum women.[17]

A population of women in Baltimore were studied in comparison to a group from Manila by Gray et al.[34] The Baltimore group were older, more educated, more frequently employed, and had fewer children. Women in Manila breastfed more frequently (at 10 weeks postpartum: 11.4 feeds in Manila versus 7.1 feeds in Baltimore). The mean duration of amenorrhea was 31.7 weeks versus 26.3 weeks, and mean delays before first ovulation were 38 versus 27 weeks (Manila versus Baltimore). The frequency of suckling episodes was most strongly associated with ovulation in the Baltimore population, where small declines in breastfeeding were sufficient to permit the return of ovarian activity. Women in Manila, in contrast, maintained high suckling rates even when solids were introduced. More Baltimore women (49%) than Manila women (31%) ovulated before 6 months. There was no simple algorithm, however, to predict ovulation.[31]

The effects of age at introduction of complementary foods to breastfed infants on duration of lactational amenorrhea in Honduran women were reported by Dewey et al.[21] Introducing foods at 4 months significantly affected the likelihood of amenorrhea at 6 months but not thereafter. This effect was not seen, however, if breastfeeding frequency was maintained. The most significant determination of lactational amenorrhea was time spent breastfeeding (minutes per day), which was negatively associated with the infant's energy intake from complementary foods.

CONTRACEPTION DURING LACTATION

Natural family planning

Although lactation provides protection early in the postpartum period, a woman who is not exclusively breastfeeding around the clock and who is seriously concerned about avoiding conception should be informed of her options. If she does not want to use contraceptives—medications or devices—she should be instructed in the external signs of ovulation. Most studies of lactation indicate that the initial menses occurs before the onset of adequate ovulation and the luteal phase. The risk of pregnancy during lactational amenorrhea, however, in the first 6 months is less than 1% when LAM is combined with the basal thermal method or secretion surveillance. Unplanned pregnancy rates rise among breastfeeders after menses return compared with the rates for those who use thermal or secretion surveillance methods when not lactating. The increased pregnancy rate was related to poor compliance and understanding of the "rules" of the method.[35]

The *symptothermal method* of fertility awareness during lactation was studied in Canada.[70] A special postpartum chart was designed to record

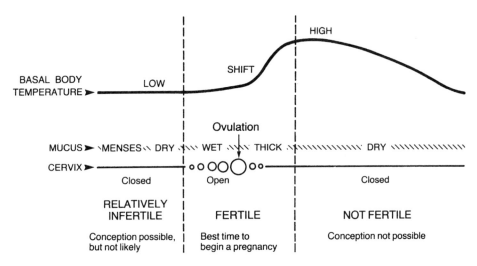

Fig. 19-8. Temperature, mucus, and cervical assessment during lactation to identify ovulation. (Courtesy National Family Planning of Rochester, NY.)

morning temperature, cervical mucus, and other signs of fertility/infertility in relation to dates and postpartum days. The intensity of the breastfeeding was also recorded. There were 54 breastfeeding experiences in 47 women whose ages ranged from 20 to 39. Parity ranged from 1 to 7 with an average of 3.3. The duration of full breastfeeding averaged 3.6 months (range 3 weeks to 8 months). The duration of partial breastfeeding ranged from 2 to 28 months with an average of 8.8 months. These mothers found that in general they could predict their fertile times with accuracy while breastfeeding. During times of weaning or change in suckling pattern, special caution was suggested during which the mothers watched for signs of first ovulation.

The effectiveness of periodic abstinence for lactating women shows that long periods of lactational infertility can be identified by either lack of mucus or continuous unchanging mucous flow.

Cervical mucus accepts, filters, prepares, and releases sperm for successful transport to the egg for fertilization. The advancing sperm must penetrate the mucous structure or the small interstices between the mucous macromolecules. The interstices are largest in the periovulatory phase of the menstrual cycle.[74] As ovulation resumes, irregular mucous patterns occur that are difficult to interpret

and therefore require prolonged abstinence. A pregnancy rate with this method was 9.1 per 100 women-years. Because two thirds of the 82 women studied were totally breastfeeding, many of the ensuing postpartum cycles may have been anovulatory or had an inadequate luteal phase, thus helping to keep the pregnancy rate low.

Studies of cervical secretions alone (mucous patterns) during lactation have indicated that the same signs in mucus are reliable during lactation. Charting is carried out in the usual manner, and feedings are also recorded. A woman who is following her pattern postpartum should be seen every 2 weeks for guidance until her pattern is well documented. The couple should make careful observations of when (1) the infant sleeps through the night, (2) the mother reduces the number of breastfeedings, (3) the infant begins solid foods, (4) the infant begins other liquids or a bottle, and (5) illness occurs in either mother or baby. Abstinence is advised until the situation is clear. If there has been no prior ovulation or menstruation when weaning begins, ovulation may occur quite quickly.[13]

Figure 19-8 illustrates temperature, mucus, and cervical assessments during lactation.

Although contraceptive methods such as barrier methods and "the pill" have a statistically better record in avoiding pregnancy, that is a moot point for the woman for whom these methods are not an option for religious, ethical, moral, or medical grounds.[4] It is therefore important that the clinician be as well informed about natural child spacing as possible so the best advice can be provided. Ideally, the woman has used natural family planning before the pregnancy, so she is familiar with her own patterns, but it is more urgent that she knows how to check her mucus, her cervix, and her temperature and is not trying to learn about her fertility signs during lactation. Natural-family-planning programs across the United States are gaining experience with lactating women using the ovulation method and are available to assist lactating women. Further information can be obtained from the National Office of Natural Family Planning, 8514 Bradmoor Drive, Bethesda, MD 20817-3810, (301) 897-9323, if no local office is available.

In a carefully designed study conducted in Chile by Perez[71] at the Pontificia Universidad Católica de Chile Department of Obstetrics and Gynecology and by members of the faculty at Johns Hopkins University School of Hygiene and Public Health, 419 postpartum women were enrolled in the Natural Family Planning Program and taught the method and how to record their observations. The purpose was to define cervical mucus patterns in relation to time since delivery, time of first bleed, frequency of feeding, introduction of supplements and solid foods, and time of weaning. The diaries of 110 women with detailed records were selected for critical evaluation. Forty-nine have been reported and the preliminary observations evaluated by Barker.[4] Two characteristics of mucus (sensation and observation) were charted each day along with the women's breastfeeding pattern. Only seven women had used natural family planning previously. No woman menstruated before 4 months postpartum, when 10% did have first menses. Fifty percent of the women detected mucus by the fourth month, and not until the seventh month had 50% had first menses. Mucus was observed about 2 months before first menses. As women moved from total breastfeeding

to partial and to complete weaning, the duration of episodes of mucus increased. Duration of mucus approached normal on weaning.

Rural women exposed to a breastfeeding education program prenatally and postpartum breastfed more and used fewer bottles than the comparison group, who had no training about lactational infertility.[78] However, no difference was seen in postpartum amenorrhea. No measures of ovulation or pregnancy were made. Rural women tend to breastfeed optimally naturally.

The natural suppression of ovulation during early lactation and the concomitant amenorrhea induced by exclusive or nearly exclusive breastfeeding provide 98% or higher protection against pregnancy. Three conditions are necessary: amenorrhea, intensive breastfeeding day and night, and up to 6 months of exclusive breastfeeding postpartum. LAM can be used to time the introduction of any complementary method (barrier, etc.) (Fig. 19-9); it is not just for users of natural family planning.

Touch sensitivity and ovulation

In search of a simple method of identifying ovulation during lactation, Drife[26] measured urinary pregnanediol and estrogen and breast sensitivity in six breastfeeding and six bottle-feeding normal women. Two-point discrimination and touch sensitivity were measured. The mean duration of amenorrhea among breastfeeders was 24.3 weeks (range 14 to 35 weeks) and among bottle feeders 7.5 weeks (range 6 to 14 weeks). Findings, however, were not diagnostic of ovulation. Touch sensitivity tended to decrease as lactation progressed over months. The change is so gradual and difficult to detect that it has no practical value in determining ovulation.[26]

Oral contraceptives and lactation

The significant issues related to lactation and the use of oral contraceptives are the potentially adverse effects of oral contraceptives on milk production, uterine involution, and growth and

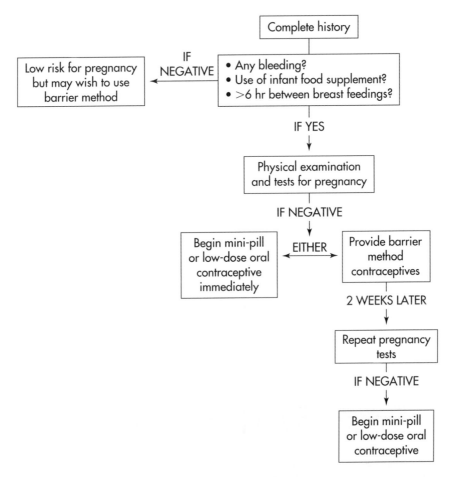

Fig. 19-9. Algorithm for initiating contraceptive treatment in a breastfeeding woman. (See references 50, 51, and 61.) (Modified from Winikoff B, Semeraro P, Zimmerman M: *Contraception during breastfeeding: a clinician's source book,* New York, 1988, Population Council; and Labbok M: *N Engl J Med* 308:51, 1983.)

development of the breastfed infant.[68] Curtis[19] reported a single case of breast enlargement in a breastfed male infant whose mother began taking norethynodrel with ethinyl estradiol 3-methyl ether (Enovid) on the third day postpartum. Breast enlargement began on the third week of life. The mother had noted her milk was not as "rich" and started supplements the second week. Nursing was discontinued at about 4 weeks of age, and the breasts of the infant returned to normal in 2 to 3 weeks. The additional risks to the mother of thromboembolism, hypertension, and cancer have

also been discussed extensively in the literature. These occurred with the early high-dose products.

The data on oral contraceptives available have been well reviewed by Vorherr.[89,90] He summarizes the information by noting that preparations containing 2.5 mg or less of a 19-norprogestogen and 50 µg or less of ethinyl estradiol or 100 µg or less of mestranol present no hazard to mother or infant. He further points out that milk yield can be decreased with larger doses of combination oral contraceptives containing estrogen and 5 to 10 mg of progestogen per dose. Only two studies of many suggest any variation in the content of the milk (protein, fat, and calcium) resulting from oral contraceptives.[77,82]

Toddywalla et al[86] reported the effect of injectable contraceptives as well as oral combinations on milk production. They found an increase in the protein content of the milk and a slight increase in quantity from the group given injection of 150 mg of medroxyprogesterone (Depo-Provera) every 3 months. The group receiving 300 mg of medroxyprogesterone every 6 months showed significant increase in quantity but a decrease in protein, fat, and calcium as compared with controls (who used mechanical means of contraception).[82] The secretion of hormones in human milk is poorly documented, with only a few infants studied in each hormone combination.[15] In all cases, a small but measurable amount was found in the milk. Unfortunately, measurements in the infant's serum are not reported.

The impact of the distribution of oral contraceptives on breastfeeding and pregnancy status in rural Haiti indicated that it did not alter breastfeeding patterns in women who began the pills at 8 to 9 months postpartum.[10] Pregnancy prevalence also decreased as a result.[95]

Implants and injections

The recommendation for contraceptive use during lactation is the progestin-only products (Norplant System, Depo-Provera injections and minipills, progestin once-only pills). Use of these methods has not been associated with adverse effects on infant growth or development and may even increase the volume of milk (Table 19-5).[2,60,92,93] It is recommended that the progestin-only method not be initiated until 6 weeks postpartum on the premise that the theoretic danger to the infant from exogenous steroids has passed by this time. The practice of injecting Depo-Provera immediately after delivery can interfere with the establishment of lactation, which depends on the dramatic natural decline in progesterone postpartum.

Steroids are not bound well in plasma and not well conjugated by the liver or excreted by the immature kidneys of the neonate. Exogenous hormones may compete for receptor sites with natural

TABLE 19-5   Effects of contraceptive agents on milk yield and infant development

Agent	Milk yield	Effect on infant
Combined estrogen/progestin	Moderate inhibitory effect Shorter breastfeeding Milk concentration unchanged Small amount of steroid in milk	Slower weight gain No long-term effects
Progestin only Minipill (Micronor, Nory-D) Other products	No effect on volume No effect on duration	No effect on weight gain No reported long-term effects
Injectable depot medroxy-progesterone acetate (DMPA), Depo-Provera and norethindrone enanthate (NET-EN, NORIS-TERAT)	Breastfeeding lasts longer ? Change in milk: protein increased, fat decreased Steroid present in milk	No long-term effects
Norplant System	No effect Small amount of steroid in milk	Normal growth No long-term effects
Vaginal rings containing natural hormone progesterone	No significant differences	No effect on growth Long-term effects under study

Modified from Winikoff B, Semeraro P, Zimmerman M: *Contraception during breastfeeding: a clinician's source book,* New York, 1987, Population Council.

ones in the liver, brain, or other tissues. As the infant's liver and kidneys mature, these issues disappear.[44] Medications that also contain estrogen suppress milk production.[94] With the many alternatives available, it should never be necessary to discontinue breastfeeding to initiate contraception.[42]

The growth and development of breastfed infants whose mothers received implants of Norplant containing levonorgestrel or injections of norethindrone enanthate were studied and compared with those whose mothers used intrauterine devices (IUDs).[37] The breastfeeding performance was similar. The infants were also similar in growth rate, development, and general health. Similarly, a group of mothers were given a vaginal ring that released 10 mg of "natural" progesterone every 24 hours, producing a maternal serum level of 4 ng/ml, which results in only a minimal amount in the milk and which is not absorbed by the infant gut. These infants also had normal growth and development and remained in good health.[80]

Ovulation method, LH-RH, and home tests

Pregnancy rates and fertility-related behavior of users of the *ovulation method* (OM) were studied prospectively in Kenya and Chile in two groups of breastfeeding women.[55] The rate of unplanned pregnancy was less than 1% in the first 6 months. The rate of unplanned pregnancies increased once menses had begun and supplementary food was added to the infant's diet. The rates were compared with the rates among nonlactating women who were also using OM to avoid pregnancy. The breastfeeding women had followed the method closely, although clients who had not used OM before the pregnancy had an increased incidence of unplanned pregnancy.

Risk of ovulation during lactation was studied by Gray et al[33] in Baltimore and in Manila. During the first 6 months postpartum, amenorrheic women had a low risk of ovulation (below 10%) with a partial breastfeeding and a 1% to 5% risk with exclusive breastfeeding with either frequent short feeds or infrequent longer feeds. This would have

resulted in a pregnancy rate of 2% and 1%, respectively.

One of the difficulties of studying the use/effectiveness and continuation of natural-family-planning methods is that terms have always been imprecise and markers have been different between studies.[76] The method is very effective when properly used (failure rate 3.4%) but unforgiving when use is imperfect (failure rate 84.2% in the first year).[41]

Luteinizing hormone–releasing hormone (LH-RH) agonist for contraception has also been tested in nine fully breastfeeding women beginning 6 weeks postpartum. They received 300 µg LH-RH agonist (buserelin) intranasally once a day for the duration of their breastfeeding. Urinary excretion of LH, estrone, and pregnanediol was compared with that of nine control breastfeeding women. No ovulation occurred in the treated group, and seven of the nine untreated controls had one to six ovulations. LH-RH has potential as a safe, acceptable method of contraception while breastfeeding, according to Fraser et al.[29]

Home tests to monitor fertility are available; however, women must be tested during lactation and especially during the transition period when breastfeeding frequency and feeding duration are changing. Ovarian follicular dynamics can be accurately monitored through the noninstrumented analysis of daily estrone conjugates in urine samples at home.[56] Readings can be affected by urine osmolarity, either high or low, giving false-positive or false-negative results, respectively. Controlling intake of fluids would guard against this.

Two algorithms for initiating contraceptive treatment are illustrated in Figs. 19-7 and 19-9.

Intrauterine devices and other contraceptive methods

Various alternatives to oral contraceptives do exist and have been observed to have different degrees of reliability. The IUDs (95% to 98% effective), cervical caps and diaphragms (85% to 88% effective), condoms (80% to 85% effective), and vaginal suppositories, jellies, or creams (80%

effective) have no known contraindication during breastfeeding, because no chemicals are absorbed. The only contraceptive that is 100% effective is abstinence.

A study of 2271 postpartum women who had IUDs inserted between 1976 and 1981 and were followed for 6 to 12 months was reported with careful attention to details of lactation.[14] Data were analyzed separately for IUDs inserted immediately after birth (within 10 minutes of placental expulsion). The results of this analysis indicate that IUD insertion for breastfeeding women would be appropriate either immediately after delivery or later (42 days or more postpartum). When inserted immediately postpartum, the Delta Loop and Delta T were modified by adding projections of chromic sutures, which help the device remain in the uterus. The sutures biodegrade in 6 weeks, leaving a standard device in place. These authors report that breastfeeding is not a contraindication to IUD insertion, with no increased expulsion rate.[37] Conversely, the presence of an IUD has no adverse effect on lactation. The appropriate time for insertion should be selected to predate anticipated ovulation but guarantee patient compliance. A study showed that the use of the TCu-380A IUD in breastfeeding women resulted in fewer insertion-related complaints and lower removal rates for bleeding and pain over 12 months postpartum than in nonbreastfeeders. No intrauterine perforations were reported in either group.[28]

A group of 32 women hospitalized for uterine perforation necessitating transperitoneal IUD removal and a matched control group of 497 women who had worn IUDs uneventfully were compared.[36] Of the women in the study, 97% were postpartum compared with 68% of the controls. Of the parous study group, 42% were lactating, and of the parous controls, 7% were lactating when the IUD was inserted. The risk of perforation was 10 times greater in the lactating than in the nonlactating women, unrelated to time of the insertion postpartum. In another group hospitalized for difficult transcervical IUD removal, the risk was 2.3 times greater for lactating women. The authors recommend caution, not abandonment of the procedure, during lactation, because they be-

lieve the IUD is the best form of artificial contraception during lactation. Because of problems with the Dalkon Shield, IUDs were generally unavailable in the United States in 1986 and 1987, although in other parts of the world they were still in use. In 1989 a copper-T device became available again. The ideal candidate is a woman who wants reversible contraception to space births or limit size of the family, especially breastfeeding parous women with a monogamous relationship.

The Technical Guidance/Competence Group of the United States Agency for International Development (USAID) and World Health Organization (WHO)[85] recommends IUD insertion immediately postpartum as soon as the placenta is removed, whether by vaginal or cesarean delivery. They point out it must be done by a specially trained physician. From 10 minutes to 48 hours after delivery, however, the expulsion rate is high. If this window of opportunity is missed or no urgency exists, it is best to wait. Although immediate insertion is possible, a copper-T device may be safely inserted 4 or more weeks postpartum in breastfeeding women. Using the withdrawal technique minimizes the risk of perforation. Other IUDs should not be inserted until 6 weeks postpartum.

Use of *barrier* and *spermicidal products* are alternative contraceptive methods during early lactation before hormonal methods or IUDs are introduced. These coital-dependent methods have no effect on lactation. The lubrication provided by the spermicidally treated condoms have the advantage of contributing lubrication when the hypoestrogenic vagina is exceptionally dry in association with lactation. A spermicide is more effective with a condom but is adequate early postpartum, when relative infertility is present. A *diaphragm* cannot be adequately fitted for 6 to 8 weeks postpartum, so it is not recommended during this period with or without lactation.

Abstinence

Many cultures and societies place taboos on sexual intercourse for the nursing mother as an effective means of spacing children. Usually there are no medical contraindications to sexual relationships during lactation. In a study on contraceptive use in the United States, Ford and Labbok[31] reported that among white women, 34% were not sexually active in the first month postpartum, 12.5% in the second month, and 4.3% during the third month. Among black women in the survey, 25% were not sexually active in the first month, 8.1% the second, and 4.2% the third. Contraceptive use among those sexually active was absent in 16% in the first postpartum month and 12.2% and 13.8%, respectively, in the second and the third postpartum month among whites. Among blacks, 27.3% used no method the first month, and 22.7% and 22.3%, respectively, used no method the second and third month.

SEX AND THE NURSING MOTHER

Sexual arousal associated with suckling

If one examines the normal adult female in regard to the menstrual cycle, sexual intercourse, pregnancy, childbirth, and lactation, one observes that these events are all influenced by the interaction of the same hormones, not only estrogen, progesterone, testosterone, FSH, and LH, but oxytocin and prolactin as well. The breast is known to respond during all these phases, enlarging before menstruation, during pregnancy, before orgasm, and during lactation. The nipples also respond during these phases. Furthermore, the uterus contracts during childbirth, orgasm, and lactation. Body temperature rises during ovulation, childbirth, orgasm, and lactation. As pointed out in Chapter 3, *oxytocin* is a critical element in the let-down reflex during lactation. Oxytocin levels also rise during orgasms and labor, and oxytocin causes the uterus to contract and the nipples to become erect. Newton and Newton[65] report other similarities in women during these events, including sensory perception and emotional reactions. The psychophysiologic similarities between lactation and coitus are as follows:

1. The uterus contracts.
2. The nipples become erect.
3. Breast stroking and nipple stimulation occur.
4. The emotions experienced involve skin changes (vascular dilatation and raised temperature).
5. Milk let-down (or ejection) reflex can be triggered.
6. The emotions experienced may be closely allied.
7. An accepting attitude toward sexuality may be related to an accepting attitude to breastfeeding (and vice versa).

Women also report hot flushes in association with some feeds, especially at night. This phenomenon has been studied by Marshall et al,[58] who looked at oxytocin effect. Initiation of breastfeeding was accompanied by an increase in skin conductance resulting in increased skin temperature, especially of the breast. The pattern is similar to menopausal hot flashes.

Given the biologic and hormonal similarities of lactation to the other events in the sexual cycle of the adult female, it is not surprising that some women experience some form of sexual gratification during suckling on certain occasions. Masters and Johnson,[59] in a study of 111 parturient women, only 24 of whom breastfed, reported that sexual arousal was experienced during suckling on some occasions. The exact incidence of this response is unknown, but it is believed to be uncommon. Nursing mothers may have an element of guilt surrounding these experiences and underreport. That guilt may lead to early weaning in some cases. For some women, the breasts are highly erogenous. The handling and manipulation of the breast necessary during lactation by both mother and infant can, in the right circumstances but unpremeditated, be stimulating. Clearly, the majority of women who enjoy breastfeeding have no feelings or responses to the stimulation of the breast that could be construed as sexual arousal, although they enjoy breastfeeding and the intimacy with their infant that it provides.

The erotic response to nursing the infant has no significance in terms of being normal or abnormal. The decline of breastfeeding because of feelings of shame, modesty, embarrassment, and distaste has been reported by Bentovin[6] and interpreted as indicating that breastfeeding is viewed as a forbidden sexual activity. For such women, any sexual allusions and excitement accompanying breast-feeding are not permissible and cause shame. Such attitudes are more common in lower social groups and need to be considered in counseling mothers about breastfeeding prepartum or when premature weaning takes place. Major changes in the number of women who breastfeed may not be possible until society can accept the breast in its relationship to nurturing the infant and also as an object of less sexual ambivalence.

The sensuousness of breastfeeding has been the topic of discussion in popular women's magazines as more has been written about women and their bodies. For the well-educated, well-read woman who breastfeeds her infant because she intellectually arrives at the decision, such discussions are an avenue of increased knowledge. Others may still be uncomfortable about breastfeeding if it is apt to be "pleasurable." The physician may sense this discomfort in a patient prenatally by her responses to bodily change during pregnancy. Cultural attitudes are an important part of this response and are deeply ingrained in an individual by the time she reaches the age of parenting. Professionals need to be sensitive to the patient and cautious about imposing cultural change on a given patient, while being alert to needs for information and openness. A woman who experiences any erogenous reaction to breastfeeding, especially with an older child who may inadvertently roll the nipple while feeding, should not be criticized, but the phenomenon should be explained and discussed openly by the physician.

Sexual activity of the nursing mother

A review of the limited data available on lactating women in the Masters and Johnson study[59] does indicate that in their group of 111 postpartum women, the nursing mothers were more eager than nonnursing mothers to resume sexual relations postpartum. The data were independent of the fear of pregnancy. They report that this interest was apparent 2 to 3 weeks postpartum. Individual reports through a questionnaire indicate that 30%

of nursing mothers believed their sexual relationships were improved and 2.5% believed they were worse postpartum. The individual testimonies of nursing mothers indicate they had a better feeling about themselves as well as their relationships with their husbands and family in general. In a study of sexual behavior during pregnancy and lactation, Kenney[46] reported that the desire returned by 4 weeks for most women, long before they thought it was safe. The longer they had been married and the more children, the sooner the interest returned and the sooner they felt it was safe. No change in interest or enjoyment occurred with weaning.

In studies of recovery after childbirth, the longer duration of breastfeeding (over 5 months) has been associated with a longer duration of awareness of perineal damage (dyspareunia) during intercourse and a longer amenorrheic period in some women.[2] High prolactin levels and decreased libido have also been observed in women with evidence of continued vaginal discomfort. In the clinical study of lactational amenorrhea in 422 women in Chile, however, Perez et al[72] recorded the incidence of intercourse to be one to two times a week, beginning 4 weeks postpartum.

The frequency of coitus during breastfeeding was studied in four sites: Birmingham, United Kingdom; Montreal, Canada; Sidney, Australia; and Manila, the Philippines. The frequency was lower than reported in other studies of married women, ranging from 4 to 30 episodes a month while averaging three to five times a month. Rates were not correlated with number of children but were related to maternal age, being slightly more frequent in younger women. The resumption of coital activity in these populations was more variable, with a median of 8 weeks postpartum, with 75% resuming activities by the end of the third postpartum month. Thus "normal" encompasses a broad range, according to the authors.[87]

More general observations indicate that although some women may have increased interest in sexual relations while nursing, others may experience no interest at all for 6 months or so. Whether this results from the satiation of the mother's needs for intimate relationship and stimulus through nursing, general fatigue, or fear of pregnancy is debatable.[65] Sexual stimulus may trigger the ejection reflex, and milk ejection may have a negative effect on some men. A practical solution to spraying milk during lovemaking is feeding the infant or expressing some milk beforehand. The total knowledge of nursing and suckling as a biologic phenomenon will help couples to understand such reactions and thus avoid inappropriate psychologic responses.

The conflict in some adult men over their role in regard to the nursing mother's breasts is usually a result of guilt or upbringing. No need exists to advise against fondling the lactating breast during lovemaking, although physicians have often imposed rigid restrictions on sexual activity in the lactating woman. No scientific basis exists for such restriction, and no difference in the incidence of infection and mastitis is associated with such activity. Unusually restrictive protocols are often imposed on patients without medical indication. Bradley[11] recommends, in fact, oral and manual manipulation of the breasts by the husband during both pregnancy and lactation to prevent sore nipples.

It is helpful to discuss with the lactating woman that the hormonal effect on the vagina may be excessive dryness with an increase in dyspareunia. With the abrupt withdrawal of gonadotropins and ovarian hormones and elevation of prolactin at the time of delivery of the infant and placenta, the vaginal epithelium becomes thin and atrophic.[84] Normally the vagina and ectocervix are lined with stratified squamous epithelium, which is multilayered and protective. It is also very responsive to ovarian hormones. The greatest maturation and thickness occur around ovulation in response to peak estrogen secretion. During pregnancy, progesterone inhibits the maturation of the epithelial cells. The vaginal lining retains its thickness, but cells do not fully mature because the effect of progesterone overtakes the effect of estrogen on the epithelium and cervical mucus; both hormones are abundant during pregnancy.

The lowered ovarian hormones during lactation cause vaginal dryness and lack of cervical mucus

as well, leading to discomfort during intercourse. The dryness responds to locally applied lubricants and tends to improve over time. A sudden change may actually reflect ovulation. The breast that is being stimulated by feeding frequently may not be as sensitive during lovemaking. Usually this, too, is only transient. The physician should perhaps remind the mother that some adjustment to attend to the father's needs may be necessary.

NURSING WHILE PREGNANT AND TANDEM NURSING

Pregnancy can and does occur while lactating. When it does occur, it produces a number of questions. There is no need to wean the first infant hastily from the breast, which is often ordered by the physician. It is possible to lactate throughout pregnancy and then to have two infants at the breast postpartum. It is now a sufficiently common event to be called *tandem nursing*.

The amount of nourishment provided the first infant at the breast depends on age and other supplements. When the infant at the breast is only a few months old when pregnancy occurs, there is some rationale to continued breastfeeding for the benefit of the infant until it is time to wean to solids and other liquids at 6 months of age or so. This child will be about a year old when the new infant arrives and, if still at the breast, may have demands in excess of the mother's ability to provide. Concern has been expressed that the older infant will take much of the nourishment needed by the new infant. In some societies, it is believed that a suckling infant will "take the spirit" from the newly conceived fetus; thus weaning is mandated once pregnancy is confirmed.

The milk produced immediately postpartum by the mother who never stopped nursing appears to be colostrum. The kangaroo has been observed to have a teat with mature milk for the older offspring and a teat for the new offspring who requires significantly different nourishment. Such a provision does not exist for the human. It has been shown by mothers who want to maintain both infants at the breast that it can be done without any apparent effect on the nourishment of the new infant. Counseling of such a mother should take into account the mother's resources to receive adequate rest, nourishment, and psychologic support to withstand the added demand on her, physically and mentally.

If the first child is older and will be well beyond a year of age when the new infant arrives, the need for physical nourishment is minimal, and continuation at the breast is more for the security and psychologic benefits. This is referred to as *comfort nursing* and may continue for several years (see Chapter 10). Abrupt weaning should be avoided, and consideration should be given to the impact of separation when the mother is confined during the birth of the new infant. This is an argument for 12-hour hospitalization for delivery for women who request it. The first few days of colostrum are most vital for the new infant, and the supply is not infinite; therefore priorities need to be set concerning the older child. The new baby should be nursed first.

The growth rate of children weaned during a subsequent pregnancy was compared with that of children weaned at the same age but from nonpregnant mothers in a longitudinal study in Bhutan by Bohler and Bergstrom,[8] who followed 113 children closely for the first 3 years of life. The period of overlap for lactation and pregnancy was 5 months (median), increasing by 1 week for each month reduction in birth interval. When a child stopped breastfeeding during the mother's subsequent pregnancy, the growth rate was reduced during the last months before termination of breastfeeding compared with children weaned at the same age from nonpregnant mothers and with children who continued to breastfeed.

In a study of 503 LaLeche League members, Newton and Theotokatos[66] reviewed breastfeeding during pregnancy practices and found that 69% of the breastfeeding children weaned spontaneously when the mother became pregnant. Many of the children probably were at an age to wean even without an intercurrent pregnancy.

Moscone and Moore[64] conducted a question-

naire survey of 57 women who were concurrently pregnant and breastfeeding. The main reasons given for continuing breastfeeding after conception involved the emotional needs of the breastfeeding child; 43% of the children continued to breastfeed throughout pregnancy and after birth of the sibling. The main reason for mother-initiated weaning was breast and nipple pain. When the child weaned during the pregnancy, it occurred during the second trimester and seemed to be associated with diminished milk production. Three pregnancies terminated in spontaneous abortions. The ages of the children at onset of pregnancy varied from 4 to 42 months. The feeding pattern was one to eight times a day for less than 5 minutes to more than 30 minutes.

The decision to continue nursing when the new pregnancy is normal with no factors for a high-risk pregnancy should rest with the comfort level of the mother and child. The breast pain can be improved by wearing a supportive bra and repositioning during breastfeeding. The decrease in volume of milk is usually not remediable, but milk usually returns toward the end of pregnancy and is completely regenerated at delivery.[67]

Many of the changes in child-rearing practices in recent years have increased the freedom and response to human needs. Carried to extremes, instant gratification becomes a right rather than a privilege. Sometimes a mother may need help in seeing that she need not feel guilty if she decides to wean the older child. If it is only an occasional feeding or suckling experience for added security, especially when security is threatened by the arrival of a new infant, it may be tolerable in terms of endurance for the mother, and she may agree willingly. When, however, continuing nursing becomes a strain or is painful or stressful, she should feel free to stop. When the mother feels real resentment toward the older child who is nursing, it is time to wean gently but firmly. If such a situation can be anticipated, it is probably easier for the older child to be weaned before delivery of the new infant.

As with any such decisions to wean, it is best for the physician to work this out in frank discussion with the mother (and father if available) so that any misgivings, resentment, or feeling of failure can be dealt with openly. Many patients automatically suspect the physician of being antagonistic to breastfeeding if the physician suggests weaning. Even when the reason is purely but urgently medical, discussion should be open and include options and alternatives and their risks. Weaning is part of the baby's growing up, but it is sometimes part of the mother's moving on as well.

The dilemma of tandem nursing and weaning the older child has been dealt with in other societies with various manipulations, such as painting the breast with pepper or bitter herbs to make it taste terrible. The mother may leave the child with other caregivers. The provision of love and affection during this difficult adaptation for the child is what makes the difference between a traumatic occasion and a step toward growing up. Equally important is the provision of some opportunity for the mother to express her concerns and doubts during the process to her physician, who should be neither judgmental nor unduly rigid in the medical care plan.

REFERENCES

1. Abdulla KA, Elwan S, Salem H et al: Effect of early postpartum use of the contraceptive implants, Norplant®, on the serum levels of immunoglobulins of the mothers and their breastfed infants, *Contraception* 32:261, 1985.
2. Abraham S, Child A, Ferry J et al: Childbirth recovery, *Med J Aust* 152:9, 1990.
3. Adnan AM, Bakr SA: Postpartum lactational amenorrhoea as a means of family planning in the Sudan: a study of 500 cases, *J Biosoc Sci* 15:9, 1983.
4. Barker DC: Use of natural family planning by breastfeeding women. In Shivanandan M, editor: *Breastfeeding and natural family planning,* Fourth International Symposium on Natural Family Planning, Chevy Chase, Md, 1985, KM Associate Publishers.
5. Beling CG, Frandsen VA, Josimovich JB: Pituitary and ovarian hormone levels during lactation, *Acta Endocrinol* 155(suppl):40, 1971.
6. Bentovin A: Shame and other anxieties associated with breastfeeding. In Ciba Foundation Symposium no 45: *Breastfeeding and the mother,* Amsterdam, 1976, Elsevier.
7. Berman ML, Hanson K, Hellman IL: Effect of breastfeeding on postpartum menstruation, ovulation and pregnancy on Alaskan Eskimos, *Am J Obstet Gynecol* 114:524, 1972.
8. Bohler E, Bergstrom S: Child growth during weaning depends on whether mother is pregnant again, *J Trop Pediatr* 42:104, 1996.
9. Bonte M, van Balen H: Prolonged lactation and family spacing in Rwanda, *J Biosoc Sci* 1:97, 1969.
10. Bordes A, Allman J, Verly A: The impact on breastfeeding and pregnancy status of household contraceptive distribution in rural Haiti, *Am J Public Health* 72:835, 1982.
11. Bradley RA: *Husband-coached childbirth,* New York, 1965, Harper & Row.
12. Brambilla F, Sirtori CM: Gonadotropin-inhibiting factor in pregnancy, lactation and menopause, *Am J Obstet Gynecol* 109:599, 1971.
13. Brown RE: Breast-feeding and family planning: a review of relationships between breast-feeding and family planning, *Am J Clin Nutr* 35:162, 1982.
14. Cole LP, McCann MF, Higgins JE et al: Effects of breastfeeding on IUD performance, *Am J Public Health* 73:384, 1983.
15. Committee on Drugs, American Academy of Pediatrics: Breastfeeding and contraception, *Pediatrics* 68:138, 1981.
16. Consensus statement: Breastfeeding as a family planning method, *Lancet* 2:1204, 1988.
17. Cooney KA, Koniz-Booher P, Coly S: *Taking the first steps: the lactational amenorrhea method, a decade of experience,* Georgetown University, Washington, DC, 1997, Institute for Reproductive Health.
18. Cooney KA, Nahmias SR: *Bellagio and beyond: breastfeeding and LAM in reproductive health,* Georgetown University, Washington, DC, 1997, Institute for Reproductive Health.
19. Curtis EM: Oral-contraceptive feminization of a normal male infant, *Obstet Gynecol* 23:295, 1964.
20. Delvoye P, Demaegd M, Nyampeta U et al: Serum prolactin, gonadotropins, and estradiol in menstruating and amenorrheic mothers during two years' lactation, *Am J Obstet Gynecol* 130:635, 1978.
21. Dewey KG, Cohen RJ, Rivera LL et al: Effects of age at introduction of complementary foods to breast-fed infants on duration of lactational amenorrhea in Honduran women, *Am J Clin Nutr* 65:1403, 1997.
22. Diaz S, Aravena R, Cardenas ME et al: Contraceptive efficacy of lactational amenorrhea in urban Chilean women, *Contraception* 43:335, 1991.
23. Diaz S, Cardenas H, Brandeis A et al: Early difference in the endocrine profile of long and short lactational amenorrhea, *J Clin Endocrinol Metab* 72:196, 1991.

24. Diaz S, Jackanicz TM, Herreros C et al: Fertility regulation in nursing women. VIII. Progesterone plasma levels and contraception efficacy of a progesterone-releasing vaginal ring, *Contraception* 32:603, 1985.

25. Diaz S, Peralta O, Juez G et al: Fertility regulation in nursing women. I. The probability of conception in full nursing women living in an urban setting, *J Biosoc Sci* 14:329, 1982.

26. Drife JO: Breast sensitivity and lactational amenorrhoea, *Br J Obstet Gynecol* 95:824, 1988.

27. Eslami SS, Gray RH, Apelo R et al: The reliability of menses to indicate the return of ovulation in breastfeeding women in Manila, the Philippines, *Stud Fam Plann* 21:243, 1990.

28. Farr G, Rivera R: Interactions between intrauterine contraceptive device use and breastfeeding status at time of intrauterine contraceptive device insertion: analysis of TCu-380A acceptors in developing countries, *Am J Obstet Gynecol* 167:144, 1992.

29. Fraser HM, Dewart PJ, Smith SK et al: Luteinizing hormone releasing hormone agonist for contraception in breastfeeding women, *J Clin Endocrinol Metab* 69:996, 1989.

30. Frisch RE, McArthur JW: Difference between postpartum and nutritional amenorrhea, *Science* 203:921, 1979.

31. Ford K, Labbok M: Contraceptive usage during lactation in the United States: an update, *Am J Public Health* 77:79, 1987.

32. Gioiosa R: Incidence of pregnancy during lactation in 500 cases, *Am J Obstet Gynecol* 70:162, 1955.

33. Gray RH, Campbell OM, Apelo R et al: Risk of ovulation during lactation, *Lancet* 335:25, 1990.

34. Gray RH, Campbell O, Eslamic S et al: The return of ovarian function during lactation: results of studies from the United States and the Philippines. In *Biomedical demographic determinants,* Oxford, 1993, Clarendon.

35. Gross BA: Is the lactational amenorrhea method a part of natural family planning? Biology and policy, *Am J Obstet Gynecol* 165:2014, 1991.

36. Hartwell S, Schlesselman S: Risk of uterine perforation among users of IUD, *Obstet Gynecol* 61:31, 1983.

37. Heikkila M, Luukkainen T: Duration of breastfeeding and development of children after insertion of a levonorgestrel-releasing intrauterine contraceptive device, *Contraception* 25:279, 1982.

38. Howie P, McNeilly A, Houston M et al: Fertility after childbirth: infant feeding patterns, basal PRL levels, and postpartum ovulation, *Clin Endocrinol* 17:315, 1982.

39. Howie P, McNeilly A, Houston M et al: Fertility after childbirth: postpartum ovulation and menstruation in bottle and breastfeeding mothers, *Clin Endocrinol* 17:323, 1982.

40. Hull VJ: The effects of hormonal contraceptives on lactation: current findings, methodological considerations and future priorities, *Stud Fam Plann* 12:134, 1981.

41. Kambic RT: Natural family planning use—effectiveness and continuation, *Am J Obstet Gynecol* 165:2046, 1991.

42. Kennedy KI, Labbok MH, Van Look PFA: Consensus statement: lactational amenorrhea method for family planning, *Int J Gynecol Obstet* 54:55, 1996.

43. Kennedy KI, Rivera R, McNeilly AS: Consensus statement on the use of breastfeeding as a family planning method, *Contraception* 39:477, 1989.

44. Kennedy KI, Short RV, Tully MR: Premature introduction of progestin-only contraceptive methods during lactation, *Contraception* 55:347, 1997.

45. Kennedy KI, Visness CM: Contraceptive efficacy of lactational amenorrhoea, *Lancet* 339:227, 1992.

46. Kenney JA: Sexuality of pregnant and breastfeeding women, *Arch Sex Behav* 2:215, 1973.

47. Kippley S: *Breastfeeding and natural child spacing,* New York, 1976, Harper & Row.

48. Konner M, Worthman C: Nursing frequency, gonadal function, and birth spacing among !Kung hunter-gatherers, *Science* 207:788, 1980.

49. Kurz KM, Habicht J-P, Rasmussen KM: Influences of maternal nutrition and lactation on length of postpartum amenorrhoea, *J Trop Pediatr* 37(suppl):15, 1991.

50. Labbok M: Breastfeeding and contraception, *N Engl J Med* 308:51, 1983.

51. Labbok M: Contraception during lactation: considerations in advising the individual and in formulating program guidelines. In Potts M, Thapa S, Herbertson MA: Breastfeeding and fertility, *J Biosoc Sci,* suppl 9, 1985, Galton Foundation.

52. Labbok M, Koniz-Booker P, Goney K et al: *Guidelines for breastfeeding, LAM, and family planning,* Washington, DC, 1992, Institute for Reproductive Health.

53. Labbok MH, Laukaran VH: Breastfeeding and family planning. In Sciarra JJ: *Gynecology and obstetrics,* Philadelphia, 1994, Lippincott.

54. Labbok MH, Peréz A, Valdés F, et al: The lactational amenorrhea method (LAM): a postpartum introductory family planning method with policy and program implications, *Adv Contracept* 10:93, 1994.

55. Labbok MH, Stallings RY, Shah F et al: Ovulation method use during breastfeeding: is there an increased risk of unplanned pregnancy? *Am J Obstet Gynecol* 165:2031, 1991.

56. Lasley BL, Shideler SE, Munrol CJ: A prototype for ovulation detection: pros and cons, *Am J Obstet Gynecol* 165:2003, 1991.

57. Lewis PR, Brown JB, Renfree MB et al: The resumption of ovulation and menstruation in a well-nourished population of women breastfeeding for an extended period of time, *Fertil Steril* 55:529, 1991.

58. Marshall WM, Cumming DC, Fitzsimmons GW: Hot flushes during breastfeeding? *Fertil Steril* 57:1349, 1992.

59. Masters WH, Johnson VE: *Human sexual response,* Boston, 1966, Little, Brown.

60. McCann MF, Potter LS: Progestin-only oral contraception: a comprehensive review, *Contraception* 50:S1, 1994.

61. McCann M et al: Breastfeeding, fertility, and family planning, *Popul Rep J* 24:J-552, revised March, 1984.

62. McNeilly AS, Glasier AF, Howie PW et al: Fertility after childbirth: pregnancy associated with breastfeeding, *Clin Endocrinol* 18:167, 1983.

63. McNeilly AS, Glasier AF, Howie PW: Endocrine control of lactational infertility. In Dobbin J, editor: *Maternal nutrition and lactational infertility,* New York, 1985, Nestle Nutrition, Vevey/Raven.

64. Moscone SR, Moore MJ: Breastfeeding during pregnancy, *J Hum Lact* 9:83, 1993.

65. Newton N, Newton M: Psychologic aspects of lactation, *N Engl J Med* 277:1179, 1967.

66. Newton N, Theotokatos M: Breast-feeding during pregnancy in 503 women: does psychobiological weaning mechanism exist in humans? *Emotion Reprod* 20B:845, 1979.

67. Nichols-Johnson V: Tandem nursing: before and after, *ABM News Views* 2:6, 1996.

68. Nilsson S, Mellbin T, Hofvander Y et al: Long-term follow-up of children breastfed by mothers using oral contraceptives, *Contraception* 34:443, 1986.

69. Ojofeitimi EO: Effect of duration and frequency of breastfeeding on postpartum amenorrhea, *Pediatrics* 69:164, 1982.

70. Perez A: Lactational amenorrhea and natural family planning. In Hafez ESE, editor: *Human ovulation: mechanisms, prediction, detection, and induction,* Amsterdam, 1979, North-Holland.

71. Perez A: Natural family planning: postpartum period, *Int J Fertil* 26:219, 1981.

72. Perez A, Labbok MH, Queenan JT: Clinical study of the lactational amenorrhoea method for family planning, *Lancet* 339:968, 1992.

73. Prema K, Naidu AN, Kumari SN: Lactation and fertility, *Am J Clin Nutr* 32:1298, 1979.

74. Queenan JT, Jennings VH, Spieler JM et al: Natural family planning: current knowledge and new strategies for the 1990s, Georgetown University, Washington, DC, 1993, Institute for Reproductive Health.

75. Rosner AE, Schulman SK: Birth interval among breastfeeding women not using contraceptives, *Pediatrics* 86:747, 1990.

76. Saadeh R, Benboozid D: Breastfeeding and child-spacing: importance of information collection for public health policy, *Bull World Health Organ* 68:625, 1990.

77. Sas M, Gellen JJ, Dusitsin N et al: An investigation on the influence of steroidal contraceptives on milk lipid and fatty acids in Hungary and Thailand, *Contraception* 33:159, 1986.

78. Savina G, Kennedy K: The effect of a breastfeeding educational program on lactational amenorrhea in the Philippines, *Stud Fam Plann* 20:203, 1989.

79. Selye H, McKeown T: The effect of mechanical stimulation of the nipples on the ovary and the sexual cycle, *Surg Gynecol Obstet* 59:856, 1934.

80. Shaaban MM: Contraception with progestogens and progesterone during lactation, *J Steroid Biochem Molec Biol* 40:705, 1991.

81. Short RV, Lewis PR, Renfree MB et al: Contraceptive effects of extended lactational amenorrhoea: beyond the Bellagio consensus, *Lancet* 337:715, 1991.

82. Tankeyoon M, Dusitsin N, Chalapati S et al: Effects of hormonal contraceptives on milk volume and infant growth, *Contraception* 30:505, 1984.

83. Tay CCK, Glasier AF, McNeilly AS: Twenty-four-hour patterns of prolactin secretion during lactation and the relationship to suckling and the resumption of fertility in breast-feeding women, *Hum Reprod* 11:950, 1996.

84. Taylor RS: Physiology of the vagina and cervix in breastfeeding women. In Shivanandan M, editor: *Breastfeeding and natural family planning,* Fourth International Symposium on Natural Family Planning, Chevy Chase, Md, 1985, KM Associate Publishers.

85. Technical Guidance/Competence Group, USAID/WHO: Family planning methods: new guidance, *Popul Rep* XXIV, no 2, Baltimore, 1996, Johns Hopkins School of Public Health.

86. Toddywalla VS, Joshi L, Virkar K: Effect of contraceptive steroids on human lactation, *Am J Obstet Gynecol* 127:245, 1977.

87. Visness CM, Kennedy KI: The frequency of coitus during breastfeeding, *Birth* 24:253, 1997.

88. Visness CM, Kennedy KI, Gross BA et al: Fertility of fully breast-feeding women in the early postpartum period, *Obstet Gynecol* 89:164, 1997.

89. Vorherr H: *The breast: morphology, physiology and lactation,* New York, 1974, Academic Press.

90. Vorherr H: Human lactation and breast feeding. In Larson BL, editor: *Lactation: a comprehensive treatise,* New York, 1978, Academic Press.

91. Wade K, Sevilla F, Labbok M: Integrating the lactational amenorrhea method into a family planning program in Ecuador, *Stud Fam Plann* 25:162, 1994.

92. World Health Organization Task Force for Epidemiological Research on Reproductive Health: Progestogen-only contraceptives during lactation. I and II. Infant development, *Contraception* 50:55, 1994.

93. Winikoff B, Semeraro P, Zimmerman M: *Contraception during breastfeeding: a clinician's source book,* New York, 1988, Population Council.

94. Zacharias S, Aguilera E, Assenzo JR et al: Effects of hormonal and nonhormonal contraceptives on lactation and incidence of pregnancy, *Contraception* 33:203, 1986.

95. Zarate A, Canales ES, Soria J et al: Ovarian refractoriness during lactation in women: effect of gonadotropin stimulation, *Am J Obstet Gynecol* 112:1130, 1972.

20

The collection and storage of human milk and human milk banking

The human milk bank has entered another era. The interest in providing human milk for human infants with special needs, especially premature infants, has increased, but the concerns regarding donor milk have also escalated. Most neonatologists strongly believe that donor human milk must be pasteurized before use in an infant, and only the mother's own milk may be used fresh in a sick neonate. In addition, donors must be carefully screened and women at high risk for certain infection eliminated.

When there are risks associated with using even the mother's own milk for a given baby, the risk/benefit ratio is determined. Because of the effects of heating, cooling, freezing, and storing milk, some of the most valued and precious qualities are diminished or destroyed; feeding the milk fresh or at least fresh frozen and not heated preserves most of the constituents. The value of the milk produced by women who deliver prematurely has been discussed in Chapter 14. There are no reported cases of infection acquired from milk provided by a milk bank in compliance with the standards prescribed by the Human Milk Banking Association of North America (HMBANA).

HISTORIC PERSPECTIVE

When wet nursing was the immediate alternative feeding to replace the mother's own milk and no safe ways were available to store milk of any species, no human milk banks existed. As pasteurization became available and formulas based on milk from other species increased in popularity, the pool of human milk diminished. "Wet nurses" were increasingly difficult to locate and often were not safe sources because of wet-nurse lifestyle, risk of infections, and poor nutrition. It had already been clearly demonstrated in the early twentieth century that infants who did not receive their mother's milk had six times the risk of dying in the first year of life (see Chapter 1).

The impetus behind milk banks at the turn of the twentieth century was actually the medical profession's desire to remove the control of infant feeding from wet nurses and separate the product (human milk) from the producer. Pediatricians anxious to improve the prognosis for infants deprived of human milk for medical and social reasons developed a means of storing human milk for general use with sick infants. The first milk bank was opened in Vienna in 1900. The first one in the United States was established 10 years later at the Massachusetts Infant Asylum, where wet nurses had been the only sources of human milk.[30] In 1919 the first human milk bank was founded in Germany in Magdeburg by Dr. Marie-Elise Kayser. In 1934 she wrote guidelines that were used throughout Europe for the creation and operation of milk banks.[58]

Early attempts at providing donor milk depended on casual screening of donors for tuberculosis, syphilis, and various acute contagious diseases.[43] There was little investigation of human milk, but the dairy industry was rigorous in its attempt to store and market bovine and other mammalian milks. This technology was applied on a small scale, but other human milk banks appeared after Denny and Talbot created the one in Boston. The American Academy of Pediatrics (AAP) established its first formal guidelines for human milk banks in 1943.[12,13] Similar guidelines were provided in other countries. After World War II, milk banks were mandated on both sides of the Berlin Wall. In 1959 the Federal Republic of Germany (West Germany) had 24 milk banks and the German Democratic Republic had 62.[58] The numbers gradually decreased.

As technology advanced in newborn care and in infant nutrition, science replaced nature. The interest in human milk faded and with it the call for banked human milk in the 1960s and into the 1970s. Experience in Rochester with short-gut syndrome and malabsorption syndromes, however, resulted in the development of a registry of lactating women who donated fresh milk when needed. A milk bank was developed with donors providing frozen milk on a regular basis. By 1975, five large commercial milk banks were operating in Britain. Milk banks also sprang up across the United States. The system thrived with the establishment in 1985 of the HMBANA, which not only facilitated communications among banks, but also began to investigate processes, develop uniform policies, and most important, provide professional and public education.[4]

The threat of human immunodeficiency virus (HIV) and hepatitis, the return of tuberculosis, and drug abuse have cast a long shadow on milk banks in the United States, resulting in the closure of all but seven in North America and five in the United States (see Appendix H). In Europe, milk banking has been key in the nourishment of premature and other high-risk infants. The Sorrento Maternity Hospital has supplied 50,000 liters of milk from 10,000 donors over 40 years and now provides 700 liters a year both locally and across Britain.[6] In 1994 the remaining 18 milk banks in unified Germany supplied about 15,000 liters.

Many developing countries, especially in Central and South America, are establishing milk banks as part of national efforts to promote breastfeeding. Studies done in nurseries in Guatemala have shown a marked decrease in mortality and morbidity by providing every infant with human milk.[14] The United Nation's Children's Fund (UNICEF) has encouraged and supported such efforts.[67]

STORING HUMAN MILK

It is often necessary to store milk for infants, especially in the hospital. The storage of human milk involves two types of milk: mother's milk and donor milk. The distinction becomes important in how the milk is stored and prepared for the infant. It is also important because many states have developed codes for donor milk but fortunately have not regulated mother's milk as yet. Certain guidelines are appropriate for each milk. Indications for use of such milk were alluded to in other chapters but are briefly summarized here.

Mother's milk for a healthy infant

The conditions under which a mother collects and stores milk while at work are not always ideal. At home, at work, or at school, milk should be collected with clean equipment, stored in sterile containers (dishwasher cleaned and dried suffices), and handled with just-washed hands. The limits of temperature and time are an important consideration.

To assess microbial growth and stability of milk protein and lipid at varying temperatures and for varying lengths of time, Hamosh et al[32] collected samples from 16 healthy women with healthy babies who were exclusively breastfed. Sampling was done early in lactation (1 month postpartum) and late in lactation (5 to 6 months postpartum). The milk pH decreased from 7.02 ± 0.20 to 5.16 ± 0.26 after 24 hours of storage at 38° C (100° F), and significant differences in pH occurred at all temperatures at 24 hours or longer. Proteolysis was minimal at 15° C (59° F) and 25° C and 25° (77° F) but became apparent at 38° C at 24 hours. Lipolysis was marked in the first 24 hours at all temperatures compared with freshly expressed milk. Bacterial growth or normal flora was minimal at 15° C at 24 hours, low at 25° C at 8 hours, and higher at 38° C by 4 hours.

The authors concluded that storage of human milk is safe at 15° C for 24 hours and 25° C room temperature for 4 hours and should not be stored at 38° C. Proteins appear to maintain their structure and function in short-term storage. The marked lipolysis appears to slow bacterial growth at the same time.[32]

Mother's milk for a sick infant

1. The mother plans to breastfeed the infant ultimately but needs to provide pumped milk until the infant can be put to the breast.
2. The infant requires the special nutritional benefits of human milk (as with those infants who are recovering from intestinal surgery) but cannot nurse at the breast.
3. The infant weighs 1500 g or less and has difficulty digesting and absorbing other milks and is usually fed by nasogastric tube.

Appendix H lists guidelines for handling mother's milk for hospital use.

Donor milk

1. The infant is at risk of infection or necrotizing enterocolitis. Although effects are not clearly demonstrated with mature milk, fresh colostrum is held to be especially protective and may be collected from low-risk, carefully screened mothers.
2. The physician believes the infant would benefit from the nourishment in human milk because of prematurity, especially if the infant weighs less than 1500 g.
3. The mother is temporarily unable to nourish a breastfed infant completely. It may be that the mother's supply is inadequate when she first puts the infant to the breast after weeks of pumping or when the mother has been ill or hospitalized. Usually these infants are already at home.
4. Donor milk is an excellent transition from parenteral nutrition when mother's milk is not available. It allows earlier weaning from parenteral solution, earlier than formula is known to be tolerated.
5. Metabolic disorders, especially amino acid disorders, respond well because of the physiologic profile of human milk (decreased casein, tyrosine, and phenylalanine). In addition, human milk is protective against infection, which may be a serious complication of these disorders.
6. Pooled samples of donor milk are prepared as a dried preparation for addition to fresh mother's milk to increase the calorie and nutrient value for high-risk premature infants whose requirements exceed those available with unsupplemented human milk.
7. The older infant or child has unique feeding difficulties usually characterized by an inability to tolerate any oral nourishment except human milk (e.g., the child dying of HIV infection).

Structure of a milk bank

Most informal and casual milk banks operating in conjunction with a neonatal intensive care unit (NICU) have disappeared.[53] NICUs may provide a deep freeze for storage of mother's own milk for use by her infant. They store it for feeding of the infant and do not process it at all except to culture random samples for contamination. Most do not permit "donating" milk to other infants except by private arrangements between the two mothers with physician's approval. No feeding is given an infant in the hospital without a physician's order. Smaller public milk banks have phased out since state legislation or local medical practice standards have mandated strict surveillance of samples and pasteurization.

A few large, well-established banks continue to operate in the United States and around the world. A network of these milk banks that meets and shares information through the HMBANA.[4,5,*] Copies of the association's guidelines for milk storage are available for a fee. HMBANA works closely with the Food and Drug Administration (FDA) concerning FDA regulations for human tissues and fluids. Appendix H provides the 1997 guidelines.

*8 Jan Sebastian Way #13, Sandwich, MA 02563 USA.

Fig. 20-1. Flowchart of human milk bank process.

The Mother's Milk Bank (MMB) of the Institute for Medical Research in San Jose, Calif, was established in 1974. It has a full-time coordinator and a medical director, provides milk for hundreds of infants, and contributes to the fund of knowledge on human milk. Because the milk is provided to patients only by physician's prescription, it is reimbursable by health insurance carriers of California. MMB has developed procedures and policies regarding milk collection, storage, and processing. This is described in detail by Asquith et al[5] and documented with an extensive bibliography. The MMB has prepared and keeps current a comprehensive manual for the organization and operation of a modern human milk bank, which is available to health care facilities. It is also a member of HMBANA, which can provide the names and addresses of other centers (Fig. 20-1).

The state of New York passed an amendment to the public health law in 1980 in which it was declared policy that any and all infants requiring human breast milk be assured access to sufficient quantities of wholesome human breast milk donated by concerned lactating mothers on a continued and systematic basis (see Appendix L for entire law). This law resulted in an addition to the rules and regulations of the hospitals' minimum standards, because it was anticipated that the greatest number of infants requiring human milk would be hospitalized in tertiary neonatal units. The administrative rules and regulations were developed with the consultation of experts in milk banking and neonatal care. Because the items cover all the considerations known to be necessary to provide the safest and most effective human milk for recipients, the regulations are duplicated in Appendix H for reference.

The recommendations for the expansion of the human-milk-banking system have not gone without challenge from neonatologists. They offer sincere concerns about the risk/benefit ratio because alteration during storage and contamination may detract from the value of the original product for the mother's own infant. They caution that the cavalier feeding of unsterile unsupplemented breast milk to premature infants may produce iatrogenic problems.

Qualifications of donors

A mother who is willing to donate milk should be healthy and fulfill the following qualifications (Box 20-1):

1. Normal pregnancy and delivery
2. Serologically negative for syphilis, hepatitis B surface antigen (HBsAg), cytomegalovirus (CMV), and HIV
3. No infection, acute or chronic (i.e., not at high risk)
4. Not taking medications, smoking, or using excessive alcohol
5. Capable of carrying out sterile technique
6. If donating for other infants, own child is healthy and without jaundice

A directive from the Department of Health and Social Security (DHSS) in Great Britain mandated HIV testing for donors to milk banks, and it was observed that the list of 19 established milk banks dwindled to six.[6] The Sorrento Maternity Hospital, however, in accordance with the DHSS directive, screened all donors for HIV antibodies. Only four mothers of 470 potential donors have refused to be tested, contrary to fears that the ruling would discourage donating.[6]

The donor should not be taking medications, including certain oral contraceptives and any nonprescription medications regularly, such as aspirin or acetaminophen. Her infant should be well and should not have had neonatal jaundice. If the mother is donating only for her own infant, the state of the infant's health does not prevent her from donating. Any time the donor becomes ill, however, she should discard milk from the previous 24-hour period and not save milk until the illness is over if the milk is to be donated.

Discarding milk during maternal illness is the most difficult regulation to which a mother must adhere. The desire to contribute may overshadow the mother's understanding of the risk it poses for an infant not her own receiving such milk.

The one limiting factor in donating milk is that the woman must be lactating. Becoming a professional donor of milk today is highly unlikely. The amount of protein has been noted to be lower after

Donor screening procedures

1. Donors answer questions on a verbal health history screening form. Primary health care providers for the prospective donor and her infant are asked for verification of health.
2. Donors are tested serologically for:
   a. HIV-1 and HIV-2
   b. HTLV-I and HTLV-II
   c. Hepatitis B
   d. Hepatitis C
   e. Syphilis
3. Repeat donors are treated as new donors with each pregnancy.
4. Milk banks will cover the cost of the serologic screening if the tests are done by the milk bank.

Reasons for excluding a donor

- Receipt of a blood transfusion or blood products within last 12 months
- Receipt of an organ or tissue transplant within last 12 months
- Regular use of more than 2 ounces of hard liquor or its equivalent in a 24-hour period
- Regular use of over-the-counter medications or systemic prescriptions (replacement hormones and some birth control hormones are acceptable)
- Use of megadose vitamins or pharmacologically active herbal preparations
- Total vegetarians (vegans) who do not supplement their diet with vitamins
- Use of illegal drugs
- Use of tobacco products
- Silicone breast implants
- History of hepatitis, systemic disorders of any kind, or chronic infections (e.g., HIV, HTLV, TB)

Modified from Arnold LDW: *J Hum Lact* 13:159, 1997.
HIV, Human immunodeficiency virus; *HTLV,* human T-cell leukemia virus; *TB,* tuberculosis.

6 months of lactation; thus it is advisable to limit a given mother's contributions to 6 months or, at most, 8 months postpartum.

Technique for collection

Whether collecting for a mother's own infant or for other uses, it is of prime importance to maintain cleanliness and minimize bacteria in the process of collection. The mother should be instructed in washing her hands and her breasts before handling the equipment or pumping.

The two major ways of collecting are letting the milk drip while the infant nurses on the other side and pumping or manually expressing the milk.[27,29,60] Drip milk is acceptable for one's own infant when it is used as an occasional tide-over feeding in the mother's temporary absence; however, it is not appropriate for donor milk. Dripped milk has been found to have lower caloric value and a much higher incidence of contamination. Pumped milk has a higher fat content than dripped or manually expressed milk, and in most individuals the volume is also greater. Any equipment used, such as hand pumps, tubing, and collecting bottles, should be sterile. If an electric pump is used, the parts that come in contact with the milk should be sterile and/or disposable (Fig. 20-2). Many hospi-

Fig. 20-2. Purse-sized electric pump. Serviceable for women who are fully lactating.

tals own electric pumps, or one may be rented from a local rental company. Some women can pump large volumes of fat-rich milk manually, and for them, manual expression would be acceptable on a case-by-case basis.

The hospital or the bank should provide a program of education for the donors. Milk samples should be cultured initially to ensure proper technique and the absence of significant contamination. Then samples should be sent for culture on a random basis. Studies have shown that milk collected at home has a higher contamination rate than that collected while the donor is hospitalized or with equipment maintained by the hospital. Collection at the hospital also avoids the transportation problem.

Many hospitals use the 4-oz sterile water-nursing bottles packaged by formula companies for collections by discarding the water at the time of collection and then filling them with milk. Other programs suggest the use of 50-ml plastic centrifuge tubes,* which are presterilized and have tight-fitting tops. These tubes have the advantage of more appropriate volume and easy measurability and sterility. Ideally the hospital or milk bank provides a uniform container. Soft plastic bags are not recommended. If a woman wants to donate a large amount of previously collected and frozen milk that suddenly becomes available (infant weans or dies), this milk is a valuable resource and can be handled separately with culturing and pasteurization.[1-3]

Zinaman et al[73] evaluated the efficacy of various methods of removing milk from the breast. Electric pumping (White River model) was clearly more effective in raising the maternal prolactin levels and increasing the volume of milk when compared with hand pumping and manual expression. The study did not compare various brands of pumps. A hospital may own a breast pump that is 10 or 20 years old, however, which may not have safety features that are built into current models. Problems of contamination are a significant issue because old models may not protect against milk

backing up into the motor or tubing normally thought to be free of milk and of potential contamination. Care must be taken to check each machine and follow directions for its proper use.

The use of most of the modern electric pumps with their disposable tubing and collecting vessels makes mechanical pumping the most efficient and cleanest of the methods. In addition, the milking action of an electric pump produces more physiologic stimulus to the breast. When a Y-connector is used and both breasts are pumped simultaneously, overall production is increased, and time for pumping may be cut in half.

Bank milk collected by manual expression is less likely to be contaminated than that collected by hand pumps, even when pumps are boiled or placed in an electric dishwasher.[38,63] The rubber bulb of the hand pump, resembling a bicycle horn, retains milk and bacteria and should not be used. "Nesty cups," which are placed inside the brassiere to collect milk drippings between feedings, have been associated with the greatest contamination and are not recommended.

Donowitz et al[16] reported contaminated breast milk as the source of *Klebsiella* bacteremia in an NICU. Unpasteurized human milk from a single donor fed through nasogastric and nasoduodenal tubes to sick newborns was found to be contaminated from the safety overflow bottle and tubing of the electric breast pump maintained in the NICU. This part of the tubing and equipment should be sterilized or disposed of between collections according to the manufacturer's instructions. Strict attention to sterilization of equipment is imperative. Older electric pumps that do not have a built-in mechanism to prevent milk from getting into the permanent "works" should be discarded, and only pumps with disposable and/or cleanable parts and a safety valve should be used.

The bacteriologic benefit to discarding the first 5 to 10 ml of milk pumped from the breast remains disputed.[10] Some banks require that their donors follow instruction for discarding the first 5 to 10 ml of milk expressed at each pumping and each breast. When a donor is collecting for long-term storage, this may be appropriate. When a mother is collect-

---

*No. 25330, manufactured by Corning Glass Works.

ing for her own baby and her volume is meager, discarding 10 ml may be counterproductive. This is particularly important initially, when early colostrum and milk are less in total volume but high in value to the infant. At home, later, when production is abundant and technique may be less stringent, discarding 2 to 3 ml might be appropriate. This will allow a clean collection without washing the breast before pumping, which is associated with sore nipples in some women.

Collection and storage containers

Colostrum was reported by Goldblum et al[29] to impart greater stability to its components than did mature milk. None of the cellular or humoral immunologic factors investigated was diminished when colostrum was stored at 4° C (39° F) for 24 hours in any of the containers (Table 20-1).

The effect of the container on the stability of the constituents of milk was investigated by Garza et al.[26] Pyrex and polypropylene containers were found not to interact with water-soluble and fat-soluble nutrients such as vitamin A, zinc, iron, copper, sodium, and protein nitrogen. Polyethylene bags were found to spill easily, to be harder for mothers to fill without contamination, and to be difficult to handle in the nursery. The containers also leaked and punctured easily, resulting in 60% lower secretory immunoglobulin A (sIgA) levels because of adherence to the material. It appears

that rigid polypropylene plastic containers may have a significant advantage in maintaining the stability of all constituents in human milk collections and may be easier and safer to handle.

Paxson and Cress[50] have reported a significant difference in the survival of the leukocytes when the milk is collected and stored in plastic containers rather than glass, because the cells apparently stick to the glass. The phagocytosis of these cells, however, is not affected by the container. The researchers further demonstrated that varying the osmolarity or protein concentration does not alter the number or the phagocytosis of the cells. Because they believe the main reason for feeding preterm infants human milk is for the protection against infection, they suggest nasogastric feedings instead of nasojejunal feeding (to maintain pH in the acid range; in the small bowel, the pH is 6.5 to 8). The milk is collected in sterile plastic containers and maintained in the refrigerator until it is fed to the infant, avoiding heating, freezing, and alkaline solutions (Table 20-1).

Storage and testing of milk samples

Fresh refrigerated unsterilized mother's milk can be used for 48 hours following collection. If the milk is to be used fresh chilled, it should be refrigerated at home and brought in promptly for use within 48 hours. If it is to be frozen, this should be done immediately at −18° C (0° F) (standard

---

TABLE 20-1   Effect of container type on milk constituents

Constituent	Pyrex	Polypropylene	Polyethylene bags	Polyethylene (rigid)
Colostrum	Constituents stable	When refrigerated	24 hours in all	Containers
Mature milk				
Cells	Stick to glass	Maintain phagocytosis	Stable	Stable
Fat-soluble vitamins	No effect	No effect	—	—
Micronutrients	No effect	No effect	—	—
Secretory IgA	—	—	Lower	Stable
Difficult to handle	—	—	Very	—
			Spill easily	
Recommend for donor milk	Highly	No	No	Yes

home freezer) or in top of a refrigerator freezer. The milk stored in the latter should be deep frozen within 24 hours if it is to be stored any length of time. The milk kept at $-18°$ C can be kept for 6 months. Freezing and thawing, which can occur in a freezer that is part of a refrigerator, significantly alter the energy content and predispose to separation of the fat layer. Therefore milk stored in the freezer compartment of a refrigerator-freezer with separate doors should be placed well back in the freezer (not in door) and stored only 1 month. In the hospital or at a bank, all samples should be labeled with name of donor, date, and time. Milk is stored in the freezer in such a way that the oldest milk is used first, and all milk of a single donor is kept together and used only for the infant of that mother.

When a hospitalized mother is contributing fresh milk to her own infant, it is usually not cultured. Pumping is usually done with the help of the nursing staff, and colostrum seems to be more resistant to contamination.[15] Once a mother has been discharged home and she is producing mature milk, however, random sample culturing of mother's milk samples every week or two is a mechanism for checking milk-expression technique.[20] NICUs have found that random testing improves technique in general.

Because using the fresh milk from the mother to feed a premature infant is becoming commonplace, it is important to be aware of the bacteria cultured from fresh samples during refrigeration.[7] Samples pumped by hand pump and manually expressed were cultured at zero time and after 48 and 120 hours of refrigeration by Sosa and Barness.[57] Although 8 of 41 samples had no growth, the others had the same bacteria on skin and nipple as appeared in the milk (Table 20-2). Concentration was low and decreased over time (Table 20-3), which is attributed to the bacterial inhibitory factors present in milk and suggests that refrigeration of carefully collected breast milk is a safe method for over 48 hours. Guidelines for collection and use of mother's own milk appear in Appendix H.

Standards for raw donor milk

The FDA and the Centers for Disease Control and Prevention (CDC) do not recommend use of donor milk without heat treatment.[4] Rare children, however, require fresh donor milk and cannot tolerate the heat-treated product. For these infants, the guidelines should be carefully followed. These special donors must be meticulously screened and monitored for high-risk behaviors. Parents of the infant recipient should sign an informed consent.

All raw donor milk should be screened microbiologically before use. No generally accepted microbiologic criteria exist for such milk except that no potential pathogens should be present.[11] Such pathogens include *Staphylococcus aureus,* β-hemolytic streptococci, *Pseudomonas* species,

TABLE 20-2   **Positive bacterial cultures from 41 breastfeeding mothers**

	No. (%) of cultures	
Bacterial groups*	Skin and nipple	Milk
Staphylococcus epidermidis	77 (94)	29 (71)
Streptococcus	17 (21)	6 (15)
Propionibacterium	10 (12)	5 (12)
Staphylococcus aureus	4 (5)	—
Pseudomonas aeruginosa	2 (2)	—
Klebsiella pneumoniae	1 (1)	2 (5)

*Two or more organisms were identified in several skin, nipple, and milk cultures.

TABLE 20-3   **Positive rate of breast milk cultures over time**

	Time of refrigeration (hr)		
Cultures	0	48	120
Positive	33	27	11
Negative	8	14	30
TOTAL	41	41	41

From Sosa R, Barness L: *Am J Dis Child* 141:111, 1987.

Factor	Shown in vitro to be active against	Effect of heat
Bifid* growth factor	Enterobacteriaceae, enteric pathogens	Stable to boiling
Secretory IgA	*Escherichia coli, E. coli* enterotoxin; *Clostridium tetani, Corynebacterium diphtheriae, Streptococcus pneumoniae, Salmonella, Shigella*	Stable at 56° C for 30 min; some loss (0%-30%) at 62.5° C for 30 min; destroyed by boiling
C1 to C9	Effect not known	Destroyed by heating at 56° C for 30 min
Lactoferrin	*E. coli, Candida albicans*	Two thirds destroyed at 62.5° C for 30 min
Lactoperoxidase	*Streptococcus, Pseudomonas, E. coli, Salmonella typhimurium*	Not known; presumably destroyed by boiling
Lysozyme	*E. coli, Salmonella, M. lysodeikticus*	Stable at 62.5° C for 30 min; activity reduced 97% by boiling for 15 min
Lipid (unsaturated fatty acid)	*Staphylococcus aureus*	Stable to boiling
Milk cells	By phagocytosis: *E. coli, C. albicans* By sensitized lymphocytes: *E. coli*	Destroyed at 62.5° C for 30 min

TABLE 20-4 Antibacterial factors in breast milk

From Welsh JK, May JT: *J Pediatr* 93:1, 1979.
Lactobacillus bifidus/Bifidobacterium bifidum.

Proteus species, and *Streptococcus faecalis*. Some milk that cannot be fed raw can be pasteurized.[69]
Other guidelines include the following:
1. A total aerobic mesophilic colony count of less than 2.5×10^6 colony-forming units (CFUs)/ml with a predominance of normal skin flora
2. A count of staphylococci of less than 1×10^5 CFUs/ml
3. No enterobacteria

Standards for pasteurization of donor milk

Milk suitable for pasteurization should meet the following minimum standards[69]:
1. A total aerobic count that does not exceed 1×10^6 CFUs/ml
2. *S. aureus* that does not exceed 1×10^3 CFUs/ml; risk of feeding heat-treated enterotoxins when *S. aureus* exceeds 1×10^6 CFUs/ml
3. Presence of organisms defined as being of fecal origin not exceeding 1×10^4 CFUs/ml

4. Presence of organisms not part of normal flora not exceeding 1×10^7 CFUs/ml
5. Presence of no unusual organisms such as *Pseudomonas aeruginosa*, spore-bearing aerobes, or spore-bearing anaerobes

Heat treatment

When human milk was pasteurized at 73° C (163° F) for 30 minutes, minimal immunoglobulins A and G (IgA, IgG), lactoferrin, lysozyme, and C3 complement remained. When the temperature was kept at 62.5° C (144.5° F) for 30 minutes, there was a loss of 23.7% of the lysozyme, 56.8% of the lactoferrin, and 34% of the IgG, but no loss of IgA, according to work done by Evans et al.[21] Similar studies of heat treatments of graded severity were carried out by Ford et al.[22] The findings were similar. Pasteurization at 62.5° C for 30 minutes *(Holder method)* reduced IgA by 20% and destroyed IgM and lactoferrin. Lysozyme was stable at 62.5° C but destroyed at 100° C, as was lactoperoxidase and the ability to bind folic acid

TABLE 20-5	Antiviral factors in breast milk	
Factor	Shown in vitro to be active against	Effect of heat
Secretory IgA	Polio virus types 1, 2, 3; coxsackievirus types A9, B3, B5; Echo virus types 6, 9; Semliki Forest virus, Ross River virus, rotavirus	Stable at 56° C for 30 min; some loss (0%-30%) at 62.5° for 30 min; destroyed by boiling
Lipid (unsaturated fatty acids and monoglycerides)	Herpes simplex, Semliki Forest virus, influenza, dengue, Ross River virus, murine leukemia virus, Japanese B encephalitis virus	Stable to boiling for 30 min
Nonimmunoglobulin macromolecules	Herpes simplex, vesicular stomatitis virus	Destroyed at 60° C; stable at 56° C for 30 min; destroyed by boiling for 30 min
	Rotavirus	Unknown
Milk cells	Induced interferon activity against Sendai virus; ? sensitized lymphocytes; ? phagocytosis	Destroyed at 62.5° C for 30 min

From Welsh JK, May JT: *J Pediatr* 93:1, 1979.

against bacterial uptake. Growth of *Escherichia coli* increased when introduced into heated milk. Vitamin B_{12}–binding capacity declined progressively with increasing temperature of the heat treatment.[24]

The effects of the Holder method on antiinfective agents were reviewed by Orloff et al,[49] who concluded that high temperatures destroyed much of the bacteriostatic effect of human milk, thus decreasing the benefit to the infant. These data raise the question of whether any heat treatment might not increase the risk of enteric infection in the infant. Ford et al[22] suggest that for batch processing, however, 62.5° C for 30 minutes may be the method of choice.

The alterations of the lymphocyte and antibody content after processing were studied by Liebhaber et al.[37,38] They, too, found significant changes with heat, including a decrease in total lymphocyte count and in specific antibody titer to *E. coli*.

Welsh and May[66] discuss antiinfective properties of breast milk and provide two tables (Tables 20-4 and 20-5) to demonstrate the stability of the antibacterial and antiviral properties of human milk.

TABLE 20-6	Remaining activity of antimicrobial proteins after pasteurization of human milk		
Temperature/time	IgA (%)	Lactoferrin (%)	Lysozyme (%)
72.0/15 sec	67	27	67
62.5° C/5 min	77	59	96
56.0° C/15 min	90	91	100

Low-temperature short-time pasteurization of human milk was reported by Wills et al[70] using the Oxford human milk pasteurizer. Heating at 56.0° C for 15 minutes destroyed over 99% of the inoculated organisms, which included *E. coli, S. aureus,* and group B β-hemolytic streptococci. The remaining activity of antimicrobial proteins after different time/temperature treatments is shown in Table 20-6.

High-temperature short-time (HTST) (72° or 87° C up to 15 seconds) treatment of human milk inoculated with endogenous bacteria and CMV rendered the milk bacteria free in 5 seconds and CMV free in 15 seconds.[28] Folic acid and vitamins B_1, B_2, B_6, and C were not affected. Bile salt–stimulated lipase (BSSL) was inactivated by these conditions. Lactoferrin and IgA and sIgA antibody activity were stable at 72° C (162° F) for 15 seconds. Lysozyme concentration and enzymatic activity were increased, suggesting that lysozyme may be sequestered in the milk (Tables 20-7 and 20-8).

Viruses in human milk

The dilemma of CMV is a significant one, because the virus does pass into the milk. In a study of postpartum women, CMV was recovered from the genital tract in 10%, from the urine in 7%, from the saliva in 2%, and from the breast milk in 30%. CMV does persist after storage at 4° C and −20° C (39° and −4° F) in some specimens.[59] It is destroyed at 62.5° C after 30 minutes.[17] Donor milk should be accepted only from CMV-negative mothers. Mothers who are seropositive may be permitted to provide for their own infants because they continue to provide the antibody protection as well.

Hepatitis virus also passes into milk, and donors should therefore be screened and be seronegative. The question of having seropositive women feed their own infants is discussed in Chapter 16.

The acquired immunodeficiency syndrome (AIDS) virus has been identified in human milk.[62,71] Most banks require that donors be HIV negative, but because seropositivity may take months to develop, some mechanism for excluding high-risk donors should be in place. On the other hand, some think that donors should not be screened. Holding all milk samples for several months may not be practical, and pasteurizing all milk may decrease the value of the nutrient. Some AIDS experts are concerned that the threat may seriously alter the future of milk banks.[39] It has been demonstrated that heat treatment kills the virus when milk is inoculated experimentally.[18]

The virus associated with HIV and human T-cell leukemia virus (HTLV) were incubated at temperatures from 37° to 60° C, and the virus titer was determined over time by a microculture infectivity assay. It required 32 minutes at 60° C to reduce the

virus titer.[42] Using the HMBANA standard of 62.5° C for 30 minutes totally destroyed the viruses. No virus could be recovered after the process even with repeated subculturing. Human milk contains one or more components that inactivate HIV-1 but that are not toxic for the cells in which the virus replicates.[49] These components are under study and are probably lipids.

Lyophilization and freezing

The impact of lyophilization was similar to that of heating, showing a decrease in total lymphocyte count and in immunoglobulin concentration and specific antibody titer to *E. coli*. (Lyophilization is the creation of a stable preparation of a biologic substance by rapid freezing and dehydration of the frozen product under high-vacuum freeze drying.)

Freezing specimens up to 4 weeks showed no change in IgA or *E. coli* antibody titer, although the lymphocyte count was decreased. The technique involved freezing to −23° C (−9° F) and thawing at 1, 2, 3, and 4 weeks. Although cells were present after freezing, they showed no viability when tested with the trypan blue stain exclusion method.

The storage of human milk at 4° C (39° F) for 48 hours caused a decrease in the concentration of milk macrophages and neutrophils but not of the lymphocytes, which also maintained their activity, according to Pittard and Bill.[51] The loss of cells may be desirable if the graft versus host reaction in a premature infant who is possibly immunodeficient is of concern.

Evans et al[21] reported their results with 3-month storage at −20° C and of freeze drying and reconstitution (lyophilization). They found no significant change in lactoferrin, lysozyme, IgA, IgG, and C3 after 3-month freezing but a small loss of IgG after lyophilization (Table 20-9).

Nutritional consequences

Initially the focus in processing human milk was the effect on its unique antiinfective properties,[29,33] but attention has been given to the nutritional consequences as well.[54] Storage for 24 hours did

TABLE 20-7   Effect of high-temperature short-time (HTST) pasteurization on selected vitamins in human milk

	Time (sec)							
	0		**1**		**3**		**15**	
	$\overline{X} \pm SD$	n	$\overline{X} \pm SD$	n	$\overline{X} \pm SD$	n	$\overline{X} \pm SD$	n
Vitamin B$_1$ (μg/ml)								
72° C	0.104 ± 0.013	9	0.098 ± 0.005	3	0.091 ± 0.008	3	0.088 ± 0.009	3
87° C			0.084 ± 0.011*	3	0.095 ± 0.027	3	ND	3
Vitamin B$_2$ (μg/ml)								
72° C	0.724 ± 0.132	9	0.75 ± 0.08	3	0.70 ± 0.09	3	0.56 ± 0.07	3
87° C			0.66 ± 0.13†	3	0.72 ± 0.22	3	ND	3
Vitamin B$_6$ (μg/ml)								
72° C	0.237 ± 0.081	9	0.27 ± 0.05	3	0.26 ± 0.025	3	0.22 ± 0.012	3
87° C			0.25 ± 0.07	3	0.26 ± 0.02	3	ND	3
Folic acid (μg/ml)								
72° C	0.106 ± 0.020	9	0.089 ± 0.005‡	3*	0.065 ± 0.018	3	0.101 ± 0.012	3
87° C			0.088 ± 0.008	3	0.080 ± 0.023	3	ND	3
Vitamin C (μg/ml)								
72° C	9.2 ± 2.4	9	11.2 ± 1.2	3	21.5 ± 3.0*	3	8.7 ± 1.7	3
87° C			16.0 ± 4.9*	3	22.5 ± 13.3	3	ND	3

From Goldblum RM, Dill CW, Albrecht TB et al: *J Pediatr* 104:380, 1984.
*$p < 0.07$.
†$p < 0.001$.
‡$p < 0.04$.

TABLE 20-8   Effect of high-temperature short-time (HTST) pasteurization on immunologic proteins in human milk

	Time (sec)							
	0		**1**		**3**		**15**	
	$\overline{X} \pm SD$	**n**	$\overline{X} \pm SD$	**n**	$\overline{X} \pm SD$	**n**	$\overline{X} \pm SD$	**n**
Lactoferrin (mg/ml)	0.67 ± 0.10	8						
72° C			0.95 ± 0.21	2	0.58 ± 0.2	3	0.83 ± 0.05	3
87° C			0.50 ± 0.02	3	0.50 ± 0.2	3	0.47 ± 0.17	2
Lysozyme (µg/ml)	15.0 ± 8.7	8						
72° C			$86.0 \pm 3.5^*$	2	78.0 ± 16.0	3†	$59.0 \pm 7.0^*$	3
87° C			$86.0 \pm 9.1^*$	3	59.0 ± 9.0	3†	36.0 ± 7.7	2
Total IgA (mg/ml)	0.37 ± 0.08	8						
72° C			0.37 ± 0.07	2	0.25 ± 0.06	3	0.3 ± 0.04	3
87° C			$0.06 \pm 0.04^*$	3	0.04 ± 0.02	3†	0.05 ± 0.03	2
sIgA Ab (reciprocal titer)	10.0 ± 4.8	7						
72° C			10.2 ± 12.4	2	10.6 ± 4.8	2	15.0 ± 3.5	3
87° C			<1	3	<1	2	<1	2

From Goldblum RM, Dill CW, Albrecht TB et al: *J Pediatr* 104:380, 1984.
n, Number of experiments.
$^*p < 0.01$.
$^†p < 0.05$.

TABLE 20-9   Effect of deep freezing (3 mo) at −20° C and lyophilization of human milk proteins (mg/dl milk)

	Raw milk (mean ± SE)	Deep-frozen milk			Lyophilized milk		
		Mean ± SE	Mean as % raw	p	Mean ± SE	Mean as % raw	p
α_1-Antitrypsin (16 samples)	2.38 ± 0.3	1.98 ± 0.2	83.2	<0.05	2.22 ± 0.3	93.3	>0.1
IgA (8 samples)	9.55 ± 0.84	9.25 ± 0.83	96.9	>0.1	9.33 ± 0.74	97.7	>0.1
IgG (16 samples)	0.42 ± 0.05	0.42 ± 0.04	100	>0.1	0.33 ± 0.04	78.6	<0.05
Lactoferrin (11 samples)	332 ± 71.7	338 ± 57.4	102	>0.1	363 ± 79	109.3	>0.1
Lysozymes (11 samples)	5.1 ± 1.26	4.6 ± 0.67	90.2	>0.1	4.8 ± 1.19	94.1	>0.1
C3 (16 samples)	1.35 ± 0.13	1.26 ± 0.11	93.3	>0.1	1.27 ± 0.13	94.1	>0.1

From Evans TJ, Ryley HC, Neale LM et al: *Arch Dis Child* 53:239, 1978.

TABLE 20-10   **Storage of human milk and protein N concentrations (mg N/dl)**

	Storage temperature		
Storage time (hr)	37° C	4° C	−72° C
4	187 ± 8*	181 ± 7*	
24	183 ± 7*†	178 ± 5*†	186 ± 8†
48	189 ± 8*	178 ± 5*	

From Garza C, Johnson CA, Harrist R et al: *Early Hum Dev* 6:295, 1982.
Mean ± 1 SM (n = 11).
*Effects from temperature significant when samples stored at 37° and 4° C are compared ($p < 0.05$, $F = 9.3$).
†Comparison of storage temperature effects on samples stored only for 24 hr not significant ($p > 0.05$, $F = 1.4$).

not affect vitamin A, zinc, iron, copper, sodium, or protein nitrogen concentrations at 37° C.[61,68] Ascorbic acid levels decreased greatly when stored at 37° C and 4° C at 24 and 48 hours. (They remained stable for 4 hours.) Other investigators have found that ascorbic acid levels drop 40% with heating.[26,61]

Levels of unsaturated fatty acids apparently are also affected by heating and cold storage, but the data need clarification.[45] It is anticipated that heating or freezing and thawing are capable of damaging membranes surrounding milk fat globules.[54] The fat globule could then undergo fragmentation and allow greater access of milk lipases to triglycerides. The percentages of polyunsaturated fatty acids, linoleic ($C_{18:2}$) and linolenate ($C_{18:3}$), decreased after both heating and freezing, while monounsaturates and saturated fatty acids were unaffected.[65] When milk is stored at −11° C over 48 hours, release of fatty acids progresses over time with an increase in the proportion of free $C_{18:2}$, $C_{20:4}$, and other long-chain polyenic acids. No measurable lipolysis occurred when milk was stored at −70° C. The higher the temperature and the longer the time, the greater is the accumulation of free fatty acids.[35] Other investigators have confirmed this, concluding the lipoprotein lipase and BSSL remain fully active at −20° C but not −70° C with or without presence of serum. Berkow et al[8] therefore recommend that milk be stored at −70° C. Other enzymes were not affected by freezing and storing except lactoperoxidase, which lost activity (Tables 20-10 and 20-11).

TABLE 20-11   **Thermal destruction of milk components (follows first-order reaction kinetics)**

	D value* at 60° C (sec)	Z value†
IgA	4.9×10^4	5.5°C
Lactoferrin	2.4×10^3	4.7°C
Thiamine	7.7×10^5	28.4°C
Folic acid	1.9×10^4	6.4°C

Modified from Morgan JN, Toledo RT, Eitenmiller RR et al: *J Food Sci* 51:348, 1986.
*90% degradation at 60° C in seconds.
†Temperature change to alter degradation rate by a factor of 10.

Because the nourishment of low-birthweight (LBW) infants has been the purpose of many milk banks, the ability of preterm infants to utilize treated bank milk is relative. Pasteurization at 62.5° C for 30 minutes was reported not to influence nitrogen absorption or retention in LBW infants.[54] When raw, pasteurized, and boiled human milks were fed to very-LBW (VLBW) (less than 1.3 kg) preterm infants in three separate consecutive weeks, fat absorption was reduced by one third in the heat-treated group. There was a reduction in the amount of nitrogen retained in the heat-treated group as well, although the absorption was unaffected. The absorption and retention of calcium, phosphorus, and sodium were unaffected by heating or freezing. The mean weight gain was greater by one third when the infants were fed raw human milk.[68,69]

Pasteurization decreased vitamin B_{12} by about 50% and folate-binding capacity by 10%[47] (Table 20-11). Sterilization (100° C for 20 minutes), on the other hand, had similar effects on B_{12} binding and completely inactivated folate binding.[61] Vitamins A, D, E, B_2, and B_6, choline, niacin, and pantothenic acid were barely affected by pasteurization, whereas thiamine was reduced up to 25%, biotin up to 10%, and vitamin C up to 35%.[64]

Refrigeration at 4° to 6° C for 72 hours allows little bacterial growth and causes no change in nutrients or infection-protective properties. Freezing does have some effect on both, and the milk can be kept for months, whereas heating has significant effect, and the milk still requires freezing for storage. Experience feeding donated raw milk to newborns has shown no ill effects if carefully monitored, according to Björksten et al.[9] Quick freezing and frozen storage do not significantly affect levels of biotin, niacin, folic acid, vitamin E, and the fat-soluble vitamins. Photooxidation and absorption by the container or tubing are always a consideration. Vitamin C is reduced by both these processes.[25]

The effect of heating and freezing on the various constituents of human milk has been studied by a number of investigators. Their data should be considered before deciding how to store milk for special purposes.

Routine analysis of the nutrient value of milk samples is often not practical, so gross screening by creamatocrit has been done by some banks and nurseries. A method of infrared (IR) analysis using a Milko-Scan 104 IR Analyzer (A/S Foss Electric) has been described by Michaelsen et al.[44] It is simpler and more rapid than previous methods. These investigators found a linear correlation between IR results and the standard reference methods of Kjeldahl for nitrogen (protein), Roese Gottlieb for fat, and bomb calorimetry for energy. These techniques were used on all incoming milk and on the outgoing pooled milk.

All the milk from the same mother was thawed, pooled, and stirred vigorously on arrival at the bank. A 10-ml sample was taken and stored at −25° C until analysis. Samples were collected every 2 weeks and were analyzed up to 2 to 3 weeks after expression. For the 2554 collections of milk contributed by 224 women, the mean protein content was 9 g/L and the fat was 39 g/L. The greater the body mass index of the mother, the greater was the protein and fat content.

The authors suggest that by selecting the milk with the highest protein content (12 g/L), a high-protein milk can be created with a higher energy content (725 kcal/L) for use in the VLBW infant. Furthermore, they recommend pooling milk from up to five mothers to decrease the variability in nutrient levels.[44]

At the Hvidovre Milk Bank in Copenhagen, monitoring of the macronutrients in donor milk is part of the bank's quality assurance standards, and donors are discontinued if their milk protein content falls below 8 g/L. Their milk was viewed adequate for their own baby but not for high-risk infants, especially premature infants.

Creamatocrit

Testing milk for protein, fat, and carbohydrate is not necessary and is costly and time consuming. However, Lucas et al[40] have suggested a quick method of analysis. It involves standard hematocrit microtubes and a centrifuge. The percentage of cream, or "creamatocrit," is read from the capillary tube. Fat and energy content have a linear relationship, as follows:

$$\text{Fat (g/L)} = \frac{(\text{Creamatocrit [\%]}) - 0.59}{0.146}$$

$$\text{kcal/L} = 290 + (66.8 \times \text{Creamatocrit [\%]})$$

Accuracy is within 10%.

The Research Institute for Health Sciences provides the following formula for calculating the fat and energy content of milk using the measurement of the creamatocrit (%)[55]:

$$\text{Fat (g/L)} = (6.24 \times \text{Creamatocrit [\%]}) - 3.08$$

$$[r = 0.98, 95\% \text{ confidence limit} = \pm 4.39 \text{ g/L}]$$

$$\text{kcal/dl} = (5.57 \times \text{Creamatocrit [\%]}) + 45.13$$

$$[r = 0.92, 95\% \text{ confidence limit} = \pm 12.61 \text{ kcal/dl}]$$

Studies done comparing energy value calculated by creamatocrit with energy value from percentage of carbon, as measured by Manchester Bomb Calorimeter using pooled pasteurized milk samples, were somewhat inaccurate compared with data obtained by creamatocrit on fresh or fresh-frozen samples.[56]

The methodology was validated with further analysis by Lemons et al,[36] who repeated the studies and confirmed actual measurements of total fat and caloric content. Because the protein and lactose content remains relatively constant over time, the variation in fat content is the primary constituent affecting caloric value of the milk. Neither freezing for up to 2 months nor pasteurization affected the creamatocrit. There was no evidence of fat globule degradation during storage that affected the test.

Special cautions while performing this simple test should include the following:
- Use a representative, well-mixed sample.
- Complete a sample of pumping from at least one breast; do not take just a spot sample.
- Use a well-mixed 24-hour sample.
- Use tube at least three-fourths filled; seal one end.
- Centrifuge for 15 minutes in standard table-top centrifuge.
- Do not include the occasional small layer of liquid fat on top (free fatty acids).
- Keep tube vertical.
- Make measurement within 1 hour of centrifugation.

Ultrasonic homogenization

Pooling specimens of human milk may not result in a milk of uniform fat content after storage. The separation of fat during processing, storage, and administration by continuous nasogastric infusion, whether by gravity flow or continuous mechanical pump, results in significant loss of fat and variation in the milk received (47.4% of fat with slow infusion and 16.8% with fast infusion).

Homogenization by ultrasonic treatment was studied by Martinez et al,[41] who found that changes in fat concentration during infusion and loss of fat during administration, caused by the fat

sticking to the container and tubes, were eliminated. Furthermore, the fat-soluble vitamins are preserved. Because 31% of iron, 15% of copper, 12% of zinc, 10% of calcium, and 2% of magnesium sulfate are in the fat fraction of both human and cow's milk, preserving the fat is essential to maximizing nutrient intake from human milk, especially in compromised infants. Tube feedings have been noted to reduce vitamins B_2, B_6, A, and C in human milk.

Ultrasonic homogenization was accomplished in this study by subjecting the milk to treatment in a Tekmar Sonic Disruptor TSD-P 250 (Tekmar Co., Cincinnati, Ohio). The homogenization time (2, 4, or 8 minutes) is a function of the volume of milk and intensity of vibration. The procedure should be done with milk in an ice bath.

Microwave effects

The milk should be thawed in the refrigerator, and each bottle should be used completely within 24 hours. Defrosting in the microwave oven may lead to separation of layers, and microwaves decrease vitamin C content. The greatest danger of microwaving is that the milk heats and the container does not, so that an infant could be burned or the milk significantly overheated.

The effects of microwave radiation on human milk have been much debated. The only nutritional effect identified has been the lowering of the vitamin C level. Lysozyme activity, total IgA, and specific IgA to *E. coli* serotypes 01, 04, and 06 were tested in 22 freshly frozen milk samples before and after heating for 30 seconds at low-power and high-power settings of the microwave oven.[52] Additional samples were tested at microwave low (20° to 25° C), medium (60° to 70° C), and high (98° C or higher) powers before the addition of *E. coli* suspension. Microwaving at high temperatures (72° to 98° C) greatly decreased all the tested antiinfective factors (Table 20-12). *E. coli* growth at 98° C or higher was 18 times that of untreated thawed human milk. Low temperatures did not affect total IgA or specifics IgA to *E. coli* serotypes 01 and 04 or specifics IgA to *E. coli* serotype 06. At only 20° to 25° C, the

TABLE 20-12   Impact of microwaving on antiinfective factors in human milk*

	No.	Control	Low microwave	High microwave
Lysozyme activity (μg/ml)	22	23.7 ± 4.0	19.2 ± 3.4 $p < .005$	0.9 ± 0.72 $p < .0005$
Total IgA (mg/dl)	22	73.3 ± 16.1	48.9 ± 15.8 NS†	1.55 ± 1.54 $p < 0.0005$
Antigen-specific antigen to *E. coli* serotype				
01	22	100%	91 ± 9.2‡	24.9 ± 10.0‡
04	22	100%	90.3 ± 6.5‡	12.3 ± 3.7‡
06	22	100%	79.8 ± 5.7‡ $p < 0.005$	17.1 ± 3.6‡ $p < 0.0005$

From Quan R, Yang C, Rubinstein S et al: *Pediatrics* 89:667, 1992.
*Results are mean ± SE. All significant differences were also confirmed by the Fisher's protected least significant difference test.
†Not significant.
‡Percent of control.

TABLE 20-13   Impact of microwaving on *Escherichia coli* growth in human milk at 3½ hours*

	No.	Colony count
Control	10	$8.4 \pm 2.7 \times 10^7$
Low microwave	10	$43.9 \pm 11.4 \times 10^7$†
Medium microwave	10	$90.1 \pm 24.1 \times 10^7$‡
High microwave	10	$152 \pm 43 \times 10^7$‡

From Quan R, Yang C, Rubinstein S et al: *Pediatrics* 89:667, 1992.
*Results are mean ± SE. All significant differences were also confirmed by the Fisher's protected least significant difference test.
†$p = 0.005$ compared with control.
‡$p = 0.001$ compared with control.

growth of *E. coli* was five times that of the untreated thawed milk.[52]

Microwaving clearly interferes with the antiinfective properties of human milk: the higher the temperature, the greater the effect (Table 20-13).

Specialty milks

New technologies offer the potential for providing specialty milks. Simple homogenization would preserve the fat, as noted; however, because of the presence of active enzymes, once the fat membrane is ruptured by homogenization, the milk should be used promptly to prevent excessive fat breakdown. Lyophilization or freeze drying is an opportunity to concentrate the nutrients without increasing the volume. Adding a freeze-dried aliquot to liquid human milk would be preferable to using the commercial bovine-based products. In Denmark, infrared analysis of milk donations is used to provide high-protein or high-fat pools of milk. In Canada and the United States, some banks identify donors with dairy-free diets for specific infants.[1-3]

Contamination with cow's milk

Donor milk is at risk for being contaminated with cow's milk by the donor. The California Mother's Milk Bank checks its contributions with a simple test directed at precipitating the casein. They mix 1 ml of donor milk with 1 ml of $8N$ sulfuric acid and 8 ml of water, and let it sit at room temperature for 5 hours. If cow's milk is present, it will precipitate.[48]

Changing flavors of stored milk

Women have reported to the Lactation Study Center that their fresh-frozen breast milk smells sour and even rancid and is rejected by their infant. Although a slightly soapy odor had sometimes been noted, it had never been reported to be harmful or to be rejected by the infant. This soapy smell has been attributed to a change in the lipid structure associated with the freeze-thaw effects of the self-defrost cycle in the freezer-refrigerator.

The cases reported to the center, however, have suggested true lipid breakdown is associated with the rancid smell. The speculation was that some women have more lipase activity than others, as noted in the study of lipase and hyperbilirubinemia. Some mothers reported that their milk began to smell as soon as it cooled, whether refrigerated or frozen. Others have noted that their stockpile of milk, meticulously stored in anticipation of returning to work, was rancid and rejected by their infant. When these mothers heated their milk to a scald (not boiling) immediately after collection and then quickly cooled and froze it, the effect was not apparent, and their infants accepted the heat-treated milk. That process inactivated the lipase and halted the process of fat digestion. On the other hand, scalding rancid milk will not improve the flavor or smell.

Financial aspects

Established milk banks have various financial structures.[6] Charges can include fees for equipment rental and for processing milk. Certainly the hospital should recover costs of collecting and processing. Precedent for this has been set in the United States. Because some states have passed legislation mandating the availability of human milk for all babies who need it, reimbursement and funds must be available for its proper handling.

All banks have a minimal charge that partially covers the cost of processing, such as labor, equipment, and supplies. As with blood banks, the recipient is not charged for the milk itself. Third-party payers do reimburse for this, and Women, Infants, and Children (WIC) programs also provide this reimbursement in more and more states.

The recommendations from the State of New York (see Appendix L) suggest that the monitoring of standards of a hospital-based bank be absorbed into existing hospital surveillance. Free-standing banks would be monitored by the state and local health departments. Economic analysis indicates that the primary costs would be administrative overhead costs. The human milk supply is considered a donated product. Also acknowledged are staff costs, minimal equipment costs, and laboratory costs, as well as costs to the state health department to administer the system. Much consideration is being given to limiting banks to hospital settings, where health professionals and equipment are readily available.

The average processing fee charged by milk banks in the United States has been $2.50 per ounce for several years, although it does not totally cover costs.[3] No infant is refused access for lack of funds, and banks cover their costs by various methods, including donations, subsidies, and grants.

BREAST-PUMPING EQUIPMENT

As noted earlier, several types of breast-pumping devices have provoked questions of the sterility of milk collected. Additional issues need to be considered, including efficiency, ease of use, potential for breast trauma, availability, and cost. A good pump should be capable of completely emptying the breast and of stimulating production. It should be clean, contamination free, easy to use, and atraumatic.

Hand pumps

The "bicycle horn" pump has been marketed in drugstores for years without instructions for use or cleaning. At the museum at the Corning Glass Works in Corning, NY, a glass and rubber hand pump made by Davol circa 1830 is on display next to glass baby bottles and pewter nipples. The current model is the same, except the glass has been replaced by plastic. The dangers of this pump are legion but can be summarized by saying the milk is contaminated, a spray of milk can go directly into the bulb, the pump requires constant emptying, and it can be quite traumatic to the nipple, areola, and breast.

Modifications of the bicycle horn pump insert a removable collecting bottle in place of the well. The modification permits feeding the infant directly from the collecting vessel by placing a nipple on it. Milk does not wash back over the breast, and pumping is not interrupted for emptying. The bulb still may harbor bacteria because it is difficult to clean. The limitations of the effect of creating a simple vacuum and applying a simple, rigid, sharp-edged flange against the breast are still present. This pump is satisfactory for temporary use, but it takes time to become proficient in its use, and it may never create enough pressure to be effective. Another model (Nurture) with a special flexible silicone funnel overcomes these problems and is available from White River Natural Technologies, Inc. Figure 20-3 illustrates application of the flange. This model uses a cylinder for suction and collection.

The cylindric pumps are two all-plastic cylindric tubes that fit inside one another to create a vacuum. A rigid flange to accommodate the nipple and areola is at the top of the inner tube, which also has a gasket for tight fit at the other end. The outer tube collects the milk and is adapted for use as a feeding unit when a nipple is screwed on top. The mother creates the vacuum by pulling the outer tube and creates rhythm by alternating pushing the outer tube in and out (Fig. 20-4). It is simple, easy to clean, and the milk is usable directly from the collecting cylinder with a nipple attached. This pump is excellent in the hands of an experienced, dextrous mother. The product has several manufacturers, and models differ slightly. Some have a choice of flanges. The only precaution is that 220 mm Hg of negative pressure can be produced if the cylinder is drawn at least three quarters of the

way out when empty or when there is fluid (pumped milk) in the cylinder. The pressure desired can be achieved by pulling out the cylinder only a fraction. Most cylinder pumps are marked by the manufacturer to indicate degree of a cycle.

The Lloyd-B pump has a trigger handle adapted to a flange mechanism that empties into a collection jar the size of a baby-food jar (not a baby bottle). It does have a vacuum relief switch; however, the entire mechanism requires a certain dexterity and a rather large hand to operate. It is portable and also easily cleaned. No parts harbor bacteria.

Electric mechanical pumps

Battery-operated pumps are available, but they have all the disadvantages of most battery-operated devices and in most cases are not sufficiently powerful to stimulate the breast adequately. They are ineffective for women whose infants are not feeding at the breast, such as premature infants or those hospitalized in an NICU. These small hand pumps work for some fully lactating women who need a pump that fits in their purse for use while at work or school.

Small, purse-size electric pumps may be effective for the fully lactating woman (Fig. 20-2). They have an advantage over a manually powered hand pump in that the electric power frees one hand for the mother to stroke the breast and encourage let-down. If flow is going well, the hand is free to perform other tasks, such as read, telephone, or write, not an insignificant advantage for a busy, working, breastfeeding woman. The small electric models have a small hole in the flange base that must be closed with a finger to develop the suction, as in most hospital suctioning devices. This gives the mother control over the pressure. By rhythmically opening and closing the hole with the finger, the operator can simulate milking action that is very effective in extracting milk. The manufacturers, unfortunately, do not always point this out.

Hand-held mechanical devices may not be enough for the woman trying to build up a supply when the infant cannot stimulate the breast

Fig. 20-3.   A, *Step 1*. Apply soft flange to ensure proper positioning and comfort. Evert flange back over base. Soft flange has advantage of close application and gentle massaging (milking) of areola and nipple to create a teat. **B,** *Step 2*. Apply everted flange squarely over nipple for careful placement, and fold flange back over areola. **C,** *Step 3*. Attach flange to hand pump or electric pump.

directly. A new mother may become quite discouraged at the low volume of her production and discontinue the process. Part of the management of a sick infant is to be sure that the mother's milk production is also progressing. Most hospitals provide a lactation consultant for lactating women with babies in the NICU or have trained the unit's nursing staff to provide assistance. Large NICUs in the United States provide a room with electric pumps for the mothers of NICU infants to learn

Fig. 20-4. Cylindric pump in use.

how to pump their milk and breastfeed their infants.

Full-size electric pumps are the most efficient because the motor applies the mechanical effort. The mother can concentrate on applying the cup to her breast, massaging the breast, and relaxing so that adequate let-down can take place. All electric pumps are not equal, and some guidance is needed to be sure that the mother understands the principles involved. Nursery staff should be familiar with the equipment. The pumps are no challenge to skilled NICU nurses, who are adept at handling much more complicated electronic equipment.

A pump that cycles pressure instead of maintaining constant negative pressure will be less likely to cause petechiae or internal trauma to the breast. The ultimate effect of pressure also depends on the length of time the pressure is applied. Tissue cannot withstand sustained high pressure. Pressure sustained for 2 seconds or at a rate of 30 pumps per minute is considered maximum time or minimum rate.[19] Negative pressures should have a governing mechanism to avoid excessive pressures. Mean sucking pressures of most normal full-term infants range from −50 to −155, with a maximum up to −220 mm Hg/in^2. Manufacturers recommend

about 200 mm Hg/in^2 to initiate flow in most women.

A careful study by Johnson[34] of over 1000 patients at the University of Texas using a variety of pumps has confirmed some facts about pumps. The amount of negative pressure possible and the control mechanisms were recorded (Tables 20-14 and 20-15).

An increasing number of pumps on the market have similar designs, but each has its special nuances. A standard electric pump capable of cycling pressures to 220 mm Hg (2.5 to 8.5 psi/Hg) is usually required to stimulate production de novo, that is, when infant is unavailable to suckle directly as a small premature infant on a ventilator in the NICU. Smaller electric pumps are effective in pumping milk at work when this is done daily. The various hand models can be used for the occasional pumping.[23]

Breast pumps have been identified repeatedly as the source of infection.[46] Improvement in design with a safety trap between the collecting vessel and the machine to prevent milk getting into the mechanism is important. In addition, all equipment that comes in contact with milk or the breast should be sterilizable and/or disposable. The well-designed electric pump properly used is the best system for stimulating lactation and increasing volume.

In the hospital, as with all special equipment, it is advisable to select the best equipment to fill the needs of that hospital and then purchase the same model so that staff can learn how to use it properly and can instruct the patient.

Similarly, the equipment should be checked on a routine basis, cleaned, and bacteriologically tested. Accessory equipment (disposable) can be resterilized for the same patient but not for a second patient.

Although attention is usually given to the pressure mechanisms, equally important is the cup or flange that is applied to the breast. The diameter and depth of the flare are fixed for the hand pumps and the Gomco electric pump, but a choice is offered for the Egnell, Medela, and White River pumps (Fig. 20-5). The nipple should have room to be drawn out, and the flange should be adequate

TABLE 20-14	**Electric pumping devices**	
Mechanical pump	**Advantages**	**Disadvantages**
All mechanical pumps	More efficient than hand or battery powered Can rent Should be covered by insurance Well serviced by company	Expensive
Hollister-Egnell	Rhythmic vacuum Stimulates nursing Helpful in initiating let-down Simulates rhythm of suckling Disposable tubing and collecting cups Has double-pumping capability Accessory equipment readily available	

Gomco/Sorenson	Good visibility
	Good collection vessel
		Adapted from suction
		  apparatus
		Poor cup design—painful
		Operates on negative
		  pressure
		Continuous negative pressure
		  can run too high
		Finger control of T-tube
		  needed to cycle vacuum
		Hard to control
		Not good for long use
		Noisy

TABLE 20-14	Electric pumping devices—cont'd	
Mechanical pump	**Advantages**	**Disadvantages**
Medela	Comfortable Automatic cycling Adjustable vacuum Double or single pump	
Classic electric breast pump Heavy duty for hospital use (available to rent)		
Lactina Select electric breast pump Light, portable, economical		

Continued

TABLE 20-14   **Electric pumping devices—cont'd**

Mechanical pump	Advantages	Disadvantages
White River Concepts electric breast pump	Flexible silastin flange (Soft-Cup Funnel) Automatic cycling Variable vacuum control Minimal assembly Sturdy carrying case Hospital grade/rental grade Single or double pump kits Easy to clean between rentals Model 9050	Simple appearance

Attachment for double pumping also available

to transmit pressure or milking action to the collecting ampullae under the areola. The hand pumps are too small; however, bigger is not always better, and a mother may find that the smaller model of the two offered may be more suited physiologically to her anatomy. This feature does not corre-

late directly with overall size of breast. The ideal range is 68- to 82-mm outer diameter and 35- to 40-mm depth of flare[34] (Fig. 20-5). The White River and the Nurture silicone funnels adapt well to all sizes and shapes because of their flexibility. Instructions for the White River soft flange sug-

TABLE 20-14	Electric pumping devices—cont'd	
Mechanical pump	**Advantages**	**Disadvantages**
Automatic breast pump (for use with hospital wall suction)	Flexible silastin flange (Soft-Cup Funnel) Automatic cycling, variable vacuum Single patient use at bedside Minimizes possibility of user cross contamination Single or double pumping capability Adjustable from low to high levels Low maintenance Impact-resistant internal components Convenient and sanitary bedside pumping Can be rented in most countries	Limited to hospital use

gests moistening the flange with milk or water to allow the nipple and areola to adapt well to the flange and the shaft.

The relative efficacy of four methods of human milk expression was measured by Green et al.[31] The electric pump (Egnell) enabled mothers to pump significantly more milk with higher fat content in the 10-minute time allotted for the study than did the Lloyd-B, the Evenflo hand pump, or manual expression, all three of which were about equal in efficacy.

To understand the ability of various pumps to

TABLE 20-15   Hand pumping devices

Hand pump	Advantages	Disadvantages
Bicycle horn	Inexpensive Portable	Difficult to clean Bulb retains bacteria Works as vacuum No instructions Can cause trauma Not appropriate for donor milk Milk washes back over nipple Requires constant emptying Not recommended
Evenflo	Inexpensive	Difficult to clean; bulb harbors bacteria even when boiled

White River	Pliable flange Can feed baby from collecting container Works well for less experienced mother with good let-down No milk contacts mechanism	

TABLE 20-15 Hand pumping devices—cont'd		
Hand pump	**Advantages**	**Disadvantages**
Cylindric: two all-plastic cylindric tubes fit inside one another to create vacuum; inner tube has flange at top and rubber or nylon gasket	Less expensive than electric Portable Can feed baby from collecting container Easily cleaned and sterilized	Requires some dexterity Works as vacuum with some rhythm Rigid flange Can achieve >220 mm Hg of pressure Must follow instructions

Lloyd: glass flange attached to collecting jar; trigger handle mechanism creates vacuum; has vacuum relief switch	Less expensive than electric Portable Can be cleaned No milk contacts mechanism	Handle difficult to squeeze Hand becomes cramped Awkward Large breast and nipple may hit flange Transfer of milk to feeding unit necessary

Continued

Hand pump	Advantages	Disadvantages
Ameda-Egnell, one handed	Spring-loaded handle Each pumping action requires only one motion of energy per pump Squeeze provides suction "Ergonomically" correct Avoids muscle cramping Cleans easily	Awkward
Battery operated (several brands available)	One-handed operation Portable Milk collected in feeding container Intermittent suction release bar Adequate in good lactator who wants to pump a little once a day or less	Not adequate to stimulate production Limited pressure curve Need infant to be feeding at most feeds to stimulate breast

TABLE 20-15 Hand pumping devices—cont'd

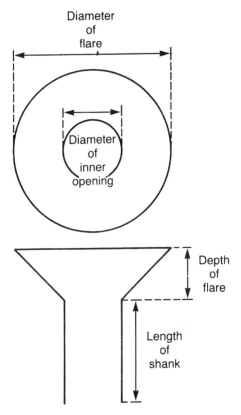

Fig. 20-5. Measurement of nipple cups. (From Johnson CA: *Clin Pediatr* 22:40, 1983.)

Fig. 20-6. Mean serum prolactin (PRL) levels for each of five expression methods. Data given as mean ± SEM. ▲, Infant; □, White River Electric; ○, Medela Manualelectric; ■, hand expression; △, Gentle Expression Battery. (Modified from Zinaman MJ, Hughes V, Queenan JT et al: *Pediatrics* 89:437, 1992.)

stimulate lactation and enhance milk volume in the maintenance of lactation, Zinaman[72] et al[73] studied milk yield, prolactin levels, and oxytocin. Twenty-three women exclusively breastfeeding were randomly assigned to use three different pumping methods serially and compare them with the suckling effectiveness of their infants. Blood samples were collected every 10 minutes from a previously inserted intravenous line controlled with a heparin lock. An electric pump (White River), pulsatile on medium settings of 180 mm Hg and autocycled at 40 pumps per minute, was used with double setup. The Medela manual pump was cycled by the user at 40 times per minute; pressures of 220 mm Hg were used 15 minutes on both breasts simultaneously. The Gentle Expressions battery-operated pump achieved suction levels of 110 mm Hg and

was cycled 6 to 10 times per minute by the subject, individually pumping each side for 15 minutes. Hand expression was performed by the Marmet method (see Appendix G). Testing was done over 7 days, at 10 AM, at least 2½ hours after the infant's last feeding. Blood was collected at −15, 0, 10, 20, 30, 40, 50, and 60 minutes. Serum prolactin and plasma oxytocin tests were performed simultaneously on all samples, which had been previously separated and frozen.

Prolactin levels were highest with the pulsatile electric pump compared with those of the infant's suckling, actually exceeding levels created by the infant. The hand pumps were similar to hand expression, with the battery-operated pump achieving the lowest levels (Figs. 20-6 and 20-7). No difference was seen in the oxytocin response, although the levels increased before feeding when the baby fed but not when the breast was pumped (Table 20-16). The mean volumes obtained were similar, with the pulsatile electric pump reaching 175 ml over 60 minutes, the manual pump 125 ml over 60 minutes, the battery-operated pump 110 ml over 60 minutes, and hand expression 75 ml over 60 minutes. Marked differences were seen in the

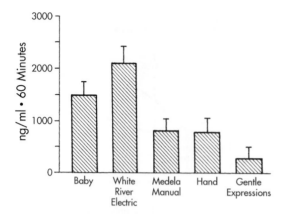

Fig. 20-7. Serum prolactin results, with breast stimulation calculated as mean net area under curves for each of five methods. Data given as mean ± SEM. (Modified from Zinaman MJ, Hughes V, Queenan JT et al: *Pediatrics* 89:437, 1992.)

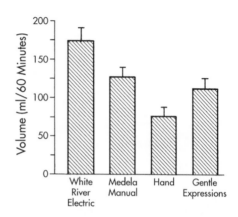

Fig. 20-8. Mean milk volumes obtained with breast stimulation for four of the five expression methods (infant not included). Data given as mean ± SEM. (Modified from Zinaman MJ, Hughes V, Queenan JT et al: *Pediatrics* 89:437, 1992.)

TABLE 20-16	**Oxytocin results***	
Method	**Mean net AUC**	**SEM**
Infant	224.7	75.4
White River Electric	174.1	41.3
Medela Manual	218.5	157.5
Hand expression	140.5	66.5
Gentle Expression Battery	186.7	67.6

*Levels of plasma oxytocin with breast stimulation calculated as mean net area under the curves (AUC) for each of the five methods over the 60-minute sampling session. No significant differences were noted. (From Zinaman M, Hughes V, Queenan JT et al: *Pediatrics* 89:437, 1992.)

pumps' ability to produce an acute and sustained response, and differences in time were required to achieve the ultimate volume (Fig. 20-8). The differences were related to the method of pumping (i.e., electric, battery operated, manual) and not to comparison of brands.

A complete assessment of all the pumps readily available on the market and details about other equipment for breastfeeding are provided in the *Breastfeeding Product Guide* by Kittie Frantz.*

*Geddes Productions, 10546 McVine Ave., Sunland, CA 91040 USA.

REFERENCES

1. Arnold LDW: The statistical state of human milk banking and what's in the future, *J Hum Lact* 7:25, 1991.
2. Arnold LDW: How North American donor milk banks operate: results of a survey. I, *J Hum Lact* 13:159, 1997.
3. Arnold LDW: How North American donor milk banks operate: results of a survey. II, *J Hum Lact* 13:234, 1997.
4. Arnold LDW, Tully MR: *Guidelines for the establishment and operation of a human milk bank,* West Hartford, Conn, 1992, Human Milk Bank Association of North America.

5. Asquith MT, Pedrotti PW, Stevenson DK et al: Clinical uses, collection, and banking of human milk, *Clin Perinatol* 14:173, 1987.
6. Balmer SE, Wharton BA: Human milk banking at Sorrento Maternity Hospital, Birmingham, *Arch Dis Child* 67:556, 1992.
7. Beerens H, Romond C, Neut C: Influence of breastfeeding on the bifid flora of the newborn intestine, *Am J Clin Nutr* 33:2434, 1980.

8. Berkow SE, Freed LM, Hamosh M et al: Lipases and lipids in human milk: effects of freeze-thawing and storage, *Pediatr Res* 18:1257, 1984.

9. Björksten B, Burman LG, DeChateau P et al: Collecting and banking human milk: to heat or not to heat? *Br Med J* 281:765, 1980.

10. Carroll L, Osman M, Davies DP: Does discarding the first few milliliters of breast milk improve the bacteriological quality of bank breast milk? *Arch Dis Child* 55:898, 1980.

11. Carroll L, Osman M, Davies DP et al: Bacteriological criteria for feeding raw breast-milk to babies on neonatal units, *Lancet* 2:732, 1979.

12. Committee on Mother's Milk, American Academy of Pediatrics: Operation of mother's milk bureaus, *J Pediatr* 23:112, 1943.

13. Committee on Nutrition, American Academy of Pediatrics: Human milk banking, *Pediatrics* 68:854, 1980.

14. Cruz JR, Gil L, Cano F et al: Protection by breastfeeding against gastrointestinal infection and disease in infancy. In Atkinson SA, Hanson LA, Chandra RK, editors: *Nutrition, infection and infant growth in developed and emerging countries,* Saint John's, Newfoundland, Canada, 1990, Arts Biomedical Publishers.

15. Davidson DC, Poll RA, Roberts G: Bacteriological monitoring of unheated human milk, *Arch Dis Child* 54:760, 1979.

16. Donowitz LG, Marsik FJ, Fisher KA et al: Contaminated breast milk: a source of *Klebsiella* bacteremia in a newborn intensive care unit, *Rev Infect Dis* 3:716, 1981.

17. Dworsky M, Stagno S, Pass RF et al: Persistence of cytomegalovirus in human milk after storage, *J Pediatr* 101:440, 1982.

18. Eglin RP, Wilkinson AR: HIV infection and pasteurization of breast milk, *Lancet* 1:1093, 1987.

19. Egnell E: The mechanics of different methods of emptying the female breast, *J Swedish Med Assoc* 40:1, 1956.

20. Eidelman AI, Szilagyi G: Patterns of bacterial colonization of human milk, *Obstet Gynecol* 53:550, 1979.

21. Evans TJ, Ryley HC, Neale LM et al: Effect of storage and heat on antimicrobial proteins in human milk, *Arch Dis Child* 53:239, 1978.

22. Ford JE, Law BA, Marshall VM et al: Influence of heat treatment of human milk on some of its protective constituents, *J Pediatr* 90:29, 1977.

23. Frantz K: *Breastfeeding product guide,* Sunland, Calif, 1994, Geddes Productions.

24. Freier S, Faber J: Loss of immune components during the processing of human milk. In Williams AF, Baum J, editors: *Human milk banking,* New York, 1984, Nestle Nutrition, Vevey/Raven.

25. Friend BA, Shahani KM, Long CA et al: The effect of processing and storage on key enzymes, B vitamins, and lipids of mature human milk. I. Evaluation of fresh samples and effects of freezing and frozen storage, *Pediatr Res* 17:61, 1983.

26. Garza C, Johnson CA, Harrist R et al: Effects of methods of collection and storage on nutrients in human milk, *Early Hum Dev* 6:295, 1982.

27. Gibbs JH, Fisher C, Bhattacharya S et al: Drip breast milk: its composition, collection and pasteurization, *Early Hum Dev* 1:227, 1977.

28. Goldblum RM, Dill CW, Albrecht TB et al: Rapid high-temperature treatment of human milk, *J Pediatr* 104:380, 1984.

29. Goldblum RM, Goldblum AS, Garza C et al: Human milk banking. II. Relative stability of immunologic factors in stored colostrum, *Acta Paediatr Scand* 71:143, 1982.

30. Golden J: From wet nurse directory to milk bank: the delivery of human milk in Boston, 1909-1927, *Bull His Med* 62:589, 1988.

31. Green D, Moye L, Schreiner RL et al: The relative efficacy of four methods of human milk expression, *Early Hum Dev* 6:153, 1982.

32. Hamosh M, Ellis LA, Pollock DR et al: Breastfeeding and the working mother: effect of time and temperature of short-term storage on proteolysis, lipolysis, and bacterial growth in milk, *Pediatrics* 97:492, 1996.

33. Hernandez J, Lemons P, Lemons J et al: Effect of storage processes on the bacterial growth-inhibiting activity of human breast milk, *Pediatrics* 63:597, 1979.

34. Johnson CA: An evaluation of breast pumps currently available on the American market, *Clin Pediatr* 22:40, 1983.

35. Lavine M, Clark RM: Changing patterns of free fatty acids in breast milk during storage, *J Pediatr Gastroenterol Nutr* 6:769, 1987.

36. Lemons JA, Schreiner RL, Gresham EL: Simple method for determining the caloric and fat content of human milk, *Pediatrics* 66:626, 1980.

37. Liebhaber M, Lewiston NJ, Asquith MT et al: Alterations of lymphocytes and antibody content of human milk after processing, *J Pediatr* 91:897, 1977.

38. Liebhaber M, Lewiston NJ, Asquith MT et al: Comparison of bacterial contamination with two methods of human milk collection, *J Pediatr* 92:236, 1978.

39. Lucas A: Human milk banks, *Lancet* 1:103, 1982.

40. Lucas A, Gibbs JAH, Lyster RLJ et al: Creamatocrit: simple clinical technique for estimating fat concentration and energy value of human milk, *Br Med J* 1:1018, 1978.

41. Martinez FE, Desai ID, Davidson AGF et al: Ultrasonic homogenization of expressed human milk to prevent fat loss during tube feeding, *J Pediatr Gastroenterol Nutr* 6:593, 1987.

42. McDougal JS, Martin LS, Cort SP et al: Thermal inactivation of the acquired immunodeficiency syndrome virus, human T lymphotropic virus-III/lymphadenopathy-associated virus, with special reference to antihemophilic factor, *J Clin Invest* 76:875, 1985.

43. McEnery G, Chattopadhyay B: Human milk bank in a district general hospital, *Br Med J* 2:794, 1978.

44. Michaelsen KF, Skafte L, Badsberg JH et al: Variation in macronutrients in human bank milk: influencing factors and implications for human milk banking, *J Pediatr Gastroenterol Nutr* 11:229, 1990.

45. Moffatt PA, Lammi-Keefe CJ, Ferris AM et al: Alpha and gamma tocopherols in pooled mature human milk after storage, *J Pediatr Gastroenterol Nutr* 6:225, 1987.

46. Moloney AC, Quoraishi AH, Parry P et al: A bacteriological examination of breast pumps, *J Hosp Infect* 9:169, 1987.

47. Morgan JN, Toledo RT, Eitenmiller RR et al: Thermal destruction of immunoglobulin A, lactoferrin, thiamin, and folic acid in human milk, *J Food Sci* 51:348, 1986.

48. Mother's Milk Unit, California Transplant Bank: *Procedures and protocols,* San Jose, Calif, 1988, The Mother's Milk Bank, The Institute for Medical Research.

49. Orloff SL, Wallingford JC, McDougal JS: Inactivation of human immunodeficiency virus type I in human milk: effects of intrinsic factors in human milk and of pasteurization, *J Hum Lact* 9:300, 1993.

50. Paxson CI, Cress CC: Survival of human milk leukocytes, *J Pediatr* 94:61, 1979.

51. Pittard WB, Bill K: Human milk banking: effect of refrigeration on cellular components, *Clin Pediatr* 20:31, 1981.

52. Quan R, Yang C, Rubinstein S et al: Effects of microwave radiation on anti-infective factors in human milk, *Pediatrics* 89:667, 1992.

53. Reynolds GJ, Lewis-Jones DI, Isherwood DM et al: A simplified system of human milk banking, *Early Hum Dev* 7:281, 1982.

54. Schmidt E: Effects of varying degrees of heat treatment on milk protein and its nutritional consequences, *Acta Paediatr Scand Suppl* 296:41, 1982.

55. Silprasert A, Dejsarai W, Keawvichit R et al: Effect of storage on the creamatocrit and total energy content of human milk, *Hum Nutr Clin Nutr* 40C:31, 1986.

56. Smith L, Bickerton J, Pilcher G et al: Creamatocrit, carbon content, and energy value of pooled banked human milk: implications for feeding preterm infants, *Early Hum Dev* 11:75, 1985.

57. Sosa R, Barness L: Bacterial growth in refrigerated human milk, *Am J Dis Child* 141:111, 1987.

58. Springer S: Human milk banking Germany, *J Hum Lact* 13:65, 1997.

59. Stagno S, Reynolds DW, Pass RF: Breast milk and the risk of cytomegalovirus infection, *N Engl J Med* 302:1073, 1980.

60. Stocks RJ, Davies DP, Carroll LP et al: A simple method to improve the energy value of bank human milk, *Early Hum Dev* 8:175, 1983.

61. Sunshine P, Asquith MT, Liebhaber M: The effects of collection and processing on various components of human milk. In Frier S, Eidelman AI, editors: *Human milk: its biological and social value,* Amsterdam, 1980, Excerpta Medica.

62. Thiry L, Sprecher-Goldberger S, Jonckheer T et al: Isolation of AIDS virus from cell-free breast milk of three healthy virus carriers, *Lancet* 2:891, 1985.

63. Tyson JE, Edwards WH, Rosenfeld AM et al: Collection methods and contamination of bank milk, *Arch Dis Child* 57:396, 1982.

64. Van Zoeren-Grobben D, Schrijver J, Van Den Berg H et al: Human milk vitamin content after pasteurisation, storage or tube feeding, *Arch Dis Child* 62:161, 1987.

65. Wardell JM, Hill CM, D'Souza SW: Effect of pasteurization and of freezing and thawing human milk on its triglyceride content, *Acta Paediatr Scand* 70:467, 1981.

66. Welsh JK, May JT: Anti-infective properties of breast milk, *J Pediatr* 93:1, 1979.

67. WHO/UNICEF joint statement: Meeting on infant and young child feedings, *J Nurs Midwife* 25:31, 1980.

68. Williamson S, Finucane E, Ellis H et al: Effect of heat treatment of human milk on absorption of nitrogen, fat, sodium, calcium, and phosphorus by preterm infants, *Arch Dis Child* 53:555, 1978.

69. Williamson S, Hewitt JH, Finucane E et al: Organisation of bank of raw and pasteurised human milk for neonatal intensive care, *Br Med J* 1:393, 1978.

70. Wills ME, Han VEM, Harris DA et al: Short-time low-temperature pasteurisation of human milk, *Early Hum Dev* 7:71, 1980.

71. Ziegler JB, Cooper DA, Johnson RO et al: Post-natal transmission of AIDS-associated retrovirus from mother to infant, *Lancet* 1:896, 1985.

72. Zinaman MJ: Breast pumps: ensuring mother's success, *Contemp Obstet Gynecol* 32:55, 1988.

73. Zinaman MJ, Hughes V, Queenan JT et al: Acute prolactin, oxytocin responses and milk yield to infant suckling and artificial methods of expression in lactating women, *Pediatrics* 89:437, 1992.

21

$\mathcal{B}$reastfeeding support groups and community resources

Certain changes in cultural aspects of Western civilization have contributed to the widespread use of artificial feedings for human infants as well as to the changing structure of the family. Urbanization has been associated not only with industrialization but also with the separation of generations. This has produced the nuclear family. *Nuclear families* are smaller, mobile, isolated families often stranded in a large urban population. The young couple and their new infant are totally without personal human resources. That is, no one cares enough to give individual support to the family. There is no one to turn to and from whom to receive advice, encouragement, and support.

HISTORIC PERSPECTIVE

Rites de passage were described by the French author Van Gennep[28] as the ceremonies and rituals that mark special changes in people's lives. The list includes marriage, motherhood, birth, death, circumcision, graduation, ordination, and retirement. In our present culture, support exists for most of these events except birth and motherhood. The most critical rite of passage in a woman's life, Raphael[19] points out, is when she becomes a mother. Raphael further distinguishes this period of transition with the term *matrescence*, "to empha-

size the mother and to focus on her new life-style." Traditional cultures herald a mother giving birth, whereas our culture announces the birth of an infant. The former highlights the mother, the latter the infant. Matrescence is a time of coddling. In preindustrial societies, the mother is coddled for some time after birth, having only the responsibility of the infant's care while the mother's needs are met by doulas. Mothering the mother should be part of the postpartum support for a new mother.

A number of other forces added momentum to the bottle-feeding trend that began in the 1920s, when manufacturers finally were able to mass-produce an inexpensive container and rubber nipple with which to feed infants inexpensively. *Pediatrics* was a new specialty to guard the health of children. The stress was on measuring and calculating. Physicians seemed more secure when they could prescribe nutrition. The rise in the female labor force has also been credited with having an impact on the method of feeding infants, who were no longer brought everywhere with the mother to be nursed but instead were left behind to be bottle fed. The technology of the infant food industry was a continuing influence on nutritional thinking of both medical and lay groups.

Breastfeeding was never totally abandoned. There was always a group of women who prepared themselves for childbirth and read and researched feeding and nutrition and chose to breastfeed.[17] In the mid-1940s, Dr. Edith Jackson began the Rooming-In Project in New Haven, Conn. Families in New Haven who sought "childbirth without fear" and an opportunity to room-in with their infants usually chose to breastfeed. In the rooming-in unit, breastfeeding was often "contagious" because one mother successfully nursing would encourage others to try. Hospital stays averaged 5 to 7 days, during which time the mother-infant couple was cared for as a pair. About 70% of the patients left the hospital breastfeeding.

Students and staff who were exposed to the philosophy of this unit went to many parts of the country, taking with them tremendous commitment to prepared childbirth and nurturing through breastfeeding. The classic article on the management of breastfeeding by Barnes et al[2] was published as a result of counseling hundreds of nursing mothers. The students of Jackson inoculated many hundreds of hospitals and communities with a zeal for breastfeeding.

DEVELOPMENT OF MOTHER SUPPORT GROUPS

The need remained for nuclear families to have access to support and conversation about healthy infants, mothering, and breastfeeding.[6] The La Leche League, developed by a group of seven mothers to meet these needs, was established in Franklin Park, Ill, in 1957. The original intent was to provide other nursing mothers with information, encouragement, and moral support. There are now thousands of local chapters and a network of 32,000 state and regional coordinators who all synchronize their activities with the headquarters now in Schaumburg, Ill. La Leche League International's 4000 groups are in 66 countries, including the United States, Canada, parts of Europe, New Zealand, and Africa, and other parts of the world.[10]

An excellent publication, *The Womanly Art of Breastfeeding*,[10] was prepared by the original group of mothers involved in the La Leche League.

The publication was revised for the twenty-fifth anniversary of the organization in 1982 and is now in its sixth edition in celebration of the fortieth anniversary in 1997. La Leche League continues to provide information and updated publications about common questions that arise during lactation. Local groups offer classes to prepare mothers to breastfeed. They help with suggestions about the nitty-gritty details of preparation, nutrition, clothing, and mothering in general. They also provide every mother with a telephone counselor. To be qualified to serve as a counselor to another mother, a member must demonstrate knowledge and expertise in breastfeeding as well as an understanding of how to counsel and render support. "Telephone mothers" do not give medical advice and are instructed to tell a troubled mother to call her own physician for such advice. Interested local physicians provide medical expertise for the group when a medical opinion is appropriate. The league provides support for mothers to reduce the time the physician needs to spend counseling on the nonmedical aspects of lactation. Most information needed by the new mother is not medical.

In the decades that this support system has been in place, no good substitute for this mother-to-mother program has evolved, because a woman needs a true *doula*.

Similar programs have been developed in more than 70 other countries. A well-established and respected program in Norway is Ammehjelpen International Group; in Australia, the Nursing Mothers' Association of Australia; and in the United Kingdom, The National Childbirth Trust.

Sociologist Alice Ladas[11] studied women who attended La Leche League preparation classes and compared them with a similar group who attempted to breastfeed but did not have this preparation. She was able to demonstrate clearly that the women who attended such programs had more confidence and seemed to benefit from receiving accurate, up-to-date and relevant information as well as receiving individual and group support.[12]

Silverman and Murrow[24] studied league activities and concluded that group dynamics are important and feelings of normalcy are reinforced. The information and experience were shown to be important, but the support from the group had far greater influence on success in breastfeeding.[27] Meara[15] reports similar observations on league activities in a nonsupportive culture.

A follow-up study of breastfeeding in Oxford was carried out by Sloper et al.[25] They observed that significantly more mothers went home breast-feeding, mothers nursed longer, and solid foods were started later when support was provided. The authors attribute this shift to the change in advice and support given in the hospital and at home visits.

The Breastfeeding Association of South Africa is a nongovernmental, nonprofit voluntary organization founded in 1978 by South Africans for the express needs of South African women. Their special problems and solutions are well described by Bergh.[3] Support groups for all of life's events, especially those covering health, have become a common feature (there are more than 150 parent support groups). In the field of perinatal care, there are groups for infertile couples; couples who are expecting; those who have experienced pregnancy loss, loss of a premature infant, or loss of a term baby; those who had a cesarean birth; and so on. Physicians should be aware of the groups that function in their community and the policies and philosophies they embrace.

The International Childbirth Education Association also provides resources for the new family in many countries. Its program makes preparation and training available for couples during pregnancy and afterward as parents. Its scope embraces the entire childbirth concept, of which breastfeeding is part.

Some carefully researched and accurate video-tapes cover the subject of perinatal experiences, including breastfeeding (e.g., VIDA's tape, entitled "Baby"). Some done by popular TV personalities, however, reflect only an individual's experience, with little substance. For an up-to-date list of resources contact the Lactation Study Center, (716) 275-0088.

COMMUNITY RESOURCES

Most hospitals provide training in preparation for childbirth. Part of the program is about the new infant and how to plan for neonatal care. These programs often serve as the initial stimulus to consider breastfeeding.

Because hospitals have become competitive and are marketing their services, many are developing birthing centers and are trying to capture the attention of the childbearing public with special services. These services often include classes on child rearing, including breastfeeding. The physician should investigate the programs and printed materials distributed by the hospitals where their patients deliver. Many pediatricians are coping with the flood of patient information from conflicting sources by printing up an office manual (desktop printers make this quite feasible). This is especially helpful if the patients are born at more than one hospital or more than one lay advocacy group are active in the community. Hospital procedures and policies can influence the success or failure of breastfeeding mothers[23] (Table 21-1). Pediatricians should be aware of the policies at the hospital(s) with which they are associated.

In a few short decades, we have gone from a paucity of support groups and resource literature to an overwhelming flood. Health care books and childbearing and family-rearing advice books are cascading off the press, written by everyone from qualified experts to poorly informed freelance writers. Some are written by health care professionals who have a personal experience in childbearing and write about it. The pediatrician should be familiar with a few good references for parents and provide a list for patients in the practice.

The Young Women's Christian Association (YWCA) in most communities provides preparation for childbirth. Its classes usually provide programming that appeals to young and unwed women, a group in need of services rarely provided by other sources.

The Visiting Nurses Association and the public health nurses on the staff of the local county health

TABLE 21-1   Hospital practices that influence breastfeeding initiation

	Strongly encouraging	Encouraging	Discouraging	Strongly discouraging
Physical contact	• Baby put to breast immediately in delivery room • Baby not taken from mother after delivery • Woman helped by staff to suckle baby in recovery room • Rooming-in, staff help with baby care in room, not only in nursery	• Staff sensitivity to cultural norms and expectations of woman	• Scheduled feedings regardless of mother's breastfeeding wishes	• Mother-infant separation at birth • Mother/infant housed on separate floors in postpartum period • Mother separated from baby because of bilirubin problem • No rooming-in policy
Verbal communication	• Staff initiate discussion on woman's intention to breastfeed prepartum and intrapartum • Staff encourage and reinforce breastfeeding immediately on labor and delivery • Staff discuss breast pump, realities of separation from baby in relation to breastfeeding	• Appropriate language skills of staff, teaching how to handle breast engorgement and nipple problem • Staff's own skills and comfort with art of breastfeeding and time to teach woman on one-to-one basis	• Staff instruct woman "to get good night's rest and miss the feed" • Strict times allotted for breastfeeding regardless of mother/baby's feeding "cycle"	• Woman told to "take it easy," "get your rest" . . . impression that breastfeeding is effortful/tiring • Woman told she "doesn't do it right"; staff interrupt her efforts; corrects her on positions, etc.

Nonverbal communication
- Pictures of woman breastfeeding

- Literature on breastfeeding in understandable terms
- Staff (physicians as well as nurses) give reinforcement for breastfeeding (respect; smiles; affirmation)
- Nurse (or any attendant) making mother comfortable and helping to arrange baby at breast for nursing

- Woman sees others breastfeeding in hospital

Experiential
- If breastfeeding not *immediately* successful, staff continue to be supportive
- Previous success with breastfeeding experience in hospital

- Closed-circuit TV program in hospital on breastfeeding

- Pictures of woman bottle feeding

- Staff interrupt breastfeeding session for tests, etc.

- Woman does not see others breastfeeding

- Woman given infant formula kit and infant food literature

- Woman sees officious nurses authoritatively caring for babies by bottle feeding (leads to woman's insecurities about own care capability)

- Previous failure with breastfeeding experience in hospital

Modified from Scrimshaw SMC: *The cultural context of breastfeeding in the United States,* Report of the Surgeon General's Workshop on Breastfeeding and Human Lactation, DHHS Pub No HRS-D-MC-84-2, Washington, DC, 1984, US Government Printing Office.

department are special resources particularly skilled at counseling new mothers with their infants. They can provide valuable information to the physician who is working with an infant who fails to thrive at the breast by witnessing the breastfeeding scene at home. As discharge from the hospital occurs earlier and earlier, the pediatrician should consider employing nurse practitioners who will make housecalls immediately after birth.

Many other organizations, local and national in scope, have the perinatal period and the family as their focus. Many of these are also interested in promoting breastfeeding as part of their overall goals.

The World Health Organization (WHO) and United Nations International Children's Education Fund (UNICEF) have joined in an international effort to create a supportive atmosphere in hospitals around the world by developing the Baby Friendly Hospital Initiative (see Chapter 1 and Appendix K). Both WHO and UNICEF provide international support for breastfeeding, especially in developing countries.

Government organizations

The U.S. government has taken an active interest in the promotion of breastfeeding as well. In the goals for national health prepared by a multidisciplinary task force in 1978, it is stated that by 1990, 75% of infants leaving the hospital shall be breastfed and at 6 months of age at least 35% will still be breastfeeding.[18] The rates in 1990 fell short of the goals and were thus restated to be achieved by the year 2000, extending to 50% the number to still be breastfeeding at 5 to 6 months.

The plan of action to reach these goals has included the development of a Healthy Mothers–Healthy Babies Program. Also, a national committee for the promotion of breastfeeding includes representation from major professional organizations of physicians, dietitians, social service workers, nurses, nurse midwives, and hospital administrators. A major thrust of the national effort has been through the Women, Infants, and Children program (WIC), in which mothers are being encouraged to breastfeed and are given nutrition and practical lactation management instruction and support. An instruction manual is available for WIC workers.[7]

The surgeon general conducted a national workshop on breastfeeding and human lactation in Rochester, NY, in June 1984 to develop recommendations for national policy. A publication from the workshop is available from the U.S. Government Printing Office in Washington, DC. A follow-up workshop was held in Washington, DC, in 1985, gathering the representatives of the major official national organizations for obstetrics, pediatrics, and family physicians, including the credential organizations for physicians, nurses, nurse midwives, and dietitians. The organizations responded to a request to have each approve a model statement in support of breastfeeding. This was accomplished by January 1987. The organizations have also undertaken a review of curriculum within their discipline to ensure adequate education, training, and accreditation regarding human lactation and breastfeeding for their members. There has been a significant increase in the number of highly skilled and specialized healthcare professionals available to support breastfeeding.

Issues of rural health have begun to include those surrounding birth and the infant's welfare. Programs are being developed to increase breastfeeding among rural women. Although the incidence of breastfeeding has increased among well-educated, self-motivated middle Americans, the number of impoverished, less well-educated women who breastfeed remains small. Progress is being made, community by community, by dedicated health care workers, dietitians, and WIC staff. Health professionals often serve as a catalyst in developing such programs but should always be ready to serve as knowledgeable, supportive consultants to the effort of others.[8]

Grants and other incentives provided by public and private sources have enlarged the communications network in states where breastfeeding remains minimal. Groups such as the Healthy Mothers–Healthy Babies Program maximize communications between resource programs and offer opportunities to share ideas, logos, publications, and strategies that work. Information about these resources is available from The Healthy Mothers–Healthy Babies Coalition.

The U.S. Department of Agriculture's breast-feeding program, through the WIC's Nutrition Program, has launched a major effort, announced during International Breastfeeding Week in August 1997 in Washington, DC, to increase breastfeeding initiation and duration throughout the 50 states. The program, Best Start, includes social marketing research, a media campaign, a staff support kit, a breastfeeding resource guide, a training conference (held April 1997), and continuing education and technical assistance. Legislative support has come through special 2-year fundings; WIC has been made a permanent national health and nutrition program; and breastfeeding was written into the legislation (see Chapter 1). The program even mandates that every WIC agency must have accommodations for employees breastfeeding their infants to pump and store their milk.[22] A major policy forum was conducted in November 1998 to continue the plans developed in 1984 to enhance government's role in breastfeeding.

Wellstart International

A program to extend the scope of global breast-feeding promotion was launched by Wellstart International in a cooperative agreement with U.S. Agency for International Development (AID). Wellstart International, a private, nonprofit organization headquartered in San Diego, grew out of clinical and teaching experiences at the University of California, San Diego Medical Center in the late 1970s.[16] In 1983, in response to a clear need to improve the breastfeeding knowledge of health professionals, a *Lactation Management Education* (LME) program was initiated with funding from AID. Almost 400 participants of the LME program now form a network of Wellstart Associates in 28 countries.

In late 1991, Wellstart joined in a cooperative agreement with AID to expand and diversify its global breastfeeding promotion activities.[16] The Expanded Promotion of Breastfeeding (EPB) can work in any country at the request of the local AID mission.

Other lactation centers have been created in health care facilities such as the program developed by Neifert in Denver. The purpose of these programs is to provide consultation services for mothers as well as education, training, and information for healthcare workers. Efforts have been made to change hospital policy regarding breastfeeding to increase the success rate.[14] A very impressive program was initiated in the Philippines by Relucio-Clavano.[20] She has not only increased the incidence of breastfeeding but also improved the morbidity from sepsis, diarrhea, and malnutrition.

Best Start—the concept of social marketing

Using the concept of social marketing, Bryant et al[4] have designed an approach to promoting breast-feeding that utilizes the counseling strategies, educational materials, policies, and community-based activities that form the Best Start Program. *Social marketing* "combines the principles of commercial marketing with health education to promote a socially beneficial idea, practice or product."[4] Typically, a well-articulated program involves a combination of mass media, print materials, personal counseling, and community-based activities.

Best Start is an innovative program that grew out of a project involving focus-group interviews, which were used to identify the determinants of infant-feeding decisions and the most effective strategies. Focus-group interviews, according to Bryant et al,[4] "are small group discussions, guided by a trained moderator, which provide insights into the participants' perceptions, attitudes, and opinions on a designated topic." The composition of the group and the discussions are carefully planned to encourage relationships and disclosure by creating a permissive, nonthreatening environment. Motivations and perceived barriers related to breastfeeding as well as social network influences on feeding choice were identified.

From these findings, a multifaceted breastfeeding promotion campaign was designed for new mothers, family members, health professionals, and the community at large. The Best Start Program has proved to be extremely successful (see Appendixes K and M) and has been replicated by others very successfully using the materials developed by Best Start, which are available for an at-cost fee.

Utilizing strategies developed in social marketing and segmentation modeling for health communication, Best Start developed a multimedia program, Loving Support Makes Breastfeeding Work, and have provided a training manual to educate staff in the use of the Best Start visual resources. These materials are also available for a small fee. This program was the substance of the WIC National Breastfeeding Promotion Project launched in April 1997.[1,5]

Breastfeeding and human lactation study center

The Lactation Study Center of the University of Rochester School of Medicine and Dentistry (NY) encourages and promotes human lactation and breastfeeding through physician education and support. The goal is to provide information that will help the practitioner encourage and support breastfeeding for all patients. Information is available to the health care professional by telephone (see Appendix K). Originally federally funded and established at the request of the surgeon general in 1984, the center now depends on private grants and donations from users.

LACTATION CONSULTANTS

For years, many medical and nursing professionals have served as lactation consultants ready to respond to any colleague's request for knowledge and expertise. With the great national movement to embrace breastfeeding, however, a new type of lactation consultant is evolving from the vast pool of women who have served in local mother-to-

mother programs to help others breastfeed. The health care professional needs to ensure that the lactation resources available in the community are truly of professional quality and background and that the individuals have obtained the proper certification and licensure. Counseling on any topic is a special skill requiring more than personal experience with the situation.

The International Board of Lactation Consultant Examiners (IBLCE)* was developed as a separate organization by the La Leche League International to credential individuals who want to counsel about breastfeeding.[9] Those who successfully complete the IBLCE certification process are entitled to use the designation *IBCLC* (International Board Certified Lactation Consultant) after their names. The IBLCE has defined lactation consultants as "allied health care providers who possess the necessary skills, knowledge, and attitudes to facilitate breastfeeding." These lactation consultants perform as employees in some situations and as independent contractors in states where the medical practice act allows such activity. A lactation consultant should have professional liability insurance coverage and a license to practice in the health field in the state.

More recently, the International Lactation Consultants Association (ILCA) states, "A lactation consultant is a health care professional whose scope of practice is focused upon providing education and management to prevent and solve breastfeeding problems and to encourage a social environment that effectively supports the breastfeeding mother/infant dyad." ILCA has published Standards of Practice for Lactation Consultants, which is available in print (see Appendix K).

Lactation specialist as member of health care team

Modern medicine has developed a team approach to the management of many patient populations, such as elderly or handicapped persons.[13] A team

---

*PO Box 2348, Falls Church, VA 22042-0348 USA; 703-560-7330 (tel), 703-560-7332 (fax).

approach also is used in the management of many categories of diseases, such as cancer and diabetes. A health care team provides medical service for the family during the perinatal period. This team includes an obstetrician and a pediatrician or a family physician; nurse midwives; nurses working in prenatal care, obstetrics, neonatal care, and public health; social workers; dietitians; and, when a problem develops, perinatologists, neonatologists, and the skilled team from the perinatal center. These team members are well-educated and extensively trained professionals. Together they have improved the morbidity and mortality rates of childbirth. The long-range prognosis for the intact survival of infants has been significantly improved.

Thus medical progress has occurred concomitantly with the isolation of the nuclear family. The result is a medically successful birth to a family poorly prepared emotionally and socially to cope. The family is inadequately prepared to take over when the mother and infant are discharged from the hospital and instantly placed on their own without a transitional period of adjustment with close support and supervision.

Lactation specialists become a very important addition to the health care team, replacing the traditional family support system. Specialists not only must know their role as counselor interacting with the family, but also must understand how they interface with other members of the health care team. The professional team members are beginning to understand the importance of lactation specialists and how to work most effectively with them. Some physicians, however, provide a nurse practitioner, whose role is to fill that gap between medical care and family support. The nurse practitioner is usually skilled in well-baby care, especially breastfeeding, and in the era of early postpartum discharge home, may make housecalls within 48 hours of arrival home.

Lactation consultants will quickly earn the respect of the health care team if they communicate openly with them, support the mother in a positive manner, and encourage a relationship of mutual trust and respect between the mother and the team.[13]

PEER COUNSELING

Peer counseling is part of a system developed by health care providers and health educators to change personal health behavior.[26] It is an adaptation of a cultural technique that has been used for generations, wherein the family provided a personal advocate or omsbudsman to help the individual carry out good health practices. In lay midwifery, for example, members of the group attended a woman throughout pregnancy, delivery, and postpartum. The important point is that the peer counselor is a member of the *same* sociocultural group as the recipient, is selected for leadership qualities and experience, and is trained in the special issues.

Public health programs have used peer counselors to encourage women to seek prenatal care or well-child care for their children. Other programs have provided peer counselors for individuals with hypertension, diabetes, or other chronic diseases to help the patient access health care and carry out instructions for treatment. This concept has been applied to the WIC program.[26] A model program was developed in south Georgia in the mid-1980s by Wanda Grogan, PhD, which was very effective in encouraging women to carry out the health care advice, to keep appointments for health care, and appropriately to breastfeed their infants.[21] This system has been expanded to many parts of the country.

The most successful programs involve the peer in all health issues so that the relationship between counselor and client continues. These peer programs are integrated with efforts to improve health habits in general and especially those associated with child bearing. The best programs train community counselors to support women through pregnancy, delivery, and early child rearing, of which breastfeeding is a part. This type of program encourages the development of a relationship that lasts several years.

Because the lowest incidence and duration of breastfeeding are among low-income women and among black mothers, a peer-support program among these clients would have the highest probability of success.[21] Using the same model for training candidates that has been developed for other health projects will facilitate initiating the program. The local WIC program or health department is ideal to undertake a peer-support program because the permanent, full-time staff are knowledgeable about nutrition and lactation and can provide continuity when peer counselors leave the program and new ones need training. This stability is essential to developing some consistency and permanency for the system. The WIC program supports women from early pregnancy through postpartum and early infancy.

Because a peer counselor is an individual from the social or cultural community who is selected because of good health behaviors and an innate ability to help others and gain respect, a peer counselor for breastfeeding is a respected member of the community or neighborhood, is of the same or similar ethnic background and of similar educational and economic level, and has breastfed one or more children. The tremendous success of the La Leche League was based on peer counseling among well-educated, white, middle-class American women.

To effect a change among WIC women and the target populations of the U.S. health goals for the year 2000 (low-income, black, and minority women), peer counselors will have to come from these groups. The WIC programs have developed a means to identify and train women from the neighborhood to serve as models of successful breastfeeding. A program limited to breastfeeding has the disadvantage of being very limited in scope; the client has to have several other individuals with whom to relate about nonbreastfeeding issues.

Some physician practices have employed (yes, peer counselors *should* be trained and paid) peer counselors very successfully to take over some of the role of the health care professional who lacks the time to relate on an even plane with a client of different educational or socioeconomic status. Well-established peer-counseling programs may even inspire the counselors to obtain further training as nurses' aides or licensed practical nurses.

The peer counselor will complement the work of the health professionals but should never replace the role of the health care provider.

Who shall counsel?

Among those working closely with people in critical life situations, some people make good counselors and some equally good people are not appropriate as counselors and should have other jobs in the organization.[13]

Counseling is a profession, and professional counselors are carefully screened, educated, and trained. Therefore individuals who help mothers breastfeed should be screened, educated, and trained as well. They should have the following special abilities:

To *listen*
To avoid judgment
To understand other lifestyles
To admit it when they do not know
To seek appropriate help from professionals
To recognize incompatibility in a given relationship

In the past few decades, peer counseling has become widespread and has been successful, not only with breastfeeding and childbirth, but also with chronic disease such as cystic fibrosis and with devastating illnesses such as cancer. The first fact all these groups have had to acknowledge is that just because one has experienced a life event, one is not automatically qualified to counsel others experiencing similar situations.

The candidate must first put personal experiences into perspective and understand the motivation for seeking this counseling role. Counseling is an opportunity to help by listening, and being a *sympathetic listener* is the most important quality. This is not a time to talk about the counselor's pregnancies. The counselor cannot have a personal agenda and press personal views or lifestyle on the mother being counseled, nor should counseling be used as a personal platform to promote organizational biases.

The counselor must understand that assuming a place on the health care team demands time and effort. One must be available at the convenience and need of the client, even when this is inconvenient to the counselor.

Learning to help mothers

The suggestions to guide a counselor in training must be general guidelines about *attitude.* The emphasis is on listening, encouraging a mother to talk, and ultimately helping her to solve her own problem by understanding it. Professional counselors are trained using didactic sessions, role play, and supervisory sessions until skills are developed. Continued reinforcement of philosophy and techniques forms the basis of growth and improvement. The lay counselor should attend counselor-training sessions provided by the parent organization and work closely with the supervisor. Sharing counseling situations with others with more experience will give further insight. Returning to the reference materials again and again will bring to light new thoughts that have been read before but not truly assimilated initially because of lack of experience.

The peer counselor does not provide medical advice. The counselor can encourage the mother to contact her physician. When the infant is doing poorly or is sick, the pediatrician should be consulted promptly. The rare condition of failure to thrive while breastfeeding is increasing in frequency, paralleling the increased incidence of breastfeeding. It has serious implications for the infant and for the continuation of breastfeeding unless treatment is initiated promptly by the physician. The physician is powerless to help if not consulted. When the infant's problem is identified and it is prudent to continue breastfeeding, the counselor can be an invaluable asset in supporting and reassuring the mother.

Maternal problems such as mastitis should respond well if treated early, but recurrent mastitis may develop when home remedies are substituted for proper treatment. The role of the counselor in such situations is significant. Encouraging the mother to seek medical care promptly is most important. Reinforcing medical advice will further enhance its effectiveness. For example, if rest is prescribed, the counselor can help the mother to understand how critical rest is to recovery and then help her determine how she is going to cope at home with family responsibilities and a newborn and still rest.

The role of the counselor is support of the mother. The counselor should work in concert with the medical health care team as a team player, not as a competitor or as an adversary, but as a *facilitator.* The mission of the team is successful lactation, a satisfying mothering experience, and a healthy infant. The health care team will continue to be responsible for the family long after lactation has been discontinued. The confidence and trust developed between the health team and family will be critical to lasting success. The counselor should be remembered as a gentle facilitator and a caring support person who was there through the rite of passage of matrescence.

A physician working with a lactation counselor or consultant needs to recognize this specialist's skills and limitations. As in other, similar situations, the physician is the leader of the health care team and carries the ultimate responsibility.

REFERENCES

1. Albreht TL, Bryant C: Advances in segmentation modeling for health communication and social marketing campaigns, *J Health Communications* 1:65, 1996.
2. Barnes GR, Lethin AN, Jackson EB et al: Management of breastfeeding, *JAMA* 151:192, 1953.
3. Bergh A-M: The role of a nongovernmental organization in breast feeding education, *J Nutr Educ* 19:117, 1987.
4. Bryant CA, Coreil J, D'Angelo SL et al: A strategy for promoting breastfeeding among economically disadvantaged women and adolescents, *NAACOGS Clinical Issues in Perinatal & Women's Health Nursing* 3:723, 1992.
5. Bryant CA, Verbal M: *The Best Start approach to breastfeeding promotion: training manual,* Tampa, Fla, 1997, Best Start.

6. Ciba Foundation: *Breast feeding and the mother:* Symposium no 45, Amsterdam, 1976, Elsevier.

7. Food and Nutrition Service, US Department of Agriculture: *Promoting breastfeeding: a guide for health professionals working in the WIC and CSF programs,* Washington, DC, 1983, USDA.

8. Gussler J, Bryant C: *Helping mothers breastfeed: program strategies for minority communities,* Health Action Papers, vol I, Lexington Ky, 1984, Lexington Fayette County Health Department, University of Kentucky Medical Behavioral Sciences Department.

9. International Board of Lactation Consultant Examiners, 2315 Wickersham Cove, Germantown, TN 38138.

10. La Leche League International: *The womanly art of breastfeeding,* ed 7, Franklin Park, Ill, 1997, The League.

11. Ladas AK: How to help mothers breast feed, *Clin Pediatr* 9:702, 1970.

12. Ladas AK: Breastfeeding: the less viable option, *J Trop Pediatr* 18:318, 1972.

13. Lawrence RA: Introduction. In Lauwers J, Woessner C, editors: *Counseling the nursing mother: a reference handbook for health care providers and lay counselors,* Wayne, NJ, 1983, Avery.

14. Lewis L: Successful breastfeeding programs for low-income, minority mothers, *Public Health Currents* 22:1, 1982.

15. Meara H: A key to successful breastfeeding in a nonsupportive culture, *J Nurse Midwifery* 21:20, 1976.

16. Naylor A, Wester R: Providing professional lactation management consultation, *Clin Perinatol* 14:33, 1987.

17. Pryor K: *Nursing your baby,* New York, 1973, Harper & Row.

18. Public Health Service: Implementation plans for attaining the objectives for the nation. In *Healthy people 2000: national health promotion and disease prevention objectives,* DHHS Pub No (PHS) 91-50213, Washington, DC, 1991, US Government Printing Office.

19. Raphael D: *The tender gift: breast feeding,* New York, 1976, Schocken.

20. Relucio-Clavano N: The results of a change in hospital practices, *Assignment Child* 55/56:139, 1981.

21. *Report of the Surgeon General's Workshop on Breastfeeding and Human Lactation,* DHHS Pub No HRS-D-MC 84-2, Washington, DC, 1984, US Government Printing Office.

22. Schwartz JB, Popkins BA, Tognetti J et al: Does WIC participation improve breastfeeding practices? *Am J Public Health* 85:729, 1995.

23. Scrimshaw SCM: The cultural context of breastfeeding in the United States. In *Report of the Surgeon General's Workshop on Breastfeeding and Human Lactation,* DHHS Pub No HRS-D-MC 84-2, Washington, DC, 1984, US Government Printing Office.

24. Silverman PR, Murrow HG: *Caregiver during critical role in the normal life cycle,* unpublished report, 1978, Harvard Medical School.

25. Sloper KS, Elsden E, Baum JD: Increasing breast feeding in a community, *Arch Dis Child* 52:700, 1977.

26. Spisak S, Gross SS: *Second follow-up report: the Surgeon General's Workshop on Breastfeeding and Human Lactation,* Washington, DC, 1991, National Center for Education in Maternal and Child Health.

27. Thompson M: The effectiveness of mother-to-mother help: research on the La Leche League International program, *Birth Fam J* 3:1, Winter, 1976-1977.

28. Van Gennep A: *Rites of passage,* London, 1960, Rutledge & Kegan Paul (Translated by MB Vizedom and GL Caffee).

22

$\mathcal{E}$ducating and training
the medical professional

The 1984 Surgeon General's Workshop on Breastfeeding and Human Lactation[15] was the first national meeting to focus exclusively on breastfeeding. The breastfeeding strategies developed at that workshop are still being used as the United States and the world move toward the breastfeeding objectives set in *Healthy People 2000: National Health Promotion and Disease Prevention Objectives.*[9]

Although many of the objectives have been addressed, the education of the health care professional remains a challenge.[11] A second meeting of the National Planning Committee of the Surgeon General's Workshop convened in Washington, DC, in 1985 to address the issue of that education.[17] The leaders of major professional organizations attended, including the American College of Obstetricians and Gynecologists, American Academy of Pediatrics; American Academy of Family Physicians, National Association of Pediatric Nurse Practitioners, American Dietetic Association, Nurses of American College of Obstetrics and Gynecology, National Association of Nurse-Midwives, and National Board of Medical Examiners. These organizations developed and ratified a policy in support of educating and certifying its membership in human lactation and breastfeeding. Discussion was initiated about developing a curriculum appropriate to each professional level of training and specialization.

CONTINUING EFFORTS

Work continues in scattered ad hoc special presentations that may or may not have some affiliation with a medical school or hospital. However, no central unified program has been developed to change the curriculum at the seat of learning: U.S. medical schools and nursing schools.

The second follow-up report of the surgeon general's workshop in 1991 noted several accomplishments.[17] Although many respondents thought that lack of support or encouragement from physicians and nurses was a continuing barrier, no substantive progress had been made in developing curricula or credentialing. Excellent programs have been provided by Wellstart International[19,21] for teams consisting of a physician, a nurse, and a nutritionist from the same institution with co-sponsorship by the University of California at San Diego or the University of Hawaii. Wellstart's programs are international, and they provide resources around the world. Many other universities have served as co-sponsors for a program, seminar, or workshop in their own geographic area. However, the programs have not been integrated into the total medical school curriculum or the training in a residency program, and they are not taught by any medical school faculty at all levels of training.

The failure of medical schools to address the issue of education about the breast and training in the clinical issues of breastfeeding has been addressed at the University of Texas at San Antonio by Newton.[13] He initiated a program on the obstetric service for medical students and residents. He also reported the results of his national survey of medical schools' curricula: 55% of the 127 U.S. obstetric and pediatric departments had no didactic lectures for medical students. Of obstetric and pediatric residencies, 30% provided no didactic lectures to their students. Most programs relied on clinical opportunities for learning.

When Freed et al[8] investigated the attitudes and education of pediatric house staff concerning breastfeeding, they found that third-year residents did not know any more than interns about the subject. Furthermore, only personal experience seemed to provide any in-depth knowledge about simple problems, such as sore nipples. Freed[4] suggests that we "preach what we teach": that breastfeeding education for physicians should focus on (1) *knowledge* regarding techniques and problem solving to become a good counselor; (2) *outcome expectations,* that is, breastfeeding results in healthier children; and (3) *efficacy expectations,* the confidence that physicians themselves can be effective counselors and influence the incidence and duration of breastfeeding.

THE PROBLEM

Breastfeeding is important to infants and their mothers for nutritional, immunologic, psychologic, and other health reasons. U.S. health goals strive to increase the incidence and duration of breastfeeding. Little formal education is provided on the topic in medical schools and residency training programs. No planned curricula or testing mechanisms are available.

Breastfeeding has another unique problem of interest to the lay public, who have become very involved. Many nonphysicians have become involved in training. Some attempts at educating physicians have been made by nonphysicians and sometimes by non–health care professionals.[2,3] The message to the medical student is that under-

standing and encouraging breastfeeding are not in the physician's job description. When other care providers give presentations to medical students or residents, it is assumed the provider is describing the work for information only and not for its role in the physician's work. Childbirth is of great interest to the lay public and to consumer advocacy groups as well, but they do not provide the physician's training in childbirth. This training is provided by skilled specialists who have doctoral degrees, residency training, board certification, and in many cases, additional fellowship training and subspecialty certification, which are minimal qualifications for medical school faculty.

How much do residents and physicians know about managing breastfeeding? The data suggest the answer is "very little." In a study of obstetric residents, Freed et al[5] mailed a survey to more than 600 residents, and 64% responded. Only 38% had any education from the faculty about breastfeeding and indicated what little they knew came from other residents and nurses. All participants agreed, however, that they should have a role in the management of breastfeeding for their patients. A survey of 87 of a possible 108 (81%) pediatric residents evenly distributed among levels I, II, and III in a large hospital reported that level III residents were no more competent than their PL-1 counterparts.[7] If they or their spouse breastfed, they were more confident in their knowledge base. No differences were found between men and women or between those breastfed or not breastfed as an infant.[7,8]

A subsequent study confirmed that residents' knowledge was low and their misinformation disturbingly high.[7] The authors concluded that residency training programs must provide comprehensive education on breastfeeding to prepare them to meet the needs of patients and other parents. Another study of pediatricians in training given a 15-minute self-administered and anonymous questionnaire resulted in 53% participation (29 respondents).[20] On a 6-point scale of support of breastfeeding, the group achieved 2.6 (1 being most supportive), revealing an attitude barely above neutral. They only achieved 53% on the management questions, and their confidence in their skills was low, confirming the need for didactic and clinical training in breastfeeding. A national survey of 1099 family medicine residents, 71% of whom responded, indicated that they thought they should be involved in breastfeeding promotion and support.[6] They demonstrated significant deficits, however, in knowledge about benefits and clinical management. These same investigators also polled practitioners regarding their beliefs and knowledge base.[7] The results indicated a similar level of support and lack of knowledge.

Others have investigated the level of knowledge of physicians in training in other countries. A self-administered questionnaire was returned by 76 (84%) of obstetric residents in metropolitan areas of South Korea.[10] Korean breastfeeding rates have decreased, especially among well-educated women, and the rate was only 17% in 1994. The questionnaire responses indicated the residents were neutral about breastfeeding. On the other hand, they considered themselves very competent to handle breastfeeding situations. They scored, however, only 38% on the management quiz.

Improved breastfeeding education clearly is needed in obstetrics, pediatrics, and family medicine, the physicians who should be most involved in supporting and promoting breastfeeding.

THE SOLUTION

To begin to solve this educational problem, a curriculum should be developed. It should span all four years of medical school and be carefully woven into the fabric of medical school for all students and of the residency years for those specializing in obstetrics, pediatrics, and family medicine.

The program should be taught by physicians who are qualified faculty members recognized by their peer group and certified by specialty examining boards. The classes should be part of the total curriculum and not something a student can elect to do only in the fourth year, when most of the assignments are by electives. Graduate physicians in practice rarely will go to a teaching day

exclusively on breastfeeding, and they rarely attend programs directed at a broad-based audience of nonphysicians. It does not serve their educational needs when they are also responsible for keeping abreast of the constant flow of advancements in every branch of medicine.

Breastfeeding topics should become part of a well-rounded continuing education program that includes a number of other important issues, such as infectious diseases, endocrine problems, growth, development, and perinatology. When breastfeeding is included in programs on infant nutrition and presented by a physician, it will gain the status it needs.

SUGGESTED CURRICULUM FOR MEDICAL STUDENTS

Utilizing as a model the present program at the University of Rochester School of Medicine, Rochester, NY, the following schedule is suggested as a starting point for instilling knowledge about human lactation and breastfeeding into the traditional curriculum of all medical students.

First-year students have a 16-week program in *human nutrition,* which meets weekly for a 2-hour session. Breastfeeding is presented in the section on child nutrition, and the discussion provides information about the reasons breastfeeding and human milk are superior to formula feeding. The lecture is didactic but is followed by discussion. At least two questions about the composition and benefits of human milk are on the final examination.

Second-year students have a 12-week program in the last half of the year on *women's health issues.* The class meets for 4 hours once a week to explore a variety of topics, including hormonal maturation, menarche, sex, contraception, childbearing, menopause, and the breast. A 4-hour session is about the breast. The first 2 hours of the session are dedicated to the use of the breast, that is, the anatomy and physiology of lactation. At least two questions on the final examination for this course are about lactation. The second 2 hours cover pathology, including augmentation mammo-plasty, reduction mammoplasty, and benign and malignant tumors.

The third year begins with the general clerkship, wherein skills in history taking and physical examination are sharpened. A separate session taught by faculty from obstetrics and gynecology concentrates on *breast and pelvic examinations.* It is expected that all students, residents, and practi-tioners will always make these examinations part of the physical examination of women.

Third-year medical students spend 6 weeks on *obstetrics and gynecology,* usually half of which is spent on obstetrics, treating patients prenatally, intrapartum, at delivery, and postpartum. Breast-feeding is part of that continuum, from the discussion of infant feeding prenatally through the postpartum checks for physiologic engorgement and the mother's questions about, for example, her afterpains.

The third-year student also spends 6 weeks on the *pediatric service,* half on the ward and half in the outpatient and emergency service. While in clinic, each student spends a week of mornings in the newborn nursery going crib to crib, check-ing the newborn's adaptation to extrauterine life. The student also examines infants and talks to mothers. Observing a feeding is part of all dis-charge examinations and mandatory if the infant is breastfed. The student learns about the breastfed infants' feeding and weight patterns and early lactation. The student learns to identify problems and treat them.

The weeks in the clinic provide additional experience when seeing well babies. The students are exposed to the early weeks and months of breastfeeding and learn about infant weight gain and any problems that arise. The preceptors are experienced, board-certified pediatricians. The daily lecture series, which starts the day for all the residents and students assigned to the outpatient service, is directed at reviewing routine clinical issues. At least one in ten lectures is about breastfeeding. Students are encouraged to visit their patients while they breastfeed and to accom-pany the mother-baby nurse when assisting the nursing dyad. They also attend the breastfeeding classes for mothers given by the lactation consul-tants, who are the health educators. The student also makes rounds with the lactation consultant.

Fourth-year medical students have a few re-quired courses—a surgical subspecialty, emer-gency medicine, and a clinical clerkship—but the rest of the year is given to electives. A student may elect extra time in the newborn nursery or the outpatient service or even at the Lactation Study Center. Summer fellowships are available to medi-cal students throughout the 4 years to do a research project with a faculty member. One or two students a year are selected to work with the Lactation Study Center. A small stipend, which covers their living expenses, is provided by the medical school. Reports of the questions on the national board examination confirm that human lactation and breastfeeding are included. (The recent FLEX examination had nine questions about breastfeed-ing and human lactation.)

Residents in obstetrics and pediatrics are as-signed to the nursery and receive experience in managing the breastfeeding newborn. The obstetric house officer receives additional experiences by following patients prenatally and postpartum. For-mal lectures are also provided in the Grand Round Series of both departments. Special lectures di-rected specifically at the house officer on topics in breastfeeding and lactation are scheduled (e.g., drugs in breast milk, mastitis, failure to thrive).

The curriculum for the medical student is not unlike the approach to studying other organ sys-tems, such as the cardiovascular system or the renal system. It includes the anatomy, physiology, biochemistry, pharmacology, normal function, pa-thology, and finally the clinical application in a wide range of clinical settings.

Expertise and leadership issues

As in other medical issues, the physician also learns about interacting with the patient and the family and studies all the psychosocial implica-tions. When a medical school offers a visible clinical and research program that focuses atten-tion on a subject, it improves the image of the subject matter. Cancer centers, poison centers, and sports medicine clinics are examples of how certain medical problems have been elevated to positions of importance in education and training by pooling resources and expertise. The Breast-feeding and Human Lactation Study Center at the University of Rochester School of Medicine has served as an information center, a resource of expertise for the educational matrix, and an ongoing research program that allows students, residents, and fellows to develop their own investigational work. Wellstart provides a similar focus of resources at the University of California at San Diego. Newton's work in East Carolina Medical School, Neifert's at the University of Colorado at Denver, and that of many others are examples of medical school–based programs that are developing models for physician training.

The greatest obstacle to initiating a self-sustaining program on human lactation in medical schools is the need for *leadership* among the faculty. At least one interested, knowledgeable, credible faculty member must emerge to develop the curriculum so that it becomes part of the permanent learning plan. Faculty more recently trained are more interested in breastfeeding than senior faculty trained in the heyday of formula feeding. If there is a parallel training program in the nursing school, an appropriate division of labor can occur at the clinical interface.

The physician does not put the infant to the breast; that is the responsibility of the mother-baby nurse. The physician does, however, have to understand the process so that problems in clinical outcome can be solved. The nurse does not choose the medications prescribed to a lactating woman, but should understand the importance of lactation in those selections. The mother should be reminded to notify her internist that she is lactating. The health management of breastfeeding and lactation is a team effort, and it is the job of the physicians, nurses, and nutritionists working in perinatal medicine to assist in the process.

Wellstart program

Wellstart International[21] has developed a multidisciplinary approach to breastfeeding education that includes various health professionals, such as nurses, midwives, nutritionists, and physicians. The training materials are predicated on training the team together. This model works well when an institution can send a team simultaneously to the training with the intent that the team members will return and each train members of their own discipline, thus ensuring credible expertise across medicine, nursing, and nutrition. Naylor et al[12] point out that "for the continuum of health care and the safety of the mother and infant, the physician has the final responsibility for diagnosis and medical management, including the treatment of illnesses, lactation problems and growth abnormalities." The authors agree that the material must be integrated into courses that already exist, whether in traditional didactic curriculum or problem-based models. Table 22-1 presents the curriculum recommended in the Wellstart model, and Box 22-1 provides the model's breastfeeding policy for hospitals.

CURRICULUM FOR NURSES' TRAINING IN BREASTFEEDING AND LACTATION

A number of programs have been developed for the training of the health professional.[16,18] According to their titles, they have been developed by nurses for nurses or by nutritionists for nutritionists. Several of these programs were sponsored by the Maternal and Child Health Bureau, and their materials are available through the National Center for Education in Maternal and Child Health. *Lactation Education for Health Professionals,* edited by Rodriguez-Garcia, Schaefer, and Yunes of the Pan American Health Organization of the World Health Organization, is an excellent description of such a program.[16] This text is directed at nursing school faculty. The target audience is undergraduate nursing students, although the text could serve as a guide for postgraduate and continuing education programs. The well-trained student will be able to teach the mother optimal breastfeeding and weaning techniques. The student will also be able, within the scope of the total

Text continued on p. 732

TABLE 22-1	Wellstart International curriculum for breastfeeding management		
Level I (awareness)	**Level II (generalist)**	**Level III (specialist)**

Module A: scientific basis

Discuss, in general terms, findings from basic and social sciences of lactation	*Apply findings from basic and social sciences to breastfeeding and lactation issues:*	*Critique findings from basic and social sciences and evaluate their applicability to clinical management issues:*
1. Describe general benefits of breastfeeding for infant.	1.1 Describe unique properties of human milk for human infants.	1.1 Discuss in detail components of human milk and their functions.
	1.2 Describe advantages of preterm milk for preterm infant.	1.2 Describe in detail suitability of preterm human milk for preterm infant.
2.1 Describe general benefits of breastfeeding for mother.	2.1 Summarize impact of lactation on maternal nutritional status.	2.1 Critically review current literature on impact of lactation on maternal health status.
2.2 Describe benefits of breastfeeding for community.	2.2 Discuss effect of lactation on fertility.	2.2 Discuss current research and controversies related to lactational infertility.
3. Identify mammary structures involved in milk production and transfer.	3.1 Diagram anatomic structures of breast.	3. Describe normal and abnormal development of breast from fetal life through lactation and involution.
	3.2 Describe structural changes in breast during pregnancy and lactation.	
4. Describe process of milk production and removal.	4. Describe physiology of milk production, removal, and involution.	4. Describe synthesis of human milk at cellular level.
5. Describe ways that suckling process differs between breastfeeding and bottle feeding.	5. Describe anatomic development and physiology of suckling process.	5. Describe structural and functional factors related to oral-motor dysfunction.
6. Describe, in general terms, impact of maternal nutrition on lactation.	6. Describe specific impact of maternal diet and nutritional status on quantity and quality of milk produced.	6. Critically review current literature on impact of maternal nutrition on lactation.
7. Describe growth pattern of breastfed infant.	7. Summarize current knowledge on normal growth parameters of breastfed infants.	7. Critique scientific literature on infant growth and its applicability to breastfed infants.

From Wellstart International and the University of California, San Diego: *Lactation management curriculum: a faculty guide for schools of medicine, nursing and nutrition,* ed 4, San Diego, 1998, Wellstart International.

TABLE 22-1	Wellstart International curriculum for breastfeeding management—cont'd		
Level I (awareness)	**Level II (generalist)**	**Level III (specialist)**	

Module A: scientific basis—cont'd

8. Describe relative impact of age, ethnicity, socioeconomic status, and geographic region on breastfeeding rates in your country.	8. Identify local sources of data on breastfeeding trends.	8. Identify and interpret national and international trends in breastfeeding incidence and duration.
9. Identify cultural and psychosocial factors that impact breastfeeding rates.	9. Describe ways in which cultural beliefs, societal influences, and community practices impact breastfeeding in local community.	9. Critique and interpret research on cultural and psychosocial aspects of breastfeeding.

Module B: clinical management

Provide clinical care consistent with initiation and maintenance of lactation:	*Provide routine clinical support for successful initiation and maintenance of lactation and prevention and management of common clinical problems:*	*Provide clinical support/develop protocols for successful initiation and maintenance of lactation in high-risk/complicated situations:*
1. Identify factors that contribute to breastfeeding decision.	1.1 Provide breastfeeding care that is sensitive to cultural influences.	1.1 Same as level II.
	1.2 Assist expectant mother with breastfeeding decision.	1.2 Same as level II.
2. Conduct breastfeeding history and examination of breasts.	2. Use breast examination as opportunity to reassure woman she can breastfeed her infant.	2. Same as level II.
3.1 Identify components of anticipatory guidance for all women.	3. Provide anticipatory guidance targeted to specific needs of expectant mother and breastfeeding dyad.	3. Provide anticipatory guidance to pregnant women with unusual or high-risk conditions.
3.2 Identify components of anticipatory guidance and support for women with special needs.		
4. Recognize impact of intrapartum and immediate postpartum procedures/ medications on lactation.	4. Provide intrapartum and immediate postpartum care that supports successful lactation.	4. Develop and implement intrapartum care protocols that facilitate breastfeeding for high-risk mother-infant dyads.
5. Recognize correct attachment and effective suckling at breast.	5. Provide postpartum care that supports successful lactation.	5. Same as level II.

Continued

TABLE 22-1	Wellstart International curriculum for breastfeeding management—cont'd	
Level I (awareness)	Level II (generalist)	Level III (specialist)

Module B: clinical management—cont'd

6. Recognize when and how lactation needs to be maintained during separation, and refer mother for assistance.	6. Assist mother to maintain lactation during separation from her infant.	6. Provide consultation regarding banking and use of human milk in special circumstances.
7. Discuss basic nutrition recommendations for lactating woman.	7. Assess lactating woman for nutritional risk and refer appropriately.	7. Assess and manage breastfeeding mother with complicated nutritional needs.
8. Describe current recommendations for introducing complementary foods and supplements.	8. Provide guidance regarding introduction of complementary foods.	8. Manage complex lactation-related issues associated with introduction of complementary foods.
9. Discuss causes and prevention of common breastfeeding problems.	9. Manage uncomplicated problems seen in breastfed infant.	9.1 Assess and manage complex dysfunctional suckling patterns.
		9.2 Assess and manage lactation in infants with persistent slow growth.
10. Recognize that infants with special health care needs can breastfeed.	10. Facilitate breastfeeding for infant with special health care needs.	10. Facilitate successful lactation in infant with complex health care needs.
11. Same as 9.	11. Manage uncomplicated breastfeeding problems of mother.	11. Facilitate successful lactation in mother with complex breastfeeding problems.
12. Prescribe/recommend medications and treatment options compatible with lactation.	12. Facilitate successful lactation in mother with medical conditions or receiving treatments.	12. Provide consultation to colleagues and breastfeeding mothers regarding support of breastfeeding for mothers with complex health problems.
13. Discuss family-planning options for lactating woman.	13.1 Counsel lactating woman about contraceptive options.	13.1 Same as level II.
	13.2 Provide anticipatory guidance and problem solving regarding lactation and sexuality.	13.2 Same as level II.
14. Same as 6.	14. Counsel woman about maintaining lactation while returning to work/school.	14. Same as level II.

From Wellstart International and the University of California, San Diego: *Lactation management curriculum: a faculty guide for schools of medicine, nursing and nutrition*, ed 4, San Diego, 1998, Wellstart International.

TABLE 22-1   Wellstart International curriculum for breastfeeding management—cont'd

Level I (awareness)	Level II (generalist)	Level III (specialist)
Module C: professional practice issues		
1.0 Coordinate services with, and provide appropriate referral to, other professionals, lay persons, and community groups:	*1.0 Coordinate care consistent with multidisciplinary approach:*	*1.0 Provide leadership in development and implementation of a team approach to lactation management:*
1.1 Identify various professionals who contribute to support and management of breastfeeding mother/infant pair.	1.1 Describe and explain philosophy of multidisciplinary approach to care.	1.1 Evaluate own team situation in terms of philosophy and decision-making structure.
1.2 Discuss, in general terms, roles of various professionals as members of lactation management team.	1.2 Define one's own role on lactation management team.	1.2 Identify specific strategies for change in own team activities.
1.3 Identify community and professional groups and activities that promote breastfeeding.	1.3 Work within team to coordinate lactation services and ensure continuity of care.	1.3 Provide leadership for multidisciplinary lactation management team.
1.4 Make appropriate referrals for women needing assistance with breastfeeding.	1.4 Develop linkages among appropriate community and professional groups to support breastfeeding.	1.4 Develop team protocols to promote accurate, consistent, and continuous care to breastfeeding families at critical periods.
2.0 Support policies that promote breastfeeding:	*2.0 Advocate for policies that support breastfeeding:*	*2.0 Develop policies/positions on breastfeeding-related issues:*
2.1 Discuss your professional organization's policy statements regarding breastfeeding.	2.1 Debate ethical issues affecting breastfeeding promotion and support.	2.1 Formulate a position on ethical issues that affect breastfeeding.
2.2 Discuss your country's policies and goals for breastfeeding.	2.2 Analyze effect of hospital and health service policies on actual breastfeeding practice.	2.2 Formulate positions on current national or international policies/initiatives that affect breastfeeding.
	2.3 Analyze local, state, or national policy issues affecting breastfeeding promotion and support.	2.3 Participate in effecting policy changes.

Continued

TABLE 22-1	Wellstart International curriculum for breastfeeding management—cont'd	
Level I (awareness)	Level II (generalist)	Level III (specialist)
Module C: professional practice issues—cont'd		
	3.0 *Apply change theory and adult learning principles to breastfeeding promotion:*	3.0 *Provide leadership in development, implementation, and evaluation of programs that support and promote breastfeeding:*
	3.1 Discuss strategies for overcoming resistance to change.	3.1 Compare and contrast change theories.
	3.2 Apply principles of adult learning to development of educational session on breastfeeding.	3.2 Describe program planning process and program evaluation techniques as they pertain to lactation programs.
	3.3 Plan a teaching session on breastfeeding.	3.3 Apply adult learning principles, change theory, and program planning principles to development of lactation programs in any of following areas: • Health professional education and training • Health care practice • Population/community level interventions
	3.4 Critique breastfeeding-related teaching materials.	

From Wellstart International and the University of California, San Diego: *Lactation management curriculum: a faculty guide for schools of medicine, nursing and nutrition,* ed 4, San Diego, 1998, Wellstart International.

health team, to promote, maintain, and protect breastfeeding.[14]

The learning objectives for the nurse include being able to do the following:
• Apply acquired knowledge and skills.
• Assist mothers in initiating and continuing breastfeeding.
• Promote breastfeeding.
• Organize and conduct breastfeeding education seminars for other members of the nursing staff.
• Plan and implement breastfeeding services in clinical sites.

A training guide for experienced health care professionals has been prepared by Best Start and

Bryant and Roy.[1] The work is culturally sensitive and is based on a thorough study of social marketing. Using this guide, health care professionals will be able to do the following:
• Identify the common factors that deter disadvantaged women from breastfeeding.
• Develop strategies for helping these women overcome these barriers.
• Develop strategies for identifying and building on the factors that make breastfeeding appealing to these women.

Other resources for the education and training are listed in Appendix O. Nursing schools should seek the same quality in their lactation resources as

---

BOX 22-1   Wellstart International model hospital breastfeeding policies for full-term normal newborn infants

---

Definition and purpose: To promote a philosophy of maternal and infant care that advocates breastfeeding and supports the normal physiologic functions involved in this maternal-infant process. The goal is to ensure that all families who elect to breastfeed their infants will have a successful and satisfying experience.

1. Hospital administrative, medical, nursing and nutrition staff should establish a strategy that promotes and supports breastfeeding through the formation of an interdisciplinary team responsible for the implementation of hospital policies and provision of ongoing educational activities.

2. All pregnant women should receive information before delivery regarding the benefits and management of breastfeeding.

3. Every mother should be allowed to have a close companion stay with her continuously throughout labor.

4. Infants are to be put to breast as soon after birth as feasible for both mother and infant. This is to be initiated in either the delivery room or the recovery room, and every mother is to be instructed in proper breastfeeding technique and reevaluated before discharge.

5. Breastfeeding mother-infant couples are to room-in together on a 24-hour basis.

6. The infant is to be encouraged to nurse *at least* 8 to 12 times or more in 24 hours, for a minimum of 8 feedings per 24 hours.

7. Specific timing at the breast is not necessary. Infants usually fall asleep or release the nipple spontaneously when satiated.

8. Infants should spontaneously finish at the first breast, then should be encouraged to try the second breast at each feed.

9. If a feeding at the breast is incomplete or ineffective, the mother should be instructed to begin regular expression of her breasts in conjunction with continued assistance by an experienced staff member. The colostrum or milk obtained by expression should be given to the baby.

10. No supplementary water or milk is to be given unless specifically ordered by a physician or nurse practitioner.

11. Pacifiers are not to be given to any breastfeeding infant unless specifically ordered by a physician or nurse practitioner. The use of bottle nipples and nipple shields should be discouraged.

12. Breastfeeding mothers are to have breasts examined for evidence of lactation or breastfeeding problems at least once every nursing staff shift.

13. Discharge gift packs offered to breastfeeding mothers should contain only noncommercial materials that provide educational information and promote breastfeeding.

14. All breastfeeding mothers are to be advised to arrange for an appointment for their baby's first checkup within 1 week after discharge.

15. At discharge, each mother is to be given a phone number to call for breastfeeding assistance.

16. Policies 1, 2, 4, and 10 through 15 apply when mothers and babies are separated. Mothers who are separated from their babies are to be instructed on how to maintain lactation.

From Naylor AJ, Creer AE, Woodward-Lopez G et al: *Semin Perinatol* 18:525, 1994.

they have in all other phases of nursing. When the professional nursing certifying organizations develop appropriate certification for lactation throughout perinatal nursing to accompany the certification already established for labor and delivery, normal newborn, postpartum care, and other areas, the curriculum will come into place quickly.

Postgraduate learning opportunities for nurses and lactation consultants

Numerous programs across the United States are geared toward nurses and often are provided by nurses. Many of these focus on curricula designed to assist the participant in passing the certifying examination provided by the International Board of Lactation Consultant Examiners (IBLCE). Postgraduate teaching for lactation consultants is provided by the International Lactation Consultants Association (ILCA) and by independent professional groups. La Leche League International also provides programs for all levels of interest, from the lay public to professionals, including a physician's seminar (see Chapter 21).

Postgraduate learning opportunities by medical groups for physicians

Postgraduate educational opportunities are one of the major goals of the Academy of Breastfeeding Medicine (ABM), an international organization founded in 1992 and limited to physicians from all disciplines and physician trainees. The ABM holds an annual meeting with plenary sessions, workshops, and submitted papers and posters on the wide range of topics involving breastfeeding and human lactation. ABM's mission is to encourage and support breastfeeding, especially through physician education.

The Milk Club is a group that meets in conjunction with the American Pediatric Society, Society for Pediatric Research, and Ambulatory Pediatric Association. Their mission is to bring new science in the field to the attention of all investigators. The format is usually a symposium with discussion and a poster session.

The International Society for Research in Human Milk and Lactation is an organization of investigators who meet annually in conjunction with the Federation of American Societies for Experimental Biology and meet biannually and independently at international sites to discuss current knowledge of laboratory and clinical research. Membership is limited to qualified investigators in the field. Appendix K provides the addresses for these organizations.

The American Academy of Pediatrics (AAP), American College of Obstetricians and Gynecologists, and American Academy of Family Practice all have increased their programming about human lactation at their annual and regional meetings. The AAP established a Work Group

on Breastfeeding and approved its statement in support of breastfeeding, published in *Pediatrics* in December 1997. The work group makes the following 12 major recommendations for pediatricians[22]:

1. Promote and support breastfeeding enthusiastically. In consideration of the extensive published evidence for improved outcomes in breastfed infants and their mothers, a strong position on behalf of breastfeeding is justified.

2. Become knowledgeable and skilled in both the physiology and the clinical management of breastfeeding.

3. Work collaboratively with the obstetric community to ensure that women receive adequate information throughout the perinatal period to make a fully informed decision about infant feeding. Pediatricians should also use opportunities to provide age-appropriate breastfeeding education to children and adults.

4. Promote hospital policies and procedures that facilitate breastfeeding. Electric breast pumps and private lactation areas should be available to all breastfeeding mothers in the hospital, on both ambulatory and inpatient services. Pediatricians are encouraged to work actively toward eliminating hospital practices that discourage breastfeeding (e.g., infant formula discharge packs, separation of mother and infant).

5. Become familiar with local breastfeeding resources (e.g., Special Supplemental Nutrition Program for Women, Infants, and Children clinics; lactation educators and consultants; lay support groups; breast pump rental stations) so that patients can be referred appropriately. When specialized breastfeeding services are used, pediatricians need to clarify for mothers their essential role as the infant's primary medical caregiver. Effective communication among the various counselors who advise breastfeeding women is essential.

6. Encourage routine insurance coverage for necessary breastfeeding services and supplies, including breast pump rental and the time required by pediatricians and other licensed

health care professionals to assess and manage breastfeeding.

7. Promote breastfeeding as a normal part of daily life, and encourage family and societal support for breastfeeding.

8. Develop and maintain effective communications and collaboration with other health care providers to ensure optimal breastfeeding education, support, and counseling for mother and infant.

9. Advise mothers to return to their physician for a thorough breast examination when breastfeeding is terminated.

10. Promote breastfeeding education as a routine component of medical school and residency education.

11. Encourage the media to portray breastfeeding as positive and the norm.

12. Encourage employers to provide appropriate facilities and adequate time in the workplace for breast pumping.

SUMMARY

To establish breastfeeding and human lactation as an integral part of medical student education, they should be inserted into the present curriculum at the appropriate natural points, whether it is a class on anatomy, physiology, nutrition, endocrinology, women's health, or infant care. The class should be taught by recognized faculty who also teach the rest of the subject material. Finally, the material should be included in the examination for the subject. Much remains to be learned in modern medicine, and lactation should be part of it.

REFERENCES

1. Bryant CA, Roy M: *Best Start training manual: breastfeeding for healthy mothers, healthy babies,* Tampa, Fla, 1990, Best Start.

2. Department of Human Services, District of Columbia, WIC State Agency: *District of Columbia Breastfeeding Peer Counselor Program: training manual,* Washington, DC, 1990, The Department.

3. Food and Nutrition Service, US Department of Agriculture: *Promoting breastfeeding in WIC: a compendium of practical approaches,* Alexandria, Va, 1988, Nutrition and Technical Services Division, USDA.

4. Freed GL: Breastfeeding: time to teach what we preach, *JAMA* 269:243, 1993.

5. Freed GL, Clark SJ, Cefalo RC et al: Breast-feeding education of obstetrics-gynecology residents and practitioners, *Am J Obstet Gynecol* 173:1607, 1995.

6. Freed GL, Clark SJ, Curtis P et al: Breast-feeding education and practice in family medicine, *J Fam Pract* 40:263, 1995.

7. Freed GL, Clark SJ, Lohr JA et al: Pediatrician involvement in breast-feeding promotion: a national study of residents and practitioners, *Pediatrics* 96:490, 1995.

8. Freed GL, Jones MTM, Fraley JK: Attitudes and education of pediatric house staff concerning breastfeeding, *South Med J* 85:484, 1992.

9. *Healthy people 2000: national health promotion and disease prevention objectives,* DHHS Pub No (PHS) 91-50213, Washington, DC, 1991, US Government Printing Office.

10. Kim HS: Attitudes and knowledge regarding breastfeeding: a survey of obstetric residents in metropolitan areas of South Korea, *South Med J* 89:684, 1996.

11. Lawrence RA: Review of the Surgeon General's Workshop on Breastfeeding and Human Lactation. Presented at American Public Health Association meetings, San Diego, November 1984.

12. Naylor AJ, Creer AE, Woodward-Lopez G et al: Lactation management education for physicians, *Semin Perinatol* 18:525, 1994.

13. Newton E: Breastfeeding/lactation and the medical school curriculum, *J Hum Lact* 8:122, 1992.

14. Powers NG, Naylor AJ, Wester RA: Hospital policies: crucial to breastfeeding success, *Semin Perinatol* 18:517, 1994.

15. *Report of the Surgeon General's Workshop on Breastfeeding and Human Lactation,* DHHS Pub No HRS-D-MC 84-2, Washington, DC, 1984, US Government Printing Office.

16. Rodriguez-Garcia R, Schaefer LA, Yunes J: *Lactation education for health professionals,* Washington, DC, 1990, Pan American Health Organization.

17. Spisak S, Gross SS: *Second follow-up report: the Surgeon General's Workshop on Breastfeeding and Human Lactation,* Washington, DC, 1991, National Center for Education in Maternal and Child Health.

18. Tully MR, Overfield ML: *Educating health professionals for breastfeeding support,* SPRANS Grant, Athens, Ga, 1986, University of Georgia.
19. Wellstart International: *Model hospital breastfeeding policies for full-term normal newborn infants,* San Diego, 1990, Wellstart.
20. Williams EL, Hammer LD: Breastfeeding attitudes and knowledge of pediatricians-in-training, *Am J Prev Med* 11:26, 1995.
21. Woodward-Lopez G, Creer AE, editors: *Lactation management curriculum: a faculty guide for schools of medicine, nursing and nutrition,* ed 4, San Diego, 1994, Wellstart International and University of California at San Diego.
22. Working Group on Breastfeeding, American Academy of Pediatrics: Breastfeeding and the use of human milk, *Pediatrics* 100:1035, 1997.

Composition of human milk

TABLE A-1	Composition of human colostrum and mature breast milk	
Constituent (per 100 ml)	Colostrum 1-5 days	Mature milk >30 days
Energy (kcal)	58	70
Total solids (g)	12.8	12.0
Lactose (g)	5.3	7.3
Total nitrogen (mg)	360	171
Protein nitrogen (mg)	313	129
Nonprotein nitrogen (mg)	47	42
Total protein (g)	2.3	0.9
Casein (mg)	140	187
α-Lactalbumin (mg)	218	161
Lactoferrin (mg)	330	167
IgA (mg)	364	142
Amino acids (total)		
Alanine (mg)	—	52
Arginine (mg)	126	49
Aspartate (mg)	—	110
Cystine (mg)	—	25
Glutamate (mg)	—	196
Glycine (mg)	—	27
Histidine (mg)	57	31
Isoleucine (mg)	121	67
Leucine (mg)	221	110
Lysine (mg)	163	79
Methionine (mg)	33	19
Phenylalanine (mg)	105	44
Proline (mg)	—	89
Serine (mg)	—	54
Threonine (mg)	148	58
Tryptophan (mg)	52	25
Tyrosine (mg)	—	38

Data from multiple references (see Chapter 4). Figures have been averaged.

Continued

TABLE A-1   Composition of human colostrum and mature breast milk—cont'd

Constituent (per 100 ml)	Colostrum 1-5 days	Mature milk >30 days
Amino acids (total)—cont'd		
Valine (mg)	169	90
Taurine (free) (mg)	—	8
Urea (mg)	10	30
Creatine (mg)	—	3.3
Total fat (g)	2.9	4.2
Fatty acids (% total fat)		
12:0 tauric	1.8	5.8
14:0 myristic	3.8	8.6
16:0 palmitic	26.2	21.0
18:0 stearic	8.8	8.0
18:1 oleic	36.6	35.5
18:2, n-6 linoleic	6.8	7.2
18:3, n-3 linolenic	—	1.0
C_{20} and C_{22} polyunsaturated	10.2	2.9
Cholesterol (mg)	27	16
Vitamins		
Fat soluble		
Vitamin A (retinol equivalents) (µg)	89	67
β-Carotene (µg)	112	23
Vitamin D (µg)	—	0.05
Vitamin E (total tocopherols) (µg)	1280	315
Vitamin K (µg)	0.23	0.21
Water soluble		
Thiamin (µg)	15	21
Riboflavin (µg)	25	35
Niacin (µg)	75	150
Folic acid (µg)	—	8.5
Vitamin B_6 (µg)	12	93
Biotin (µg)	0.1	0.6
Pantothenic acid (µg)	183	180
Vitamin B_{12} (ng)	200	26
Ascorbic acid (mg)	4.4	4.0

TABLE A-1	**Composition of human colostrum and mature breast milk—cont'd**		
Constituent (per 100 ml)	**Colostrum 1-5 days**	**Mature milk >30 days**	
Minerals			
Calcium (mg)	23	28	
Magnesium (mg)	3.4	3.0	
Sodium (mg)	48	18	
Potassium (mg)	74	58	
Chlorine (mg)	91	42	
Phosphorus (mg)	14	15	
Sulphur (mg)	22	14	
Trace elements			
Chromium (ng)	—	50	
Cobalt (μg)	—	1	
Copper (μg)	46	25	
Fluorine (μg)	—	16	
Iodine (μg)	12	11	
Iron (μg)	45	40	
Manganese (μg)	—	0.6±	
Nickel (μg)	—	2	
Selenium (μg)	—	2.0	
Zinc (μg)	540	120	

$\mathcal{D}$ietary guidance during lactation

GENERAL GUIDELINES

1. Follow nutrition guide for regular food plan during pregnancy.
2. Eat a wide variety of foods, including milk and milk products and eggs.
3. If no milk is allowed, use a supplement of 4 μg of vitamin B_{12} daily. If goat or soy milk is used, partial supplementation may be needed.
4. If no milk is taken, also use supplements of 12 mg of calcium and 400 IU of vitamin D daily. Partial supplementation will be necessary if fewer than four servings of milk and milk products are consumed.
5. Select a variety of plant foods (especially nuts, grains, legumes, and seeds) to obtain "complete" proteins by complementary combinations.
6. Use iodized salt.

Normal serum values for breastfed infants

TABLE C-1   Serum chemical values of normal breastfed infants*

Concentration/100 ml of serum	Age 28 days			Age 56 days			Age 84 days			Age 112 days		
	N	Mean	SD	N	Mean	SD	N	Mean	SD	N	Mean	SD
Males												
Total protein (g)	22	5.87	0.50	36	5.96	0.42	29	6.16	0.57	51	6.29	0.51
Albumin (g)	22	4.02	0.35	36	4.14	0.34	29	4.27	0.39	51	4.38	0.40
Globulins (g)												
alpha$_1$	22	0.14	0.03	36	0.17	0.03	29	0.18	0.03	51	0.17	0.04
alpha$_2$	22	0.53	0.10	36	0.60	0.11	29	0.74	0.14	51	0.81	0.19
beta	22	0.61	0.11	36	0.67	0.13	29	0.69	0.20	51	0.67	0.11
gamma	22	0.57	0.14	36	0.38	0.09	29	0.28	0.08	51	0.26	0.10
Cholesterol (mg)	21	139	31	32	153	34	25	133	32	47	145	26
Triglycerides (mg)	18	122	36	32	106	57	25	170	76	46	148	57
Urea nitrogen (mg)	43	8.5	3.2	49	6.6	2.1	47	7.0	2.7	51	7.3	4.2
Calcium (mg)	41	10.2	0.8	47	10.3	1.0	42	10.4	0.8	48	10.3	0.8
Phosphorus (mg)	43	6.6	0.7	49	6.4	0.7	47	6.2	0.5	49	6.2	0.7
Alkaline phosphatase†	31	22	6	40	21	7	35	21	8	44	18	7
Magnesium (mg)	40	2.0	0.2	47	2.1	0.2	45		0.2	50	2.2	0.2

Females

	N	Mean	SD	N	Mean	SD	N	Mean	SD	N	Mean	SD
Total protein (g)	18	6.04	0.40	27	5.86	0.44	21	6.21	0.57	42	6.31	0.62
Albumin (g)	18	4.07	0.27	27	4.03	0.35	21	4.29	0.37	42	4.36	0.42
Globulins (g)												
alpha$_1$	18	0.15	0.02	27	0.17	0.04	21	0.17	0.03	42	**0.19**	0.04
alpha$_2$	18	0.55	0.07	27	0.65	0.12	21	0.74	0.18	42	0.78	0.17
beta	18	0.70	0.18	27	0.63	0.11	21	0.71	0.13	42	0.67	0.16
gamma	18	0.57	0.10	27	0.38	0.10	21	0.30	0.06	42	**0.31**	0.10
Cholesterol (mg)	13	**180**	35	25	157	37	20	**155**	29	40	**165**	36
Triglycerides (mg)	9	**157**	43	24	112	53	18	195	56	38	**170**	52
Urea nitrogen (mg)	37	8.3	2.3	33	6.4	2.2	40	6.4	2.2	42	6.6	3.5
Calcium (mg)	37	10.3	0.8	33	10.3	0.8	40	10.3	0.8	42	10.7	0.7
Phosphorus (mg)	39	6.9	0.8	33	6.4	0.8	40	6.1	0.7	42	6.1	0.7
Alkaline phosphatase	31	19	5	28	17	5	32	17	5	36	17	5
Magnesium (mg)	39	2.0	0.4	32	2.0	0.2	40	2.1	0.2	41	2.1	0.3

From Fomon SJ, Filer LJ, Thomas LN et al: Growth and serum chemical values of normal breastfed infants, *Acta Paediatr Scand Suppl* 202:1, 1970.
*Bold figures indicate that value is greater than the corresponding value for infants of the opposite sex and that the difference is statistically significant at the 95% level of confidence.
†King-Armstrong units.

$\mathcal{D}$rugs in breast milk and the effect on the infant

The following list of drugs in Table D-1 is provided to assist the clinician in making judgments about management for specific drugs in an individual mother and her infant. The clinician is referred to Chapter 11 for the discussion of interpretation of risks and benefits. It is also important to point out that the significance of a given blood level would vary with the pH and the binding capacity of the maternal plasma protein, which may differ for various ethnic and racial groups. Furthermore, it is not merely a matter of understanding the pharmacokinetics of a specific drug, but also of understanding the physiology of milk production and, most critically, understanding the absorption and excretion of the drug by the newborn, which changes with conceptual and chronologic age.

The drugs have been grouped by their major use to provide an opportunity to compare therapeutic choices and select the medication that is best for both mother and infant. The drugs have also been numbered if they were rated by the Committee on Drugs of the American Academy of Pediatrics (AAP), which has published a list of drugs that may transfer into human milk.* When no Arabic number follows the drug name, the compound was not included in that list. The following numbers and definitions are used by the committee:

1. Drugs that are contraindicated during breast-feeding
2. Drugs of abuse that are contraindicated during breastfeeding
3. Radioactive compounds that require temporary cessation of breastfeeding
4. Drugs whose effect on nursing infants is unknown but may be of concern
5. Drugs that have been associated with significant effects on some nursing infants and should be given to nursing mothers with caution
6. Maternal medication usually compatible with breastfeeding
7. Food and environmental agents: effect on breastfeeding

This appendix has been grouped into drugs used in different medical situations, thus providing the physician an opportunity to select the safest drug for a specific purpose. The classifications are grouped by use. The drug can also be found in the index. Only the most significant bibliography has been included to conserve space.

The classifications of the drugs listed are as follows:

Analgesics and antiinflammatory drugs (non-narcotic), p. 746

Anesthetics, p. 754

Anticoagulants and coagulants, p. 756

---

*The Committee on Drugs, American Academy of Pediatrics: The transfer of drugs and other chemicals into human breast milk, *Pediatrics* 93:137, 1994. An update is planned by the Committee in 1999.

The continued update and expansion of the drug information resource has been carried out by Linda R. Friedman, PhD. In the interest of space, references older than 1985 have been deleted. Please refer to the fourth edition of the text to access them.

TABLE D-1	Relationship of drugs to breast milk and effect on infant			
Drug and AAP rating	% Oral availability	Peak plasma time (hr)	% Plasma protein bound	Volume of distribution (L/kg)
Analgesics and antiinflammatory (nonnarcotic)				
Acetaminophen 6	88 ± 15	0.16-1	0-25	0.8-1.36
Antipyrine	99		Negligible	
Aspirin 5	58.5 ± 12.5		49-70	0.15 ± 0.03
Auranofin	15-25	Within 2	60	0.045
Aurothioglucose 6			90-99	
Azapropazone 6		2-6	99.5	0.125 ± 0.025
Butorphanol 6	~5 44-113 nasal	0.15-1.5 nasal	80	
Colchicine 6		1.25	31	0.7

M/P ratio	% Adult dose in milk	Maximum amount in milk (mg/L)	Comments and references
0.2-1.9	0.04-1.85	15	In milk: 0.05%-0.7% of newborn therapeutic dose; mean 0.888 mg/L, peak 2 hr. Active metabolite: paracetamol. Only drug found in milk; both drug and metabolite found in the infant's urine. Brand names: Tylenol, Excedrin, Darvocet, Comtrex, etc. (68, 192, 390)
1	0.56-2.38	30	Use in ear drops. In milk: half-life 11.6 ± 5.4 hr. (123)
0.03-1.0	0.5-21	42.6	High first-pass hepatic metabolism. Exposure in utero may increase rate of maturation of metabolic process. In milk: 0.06%-25% of newborn therapeutic dose, peak 6 ± 3 hr. Brand names: Bayer, Anacin, Bufferin, Excedrin, Fiorinal, Empirin, etc. (192, 519, 558)
Found in rodent milk, and gold is excreted into human milk			Brand name: Ridaura (192, 424)
0.01-0.2	20	10.2	In milk: peak 5 ± 1 hr. Gold has been found in the infant's red blood cells and serum. Some believe it is incompatible with breastfeeding. Brand name: Solganal. (192, 406, 424, 456, 519)
	0.04-1.5		Almost completely absorbed. (30, 519)
0.7-1.9		0.004	1% of newborn dose in milk. Given during labor, it crosses the placenta. Brand name: Stadol. (424, 489, 519)
>1		0.003	One report of a woman who took drug as long-term therapy through pregnancy and 0.6 mg twice a day while lactating. No apparent effects on a 6-month-old. Brand name: ColBenemid. (192, 355, 377, 519)

Continued

TABLE D-1	**Relationship of drugs to breast milk and effect on infant—cont'd**			
Drug and AAP rating	**% Oral availability**	**Peak plasma time (hr)**	**% Plasma protein bound**	**Volume of distribution (L/kg)**
Analgesics and antiinflammatory (nonnarcotic)—cont'd				
Diclofenac	58 ± 14	0.5-4	99-99.9	0.335 ± 0.215
Diflunisal	>99	2.5 ± 0.5	99.9 ± 0.01	0.1 ± 0.01
Etodolac	At least 80	1.2-2	95->99	0.84-3.1 active S enantiomer
Fenbufen	86	1.5 ± 0.5	98-99	3
Fenoprofen	82.5 ± 2.5	1-2	99	0.08-0.1
Flufenamic acid 6		1.5-6	>90	
Flunisolide	8-78 Mean 20			1.96 ± 0.46
Fluocortolone	78-89	1.4 ± 0.2	80	0.84 ± 0.16
Flurbiprofen	Almost completely absorbed orally	0.5-4	99	0.1

M/P ratio	% Adult dose in milk	Maximum amount in milk (mg/L)	Comments and references
	1.2	0.01	Completely and rapidly absorbed with extensive first-pass metabolism. Food delays absorption but does not decrease amount taken in. Rectal and oral parameters are the same. 48% protein bound in human skim milk. Has four active metabolites whose presence in milk is unknown. Brand name: Voltaren. (18, 245, 424, 496, 538, 549, 595)
0.02-0.07			A difluorophenyl derivative of aspirin whose half-life is dose dependent. The percentage protein bound decreases at concentrations greater than 100 mg/L. Brand name: Dolobid. (192, 424, 519)
			Food delays absorption. Brand name: Lodine. (33, 247)
0.006-0.02	<0.75		Absorption delayed but not decreased when taken with food. Has two active metabolites that have longer half-lives than drug. (20, 519)
0.017			Food delays and reduces absorption. Brand name: Nalfon. (68, 424, 496, 519)
<0.01			Maternal plasma level is 50 times greater than infant's. Mean plasma concentration in nursing infant is 0.43 μg/L. Brand name: Arlef. (519)
			Extensive first-pass metabolism. Not known whether excreted into milk; other corticosteroids are. Brand names: Nasalide, AeroBid. (7, 424)
			The metabolite is less active. (496)
0.008-0.03	0.25	0.08	Metabolites are inert. Drug not detected in most milk samples. Peak plasma concentration, but not amount absorbed, reduced when taken with food. Bioavailability from suppositories similar to tablets. Brand name: Ansaid. (87, 506)

Continued

TABLE D-1	Relationship of drugs to breast milk and effect on infant—cont'd			
Drug and AAP rating	**% Oral availability**	**Peak plasma time (hr)**	**% Plasma protein bound**	**Volume of distribution (L/kg)**
Analgesics and antiinflammatory (nonnarcotic)—cont'd				
Ibuprofen 6	>80	1.5 ± 0.5	>99	0.15 ± 0.02
Indomethacin 6	85-122 37-112 rectal	2 ± 1	90-99.6	0.12-1.57
Ketoprofen	92 ± 7	1.25 ± 0.75	99.2 ± 0.1	0.15 ± 0.03
Ketorolac tromethamine 6	80-100	0.33-1	99.1-99.3	0.11-0.33
Mefenamic acid 6		1-3	High	
Nalbuphine	16 ± 8	0.3		3.8 ± 1.1
Naproxen	74-99	1-4	98.2 ± 4.5	0.16 ± 0.02
Noscapine 6	30	1.5 ± 0.5		
Olsalazine	1-3	0.5-2	99.5	
Oxaprozin	95	3-5	99.9	Large
Oxyphenbutazone			95.7 ± 3.3	Small
Pentazocine	18 ± 8	0.5-4	60-65	5.6
Phenacetin	0-49		30-52.7	1.5

M/P ratio	% Adult dose in milk	Maximum amount in milk (mg/L)	Comments and references
	<0.8	<0.05	Metabolites are inert. Food slows absorption. Half-life and % protein bound show nonlinear kinetics probably caused by saturable plasma-binding protein. Brand names: Advil, Motrin, Rufen, Dristan, Nuprin, etc. (20, 192, 506, 595)
0.01-1.48	0.07-0.98	4	Food delays absorption. In milk: 66%-133% of newborn dose. Bioavailability in premature infant: 13%. Brand name: Indocin. (39, 51, 52, 192, 303, 424, 446, 496, 519, 561, 565)
		Trace	Brand name: Orudis. (192, 424, 496, 519)
0.015-0.037	0.16-0.4	0.008	Food decreases rate but not extent of absorption. Brand name: Toradol. (7, 71, 595)
0.23	0.036-0.8		Infant able to excrete drug via urine. No evidence for drug accumulation. Brand name: Ponstel. (424, 519)
	<1		Has active metabolites. Brand name: Nubain. (192, 424, 519)
0.01	0.26-1.1	2.37	In milk: less than 0.5%-2% of newborn therapeutic, peaks at 4 hr. 0.26% of a chronic user's dose recovered in infant's urine. Food delays absorption. Brand names: Anaprox, Naprosyn. (7, 17, 20, 192, 424, 496, 545, 569)
0.15-0.88	0.5		Extensive first-pass metabolism. In milk: peak 1.5 ± 0.5 hr. (20, 266, 403)
			Two molecules of 5-aminosalicylic acid (ASA) joined by an azobond. Most of it is split into two ASA in the colon. Brand name: Dipentum. (300, 571)
			Brand name: Daypro. (424)
0.1-0.8			Drug was found in the milk of 2 of 55 women. No known effect of drug in milk. (192, 519)
			Well absorbed from GI tract with extensive first-pass metabolism. Brand names: Talacen, Talwin. (7, 424, 496, 519)
0.16-1.02	0.05		Active metabolite: acetaminophen. Average amount in milk: 0.071 mg/L. (68, 496, 519)

Continued

TABLE D-1	Relationship of drugs to breast milk and effect on infant—cont'd			
Drug and AAP rating	% Oral availability	Peak plasma time (hr)	% Plasma protein bound	Volume of distribution (L/kg)
Analgesics and antiinflammatory (nonnarcotic)—cont'd				
Phenylbutazone 6	80-100 rectal availability 77% of oral availability	2.5 ± 1.4	97 ± 2	0.14 ± 0.05
Piroxicam 6	99	2-3 after oral dose 5-6 after rectal dose	99.3 ± 0.2	0.12-0.15
Propoxyphene 6	23-35	2.25 ± 0.25		
Salicylic acid	95 ± 6	2.3 ± 0.1	70 ± 20	0.13-0.2
Sulindac	89 ± 1	1-4	92-96	2
Suprofen 6	92	1.25 ± 0.75	99.2 ± 0.2	
Tolmetin 6	>90	0.34-1	99.6 ± 0.1	0.54 ± 0.07
Tramadol	68 after single dose 90-100 after multiple doses	1.6-2	4-20	3.3

M/P ratio	% Adult dose in milk	Maximum amount in milk (mg/L)	Comments and references
0.1-0.91	0.4	6.3	Two active metabolites; dose-dependent kinetics. In newborn, plasma protein bound: 85%-90%, volume of distribution 0.2-0.25 L/kg, plasma half-life 21-34 hr. Brand name: Butazolidin. (68, 192, 424)
0.01-0.03	6.75 ± 3.25	0.22	One nursing infant was studied; drug not detected in infant's plasma. In milk: peak 4 hr. Brand name: Feldene. (20, 405, 424, 496)
0.5		1	Extensive hepatic first-pass metabolism. In milk: less than 0.3% of newborn therapeutic dose, maximum amount of active metabolite, norpropoxyphene: 169.1 μg/ml. M/P ratio based on one mother-infant pair. Brand names: Darvon, Wygesic. (68, 424, 496)
0.03-0.4	11.6 ± 9.4	38	Aspirin metabolite with dose-dependent kinetics. Amount bound to plasma protein decreases as amount in plasma increases. In neonate: half-life greater than 7 hr. In milk: average amount 0.924 mg/L, peaks at 3 hr; 0.1% of maternal dose excreted in 12 hr. Metabolic acidosis reported in 16-day-old when mother took drug every 4 hr. Brand names: Viranol, Salactic, Sal-Plant, Paplex, SalAc, Occlusal, etc. (20, 51, 192, 496)
Excreted into rat's milk			Food decreases rate and extent of absorption. Brand name: Clinoril. (192, 424, 496, 519)
0.005-0.014	0.7	0.23	On empty stomach, rapidly and completely absorbed. With food, oral availability is less. Does not accumulate to any extent. In milk: peak 1.5 ± 0.5 hr, 10% is bound to milk proteins. (20, 424, 496)
0.005-0.007	0.3	0.18	Completely absorbed. In milk: peak 0.67-1 hr. Active metabolite formed. Brand name: Tolectin. (20, 68, 192, 424)
	0.1		% availability: IM 100; rectal 78. Brand name: Ultram. (306)

Continued

TABLE D-1	Relationship of drugs to breast milk and effect on infant—cont'd			
Drug and AAP rating	% Oral availability	Peak plasma time (hr)	% Plasma protein bound	Volume of distribution (L/kg)
Anesthetics				
Alfentanil			80.9-96.3	0.8 ± 0.3
Bupivacaine		0.15-1.5	90 ± 5	1.2 ± 0.4
Fentanyl 6	0-49	0.33-3	84 ± 2	4 ± 0.4
Halothane 6				
Ketamine	20 ± 7		12	1.8 ± 0.7
Lidocaine 6	34 ± 12	0.5	55-80	0.2-1.8
Meperidine	54 ± 19	1.25 ± 0.75	54.5 ± 15.5	4.4 ± 0.9
Methohexital				2.2 ± 0.7
Midazolam 4	28-72	1.22 ± 0.88	93-97	0.6-6.6
Procaine	When given as a local for dental work, it is usually confined to the local area by the addition of adrenalin			
Propofol			97-99	2.46-8.09
Sufentanil		0.05-1.5	93 ± 1	2.5 ± 1.6

M/P ratio	% Adult dose in milk	Maximum amount in milk (mg/L)	Comments and references
		0.00156	Used in premature infants. Brand name: Alfenta. (111, 192, 309, 310)
	0.1	0.45	Infant exposed during C-section. No drug isolated from the blood of infant whose mother had 0.1% of the dose in her milk. Brand names: Marcaine, Sensorcaine. (28, 66, 240, 424)
2.1			In colostrum: at peak 0.08-0.97 ng/ml. In milk: peak 0.75 hr. Brand names: Duragesic, Innovar, Sublimaze. (7, 192, 519, 526, 530)
3.5		0.002	In milk: 2 ppm. No symptoms in infants. Mother's exposure may be in working environment (i.e., operating room). Brand name: Fluothane. (427)
			Has metabolites with possible metabolic activity. Brand name: Ketalar. (192, 519)
0.4	0.34	16	Rapidly metabolized in liver. Given to neonates. Depresses prolactin secretion. Brand names: Anestacon, Decadron, Xylocaine. (20, 51, 192, 356, 496, 519, 580, 613)
1-2.5		0.571	In milk: peak 2 hr, less than 3.3% newborn therapeutic dose. Renal excretion of drug and metabolite, which is half as active as drug, is pH dependent. Brand names: Demerol, Mepergan. (68, 192, 380, 388, 522)
0.4-2.5		0.407	Brand name: Brevital. (192, 519)
0.09-0.21		0.7	Undergoes first-pass metabolism. Active metabolite: hydroxymidazolam is less active than the drug and is found in milk in the same amount as parent drug. Drug used in C-sections and in critically ill neonates. Brand name: Versed. (7, 23, 192, 252, 334, 519)
			Brand name: Novocaine.
0.6-1.3		0.97	May not have good oral availability in infant. Exposure through breast milk is negligible compared to placental transfer during C-section. Brand name: Diprivan. (106, 193)
Not detected in breast milk after a single dose			80% excreted in 24 hr with only 2% eliminated as unchanged drug. Volume of distribution and half-life increase in neonate. Very lipid soluble. (192, 218, 424)

Continued

TABLE D-1	Relationship of drugs to breast milk and effect on infant—cont'd			
Drug and AAP rating	% Oral availability	Peak plasma time (hr)	% Plasma protein bound	Volume of distribution (L/kg)
Anesthetics—cont'd				
Thiopental 6			87 ± 6	2.3 ± 0.5
Vecuronium bromide			60-90	0.19-0.51
Anticoagulants and coagulants				
Acenocoumarol		1-4	98.5	
Aminocaproic acid		2	0	0.4
Dicumarol 6	Slow and incomplete		95-99	0.15
Enoxaparin	Inactivated in the GI tract			
Ethyl biscoumacetate			90	0.079 ± 0.021
Heparin	0		95	0.058 ± 0.010
Phenindione				
Tranexamic acid	34-38.5 Low absorption through rectum			
Warfarin 6	93 ± 8	1-9	97-99	0.14 ± 0.06

M/P ratio	% Adult dose in milk	Maximum amount in milk (mg/L)	Comments and references
0.4-0.5		20	Used for C-sections. (23, 192)
			Half-life in maternal plasma: 0.52-1.92 hr. Metabolite has 50%-70% of the activity of the drug. Brand name: Norcuron. (2, 7, 192, 424, 480)
Not detected in milk of 20 mothers (sensitivity 15 ng/ml)			Food delays absorption. Brand name: Sintrom. (165)
			Completely absorbed from GI tract. Brand name: Amicar. (7, 519)
0.01-0.02	0.5	2	Not measurable in all milk samples. Has been associated with bleeding in breastfed infants. (192, 424)
			A heparin of 4500 average molecular weight. Brand name: Lovenox. (68, 424)
0.013-0.8	0.1	1.7	Hemorrhage around umbilical stump and cephalhematoma reported. No adverse effects found in the nursing infants of 22 mothers taking the drug. Brand name: Tromexan. (68, 519)
Not excreted into human milk			(192, 424, 519)
		5	Not used in US. Amount in milk dose related. Breast milk a major route of excretion. Reports of serious hemorrhaging in the infant. (68)
	0.018 ± 0.006		Brand name: Cyklokapron. (496, 519)
<0.2	<4.4		Excretion into milk varies. In 13 mothers taking 2-12 mg/day, less than 25 ng/ml found in milk. Brand name: Coumadin. (17, 192, 358, 424, 519)

Continued

TABLE D-1	Relationship of drugs to breast milk and effect on infant—cont'd				
Drug and AAP rating	**% Oral availability**	**Peak plasma time (hr)**	**% Plasma protein bound**	**Volume of distribution (L/kg)**
Anticonvulsants and sedatives				
Carbamazepine 6	70-85	4-8	73-90	1.4 ± 0.4
Clonazepam	98 ± 31	1.5 ± 0.5	86 ± 0.5	1.5-4.4
Divalproex	Drug dissociates into valproic acid in the GI tract			
Ethosuximide 6	100 ± 10	3 ± 1	0	0.72 ± 0.16
Gabapentin	53-60	2-3.2	<3	0.7-1
Glutethimide	Erratic	1-6	47.3-59.3	
Lamotrigine	98 ± 5	2.75 ± 1.2	55	1.15 ± 0.25
Magnesium sulfate 6	25-40		30	
Oxcarbazepine		1-4	67	

M/P ratio	% Adult dose in milk	Maximum amount in milk (mg/L)	Comments and references
0.2-0.69	2.5-4.9	4.8	Amount in nursing infant's serum about 0.004 mg/L. One report of transient cholestatic hepatitis in a nursing baby. Plasma level of metabolite, carbamazepine 10, 11 epoxide is 10%-50% that of the drug. Metabolite's kinetics are oral availability: 90% ± 11%; M/P ratio: 0.53-1.8; maximum amount in breast milk: 2 mg/L. Brand name: Tegretol. (20, 49, 68, 125, 172, 192, 342, 424, 446, 592)
0.33	2.5	0.013	In milk: peak 4 hr. Brand name: Klonopin. (192, 424, 509, 519)
			Brand name: Depakote. (424)
0.5-1.1	13-30	80	Half-life lower in children; varies in neonates. In nursing infant's serum: 15-40 mg/L. Drug not bound to protein in milk. Infants may be sedated. Brand name: Zarontin. (17, 20, 38, 68, 192, 342, 446, 496, 519)
			Brand name: Neurontin. (54, 439)
1	0.5	0.27	In milk: peak 8-12 hr. Active metabolite: 4-hydroxygluthimide. Brand name: Doriden. (20, 424, 519)
			Brand name: Lamictal. (54, 196, 439)
0.6-2.1	0.5		M/P ratio in women not taking the drug: 2.1; in women taking the drug: 1.9. Brand names: Eldertonic, Vicon Forte. (20, 68)
0.5			Amount in milk comes from the study of one patient. Active metabolite, 10-hydroxy-carbazepine, is 30%-47% protein bound, systemic availability of metabolite increases 17% when the drug is taken with food. (81, 136)

Continued

TABLE D-1	Relationship of drugs to breast milk and effect on infant—cont'd			
Drug and AAP rating	% Oral availability	Peak plasma time (hr)	% Plasma protein bound	Volume of distribution (L/kg)
Anticonvulsants and sedatives—cont'd				
Pentobarbital	94 ± 11		55	1
Phenobarbital 5	97 ± 14	3 ± 1	20-60	0.63 ± 0.12
Phenylethylmalonamide	91 ± 4		8 ± 1	0.69 ± 0.1
Phenytoin 6	89 ± 16		89 ± 23	0.675 ± 0.075
Primidone 5	92 ± 18		19	0.67 ± 0.6
Sodium bromide 6,7				
Topiramate	75-80	1.8-4.3	9-17	0.6-0.8
Valproic acid 6	100 ± 10	1-4	80-95	0.22 ± 0.07

M/P ratio	% Adult dose in milk	Maximum amount in milk (mg/L)	Comments and references
	Excreted into human milk		0.17 mg/L was detected in milk 19 hr after a 100-mg dose taken daily for 32 days. Depends on the liver for detoxification, so may accumulate in newborn. Plasma half-life is dose dependent. Brand name: Nembutal. (68, 424, 496, 519)
0.2-1	1.5	33	In milk: 4%-100% of newborn therapeutic dose. If mother's plasma level >30 mg/L, infant may be excessively sleepy. One case of methemoglobinemia reported. Drug is active metabolite of primidone. Brand names: Donnatal, Kinesed, Tedral, Quadrinal. (41, 125, 342, 496, 519)
0.5-1			Active metabolite of primidone with increased half-life in neonate. (125, 192)
0.13-2	1.4-7.2	18	No problem breastfeeding if mother's plasma concentration is in therapeutic range. Decreased oral availability in newborn. In milk: peak 3.5 ± 0.5 hr; 2%-40% of newborn therapeutic dose. Brand name: Dilantin. (17, 20, 52, 68, 125, 192, 342, 356, 389, 424, 427, 446, 458, 496, 509)
0.18-1	2.1 ± 0.7	10	15%-25% of dose converted to phenobarbital. Phenylethylmalonamide also a metabolite. Infant may be drowsy. Bleeding may result from hypoprothrombinemia. Brand name: Mysoline. (20, 136, 192, 342, 358, 446, 519)
		66	No longer available in the US. Rash and drowsiness reported after breastfeeding. Absorption through skin and transfer to milk is a concern if mother works in a photographic laboratory. (39, 68)
	Excreted in rat's milk		Elimination is faster in children. Brand name: Topamax. (54)
0.05-0.42	1.8	12	In milk: 0.05%-11.3% of newborn therapeutic dose. Neonate has good clearance and poorly absorbs drug orally. Brand name: Depakene. (20, 68, 125, 192, 277, 342, 397, 592)

Continued

TABLE D-1   Relationship of drugs to breast milk and effect on infant—cont'd

Drug and AAP rating	% Oral availability	Peak plasma time (hr)	% Plasma protein bound	Volume of distribution (L/kg)
Anticonvulsants and sedatives—cont'd				
Valpromide				1
Antihistamines	Anticholinergic action may suppress lactation; administer after nursing			
Azatadine		4		
Brompheniramine		3.1 ± 1.1		11.7 ± 3.1
Brompheniramine maleate		1-5		11.7
Cetirizine		0.5-1.2	93	0.7
Chlorpheniramine	41 ± 16	4.25 ± 1.75	70 ± 3	3.2 ± 0.3
Chlorpheniramine maleate	25-60	4 ± 2	69-72	2.5-3.2
Clemastine 5		3.5 ± 1.5		
Dexbrompheniramine 6	Dexbrompheniramine maleate is well absorbed from GI tract			
Diphenhydramine	72 ± 25	1-4	75-98.5	6.2 ± 2.9
Fexofenadine				
Flunarizine	85-86	2-4	90-99	43-78

M/P ratio	% Adult dose in milk	Maximum amount in milk (mg/L)	Comments and references
			81% ± 11% metabolized to valproic acid. If taken orally, not found in the plasma, only metabolite is. (53)
			Readily absorbed from GI tract. Brand name: Trinalin (7, 424)
	Half-life in milk: 24.9 ± 9.3 hr		Has two active metabolites.
			Well absorbed from GI tract. Active metabolite: brompheniramine. Brand names: Bromfed, Dimetane, Dristan. (7)
			Does not have anticholinergic activity. Half-life is shorter in children. Brand name: Zyrtec. (85, 122, 520)
	Excreted into human milk		Clearance negatively correlated with age. Other reports of volume of distribution: children 4.3-7 L/kg, adults 5.9-11.7 L/kg. (192, 519, 542)
			Oral availability: tablets, 25%-45%; solution, 35%-60%. Volume of distribution in children: 3.8 L/kg. Brand name: Chlor-Pro. (7)
0.25-0.5	29.5 ± 20.5	0.01	Drug not detected in infant's plasma. Infant may be irritable and drowsy. Brand name: Tavist. (68, 424, 519)
			Related to brompheniramine. (7, 424)
	Excreted into human milk		Metabolism shows ethnic variation. Volume of distribution greater and amount protein bound less in Orientals than Caucasians. In rats, amount received through milk is quite low, but the M/P ratio varies from 3.85 to 9.54. Brand name: Benadryl. (7, 68, 129, 192, 444, 496, 519)
0.04-0.77			In milk: peak 4.25 ± 2.36 hr; half life 14.15 ± 5.44 hr. Brand name: Allegra. (325)
	Excreted into dog's milk		Elimination half-life after one dose is 17-18 days. (519)

Continued

TABLE D-1   Relationship of drugs to breast milk and effect on infant—cont'd

Drug and AAP rating	% Oral availability	Peak plasma time (hr)	% Plasma protein bound	Volume of distribution (L/kg)
Antihistamines—cont'd				
Levocabastine	100-120	2	55	1.14
Loratadine				
Promethazine	25 ± 10 Well absorbed from GI tract; rapidly metabolized	2.8 ± 1.4	76-80	13.4 ± 3.6
Roxatidine		1.3 ± 0.7		1.7-3.2
Trimeprazine				
Tripelennamine		2-3		
Triprolidine 6	Erratic	2 ± 1.2		
Antiinfective agents	May change intestinal flora of baby and sensitize for later allergic reaction			
Acyclovir 6	15-50	1.5-2.5	9-33	0.69 ± 0.19
Amantadine	50-100	4	67	6.6 ± 1.5
Amikacin	Poor absorption	1 after IM	<10	0.08-0.48
Aminosalicylic acid (para)		1.5-2	15	0.2
Amoxicillin 6	70.9-105.5	1.5 ± 0.5	17-20	0.29 ± 0.11
Amphotericin B	<10 Poor absorption		90-95	3-4.4

M/P ratio	% Adult dose in milk	Maximum amount in milk (mg/L)	Comments and references
			Availability: intranasal 60%-80%; ocular, 30%-60%; topically absorption incomplete. As nasal spray, amount in milk <3.5 μg/day. (116)
1.2	0.01	0.0292	In milk: worst case, drug + metabolite, 1.1% of adult dose on mg/kg basis. Brand name: Claritin. (229)
Passage into human milk expected			Increases serum prolactin level. Brand names: Phenergan, Mepergan. (68, 496)
			Taken as roxatidine acetate. Greater than 95% orally absorbed; almost completely deacetylated to roxatidine. In vitro, 6%-7% plasma protein bound. (318, 373)
Low level found in human milk			May cause galactorrhea. Brand name: Temaril. (68)
Has been isolated from bovine milk			Well absorbed orally. Brand name: PBZ. (7, 68)
0.5-1.2	0.06-0.2	0.004	In milk: peak 1.5 ± 0.5 hr. Transdermal patch: plasma peak 14.4 ± 9.9 hr. Brand name: Actifed. (20, 353)
0.6-4.1	5.6 ± 4.4	5.81	Oral availability decreases with dose. Baby gets <1-2 mg/day. In milk: peak 3-10 hr, half-life 2.8 hr. Minimal absorption through skin. Brand name: Zovirax. (20, 68, 126, 192, 298, 350, 364, 496, 534, 573)
Excreted into human milk in low amounts			May lower maternal prolactin levels. Brand name: Symmetrel. (68, 192, 424, 496, 519)
Trace			In milk: peak 5 ± 1 hr. Given to prematures. Renal function most significant factor in drug elimination. Brand name: Amikin. (20, 68, 192, 276, 407, 519, 612)
0.016	0.25-0.5	1.1	In milk: peak 3 hr. (20, 192, 519)
0.013-0.043	0.7	1.3	In milk: 0.18% of calculated newborn therapeutic dose. Dose-dependent oral availability. Brand names: Amoxil, Augmentin. (7, 20, 192, 446, 519, 583)
			Used in infants. Brand names: Abelect, Amphotec, Fungizone. (7, 32, 192, 446, 471, 496, 519)

Continued

TABLE D-1   Relationship of drugs to breast milk and effect on infant—cont'd

Drug and AAP rating	% Oral availability	Peak plasma time (hr)	% Plasma protein bound	Volume of distribution (L/kg)
Antiinfective agents—cont'd				
Ampicillin	62 ± 17	1.5	22 ± 7	0.21-0.7
Azithromycin	37-40	1-4	7-50 Negatively correlated with serum concentration	23-31
Azlocillin	Poor absorption		28 ± 6	0.22 ± 0.06
Aztreonam 6	Poor absorption	1.5 after IM	56	0.21
Bacampicillin	87 ± 22	0.8 ± 0.1		
Carbenicillin	<10		50-60	0.18-0.2
Cefaclor	90	0.5-2	25	0.36
Cefadroxil 6	78-90	1-3	18-20	0.17-0.3
Cefamandole nafate	Not absorbed orally	1.25 ± 0.75	73.5 ± 6.5	0.16 ± 0.05
Cefatrizine	55-77	2	58	
Cefazolin 6	Not absorbed orally	1.5 ± 0.5 after IM	77.5 ± 7.5	0.12 ± 0.03

M/P ratio	% Adult dose in milk	Maximum amount in milk (mg/L)	Comments and references
0.01-0.58	0.05-0.4	1	In milk: 0.14%-0.4% newborn therapeutic dose, reaches a plateau at 2-6 hr. In neonates: half-life increases, 7%-12% plasma protein bound, oral availability increases. An active metabolite of pivampicillin and bacampicillin. Brand name: Unasyn. (51, 64, 68, 192, 336, 446)
		2.8	Average tissue half-life is 1-4 days. Given directly to 20 children between the ages of 7 months and 2 years. No side effects were noted. Brand name: Zithromax. (99, 236, 275, 289, 321, 423, 593)
	Low		Half-life dose dependent, increases from beginning to end of treatment. Given to neonates and prematures. Brand name: Azlin. (192, 407, 424, 519)
0.002-0.009	2.35 ± 0.35	0.4	In milk: peak 3-6 hr. Used in prematures. Brand name: Azactam. (20, 104, 379)
			In GI tract, converted to ampicillin. Brand name: Spectrobid. (424, 496)
0.02	0.001		Not well absorbed from GI tract. Given to neonates. In milk: 0.03% of newborn dose, peak 4 hr, 1 hr after 1-g dose, 0.265 µg/ml found. Brand name: Geocillin. (19, 20, 192, 407, 446, 496, 519)
		0.21	Food delays absorption. Brand name: Ceclor. (68, 192, 394, 424, 496)
0.009-0.02	0.4	2.4	Saturable GI and renal tubular reabsorption; both affect amount of drug in the system. In milk: peak 5-7 hr; larger doses peak later. Brand name: Duricef. (7, 68, 188, 192, 363, 424, 519)
0.02		0.46	85%-89% rapidly hydrolyzed to cefamandole. Half-life longer in neonates. Brand name: Mandol. (7, 68, 192, 407, 424, 519)
	Excreted into human milk		(496, 542)
0.02-0.023	0.075	1.5	Detected in milk, when given IV not IM. Given to prematures. In milk: maximum amount 0.9% of newborn therapeutic dose; peak 3 hr. Brand names: Ancef, Kefzol. (20, 68, 192, 407, 424)

Continued

| TABLE D-1 | Relationship of drugs to breast milk and effect on infant—cont'd | | | |

Drug and AAP rating	% Oral availability	Peak plasma time (hr)	% Plasma protein bound	Volume of distribution (L/kg)
Antiinfective agents—cont'd				
Cefixime	30-50	2-6	65-70	0.103 ± 0.008
Cefmenoxine	Not absorbed orally			0.12
Cefpodoxime		2.9 ± 0.8	18-50	
Cefpodoxime proxetil	Food increases bioavailability; esterases in the intestinal wall convert this prodrug to the active compound cefpodoxime (see above)			
Cefonicid	Not absorbed orally		96-98	0.11 ± 0.01
Cefoperazone	<10		77.5 ± 12.5	0.25 ± 0.15
Ceforanide	Not absorbed orally	1 after IM	80-82	0.14 ± 0.04
Cefotaxime 6		0.5	40 ± 10	0.33 ± 0.12
Cefotetan	Not absorbed orally	1.5-3 after IM	76-91	0.194
Cefotiam hexitil			40	0.3
Cefoxitin 6	Not absorbed orally		61.5 ± 11.5	0.31 ± 0.12
Cefprozil 6	90	1-3.5	36-45	
Ceftazidime 6	<10		21 ± 6	0.23 ± 0.02
Ceftibuten	90-94	1.96 ± 1.12	63	0.21 ± 0.03

M/P ratio	% Adult dose in milk	Maximum amount in milk (mg/L)	Comments and references
	Excreted into human milk		Absorption limited, food delays it. Given to 2-month-olds. Brand name: Suprax. (7, 363, 424, 542)
1.1-1.6			Competes with bilirubin. (404)
		0.12	Used in infants 6 months old. (24, 466)
			Brand name: Vantin. (466)
0.002		0.3	In milk: average amount 0.16 mg/L. Brand name: Monocid. (192)
	0.9		Brand name: Cefobid. (68, 192, 407, 519)
	Excreted into human milk		Brand name: Precef. (68, 192, 424, 542)
0.02-0.21	0.3	1.6	In milk: maximum found, 0.1%-0.2% of the newborn dose; peak 2.5 ± 0.5 hr. Brand name: Claforan. (20, 21, 272, 424)
		0.59	Plasma protein binding inversely related to plasma drug concentration. In milk: peak 4 hr. Brand name: Cefotan. (7, 68, 192, 424)
			Hydrolyzed in the GI tract to cefotiam (plasma protein bound: 44.5% ± 2.1%) with the main metabolite being cyclohexanol (plasma protein bound: 53.1% ± 0.8%). (35, 435, 519)
	0.16	2	Not all women excrete drug into milk. In milk: peak 4 ± 3 hr. Given to neonates. Brand name: Mefoxin. (19, 20, 68, 192, 407, 424)
0.05-5.67	0.3	3.4	About 95% absorbed. Food does not affect absorption. In milk: peak 6 hr. Brand name: Cefzil. (424, 487, 490, 491, 492, 493, 596)
		7.6	In milk: peak 1 hr. In prematures and neonates: half-life 2.9-14.2 hr, volume of distribution 0.53 ± 0.12 L/kg. Brand names: Ceptaz, Fortaz, Tazicef, Tazidime. (192, 368, 407, 424, 496, 519, 539)
			Absorption slightly decreased by food. Six women given 200 mg, no drug detected in milk; assay limit of 1 mg/L. (35, 152, 273)

Continued

TABLE D-1	Relationship of drugs to breast milk and effect on infant—cont'd			
Drug and AAP rating	**% Oral availability**	**Peak plasma time (hr)**	**% Plasma protein bound**	**Volume of distribution (L/kg)**
Antiinfective agents—cont'd				
Ceftizoxime	1		23-65	0.36 ± 0.19
Ceftriaxone 6		0.5-1	<60-95 Saturable	0.1-0.2
Cefuroxime	Poor		27-50	0.19 ± 0.04
Cefuroxime axetil	38 ± 17	2.5 ± 1.5		
Cephacetrile	Not absorbed orally		23 ± 3	0.6
Cephalexin	90 ± 9	1-2	13.5 ± 3.5	0.26 ± 0.03
Cephaloridine	Poor oral absorption	1 after IM	10-30	0.2
Cephalothin	Negligible	0.75 ± 0.25 after IM	66 ± 6	0.26 ± 0.11
Cephapirin	0	0.75 ± 0.25	55 ± 11	0.21 ± 0.06
Cephradine	85 ± 29	0.75	11.5 ± 5.5	0.25 ± 0.01
Chloramphenicol 4	75-90	1	53 ± 5	0.94 ± 0.06

M/P ratio	% Adult dose in milk	Maximum amount in milk (mg/L)	Comments and references
0.01		0.35 ± 0.08	Brand name: Cefizox. (68, 192, 446, 496)
0.03-0.04	0.7	7.89	Saturable plasma protein binding. In milk: half-life IM 17.3 hr, IV 12.8 hr, peak 5.5 ± 1.5 hr. Brand names: Rocephin, Bourqet. (19, 20, 62, 68, 192, 407, 424, 519)
	Excreted into human milk		Brand names: Kefurox, Zinacef. (7, 68, 192, 283, 407, 424)
	A prodrug for cefuroxime		Food and milk increase absorption by 50%. Brand name: Ceftin. (7, 35, 253, 424, 542)
	Excreted into human milk		Given to premature infants. (7, 542)
0.008-0.14	0.85 ± 0.35	5.23	In milk: peak 4.5 ± 0.5 hr, completely gone by 8 hr, maximum 0.04%-0.4% newborn therapeutic dose. Absorption less in the first few months of life. Food lowers plasma peak at 2 hr. Brand name: Keflex. (20, 35, 68, 192, 363, 424, 519)
	Excreted into human milk		Serum bioavailability: 76%. Not metabolized. (519, 542)
0.051-0.57	0.4	0.62	Higher volume of distribution in baby. In milk: maximum 0.05%-0.09% of newborn dose. Peak: 1-2 hr. (20, 51, 68, 192, 424, 446)
0.068-0.5		0.64	Amount in cow's milk: 5 ppb. (90, 192, 424, 519)
0.12-1.3	0.005	0.7	Food in GI tract delays uptake; amount absorbed is the same. Over 90% of drug excreted by kidneys within 6 hr. In milk: peak 1 hr. Brand names: Anspor, Velosef. (20, 192, 363, 424, 496, 519)
0.05-0.73	1.3-7.4	26	In milk: 0.2%-25% of newborn dose, peak 3.5 ± 2.5 hr. Possible idiosyncratic bone marrow depression. Brand name: Chloromycetin. (19, 20, 51, 68, 90, 192, 424)

Continued

TABLE D-1   **Relationship of drugs to breast milk and effect on infant—cont'd**

Drug and AAP rating	% Oral availability	Peak plasma time (hr)	% Plasma protein bound	Volume of distribution (L/kg)
Antiinfective agents—cont'd				
Chloroquine 6	67-114 Absorption not complete	1.6-5.3	61 ± 9	100-1000
Chlortetracycline	25-30		55	1.2
Cilastatin			35-40	0.2 ± 0.03
Cinoxacin			63	0.25-0.33
Ciprofloxacin	52-86	1-2.4	20-40	1.74-5
Clarithromycin	50-55	0.5-6	42-70	
Clavulanic acid	31-99	0.75-2	19.5 ± 9.5	0.2
Clindamycin 6	86 ± 1	0.5-1.5	93.6 ± 0.2	1.1 ± 0.3
Cloxacillin	41.5 ± 17.5	1.25 ± 0.25	94.1 ± 1.1	0.094 ± 0.015
Colistimethate	Not absorbed orally			
Colistin	GI absorption negligible			

M/P ratio	% Adult dose in milk	Maximum amount in milk (mg/L)	Comments and references
0.268-9	0.55-4.2	0.319	In milk: peak 2.2-7 hr, half-life 5.5 ± 0.7 days, upper limit is 4.2% of maternal dose. Metabolite also found in milk. Level in maternal saliva about the same as in milk. Brand name: Aralen. (4, 7, 20, 68, 148, 192, 395, 540)
0.125-1	0.7 ± 0.2	4.1	Oral availability reflects GI absorption. In cow's milk: 2000 ppb. Brand name: Aureomycin. (20, 68, 90, 496, 505, 519)
			Combined with antibiotics because it is an inhibitor of renal dipepidase. (76, 192, 424)
			(192, 424, 519)
0.85-2.14		3.79	Four less active metabolites from 15% of dose. Milk decreases uptake. Causes arthropathy in immature animals and teens with cystic fibrosis. Has been given directly to two preterm infants. In milk: plateaus at 4-12 hr. Pump 4 hr after last pill, feed 6 hr after last pill. Brand name: Cipro. (102, 180, 190, 291, 323, 332, 384, 424, 559, 577)
	Excreted into animal milk		Food slightly delays absorption and metabolism but does not affect overall availability. Higher doses have longer half-lives. Kinetics in infants published. Brand name: Biaxin. (93, 170, 185, 424)
	Excreted into human milk		Brand name: Augmentin. (109, 496, 519, 579)
0.1-3	4.1 ± 1.3	4	Absorption not decreased by food. 400 ppb in cow's milk. In milk: 1%-7.6% of newborn therapeutic dose; peak 2-4 hr. Brand name: Cleocin. (7, 20, 68, 90, 192, 424, 496, 519)
	9		Oral absorption delayed if taken with food. 100 ppb in cow's milk. Brand names: Cloxapen, Tegopen. (90, 192, 378, 379, 389, 424, 496, 519)
0.17-0.18			Brand name: Coly-Mycin. Hydrolized to colistin in vitro and in vivo. (68)
0.17-0.18	0.07	0.9	Brand name: Coly-Mycin. (424)

Continued

TABLE D-1	Relationship of drugs to breast milk and effect on infant—cont'd			
Drug and AAP rating	**% Oral availability**	**Peak plasma time (hr)**	**% Plasma protein bound**	**Volume of distribution (L/kg)**
Antiinfective agents—cont'd				
Cycloserine 6				
Dapsone 6	93 ± 8	6 ± 2	70-80	1.09 ± 0.18
Demeclocycline	66		70-95	1.8
Dicloxacillin	38-85	1 ± 0.8	89-96	0.095 ± 0.026
Didanosine	19-43	0.25-2	<5	0.87 ± 0.33
Dirithromycin	6-14	4.8 ± 2.6	15-30	109 ± 69
Doxycycline	94 ± 1	2.9 ± 0.9	88 ± 5	0.75 ± 0.32
Enoxacin	70-90	1.9 ± 1	18-54	1.6-2.9
Erythromycin 6	37.5 ± 27.5	3	66 ± 24	0.89 ± 0.55
Ethambutol 6	77 ± 8	2-4	<5-22	1.6 ± 0.2
Famciclovir	77 ± 8	Not detected in plasma or urine		
Fleroxacin	99 ± 14	0.2-6	27.5 ± 4.5	1.4 ± 0.34

M/P ratio	% Adult dose in milk	Maximum amount in milk (mg/L)	Comments and references
0.31-1.18	0.6	19	From milk, a nursing infant would ingest up to 11.3% of the usual pediatric dose. The average M/P ratio is 0.72. Brand name: Seromycin.
0.22-0.67	11.95 ± 2.35		Two acetylation phenotypes in the population. Drug and primary metabolite found in milk. One case report in which both mother and baby had compensating hemolytic anemia. (20, 140, 142, 192, 424, 494, 519)
0.7		1.4	Oral availability reflects absorption through GI tract. Drug is given to infants. Drug remains in milk for 3 days after dose. Brand name: Declomycin. (496, 505, 519)
Small amount found in human milk			Has been used to treat mastitis without stopping nursing. Brand names: Dynapen, Dycill, Pathocil. (192, 378, 496, 519)
			Bioavailability reduced twofold when taken with food. Brand name: Videx. (7, 155, 247, 281, 488)
	65		Brand name: Dynabac. (495)
0.3-0.4		0.77	Bioavailability not altered by food. Brand names: Doryx, Vibramycin, Monodox. (68, 192, 465, 519)
			Absorption not decreased by food. Brand name: Penetrex. (237, 291, 323, 560, 576)
0.02-1.6	0.1-2.1	6.2	Maximum absorption on an empty stomach. Possible jaundice if infant less than 1 month old. In milk: peak 4 hr, 0.1%-0.25% of newborn therapeutic dose. Brand names: Benzamycin, E-Mycin, Pediazole. (20, 67, 68, 192, 469, 496, 519)
1		4.6	In milk: 1%-5.7% of newborn therapeutic dose. Brand name: Myambutol. (192, 424, 519)
See active metabolite, penciclovir, p. 782			Brand name: Famvir. (424, 434)
0.62		4.5	Food does not affect absorption. In milk: peak 2-6 hr, half-life 7.18-8.97 hr. (107, 323, 502, 531, 600)

Continued

TABLE D-1 Relationship of drugs to breast milk and effect on infant—cont'd

Drug and AAP rating	% Oral availability	Peak plasma time (hr)	% Plasma protein bound	Volume of distribution (L/kg)
Antiinfective agents—cont'd				
Fluconazole	90	1-3	10-15	0.85 ± 0.15
Flucytosine	88.5 ± 10.5	1-2	2-4	0.68 ± 0.04
Fosfomycin	10-58	2.2 ± 0.9	0	1.5
Gentamicin	Negligible		0-30	0.34 ± 0.15
Griseofulvin	95	4 when fasting		1.5
Halofantrine	Oral absorption poor and variable	3-27	>98	1.1-9.7
Hydroxychloroquine 6	Absorption 25%-100% from tablet; mean: 70	2.3-6	62.5 ± 2.5	
Imipenem	Not absorbed orally		<10-20	0.23 ± 0.05
Isoniazid 6	90	1-2	0	0.67 ± 0.15
Ivermectin		3-6	93.2 ± 4.4	11.1 ± 4.2

M/P ratio	% Adult dose in milk	Maximum amount in milk (mg/L)	Comments and references
0.46-1		2.93	80% of dose recovered in urine unchanged. Oral availability independent of pH of stomach and food in GI tract. In milk: peaks by 2 hr. In premature infants: half-life 43.3-187.3 hr; volume of distribution 1.05-1.48 L/kg. Brand name: Diflucan. (7, 57, 112, 167, 184, 202, 227, 424, 445, 582, 588)
			Half-life slightly longer in premature infants. Given to neonates. Brand name: Ancobon. (7, 32, 192, 496)
0.1			Drug has poor solubility and is degraded by stomach acid. Food significantly reduces oral absorption. Brand name: Monural. (46, 519)
0.08-0.57		0.78	In neonate may see appreciable GI absorption. In milk: 0.012%-0.9% of the newborn therapeutic dose. Brand names: Garamycin, G-myticin. (7, 51, 88, 183, 192, 407, 424, 429, 446)
Not excreted into human milk			Absorption from GI tract varies considerably. There are good and poor absorbers. Brand names: Fulvicin, Grisactin. (7, 424, 496, 519)
			Oral availability increased by food. (75, 265, 285)
5.5	0.0003-2	1.46	If chronically used by mother, may cause retinal damage in infant. Percentage of adult dose in chart based on data from two women. Brand name: Plaquenil. (540)
			Brand name: Primaxin. (192, 497, 519)
0.5-3	2.3	16.6	In milk: 6.3%-25% newborn therapeutic dose, peak 3 hr. Not detected in infant's blood, but found in urine. Oral absorption decreased by food. Active metabolite: M/P ratio 1; peaks in milk at 5 hr. Brand names: INH, Rifamate. (51, 68, 192)
0.18-0.97 at peak: 0.18-0.37		0.0206	Bioavailability of tablet vs. solution is 60%. Mean amount in milk: 9.85 ± 0.38 ng/ml. Brand name: Stromectol. (192, 195, 393, 400)

Continued

TABLE D-1   Relationship of drugs to breast milk and effect on infant—cont'd

Drug and AAP rating	% Oral availability	Peak plasma time (hr)	% Plasma protein bound	Volume of distribution (L/kg)
Antiinfective agents—cont'd				
Kanamycin 6	Oral absorption poor		0	0.26 ± 0.05
Ketoconazole		1.5 ± 0.5	99 ± 0.1	2.4 ± 1.6
Levofloxacin	99	1-2	24-38	1.25
Lincomycin		3 ± 1	72	0.5
Lindane		6-8		
Lomefloxacin	50-76 95%-100% absorbed	0.7-2	17.5 ± 7	1.5-2.5
Mebendazole	2-22	0.5-7.25	90	2
Mefloquine	85-89	33.6 ± 12	98.2-98.4	25.27 ± 9.75
Methacycline	58	2-3	80-95	
Methenamine		1.5 ± 0.5		0.63 ± 0.12
Methicillin	Negligible		39 ± 2	0.43 ± 0.1

M/P ratio	% Adult dose in milk	Maximum amount in milk (mg/L)	Comments and references
0.05->1	0.95	18.4	IM serum peak: 1 hr with 100% bioavailability. In milk: 30% of newborn therapeutic dose, peak 1 hr. Serum half-life in infant is inversely related to age. Brand name: Kantrex. (68, 192, 407)
0.38	0.3-1.4	0.22	Oral absorption varies considerably. Extensively metabolized in the liver to inactive products. Oral availability decreases as pH of stomach increases. Brand name: Nizoral. (7, 57, 184, 192, 302, 362, 420, 424)
Secretion into breast milk is expected as with other fluoroquinolones			Brand name: Levaquin. (424)
0.13-2.25	0.026-0.6	2.4	Brand name: Lincocin. (20, 68, 90, 424, 519)
		0.08	Used as a cream, lotion, or shampoo. Through milk, maximum daily intake 62.07 µg/kg. Brand name: Kwell. (68, 254, 255, 424)
			Food decreases rate but not amount absorbed. Amount in serum proportional to dose. Brand name: Maxaquin. (237, 308, 516, 572, 600)
		0.005	May inhibit lactation (one case, with circumstantial evidence). Brand name: Vermox. (7, 192, 496, 519)
0.13-0.27	3.2 ± 0.6	0.31	In milk: maximum 0.14 mg/kg. During lactation, plasma clearance and volume of distribution about 50% less than after weaning. Elimination half-life of drug: 6-28 days. Brand name: Lariam. (61, 141, 264, 409, 496, 519)
0.5		2.6	Oral absorption about 60% in a fasting adult. Food and/or milk reduces normal GI absorption by 50% or more. (7, 192, 496, 505)
0.88-1.08	8.3	1.1	In milk: 0.07%-0.6% of the newborn therapeutic dose, peak 1 hr. Brand names: Hiprex, Urex. (20)
A small amount found in milk			Brand name: Staphcillin. (51, 192, 446, 519)

Continued

TABLE D-1	Relationship of drugs to breast milk and effect on infant—cont'd			
Drug and AAP rating	**% Oral availability**	**Peak plasma time (hr)**	**% Plasma protein bound**	**Volume of distribution (L/kg)**
Antiinfective agents—cont'd				
Metronidazole 4	80-100 Availability: intravaginally 19-81, usually 20; ointment 3-10	0.25-4 oral 4-24 vaginal 17 ± 9.6 ointment	<1-20	0.52-1.1
Mezlocillin	Negligible		16-42	0.25
Miconazole	25-30		90-99	20
Minocycline	95-100	2	70-76	1.3 ± 0.2
Moxalactam 6	Negligible	0.5-2	45-67	0.25 ± 0.08
Nafcillin	33 ± 3		87-90	0.63 ± 0.3
Nalidixic acid 6	60 50%-100% absorbed	1-2	82-97	1
Netilmicin			<10	0.2 ± 0.02
Nitrofurantoin 6	99 Food increases absorption		20-60	0.8
Norfloxacin	30-80 Milk reduces absorption	1-2	10-15	3.2 ± 1.4
Novobiocin		2.5 ± 0.5		

M/P ratio	% Adult dose in milk	Maximum amount in milk (mg/L)	Comments and references
0.45-1.8	0.13-36	60	In milk: 1.3%-75% newborn therapeutic dose, amount secreted is dose dependent, peak 2.25 ± 1.75 hr. AAP says mother take 2 g orally, discard milk for 12-24 hr. Brand names: Flagyl, MetroGel, Protostat. (7, 20, 68, 131, 192, 297, 414, 496, 614)
Low amount detected in human milk			Given to neonates. Brand name: Mezlin. (192, 261, 407, 424, 519)
			About 50% of oral dose is absorbed from GI tract. Used in infants. Brand name: Monistat. (7, 424, 496, 519)
		0.8	May turn milk black. Brand name: Minocin. (192, 505, 519)
	0.6	6	IM availability 70%-100%. In milk: up to 1.7% of newborn therapeutic dose. Brand name: Moxam. (7, 20, 192, 407, 446, 519)
A small amount found in milk			Variable oral absorption. Increased oral availability in neonates. Brand name: Unipen. (192, 407, 496, 519)
0.08-0.13	0.3	4	Decreased oral availability in neonate. Caution needed in G6PD-deficient infants. Brand name: NegGram. (20, 68, 424, 576)
Small amount found in human milk			Given to neonates. Brand name: Netromycin. (192, 407, 424)
0.3-2	0.6	0.5	Caution needed in G6PD-deficient infants. Brand name: Macrodantin, Furadantin. (20, 192, 424)
In milk, not detected after a single 200-mg dose			Food may delay, not reduce absorption. Brand names: Chibroxin, Noroxin. (7, 192, 291, 323, 576)
0.1-0.25	0.15	7	Drug may be given to infants directly. In cow's milk: 50 ppb. Brand name: Albamycin. (7, 68)

Continued

TABLE D-1 **Relationship of drugs to breast milk and effect on infant—cont'd**

Drug and AAP rating	% Oral availability	Peak plasma time (hr)	% Plasma protein bound	Volume of distribution (L/kg)
Antiinfective agents—cont'd				
Nystatin	Sparingly absorbed in GI tract			
Ofloxacin	70-100	1.5-3	8-30	1.25 ± 0.25
Oxacillin	55 ± 25		91.6-96	0.33 ± 0.09
Oxytetracycline	58		20-40	1.5
Pefloxacin	80-110	1-3	20-30	1.4 ± 0.3
Penciclovir		0.9 ± 0.5	<20	1.08 ± 0.17
Penicillin G	15-30	0.75 ± 0.25	60 ± 10	0.1-0.3
Penicillin V	60 Oral absorption 60%-73%	0.75	75-89	0.25-0.51
Pentamidine	Negligible Poor GI absorption			16 ± 9
Permethrin	Used as a topically applied 5% cream; 2% or less is absorbed through the skin			
Piperacillin	Not absorbed orally		16-48	0.17-0.37
Praziquantel	80	2 ± 1		
Pyrazinamide	Well absorbed orally	2	50	

M/P ratio	% Adult dose in milk	Maximum amount in milk (mg/L)	Comments and references
Not excreted into human milk			Can be given to infants directly. Brand names: Mycolog, Mycostatin, Mytrex. (424)
0.98-1.66		2.41	Food delays peak plasma time. Brand names: Floxin, Ocuflox. (132, 190, 207, 291, 323, 546, 576, 577, 601)
Excreted into human milk in low concentrations			Displaces bilirubin from albumin in neonates. Brand names: Bactocill, Prostaphlin. (68, 407, 519)
		3	In cow's milk: 2000 ppb. Oral availability reflects absorption from GI tract. Brand names: Terra-Cortril, Terramycin, Urobiotic. (90, 496, 505, 519)
0.75-1.04		3.54	Norfloxacin is the active metabolite. (190, 237, 244, 291, 323, 496)
Drug is concentrated in rat's milk			Drug given IV. A metabolite of famciclovir. (169, 424)
0.016-0.37	0.8	0.036	Oral availability: best on empty stomach, increased in neonate. In milk: 0.005%-0.4% of newborn therapeutic dose, peak 2-4 hr. Brand name: Bicillin. (20, 90, 192, 389, 407, 424, 446, 496, 519)
0.016-0.13	0.2		Kinetics may differ in woman with mastitis. In neonate: 65% plasma protein bound. Brand name: Pen-Vee. (51, 335, 378, 424, 496, 519)
			Has been detected in some tissues for up to a year. Brand names: Pentam, Nebupent. (192, 360)
			Rapidly metabolized in the body to inactive products. (424)
Passage into human milk after IM is minute			Amount in milk is below any therapeutic or toxic level. Brand names: Pipracil, Zosyn. (278, 407, 424)
0.25-0.28	0.13		Infant receives, through milk, 69 µg/kg/day. In milk: peak 6 ± 4 hr. Brand name: Biltricide. (20, 519)
0.036	0.5-1.4	1.5	In milk: peak 3 hr. (20, 519)

Continued

TABLE D-1	Relationship of drugs to breast milk and effect on infant—cont'd			
Drug and AAP rating	**% Oral availability**	**Peak plasma time (hr)**	**% Plasma protein bound**	**Volume of distribution (L/kg)**
Antiinfective agents—cont'd				
Pyrethrin	Poorly absorbed through the skin and metabolized rapidly			
Pyrimethamine 6	Well absorbed orally	4.75 ± 3.25	87 ± 1	2.9 ± 0.5
Quinine 6	99 ± 10	1-6	93 ± 3	1.8 ± 0.4
Rifampin 6	99	3 ± 1	80-90	0.97 ± 0.36
Rosaramicin				3.78
Roxithromycin		2-2.5	96	
Streptomycin 6	GI absorption poor	1 after IM	48 ± 14	0.18 ± 0.11
Sulfacetamide	Readily absorbed from GI tract			
Sulfadiazine	99		54 ± 4	0.29 ± 0.04
Sulfamethazine		2-4	80	0.2
Sulfamethoxazole 6	96 ± 14	2.5 ± 1.5	63.5 ± 6.5	0.21 ± 0.02
Sulfanilamide				

M/P ratio	% Adult dose in milk	Maximum amount in milk (mg/L)	Comments and references
			Brand name: RID. (192)
0.2-0.66	31.2 ± 14.4	3.3	In milk: peak 6 hr, found up to 48 hr after last dose, enough drug to cure an infant less than 6 months old, 62%-66% of the newborn therapeutic dose. Brand names: Daraprim, Fansidar. (68, 142, 192, 424, 519)
0.14	0.05	2.2	In milk: peak 0.5-6 hr. At therapeutic doses, no effect on infant except rare thrombocytopenia. If at risk for G6PD, do not breastfeed until it is ruled out. Brand name: Quinamm. (68, 192, 496, 585)
0.19-0.6	0.05	4.9	Given to infants. In milk: 0.57%-60% of therapeutic dose. If taken with food, plasma peak is delayed 1-2 hr. May turn milk orange. Brand names: Rifadin, Rifamate, Rimactane. (68, 192, 519)
0.12	0.0025-0.2		In milk: peak 3 ± 1 hr. Positive correlation between breast milk volume and milk clearance. Infant gets 6.7 µg/kg/day. (20)
	<0.05		In milk: drug appears by 2 hr. Within 12 hr, 0.14 mg of a 300-mg dose is found in milk. (58, 84, 295, 386)
0.12-1	0.5	30	In milk: 0.3%-1.3% newborn dose. (68, 192)
0.08-1.3		66	(424)
0.21			An infant over 1 month can better clear the drug. Brand name: Microsulfon. (68, 192, 519)
	Excreted into human milk		Food delays absorption. (7, 519)
0.06	0.45		In milk: about 1.2% of newborn dose. In first month, displaces bilirubin. Contraindicated in G6PD-deficient infants. Cow's milk: 50 ppb. Brand names: Gantanol, Bactrim, Septra. (68, 90, 96, 192, 519)
0.5-1.2	1.6	94	In milk: may persist several days after mother stops taking it. Avoid in first month as it displaces bilirubin. Significant therapeutic doses not found in milk. Brand name: AVC. (68)

Continued

				Volume of
TABLE D-1 **Relationship of drugs to breast milk and effect on infant—cont'd**				
Drug and AAP rating	**% Oral availability**	**Peak plasma time (hr)**	**% Plasma protein bound**	**Volume of distribution (L/kg)**
Antiinfective agents—cont'd				
Sulfapyridine				
Sulfasalazine 5	10%-30% absorbed in small intestine	1.5-6		1
Sulfathiazole				
Sulfisoxazole 6	96 ± 14	2.5 ± 1.5	88-92.6	0.13-0.35
Teicoplanin	Not absorbed orally		87.6-90.8	0.6-2.78
Temafloxacin HCl	62-93	2.7 ± 1.9	26	1.53-1.83
Terconazole				
Tetracycline 6	72.5 ± 22.5	2	20-75	1.5 ± 0.08
Thiabendazole		1-2		
Ticarcillin 6	0	0.5-1.25 after IM	45-65	0.21 ± 0.03
Tinidazole 4	108 ± 47			
Tobramycin	GI absorption poor	1 ± 0.5	<10	0.25-0.33

M/P ratio	% Adult dose in milk	Maximum amount in milk (mg/L)	Comments and references
0.4-1	0.12	130	A metabolite of sulfasalazine. Caution in infant with jaundice or G6PD. (28, 40, 519)
0.3-0.6	4.1 ± 2.9	2.5	Active metabolites: sulfapyridine and 5-amino salicylic acid. If jaundice develops, postpone nursing til it clears. Bloody diarrhea can develop. Brand name: Azulfidine. (20, 65, 68, 300, 424, 519, 540)
0.33-0.7		77	A vaginal cream or tablet. In milk: 5 mg/L after maternal dose of 3 g/day. Some reports of diarrhea and rash in infants when mother took drug. Brand names: Sultrin, Trysul. (68, 424, 519)
0.06-1	0.45	1.1	In milk: 33%-50% of newborn therapeutic dose. Jaundice may develop. Avoid in infants with G6PD. Brand names: Gantrisin, Pediazole. (51, 68, 90, 192, 424, 519)
			Given to newborns. (11, 37, 118, 322, 508)
			Absorption not affected by food. (201, 413, 424, 517)
	Excreted into rat's milk		As vaginal suppository amount absorbed, 5%-16%, is proportional to dose. Does not accumulate in body. Brand name: Terazol. (7, 424)
0.2-1.5	0.03-4.8	8	In infant: drug negligibly absorbed, undetected in serum. In milk: probably chelated by calcium, peak 4 hr. In cow's milk: 2000 ppb. Brand name: Achromycin. (7, 20, 68, 90, 192, 424, 496, 505, 519)
	Excreted into cow's milk		Brand name: Mintezol. (7, 13, 192)
	<0.09		Brand names: Timentin, Ticar. (7, 20, 192, 209, 407, 424, 519, 579)
0.62-1.39	1		(20, 496)
		0.6	In milk: 0%-2.4% of newborn therapeutic dose, peak 4 hr. Brand name: TobraDex. (68, 192, 407, 424, 519)

Continued

TABLE D-1	Relationship of drugs to breast milk and effect on infant—cont'd			
Drug and AAP rating	% Oral availability	Peak plasma time (hr)	% Plasma protein bound	Volume of distribution (L/kg)
Antiinfective agents—cont'd				
Trimethoprim 6	99	2.5 ± 1.5	44-45	1.8 ± 0.2
Valacyclovir	Converted to acyclovir, the active compound (see p. 764)			
Vancomycin	Not absorbed orally		10-55	0.39 ± 0.06
Zidovudine	63 ± 13	0.1-2 Food delays peak	<25-38	1.6 ± 0.6
Antineoplastics and antimetabolites				
Allopurinol 6	90 ± 9			0.6
Azathioprine	60 ± 31		30	0.81 ± 0.65
Bleomycin				0.27 ± 0.09
Busulfan	Oral absorption is slow and almost complete			0.99 ± 0.23
Carmustine	Rapidly absorbed			3.3 ± 1.7
Chlorambucil	87 ± 20	1	99	0.86 ± 0.81

M/P ratio	% Adult dose in milk	Maximum amount in milk (mg/L)	Comments and references
1.25		5.5	In children: decreased half-life. In milk: peak 2.5 ± 0.5 hr, amount related to dose. Newborn absorbs 0.75-1 mg daily. Brand names: Bactrim, Septra, Trimpex. (68, 192, 519)
			Compared with taking acyclovir, the relative bioavailability of acyclovir from taking this drug is 3.3-5.5 times greater. Brand name: Valtrex (424)
Approximately 1		12.7	Given to newborns. Brand name: Vancocin. (68, 192, 312, 322, 407, 424, 519)
			Brand name: Retrovir. (192, 200, 424, 463, 590)
0.9-1.4		1.4	Drug not found in infant's plasma. Active metabolite, alloxanthine (oxipurinol): maternal plasma peak 4.5 hr; M/P ratio 2.4-3.89; maximum in milk 53.7 mg/L; 6.6 mg/L found in infant's plasma. Brand name: Zyloprim. (262, 482, 496, 519)
Small amount excreted into human milk			Metabolite: mercaptopurine. Brand name: Imuran. (42, 192, 424)
			Brand name: Blenoxane. (192, 424, 519)
			Brand name: Myleran. (192, 424, 519)
			Brand names: BiCNU, Gliadel. (192, 424, 519)
			When taken with food, peak value reduced by 50%, the extent of absorption by 25%. Brand name: Leukeran. (192, 383, 424, 519)

Continued

TABLE D-1	Relationship of drugs to breast milk and effect on infant—cont'd			
Drug and AAP rating	**% Oral availability**	**Peak plasma time (hr)**	**% Plasma protein bound**	**Volume of distribution (L/kg)**
Antineoplastics and antimetabolites—cont'd				
Cisplatin	Negligible		Extensive	0.28 ± 0.07
Cyclophosphamide 1	74 ± 22	1	13-20	0.78 ± 0.57
Cytarabine	20 ± 1		13	3 ± 1.9
Dacarbazine	Oral absorption poor			0.88-1.74
Doxorubicin 1	5	0.5	50-85	9-66
Estramustine phosphate	44 ± 5	2.2 ± 0.2		
Etoposide	17-72	0.5-4	96 ± 0.4	0.36 ± 0.15
Fluorouracil	0-74		8-12	0.25 ± 0.12
Gallium nitrate	5			1.27
Hydroxyurea	>80			
Idarubicin	30.5 ± 18.5	1-6	97	63.9
Ifosfamide	85-100	1-2		0.34-0.64
Melphalan	71 ± 23			0.45 ± 0.15

M/P ratio	% Adult dose in milk	Maximum amount in milk (mg/L)	Comments and references
1.1		0.9	Brand name: Platinol. (20, 68, 192, 317, 446, 519)
	Excreted into human milk		Is activated in liver. Metabolites in maternal plasma for up to 72 hr. Brand name: Cytoxan. (192, 361, 424, 519)
			Brand name: Cytosar-U. (192, 424, 519)
			Brand name: DTIC-Dome. (7, 79, 424, 519)
4.4	1.3	0.24	In milk: detectable up to 72 hr, peak 24 hr, no platinum found. Brand name: Adriamycin. (7, 20, 68, 192, 446, 521)
			Metabolically activated by extensive first-pass metabolism. Brand name: Emcyt. (424)
			Oral availability decreases at doses greater than 200 mg. Brand name: VePesid. (192, 269, 519)
			When used topically, <5%-10% absorbed. Brand names: Efudex, Fluoroplex. (7, 192, 431, 496, 519)
			Brand name: Ganite. (247, 548)
		8.4	Brand name: Hydrea. (68, 424, 532)
			Pharmacokinetics not affected by food. Not detected in plasma after 72 hr. Active metabolite, idarubicinol, detected for up to 7 days. Brand name: Idamycin. (83, 145, 234, 448, 528)
	Excreted into human milk		Metabolically activated in liver. Some evidence that drug has dose-dependent kinetics. Brand name: Ifex. (113, 314, 424, 496)
			Food reduces absorption. Brand name: Alkeran. (192, 383, 519)

Continued

TABLE D-1   **Relationship of drugs to breast milk and effect on infant—cont'd**

Drug and AAP rating	% Oral availability	Peak plasma time (hr)	% Plasma protein bound	Volume of distribution (L/kg)
Antineoplastics and antimetabolites—cont'd				
Mercaptopurine	5-37	2-2.5	19	0.56 ± 0.38
Methotrexate 1	36-88 Can be saturated	1.5 ± 0.5		0.55 ± 0.19
Tamoxifen	30	3-7	>99	~20
Autonomic				
Acebutolol 4	37 ± 12	1-4	11-29	1-3.8
Albuterol	50	1-4	7-8	2.5
Alprenolol	1-15	1 ± 0.5	85 ± 3	3.3 ± 1.2
Amphetamine 2	>95		15	0.6
Atropine 6	50		14-50	3-3.3
Dobutamine				0.2 ± 0.8
Domperidone 6	12-18	0.5-1	92	5-6

M/P ratio	% Adult dose in milk	Maximum amount in milk (mg/L)	Comments and references
	It is excreted into breast milk		Active metabolite of azathioprine. Food reduces absorption. When first-pass metabolism inhibited by allopurinol, oral availability is 60%. Brand name: Purinethol. (7, 9, 192, 311, 317, 383, 496)
0.04-0.1	0.93	0.003	Food delays absorption. In milk: peak 10 hr. Brand names: Folex, Rheumatrex. (20, 192, 383, 424, 496, 519)
			Brand name: Nolvadex. (7, 160, 226, 324, 424)
1.9-10 mean: 7.1	3.5	4.123	One beta blocker affect seen in a nursing infant. Oral availability unchanged if taken with food. Active metabolite, diacetolol: poorly absorbed from GI tract; M/P ratio 1.5-24.7 (mean 12.2). If mother's dose exceeds 400 mg/day or her renal function is impaired, baby may receive a therapeutic dose through the milk. Brand name: Sectral. (7, 20, 63, 101, 192, 279, 442, 474)
			As an inhaler, bioavailability is 2%-15%. Brand names: Airet, Proventil, Ventolin. (7, 232, 365, 424, 519)
			Extensive hepatic first-pass metabolism, which exhibits debrisoquine polymorphism. Dose-dependent bioavailability. (137, 192, 211, 389, 536)
2.8-7.5	6.1 ± 0.1	0.138	Baby's urinary excretion 0.001%-0.003% of mother's. Stimulation (jitteriness, irritability, sleepiness) may be seen in nursing infants. Half-life depends on pH of urine. Brand name: Adderall. (20, 446, 519)
		1	Drug is racemic mixture of S (active) and R (inactive) isomers. May inhibit lactation. Brand names: Arco-Lase, Donnatal, Lomotil, Urised. (5, 51, 192, 519)
			Not effective orally; rapidly metabolized in liver to inactive products. Brand name: Dobutrex. (20, 299)
0.03-0.6	0.05	2.6	(20, 299)

Continued

TABLE D-1   **Relationship of drugs to breast milk and effect on infant—cont'd**

Drug and AAP rating	% Oral availability	Peak plasma time (hr)	% Plasma protein bound	Volume of distribution (L/kg)
Autonomic—cont'd				
Dopamine	Oral drug rapidly metabolized in GI tract			
Edrophonium				1.1 ± 0.2
Ephedrine		2.12 ± 0.75		
Ergonovine				
Ergotamine 1	2-5	0.5-3		1.8
Hyoscyamine	Well absorbed		50	
Labetalol 6	10-80	0.33-2	45-55	2-16
Mepenzolate bromide	Completely ionized in GI tract and not absorbed			
Mepindolol	82 ± 11		40-60	
Methylergonovine (methylergometrine)	60	0.5-3	36	
Neostigmine	1-20	0.5	15-25	0.7 ± 0.3

M/P ratio	% Adult dose in milk	Maximum amount in milk (mg/L)	Comments and references
			Given to pediatric patients. Suggested to inhibit prolactin release. (7, 424, 476)
			Given by injection. Ionized at physiologic pH; not expected to be excreted into milk. Brand names: Enlon-Plus, Tensilon. (68, 192, 424)
	Excreted into human milk		Case report of mother with a 3-month-old who took a long-acting preparation. Child became irritable and changed sleeping pattern; returned to normal after mother stopped taking the drug. Brand name: Marax. (68)
	Excreted into human milk		Abrupt drop in prolactin levels at 30 min with normal levels returning by 2.5 hr. Brand name: Ergotrate. (542)
	Excreted into human milk		Vomiting, diarrhea, convulsions in infant when mother took drug for migraines. May inhibit lactation. Caffeine increases absorption and peak plasma concentration by a factor of 2. Brand names: Cafergot, Ergomar, Wigraine. (7, 192, 424, 496, 519)
	Traces found in breast milk		Food does not affect absorption. Brand names: Cystospaz, Urised. (7)
0.4-2.6	0.004-0.07	0.662	Food increases oral availability. Extensive first-pass metabolism. If mother takes 330-800 mg/day, a mean of 33 ng/ml in milk. Recovered in some infants, not all. In milk: peak 2.7 ± 0.6 hr. Brand names: Normodyne, Trandate. (20, 47, 68, 128, 177, 192, 383, 424, 446, 496)
			Brand name: Cantil. (7, 424)
0.35-0.61	0.1-1.1	0.095	Recovered in 20% of nursing infants whose mothers took the drug. (20, 424, 496)
0.3	4.6		Quickly disappears into the tissues. Brand name: Methergine. (20, 496)
	Not detected in breast milk		Poorly absorbed from GI tract. Ionized at physiologic pH. Brand name: Prostigmin. (7, 192, 496, 519)

Continued

TABLE D-1   **Relationship of drugs to breast milk and effect on infant—cont'd**

Drug and AAP rating	% Oral availability	Peak plasma time (hr)	% Plasma protein bound	Volume of distribution (L/kg)
Autonomic—cont'd				
Oxprenolol 6	24-60 About 90% absorbed	0.75 ± 0.25	80-92	1.1-1.3
Pindolol	86 ± 21	1.75 ± 0.25	47 ± 7	2.3 ± 0.9
Propantheline bromide		1		
Propranolol 6	2-54	2.5 ± 0.5	87 ± 6	2.8-4.9
Pseudoephedrine 6	Almost 100% absorbed	1		
Pyridostigmine 6	19 ± 15			1.1 ± 0.3
Salbutamol	See albuterol; it is the same drug with two different names			
Scopolamine 6	27 ± 12	0.88 ± 0.13		1.4 ± 0.7
Sumatriptan succinate	14		14-21	1.34-2.34
Terbutaline 6	12-40 52% absorbed from GI tract	1-4	14-25	1.4 ± 0.4
Timolol 6	30-95	1-3	60 ± 3	2.4 ± 1.2

M/P ratio	% Adult dose in milk	Maximum amount in milk (mg/L)	Comments and references
0.14-0.49	0.45-1.5	0.47	(20, 177, 496, 519)
1.6			Food does not alter oral availability. Brand name: Visken. (177, 192, 279, 424, 442, 474, 496)
			Rapidly metabolized to inactive products. Uncontrolled data: no measurable amounts found in human milk. Activity of long-acting dose not studied. Brand name: Pro-Banthine. (424, 519)
0.05-2	0.05-1	0.16	99% absorbed from GI tract. More available if taken with food. In milk: peak 3.5 ± 1.5 hr; 0.4%-6% newborn therapeutic dose; risk of an effect dose almost nonexistent. 5%-10% of Caucasians poor metabolizers. Brand names: Inderal, Inderide. (17, 20, 51, 164, 166, 192, 496)
2-3.9	3.2 ± 2.8	0.33	Report of a 3-month-old with excessive irritability that cleared up when mother stopped taking a decongestant with this and dexbrompheniramine in it. In milk: peak 1.25 ± 0.25 hr. Brand names: Actifed, Advil, Dristan, etc. (20, 68, 424)
0.22-4	0.05-0.12	0.025	Poor absorption from gut. In milk: peak 3.75 ± 0.25 hr. Drug not detected in nursing infants. Brand names: Mestinon, Regonol. (20, 192, 496)
Excreted into human milk in minute amounts			Brand names: Atrohist, Ballatal, Donnatal. (192)
4.1-5.7	0.21	0.113	An ergotamine derivative. In milk: peak 1.7-3.5 hr. By 8 hours, almost no drug in milk. (115, 424, 563, 598)
1.04-2.9	0.45 ± 0.25	0.005	Food decreases oral availability. Substantial first-pass metabolism. In milk: peak 4 hr. Not detected in nursing infant. Brand names: Brethine, Bricanyl. (20, 94, 192, 424, 479, 496)
0.25-1.73	3.3	0.088	Poor and extensive metabolizers exist. When used as eyedrop solution, 1.5 hr after dose, M/P ratio is 6.02. Brand names: Blocadren, Timoptic. (20, 177, 192, 424, 496, 519)

Continued

TABLE D-1	Relationship of drugs to breast milk and effect on infant—cont'd			
Drug and AAP rating	**% Oral availability**	**Peak plasma time (hr)**	**% Plasma protein bound**	**Volume of distribution (L/kg)**
Cardiovascular drugs				
Amiodarone	3-100 Incomplete absorption	1.5-10	95-99	66 ± 44
Amlodipine besylate	52-88 Completely absorbed from GI tract	8.9 ± 3.7	95.5-98	21.4 ±4.4
Amrinone	93 ± 12	0.5-2	35-49	1.3 ± 0.3
Aprindine	85-95		96	4-16
Atenolol 4	56 ± 30	1-4	5-16	0.95 ± 0.15
Benazepril	17	0.5-0.7 in fasting state 2-4 with food	95-97	
Betaxolol	80-90	2-4	45-60	4.9-9.8
Bretylium	12-37		0-8	5.9 ± 0.8
Cadralazine	80	0.5-1.3	25.9	0.7-1
Captopril 6	63.5 ± 1.5 60%-75% orally absorbed	1 ± 0.5	30 ± 6	0.81 ± 0.18
Carteolol HCl	85-90	2 ± 1	20-30	
Cibenzoline (cifenline)	83-90	1-3	50-60	4.1-7.3

M/P ratio	% Adult dose in milk	Maximum amount in milk (mg/L)	Comments and references
0.4-13	37	16.4	Terminal half-life: 8-120 days. In milk: 8%-50% newborn dose. Concern: 37% iodine level might affect infant's thyroid. Brand name: Cordarone. (20, 41, 68, 171, 191, 192, 424, 426, 496, 510, 557)
			Food does not alter oral availability. Extensively metabolized in the liver. Brand names: Norvasc, Lotrel. (158, 248, 274, 349, 372)
			There are fast and slow acetylators. Brand name: Inocor. (192, 479)
			Dose-dependent half-life. Exhibits debrisoquine polymorphic metabolism. (48, 296, 496, 519)
1.3-6.8	12.45 ± 6.75	1.8	In milk: peak 5 ± 3 hr. In serum and urine of some breastfed infants. Serum level 0.1% of mothers. Limited absorption decreased by food. One report of beta blocker effect in infant. Brand names: Tenoretic, Tenormin. (7, 17, 20, 192, 267, 347, 356, 474, 496, 519)
0.01 drug and metabolite	0.04 of drug 0.1 of active metabolite		At least 37% of this prodrug is absorbed from GI tract. Brand name: Lotensin. (34, 327, 328, 486)
2.5-3.0			Food does not alter rate or extent of absorption. When used opthalmically risk of effective intake by breastfed infant extremely low. Brand names: Betoptic, Kerlone. (7, 77, 101, 441, 524)
	Excreted into human milk		Brand name: Bretylol. (9, 192, 296, 496)
			Slow and fast acetylators. Has active metabolite. (73, 215, 305, 345)
0.006-0.6	0.002-0.014	0.008	Food decreases absorption by 30%-40%. In milk: peak 3.8 ± 0.6 hr; 0.1% of newborn dose. Brand names: Capoten, Capozide. (20, 176, 192, 392, 424, 496, 519, 570)
	Excreted into rat's milk		Food in GI tract slows absorption but does not affect extent. Brand name: Cartrol. (177, 424)
			(220, 296, 333, 351, 382)

Continued

TABLE D-1	**Relationship of drugs to breast milk and effect on infant—cont'd**			
Drug and AAP rating	% Oral availability	Peak plasma time (hr)	% Plasma protein bound	Volume of distribution (L/kg)
Cardiovascular drugs—cont'd				
Clofibrate	95 ± 10	4-6	95-98 Lower when plasma concentration is >200 mg/L	0.11 ± 0.02
Clonidine	87 ± 12	3-5	20	3.32 ± 1.5
Deserpidine				
Diazoxide	86-96		94 ± 14 Can be saturated	0.21 ± 0.02
Digitoxin	84-93		90-97	0.54 ± 0.14
Digoxin 6	40-100	1.5-3	20-40	5.17-7.35
Dilevalol	10-33	0.85 ± 0.15	68-77	17-25
Diltiazem 6	24-90 80%-90% absorbed orally	2-4	70-86	3-8
Diprafenone	50-mg dose 11 ± 1 150-mg dose 33 ± 26	1.35 ± 0.15	98.45 ± 0.55	1.23 ± 0.28
Dipyridamole	52 ± 23		95-99	

M/P ratio	% Adult dose in milk	Maximum amount in milk (mg/L)	Comments and references
	Excreted into animal milk		Data are for active metabolite. Drug used in neonates to treat jaundice. Brand name: Atromid-S. (7, 182, 192, 424, 519)
1.5-4.0	7.9 ± 0.1	0.002	In milk: up to 10% of newborn therapeutic dose. Hypotension not observed in nursing infants; drug found in their serum at mean levels less than in mother's serum. Brand names: Catapres, Combipres, Duraclon. (20, 68, 157, 192, 221, 424, 496, 519)
	Excreted into human milk		Predicted that may cause prolactin increases. Brand names: Enduronyl, Harmonyl, Oreticyl. (424)
			Brand names: Hyperstat, Proglycem. (192, 424, 519)
			Active metabolite: digoxin. Brand name: Crystodigin. (192, 356, 496)
0.45-1.0	0.07-14	0.0019	In milk: 0.06%-0.3% newborn therapeutic dose, peak 4-6 hr. Not detected in nursing infant's plasma. Brand name: Lanoxin. (19, 20, 47, 51, 259, 356, 446, 479, 494)
0.31-0.46		0.149	Optical isomer of labetalol. Absorption through GI tract 100% with dose-dependent hepatic metabolism. In milk: peak 1 hr. (128, 177, 178, 179, 438)
0.98-1.0	0.9	0.22	Drug undergoes hepatic metabolism. In milk: peak 2.5 ± 0.5 hr. Brand names: Cardizem, Dilacor, Tiazac. (7, 20, 78, 192, 356, 424, 446, 449, 496, 541)
			First-pass metabolism can be saturated, so oral availability is dose dependent. (554)
	Amount in human milk too low to measure		Brand name: Persantine. (68, 330, 496)

Continued

TABLE D-1	**Relationship of drugs to breast milk and effect on infant—cont'd**			
Drug and AAP rating	% Oral availability	Peak plasma time (hr)	% Plasma protein bound	Volume of distribution (L/kg)
Cardiovascular drugs—cont'd				
Disopyramide 6	83 ± 11	0.5-3	35-95	0.59 ± 0.15
Doxazosin	65 ± 14	3 ± 2.1	98-99	0.97
Enalapril 6	41 ± 15 53%-74% of dose absorbed	0.5-1.5	<50	1.7 ± 0.7
Enalaprilat	5%-12% orally absorbed	2-5	5	
Encainide	30 ± 19	1.1 ± 0.6	70 ± 6	3.6 ± 1
Enoximone	53-60	0.75-6	1-15	9.23 ± 6.84
Esmolol			55	1.9 ± 1.3
Felodipine	4.4-36	0.34-3	99.64 ± 0.08	9.7 ± 4
Flecainide 6	60-95	0.5-6	32-60	5-13.4

M/P ratio	% Adult dose in milk	Maximum amount in milk (mg/L)	Comments and references
0.4-1.07	6.8 ± 0.2	4.4	Active metabolite, N-monodesalkyl disopyramide: M/P ratio 2.7-8.5, maternal plasma level 10% that of drug. Drug found in blood of some nursing infants. Both drug and metabolite found in the infant's urine. Amount protein bound in milk and plasma is concentration dependent. Brand name: Norpace. (17, 20, 68, 192, 238, 268, 356, 424, 441, 443, 479, 496)
			Completely absorbed with first-pass metabolism. Significant accumulation during chronic administration. Brand name: Cardura. (127, 271, 402, 441)
0.14-0.78		0.002 Not found in all milk samples	Food does not influence absorption. A prodrug for enalaprilat (see below). Brand names: Vasotec, Vaseretic. (68, 124, 176, 192, 249, 329, 424, 496)
0.02-0.11		0.00172	Active metabolite of enalapril. (68, 328, 424)
		0.4	Tabular data for the 93% of U.S. population who are fast metabolizers. Slow metabolizers: oral availability 83% ± 19%, plasma level 20 times that of fast metabolizers. Metabolites formed are more active than the drug. Maximum amount of one of the metabolites (ODE) in milk is 0.2 mg/L. Brand name: Enkaid. (68, 351, 452, 453, 519, 581, 584)
			Rapidly absorbed orally with significant first-pass metabolism. Food increases absorption, with peak being achieved earlier. (504, 507, 568)
			Available IV. Brand name: Brevibloc. (267, 424)
			Complete absorption; first-pass metabolism. Flavonoids in grapefruit juice inhibit its oxidation; oral availability when taken with grapefruit juice instead of water or orange juice: 164%-469%. Brand name: Plendil. (25, 133, 139, 212)
0.8-4.6		1.68	In milk: peak 3-6 hr. Exhibits debrisoquine polymorphic metabolism. Brand name: Tambocor. (7, 268, 344, 424, 519, 544, 604)

Continued

TABLE D-1				
Relationship of drugs to breast milk and effect on infant—cont'd				
Drug and AAP rating	**% Oral availability**	**Peak plasma time (hr)**	**% Plasma protein bound**	**Volume of distribution (L/kg)**
Cardiovascular drugs—cont'd				
Fosinopril	29-36	3	95	
Guanabenz	70%-80% absorbed with extensive hepatic metabolism	2-5	90	93-191
Guanethidine	Individual variation in absorption and metabolism			
Hydralazine 6	26-55	0.5-2	85-89	5.45 ± 5.15
Ketanserin	50	0.5-2	95.1 ± 0.36	3.3-6.2
Lorcainide	1-65	1-2	85 ± 5	11.79 ± 7.15
Losartan	25-35	About 1	98.7	
Methyldopa 6	8-62 Due to absorption parameters	1-4	1-16	0.28-1.4
Metoprolol 6	42.5 ± 18.5	0.5-2	8-12	4.55 ± 1.05

M/P ratio	% Adult dose in milk	Maximum amount in milk (mg/L)	Comments and references
Excreted into human milk			Almost completely hydrolyzed to active metabolite whose oral availability is 25%-29%. Brand name: Monopril. (103, 243, 247, 248, 374, 500)
			Prolactin level in serum not affected. Brand name: Wytensin. (7, 519)
Not in significant therapeutic doses in human milk			Brand names: Esimil, Ismelin. (424, 519)
0.49-1.4	0.8	0.76	In milk: 0.3%-3% of newborn therapeutic dose, peak 2 hr. Oral availability higher in slow acetylators. First-pass metabolism may be saturated in rapid acetylators. Brand names: Apresazide, Apresoline, Ser-Ap-Es. (20, 68, 192, 496, 519)
			Absorption not affected by food in GI tract. (224, 421, 519)
			Saturable first-pass metabolism gives dose-dependent oral availability: 100 mg 1%-4%; 200 mg 35%-65%. (192, 511, 519)
Both drug and potent metabolite appear in rat's milk at a significant level			Brand name: Cozaar. (370)
0.19-0.34	0.02-0.09	1.36	In milk: peak 3-6 hr, 0.04%-2.7% of newborn dose. With maternal dose of 750-2000 mg/day, 0.1-0.9 mg/ml excreted into milk. Found in plasma in 1 of 3 infants. Recovered from infant's urine. Brand names: Aldoclor, Aldomet, Aldoril. (20, 192, 424, 446, 519)
2-4.8	1.7-5	0.225	Near complete absorption with first-pass metabolism; metabolites active. Food increases oral availability. Shows debrisoquine-type polymorphism. Increase half-life in neonate. In milk: peak 4 ± 2 hr. Brand name: Toprol. (159, 260, 280)

Continued

TABLE D-1	Relationship of drugs to breast milk and effect on infant—cont'd			
Drug and AAP rating	% Oral availability	Peak plasma time (hr)	% Plasma protein bound	Volume of distribution (L/kg)
Cardiovascular drugs—cont'd				
Mexiletine 6	87 ± 13	2-4	50-75	4.9-9.5
Minoxidil 6	90	Within 1	0	2.7 ± 0.7
Moricizine	30-40	0.5-3	88 ± 7	11.6 ± 6.71
Nadolol 6	34 ± 5	2-4	16-30	2.1 ± 1
Nicardipine	8.7-45	0.5-2.25	89-99.5	1.13 ± 0.51
Nifedipine 6	31-92		90-98	1.45 ± 0.75
Nimodipine	10-20	0.5-1.5	98	0.94-2.3
Nitrendipine	5-30 Increased when taken with grapefruit juice	0.33-3	98	2.3-9.5
Nitroglycerin	<1			3.3 ± 1.2
Penbutolol	92.5 ± 2.5	2-3	89 ± 9	
Pentoxifylline	19 ± 13 Nearly completely absorbed from the GI tract	1 ± 0.6	0	2.4 ± 1.2

M/P ratio	% Adult dose in milk	Maximum amount in milk (mg/L)	Comments and references
0.78-2	0.6-2.8	0.959	10% of Caucasians lack enzyme to metabolize drug. Food delays absorption, lowers peak level. In milk: 0.6%-2.4% newborn dose. Brand name: Mexitil. (20, 192, 356, 424, 447, 556)
0.67-1.13	2.5	0.042	In milk: peak 1 hr. Brand name: Loniten. (19, 20, 192, 424, 446, 519)
			Some active metabolites. Well absorbed with extensive first-pass metabolism. Brand name: Ethmozine. (1, 161, 241, 494, 605)
2-8	4.5 ± 2.5	0.44	In milk: 2%-7% of newborn dose, peak 6 hr. Brand names: Corgard, Corzide. (19, 20, 68, 192, 267, 356, 424, 446, 474)
	Excreted into rat's milk		90%-100% absorbed; extensive first-pass metabolism. Food in GI tract lowers availability, delays plasma peak. Brand name: Cardene. (176, 208, 357, 424, 496)
1	0.00163 ± 0.00125	0.053	In milk: less than 5% of effective dose, peak 0.75 ± 0.25 hr. In rapid absorber, drug peak 0.5 hr; in slow absorber, peak 4 hr. Total amount absorbed is the same. Oral availability when taken with grapefruit juice. 108%-169% of oral availability when taken with water. Brand names: Adalat, Procardia. (44, 68, 123, 143, 192, 216, 407, 418, 424, 478, 496)
~1	0.008-0.3	0.0047	Complete absorption with first-pass metabolism. Brand name: Nimotop. (7, 216, 274, 424, 537, 551)
0.5-1.4	0.095	0.007	In milk: peak 2.5 ± 1.5 hr. (26, 197, 216, 513, 514, 586)
			Half-life in maternal plasma: 1-4 min. (68, 550)
			Brand name: Levatol. (101, 177, 424, 496, 519)
0.25-1.49	0.17	0.074	In milk: peak 2 hr. Metabolites I, IV, V appear in milk. M/P ratio: I, 0.53-0.99; IV, 0.27-0.81; V, 0.64-1.62. Drug and metabolites stable in breast milk frozen for 3 weeks. Brand name: Trental. (20, 68, 192)

Continued

| TABLE D-1 | Relationship of drugs to breast milk and effect on infant—cont'd |||

Drug and AAP rating	% Oral availability	Peak plasma time (hr)	% Plasma protein bound	Volume of distribution (L/kg)
Cardiovascular drugs—cont'd				
Perindopril	66-95 Food decreases it by 35%	0.6-1.2	60	0.22
Pinacidil	57.1 ± 13.7	1 and 4-6	39-65	1.25 ± 0.25
Pindolol	86 ± 21	1.75 ± 0.25	47 ± 7	2.3 ± 0.9
Pirmenol	83 ± 24	1-2	83-90	1.93 ± 1.17
Prazosin	43-82	1-3	94 ± 3.1	0.6 ± 0.13
Procainamide 6	83 ± 16	0.66-2	16 ± 5	1.9 ± 0.3
Propafenone	5-50	1-5.68	77-97	3 ± 1.4
Quinidine 6			72.5 ± 22.5	2.7 ± 1.2
Recainam	39-106	1.2-5.4		1.4 ± 0.4
Sotalol 6	77.5 ± 17.5	2-4	0	1.3-2.4
Terazosin	82-90	1.3 ± 0.9	90-94	0.8 ± 0.18

M/P ratio	% Adult dose in milk	Maximum amount in milk (mg/L)	Comments and references
	<0.02		Drug has weak activity; metabolite, perindoprilat, potent. Metabolite: poorly absorbed from GI tract; plasma peak 3-4 hr; plasma protein bound 10%-20%; volume of distribution 0.16 L/kg. In plasma, 19% ± 7% of drug is metabolite. Brand name: Aceon. (307, 440, 547)
			Available in a control-release tablet. (174, 199)
1.6			Bioavailability not altered if taken with food. Brand name: Visken. (177, 192, 279, 424, 442, 474, 496)
			(187, 258, 351, 382)
		0.018	Bioavailability unchanged if taken with food. Extensive first-pass metabolism. In milk: 1%-4% of newborn therapeutic dose. Brand name: Minizide. (7, 192, 279, 424, 564)
1-7.3	1.5 ± 0.5	10.2	Rapid acetylators make N-acetylprocainamide. M/P ratio 1:6.2. Half-life of drug and metabolite 3-4 times longer in infant than adult. In milk: 2.2% of newborn therapeutic dose. Brand name: Procanbid. (192, 356, 441, 443, 446, 479, 519)
	0.03	0.032	Bioavailability increased greatly by food. Over 95% absorbed. Good and poor metabolizers. In milk: 47 ng/ml of active metabolite. Brand name: Rythmol. (181, 214, 228, 316, 351, 382, 383, 424, 475, 496)
0.71-0.91	4.1	8.2	In milk: 3.5%-10% of newborn therapeutic dose. Sulfate peaks in plasma at 1-1.5 hr, with oral availability of 80% ± 15%. Gluconate peaks at 3-4 hr, with oral availability of 71% ± 17%. May suppress prolactin secretion. Brand names: Quinaglute, Quinidex. (20, 120, 154, 192, 356, 424, 479, 580, 604)
			(110, 296, 555)
2.2-8.8	20-30	20.2	Food alters availability. Brand name: Betapace. (101, 163, 213, 296, 396, 468, 519)
			Plasma peak when taken with food: 2.2 ± 1.1 hr. Total amount absorbed is unaffected. Brand name: Hytrin. (192, 343, 424, 512, 543)

Continued

TABLE D-1	Relationship of drugs to breast milk and effect on infant—cont'd			
Drug and AAP rating	**% Oral availability**	**Peak plasma time (hr)**	**% Plasma protein bound**	**Volume of distribution (L/kg)**
Cardiovascular drugs—cont'd				
Tocainide	89 ± 5	0.5-2	2-22	1.6-3.8
Urapidil	78 ± 6	0.75 ± 0.25	76-80	0.87 ± 0.29
Verapamil 6	10-27 Oral absorption >90%	0.5-2	84-91.3	4.7 ± 2.5
Diagnostic materials and procedures				
Diatrizoate meglumine	Poorly absorbed from GI tract		<5	
Fluorescein 6	99			
Iohexol		4 ± 2	<5	0.35-0.83
Ipanoic acid 6				
Iothalamate				

Radioactive isotopes   Nursing should be discontinued until radioactivity is no longer excreted into the milk. Have milk tested if possible. Times to stop breastfeeding are advisory.

Gallium 67 3				

Iodine is concentrated in human milk. Always potential for interference with normal thyroid function.

Iodine 123				
Iodine 123 hippuran			5 ± 1.9	

M/P ratio	% Adult dose in milk	Maximum amount in milk (mg/L)	Comments and references
2.143-3.043			Food delays absorption and decreases peak values. Brand name: Tonocard. (7, 192, 382, 447, 479, 496, 519, 594, 603)
			100% absorbed orally. (60, 279, 433, 484, 529)
0.23-0.94	0.01-0.835	0.026	In milk: peak 1.25 ± 0.25 hr, not detected 38 hr after treatment stopped. Active metabolite: norverapamil. Brand names: Calan, Isoptin, Verelan. (7, 8, 20, 192, 219, 257, 296, 351, 356, 424, 472, 519)
	Not found in human breast milk		Used on newborn eyes. Brand names: Gastrografin, Renovist, Hypaque, Angiovist. (7)
0.5		8.826	In milk: peak 6 hr; half-life 62 hr. Decrease in neonatal renal clearance along with accumulation in milk may present toxic problems for infant. (331, 339, 496)
	0.5		In milk: 0.2% of pediatric dose, half-life 33.5 ± 18.5 hr. Brand name: Omnipaque. (385, 424)
	0.08	29.9	In milk: peak 5-19 hr; compound is inert. Brand name: Telepaque. (68)
	Contains iodine, which appears in human milk		Used in organ-specific tests. May cause transient metabolic taste in milk.
	Excreted into human milk		Discontinuing nursing for 72 hr usually sufficient. (461)
	<10		May contain up to 4.6% of I^{124}, whose physical half-life is 4.2 days with a half-life in milk of 3.5 days. See References for debate on how long to stop nursing, or have milk tested. (135, 225)
	1.2-3.5		In milk: half-life 3.5 hr. Effective secretion half-life is 2.2-5.8 hr. Breast should be pumped for 24 hr. (367, 457)

Continued

| TABLE D-1 | Relationship of drugs to breast milk and effect on infant—cont'd | | | |

Drug and AAP rating	% Oral availability	Peak plasma time (hr)	% Plasma protein bound	Volume of distribution (L/kg)
Diagnostic materials and procedures—cont'd				
Iodine 125 3				
Iodine 131 3				
Iodine 131 hippuran				
Iodine 131 macroaggregate				
Metrizamide 6		0-7	0	
Radioactive sodium 3				
Technetium 99m Tc 3				
Technetium 99m MMA			22	
Technetium pertechnetate				
Technetium 99m plasmin				
Technetium 99m RBC				

M/P ratio	% Adult dose in milk	Maximum amount in milk (mg/L)	Comments and references
	Excreted into human milk		Radioactivity may be found in milk for 2 weeks. Some say stop breastfeeding for 3-4 weeks. Have milk tested for isotope. (339)
40-65	2-46		In milk: half-life 4 ± 1.8 hr; peak 6 hr; excreted for 2-14 days. Suggestions: (1) give infant 60-100 mg KI, nurse, give mother isotope, discard next three pumpings of milk; (2) discard milk for 8 days; (3) if test dose used, discard milk for 36 hr; if diagnostic dose used, discard milk for 2 weeks. (135, 358, 460)
	1.8-4.9		In milk: peak first day at an average of 0.37 nCi/ml. Discontinue breastfeeding for 24 hr. (457)
	Excreted into human milk Half-life in milk: 20 hr		4.2-2.8 nCi/ml peaking in milk probably at 24 hr after dose. Discontinue breastfeeding for 10-12 days.
	0.02	214	In milk: 0.02% of dose recovered in 44.3 hr. If given to mother IV, 94% excreted in her urine in 24 hr. (7, 68, 424, 599)
	Can be detected in milk after 96 hr		In milk: 0.5%-1.3% of dose/L, peak 2 hr. (358)
3-5.2			In milk: half-life 35 ± 0.5 hr; amount and its kinetics depend on what molecule carries the label. (225)
	0.2-5.4		In milk: half-life 4.6 hr; peak 4 hr; maximum amount found 150 nCi/ml. If infant nursed just before dose, 4 hr later the milk will contain 60% of total activity. Suggestions: (1) feed just before dose, discard the next three fractions, (2) stop breastfeeding for 24 hr. (367, 457)
	0.07%-33% of the radioactivity found in milk		In milk: from mother who got 10 mCi: 6.5% after 24 hr, 0.177% after 46 hr, none after 70 hr. (366, 462)
	1.75 ± 0.25		
	0.006-1		Binding to maternal RBC very stable. 0.000005 of ingested activity excreted into breast milk. (457)

Continued

TABLE D-1	Relationship of drugs to breast milk and effect on infant—cont'd

Drug and AAP rating	% Oral availability	Peak plasma time (hr)	% Plasma protein bound	Volume of distribution (L/kg)
Diagnostic materials and procedures—cont'd				
Thallium 201				
Tuberculin test		OK to do when mother is lactating		
X-rays		No effect on breastfeeding and lactation		
Diuretics May suppress lactation				
Amiloride	54 ± 7	3-4	40	17 ± 4
Bendroflumethiazide 6		2.3	94	1.18 ± 0.31
Bumetanide	66 ± 11	0.5-2	94-97	0.19 ± 0.09
Canrenone		2-4	94 ± 4	
Chlorothiazide 6	9-56		94.6 ± 1.3	0.2 ± 0.08
Chlorthalidone 6	64 ± 10		75 ± 1	3.9 ± 0.8
Dyphylline 6		0.75		
Ethacrynic acid	Well absorbed from GI tract		Largely bound to plasma proteins	
Furosemide	11-90	1-5	91-99	0.07-0.35

M/P ratio	% Adult dose in milk	Maximum amount in milk (mg/L)	Comments and references
	Concentrated in human milk		In milk: effective half-life has two components: 1.13 and 15.1 days. Infant gets radiation by being held by mother. (376)
			Tuberculin-sensitive mothers can immunize their infants through breast milk. Immunity may last several years.
	Excreted into animal milk		Food interferes with oral absorption. Brand names: Midamor, Moduretic. (7, 192, 424, 519)
	Excreted into human milk		Used to suppress lactation. Brand name: Corzide. (39, 519)
			Brand name: Bumex. (51, 175, 192, 424, 494, 519)
0.51-0.72	0.2	0.2	Active metabolite of spironolactone and potassium canrenoate. (68, 424)
0.05-0.25		1	Absorption from GI tract incomplete, dose dependent, and saturable. In milk: peak 7.5 ± 2.5 hr, 0.4%-1% of newborn therapeutic dose. Brand names: Aldoclor, Diupres, Diuril. (7, 68, 192, 519)
0.03-0.05	6.7	36	Drug sequestered in RBC. In milk: excreted slowly, 0.75%-7.5% of newborn therapeutic dose. Term baby might get 180 µg/day. Brand names: Combipres, Tenoretic, Thalitone. (6, 20, 192, 519)
2			Brand names: Dylline, Lufyllin. (424)
			Brand name: Edecrin. (424, 519)
	Excreted into some human milk		Food delays absorption. In milk: not found in all samples. Given to neonates. Brand name: Lasix. (42, 52, 68, 175, 192, 424, 479, 519)

Continued

TABLE D-1	Relationship of drugs to breast milk and effect on infant—cont'd			
Drug and AAP rating	**% Oral availability**	**Peak plasma time (hr)**	**% Plasma protein bound**	**Volume of distribution (L/kg)**
Diuretics—cont'd				
Hydrochlorothiazide 6	72 ± 17	1.5-5	58 ± 17	1.53-4.19
Hydroflumethiazide	50		95	
Spironolactone 6	25 ± 9		94 ± 4	
Torsemide (Torasemide)	76-92	1	97-99	0.09-0.31
Triamterene	52 ± 18	3	61 ± 2	13.4 ± 4.9
Environmental agents				
Cadmium 7				
Carbon disulfide				
Chlordane 7				
DDE				
DDT 7				

M/P ratio	% Adult dose in milk	Maximum amount in milk (mg/L)	Comments and references
0.25-0.43		0.43	In milk: average amount 80 ng/ml, <0.02%-4% of newborn therapeutic dose, peak 7.5 ± 2.5 hr. Food in GI tract increases absorption. No drug found in infant (<1 ng/ml) when mother took 50 mg. Brand names: Aldactazide, Aldoril, Apresazide, Capozide, Esimil, HydroDIURIL, Inderide, Lopressor, Maxzide, etc. (68, 92, 192, 496, 519)
	Excreted into human milk		Brand name: Diucardin. (424, 496, 519)
		0.104	80% of drug converted to canrenone (see p. 814). In milk: 0.3%-6% of newborn therapeutic dose. Oral availability of film-coated tablets 25%-30% higher than uncoated ones. Brand names: Aldactazide, Aldactone. (20, 42, 68, 424, 496, 611)
			(175 496, 518)
	Excreted into animal milk		(192, 424, 496, 519)
0.1		0.786	About 10 times more absorbed through GI tract by neonate than by adult. Smokers have 2-3 times more in their milk than nonsmokers. Exposure of infants of smoking or nonsmoking mothers is far below that of formula-fed infants. (427, 437, 498)
1		0.306	Neurovascular and cardiovascular volatile solvent toxin that can be found on the hands and clothes of mother. (427)
Range in human milk is 0-66 ng/g, mean 6 ng/g			Metabolized to oxychlordane. In milk: peak 1-7 weeks after exposure.
6-7			A stable metabolite of DDT. In colostrum: 0.168-3.175 mg/kg. In mature milk: 0.011-2.86 mg/kg. (263, 416, 427, 454)
6-7		0.83	In milk: in general population, 20-830 µg/L, mean 100 µg/L or 4 mg/kg. Maximum daily intake of infant: 33.78 µg/kg of body weight. No need to test milk unless inordinate exposure. (254, 255, 340, 454, 553)

Continued

TABLE D-1	Relationship of drugs to breast milk and effect on infant—cont'd			
Drug and AAP rating	**% Oral availability**	**Peak plasma time (hr)**	**% Plasma protein bound**	**Volume of distribution (L/kg)**
Environmental agents—cont'd				
Dieldrin 7				
Heptachlor				
Heptachlorepoxide 7				
Hexachlorobenzene 7				
Methylmercury				
Polybrominated biphenyl 7				
Polychlorinated biphenyl 7				
Tetrachloroethylene 7				
Gastrointestinal agents				
Bisacodyl	Not absorbed from the GI tract			
Casanthranol				
Cascara sagrada 6				

M/P ratio	% Adult dose in milk	Maximum amount in milk (mg/L)	Comments and references
6		0.007	Found in permanently mothproofed garments. In milk: in general population, 2-7 µg/L or 0.05 mg/kg. Still found in milk in usual quantities months after spraying. (340, 553)
Range in human milk is 0-13 ng/g, mean 1 ng/g			In milk: peak 1 day after spraying. The 1970 FOA/WHO level for amount allowed in cow's milk is 5 times higher than the mean level in human milk reported by Matuo of 0.001 mg/kg. (340, 553)
		0.07	Amount generally found in human milk is 2-9 µg/L. In milk: peak 4-5 weeks after spraying. (553)
Excreted into human milk			Allowed in cow's milk at 0.02 ppm. Significant amount found in milk of Turkish women 25 years after massive contamination of grain seeds. Symptoms in nursing infants: skin rash, diarrhea, vomiting, dark urine, neurotoxicity, and death. (6, 416, 553)
0.086-0.9			In milk: half-life 70 days. (358)
3-131.7		0.036	Concentrated in fat. The more in mother's milk, the greater the amount in the child's adipose tissue. If mother at risk, milk should be tested. (427)
4-10		4.091	Concentrated in fat. The more in mother's milk, the greater the amount in the child's adipose tissue. If mother at risk, milk should be tested. (130, 427, 436, 553)
3.3		0.01	1 hour after exposure at a cleaning plant, mother had 10 ppm in milk, child developed severe jaundice. Detectable in milk for 2 weeks. (427, 599)
			Brand name: Dulcolax. (9)
Low amount found in human milk; can cause colic and diarrhea in infant			Brand name: Peri-Colace. (68)
High			May increase bowel activity in infant. Brand name: Milk of Magnesia. (424)

Continued

TABLE D-1	Relationship of drugs to breast milk and effect on infant—cont'd			
Drug and AAP rating	**% Oral availability**	**Peak plasma time (hr)**	**% Plasma protein bound**	**Volume of distribution (L/kg)**
Gastrointestinal agents—cont'd				
Cimetidine 6	58-89	0.75-1.5	19 ± 6	2.85 ± 1.45
Cisapride 6	40-50	1-2	98	2.4
Danthron 6				
Diphenoxylate HCl		2-3		4.6
Famotidine	45 ± 14	1-4	17 ± 7	0.94-1.42
Lansoprazole	>85 Absolute bioavailability	1.48 ± 0.99		
Loperamide 6	40	2.5-5	97	
Metoclopramide 4	32-97	1.6-3	13-44	3.4 ± 1.3
Nizatidine	70-90	1-3	35 ± 3	1.2 ± 0.5
Omeprazole	25-100		95.5 ± 0.5	0.19-0.45

M/P ratio	% Adult dose in milk	Maximum amount in milk (mg/L)	Comments and references
1.6-12	5.2 ± 0.2	6	In milk: 2%-2.5% of newborn therapeutic dose. Has produced galactorrhea. Theoretically may suppress infant's gastric activity, inhibit drug metabolism, and produce CNS stimulation. These effects not reported. Time taking drug and nursing. Brand name: Tagamet. (20, 86, 144, 299, 318)
0.05-0.063	0.1		Food slighlty enhances absorption. Nursing infant gets 600-800 times lower dose through milk than the normal therapeutic dose for infants. Brand name: Propulsid. (233, 299)
Excreted into human milk			Absorbed to a limited extent. May increase bowel activity in infant.
Rapidly produced active metabolite excreted into human milk			Bioavailability of tablet is 90% of liquid. Brand names: Lomotil, Lonox. (7, 68, 300, 424, 519)
0.41-1.78		0.072	Minimal first-pass metabolism. Decreased oral availability because of incomplete absorption. Calculated amount in milk (assuming intake of 600-800 ml) is 0.14 mg/day. Brand names: Pepcid, Mylanta. (68, 86, 138, 192, 299, 318, 320, 424)
			Acid liable, extensively degraded in stomach, so enteric capsules are used. Brand name: Prevacid. (119)
			Brand name: Imodium. (7, 300, 424, 519)
0.543-4.062	8 ± 3.3	0.157	In milk: peak 1-2 hr 10%-31% newborn therapeutic dose. Found in plasma of 1 of 5 infants studied. May see sedation, poor feeding. Brand name: Reglan. (7, 20, 192, 299, 346, 424)
	<0.1		Metabolite 60% as active as drug. In milk: peak 1-2 hr; mean amount at 12 hr 96.1 ± 31 mg. Experiments in rats show growth depression in pups. Brand names: Nizatidine, Axid. (192, 299, 318, 320, 391, 424)
			Undergoes first-pass metabolism to active compound. Brand name: Prilosec. (95, 239, 246, 338, 459, 496, 515)

Continued

TABLE D-1	Relationship of drugs to breast milk and effect on infant—cont'd				
Drug and AAP rating	**% Oral availability**	**Peak plasma time (hr)**	**% Plasma protein bound**	**Volume of distribution (L/kg)**
Gastrointestinal agents—cont'd				
Ondansetron	52-62	0.75-3	4-10	
Prochlorperazine	4.8-25.3	3.4-9.9		5.8-17.1
Ranitidine	39-87	0.5-3	10-19	1.3 ± 0.4
Senna 6	Drug not absorbed from GI tract; active metabolite is			
Trimethobenzamide	60% of IM			
Heavy metals and other elements				
Aluminum	Greater than 95% ingested aluminum is excreted in feces			
Chromium				
Copper				
Fluorine		2		
Iron				
Lead				
Mercury 7				
Zinc				

M/P ratio	% Adult dose in milk	Maximum amount in milk (mg/L)	Comments and references
			Brand name: Zofran. (97, 354)
	Excretion into milk not significant after therapeutic dose		Galactorrhea reported in some women. Increases serum prolactin levels. Brand name: Compazine. (250, 519)
0.25-7		3	Decreases gastric acidity. Amount in milk varies widely. IM availability: 90%-100%. Cimetidine is rated "6." Brand name: Zantac. (7, 68, 86, 192, 299, 318, 424, 519)
			Active metabolite, rhein, found in milk at 27 ng/ml or 0-4086 ng/day. Some suggestion that older preps might affect the infant's bowel function. Brand names: Perdiem, Senokot. (68, 149)
			Brand name: Tigan. (7)
			Amount in breast milk less than in drinking water and soy or cow's-milk–based formula. (55, 427, 575)
	Excreted into human milk		In multiple vitamins. In milk: about 0.4 µg/L, half-life 6 ± 1 hr. Allowable daily intake is 5-15 µg/day.
	Excreted into human milk		Maternal elimination fairly rapid. Maternal homeostatic mechanisms should prevent excess transfer during lactation. Prolactin levels increase.
0.21-0.32	0.19	0.008	In milk: peak 2 hr, 0-0.35 ppm reflects level in local water supply. Frequency of dental caries equal in breastfed infants and infants receiving formula diluted with fluorinated water. (20, 576)
	Excreted into human milk		
0.02-1		0.35	Higher uptake in infant than mother. Strongly bound to hemoglobin so not much gets into milk. Formula may have higher concentration. (6, 217, 358, 416, 496, 599)
0.03-1		0.54	Toxicity caused by lactation transfer reported. In milk: 0.93 ± 0.23 ppb. (358, 416)
	Excreted into human milk		Essential dietary element. Homeostatic mechanisms of mother prevent excess transfer to milk.

Continued

TABLE D-1	Relationship of drugs to breast milk and effect on infant—cont'd			
Drug and AAP rating	**% Oral availability**	**Peak plasma time (hr)**	**% Plasma protein bound**	**Volume of distribution (L/kg)**
Hormones, antithyroid, contraceptive, steroids				
Acetohexamide			75	0.2
Beclomethasone dipropionate			87	
Betamethasone	72	1-3	64 ± 6	1.4 ± 0.3
Carbimazole 6				
Chlormethiazole	12 ± 3		64	
Chlorotrianisene				
Chlorpropamide	99 ± 9	3 ± 1	90-96.6	0.09-0.27
Clomiphene				Large
Cortisone				
Cyclosporine 1	2-89 Mean: 30 More absorbed if taken with food	1-8	91-98	2.9-8
Dexamethasone	53 ± 40		68 ± 3	1.163 ± 0.88
Dienestrol	Possible decrease in milk volume and its nitrogen and protein content			
Diethylstilbestrol	Possible decrease in milk volume and its nitrogen and protein content			

M/P ratio	% Adult dose in milk	Maximum amount in milk (mg/L)	Comments and references
			Brand name: Dymelor (7, 424, 519)
			Given to neonates. Brand name: Vancenase. (7, 9, 417, 424)
Half-life in human milk is 5.6 ± 0.8 hr			Can use in a limited area as a cream. (192, 287)
0.58-0.9	27		Active metabolite: methimazole (see p. 828). Average concentration in milk: 182 ± 25 µg/L. Dose of 5-15 mg/day appears safe for nursing. In milk: peak 1 hr. (20, 98, 464)
0.73		3.23	Extensive first-pass metabolism. Detected in blood of 3 of 27 infants. (496, 519)
	Excreted into human milk		Has estrogenic effect but does not change consistency of milk. May suppress lactation. Brand name: Tace.
	Excreted into human milk		In milk: after 5 hr, 5 mg/L. How quickly mother eliminates it depends on pH of urine. Brand name: Diabinese. (192, 424, 496, 519)
			Taking fertility drug and nursing gives the body two opposite stimuli. Brand name: Serophene, Clomid. (352, 533)
	Excreted into human milk		Probably okay to use as replacement therapy in Addison's disease or if used as a one-time shot in a joint (it is depot, not systemic). Brand name: Cortone. (519)
0.17-0.4		0.263	Drug extensively metabolized. It consists of 11 amino acids. Not absorbed if given by enema. 16 µg/L found in breast milk 22 hr after last dose. Brand name: Sandimmune. (3, 150, 156, 192, 282, 315, 319, 424, 470, 608)
	Excreted into human milk		Some, not all, studies show drug induces prolactin suppression. Concern about interface with endogenous steroid production. Brand name: Decadron. (36, 192, 424)
			(68, 424)
			(15, 68)

Continued

TABLE D-1   Relationship of drugs to breast milk and effect on infant—cont'd

Drug and AAP rating	% Oral availability	Peak plasma time (hr)	% Plasma protein bound	Volume of distribution (L/kg)
Hormones, antithyroid, contraceptive, steroids—cont'd				
Epinephrine				
Estradiol 6				
Estrogen 6				
Ethinyl estradiol 6	20-65	2.1 ± 0.99		3.79 ± 0.83
Ethynodiol	(Data for active metabolite: norethisterone)			
Fluoxymesterone				
Fluticasone propionate	<1			
Glipizide	95-99	1.95 ± 1.45	98.5 ± 0.5	0.17 ± 0.02
Halobetasol propionate	In 96 hr, approximately 3% enters the circulation after topical application			
Hydrocortisone	96 ± 20	1.2 ± 0.4	75-95	0.4 ± 0.1
Insulin			5	
Leuprolide	Not active when given orally; it is a modified 10 amino acid compound			
Levonorgestrel 6	87 ± 9	1-4	50	1.75 ± 0.45
Levothyroxine	50-80			
Liothyronine	95		>99	0.5
Medroxyprogesterone 6	<10		94	0.6
Mestranol				

M/P ratio	% Adult dose in milk	Maximum amount in milk (mg/L)	Comments and references
	Destroyed in GI tract of infant		Brand names: EpiPen, Sensorcaine. (424)
	0.004-<10		In milk: peak 7 ± 4 hr. Brand names: Emcyt, Estrace. (20, 68)
	0.1		May alter the quality and quantity of milk.
0.25	0.16 ± 0.14		In milk: peak 2 hr. May alter the quality and quantity of milk. In many birth control medications. (20, 424, 483)
	0.02-0.07	0.00084	Rapidly metabolized to norethisterone, which peaks in milk at 4-8 hr. Brand name: Demulen.
	Suppresses lactation		Brand name: Halotestin. (424)
			87%-100% excreted in the feces. 3%-40% as inactive metabolite. Brand name: Flonase. (10, 74)
			Brand name: Glucotrol. (192, 424, 519)
			Brand name: Ultravate. (424)
	Excreted into human milk		Drug exhibits dose-dependent kinetics. Rectal availability: $2 \pm 1\%$. Brand name: Westcort. (121, 359, 519)
	Not excreted into human milk		(148, 519)
			Brand name: Lupron. (192, 424)
0.072-0.365	1.1	0.0005	Does not undergo first-pass metabolism or affect milk production. Brand names: Norplant, Levlen, Triphasil. (20, 168, 341, 483, 485, 496, 519)
		0.043	May increase milk production. Brand names: Levothroid, Synthroid. (7, 68)
0.36		0.005	Brand names: Cytomel, Triostat. (68, 424, 519)
0.2-1	0.86-5		Increased prolactin level before and after sucking. When 3-month injection given, no decrease in amount of milk produced; 6-month injection had a strong negative effect. Brand names: Amen, Cycrin, Depo-Provera. (20, 147, 256, 519)
	1.4		May interfere with quality and quantity of milk. Brand names: Norethin, Norinyl, Ortho-Novum. (20, 424)

Continued

| TABLE D-1 | Relationship of drugs to breast milk and effect on infant—cont'd | | | |

Drug and AAP rating	% Oral availability	Peak plasma time (hr)	% Plasma protein bound	Volume of distribution (L/kg)
Hormones, antithyroid, contraceptive, steroids—cont'd				
Methimazole 6	93	1.5 ± 0.5	0	0.6
Methylprednisolone	49-81		78 ± 3	1.2 ± 0.2
Mometasone furoate	When used as a topical ointment, after 8 hr of contact, about 0.7% is systemically absorbed of the 0.1% ointment			
Norethindrone	64 ± 8		80	4
Norethynodrel 6				
Norgestrel		2		
Oxycodone	60 ± 20	0.75-4.17		1.83-3.65
Oxytocin	Destroyed in the stomach			
Phenformin			12-20	5-10
Prednisolone 6	82 ± 13	1-4 Drug concentration dependent	65-95	0.2-1.3
Prednisone 6	80 ± 11		75 ± 2	0.97 ± 0.11
Propylthiouracil 6	78 ± 15		80	0.4
Tolbutamide 6	93 ± 10	3.5 ± 0.5	93 ± 4	0.1-0.25

M/P ratio	% Adult dose in milk	Maximum amount in milk (mg/L)	Comments and references
0.3-1.28	0.47-16.6	0.207	In milk: peak 2.5 ± 1.5 hr. Brand name: Tapazole. (20, 68, 98, 192, 496)
			Oral availability may be saturated. Brand name: Solu-Medrol. (192, 230, 496, 519)
			Brand name: Elocon. (424)
0.1-0.26	0.02-2.12	0.016	Higher levels in milk when taken with norgestrel. In milk: peak 6 ± 2 hr, some decrease of fat and calcium. Brand name: Micronor. (20, 68, 424, 446, 467, 496, 519)
	1.1		May decrease quality and quantity of milk. (424)
0.1-0.2	2.8	0.5	In milk: peak 2 hr; if taken alone, below detection level by 4 hr; if taken with norethisterone, high level in milk for 24 hr. Brand names: Lo/Ovral, Ovrette. (20, 68, 424)
3.4		0.226	In milk: peak 1.75 ± 0.25 hr. Structurally related to codeine and morphine. (68, 192, 432)
	Excreted into human milk		Enhances let-down reflex; does not necessarily increase amount of milk. Brand names: Pitocin, Syntocinon. (424)
	Minimal amount excreted into human milk		No effects seen in infants. Fast and slow metabolizers exist. (519)
0.05-0.25	0.06-3.6	0.3	Active form of prednisone. In milk: peak 1 hr, half-life 23 hr. At a high dose of 80 mg/day, infant gets less than 0.1% of dose, less than 10% of the child's own endogenous cortisol production. Brand names: Blephamide, Pediapred. (20, 68, 192, 424, 446, 519)
0.05-0.25	0.15 ± 0.11	0.042	Active metabolite: prednisolone. Brand name: Deltasone. (20, 68, 173, 192)
0.1-0.77	0.03-2.6	0.9	In milk: peak 1.5 hr. In infant, get baseline levels of T3, T4, TSH before and 6 weeks after mother starts taking medication. (20, 68, 98, 192, 496, 519)
0.09-0.4	18	20	Fast and slow metabolizers exist. Percent plasma protein bound is concentration dependent. Watch for jaundice. Brand name: Orinase. (20, 192, 408, 424, 519)

Continued

TABLE D-1	Relationship of drugs to breast milk and effect on infant—cont'd

Drug and AAP rating	% Oral availability	Peak plasma time (hr)	% Plasma protein bound	Volume of distribution (L/kg)
Hormones, antithyroid, contraceptive, steroids—cont'd				
Triamcinolone				1.39-2.11 The higher the dose, the lower the volume of distribution
Vasopressin	Negligible			
Narcotics and antiaddiction drugs				
Cocaine 1 and 2	30-40	0.5-2	91	1.2-3
Codeine 6	12-84	0.5-2	7	1.1-3.3
Dextromethorphan		1.6		
Disulfiram	80%-95% absorbed from the GI tract			8.2
Heroin 2	Excreted into human milk in sufficient quantities to cause addiction in the infant			
Hydrocodone bitartrate	Well absorbed from GI tract	1.3		
Hydromorphone	51-52 Rectal availability 36			
LSD	Expected to be excreted into human milk; ergot, a structurally related compound, is found in milk			
Marijuana 2				

M/P ratio	% Adult dose in milk	Maximum amount in milk (mg/L)	Comments and references
	Excreted into human milk		Brand names: Aristocort, Azmacort, Kenalog, Mycolog, Mytrex, Nasacort. (519)
		0.001	Brand name: Pitressin. (68, 446)
	Significant level excreted into human milk		57% ± 19% intranasally available. No drug or metabolite found in milk after 36 hr or in infant's urine after 60 hr. In rats, M/P ratio >1. (45, 91, 192, 481, 589)
1.3-2.5	5 ± 2	179	About 10% metabolized to morphine. Chinese metabolize less drug than Caucasians. In milk: half-life 2-2.5 hr, peak 1.25 ± 0.25 hr, 1.5% of newborn therapeutic dose, average amount 0.14 mg/L. Brand name: Calcidrine. (20, 192, 422, 496, 599, 609, 610)
			The *d* isomer of codeine analog levorphanol. 5%-10% of Caucasians are poor metabolizers. (192, 499)
			Brand name: Antabase. (7, 424, 519)
			(68)
			Chemically related to codeine and morphine. (7, 424, 519)
			Very closely related to morphine. Brand name: Dilaudid. (424, 496)
			Lysergic acid diethylamide. Rapidly absorbed and distributed throughout body. Half-life is not dose dependent. (68, 192)
>1			Metabolite: THC (see p. 832). In infants: found in urine and stool, at risk of inhaling smoke when held while mother is smoking. In animals, makes structural changes in nurslings' brain cells. (14, 358)

Continued

TABLE D-1   Relationship of drugs to breast milk and effect on infant—cont'd

Drug and AAP rating	% Oral availability	Peak plasma time (hr)	% Plasma protein bound	Volume of distribution (L/kg)
Narcotics and antiaddiction drugs—cont'd				
Methadone 6	79 ± 21	1.8-3.8	89 ± 1.4	4.13-13.4
Morphine 6	15-64		38 ± 5	2.2-5.5
Naloxone	2 91% of drug absorbed			2.1-3
Naltrexone	5-40	0.8 ± 0.2	20-21	16.1 ± 5.2
Nicotine 2	30->90		4.9 ± 2.8	2.6 ± 0.9
Phencyclidine (PCP) 1	72			
THC	4-12 2%-50% availability if smoked		95	8.9 ± 4.2
Psychotropic and mood-altering drugs				
Alprazolam	92 ± 17	0.3-6	71 ± 3	0.72 ± 0.12
Amitriptyline 4	48 ± 11 High hepatic metabolism	4	98.8 ± 0.8	15 ± 3

M/P ratio	% Adult dose in milk	Maximum amount in milk (mg/L)	Comments and references
0.3-1.5	2.2	5.6	In milk: peak 2-6 hr. No signs in infants if mother getting less than 20 mg/24 hr. Above that, withdrawal may be a problem. Suggested that mother get her daily dose after the evening feeding, supplement with a bottle at the next feeding. (6, 19, 67, 68, 192, 424, 496, 519, 599)
0.23-5.07	0.8-12	0.1	High first-pass metabolism. In infant: found in plasma when not detected in milk 108 hr after mother's last dose; elimination half-life is increased. Amount in milk too variable to treat withdrawal symptoms. May cause galactorrhea and prolactin increase. Brand names: Astramorph, MSIR, Roxanol. (7, 51, 192, 223, 380, 450, 496, 536)
			91% of drug is absorbed, but hepatic metabolism destroys most of it. Brand names: Narcan, Talwin. (192, 424, 519)
			Brand name: Trexan. (192, 424)
0.3-9.6		0.6	In milk: peak 0.165 hr; half-life 1.53 ± 0.25 hr. May suppress lactation. Decreased response of prolactin and oxytocin to suckling. Active metabolite, continine, excreted into milk. (6, 20, 105, 192, 326, 477, 527, 602)
	Excreted into human milk		Animal studies show M/P ratio as 10. In one case, mother's last dose was 40 days previous and milk had 3.9 ng/ml. (496)
8-8.4		0.34	Δ-9-Tetrahydrocannabinol, an active metabolite of marijuana. Infants may have decreased motor development. (14, 16, 68)
	Excreted into human milk		Withdrawal symptoms seen in an infant when mom stopped taking the drug. Metabolite is half as active as drug. Brand name: Xanax. (7, 192, 205, 424, 519, 542)
0.5-1.69	0.8 ± 0.2	0.15	Galactorrhea or prolactin increase reported. Not detected in infant's urine or serum detection limit, 5 ng/ml. In milk: peak 1.5 hr. Brand names: Elavil, Etrafon, Limbitrol, Triavil. (20, 68, 72, 80, 192, 424, 425)

Continued

TABLE D-1	Relationship of drugs to breast milk and effect on infant—cont'd			
Drug and AAP rating	**% Oral availability**	**Peak plasma time (hr)**	**% Plasma protein bound**	**Volume of distribution (L/kg)**
Psychotropic and mood-altering drugs—cont'd				
Amoxapine 4	99	1.5	90	
Bupropion	60-80 Extensive hepatic metabolism	1-2	>80	Very large
Buspirone	7.25 ± 5.75	1.1 ± 0.4	95	5.31
Caffeine 6	99 ± 14	0.5 ± 0.25	29 ± 14	0.5 ± 0.1
Chloral hydrate 6		0.5		1.5 ± 0.5
Chlordiazepoxide	100		96 ± 5.8	0.3 ± 0.03
Chlorpromazine 4	32 ± 19	2	95-98	9.9-254.3
Chlorprothixene 4	41 ± 21			
Clomipramine	36-68	3-5	96.5-98.6	16.6 ± 4.9
Clorazepate				0.33 ± 0.17

M/P ratio	% Adult dose in milk	Maximum amount in milk (mg/L)	Comments and references
0.21	<0.07	<0.02	Active metabolite, in milk: maximum amount 168 ng/ml, M/P ratio 0.45-0.86. Brand name: Asendin. (20, 68, 424)
2.49-8.72		0.189	One report of a woman taking the drug and no drug or metabolite found in the infant's plasma. Brand name: Wellbutrin. (69, 246, 424, 496)
Excreted in rat's milk			Extensively metabolized. Brand name: BuSpar. (424)
0.48-0.9	0.66-2.3	28.6	In milk: peak 0.5-2 hr, average amount 0.846 mg/L, half-life 6.1 ± 4.4 hr. Ability to metabolize it developed by 3-4.5 months of age. After 1 cup, not found in baby's urine. (20, 51, 68, 189, 192, 313, 381, 574)
0.09-3	0.6-2	15	Trichloroethanol is metabolite to which effects are attributed (see p. 844). In milk: 0%-15% newborn therapeutic dose, peak 0.75 hr, trace amounts after 10 hr. (12, 20, 68, 192, 290)
Excreted into human milk			In first weeks of life, may contribute to jaundice. Conflicting reports of drowsiness. Brand names: Libritabs, Limbitrol, Librium, Menrium. (39, 192, 424, 446, 519)
0.3 ≥ 1	0.07-0.2	0.3	Rapidly and completely absorbed; high hepatic metabolism. Galactorrhea, increase in serum prolactin level reported. Drowsiness and lethargy in infant. In 11 mothers taking an average of 200 mg/day, no ill effects were seen in the infants. In milk: 0.05%-0.26% of newborn therapeutic dose, peak 2 hr. Brand name: Thorazine. (6, 20, 72, 192, 203, 288, 446, 519)
1.2-2.6	0.12 ± 0.04	18.75	In milk: peak 4.25 ± 0.25 hr. Active metabolite M/P ratio 0.5-0.8. Causes galactorrhea, prolactin increase. Brand name: Taractan. (20, 68, 496)
0.76-1.62	0.4	0.624	Well absorbed from GI tract. Up to 50% first-pass metabolism yielding active metabolite. Hydroxylation of drug and metabolite under debrisoquin/sparteine control; 10%-20% of Caucasians cannot break down either. Not detected in infant's serum. Brand name: Anafranil. (7, 29)
Excreted into human milk			A prodrug for desmethyldiazepam (see p. 836). Brand name: Tranxene. (192, 424, 542)

Continued

TABLE D-1   Relationship of drugs to breast milk and effect on infant—cont'd

Drug and AAP rating	% Oral availability	Peak plasma time (hr)	% Plasma protein bound	Volume of distribution (L/kg)
Psychotropic and mood-altering drugs—cont'd				
Clozapine	12-90 Mean 50-60	1-6	95	5
Desipramine 4	33-68 Well absorbed, high first-pass metabolism	4-6	86.55 ± 4.45	20 ± 3
Desmethyldiazepam	99 ± 6		97.25 ± 0.25	0.78 ± 0.12
Dextroamphetamine		2		
Diazepam 4	100 ± 14		90-98	0.7-4.7
Dichloralphenazone	Body reduces drug to trichloroethanol (see p. 844), which produces CNS effect			
Dothiepin 4				70
Doxepin 4	13-45			20 ± 8
Ethanol 6	90 ± 10			0.54 ± 0.05
Fenfluramine	89 ± 10		34	
Flunitrazepam	85		77-79	3.3 ± 0.6

M/P ratio	% Adult dose in milk	Maximum amount in milk (mg/L)	Comments and references
2.79-4.32		0.116	High first-pass hepatic metabolism. Produces little or no prolactin increase. Brand name: Clozaril. (31, 424)
0.4-1.2	1	0.328	Neither drug nor metabolite recovered from nursing infant's serum or urine. 5%-10% of Caucasians are poor metabolizers. Metabolite of imipramine. Its metabolite is excreted into milk; M/P ratio 1.63; maximum amount found 327 ng/ml. Brand name: Norpramin. (7, 20, 68, 80, 166, 192, 424, 496, 519, 525, 597)
0.08-0.53		0.085	A metabolite of clorazepate, pinazepam, prazepam, and diazepam. Metabolizes to oxazepam (see p. 840). Higher in evening milk and morning plasma. (192, 446, 522)
2.8-7.5			In infant: amphetamine in the urine, insomnia, or stimulation not seen. Brand names: Biphetamine, Dexedrine. (68, 424)
0.1-2.7	2-12	0.6	In infant: sedation if fed 4 hr but not 8 hr after dose. More in evening milk when plasma levels are lower. In milk: 1.7%-3.8% therapeutic pediatric dose. Brand name: Valium. (17, 20, 51, 59, 68, 342, 446, 519, 522)
			(68)
0.33-1.59	0.15-0.58	0.475	Drug not detected in infant's serum. (20, 68, 519, 597)
0.3-2.39	0.01-2.2	0.029	Estimated that infant gets 71 µg/day. One report of a very sedated infant when mother took 25 mg 3 times a day. In milk: peak 4-5 hr. Active metabolite: M/P ratio 0.12:2.35; 11 ng/ml found in milk. Brand names: Adapin, Sinequan. (7, 20, 68, 192, 446, 496)
0.777-1.41	1-19.5	5600	Milk may smell of it. High amounts may suppress lactation. Infant can't metabolize it. Metabolite, acetaldehyde, not excreted into milk. In milk: peak 0.5-1 hr. (19, 20, 68, 192, 292, 348, 427)
			Mediates release of prolactin. Excreted rapidly if urine pH less than 5. Brand name: Pondimin. (424, 496, 519)
0.6-0.9			No significant binding to milk proteins. (18, 192, 519, 606)

Continued

TABLE D-1   Relationship of drugs to breast milk and effect on infant—cont'd

Drug and AAP rating	% Oral availability	Peak plasma time (hr)	% Plasma protein bound	Volume of distribution (L/kg)
Psychotropic and mood-altering drugs—cont'd				
Fluoxetine 4	>60-80 Drug almost completely absorbed	6-8	80-95	35 ± 21
Fluphenazine		1.5-2	>99	20->30
Flurazepam		0.75 ± 0.25	97	
Fluvoxamine maleate 4	94	2-12	77	5.1
Haloperidol 4	60 ± 18		92 ± 2	18 ± 7
Hydroxyzine		2 ± 0.9		19.5 ± 9.7
Imipramine 4	19-68	1-2	85-95	20-40
Lithium 1	95 ± 5	2-4	0	0.79 ± 0.34
Lorazepam 4	64-109	2	91 ± 2	1.3 ± 0.2
Lormetazepam	70-80			
Maprotiline	36-67	9-16	88	22.6-52

M/P ratio	% Adult dose in milk	Maximum amount in milk (mg/L)	Comments and references
0.29-0.88	3.3-13.9	0.181	In milk: maximum of active metabolite 0.199 mg/L. Recovered from infant's blood: drug 0-61 ng/ml, metabolite 57-58 ng/ml. Twelve reports of mothers taking the drug and breastfeeding. Possible connection with one case of colic. Otherwise, no adverse effects reported. Brand name: Prozac. (82, 192, 210, 235, 251, 415, 424, 523)
Excreted into human milk			Galactorrhea seen.
			Brand name: Dalmane. (7, 192, 424)
0.29	0.5	0.09	Not metabolized to active products. One case report of nursing mother taking the drug; no unwanted effects seen in infant. Brand name: Luvox. (210, 591, 607)
0.6-0.7	0.15-2	0.032	In milk: 1.3%-10% of newborn calculated dose, 2-5 ng/ml if mother has 12-30 mg/day. Causes prolactin increase. In animals if dose 1 mg/kg, nurslings have behavioral abnormalities. These effects not seen in humans. Brand name: Haldol. (20, 68, 192, 398, 566)
			Half-life is shorter in children. Active metabolite is cetirizine (see p. 762). Brand name: Atarax, Vistaril. (424)
0.08-1.0	0.1	1	Active metabolite: desipramine (see p. 836). Reported to cause galactorrhea and prolactin increase. Completely absorbed from GI tract. Brand name: Tofranil. (7, 20, 80, 192, 446, 496)
0.24-0.66	1.8	4	Infant's serum level: 10%-50% of mother. Inhibits cAMP, which is significant for brain growth. Cyanosis, poor muscle tone, and ECG changes seen in nursing infants. Brand names: Eskalith, Lithobid. (20, 80, 192, 496)
0.148-0.257	2.2	0.082	Infant toxicity observed at times. Increased half-life in neonate. Brand name: Ativan. (20, 192, 424, 446, 496)
Est. 0.06	<0.1-0.35		Drug and metabolite found in infant's plasma. Metabolite: M/P ratio 0.04. (20, 496)
1-1.5		0.2	Slowly but completely absorbed from GI tract. In milk: peak 8 hr. Brand name: Ludiomil. (7, 68, 424, 496, 519)

Continued

| TABLE D-1 | Relationship of drugs to breast milk and effect on infant—cont'd | | | |

Drug and AAP rating	% Oral availability	Peak plasma time (hr)	% Plasma protein bound	Volume of distribution (L/kg)
Psychotropic and mood-altering drugs—cont'd				
Meprobamate		2		
Mesoridazine 4				>30
Methyprylon 6		1.5 ± 0.5	60	
Mirtazapine	50 Complete absorbed	2	85	
Moclobemide	27-70	0.58-3.17	50	0.81-1.5
Nefazodone	20 Completely absorbed; decreased 20% by food	1	>99	0.22-0.87
Nitrazepam	78 ± 16		87 ± 1	1.9 ± 0.3
Nortriptyline	46-59	10	92 ± 2	18 ± 4
Oxazepam	97 ± 11		97.8 ± 2.3	0.6 ± 0.2
Paroxetine		0.5-11	95	
Perphenazine 4				
Pinazepam	Active metabolite desmethyldiazepam (see p. 836), not drug, found in human milk			

M/P ratio	% Adult dose in milk	Maximum amount in milk (mg/L)	Comments and references
2-4			In milk: 96% of newborn dose; peak 4 hr. Galactorrhea seen in some women. Brand names: Equagesic, Miltown, PMB, Equanil. (424, 519)
Minimal amount excreted into human milk			May cause galactorrhea or prolactin increase. Brand name: Serentil.
Excreted into human milk			May see sedation and poor feeding in infant. Brand name: Noludar. (192, 358)
			Brand name: Remeron. (424)
0.69-0.72	0.057 ± 0.02		In milk: peak 3 hr. More than 95% absorbed with hepatic metabolism. Stimulates the release of prolactin in men. (43, 430, 473)
			Brand name: Serzone. (424, 578)
0.18-0.6	<1	0.015	Not detected in infant's plasma. (81, 192, 334, 606)
0.6-3.71	0.53	0.404	Extensive first-pass metabolism; 5%-10% of Caucasians are poor metabolizers. Not detected in infant's serum. Brand names: Pamelor, Aventyl. (20, 68, 70, 166, 192, 296)
0.1-0.33	0.001	0.03	Also metabolite of prazepam and diazepam. Detected in urine of infant exposed to high doses through milk. In milk: half-life 12 hr. Brand name: Serax. (68, 80, 134, 192, 446, 519, 606)
1			Extensive first-pass metabolism; can be partially saturated. Absorption not affected by food. Usual plasma peak: 4.8-5.6 hr. Brand name: Paxil. (114, 562)
0.7-1.1	0.1	0.003	Increases serum prolactin levels. One report: mother taking drug, infant grew normally. Brand names: Etrafon, Triavil, Trilafon. (401, 519)

TABLE D-1   Relationship of drugs to breast milk and effect on infant—cont'd

Drug and AAP rating	% Oral availability	Peak plasma time (hr)	% Plasma protein bound	Volume of distribution (L/kg)
Psychotropic and mood-altering drugs—cont'd				
Prazepam 4				14.4 ± 5.1
Protriptyline	77-93		92 ± 0.6	22 ± 1
Quazepam 4		2.5 ± 0.5		
Raclopride	65 ± 15	0.45 ± 0.2	94-96	1.1 ± 0.4
Remoxipride	96	1.25 ± 0.75	81 ± 3	0.41 ± 0.31
Risperidone	66-70	0.8 ± 0.3	90	1.1
Secobarbital 6		2-4	30-50	1.5
Sertraline		4-8.5	98-99	>20
Temazepam 4	98.4 ± 15.6	1-3	96-97.6	1.06 ± 0.31
Theobromine 7		2.3 ± 0.8	20 ± 5	0.63 ± 0.19
Thioridazine			99	>30
Tranylcypromine	Inhibits lactation			

M/P ratio	% Adult dose in milk	Maximum amount in milk (mg/L)	Comments and references
>1			A prodrug for desmethyldiazepam (see p. 836). Metabolized ultimately to 3-hydroxyprazepam and oxazepam. Brand name: Centrax. (6, 192)
	Excreted into human milk		Predicted to cause galactorrhea and prolactin increase. Brand name: Vivactil. (192, 424, 542)
4.13	0.02-5.8	0.216	Levels of drug and active metabolite decline at same rate in plasma and milk. In milk: peak 3 ± 1 hr. Brand name: Doral. (20)
			Increases serum prolactin levels. (369)
			Acid urine enhances excretion; basic urine delays it. Low doses decrease prolactin concentration; high doses increase it. (22, 151, 206, 369, 587)
			Increase in prolactin levels. Data given for good metabolizers. 6%-8% Caucasians and a low percentage of Asians are poor metabolizers. Brand name: Risperdal. (242, 424)
	Small amounts excreted into human milk		Oral dose: about 90% absorbed. Brand names: Tuinal, Seconal. (7, 424, 519)
			Extensive first-pass metabolism. Metabolite has 10% the activity of the drug. Drug usually not recovered from infant's serum; metabolite found at level of <2 ng/ml. Four nursing infants had normal platelet levels of 5-hydroxytryptamine. Brand name: Zoloft. (146, 375, 424, 597)
0.09-0.63	4.7	0.028	Level of drug in infant's plasma: 7 µg/L. Metabolite of diazepam. Brand name: Restoril. (134, 192, 304, 365, 424, 519, 542)
0.6-1.06	20	7.5	Usual source is chocolate. In milk: peak 4.5 ± 2.5 hr, half-life 4-8 hr. If mother consumes more than a pound per day, may see irritability or increased bowel activity in infant. (6, 19, 20, 599)
	Excreted into human milk		Galactorrhea reported in some women. Percent plasma protein bound is concentration dependent. Brand name: Mellaril. (519)
	Excreted into human milk in insignificant amounts		Brand name: Parnate. (424)

Continued

TABLE D-1	Relationship of drugs to breast milk and effect on infant—cont'd			
Drug and AAP rating	% Oral availability	Peak plasma time (hr)	% Plasma protein bound	Volume of distribution (L/kg)
Psychotropic and mood-altering drugs—cont'd				
Trazodone 4	81 ± 29	1.34 ± 0.84 on empty stomach 2.03 ± 1.51 if taken with food	89-98	1.0 ± 0.3
Triazolam	44	1.25 ± 0.32	80-91.6	1.1 ± 0.4
Trichloroethanol			38 ± 3	
Trifluoperazine				>30
Venlafaxine	12.6 At least 92% absorbed 45 for extended release	1-2	27 ± 2	7.5 ± 3.7
Zopiclone	75-80	0.5-4	45	1.5
Vitamins				
Acitretin 6	36-95 Food increases availability	0.9-4.6	Extensive	
Calcipotriene	Same as calcipotriol (see below)			
Calcipotriol	Less than 1% systemically absorbed; rapidly metabolized to inactive products			
Dihydrotachysterol				
Etretinate	50	2-6	98->99	2
Folic acid 6				
Isotretinoin		3.2	99.9	7

M/P ratio	% Adult dose in milk	Maximum amount in milk (mg/L)	Comments and references
0.09-0.2	0.0065-1.1		In milk: peak 2 hr. Brand name: Desyrel. (7, 20, 80, 192, 387, 424, 567)
	Excreted into human milk		Sublingual availability: 53%. Brand name: Halcion. (56, 192, 424, 451, 519, 542)
0.125-2.4		2.7	Active metabolite of dichloralphenazone and chloral hydrate. In milk (when taken as chloral hydrate): peak 3.37 ± 2.63 hr, 2.4% of the adult dose. (20, 68)
	Excreted into human milk		Excretion into milk not significant after therapeutic doses. Galactorrhea reported in some women. There is an increase in serum prolactin levels. Brand name: Stelazine. (424)
			Extensive first-pass metabolism. Active metabolite: percent plasma protein bound 30 ± 12; volume of distribution 5.7 ± 1.8 l/kg; peaks in plasma at 1-2 hr. Brand name: Effexor (424)
0.39-0.63	1.2		In milk: peak 1-6 hr; in most women 2-3 hr. (194, 337)
0.093-0.18			Steady state milk level: 30-40 ng/ml. (293, 455)
			(371)
			(371)
	Excreted into human milk		Concern about hypercalcemia. Monitor calcium in infant's serum and urine. Brand name: DHT. (68)
	Excreted into human milk		Stored in adipose tissue; absorption enhanced by milk or fatty foods. Brand name: Tegison. (68, 192, 293, 424, 519)
0.02-0.23	0.1	0.141	Preferentially excreted into milk. (68, 424)
	Concentrated in milk		Brand name: Accutane. (192, 294, 424)

Continued

TABLE D-1	Relationship of drugs to breast milk and effect on infant—cont'd			

Drug and AAP rating	% Oral availability	Peak plasma time (hr)	% Plasma protein bound	Volume of distribution (L/kg)
Pyridoxine 6				
Tretinoin	Minimal absorption occurs after topical application			
Miscellaneous				
Acetazolamide 6	>90	Within 2	91.5 ± 4.5	0.2
Aminophylline	99	1.75 ± 1.25	61 ± 12	
Azelaic acid		2		
Baclofen 6		2-3	30	
Bromocriptine 1	65 ± 25	1-3	92.5 ± 2.5	3.4
Carisoprodol				
Chlorhexidine gluconate	Poorly absorbed	0.5		
Cromolyn	1 Little gastric absorption		70	0.32 ± 0.06
Cyclobenzaprine	52	3-8	93	
Doxapram	35-86	2.4		3.5
Enprofylline	Oral absorption complete Rectal availability 89%	0.5	47	
Guaifenesin	Readily absorbed from the GI tract			

M/P ratio	% Adult dose in milk	Maximum amount in milk (mg/L)	Comments and references
0.25	Amount in milk directly proportional to mother's intake		Large amounts may inhibit lactation. In milk: peak 5.5 ± 2.5 hr. Brand names: Beelith, Mega-B, Lurline. (68, 419)
			Brand name: Retin. (68)
0.25-0.3	0.06-1.9	2.1	Amount in maternal plasma about 30 times the amount in neonate's plasma. Brand name: Diamox. (20, 470, 519)
			Active metabolite: theophylline (see p. 848). (424, 496)
			Percutaneous absorption: at 8 hr, 8.1% absorbed from gel; 3%-3.6% from aqueous solution. Mostly dissociated at physiological pH. (50, 162, 424)
0.66	0.1-5.4		In milk: peak 4 hr; half-life 5.6 hr. Absorption decreases as dose decreases. Elimination from milk delayed 3 hr in relation to serum. (20, 424, 519)
	Excreted into human milk		Suppresses prolactin secretion. Extensive first-pass metabolism. Hyperprolactinemic mothers taking drug can breastfeed successfully. Brand name: Parlodel. (198, 231, 270, 284, 519)
2-4			Brand name: Soma. (424)
			Can cause allergic reactions. Brand names: Hibiclens, Peridex, Hibistat. (399, 424)
			After eye treatment, 0.03% absorbed. 10% or less absorbed from an inhaled dose. Brand names: Intal, Gastrocrom. (192, 204, 424, 519)
			Well absorbed orally. Structurally related to tricyclic antidepressants. Concern about SIDS if it gets into milk. Brand name: Flexeril. (7, 424, 496)
			Used in premature infants where it is poorly absorbed orally. Brand name: Dopram. (27, 424, 519)
0.67-0.98	10		Some binding may occur to milk proteins, 90% excreted renally by mother. Dose to infant: 1.32 mg/kg/day. (301)
	A small, insignificant amount is excreted into milk		(424)

Continued

TABLE D-1   **Relationship of drugs to breast milk and effect on infant—cont'd**

Drug and AAP rating	% Oral availability	Peak plasma time (hr)	% Plasma protein bound	Volume of distribution (L/kg)
Miscellaneous—cont'd				
Lanolin	If used on nipples, there is a concern about the presence of pesticides			
Levodopa	35			
Methocarbamol 6	Oral absorption complete Extensive first-pass metabolism	1-2		
Metocurine iodide			35 ± 6	0.35 ± 0.04
Olopatadine	Low exposure when used as eye drops; plasma concentration <0.5-1.3 ng/ml			
Papaverine	23 ± 6	2	91 ± 4	1.5
Povidone-iodine 6				
Pravastatin	17-18	0.7-1.6	43-55	0.67 ± 0.21
Probenecid	100		89 ± 6	0.17 ± 0.03
Rubella vaccine				
Sulfinpyrazone	99		98.3 ± 0.5	0.74 ± 0.23
Theophylline 6	65-100	1.5 ± 0.5	55 ± 15	0.5 ± 0.16
Tiapamil	15-40		75	
Tubocurarine			50 ± 8	0.39 ± 0.14
Zafirlukast		2-4	>99	
Zolpidem 6	67 ± 4	0.5-2	92	

M/P ratio	% Adult dose in milk	Maximum amount in milk (mg/L)	Comments and references
			(100)
			May suppress prolactin levels. Brand names: Dopar, Sinemet, Larodopa, Atamet. (496, 519)
Minimal amount excreted into animal milk			Too little in milk to produce any effects. Brand name: Robaxin, Robaxisal. (7)
			Brand name: Metubine. (2, 192, 424)
			(424)
			Extensive first-pass metabolism. Bioavailability of slow-release tablets: 68% and 89%. (496, 519)
8-25	15		Increase of iodine in the milk and a shift in concentration of neonatal TSH when used on or by mother. Brand names: Betadine, Massengill. (89, 108, 117)
	<0.4	0.047	In milk: peak 3.3 ± 0.8 hr. Oral absorption: 34%. Food in GI tract reduces bioavailability. Brand name: Pravachol. (410, 411, 412, 424, 501)
			Dose-dependent half-life. Brand name: Benemid. (192, 519)
Live, attenuated virus gets into milk			Infant may have serologic evidence of disease but does not exhibit severe symptoms. Does not enhance or suppress subsequent response to vaccine in early childhood. (286, 424)
			Brand name: Anturane. (192)
0.45-1.08	<1-15	8	In milk: peak 1-3 hr; half-life 6 ± 2 hr; 6.7%-20% newborn therapeutic dose. Extremely low clearance in infants less than 6 months old. Brand names: Marax, Quibron, Theolair. (6, 17, 20, 51, 68, 183, 186, 192, 496, 503, 519, 535)
0.36-0.6			Is extensively bound to tissues. (222)
			(2, 192, 519)
0.2			Extensive first-pass metabolism. Food decreases mean bioavailability by 40%. Brand name: Accolate. (424)
0.11-0.18	0.005-0.019		Most of the drug excretion into milk occurs in the first 3 hr. Brand name: Ambien. (153, 428, 496)

REFERENCES

1. Abramowicz M: Moricizine for cardiac arrhythmias, *Med Lett Drugs Ther* 32:99, 1990.
2. Agoston S, Vandenbrom RHG, Wierda JMKH: Clinical pharmacokinetics of neuromuscular blocking drugs, *Clin Pharmacokinet* 22:94, 1992.
3. Akagi H, Reynolds A, Hjelm M: Cyclosporin A and its metabolites: distribution in blood and tissues, *J Int Med Res* 19:1, 1991.
4. Akintonwa A, Gbajumo SA, Mabadeje AFB: Placental and milk transfer of chloroquine in humans, *Ther Drug Monit* 10:147, 1988.
5. Ali-Melkkila T, Kanto J, Iisalo E: Pharmacokinetics and related pharmacodynamics of anticholinergic drugs, *Acta Anaesthesiol Scand* 37:633, 1993.
6. American Academy of Pediatrics Committee on Drugs: The transfer of drugs and other chemicals into human breast milk, *Pediatrics* 93:137, 1994.
7. American Hospital Formulary Service: *AHFS Drug Information,* Bethesda, Md, 1993, American Society of Hospital Pharmacists.
8. Anderson P, Bondesson U, Mattiasson I et al: Verapamil and norverapamil in plasma and breast milk during breastfeeding, *Eur J Clin Pharmacol* 31:625, 1987.
9. Anderson PO: Drug use during breast-feeding, *Clin Pharmacy* 10:594, 1991.
10. Andersson P, Brattsand R, Dahlstrom K et al: Oral availability of fluticasone propionate *Br J Clin Pharmacol* 36:135, 1993.
11. Antony KK, Lewis EW, Kenny MT et al: Pharmacokinetics and bioavailability of a new formulation of teicoplanin following intravenous and intramuscular administration to humans, *J Pharm Sci* 80:605, 1991.
12. Anyebuno MA, Rosenfeld CR: Chloral hydrate toxicity in term infant, *Dev Pharmacol Ther* 17:116, 1991.
13. Arenas RV, Johnson NA: Liquid chromatographic fluorescence method for multiresidue determination of thiabendazole and 5-hydroxythiabendazole in milk, *J AOAC Int* 78:642, 1995.
14. Asch RH, Smith CG: Effects of 9-THC, the principal psychoactive component of marijuana, during pregnancy in the rhesus monkey, *J Reprod Med* 31:1071, 1986.
15. Assies J: Hyperprolactinaemia in diethylstilboestrol-exposed women, *Lancet* 337:983, 1991.
16. Astley SJ, Little RE: Maternal marijuana use during lactation and infant development at one year, *Neurotoxicol Teratol* 12:161, 1990.
17. Atkinson HC, Begg EJ: Prediction of drug concentrations in human skim milk from plasma protein binding and acid-base characteristics, *Br J Clin Pharmac* 25:495, 1988.
18. Atkinson HC, Begg EJ: The binding of drugs to major human milk whey proteins, *Br J Clin Pharmac* 26:107, 1988.
19. Atkinson HC, Begg EJ: Prediction of drug distribution into human milk from physiochemical characteristics, *Clin Pharmacokinet* 18:151, 1990.
20. Atkinson HC, Begg EJ, Darlow BA: Drugs in human milk: clinical pharmacokinetic considerations, *Clin Pharmacokinet* 14:217, 1988.
21. Aujard Y, Brion F, Jacqz-Aigrain E et al: Pharmacokinetics of cefotaxime and desacetylcefotaxime in the newborn, *Diagn Microbiol Infect Dis* 12:87, 1989.
22. Awad AG, Lapierre YD, Jostell K-G et al: Selective dopamine D2 antagonist and prolactin response in acute schizophrenia: results from remoxipride studies, *Prog Neuropsychopharmacol Biol Psychiatry* 14:769, 1990.
23. Bach V, Carl P, Ravlo O et al: A randomized comparison between midazolam and thiopental for elective cesarean section anesthesia. III. Placental transfer and elimination in neonates, *Anesth Analg* 68:238, 1989.
24. Backhouse C, Wade A, Williamson P: Multiple dose pharmacokinetics of cefpodoxime in young adult and elderly patients, *J Antimicrob Chemother* 26(suppl E):29, 1990.
25. Bailey DG, Spence JD, Munoz C et al: Interaction of citrus juices with felodipine and nifedipine, *Lancet* 337:268, 1991.
26. Bailey DG, Arnold JMO, Strong HA et al: Effect of grapefruit juice and naringin on nisoldipine pharmacokinetics, *Clin Pharmacol Ther* 54:589, 1993.
27. Bairam A, Akramoff-Gershan L, Beharry K et al: Gastrointestinal absorption of doxapram in neonates, *Am J Perinatol* 8:110, 1991.
28. Baker PA, Schroeder D: Interpleural bupivacaine for postoperative pain during lactation, *Anesth Analg* 69:400, 1989.
29. Balant-Gorgia AE, Gex-Fabry M, Balant LP: Clinical pharmacokinetics of clomipramine, *Clin Pharmacokinet* 20:447, 1991.
30. Bald R, Bernbeck-Betthauser E-M, Spahn H et al: Excretion of azapropazone in human breast milk, *Eur J Clin Pharmacol* 39:271, 1990.
31. Baldessarini RJ, Frankenburg FR: Clozapine: a novel antipsychotic agent, *N Engl J Med* 324:746, 1991.
32. Baley JE, Meyers C, Kliegman RM et al: Pharmacokinetics, outcome of treatment, and toxic effects of amphotericin B and 5-fluorocytosine in neonates, *J Pediatr* 116:791, 1990.
33. Balfour JA, Buckley MMT: Etodolac: a reappraisal of its pharmacology and therapeutic use in rheumatic diseases and pain states, *Drugs* 42:274, 1991.
34. Balfour JA, Goa KL: Benazepril: a review of its pharmacodynamic and pharmacokinetic properties, and therapeutic efficacy in hypertension and congestive heart failure, *Drugs* 42:511, 1991.

35. Barr WH, Lin C-C, Radwanski E et al: The pharmacokinetics of ceftibuten in humans, *Diagn Microbiol Infect Dis* 14:93, 1991.

36. Bartha L, Nagy GM, Do et al: Inhibition of suckling-induced prolactin release by dexamethasone, *Endocrinology* 129:635, 1991.

37. Bassetti D, Cruciani M: Teicoplanin therapy in children: a review, *Scand J Infect Dis* 72(suppl):35, 1990.

38. Bauer J, Uhlig B, Schrell U et al: Exhaustion of postictal serum prolactin release during status epilepticus, *J Neurol* 239:175, 1992.

39. Beall MH: Advising the nursing mother about her medications, *Contemp Pediatr* 5:67, 1988.

40. Beaulac-Baillargeon L, Allard G: Distribution of indomethacin in human milk and estimation of its milk to plasma ratio in vitro, *Br J Clin Pharmac* 36:413, 1993.

41. Beckers J, Kulbertus HE: Class III drugs: amiodarone, *Eur Heart J* 8(suppl A):53, 1987.

42. Beeley L: Drugs and breastfeeding, *Clin Obstet Gynecol* 13:247, 1986.

43. Begg EJ, Atkinson HC, Duffull SB: Prospective evaluation of a model for the prediction of milk: plasma drug concentrations from physiochemical characteristics, *Br J Clin Pharmac* 33:501, 1992.

44. Bennett PN, Humphries SJ, Osborne JP et al: Use of sodium aurothiomalate during lactation, *Br J Clin Pharmacol* 29:777, 1990.

45. Benowith NL: Clinical pharmacology and toxicology of cocaine, *Pharmacol Toxicol* 72:3, 1993.

46. Bergan T, Thorsteinsson SB, Albini E: Pharmacokinetic profile of fosfomycin trometamol, *Chemotherapy* 39:297, 1993.

47. Berlin CM: Advances in pediatric pharmacology and toxicology, *Adv Pediatr* 34:411, 1987.

48. Berlin Jr CM: Drugs in breastfeeding, *Pediatrics* 95:957, 1995.

49. Bertilsson L, Tomson T: Clinical pharmacokinetics and pharmacological effects of carbamazepine and carbamazepine-10,11-epoxide: an update, *Clin Pharmacol Ther* 11:177, 1986.

50. Bertuzzi A, Gandolfi A, Salinari S et al: Pharmacokinetic analysis of azelaic acid disodium salt: a proposed substrate for total parenteral nutrition, *Clin Pharmacokinet* 20:411, 1991.

51. Besunder JB, Reed MD, Blumer JL: Principles of drug biodisposition in the neonate: a critical evaluation of the pharmacokinetic-pharmacodynamic interface, I. *Clin Pharmacokinet* 14:189, 1988.

52. Besunder JB, Reed MD, Blumer JL: Principles of drug biodisposition in the neonate: a critical evaluation of the pharmacokinetic-pharmacodynamic interface, II. *Clin Pharmacokinet* 14:261, 1988.

53. Bialer M: Clinical pharmacology of valpromide, *Clin Pharmacokinet* 20:114, 1991.

54. Bialer M: Comparative pharmacokinetics of the newer antiepileptic drugs, *Clin Pharmacokinet* 24:441, 1993.

55. Bishop NJ: Aluminum in infant feeding: is it a problem? *Eur J Clin Nutr* 46(suppl 4):S37, 1992.

56. Bixler EO, Kales A, Manfredi RL et al: Next-day memory impairment with triazolam use, *Lancet* 337:827, 1991.

57. Blum RA, D'Andrea DT, Florentino BM et al: Increased gastric pH and the bioavailability of fluconazole and ketoconazole, *Ann Intern Med* 114:755, 1991.

58. Boeckh M, Lode H, Hoffken G et al: Pharmacokinetics of roxithromycin and influence of H2-blockers and antacids on gastrointestinal absorption, *Eur J Clin Microbiol Infect Dis* 11:465, 1992.

59. Borgatta L, Jenny RW, Gruss L: Clinical significance of methohexital meperidine and diazepam in breast milk, *J Clin Pharmacol* 37:186, 1997.

60. Bottorff MB, Hoon TJ, Rodman JH et al: Pharmacokinetics and pharmacodynamics of urapidil in severe hypertension, *J Clin Pharmacol* 28:420, 1988.

61. Boudreau EF, Fleckenstein L, Pang LW et al: Mefloquine kinetics in cured and recrudescent patients with acute falciparum malaria and in healthy volunteers, *Clin Pharmacol Ther* 48:399, 1990.

62. Bourget P, Quinquis-Desmaris V, Fernandez H: Ceftriaxone distribution and protein binding between maternal blood and milk postpartum, *Ann Pharmacother* 27:294, 1993.

63. Boutroy MJ, Bianchetti G, Dubruc C et al: To nurse when receiving acebutolol: is it dangerous for the neonate? *Eur J Clin Pharmacol* 30:737, 1986.

64. Branebjerg PE, Heisterberg L: Blood and milk concentration of ampicillin in mothers treated with pivampicillin and in their infants, *J Perinat Med* 15:555, 1987.

65. Branski D, Kerem E, Gross-Kieselstein E et al: Bloody diarrhea: a possible complication of sulfasalazine transferred through human breast milk, *J Ped Gastroenterol Nutr* 5:316, 1986.

66. Brashear WT, Zuspan KJ, Lazebnik N et al: Effect of ranitidine on bupivacaine disposition, *Anesth Analg* 72:369, 1991.

67. Bree F, Houin G, Barre J et al: Binding to alpha-1-acid glycoprotein and relevant apparent volume of distribution, *Prog Clin Biol Res* 300:321, 1989.

68. Briggs GG, Freeman RK, Yaffe SJ: *Drugs in pregnancy and lactation*, ed 4, Baltimore, 1994, Williams & Wilkins.

69. Briggs GG, Samson JH, Ambrose PJ et al: Excretion of bupropion in breast milk, *Ann Pharmacother* 27:431, 1993.

70. Brixen-Rasmussen L, Halgrener J, Jorgensen A: Amitriptyline and nortriptyline excretion in human breast milk, *Psychopharmacology* (Berl) 76:94, 1982.

71. Brocks DR, Jamali F: Clinical pharmacokinetics of ketorolac tromethamine, *Clin Pharmacokinet* 23:415, 1992.

72. Brodie MJ, Feely J: Adverse drug interactions, *Br Med J* 296:845, 1988.

73. Brunel P, Lecaillon JB, Guyene TT et al: Influence of acetylator status on the haemodynamic effects and pharmacokinetics of cadralazine in healthy subjects, *Br J Clin Pharmac* 29:503, 1990.

74. Bryson HM, Faulds D: Intranasal fluticasone propionate: a review of its pharmacodynamic and pharmacokinetic properties, and therapeutic potential in allergic rhinitis, *Drugs* 43:760, 1992.

75. Bryson HM, Goa KL: Halofantrine: a review of its antimalarial activity, pharmacokinetic properties and therapeutic potential, *Drugs* 43:236, 1992.

76. Buckley MM, Brogden RN, Barradell LB, Goa KL: Imipenem/cilastatin: a reappraisal of its antibacterial activity, pharmacokinetic properties and therapeutic efficacy, *Drugs* 44:408, 1992.

77. Buckley MMT, Goa KL, Clissold SP: Ocular betaxolol: a review of its pharmacological properties, and therapeutic efficacy in glaucoma and ocular hypertension, *Drugs* 40:75, 1990.

78. Buckley MMT, Grant SM, Goa KL et al: Diltiazem: a reappraisal of its pharmacological properties and therapeutic use, *Drugs* 39:757, 1990.

79. Buesa JM, Urrechaga E: Clinical pharmacokinetics of high dose DTIC, *Cancer Chemother Pharmacol* 28:475, 1991.

80. Buist A, Norman TR, Dennerstein L: Breastfeeding and the use of psychotropic medication: a review, *J Affective Disorders* 19:197, 1990.

81. Bulau P, Paar WD, von Unruh GE: Pharmacokinetics of oxcarbazepine and 10-hydroxy-carbazepine in the newborn child of an oxcarbazepine-treated mother, *Eur J Clin Pharmacol* 34:311, 1988.

82. Burch KJ, Wells BG: Fluoxetine/norfluoxetine concentrations in human milk, *Pediatrics* 89:676, 1992.

83. Camaggi CM, Strocchi E, Carisi P et al: Idarubicin metabolism and pharmacokinetics after intravenous and oral administration in cancer patients: a crossover study, *Cancer Chemother Pharmacol* 30:307, 1992.

84. Campa M, Zolfino I, Senesi S et al: The penetration of roxithromycin into human skin, *J Antimicrobial Chemother* 26:87, 1990.

85. Campoli-Richards DM, Buckley MMT, Fitton A: Cetirizine: a review of its pharmacological properties and clinical potential in allergic rhinitis, pollen-induced asthma, and chronic urticaria, *Drugs* 40:762, 1990.

86. Campoli-Richards DM, Clissold SP: Famotidine: pharmacodynamic and pharmacokinetic properties and a preliminary review of its therapeutic use in peptic ulcer disease and Zollinger-Ellison syndrome, *Drugs* 32:197, 1986.

87. Cefali EA, Poynor WJ, Sica D et al: Pharmacokinetic comparison of flurbiprofen in end-stage renal disease subjects and subjects with normal renal function, *J Clin Pharmacol* 31:808, 1991.

88. Celiloglu M, Celiker S, Guven H et al: Gentamicin excretion and uptake from breast milk by nursing infants, *Obstet Gynecol* 84:263, 1994.

89. Chanoine JP, Boulvain M, Bourdoux P et al: Increased recall rate at screening for congenital hypothyroidism in breastfed infants born to iodine overloaded mothers, *Arch Dis Child* 63:1207, 1988.

90. Charm SE, Chi R: Microbial receptor assay for rapid detection and identification of seven families of antimicrobial drugs in milk: collaborative study, *J Assoc Off Anal Chem* 71:304, 1988.

91. Chasnoff IJ, Lewis DE, Squires L: Cocaine intoxication in a breastfed infant, *Pediatrics* 80:836, 1987.

92. Chen T-M, Chiou WL: Large differences in the biological half-life and volume of distribution of hydrochlorothiazide in normal subjects from eleven studies, *Int J Clin Pharmacol Ther Toxicol* 30:34, 1992.

93. Chu S-Y, Park Y, Locke C et al: Drug-food interaction potential of clarithromycin, a new macrolide antimicrobial, *J Clin Pharmacol* 32:32, 1992.

94. Chung KF, Barnes PJ: Treatment of asthma, *Br Med J* 294:103, 1987.

95. Clissold SP, Campoli-Richards DM: Omeprazole: a preliminary review of its pharmacodynamic and pharmacokinetic properties, and therapeutic potential in peptic ulcer disease and Zollinger-Ellison syndrome, *Drugs* 32:15, 1986.

96. Cockerill FR, Edson RS: Trimethoprim-sulfamethoxazole, *Mayo Clin Proc* 66:1260, 1991.

97. Colthup PV, Felgate CC, Palmer JL et al: Determination of ondansetron in plasma and its pharmacokinetics in the young and elderly, *J Pharm Sci* 80:868, 1991.

98. Cooper DS: Antithyroid drugs: to breast-feed or not to breast-feed, *Am J Obstet Gynecol* 157:234, 1987.

99. Cooper MA, Nye K, Andrews JM et al: The pharmacokinetics and inflammatory fluid penetration of orally administered azithromycin, *J Antimicrob Chemother* 26:533, 1990.

100. Copeland CA, Raebel MA, Wagner SL: Pesticide residue in lanolin, *JAMA* 261:242, 1989.

101. Coumel P, Leclercq JF, Escoubet B: Beta-blockers: use for arrhythmias, *Eur Heart J* 8(suppl A):41, 1987.

102. Cover DL, Mueller BA: Ciprofloxacin penetration into human breast milk: a case report, DICP, *Ann Pharmacother* 24:703, 1990.

103. Criscuoli M, Lippi A, Mengozzi G: Pharmacokinetics and pharmacodynamics of idrapril in rats, dogs, and humans, *Drug Metab Dispos* 21:835, 1993.

104. Cuzzolin L, Fanos V, Zambreri D et al: Pharmacokinetics and renal tolerance of aztreonam in premature infants, *Antimicrob Agents Chemother* 35:1726, 1991.

105. Dahlstrom A, Lundell B, Curvall M et al: Nicotine and cotinine concentrations in the nursing mother and her infant, *Acta Paediatr Scand* 79:142, 1990.

106. Dailland P, Cockshott ID, Lirzin JD et al: Intravenous propofol during cesarean section: placental transfer, concentrations in breast milk, and neonatal effects—a preliminary study, *Anesthesiology* 71:827, 1989.

107. Dan M, Weidekamm E, Sagiv R et al: Penetration of fleroxacin into breast milk and pharmacokinetics in lactating women, *Antimicrob Agents Chemother* 37:293, 1993.

108. Danziger Y, Pertzelan A, Mimouni M: Transient congenital hypothyroidism after topical iodine in pregnancy and lactation, *Arch Dis Child* 62:295, 1987.

109. Davies BE, Coates PE, Clarke JGN et al: Bioavailability and pharmacokinetics of clavulanic acid in healthy subjects, *Int J Clin Pharmacol Ther Toxicol* 23:70, 1985.

110. Davies RF, Lineberry MD, Funck-Brentano C et al: Recainam dose titration and pharmacokinetics in patients with resistant arrhythmias, *Clin Pharmacol Ther* 46:324, 1989.

111. Davis PJ, Killian A, Stiller RL et al: Pharmacokinetics of alfentanil in newborn premature infants and older children, *Dev Pharmacol Ther* 13:21, 1989.

112. Debruyne D, Ryckelynck J-P: Clinical pharmacokinetics of fluconazole, *Clin Pharmacokinet* 24:10, 1993.

113. Dechant KL, Brogden RN, Pilkington T et al: Ifosfamide/mesna: a review of its antineoplastic activity, pharmacokinetic properties and therapeutic efficacy in cancer, *Drugs* 42:428, 1991.

114. Dechant KL, Clissold SP: Paroxetine: a review of its pharmacodynamic and pharmacological properties, and therapeutic potential in depressive illness, *Drugs* 41:225, 1991.

115. Dechant KL, Clissold SP: Sumatriptan: a review of its pharmacodynamic and pharmacokinetic properties and therapeutic efficacy in the acute treatment of migraine and cluster headache, *Drugs* 43:776, 1992.

116. Dechant KL, Goa KL: Levocabastine: a review of its pharmacological properties and therapeutic potential as a topical antihistamine in allergic rhinitis and conjunctivitis, *Drugs* 41:202, 1991.

117. Delange F, Chanoine JP, Abrassart C et al: Topical iodine, breastfeeding, and neonatal hypothyroidism, *Arch Dis Child* 63:106, 1988.

118. Del Favero A, Patoia L, Rosina R et al: Pharmacokinetics and tolerability of teicoplanin in healthy volunteers after single increasing doses, *Antimicrob Agents Chemother* 35:2551, 1991.

119. Delhotal-Landes B, Flouvat B, Duchier J et al: Pharmacokinetics of lansoprazole in patients with renal or liver disease of varying severity, *Eur J Clin Pharmacol* 45:367, 1993.

120. De Mey C, Enterling D, Brendel E et al: Pharmacokinetics and pharmacodynamics of single oral doses of ibopamine, quinidine, and their combination in normal man, *Eur J Clin Pharmacol* 34:415, 1988.

121. Derendorf H, Mollmann H, Barth J et al: Pharmacokinetics and oral bioavailability of hydrocortisone, *J Clin Pharmacol* 31:473, 1991.

122. Desager JP, Horsmans Y, Harvengt C: A pharmacokinetic evaluation of the second-generation H1-receptor antagonist cetirizine in very young children, *Clin Pharmacol Ther* 53:431, 1993.

123. Dickinson TH, Egan JM, Abernethy DR: Effects of nifedipine on hepatic drug oxidation, *Pharmacology* 36:405, 1988.

124. Dickstein K: Pharmacokinetics of enalapril in congestive heart failure, *Drugs* 32(suppl 5):40, 1986.

125. Dodson WE: Special pharmacokinetic considerations in children, *Epilepsia* 28(suppl):S56, 1987.

126. Don PC, Kizner R: Excretion of acyclovir in human breast milk, *J Am Acad Dermatol* 25:342, 1991.

127. Donnelly R, Elliott HL, Meredith PA et al: Concentration-effect relationships and individual responses to doxazosin in essential hypertension, *Br J Clin Pharmacol* 28:517, 1989.

128. Donnelly R, Macphee GJA: Clinical pharmacokinetics and kinetic-dynamic relationships of dilevalol and labetalol, *Clin Pharmacokinet* 21:95, 1991.

129. Dostal LA, Schwetz BA: Determination of diphenhydramine in rat milk and plasma and its effects on milk composition and mammary gland nucleic acids, *J Pharm Sci* 78:423, 1989.

130. Drijver M, Duijkers TJ, Kromhout D et al: Determinants of polychlorinated biphenyls (PCBs) in human milk, *Acta Paediatr Scand* 77:30, 1988.

131. Drinkwater P: Metronidazole, *Aust N Z J Obstet Gynaecol* 27:288, 1987.

132. Dudley MN, Marchbanks CR, Flor SC et al: The effect of food or milk on the absorption kinetics of ofloxacin, *Eur J Clin Pharmacol* 41:569, 1991.

133. Dunselman PHJM, Edgar B: Felodipine clinical pharmacokinetics, *Clin Pharmacokinet* 21:418, 1991.

134. Dusci LJ, Good SM, Hall RW et al: Excretion of diazepam and its metabolites in human milk during withdrawal from combination high dose diazepam and oxazepam, *Br J Clin Pharmacol* 29:123, 1990.

135. Dydek GJ, Blue PW: Human breast milk excretion of iodine-131 following diagnostic and therapeutic administration to a lactating patient with Graves' disease, *J Nucl Med* 29:407, 1988.

136. Eadie MJ: Formation of active metabolites of anticonvulsant drugs: a review of their pharmacokinetic and therapeutic significance, *Clin Pharmacokinet* 21:27, 1991.

137. Ebihara A, Fujimura A: Metabolites of antihypertensive drugs: an updated review of their clinical pharmacokinetic and therapeutic implications, *Clin Pharmacokinet* 21:331, 1991.

138. Echizen H, Ishizaki T: Clinical pharmacokinetics of famotidine, *Clin Pharmacokinet* 21:178, 1991.

139. Edgar B, Bailey D, Bergstrand R et al: Acute effects of drinking grapefruit juice on the pharmacokinetics and dynamics of felodipine and its potential clinical relevance, *Eur J Clin Pharmacol* 42:313, 1992.

140. Edstein MD, Rieckmann KH: Lack of effect of proguanil on the pharmacokinetics of dapsone in healthy volunteers, *Chemotherapy* 39:235, 1993.

141. Edstein MD, Veenendaal JR, Hyslop R: Excretion of mefloquine in human breast milk, *Chemotherapy* 34:165, 1988.

142. Edstein MD, Veenendaal JR, Newman K et al: Excretion of chloroquine, dapsone, and pyrimethamine in human milk, *Br J Clin Pharmac* 22:733, 1986.

143. Ehrenkranz RA, Ackerman BA, Hulse JD: Nifedipine transfer into human milk, *J Pediatr* 114:478, 1989.

144. Ehrinpreis MN, Dhar R, Narula A: Cimetidine-induced galactorrhea, *Am J Gastroenterol* 84:563, 1989.

145. Eksborg S, Soderberg M, Nilsson B et al: Plasma pharmacokinetics of idarubicin and its 13-hydroxy-metabolite after intravenous and oral administration under fasting and non-fasting conditions, *Acta Oncologica* 29:921, 1990.

146. Epperson CN, Anderson GM, McDougle CJ: Sertraline and breast-feeding, *New Engl J Med* 336:1189, 1997.

147. Etienne M-C, Milano G, Rene N et al: Improved bioavailability of a new oral preparation of medroxyprogesterone acetate, *J Pharm Sci* 80:1130, 1991.

148. Ette EI, Essien EE, Ogonor JI et al: Chloroquine in human milk, *J Clin Pharmacol* 27:499, 1987.

149. Faber P, Strenge-Hesse A: Relevance of rhein excretion into breast milk, *Pharmacology* 36:212, 1988.

150. Fahr A: Cyclosporin clinical pharmacokinetics, *Clin Pharmacokinet* 24:472, 1993.

151. Farde L, Grind M, Nilsson MI et al: Remoxipride: a new potential antipsychotic drug, *Psychopharmacology* 95:157, 1988.

152. Fassbender M, Lode H, Schaberg T et al: Pharmacokinetics of new oral cephalosporins, including a new carbacephem, *Clin Infect Dis* 16:646, 1993.

153. Fattapposta F, Sanarelli L, Valle E et al: A double-blind study of the effects of zolpidem, a new imidazopyridine hypnotic, on contingent negative variation in patients with situational insomnia, *Curr Ther Res* 48:766, 1990.

154. Fattinger K, Vozeh S, Ha HR et al: Population pharmacokinetics of quinidine, *Br J Clin Pharmac* 31:279, 1991.

155. Faulds D, Brogden RN: Didanosine: a review of its antiviral activity, pharmacokinetic properties and therapeutic potential in human immunodeficiency virus infection, *Drugs* 44:94, 1992.

156. Faulds D, Goa KL, Benfield P: Cyclosporin: a review of its pharmacodynamic and pharmacokinetic properties, and therapeutic use in immunoregulatory disorders, *Drugs* 45:953, 1993.

157. Fauler J, Verner LJ: The pharmacokinetics of clonidine in high dosage, *Eur J Clin Pharmacol* 45:165, 1993.

158. Faulkner JK, McGibney D, Chasseaud LE et al: The pharmacokinetics of amlodipine in healthy volunteers after single intravenous and oral doses and after 14 reported oral doses given once daily, *Br J Clin Pharmac* 22:21, 1986.

159. Feliciano NR, Bouvet AA, Redalieu E et al: Pharmacokinetic and pharmacodynamic comparison of an osmotic release oral metoprolol tablet and the metoprolol conventional tablet, *Am Heart J* 120:483, 1990.

160. Fentiman IS: Tamoxifen: use in benign conditions, *Br J Clin Pract* 42:384, 1988.

161. Fitton A, Buckley MMT: Moricizine: a review of its pharmacological properties, and therapeutic efficacy in cardiac arrhythmias, *Drugs* 40:138, 1990.

162. Fitton A, Goa KL: Azelaic acid: A review of its pharmacological properties and therapeutic efficacy in acne and hyperpigmentary skin disorders, *Drugs* 41:780, 1991.

163. Fitton A, Sorkin EM: Sotalol: an updated review of its pharmacological properties and therapeutic use in cardiac arrhythmias, *Drugs* 46:678, 1993.

164. Fleishaker JC, Desai N, McNamara J: Factors affecting the milk-to-plasma drug concentration ratio in lactating women: physical interactions with protein and fat, *J Pharm Sci* 76:189, 1987.

165. Fondevila CG, Meschengieser S, Blanco A et al: Effect of acenocoumarine on the breast-fed infant, *Thromb Res* 56:29, 1989.

166. Fonne-Pfister R, Meyer UA: Xenobiotic and endobiotic inhibitors of cytochrome P-450dbl function, the target of the debrisoquine/sparteine type polymorphism, *Biochem Pharmacol* 37:3829, 1988.

167. Force RW: Fluconazole concentrations in breast milk, *Pediatr Infect Dis J* 14:235, 1995.

168. Fotherby K: Pharmacokinetics of gestagens: some problems, *Am J Obstet Gynecol* 163:323, 1990.

169. Fowles SE, Pierce DM, Prince WT et al: The tolerance to and pharmacokinetics of penciclovir (BRL 39 123A), a novel antiherpes agent, administered by intravenous infusion to healthy subjects, *Eur J Clin Pharmacol* 43:513, 1992.

170. Fraschini F, Scaglione F, Demartini G: Clarithromycin clinical pharmacokinetics, *Clin Pharmacokinet* 25:189, 1993.

171. Freedman MD, Somberg JC: Pharmacology and pharmacokinetics amiodarone, *J Clin Pharmacol* 31:1061, 1991.

172. Frey B, Schubinger G, Musy JP: Transient cholestatic hepatitis in a neonate associated with carbamazepine exposure during pregnancy and breastfeeding, *Eur J Pediatr* 150:136, 1990.

173. Frey BM, Frey FJ: Clinical pharmacokinetics of prednisone and prednisolone, *Clin Pharmacokinet* 19:126, 1990.

174. Friedel HA, Brogden RN: Pinacidil: a review of its pharmacodynamic and pharmacokinetic properties, and therapeutic potential in the treatment of hypertension, *Drugs* 39:929, 1990.

175. Friedel HA, Buckley MMT: Torasemide: a review of its pharmacological properties and therapeutic potential, *Drugs* 41:81, 1991.

176. Frishman WH: Comparative pharmacokinetic and clinical profiles of angiotensin-converting enzyme inhibitors and calcium antagonists in systemic hypertension, *Am J Cardiol* 69:17C, 1992.

177. Frishman WH, Lazar EJ, Gorodokin G: Pharmacokinetic optimisation of therapy with beta-adrenergic blocking agents, *Clin Pharmacokinet* 20:311, 1991.

178. Fujimura A, Ohashi K, Tsuru M et al: Clinical pharmacology of dilevalol. I. Comparison of the pharmacokinetic and pharmacodynamic properties of dilevalol and labetalol after a single oral administration in subjects, *J Clin Pharmacol* 29:635, 1989.

179. Fujimura A, Ohashi K, Tsuru M et al: Clinical pharmacology of dilevalol. II. The pharmacokinetic, pharmacodynamic and tolerance studies of dilevalol during repeated administration in healthy subjects, *J Clin Pharmacol* 29:643, 1989.

180. Fulton B, Moore LL: Comment: ciprofloxacin excretion into breast milk, DICP, *Ann Pharmacother* 24:1122, 1990.

181. Funck-Brentano C, Kroemer HK, Lee JT et al: Drug therapy, *N Engl J Med* 322:518, 1990.

182. Gabilan JC, Benattar C, Lindenbaum A: Clofibrate treatment of neonatal jaundice, *Pediatrics* 86:647, 1990.

183. Gal P: Therapeutic drug monitoring in neonates: problems and issues, *Drug Intell Clin Pharm* 22:317, 1988.

184. Galgiani JN: Fluconazole, a new antifungal agent, *Ann Intern Med* 113:177, 1990.

185. Gan VN, Chu S-Y, Kusmiesz HT et al: Pharmacokinetics of a clarithromycin suspension in infants and children, *Antimicrob Agents Chemother* 36:2478, 1992.

186. Gardner MJ, Schatz M, Zeiger R et al: Longitudinal effects of pregnancy on the pharmacokinetics of theophylline, *Eur J Clin Pharmacol* 31:289, 1987.

187. Garg DC, Jallad NS, Singh S et al: Efficacy and pharmacokinetics of oral pirmenol, a new anti-arrhythmic drug, *J Clin Pharmacol* 28:812, 1988.

188. Garrigues TM, Martin U, Peris-Ribera JE et al: Dose-dependent absorption and elimination of cefadroxil in man, *Eur J Clin Pharmacol* 41:179, 1991.

189. Giacoia GP, Jungbluth GL, Jusko WJ: Effect of formula feeding on oral absorption of caffeine in premature infants, *Dev Pharmacol Ther* 12:205, 1989.

190. Giamarellou H, Kolokythas E, Petrikkos G et al: Pharmacokinetics of three newer quinolones in pregnant and lactating women, *Am J Med* 87(suppl 5A):49S, 1989.

191. Gill J, Heel RC, Fitton A: Amiodarone: an overview of its pharmacological properties, and review of its therapeutic use in cardiac arrhythmias, *Drugs* 43:69, 1992.

192. Gilman AG, Rall TW, Nies AS et al, editors: *The pharmacological basis of therapeutics*, ed 8, New York, 1990, Pergamon Press.

193. Gin T, Yau G, Jong W et al: Disposition of propofol at caesarean section and in the postpartum period, *Br J Anaesth* 67:49, 1991.

194. Goa KL, Heel RC: Zopiclone: a review of its pharmacodynamic and pharmacokinetic properties and therapeutic efficacy as a hypnotic, *Drugs* 32:48, 1986.

195. Goa KL, McTavish D, Clissold SP: Ivermectin: a review of its antifilarial activity, pharmacokinetic properties and clinical efficacy in onchocerciasis, *Drugs* 42:640, 1991.

196. Goa KL, Ross SR, Chrisp P: Lamotrigine: a review of its pharmacological properties and clinical efficiency in epilepsy, *Drugs* 46:152, 1993.

197. Goa KL, Sorin EM: Nitrendipine: a review of its pharmacodynamic and pharmacokinetic properties, and therapeutic efficacy in the treatment of hypertension, *Drugs* 33:123, 1987.

198. Godo G, Koloszar S, Szilagyi I et al: Experience relating to pregnancy, lactation, and the after-weaning condition of hyperprolactinemic patients treated with bromocriptine, *Fertil Steril* 51:529, 1989.

199. Goldberg MR, Rockhold FW, Thompson WL et al: Clinical pharmacokinetics of pinacidil, a potassium channel opener, in hypertension, *J Clin Pharmacol* 29:33, 1989.

200. Good SS, Koble CS, Crouch R et al: Isolation and characterization of an ether glucoronide of zidovudine, a major metabolite in monkeys and humans, *Drug Metab Dispos* 18:321, 1990.

201. Granneman GR, Guay DRP: The influence of age on the pharmacokinetics of temafloxacin, *Am J Med* 91(suppl 6A):71S, 1991.

202. Grant SM, Clissold SP: Fluconazole: a review of its pharmacodynamic and pharmacokinetic properties, and therapeutic potential in superficial and systemic mycoses, *Drugs* 39:877, 1990.

203. Green AI, Brown WA: Prolactin and neuroleptic drugs, *Neurol Clin* 6:213, 1988.

204. Greenberger PA, Patterson R: The management of asthma during pregnancy and lactation, *Clin Rev Allergy* 5:317, 1987.

205. Greenblatt DJ, Wright CE: Clinical pharmacokinetics of alprazolam: therapeutic implications, *Clin Pharmacokinet* 24:453, 1993.

206. Grind M, Nilsson MI, Nilsson L et al: Remoxipride: a new potential antipsychotic compound, *Psychopharmacology* 98:304, 1989.

207. Guay DRP, Opsahl JA, McMahon FG et al: Safety and pharmacokinetics of multiple doses of intravenous ofloxacin in healthy volunteers, *Antimicrob Agents Chemother* 36:308, 1992.

208. Guerret M, Cheymol G, Hubert M et al: Simultaneous study of the pharmacokinetics of intravenous and oral nicardipine using a stable isotope, *Eur J Clin Pharmacol* 37:381, 1989.

209. Guglielmo BJ, Flaherty JF, Batman R et al: Comparative pharmacokinetics of low and high-dose ticarcillin, *Antimicrob Agents Chemother* 30:359, 1986.

210. Guimaraes FS: Fluoxetine and fluvoxamine, *Br J Hosp Med* 45:146, 1991.

211. Guttendorf RJ, Wedlund PJ: Genetic aspects of drug disposition and therapeutics, *J Clin Pharmacol* 32:107, 1992.

212. Haarnhielm C, Dahlback H, Skanberg I: In vivo pharmacokinetics of felodipine predicted from in vitro studies in rat, dog and man, *Acta Pharmacol Toxicol* 59:113, 1986.

213. Hackett LP, Wojnar-Horton RE, Dusci LJ et al: Excretion of sotalol in breast milk, *Br J Clin Pharmac* 29:277, 1990.

214. Haefeli EW, Vozeh S, Ha HR et al: Comparison of the pharmacodynamic effects of intravenous and oral propafenone, *Clin Pharmacol Ther* 48:245, 1990.

215. Haglund K, Dahlqvist R, Emilsson H et al: Cadralazine pharmacokinetics: a pilot study, *Eur J Clin Pharmacol* 35:571, 1988.

216. Hall ST, Harding SM, Evans GL et al: Clinical pharmacology of lacidipine, *J Cardiovasc Pharmacol* 17:S9, 1991.

217. Hallen IP, Oskarsson A: Dose dependent transfer of 203lead to milk and tissue uptake in suckling offspring studied in rats and mice, *Pharmacol Toxicol* 73:174, 1993.

218. Hansdottir V, Hedner T, Woestenborghs R et al: The CSF and plasma pharmacokinetics of sufentanil after intrathecal administration, *Anesthesiology* 74:264, 1991.

219. Harder S, Thurmann P, Siewert M et al: Pharmacodynamic profile of verapamil in relation to absolute bioavailability: investigations with a conventional and a controlled-release formulation, *J Cardiovasc Pharmacol* 17:207, 1991.

220. Harron DWG, Brogden RN, Faulds D et al: Cibenzoline: a review of its pharmacological properties and therapeutic potential in arrhythmias, *Drugs* 43:734, 1992.

221. Hartikainen-Sorri AL, Heikkinen JE, Koivisto M: Pharmacokinetics of clonidine during pregnancy and nursing, *Obstet Gynecol* 69:598, 1987.

222. Hartmann D, Lunell NO, Friedrich G et al: Excretion of tiapamil in breast milk, *Br J Clin Pharmac* 26:183, 1988.

223. Hasselstrom J, Sawe J: Morphine pharmacokinetics and metabolism in humans: enterohepatic cycling and relative contribution of metabolites to active opioid concentrations, *Clin Pharmacokinet* 24:344, 1993.

224. Hedner T, Persson B: Effects of a new serotonin antagonist, ketanserin, in experimental and clinical hypertension, *Am J Hypertens* 1:317S, 1988.

225. Hedrick WR, DiSimone RN, Keen RL: Radiation dosimetry from breast milk excretion of radioiodine and pertechnetate, *J Nucl Med* 27:1569, 1986.

226. Herrlinger C, Braunfels M, Fink E et al: Pharmacokinetics and bioavailability of tamoxifen in healthy volunteers, *Int J Clin Pharmacol Ther Toxicol* 30:487, 1992.

227. Heykants J, Van Peer A, Lavrijsen K et al: Pharmacokinetics of oral antifungals and their clinical implications, *Br J Clin Pharmac* 44(suppl 71):50, 1990.

228. Hii JTY, Duff HJ, Burgess ED: Clinical pharmacokinetics of propafenone, *Clin Pharmacokinet* 21:1, 1991.

229. Hilbert J, Radwanski E, Affrime MB et al: Excretion of loratadine in human breast milk, *J Clin Pharmacol* 28:234, 1988.

230. Hill MR, Szefler SJ, Ball BD et al: Monitoring glucocorticoid therapy: a pharmacokinetic approach, *Clin Pharmacol Ther* 48:390, 1990.

231. Ho KY, Thorner MO: Therapeutic applications of bromocriptine in endocrine and neurological diseases, *Drugs* 36:67, 1988.

232. Hochhaus G, Mollmann H: Pharmacokinetic/pharmacodynamic characteristics of the beta-2-agonists terbutaline, salbutamol and fenoterol, *Int J Clin Pharmacol Ther Toxicol* 30:342, 1992.

233. Hofmeyr GJ, Sonnendecker EWW: Secretion of the gastrokinetic agent cisapride in human milk, *Eur J Clin Pharmacol* 30:735, 1986.

234. Hollingshead LM, Faulds D: Idarubicin: a review of its pharmacodynamic and pharmacokinetic properties, and therapeutic potential in the chemotherapy of cancer, *Drugs* 42:690, 1991.

235. Hollister LE, Claghorn JL: New antidepressants, *Annu Rev Pharmacol Toxicol* 32:165, 1993.

236. Hopkins S: Clinical safety and tolerance of azithromycin in children, *J Antimicrob Chemother* 31(suppl E):111, 1993.

237. Hooper DC, Wolfson JS: Fluoroquinolone antimicrobial agents, *N Engl J Med* 324:384, 1991.

238. Hoppu K, Neuvonen PJ, Korte T: Disopyramide and breast feeding, *Br J Clin Pharmac* 21:533, 1986.

239. Howden CW: Clinical pharmacology of omeprazole, *Clin Pharmacokinet* 20:38, 1991.

240. Howell P, Davies W, Wrigley M et al: Comparison of four local extradural anaesthetic solutions for elective caesarean section, *Br J Anaesth* 65:648, 1990.

241. Howrie DL, Pieniaszek HJ, Fogoros RN et al: Disposition of moracizine (Ethomozine) in healthy subjects after oral administration of radiolabelled drug, *Eur J Clin Pharmacol* 32:607, 1987.

242. Huang M-L, Van Peer A, Woestenborghs R et al: Pharmacokinetics of the novel antipsychotic agent risperidone and the prolactin response in healthy subjects, *Clin Pharmacol Ther* 54:257, 1993.

243. Hui KK, Duchin KL, Kripalani KJ et al: Pharmacokinetics of fosinopril in patients with various degrees of renal function, *Clin Pharmacol Ther* 49:457, 1991.

244. Humbert G, Brumpt I, Montay G et al: Influence of rifampin on the pharmacokinetics of pefloxacin, *Clin Pharmacol Ther* 50:682, 1991.

245. Hussar DA: New drugs of 1988, *Am Pharm* NS29:25, 1989.

246. Hussar DA: New drugs of 1989, *Am Pharm* NS30:27, 1990.

247. Hussar DA: New drugs of 1991, *Am Pharm* NS32:37, 1992.

248. Hussar DA: New drugs of 1992, *Am Pharm* NS33:20, 1993.

249. Huttunen JK, Gronhagen-Riska C, Fybrquist F: Enalapril treatment of a nursing mother with slightly impaired renal function, *Clin Nephrol* 31:278, 1989.

250. Isah AO, Rawlins MD, Bateman DN: Clinical pharmacology of prochlorperazine in healthy young males, *Br J Clin Pharmac* 32:677, 1991.

251. Isenberg KE: Excretion of fluoxetine in human breast milk, *J Clin Psychiatry* 51:169, 1990.

252. Jacqz-Aigrain E, Daoud P, Burtin P et al: Pharmacokinetics of midazolam during continuous infusion in critically ill neonates, *Eur J Clin Pharmacol* 42:329, 1992.

253. James NC, Donn KH, Collins JJ et al: Pharmacokinetics of cefuroxime axetil and cefaclor: relationship of concentrations in serum to MICs for common respiratory pathogens, *Antimicrob Agents Chemother* 35:1860, 1991.

254. Jani JP, Patel JS, Shah MP et al: Levels of organochlorine pesticides in human milk in Ahmedabad, India, *Int Arch Occup Environ Health* 60:111, 1988.

255. Jemaa Z, Sabbah S, Bouguerra ML: Preliminary study of organochlorine residues in human milk and cord blood, *Acta Biol Hung* 38:93, 1987.

256. Johansson E, Odlind V: The passage of exogenous hormones into breast milk: possible effects, *Int J Gynecol Obstet* 25(suppl):111, 1987.

257. John DN, Fort S, Lewis MJ et al: Pharmacokinetics and pharmacodynamics of verapamil following sublingual and oral administration to healthy volunteers, *Br J Clin Pharmac* 33:623, 1992.

258. Johnson BF, Haffajee CI, Woodman T et al: The relation of the kinetics of pirmenol to its antiarrhythmic efficacy, *J Clin Pharmacol* 28:401, 1988.

259. Johnson BF, Wilson J, Johnson J et al: Digoxin pharmacokinetics and spirapril, a new ace inhibitor, *J Clin Pharmacol* 31:527, 1991.

260. Jonkers RE, Koopmans RP, Portier EJG et al: Debrisoquine phenotype and the pharmacokinetic and beta-2 receptor pharmacodynamics of metoprolol and its enantiomers, *J Pharmacol Exp Ther* 256:959, 1991.

261. Jungbluth GL, Wirth FH Jr, Rubio TT et al: Developmental pharmacokinetics of mezlocillin in 4 newborn infants, *Dev Pharmacol Ther* 11:317, 1988.

262. Kamilli I, Gresser U, Schaefer C et al: Allopurinol in breast milk, *Adv Exp Med Biol* 309A:143, 1991.

263. Kanja LW, Skaare JU, Ojwang SBO et al: A comparison of organochlorine pesticide residues in maternal adipose tissue, maternal blood, cord blood, and human milk from mother/infant pairs, *Arch Environ Contam Toxicol* 22:21, 1992.

264. Karbwang J, Bangchang KN, Bunnag D et al: Pharmacokinetics and pharmacodynamics of mefloquine in Thai patients with acute falciparum, *Bull World Health Organ* 69:207, 1991.

265. Karbwang J, Milton KA, Bangchang KN et al: Pharmacokinetics of halofantrine in Thai patients with acute uncomplicated falciparum malaria, *Br J Clin Pharmac* 31:484, 1991.

266. Karlsson MO, Dahlstrom B, Eckernas SA et al: Pharmacokinetics of oral noscapine, *Eur J Clin Pharmacol* 39:275, 1990.

267. Kassner JT: Beta blockers, *Clin Tox Rev* 12:1, 1989.

268. Kates RE: Metabolites of antiarrhythmic drugs: are they clinically important? *Rational Drug Therapy* 20:1, 1986.

269. Katoh O, Yamada H, Hiura K et al: Clinical pharmacology and toxicity of low daily administration of oral etoposide in advanced lung cancer patients, *J Clin Pharmacol* 31:1155, 1991.

270. Katz E, Schran HF, Weiss BE et al: Increased circulating levels of bromocriptine after vaginal compared with oral administration, *Fertil Steril* 55:882, 1991.

271. Kaye B, Cussans NJ, Faulkner JK et al: The metabolism and kinetics of doxazosin in man, mouse, rat and dog, *Br J Clin Pharmac* 21:19S, 1986.

272. Kearns GL, Jacobs RF, Thomas BR et al: Cefotaxime and desacetylcefotaxime pharmacokinetics in very low birth weight neonates, *J Pediatr* 114:461, 1989.

273. Kelloway JS, Awni WM, Lin CC et al: Pharmacokinetics of ceftibuten-cis and its trans metabolite in healthy volunteers and in patients with chronic renal insufficiency, *Antimicrob Agents Chemother* 35:2267, 1991.

274. Kelly JG, O'Malley K: Clinical pharmacokinetics of calcium antagonists, *Clin Pharmacokinet* 22:416, 1992.

275. Kelsey JJ, Moser LR, Jennings JC et al: Presence of azithromycin breast milk concentrations: a case report, *Am J Obstet Gynecol* 170:1375, 1994.

276. Kenyon CF, Knoppert DC, Lee SK et al: Amikacin pharmacokinetics and suggested dosage modifications for the preterm infant, *Antimicrob Agents Chemother* 34:265, 1990.

277. Kilpatrick CJ, Moulds RFW: Anticonvulsants in pregnancy, *Med J Aust* 154:199, 1991.

278. Kinzig M, Sorgel F, Brismar B et al: Pharmacokinetics and tissue penetration of tazobactam and piperacillin in patients undergoing colorectal surgery, *Antimicrob Agents Chemother* 36:1997, 1992.

279. Kirsten R, Nelson K, Molz KH et al: Influence of food intake on the bioavailability of urapidil in healthy volunteers, *Int J Clin Pharmacol* 27:298, 1989.

280. Klotz U, Ogbuokiri JE, Okonkwo PO: Ivermectin binds avidly to plasma proteins, *Eur J Clin Pharmacol* 39:607, 1990.

281. Knupp CA, Milbrath R, Barbhaiya RH: Effect of time of food administration on the bioavailability of didanosine from a chewable tablet formulation, *J Clin Pharmacol* 33:568, 1993.

282. Kolars JC, Awni WM, Merion RM et al: First-pass metabolism of cyclosporin by the gut, *Lancet* 338:1488, 1991.

283. Konishi K, Suzuki H, Hayashi M et al: Pharmacokinetics of cefuroxime axetil in patients with normal and impaired renal function, *J Antimicrob Chemother* 31:413, 1993.

284. Kremer JAM, Rolland R, Van der Heijden PFM et al: Lactation inhibition by a single injection of a new depot-bromocriptine, *Br J Obstet Gynaecol* 97:527, 1990.

285. Krishna S, ter Kuile F, Supanaranond W et al: Pharmaco-kinetics, efficacy and toxicity of parenteral halofantrine in uncomplicated malaria, *Br J Clin Pharmac* 36:585, 1993.

286. Krogh V, Duffy LC, Wong D et al: Postpartum immuni-zation with rubella virus vaccine and antibody response in breastfeeding infants, *J Lab Clin Med* 113:695, 1989.

287. Kubota K, Lo ES, Huttinot G et al: Plasma concentrations of betamethasone after topical application of betametha-sone 17-valerate: comparison with oral administration, *Br J Clin Pharmac* 37:86, 1994.

288. Lader M: Clinical pharmacology of antipsychotic drugs, *J Int Med Res* 17:1, 1989.

289. Lalak NJ, Morris DL: Azithromycin clinical pharmacoki-netics, *Clin Pharmacokinet* 25:370, 1993.

290. Lambert GH, Muraskas J, Anderson CL et al: Direct hyperbilirubinemia associated with chloral hydrate ad-ministration in the newborn, *Pediatrics* 86:277, 1990.

291. Lamp KC, Bailey EM, Rybak MJ: Ofloxacin clinical pharmacokinetics, *Clin Pharmacokinet* 22:32, 1992.

292. Lancaster FE, Selvanayagam PF, Hsu LL: Lactational ethanol exposure: brain enzymes and 3(H)spiroperidol binding, *Int J Dev Neurosci* 4:151, 1986.

293. Larsen FG, Jakobsen P, Eriksen H et al: The pharmaco-kinetics of acitretin and its 13-*cis*-metabolite in psoriatic patients, *J Clin Pharmacol* 31:477, 1991.

294. Larsen FG, Nielsen-Kudsk F, Jakobsen P et al: Pharma-cokinetics and therapeutic efficacy of retinoids in skin diseases, *Clin Pharmacokinet* 23:42, 1992.

295. Lassman HB, Puri SK, Ho I et al: Pharmacokinetics of roxithromycin (RU 965), *J Clin Pharmacol* 28:141, 1988.

296. Latini R, Maggioni AP, Cavalli A: Therapeutic drug monitoring of antiarrhythmic drugs: rationale and current status, *Clin Pharmacokinet* 18:91, 1990.

297. Lau AH, Lam NP, Piscitelli SC et al: Clinical pharmaco-kinetics of metronidazole and other nitroimidazole anti-infectives, *Clin Pharmacokinet* 23:328, 1992.

298. Lau RJ, Emery MG, Glainsky RE: Unexpected accumu-lation of acyclovir in breast milk with estimation of infant exposure, *Obstet Gynecol* 69:468, 1987.

299. Lauritsen K, Laursen LS, Rask-Madsen J: Clinical phar-macokinetics of drugs used in the treatment of gastroin-testinal diseases. I. *Clin Pharmacokinet* 19:11, 1990.

300. Lauritsen K, Laursen LS, Rask-Madsen J: Clinical phar-macokinetics of drugs used in the treatment of gastroin-testinal diseases. II. *Clin Pharmacokinet* 19:94, 1990.

301. Laursen LC, Borga O, Ljungholm K et al: Transfer of enprofylline into breast milk, *Ther Drug Monit* 10:150, 1988.

302. Leal-Cerro A, Garcia-Luna PP, Pereira JL et al: Ketocona-zole: a new type of agent in the treatment of hypercho-lesterolemia? *Horm Metab Res* 22:398, 1990.

303. Lebedevs TH, Wojnar-Horton RE, Yapp P et al: Excretion of indomethacin in breast milk, *Br J Clin Pharmac* 32:751, 1991.

304. Lebedevs TH, Wojnar-Horton RE, Yapp P et al: Excretion of temazepam in breast milk, *Br J Clin Pharmac* 33:204, 1992.

305. Lecaillon JB, Dubois JP, Darragon T et al: Pharmacoki-netics of cadralazine in a large group of hypertensive patients chronically treated with cadralazine: advantage over a conventional study in a small group of patients, *Ther Drug Monit* 13:103, 1991.

306. Lee CR, McTavish D, Sorkin EM: Tramadol: a prelimi-nary review of its pharmacodynamic and pharmacokinetic properties, and therapeutic potential in acute and chronic pain states, *Drugs* 46:313, 1993.

307. Lees KR, Green ST, Reid JL: Influence of age on the pharmacokinetics and pharmacodynamics of perindopril, *Clin Pharmacol Ther* 44:418, 1988.

308. Leigh DA, Harris C, Tait S et al: Pharmacokinetic study of lomefloxacin and its effect on the faecal flora of volun-teers, *J Antimicrob Chemother* 27:655, 1991.

309. Lemmens HJM, Burm AGL, Bovill JG et al: Pharmaco-dynamics of alfentanil, *Anesthesiology* 76:65, 1992.

310. Lemmens HJM, Burm AGL, Hennis PJ et al: Influence of age on the pharmacokinetics of alfentanil: gender depen-dence, *Clin Pharmacokinet* 19:416, 1990.

311. Lennard L: The clinical pharmacology of 6-mercaptopurine, *Eur J Clin Pharmacol* 43:329, 1992.

312. Leonard MB, Koren G, Stevenson DK et al: Vancomycin pharmacokinetics in very low birth weight neonates, *Pediatr Infect Dis J* 8:282, 1989.

313. Leonard TK, Watson RR, Mohs ME: The effects of caffeine on various body systems: a review, *J Am Diet Assoc* 87:1048, 1987.

314. Lewis LD: Ifosfamide pharmacokinetics, *Invest New Drugs* 9:305, 1991.

315. Li G, Treiber G, Meinshausen J et al: Is cyclosporin A an inhibitor of drug metabolism? *Br J Clin Pharmac* 30:71, 1990.

316. Libardoni M, Piovan D, Busato E et al: Transfer of propafenone and 5-OH-propafenone to foetal plasma and maternal milk, *Br J Clin Pharmac* 32:527, 1991.

317. Liliemark J, Peterson C: Pharmacokinetic optimisation of anticancer therapy, *Clin Pharmacokinet* 21:213, 1991.

318. Lin JH: Pharmacokinetic and pharmacodynamic proper-ties of histamine H2-receptor antagonists: relationship between intrinsic potency and effective plasma concentra-tions, *Clin Pharmacokinet* 20:218, 1991.

319. Lindholm A: Factors influencing the pharmacokinetics of cyclosporine in man, *Ther Drug Monit* 13:465, 1991.

320. Lipsy RJ, Fennerty B, Fagan TC: Clinical review of histamine-2 receptor antagonists, *Arch Intern Med* 150:745, 1990.

321. Lode H: The pharmacokinetics of azithromycin and their chemical significance, *Eur J Clin Microbiol Infect Dis* 10:807, 1991.

322. Lode H, Boeckh M, Hoffken G et al: Comparative pharmacokinetics of glycopeptide antibiotics, and the influence of teicoplanin on granulocyte function, *Scand J Infect Dis* 72(suppl):9, 1990.

323. Lode H, Hoffken G, Boeckh M et al: Quinolone pharmacokinetics and metabolism, *J Antimicrob Chemother* 26(suppl B):41, 1990.

324. Lonning PE, Lien EA, Lundgren S et al: Clinical pharmacokinetics of endocrine agents used in advanced breast cancer, *Clin Pharmacokinet* 22:327, 1992.

325. Lucas BD Jr, Purdy CY, Scarim SK et al: Terfenadine pharmacokinetics in breastmilk in lactating women, *Clin Pharmacol Ther* 57:398, 1995.

326. Luck W, Nau H: Nicotine and cotinine concentrations in the milk of smoking mothers: influence of cigarette consumption and diurnal variation, *Eur J Pediatr* 146:21, 1987.

327. MacDonald N-J, Elliot HL, Hughes DM et al: A comparison in young and elderly subjects of the pharmacokinetics and pharmacodynamics of single and multiple doses of benazepril, *Br J Clin Pharmac* 36:201, 1993.

328. MacDonald N-J, Sioufi A, Howie CA et al: The effects of age on the pharmacokinetics and pharmacodynamics of single oral doses of benazerpril and enalapril, *Br J Clin Pharmac* 36:205, 1993.

329. MacFadyen RJ, Meredith PA, Elliot HL: Enalapril clinical pharmacokinetics and pharmacokinetic-pharmacodynamic relationships, *Clin Pharmacokinet* 25: 274, 1993.

330. MacGregor TR, Sardi ED: In vitro protein binding behavior of dipyridamole, *J Pharm Sci* 80:119, 1991.

331. Maguire AM, Bennett J: Fluorescein elimination in human breast milk, *Arch Ophthalmol* 106:718, 1988.

332. Martell M, de Ben S, Weinberger M et al: Growth and development in preterm infants receiving fluoroquinolones, *J Perinat Med* 24:287, 1996.

333. Massarella JW, Khoo KC, Aogaichi K et al: Effect of renal impairment on the pharmacokinetics of cibenzoline, *Clin Pharmacol Ther* 43:317, 1988.

334. Matheson I, Lunde PKM, Bredesen JE: Midazolam and nitrazepam in the maternity ward: milk concentrations and clinical effects, *Br J Clin Pharmac* 30:787, 1990.

335. Matheson I, Samseth M, Loberg R et al: Milk transfer of phenoxymethylpenicillin during puerperal mastitis, *Br J Clin Pharmac* 25:33, 1988.

336. Matheson I, Samseth M, Sande HA: Ampicillin in breast milk during puerperal infections, *Eur J Clin Pharmacol* 34:657, 1988.

337. Matheson I, Sande HA, Gaillot J: The excretion of zopiclone into breast milk, *Br J Clin Pharmac* 30:267, 1990.

338. Maton PN: Omeprazole, *N Engl J Med* 324:965, 1991.

339. Mattern J, Mayer PR: Excretion of fluorescein into breast milk, *Am J Ophthalmol* 109:598, 1990.

340. Matuo YK, Lopes JNC, Casanova IC et al: Organochlorine pesticide residues in human milk in the Ribeirao Preto Region, State of Sao Paulo, Brazil, *Arch Environ Contam Toxicol* 22:167, 1992.

341. McCann MF, Moggia AV, Higgins JE et al: The effects of a progestin-only oral contraceptive (Levonorgestrel 0.03 mg) on breastfeeding, *Contraception* 40:635, 1989.

342. McCormick KB: Pregnancy and epilepsy: nursing implications, *J Neurosci Nurs* 19:66, 1987.

343. McNeil JJ, Drummer OH, Raymond K et al: The influence of food on the oral bioavailability of terazosin, *Br J Clin Pharmac* 32:775, 1991.

344. McQuinn RL, Pisani A, Wafa S et al: Flecainide excretion in human breast milk, *Clin Pharmacol Ther* 48:262, 1990.

345. McTavish D, Young RA, Clissold SP: Cadralazine: a review of its pharmacodynamic and pharmacokinetic properties, and therapeutic potential in the treatment of hypertension, *Drugs* 40:543, 1990.

346. Meadow WL, Bui KC, Strates E et al: Metoclopramide promotes enteral feeding in preterm infants with feeding intolerance, *Dev Pharmacol Ther* 13:38, 1989.

347. Mehvar R, Gross ME, Kreamer RN: Pharmacokinetics of atenolol enantiomers in humans and rats, *J Pharm Sci* 79:881, 1990.

348. Mennella JA, Beauchamp GK: The transfer of alcohol to human milk, *N Engl J Med* 325:981, 1991.

349. Meredith PA, Elliott HL: Clinical pharmacokinetics of amlodipine, *Clin Pharmacokinet* 22:22, 1992.

350. Meyer LJ, de Miranda P, Sheth N et al: Acyclovir in human breast milk, *Am J Obstet Gynecol* 158:586, 1988.

351. Michelson EI, Dreifus LS: Newer antiarrhythmic drugs, *Med Clin North Am* 72:275, 1988.

352. Mikkelson TJ, Kroboth PD, Cameron WJ et al: Single-dose pharmacokinetics of clomiphene citrate in normal volunteers, *Fertil Steril* 46:392, 1986.

353. Miles MV, Balasubramanian R, Pittman AW et al: Pharmacokinetics of oral and transdermal triprolidine, *J Clin Pharmacol* 30:572, 1990.

354. Milne RJ, Heel RC: Ondansetron: therapeutic use as an antiemetic, *Drugs* 41:574, 1991.

355. Milunsky JM, Milunsky A: Breast-feeding during colchicine therapy for familial Mediterranean fever, *J Pediatr* 119:164, 1991.

356. Mitani GM, Steinberg I, Lien EJ et al: The pharmacokinetics of antiarrhythmic agents in pregnancy and lactation, *Clin Pharmacokinet* 12:253, 1987.

357. Modi NB, Veng-Pedersen P, Graham DJ et al: Application of a system analysis approach to population pharmacokinetics and pharmacodynamics of nicardipine hydrochloride in healthy males, *J Pharm Sci* 82:705, 1993.

358. Mofenson HC, Caraccio TR: Lactation pharmacology 1987, *Pediatr Pharmacol Toxic News* 6:47, 1987.

359. Mollmann H, Barth J, Mollmann C et al: Pharmacokinetics and rectal bioavailability of hydrocortisone acetate, *J Pharm Sci* 80:835, 1991.

360. Monk JP, Benfield P: Inhaled pentamidine: an overview of its pharmacological properties and a review of its therapeutic use in *Pneumocystis carinii* pneumonia, *Drugs* 39:741, 1990.

361. Moore MJ: Clinical pharmacokinetics of cyclophosphamide, *Clin Pharmacokinet* 20:194, 1991.

362. Moretti ME, Ito S, Koren G: Disposition of maternal ketoconazole in breast milk, *Am J Obstet Gynecol* 173:1625, 1995.

363. Morrow JD: The oral cephalosporin: a review, *Am J Med Sci* 303:35, 1992.

364. Morse GD, Shelton MJ, O'Donnell AM: Comparative pharmacokinetics of antiviral nucleoside analogues, *Clin Pharmacokinet* 24:101, 1993.

365. Motwani JG, Lipworth BJ: Clinical pharmacokinetics of drugs administered buccally and sublingually, *Clin Pharmacokinet* 21:83, 1991.

366. Mountford PJ, Coakley AJ: Breast milk radioactivity following injection of ^{99}Tc^{m}-pertechnetate and ^{99}Tc^{m}-glucoheptonate, *Nucl Med Commun* 8:839, 1987.

367. Mountford PJ, Coakley AJ: Secretion of radioactivity in breast milk following administration in hippuran, *Br J Radiol* 62:388, 1989.

368. Mouton JW, Horrevorts AM, Mulder PGH et al: Pharmacokinetics of ceftazidime in serum and suction blister fluid during continuous and intermittent infusions in healthy volunteers, *Antimicrob Agents Chemother* 34:2307, 1990.

369. Movin-Osswald G, Nordstrom A-L, Hammarlund-Udenaes M et al: Pharmacokinetics of raclopride formulations: influence of prolactin and tolerability in healthy male volunteers, *Clin Pharmacokinet* 22:152, 1992.

370. Munafo A, Christen Y, Nussberger J et al: Drug concentration response relationships in normal volunteers after oral administration of losartan, an angiotensin II receptor antagonist, *Clin Pharmacol Ther* 51:513, 1992.

371. Murdoch D, Clissold SP: Calcipotriol: a review of its pharmacological properties and therapeutic use in psoriasis vulgaris, *Drugs* 43:415, 1992.

372. Murdoch D, Heel RC: Amlodipine: a review of its pharmacodynamic and pharmacokinetic properties, and therapeutic use in cardiovascular disease, *Drugs* 41:478, 1991.

373. Murdoch D, McTavish D: Roxatidine acetate: a review of its pharmacodynamic and pharmacokinetic properties, and its therapeutic potential in peptic ulcer disease and related disorders, *Drugs* 42:240, 1991.

374. Murdoch D, McTavish D: Fosinopril: a review of its pharmacodynamics and pharmacokinetic properties and therapeutic potential in essential hypertension, *Drugs* 43:123, 1992.

375. Murdoch D, McTavish D: Sertraline: a review of its pharmacodynamic and pharmacokinetic properties, and therapeutic potential in depression and obsessive-compulsive disorder, *Drugs* 44:604, 1992.

376. Murphy PH, Beasley CW, Moore WH et al: Thallium-201 in human milk: observations and radiological consequences, *Health Phys* 56:539, 1989.

377. Muzaffar A, Brossi A: Chemistry of colchicine, *Pharmacol Ther* 49:105, 1991.

378. Nathwani D, Wood MJ: Penicillins: a current review of their clinical pharmacology and therapeutic use, *Drugs* 45:866, 1993.

379. Nau H: Clinical pharmacokinetics in pregnancy and perinatology. II. Penicillins, *Dev Pharmacol Ther* 10:174, 1987.

380. Naumberg EG, Meny RG: Breast milk opioids and neonatal apnea, *Am J Dis Child* 142:11, 1988.

381. Nehlig A, Debry G: Consequences on the newborn of chronic maternal consumption of coffee during gestation and lactation: a review, *J Am Coll Nutr* 13:6, 1994.

382. Nestico PF, Morganroth J, Horowitz LN: New antiarrhythmic drugs, *Drugs* 35:286, 1988.

383. Neuvonen PJ, Kivisto KT: The clinical significance of food-drug interactions: a review, *Med J Aust* 150:36, 1989.

384. Neuvonen PJ, Kivisto KT, Lehto P: Interference of dairy products with the absorption of ciprofloxacin, *Clin Pharmacol Ther* 50:498, 1991.

385. Nielsen ST, Matheson I, Rasmussen JN et al: Excretion of iohexol and metrizoate in human breast milk, *Acta Radiol* 28:523, 1987.

386. Nilsen OG, Aamo T, Zahlsen K et al: Macrolide pharmacokinetics and dose scheduling of roxithromycin, *Diagn Microbiol Infect Dis* 15:71S, 1992.

387. Nilsen OG, Dale O: Single dose pharmacokinetics of trazodone in healthy subjects, *Pharmacol Toxicol* 71:150, 1992.

388. Nissen E, Widstrom A-M, Lilja G et al: Effects of routinely given pethidine during labour on infants' developing breastfeeding behaviour: effects of dose-delivery time interval and various concentrations of pethidine/norpethidine in cord plasm, *Acta Paediatr* 86:201, 1997.

389. Notarianni LJ: Plasma protein binding of drugs in pregnancy and in neonates, *Clin Pharmacokinet* 18:20, 1990.

390. Notarianni LJ, Oldham HG, Bennett PN: Passage of paracetamol into breast milk and its subsequent metabolism by the neonate, *Br J Clin Pharmac* 24:63, 1987.

391. Obermeyer BD, Bergstrom RF, Callaghan JT et al: Secretion of nizatidine into human breast milk after single and multiple doses, *Clin Pharmacol Ther* 47:724, 1990.

392. O'Dea RF, Mirkin BL, Alward CT et al: Treatment of neonatal hypertension with captopril, *J Pediatr* 113:403, 1988.

393. Ogbuokiri JE, Ozumba BC, Okonkwo PO: Ivermectin level in human breastmilk, *Eur J Clin Pharmacol* 45:389, 1993.

394. Oguma T, Yamada H, Sawaki M et al: Pharmacokinetic analysis of the effects of different foods on absorption of cefaclor, *Antimicrob Agents Chemother* 35:1729, 1991.

395. Ogunbona FA, Onyeji CO, Bolaji OO et al: Excretion of chloroquine and desethylchloroquine in human milk, *Br J Clin Pharmac* 23:473, 1987.

396. O'Hare MF, Murnaghan GA, Russell CJ et al: Sotalol as a hypotensive agent in pregnancy, *Br J Obstet Gynaecol* 87:814, 1980.

397. Ohdo S, Nakano S, Ogawa N: Circadian changes of valproate kinetics depending on meal condition in humans, *J Clin Pharmacol* 32:822, 1992.

398. Ohkubo T, Shimoyama R, Sugawara K: Measurement of haloperidol in human breast milk by high-performance liquid chromatography, *J Pharm Sci* 81:947, 1992.

399. Okano M, Nomura M, Hata S et al: Anaphylactic symptoms due to chlorhexidine gluconate, *Arch Dermatol* 125:50, 1989.

400. Okonkwo PO, Ogbuokiri JE, Ofoegbu E et al: Protein binding and ivermectin estimations in patients with onchocerciasis, *Clin Pharmacol Ther* 53:426, 1993.

401. Olesen OV, Bartels U, Poulsen JH: Perphenazine in breast milk and serum, *Am J Psychiatry* 147:1378, 1990.

402. Oliver RM, Upward JW, Dewhurst AG et al: The pharmacokinetics of doxazosin in patients with hypertension and renal impairment, *Br J Clin Pharmac* 29:417, 1990.

403. Olsson B, Bolme P, Dahlstrom B et al: Excretion of noscapine in human breast milk, *Eur J Clin Pharmacol* 30:213, 1986.

404. Onks DL, Harris JG, Robertson AF: Cefmenoxine and bilirubin: competition for albumin binding, *Pharmacol Toxicol* 68:329, 1991.

405. Ostensen M, Matheson I, Laufen H: Piroxicam in breast milk after long-term treatment, *Eur J Clin Pharmacol* 35:567, 1988.

406. Ostensen M, Skavdal K, Myklebust G et al: Excretion of gold into human breast milk, *Eur J Clin Pharmacol* 31:251, 1986.

407. Paap CM, Nahata MC: Clinical pharmacokinetics of antibacterial drugs in neonates, *Clin Pharmacokinet* 19: 280, 1990.

408. Page MA, Boutagy JS, Shenfield GM: A screening test for slow metabolisers of tolbutamide, *Br J Clin Pharmac* 31:649, 1991.

409. Palmer KJ, Holliday SM, Brogden RN: Mefloquine: a review of its antimalarial activity, pharmacokinetic properties and therapeutic efficacy, *Drugs* 45:430, 1993.

410. Pan H, Fleiss P, Moore L et al: Excretion of pravastatin, an HMG CoA reductase inhibitor, in breast milk of lactating women, *J Clin Pharmacol* 28:942, 1988.

411. Pan HY, DeVault AR, Swites BJ et al: Pharmacokinetics and pharmacodynamics of pravastatin alone and with cholestyramine in hypercholesterolemia, *Clin Pharmacol Ther* 48:201, 1990.

412. Pan HY, DeVault AR, Wang-Iverson D et al: Comparative pharmacokinetics and pharmacodynamics of pravastatin and lovastatin, *J Clin Pharmacol* 30:1128, 1990.

413. Pankey GA: Temafloxacin: an overview, *Am J Med* 91(suppl 6A):166S, 1991.

414. Passmore CM, McElnay JC, Rainey EA et al: Metronidazole excretion in human milk and its effect on the suckling neonate, *Br J Clin Pharmac* 26:45, 1988.

415. Pato MT, Murphy DL, DeVane CL: Sustained plasma concentrations of fluoxetine and/or norfluoxetine four and eight weeks after fluoxetine discontinuation, *J Clin Psychopharmacol* 11:224, 1991.

416. Paul M, Himmelstein J: Reproductive hazards in the workplace: what the practitioner needs to know about chemical exposures, *Obstet Gynecol* 71:921, 1988.

417. Pavord I, Knox A: Pharmacokinetic optimisation of inhaled steroid therapy in asthma, *Clin Pharmacokinet* 25:126, 1993.

418. Penny WJ, Lewis MJ: Nifedipine is excreted in human milk, *Eur J Clin Pharmacol* 36:427, 1989.

419. Pepperell RJ: Suppression of lactation, *Med J Aust* 144:37, 1986.

420. Pershing LK, Corlett J, Jorgensen C: In vivo pharmacokinetics and pharmacodynamics of topical ketoconazole and miconazole in human stratum corneum, *Antimicrob Agents Chemother* 38:90, 1994.

421. Persson B, Heykants J, Hedner T: Clinical pharmacokinetics of ketanserin, *Clin Pharmacokinet* 20:263, 1991.

422. Persson K, Hammarlund-Udenaes M, Mortimer O et al: The postoperative pharmacokinetics of codeine, *Eur J Clin Pharmacol* 42:663, 1992.

423. Peters DH, Friedel HA, McTavish D: Azithromycin: a review of its antimicrobial activity, pharmacokinetic properties and clinical efficacy, *Drugs* 44:750, 1992.

424. *Physicians' Desk Reference,* Montvale, NJ, 1998, Medical Economics.

425. Pittard WB, O'Neal W Jr: Amitriptyline excretion in human milk, *J Clin Psychopharmacol* 6:383, 1986.

426. Plomp TA, Vulsma T, de Vijlder JJM: Use of amiodarone during pregnancy, *Eur J Obstet Gynecol Reprod Biol* 43:201, 1992.

427. Poitrast BJ, Keller WC, Elves RG: Estimation of chemical hazards in breast milk, *Aviat Space Environ Med* 59:A87, 1988.

428. Pons G, Francoual C, Guillet P et al: Zolpidem excretion in breast milk, *Eur J Clin Pharmacol* 37:245, 1989.

429. Pons G, Rey E, d'Athis P et al: Gentamicin monitoring in neonates, *Ther Drug Monit* 10:421, 1988.

430. Pons G, Schoerlin MP, Tam YK et al: Moclobemide excretion in human breast milk, *Br J Clin Pharmac* 29:27, 1990.

431. Port RE, Edler L, Herrmann R et al: Pharmacokinetics of 5-fluorouracil after short systemic infusion: plasma level at the end of the distribution phase as an indicator of the total area under the plasma concentration-time curve, *Ther Drug Monit* 13:96, 1991.

432. Poyhia R, Seppala T, Olkkola KT et al: The pharmacokinetics and metabolism of oxycodone after intramuscular and oral administration to healthy subjects, *Br J Clin Pharmac* 33:617, 1992.

433. Prichard BNC, Tomlinson B, Renondin JC: Urapidil, a multiple-action alpha-blocking drug, *Am J Cardiol* 64: 11D, 1989.

434. Pue MA, Pratt SK, Fairless AJ et al: Linear pharmacokinetics of penciclovir following administration of single oral doses of famciclovir 125, 250, 500, and 750 mg to healthy volunteers, *J Antimicrob Chemother* 33:119, 1994.

435. Querol-Ferrer V, Zini R, Tillement J-P: The blood binding of cefotiam and cyclohexanol, metabolites of the prodrug cefotiam hexetil, in vitro, *J Pharm Pharmacol* 43:863, 1991.

436. Qureshi AM, Robertson HE: Polychlorinated biphenyls (PCB) in breast milk from Regina nursing mothers, *Can J Public Health* 78:389, 1987.

437. Radisch B, Luck W, Nau H: Cadmium concentrations in milk and blood of smoking mothers, *Toxicol Let* 36:147, 1987.

438. Radwanski E, Nagabhushan N, Affrime MB et al: Secretion of dilevalol in breast milk, *J Clin Pharmacol* 28:448, 1988.

439. Ramsay RE: Advances in the pharmacotherapy of epilepsy, *Epilepsia* 34(suppl 5):S9-S16, 1993.

440. Resplandy G, Genissel P: Pharmacokinetics of perindipril in high-risk populations, *J Cardiovasc Pharmacol* 18(suppl 7):S9, 1991.

441. Rey AM, Grauer K, Gums JG: Newer antihypertensive agents, *Postgrad Med* 89:75, 1991.

442. Riant P, Urien S, Albengres E et al: High plasma protein binding as a parameter in the selection of beta blockers for lactating women, *Biochem Pharmacol* 35:4579, 1986.

443. Ribeiro C, Longo A: Procainamide and disopyramide, *Eur Heart J* 8(suppl A):11, 1987.

444. Rinder CS, D'Amato SL, Rinder HM et al: Survival in complicated diphenhydramine overdose, *Crit Care Med* 16:1161, 1988.

445. Ripa S, Ferrante L, Prenna M: Pharmacokinetics of fluconazole in normal volunteers, *Chemotherapy* 39:6, 1993.

446. Rivera-Calimlim L: The significance of drugs in breast milk, *Clin Perinatol* 14:51, 1987.

447. Rizzon P, Di Biase M, Favale S et al: Class 1B agents lidocaine, mexiletine, tocainide, phenytoin, *Eur Heart J* 8(suppl A):21, 1987.

448. Robert J: Clinical pharmacokinetics of idarubicin, *Clin Pharmacokinet* 24:275, 1993.

449. Roberts D, Honcharik N, Sitar DS et al: Diltiazem overdose: pharmacokinetics of diltiazem and its metabolites and effect of multiple dose charcoal therapy, *Clin Toxicol* 29:45, 1991.

450. Robieux I, Koren G, Vandenbergh H et al: Morphine excretion in breast milk and resultant exposure of a nursing infant, *Clin Toxicol* 28:365, 1990.

451. Robin DW, Lee MH, Hasan SS, Wood AJJ: Triazolam in cirrhosis: pharmacokinetics and pharmacodynamics, *Clin Pharmacol Ther* 54:630, 1993.

452. Roden DM, Wood AJJ, Wilkinson GR et al: Disposition kinetics of encainide and metabolites, *Am J Cardiol* 58:4C, 1986.

453. Roden DM, Woosley RL: Clinical pharmacokinetics of encainide, *Clin Pharmacokinet* 14:141, 1988.

454. Rogan WJ, Gladen BC, McKinney JD et al: Polychlorinated biphenyls (PCBs) and dichlorodiphenyl dichloroethene (DDE) in human milk: effects on growth, morbidity, and duration of lactation, *Am J Public Health* 77:1294, 1987.

455. Rollman O, Pihl-Lundin I: Acitretin excretion into human breast milk, *Acta Derm Venereol (Stockh)* 70:487, 1990.

456. Rooney TW, Lorber A, Veng-Pedersen P et al: Gold pharmacokinetics in breast milk and serum of a lactating woman, *J Rheumatol* 14:1120, 1987.

457. Rose MR, Prescott MC, Herman KJ: Excretion of iodine-123-hippuran, technetium-99m-red blood cells, and technetium-99m-macroaggregated albumin into breast milk, *J Nucl Med* 31:978, 1990.

458. Rosenbaum DH, Rowan AJ, Tuchman L et al: Comparative bioavailability of a generic phenytoin and dilantin, *Epilepsia* 35:656, 1994.

459. Rowbotham DJ: Omeprazole: a useful new agent? *Br J Anaesth* 65:607, 1990.

460. Rubow S, Klopper J: Excretion of radioiodine in human milk following a therapeutic dose of I-131, *Eur J Nucl Med* 14:632, 1988.

461. Rubow S, Klopper J, Scholtz P: Excretion of gallium 67 in human breast milk and its inadvertent ingestion by a 9-month-old child, *Eur J Nucl Med* 18:829, 1991.

462. Rubow S, Klopper J, Wasserman H et al: The excretion of radiopharmaceuticals in human breast milk: additional data and dosimetry, *Eur J Nucl Med* 21:144, 1994.

463. Ruhnke M, Bauer FE, Seifert M et al: Effects of standard breakfast on pharmacokinetics of oral zidovudine in patients with AIDS, *Antimicrob Agents Chemother* 37: 2153, 1993.

464. Rylance GW, Woods CG, Donnelly MC et al: Carbimazole and breastfeeding, *Lancet* 1:928, 1987.

465. Saano V, Paronen P, Peura P: Bioavailability of doxycycline from dissolved doxycycline hydrochloride tablets: comparison to solid form hydrochloride tablets and dissolved monohydrate tablets, *Int J Clin Pharmacol Ther Toxicol* 28:471, 1990.

466. Saathoff N, Lode H, Neider K et al: Pharmacokinetics of cefpodoxime proxetil and interactions with an antacid and an H2 receptor antagonist, *Antimicrob Agents Chemother* 36:796, 1992.

467. Sahlberg BL: The characterization of sulphated metabolites of norethindrone in human milk after oral administration of contraceptive steroids, *J Steroid Biochem* 26:481, 1987.

468. Samoil D, Grubb BP, Temesy-Armos PN: Sotalol: a new agent for the treatment of ventricular arrhythmias, *Am J Med Sci* 307:49, 1994.

469. Samples JR, Meyer SM: Use of ophthalmic medications in pregnant and nursing women, *Am J Ophthalmol* 106:616, 1988.

470. Sandborn WJ, Strong RM, Forland SC et al: The pharmacokinetics and colonic tissue concentrations of cyclosporine after IV, oral, and enema administration, *J Clin Pharmacol* 31:76, 1991.

471. Sanders SW, Buchi KN, Goddard MS et al: Single-dose pharmacokinetics and tolerance of a cholesteryl sulfate complex of amphotericin B administered to healthy volunteers, *Antimicrob Agents Chemother* 35:1029, 1991.

472. Sasaki M, Tateishi T, Ebihara A: The effects of age and gender on the stereoselective pharmacokinetics of verapamil, *Clin Pharmacol Ther* 54:278, 1993.

473. Scheinin M, Koulu M, Karhuvaara S et al: Evidence that the reversible MAO-A inhibitor moclobemide increases prolactin secretion by a serotonergic mechanism in healthy male volunteers, *Life Sci* 47:1491, 1990.

474. Schimmel MS, Eidelman AI, Wilschanski MA et al: Toxic effects of atenolol consumed during breastfeeding, *J Pediatr* 114:476, 1989.

475. Schlepper M: Propafenaone: a review of its profile, *Eur Heart J* 8(suppl A):27, 1987.

476. Schwartz PH, Eldadah MK, Newth CJL: The pharmacokinetics of dobutamine in pediatric intensive care unit patients, *Drug Metab Dispos* 19:614, 1991.

477. Schwartz-Bickenbach D, Schulte-Hobein B, Abt S et al: Smoking and passive smoking during pregnancy and early infancy: effects on birth weight, lactation period, and cotinine concentration in mother's milk and infant's urine, *Toxicol Lett* 35:73, 1987.

478. Shaheen O, Zmeili S, Al-Qussuois Y et al: Pharmacokinetics and pharmacodynamics of two commercial oral nifedipine products, *Int J Clin Pharmacol Ther Toxicol* 29:337, 1991.

479. Shammas FV, Dickstein K: Clinical pharmacokinetics in heart failure: an updated review, *Clin Pharmacokinet* 15:94, 1988.

480. Shanks CA, Avram MJ, Fragen RJ et al: Pharmacokinetics and pharmacodynamics of vecuronium administered by bolus and infusion during halothane or balanced anesthesia, *Clin Pharmacol Ther* 42:459, 1987.

481. Shannon M, Lacouture PG, Roa H et al: Cocaine exposure among children seen at a pediatric hospital, *Pediatrics* 83:337, 1989.

482. Shapiro TA, Were JBO, Danso K et al: Pharmacokinetics and metabolism of allopurinol riboside, *Clin Pharmacol Ther* 49:506, 1991.

483. Shenfield GM, Griffin JM: Clinical pharmacokinetics of contraceptive steroids: an update, *Clin Pharmacokinet* 20:15, 1991.

484. Shepherd AMM: Human pharmacology of urapidil, *Drugs* 35:34, 1988.

485. Shikary ZK, Betrabet SS, Patel ZM et al: Transfer of levonorgestrel administered through different drug delivery systems from the maternal circulation into the newborn infant's circulation via breastmilk, *Contraception* 35:477, 1987.

486. Shionoiri H, Ueda S-I, Minamisawa K et al: Pharmacokinetics and pharmacodynamics of benazepril in hypertensive patients with normal and impaired renal function, *J Cardiovascular Pharmacol,* 20:348, 1992.

487. Shukla UA, Pittman KA, Barbhaiya RH: Pharmacokinetic interactions of cefprozil with food, propantheline, metoclopramide, and probenecid in healthy volunteers, *J Clin Pharmacol* 32:725, 1992.

488. Shyu WC, Knupp CA, Pittman KA et al: Food-induced reduction in bioavailability of didanosine, *Clin Pharmacol Ther* 50:503, 1991.

489. Shyu WC, Pittman KA, Robinson DS et al: The absolute bioavailability of transnasal butorphanol in patients experiencing rhinitis, *Eur J Clin Pharmacol* 45:559, 1993.

490. Shyu WC, Pittman KA, Wilber RB et al: Pharmacokinetics of cefprozil in healthy subjects and patients with renal impairment, *J Clin Pharmacol* 31:362, 1991.

491. Shyu WC, Shah VR, Campbell DA et al: Excretion of cefprozil into human breast milk, *Antimicrob Agents Chemother* 36:938, 1992.

492. Shyu WC, Shah VR, Campbell DA et al: Oral absolute bioavailability and intravenous dose-proportionality of cefprozil in humans, *J Clin Pharmacol* 32:798, 1992.

493. Shyu WC, Wilber RB, Pittman KA et al: Pharmacokinetics of cefprozil in healthy subjects and patients with hepatic impairment, *J Clin Pharmacol* 31:372, 1991.

494. Siddoway LA, Schwartz SL, Barbey JT et al: Clinical pharmacokinetics of moricizine, *Am J Cardiol* 65:21D, 1990.

495. Sides GD, Cerimele BJ, Black HR et al: Pharmacokinetics of dirithromycin, *J Antimicrob Chemother* 31(suppl C): 65, 1993.

496. Sietsema WK: The absolute oral bioavailability of selected drugs, *Int J Clin Pharmacol Ther Toxicol* 27:179, 1989.

497. Signs SA, Tan JS, Salstrom S-J et al: Pharmacokinetics of imipenem in serum and skin window fluid in healthy adults after intramuscular or intravenous administration, *Antimicrob Agents Chemother* 36:1400, 1992.

498. Sikorski R, Paszkowski T, Radomanski T et al: Cadmium contamination of early human milk, *Gynecol Obstet Invest* 27:91, 1989.

499. Silvasti M, Karttunen P, Happonen P et al: Pharmacokinetic comparison of a dextromethorphan-salbutamol combination tablet and a plain dextromethorphan tablet, *Int J Clin Pharmacol Ther Toxicol* 28:268, 1990.

500. Singhvi SM, Duchin KL, Morrison RA et al: Disposition of fosinopril sodium in healthy subjects, *Br J Clin Pharmac* 25:9, 1988.

501. Singhvi SM, Pan HY, Morrison RA et al: Disposition of pravastatin sodium, a tissue-selective HMG-CoA reductase inhibitor, in healthy subjects, *Br J Clin Pharmac* 29:239, 1990.

502. Singlas E, Leroy A, Sultan E et al: Disposition of fleroxacin, a new trifluoroquinolone, and its metabolites: pharmacokinetics in renal failure and influence of haemodialysis, *Clin Pharmacokinet* 19:67, 1990.

503. Skopnik H, Bergt U, Heimann G: Neonatal theophylline intoxication: pharmacokinetics and clinical evaluation, *Eur J Pediatr* 151:221, 1992.

504. Skoyles JR, Sherry KM: Pharmacology, mechanisms of action and uses of selective phosphodiesterase inhibitors, *Br J Anaesth* 68:293, 1992.

505. Smilack JD, Wilson WR, Cockerill FR: Tetracyclines, chloramphenicol, erythromycin, clindamycin, and metronidazole, *Mayo Clin Proc* 66:1270, 1991.

506. Smith IJ, Hinson JL, Johnson VA et al: Flurbiprofen in post-partum women: plasma and breast milk disposition, *J Clin Pharmacol* 29:174, 1989.

507. Smith NA, Kates RE, Lebsack C et al: Clinical pharmacology of intravenous enoximone: pharmacodynamics and pharmacokinetics in patients with heart failure, *Am Heart J* 122:755, 1991.

508. Smithers JA, Kulmala HK, Thompson GA et al: Pharmacokinetics of teicoplanin upon multiple-dose intravenous administration of 3, 12, and 30 milligrams per kilogram of body weight to healthy male volunteers, *Antimicrob Agents Chemother* 36:115, 1992.

509. Soderman P, Matheson I: Clonazepam in breast milk, *Eur J Pediatr* 147:212, 1988.

510. Somani P: Basic and clinical pharmacology of amiodarone: relationship of antiarrhythmic effects, dose and drug concentrations to intracellular inclusion bodies, *J Clin Pharmacol* 29:405, 1989.

511. Somani P, Fraker TD, Temesy-Armos PN: Pharmacokinetic implications of lorcainide therapy in patients with normal and depressed cardiac function, *J Clin Pharmacol* 27:122, 1987.

512. Somberg JC, Achari R, Laddu AR: Terazosin: pharmacokinetics and the effect of age and dose on the incidence of adverse events, *Am Heart J* 122:901, 1991.

513. Soons PA, Grib C, Breimer DD, Kirch W: Effects of acute febrile infectious diseases on the oral pharmacokinetics and effects of nitrendipine enantiomers and of bisoprolol, *Clin Pharmacokinet* 23:238, 1992.

514. Soons PA, Mulders TMT, Uchida E et al: Stereoselective pharmacokinetics of oral felodipine and nitrendipine in healthy subjects: correlation with nifedipine pharmacokinetics, *Eur J Clin Pharmacol* 44:163, 1993.

515. Soons PA, Van den Berg G, Danhof M et al: Influence of single- and multiple-dose omeprazole treatment on nifedipine pharmacokinetics and effects in healthy subjects, *Eur J Clin Pharmacol* 42:319, 1992.

516. Sorgel F, Kinzig M: Pharmacokinetics of gyrase inhibitors. I. Basic chemistry and gastrointestinal disposition, *Am J Med* 94(suppl 3A):44S-55S, 1993.

517. Sorgel F, Naber KG, Kinzig M et al: Comparative pharmacokinetics of ciprofloxacin and temafloxacin in humans: a review, *Am J Med* 91(suppl 6A): 51S, 1991.

518. Spahn H, Knauf H, Mutschler E: Pharmacokinetics of torasemide and its metabolites in healthy controls and in chronic renal failure, *Eur J Clin Pharmacol* 39:345, 1990.

519. Speight TM, Holford NHG, editors: *Avery's drug treatment,* ed 4, Auckland, 1997, Adis International.

520. Spencer CM, Faulds D, Peters DH: Cetirizine: a reappraisal of its pharmacological properties and therapeutic use in selected allergic disorders, *Drugs* 46:1055, 1993.

521. Speth PAJ, Van Hoesel QGCM, Haanen C: Clinical pharmacokinetics of doxorubicin, *Clin Pharmacokinet* 15:15, 1988.

522. Spigset O: Anaesthetic agents and excretion in breast milk, *Acta Anaesthesiol Scand* 38:94, 1991.

523. Spiller HA, Morse S, Muir C: Fluoxetine ingestion: a one year retrospective study, *Vet Hum Toxicol* 32:153, 1990.

524. Stagni G, Davis PJ, Ludden TM: Human pharmacokinetics of betaxolol enantiomers, *J Pharm Sci* 80:321, 1991.

525. Stancer HC, Reed KL: Desipramine and 2-hydroxydesipramine in human breast milk and the nursing infant's serum, *Am J Psychiatry* 143:1597, 1986.

526. Steer PL, Biddle CJ, Marley WS et al: Concentration of fentanyl in colostrum after an analgesic dose, *Can J Anaesth* 39:231, 1992.

527. Steldinger R, Luck W: Half lives of nicotine in breast milk of smoking mothers: implications for nursing, *J Perinat Med* 16:261, 1988.

528. Stewart DJ, Grewaal D, Green RM et al: Bioavailability and pharmacology of oral idarubicin, *Cancer Chemother Pharmacol* 27:308, 1991.

529. Storck J, Kirsten R: Binding of urapidil to human serum albumin: dependency on free fatty acid concentration, *Int J Clin Pharmacol Ther Toxicol* 29:204, 1991.

530. Streisand JB, Varvel JR, Stanski DR et al: Absorption and bioavailability of oral transmucosal fentanyl citrate, *Anesthesiology* 75:223, 1991.

531. Stuck AE, Kim DK, Frey FJ: Fleroxacin clinical pharmacokinetics, *Clin Pharmacokinet* 22:116, 1992.

532. Sylvester RK, Lobell M, Teresi ME et al: Excretion of hydroxyurea into milk, *Cancer* 60:2177, 1987.

533. Szutu M, Morgan DJ, McLeish M et al: Pharmacokinetics of intravenous clomiphene isomers, *Br J Clin Pharmac* 27:639, 1989.

534. Taddio A, Klein J, Koren G: Acyclovir excretion in human breast milk, *Ann Pharmacother* 28:585, 1994.

535. Takagi K, Yamaki K, Nadai M et al: Effect of a new quinolone, sparfloxacin, on the pharmacokinetics of theophylline in asthmatic patients, *Antimicrobial Agents Chemother* 35:1137, 1991.

536. Tam YK: Individual variation in first-pass metabolism, *Clin Pharmacokinet* 25:300, 1993.

537. Tartara A, Galimberti CA, Manni R et al: Differential effects of valproic acid and enzyme-inducing anticonvulsants on nimodipine pharmacokinetics in epileptic patients, *Br J Clin Pharmac* 32:335, 1991.

538. Terhaag B, Gramatte T, Hrdlcka P et al: The influence of food on the absorption of diclofenac as a pure substance, *Int J Clin Pharmacol Ther Toxicol* 29:418, 1991.

539. Tessin I, Thiringer K, Trollfors B et al: Comparison of serum concentrations of ceftazidime and tobramycin in newborn infants, *Eur J Pediatr* 147:405, 1988.

540. Tett SE: Clinical pharmacokinetics of slow-acting antirheumatic drugs, *Clin Pharmacokinet* 25:392, 1993.

541. Thiercelin JF, Necciari J, Caplain H et al: Development and pharmacokinetics of a new sustained-release formulation of diltiazem, *J Cardiovasc Pharmacol* 16(suppl): S31, 1990.

542. Thoman ME: Drug toxicology and breast-feeding, *Pediatric Basics* 57:2, 1991.

543. Titmarsh S, Monk JP: Terazosin, *Drugs* 33:461, 1987.

544. Tjandra-Maga TB, Verbesselt R, Van Hecken A et al: Flecainide: single and multiple oral dose kinetics, absolute bioavailability and effect of food and antacid in man, *Br J Clin Pharmac* 22:309, 1986.

545. Todd PA, Clissold SP: Naproxen: a reappraisal of its pharmacology, and therapeutic use in rheumatic diseases and pain states, *Drugs* 40:91, 1990.

546. Todd PA, Faulds D: Ofloxacin: a reappraisal of its antimicrobial activity, pharmacology and therapeutic use, *Drugs* 42:825, 1991.

547. Todd PA, Fitton A: Perindopril: a review of its pharmacological properties and therapeutic use in cardiovascular disorders, *Drugs* 42:90, 1991.

548. Todd PA, Fitton A: Gallium nitrate: a review of its pharmacological properties and therapeutic potential in cancer-related hypercalcaemia, *Drugs* 42:261, 1991.

549. Todd PA, Sorkin EM: Diclofenac sodium: a reappraisal of its pharmacodynamic and pharmacokinetic properties, and therapeutic efficacy, *Drugs* 35:244, 1988.

550. Todd PA, Goa KL, Langtry HD: Transdermal nitroglycerin (glyceryl trinitrate): a review of its pharmacology and therapeutic use, *Drugs* 40:880, 1990.

551. Tonks AM: Nimodipine levels in breast milk, *Aust N Z J Surg* 65:693, 1995.

552. Trautner K, Einwag J: Influence of milk and food on fluoride bioavailability from NaF and Na_2FPO_3 in man, *J Dent Res* 68:72, 1989.

553. Travis CC, Hattemer-Frey HA, Arms AD: Relationship between dietary intake of organic chemicals and their concentrations in human adipose tissue and breast milk, *Arch Environ Contam Toxicol* 17:473, 1988.

554. Trenk D, Wagner F, Sachs W et al: Pharmacokinetic characterization of the antiarrhythmic drug diprafenone in man, *Eur J Clin Pharmacol* 37:313, 1989.

555. Troy SM, Cevallos WH, Conrad KA et al: The absolute bioavailability and dose proportionality of intravenous and oral dosage regimens of recainam, *J Clin Pharmacol* 31:433, 1991.

556. Turgeon J, Fiset C, Giguere R et al: Influence of debrisoquine phenotype and of quinidine on mexiletine disposition in man, *J Pharmacol Exp Ther* 259:789, 1991.

557. Unger J, Lambert M, Jonckheer MH et al: Amiodarone and the thyroid: pharmacological, toxic and therapeutic effects, *J Intern Med* 233:435, 1993.

558. Unsworth J, d'Assis-Fonseca A, Beswick DT et al: Serum salicylate levels in a breastfed infant, *Ann Rheum Dis* 46:638, 1987.

559. Vance-Bryan K, Guay DRP, Rotschafer JC: Clinical pharmacokinetics of ciprofloxacin, *Clin Pharmacokinet* 19:434, 1990.

560. Van der Auwera P, Stolear JC, George B et al: Pharmacokinetics of enoxacin and its oxometabolite following intravenous administration to patients with different degrees of renal impairment, *Antimicrob Agents Chemother* 34:1491, 1990.

561. Vanhaesebrouck P, Thiery M, Leroy JG et al: Oligohydramnios, renal insufficiency, and ileal perforation in preterm infants after intrauterine exposure to indomethacin, *J Pediatr* 113:738, 1988.

562. van Harten J: Clinical pharmacokinetics of selective serotonin reuptake inhibitors, *Clin Pharmacokinet* 24:203, 1993.

563. Van Hecken AM, Depre M, De Schepper PJ et al: Lack of effect of flunarizine on the pharmacokinetics and pharmacodynamics of sumatriptan in healthy volunteers, *Br J Clin Pharmac* 34:82, 1992.

564. Vanholder R, Van Landschoot N, De Smet R et al: Drug protein binding in chronic renal failure: evaluation of nine drugs, *Kidney Int* 33:996, 1988.

565. van Hoogdalem EJ, de Boer AG, Breimer DD: Pharmacokinetics of rectal drug administration. II. Clinical applications of peripherally acting drugs and conclusions, *Clin Pharmacokinet* 21:110, 1991.

566. Van Putten T, Marder SR, Mintz J: Serum prolactin as a correlate response to haloperidol, *J Clin Psychopharmacol* 11:357, 1991.

567. Verbeeck RV, Ross SG, McKenna EA: Excretion of trazodone in breast milk, *Br J Clin Pharmac* 22:367, 1986.

568. Vernon MW, Heel RC, Brogden RN: Enoximone: a review of its pharmacological properties and therapeutic potential, *Drugs* 42:997, 1991.

569. Vree TB, Van den Biggelaar-Martea M, Verwey-Van Wissen CPWGM et al: The pharmacokinetics of naproxen, its metabolite O-desmethylnaproxen, and their acyl glucuronides in humans: effect of cimetidine, *Br J Clin Pharmac* 35:467, 1993.

570. Wadworth AN, Brogden RN: Quinapril: a review of its pharmacological properties, and therapeutic efficacy in cardiovascular disorders, *Drugs* 41:378, 1991.

571. Wadworth AN, Fitton A: Olsalazine: a review of its pharmacodynamic and pharmacokinetic properties, and therapeutic potential in inflammatory bowel disease, *Drugs* 41:647, 1991.

572. Wadworth AN, Goa KL: Lomefloxacin: a review of its antibacterial activity, pharmacokinetic properties and therapeutic use, *Drugs* 42:1018, 1991.

573. Wagstaff AJ, Faulds D, Goa KL: Aciclovir: a reappraisal of its antiviral activity, pharmacokinetic properties and therapeutic efficacy, *Drugs* 47:153, 1994.

574. Wakamatsu A, Umetsu M, Motoya H et al: Change of plasma half-life of caffeine during caffeine therapy for apnea in premature infants, *Acta Paediatr Jpn* 29:595, 1987.

575. Walker JA, Sherman RA, Cody RP: The effect of oral bases on enteral aluminum absorption, *Arch Intern Med* 150:2037, 1990.

576. Walker RC, Wright AJ: The quinolones, *Mayo Clin Proc* 62:1007, 1987.

577. Walker RC, Wright AJ: The fluoroquinolones, *Mayo Clin Proc* 66:1249, 1991.

578. Walsh AES, Hockney RA, Campling G et al: Neuroendocrine and temperature effects of nefazodone in healthy volunteers, *Biol Psychiatry* 33:115, 1993.

579. Walstad RA, Hellum KB, Thurmann-Nielsen E et al: Pharmacokinetics and tissue penetration of timentin: a simultaneous study of serum, urine, lymph, suction blister, and subcutaneous thread fluid, *J Antimicrob Chemother* 17(suppl C):71, 1986.

580. Wang X, Sato N, Greer MA et al: Quinidine inhibits prolactin secretion induced by thyrotropin-releasing hormone, high medium potassium or hyposmolarity in GH_4C_1 cells, *J Pharmacol Exp Ther* 256:135, 1991.

581. Wehmeyer AE, Thomas RL: Encainide: a new antiarrhythmic agent, *Drug Intell Clin Pharm* 20:9, 1986.

582. Weintrub PS, Chapman A, Piecuch R: Renal fungus ball in a premature infant successfully treated with fluconazole, *Pediatr Infect Dis J* (1994) 13:1152, 1994.

583. Westphal JF, Deslandes A, Brogard JM et al: Reappraisal of amoxycillin absorption kinetics, *J Antimicrob Chemother* 27:647, 1991.

584. Wettrel G, Anderson KE: Cardiovascular Drugs. I. Antidysrhythmic drugs, *Ther Drug Monit* 8:59, 1986.

585. White NJ: Antimalarial pharmacokinetics and treatment regimens, *Br J Clin Pharmac* 34:1, 1992.

586. White WB, Yeh SC, Krol GJ: Nitrendipine in human plasma and breast milk, *Eur J Clin Pharmacol* 36:531, 1989.

587. Widerlov E, Termander N, Nilsson MI: Effect of urinary pH on the plasma and urinary kinetics of remoxipride, *Eur J Clin Pharmacol* 37:359, 1989.

588. Wiest DB, Fowler SL, Garner SS et al: Fluconazole in neonatal disseminated candidiasis, *Arch Dis Child* 66: 1002, 1991.

589. Wiggins RC, Rolsten C, Ruiz B et al: Pharmacokinetics of cocaine: basic studies of route, dosage, pregnancy and lactation, *Neurotoxicology* 10:367, 1989.

590. Wilde MI, Langtry HD: Zidovudine: an update of its pharmacodynamic and pharmacokinetic properties, and therapeutic efficacy, *Drugs* 46:515, 1993.

591. Wilde MI, Plosker GL, Benfield P: Fluvoxamine: an updated review of its pharmacology, and therapeutic use in depressive illness, *Drugs* 46:895, 1993.

592. Wilder BJ: Pharmacokinetics of valproate and carbamazepine, *J Clin Psychopharmacol* 12:64S, 1992.

593. Wildfeuer A, Laufen H, Leitold M et al: Comparison of the pharmacokinetics of three-day and five-day regimens of azithromycin in plasma and urine, *J Antimicrob Chemother* 31(suppl E):51, 1993.

594. Wilson JH: Breast milk tocainide levels, *J Cardiovasc Pharmacol* 12:497, 1988.

595. Wischnik A, Manth SM, Lloyd J et al: The excretion of ketorolac tromethamine into breast milk after multiple oral dosing, *Eur J Clin Pharmacol* 36:521, 1989.

596. Wiseman LR, Benfield P: Cefprozil: a review of its antibacterial activity, pharmacokinetic properties, and therapeutic potential, *Drugs* 45:295, 1993.

597. Wisner KL, Perel JM, Findling RL: Antidepressant treatment during breast-feeding, *Am J Psychiat* 153:1132, 1996.

598. Wojnar-Horton RE, Hackett LP, Yapp P et al: Distribution and excretion of sumatriptan in human milk, *Br J Clin Pharmac* 41:217, 1996.

599. Wolff MS: Lactation. In Paul M, editor: *Occupational and environmental reproductive hazards: a guide for clinicians,* Baltimore, 1993, Williams & Wilkins.

600. Wolfson JS, Hooper DC: Pharmacokinetics of quinolones: newer aspects, *Eur J Clin Microbiol Infect Dis* 10:267, 1991.

601. Wong FA, Flor SC: The metabolism of ofloxacin in humans, *Drug Metab Dispos* 18:1103, 1990.

602. Woodward A, Grgurinovich N, Ryan P: Breast feeding and smoking hygiene: major influences on cotinine in urine of smokers' infants, *J Epidemiol Community Health* 40:309, 1986.

603. Woosley RL: Mexiletine and tocainide: a profile of two lidocaine analogs, *Rational Drug Therapy* 21:1, 1987.

604. Woosley RL, Funck-Brentano C: Overview of the clinical pharmacology of antiarrhythmic drugs, *Am J Cardiol* 61:61A, 1988.

605. Woosley RL, Morganroth J, Fogoros RN et al: Pharmacokinetics of moricizine HCl, *Am J Cardiol* 60:35F, 1987.

606. Wretlind M: Excretion of oxazepam in breast milk, *Eur J Clin Pharmacol* 33:209, 1987.

607. Wright S, Dawling S, Ashford JJ: Excretion of fluvoxamine in breast milk, *Br J Clin Pharmac* 31:209, 1991.

608. Yee GC, McGuire TR: Pharmacokinetic drug interactions with cyclosporin. Part I. *Clin Pharmacokinet* 19:319, 1990.

609. Yue QY, Hasselstrom J, Svensson JO et al: Pharmacokinetics of codeine and its metabolites in Caucasian healthy volunteers: comparisons between extensive and poor hydroxylators of desbrisoquine, *Br J Clin Pharmac* 31:635, 1991.

610. Yue QY, Svensson JO, Sjoqvist F et al: A comparison of the pharmacokinetics of codeine and its metabolites in healthy Chinese and Caucasian extensive hydroxylators of debrisoquine, *Br J Clin Pharmac* 31:643, 1991.

611. Yusuff NT, York P, Chrystyn H et al: Improved bioavailability from a spironolactone beta-cyclodextrin complex, *Eur J Clin Pharmacol* 40:507, 1991.

612. Zaske DE, Strate RG, Kohls PR: Amikacin pharmacokinetics: wide interpatient variation in 98 patients, *J Clin Pharmacol* 31:158, 1991.

613. Zeisler JA, Gaarder TD, DeMesquita SA: Lidocaine excretion in breast milk, *Drug Intell Clin Pharm* 20:691, 1986.

614. Zschiesche M, Focke N, Hoffmann C et al: Bioavailability of metronidazole vaginal tablets (Vagimid), *Int J Clin Pharmacol Ther Toxicol* 30:485, 1992.

Precautions and breastfeeding recommendations for selected maternal infections

TABLE E-1   Precautions and breastfeeding recommendations for selected maternal infections[a]

Organism, syndrome, or condition[b,c]	Empiric precautions[d]	Breastfeeding acceptable[e]	Compatibility of medications with breastfeeding[f]
Adenoviruses			
Conjunctivitis	Contact		
Upper/lower respiratory infections	Droplet	Yes[g]	
Gastroenteritis	Standard		
Entamoeba histolytica			
Intestinal	Standard	Yes	Iodoquinol, paromomycin, metronidazole, tinidazole
Extraintestinal	Standard	Yes	

[a]Modified from Garner JS: Hospital Infection Control Practices Advisory Committee guidelines for isolation precautions in hospitals, *Infect Control Hosp Epidemiol* 17:53-80, 1996. To ensure that appropriate empiric precautions are always implemented, hospitals must have systems in place to routinely evaluate patients according to these criteria as part of their preadmission and admission care.

[b]Patients with the syndromes or conditions listed may present with atypical signs and symptoms (e.g., pertussis in neonates and adults may not have paroxysmal or severe cough). The clinician's index of suspicion should be guided by the prevalence of specific conditions in the community, as well as clinical judgement.

[c]The organisms listed are not intended to represent the complete, or even most likely diagnoses, but rather possible etiologic agents that may require additional precautions beyond *standard precautions* until they can be excluded.

[d]These are the usual precautions (Standard, Airborne, Contact, and Droplet), outlined in the text, as proposed by the Centers for Disease Control and Prevention. Symbols for duration of precautions are *24 hours*, 24 hours of antibiotic therapy; *CN*, until off antibiotics and culture negative; *DI*, duration of the illness; *PI*, period of infectivity.

[e]Yes means that if in a hospitalized mother and infant, the proposed precautions are followed, breastfeeding is acceptable and may be beneficial to the infant. Any infant breastfeeding during a maternal infection should be observed closely for signs or symptoms of illness.

*See text for more complete explanation; *P*, prophylactic antibiotics for the infant with *H. influenzae*: rifampin 10 mg/kg/dose once daily × 4 days for infants less than 1 month of age; rifampin 20 mg/kg/dose once daily × 4 days for infants over 1 month of age (without vaccine series, two to three doses of vaccine before 12 months and one dose after 15 months or two doses between 12 and 14 months). For *Neisseria meningitidis*, give rifampin 10 mg/kg/dose every 12 hours for four doses and 5 mg/kg/dose in children less than 1 month old. Give sulfisoxazole if *N. meningitidis* isolate is sensitive. Alternatively, ceftriaxone 250 mg IM for one dose (125-mg dose for children less than 15 years old) is acceptable. For *Corynebacterium diptheriae*, give erythromycin 40-50 mg/kg/day × 7 days or a single IM dose of benzathine penicillin G (600,000 U for the child less than 30 kg of weight. For *Bordatella pertussis* or *parapertussis*, give erythromycin 40-50 mg/kg/day divided four times a day × 14 days or clarithromycin 15 mg/kg/day in two divided doses × 10 days or TMP-SMX 8 mg/kg of TMP/day and 40 mg/kg of SMX/day in two divided doses × 14 days.

BM+, although breastfeeding is not acceptable because of exposure risk, giving the mother's expressed breast milk is acceptable.

[f]See Appendix D and Chapter 11 on medications in breast milk.

[g]Adenovirus types 4 and 7 have been known to cause severe respiratory disease in premature infants or individuals with immunodeficiency or underlying respiratory disease. In certain situations, feeding of expressed breast milk to the infant may not be advisable.

[h]Breastfeed immediately if mother receives ceftriaxone intramuscularly or intravenously. Breastfed after 24-hr antibiotic therapy for other treatment regimens, with feeding of expressed breast milk for the first 24 hours.

Continued

TABLE E-1   Precautions and breastfeeding recommendations for selected maternal infections[a]—cont'd

Organism, syndrome, or condition[b,c]	Empiric precautions[d]	Breastfeeding acceptable[e]	Compatibility of medications with breastfeeding[f]
Arboviruses			
Arthropod-borne infections, meningoencephalitis, hemorrhagic fevers, hepatitis	Standard	Yes	
California encephalitis	Standard	Yes	
Colorado tick fever	Standard	Yes	
Dengue fever	Standard	Yes	
Eastern equine encephalitis	Standard	Yes	
Japanese encephalitis	Standard	Yes	
St. Louis encephalitis	Standard	Yes	
Yellow fever	Standard	Yes	
Arcanobacterium haemolyticus			
Pharyngitis, skin infections	Standard	Yes	Erythromycin, clindamycin, chloramphenicol, tetracycline
Ascaris lumbricoides			
Gastrointestinal infections, pneumonitis	Standard	Yes	Pyrantel pamoate, mebendazole, albendazole, piperazine
Aspergillosis			
Bronchopulmonary, sinus, or invasive infections	Standard	Yes	Amphotericin B, flucytosine, rifampin
Astroviruses			
Gastroenteritis	Standard, but contact for incontinent individuals	Yes	
Babesiosis			
Babesia microti			
Subacute/chronic febrile illness	Standard	Yes	Clindamycin, quinine
Blastocystis hominis			
Gastrointestinal infection	Standard	Yes	Metronidazole
Blastomyces dermatitidis			
Pulmonary, cutaneous, or invasive infection	Standard	Yes	Amphotericin B, ketoconazole, itraconazole
Borrelia			
Relapsing fever			
Borrelia hermsii	Standard (tick-borne)	Yes	Penicillin, erythromycin
Borrelia recurrentis	Contact (louse-borne)	Yes	Tetracycline, chloramphenicol
Borrelia turicatae	Standard (tick-borne)	Yes	Doxycycline

Infection/Organism	Precautions	Breastfeeding	Treatment
Botulism *Clostridium botulinum* Hypotonia, progressive weakness, toxin-mediated paralysis	Standard	Yes	
Breast abscess (see Mastitis) *Staphylococcus aureus* Enterobacteriaceae *Streptococcus pyogenes*	Contact (24 hrs)	Yes (after 24 hrs if no drainage into breast milk; discard breast milk for first 24 hours after surgery)	First-generation cephalosporin, amoxicillin/clavulanate, ampicillin/sulbactam
Brucellosis Febrile illness with variable manifestations	Standard	Yes (after 48 hrs of therapy in the mother; discard breast milk for 48 hrs)	Doxycycline, TMP-SMX, rifampin, gentamicin, streptomycin, tetracycline
Brucella abortus *Brucella melitensis* *Brucella suis*	Contact (for draining wounds)	Yes	
Caliciviruses Gastroenteritis	Standard, but contact for incontinent individuals	Yes	
Campylobacter Gastrointestinal infection *Campylobacter fetus* *Campylobacter jejuni*	Standard, but contact for incontinent individuals	Yes	Erythromycin, ciprofloxacin
Candidiasis Mucocutaneous infection, vulvovaginitis, invasive infections *Candida albicans* *Candida krusei* *Candida tropicalis*	Standard	Yes (therapy for the infant simultaneous with mother's therapy)*	Topical agents, fluconazole, ketoconazole, itraconazole, amphotericin B, flucytosine
Cat-scratch disease Skin infection, regional lymphadenitis, and rarely, invasive infection *Bartonella henselae*	Standard	Yes	TMP-SMX, rifampin, ciprofloxacin, gentamicin, doxycycline, erythromycin

Continued

TABLE E-1 Precautions and breastfeeding recommendations for selected maternal infections[a]—cont'd

Organism, syndrome, or condition[b,c]	Empiric precautions[d]	Breastfeeding acceptable[e]	Compatibility of medications with breastfeeding[f]
Chlamydia			
Chlamydia pneumoniae Pharyngitis, pneumonia	Standard	Yes	
Chlamydia psittaci Psittacosis, pneumonia, rarely invasive infection	Standard	Yes	Tetracycline, erythromycin azithromycin, clarithromycin
Chlamydia trachomatis Urethritis, vaginitis, endometritis, salpingitis, lymphogranuloma venereum (LGV), conjunctivitis, pneumonia	Standard	Yes (consider treating the infant)	Erythromycin, azithromycin, clarithromycin, doxycycline, tetracycline, sulfisoxazole
Clostridia			
Clostridium botulinum Toxin-mediated paralysis	Standard	Yes	
Clostridium difficile Antimicrobial-associated diarrhea, pseudomembranous colitis	Contact	Yes	Metronidazole, vancomycin
Clostridium perfringens Food poisoning, wound infection, gas gangrene, myonecrosis	Standard	Yes	Penicillin, chloramphenicol, clindamycin, metronidazole
Coccidioides immitis Pulmonary, invasive infections rarely, extrapulmonary	Standard, but contact for draining lesions	Yes	Amphotericin B, fluconazole, itraconazole
Conjunctivitis			
Adenovirus	Contact	Yes	
Chlamydia trachomatis	Standard	Yes	Tetracycline, doxycycline, erythromycin
Neisseria gonorrhoeae	Standard	Yes[h]	Penicillin, ceftriaxone
Cryptococcus neoformans Meningitis, pneumonia	Standard	Yes	Amphotericin B, flucytosine
Cryptosporidiosis			
Cryptosporidium parvum Diarrhea	Contact	Yes	Paromomycin, azithromycin

Infection	Precautions	Breastfeeding	Treatment
Cytomegalovirus (CMV)			
Asymptomatic infection	Standard	Yes (for full-term infants)	
Infectious mononucleosis	Standard	No (for premature or immunodeficient infants, do not give expressed breast milk)	
Dengue fever			
Acute febrile illness, hemorrhagic fever	Standard	Yes	
Diphtheria			
Corynebacterium diphtheriae			Erythromycin, penicillin
Membranous nasopharyngitis	Droplet (DI)	Yes (with infant receiving chemoprophylaxis-P)	
Obstructive laryngotracheitis	Droplet (DI)	No (only if skin lesion involves breast)	
Cutaneous infection, toxin-mediated myocarditis, or neurologic disease	Contact (cover lesions)		
Diarrhea			
Campylobacter fetus	Standard	Yes	TMP-SMX
Campylobacter jejuni	Standard	Yes	Erythromycin, ciprofloxacin
Escherichia coli (0157:H7)	Contact	Yes	None indicated
Giardia lamblia	Standard	Yes	Furazolidone, metronidazole
Rotavirus	Contact	Yes	
Salmonella enteritidis	Standard	Yes	
Shigella boydii	Contact	Yes	Ciprofloxacin, norfloxacin, TMP-SMX
Shigella dysenteriae	Contact	Yes	Ciprofloxacin, norfloxacin, TMP-SMX
Shigella flexneri	Contact	Yes	Ciprofloxacin, norfloxacin, TMP-SMX
Shigella sonnei	Contact	Yes	Ciprofloxacin, norfloxacin, TMP-SMX
Vibrio cholerae	Standard	Yes	Ciprofloxacin, doxycycline
Vibrio parahaemolyticus	Standard	Yes	None
Yersinia enterocolitica	Standard	Yes	Ciprofloxacin, norfloxacin, ceftriaxone, TMP-SMX, doxycycline
Yersinia pseudotuberculosis	Standard	Yes	
Ebola virus	Contact, droplet, and airborne	No (do not give expressed breast milk)	

Continued

874   Breastfeeding: A guide for the medical profession

TABLE E-1   Precautions and breastfeeding recommendations for selected maternal infections[a] —cont'd

Organism, syndrome, or condition[b,c]	Empiric precautions[d]	Breastfeeding acceptable[e]	Compatibility of medications with breastfeeding[f]
Encephalitis			
Enteroviruses	Standard	Yes	
Lyme disease (*Borrelia burgdorferi*)	Standard	Yes	Ceftriaxone, doxycycline, amoxicillin
Rabies	Standard	No (BM+)	Rabies immune globulin, rabies vaccine
Endometritis, pelvic inflammatory disease			
Anaerobic organisms	Standard	Yes	Clindamycin, metronidazole, cefoxitin, cefmetazole
Chlamydia trachomatis	Standard	Yes	Erythromycin, azithromycin, tetracycline
Enterobacteriaceae	Standard	Yes	Ampicillin, aminoglycosides, cephalosporins
Group B streptococci	Standard	Yes (after 24 hrs of therapy, breast milk is ok; observation)	Penicillin, cephalosporin, macrolides
Mycoplasma hominis	Standard	Yes	Clindamycin, tetracycline
Neisseria gonorrhoeae	Standard	Yes[h]	Ceftriaxone, spectinomycin, doxycycline, azithromycin
Ureaplasma urealyticum	Standard	Yes	Erythromycin, azithromycin, clarithromycin, tetracycline
Enteroviruses			
Myocarditis; respiratory, gastrointestinal, skin, central nervous system, and eye infections	Adults: standard Children: contact		
Coxsackievirus		Yes	
Echo		Yes	
Polioviruses		Yes	
Epstein-Barr virus			
Infectious mononucleosis, broad range of infections	Standard	Yes	
Erythema infectiosum			
Parvovirus B19	Standard	Yes	

Condition / Organism	Precautions	Breastfeeding	Therapy / Comments
Food poisoning			
Bacillus cereus — Toxin mediated	Standard	Yes	
Clostridium perfringens — Toxin mediated	Standard	Yes	
Escherichia coli (0157:H7) Enterohemorrhagic	Contact	Yes	
Hepatitis A	Standard	Yes (immune serum globulin and hepatitis A vaccine for the infant)	
Norwalk virus	Standard	Yes	
Salmonella enteritidis	Standard	Yes	
Shigella	Contact	Yes	Ciprofloxacin, TMP-SMX
Staphylococcus aureus Enterotoxin	Standard	Yes	
Gastroenteritis (see Diarrhea or Food Poisoning)			
Giardiasis			
Giardia lamblia	Standard, no contact with incontinent individuals	Yes	Furazolidone, metronidazole
Gonorrhea			
Genital, pharyngeal, conjunctival, or disseminated infection			
Neisseria gonorrhoeae	Standard	Yes[h]	Ceftriaxone, ciprofloxacin, spectinomycin, azithromycin, doxycycline
Haemophilus influenzae			
Meningitis, epiglottitis, pneumonia, cellulitis, sinusitis, bacteremia	Droplet	Yes (24 hrs after initiating therapy in mother; BM+; P* if infant has not been fully immunized, observation)	Cefotaxime, ceftriaxone, ampicillin
Hantavirus			
Pulmonary syndrome, hemorrhagic fever with renal syndrome	Standard	Yes	Intravenous ribavirin is investigational

Continued

TABLE E-1 Precautions and breastfeeding recommendations for selected maternal infections[a]—cont'd

Organism, syndrome, or condition[b,c]	Empiric precautions[d]	Breastfeeding acceptable[e]	Compatibility of medications with breastfeeding[f]
Hemorrhagic fevers			
African hemorrhagic fever			
Ebola virus	Contact	No	
Marburg virus			
Dengue virus (1-4)	Standard	Yes (expressed breast milk is ok)	
Hantavirus	Standard	Yes (expressed breast milk is ok)	
Lassa fever	Contact	No (no expressed breast milk)	Intravenous ribavirin
Yellow fever	Standard	Yes (expressed breast milk is ok)	Vaccine
Hepatitis*			
A Acute only	Standard, but contact for incontinent individuals	Yes (after Immune Serum Globulin [ISG] and vaccine)	
B Chronic hepatitis, cirrhosis, hepatocellular carcinoma	Standard	Yes (after HBIG and vaccine)	
C Chronic hepatitis, cirrhosis, hepatocellular carcinoma	Standard	Yes	
D Associated with Hepatitis B	Standard	Yes (after HBIG and vaccine)	
E Severe disease in pregnant women	Standard	Yes	
G	Standard	Inadequate data	
Herpes viruses			
Cytomegalovirus Asymptomatic, infectious mononucleosis-like syndrome; severe disease in the immunodeficient person	Standard	Yes for full-term infants No for premature or immunodeficient infants (infant of CMV-negative mother should not receive milk from CMV-positive mothers)	Ganciclovir, foscarnet

Infection	Precautions	Breastfeeding	Treatment
Epstein-Barr virus Asymptomatic, infectious mononucleosis, associated with chronic fatigue syndrome, African Burkitt's lymphoma, and nasopharyngeal carcinoma	Standard	Yes	
Herpes simplex Type 1, 2 ($HSV_{1,2}$) Mucocutaneous	Contact	Yes (in the absence of breast lesions)	Acyclovir, valacyclovir, famciclovir
Neonatal	Contact		
Encephalitis	Standard		
Varicella-zoster virus (VZV)* Varicella	Airborne	No (expressed breast milk is ok in the absence of lesions on the breast)	Acyclovir, valacyclovir, famciclovir
Zoster	Standard in normal patient	Yes (covered lesions, with none involving the breast)	
	Airborne/contact in immunocompromised individuals	No VZIG for the exposed infant, especially less than 1 month of age*	
Human herpes virus 6 (HHV-6) Roseola (exanthema subitum, sixth disease), acute febrile illness	Standard	Yes	
Histoplasmosis Acute pulmonary disease, disseminated	Standard	Yes	Amphotericin B, ketoconazole, fluconazole, itraconazole
Human immunodeficiency viruses (HIV)* HIV-1	Standard	Yes/no*	Little or no available information on antiretrovirals in breast milk
HIV-2	Standard	Yes/no*	
Human T-cell leukemia viruses (HTLV) HTLV-I T-cell leukemia/lymphoma, myelopathy, dermatitis, adenitis, Sjögren's syndrome	Standard	No*	
HTLV-II Myelopathy, arthritis, glomerulonephritis	Standard	No*	
Impetigo	Contact	Yes	Oxacillin, dicloxacillin, erythromycin, first-generation cephalosporins

Continued

TABLE E-1   Precautions and breastfeeding recommendations for selected maternal infections[a] —cont'd

Organism, syndrome, or condition[b,c]	Empiric precautions[d]	Breastfeeding acceptable[e]	Compatibility of medications with breastfeeding[f]
Infectious mononucleosis (see CMV, EBV)			
Influenza	Droplet	Yes	Amantadine, rimantadine
Lassa fever	Contact	No (do not give expressed breast milk)	Intravenous ribavarin
Legionnaires' disease			
Legionella pneumophila	Standard	Yes	Erythromycin, rifampin
Pneumonia ± gastrointestinal, central nervous system, or renal involvement			
Leprosy			
Mycobacterium leprae	Standard	Yes	Dapsone, rifampin, clofazimine
Chronic disease of skin, peripheral nerves, and respiratory mucosa			
Leptospirosis			
Abrupt febrile illness, often biphasic, with multiple organ involvement			
Leptospira interrogans	Standard	Yes (no mother-infant contact except for breastfeeding)	Penicillin, tetracycline, doxycycline
Leptospira icterohaemorrhagiae			
Leptospira canicola			
Listeria monocytogenes	Standard	Yes	Ampicillin, penicillin, TMP-SMZ
In adults: nonspecific febrile illness; in neonates: meningitis, pneumonia, sepsis, granulomatosis infantisepticum			
Lyme disease			
Borrelia burgdorferi	Standard	Yes, with informed discussion	Ceftriaxone, ampicillin, doxycycline
Multi-staged illness of skin, joint, and peripheral or central nervous system			
Lymphocytic choriomeningitis	Standard	Yes	
Aseptic meningitis to severe encephalitis, with variable presentation of other symptoms			
Mastitis			
Candida albicans	Standard	Yes, with simultaneous treatment of the infant	Nystatin, ketoconazole
Enterobacteriaceae	Standard	Yes	Fluconazole

	Precautions	Breastfeeding	Therapy
Staphylococcus aureus	Contact	Yes (after 24 hrs of therapy, during which milk must be discarded)	First-generation cephalosporin, dicloxacillin, oxacillin, erythromycin
Group A streptococcus	Contact		
Mycobacterium tuberculosis	Standard (unless there is also pulmonary involvement, then airborne precautions as well)	No* breastmilk or breastfeeding for 2 weeks of maternal therapy, consider prophylactic INH for the infant (see p. 573 Figures 16-1 and 16-2)	Isoniazid, rifampin, ethambutol, pyrazinamide ethionamide
Malaria	Standard	Yes	Pyrimethamine-sulfadoxine, chloroquine, quinidine, quinine, tetracycline, mefloquine
Measles Febrile illness with coryza, conjunctivitis, cough, and an erythematous maculopapular rash	Airborne	Yes (after 72 hrs of rash in the mother and after the infant receives ISG, expressed breast milk is okay)	Ribavirin is experimental
Meningitis Aseptic meningitis (nonbacterial, viral meningitis)	Standard	Yes	
Fungal meningitis	Standard	Yes	Amphotericin, itraconazole, flucytosine
Haemophilus influenzae	Droplet (for first 24 hrs of appropriate therapy and carrier eradication with ceftriaxone or rifampin)	Yes (after 24 hrs of maternal therapy, with the infant receiving prophylaxis, P); begin infant vaccination; expressed breast milk is okay	Ceftriaxone, ampicillin, chloramphenicol, rifampin
Neisseria meningitidis	Droplet (24 hrs of appropriate therapy and carrier eradication with ceftriaxone or rifampin)	Yes (after 24 hrs of maternal therapy, with the infant receiving prophylaxis, P); expressed breast milk is okay	Ceftriaxone, penicillin, chloramphenicol
Streptococcal pneumoniae	Standard	Yes	Ceftriaxone, penicillin, vancomycin

Continued

TABLE E-1 Precautions and breastfeeding recommendations for selected maternal infections[a]—cont'd

Organism, syndrome, or condition[b,c]	Empiric precautions[d]	Breastfeeding acceptable[e]	Compatibility of medications with breastfeeding[f]
Mumps	Droplet	Yes	
*Mycobacterium tuberculosis**	Standard and airborne	Yes	Antituberculous medications are acceptable during breastfeeding, pp. 570-573
Mycoplasma pneumoniae			
Bronchitis, pneumonia, pharyngitis, otitis media, and a broad range of unusual manifestations, including central nervous system, cardiac, skin, muscle, and joint involvement	Droplet	Yes	Erythromycin, clarithromycin, azithromycin, tetracycline
Neisseria meningitidis			
Meningitis, meningococcemia	Droplet (for 24 hrs of appropriate therapy and carrier eradication with ceftriaxone or rifampin)	Yes (after 24 hrs of appropriate therapy, and with prophylaxis for the infant, P)	Penicillin, ceftriaxone, chloramphenicol, rifampin
Norwalk agent			
Gastroenteritis	Standard	Yes	
Papillomaviruses			
Skin or mucous membrane warts, laryngeal papillomas	Standard	Yes (in the absence of breast involvement)	
Parainfluenzae viruses			
Laryngotracheobronchitis, upper and lower respiratory infections	Standard (contact for infants and children)	Yes	
Parvovirus B19			
Erythema infectiosum, fifth disease, aplastic crisis, arthritis	Standard with erythema infectiosum, droplet for aplastic crisis or infection in patients with hemoglobinopathy or immunodeficiency	Yes	
Pelvic inflammatory disease (see Endometritis)			

Infection	Precautions	Breastfeeding	Treatment
Pertussis Whooping cough, pneumonia, bronchitis, encephalitis *Bordetella parapertussis* and *Bordetella pertussis*	Droplet (for 5 days of appropriate therapy)	Yes (after 5 days of appropriate therapy and chemoprophylaxis for the infant, expressed breast milk is OK, P)	Erythromycin, clarithromycin, TMP-SMX
Pneumocystis carinii pneumonitis (PCP)	Standard	Yes, but suspect HIV infection if the mother develops PCP and reassess breastfeeding with HIV infection in mind	Pentamidine, TMP-SMX, atovaquone, prednisone
Pneumonia (see specific causative agents)			
Poliomyelitis	Standard	Yes	
Rabies Severe, progressive central nervous system infection, generally fatal	Standard	No when mother is clinically sick; yes (BM+); yes during postexposure immunization of the mother without symptoms; yes if both mother and infant are receiving postexposure immunization	Rabies immune globulin, rabies vaccine
Rat-bite fever *Spirillum minus*	Standard		Tetracycline, chloramphenicol, streptomycin
Streptobacillus moniliformis	Standard	Yes	Penicillin
Relapsing fever *Borrelia recurrentis*	Standard (tick-borne)	Yes	Tetracycline, doxycycline, TMP-SMX, streptomycin, rifampin
	Contact if louse infested	Yes with simultaneous treatment of mother and infant for lice	
Respiratory syncytial virus Upper respiratory infection, pneumonia, bronchiolitis	Contact	Yes	Ribavirin

Continued

TABLE E-1   Precautions and breastfeeding recommendations for selected maternal infections[a]—cont'd

Organism, syndrome, or condition[b,c]	Empiric precautions[d]	Breastfeeding acceptable[e]	Compatibility of medications with breastfeeding[f]
Retroviruses (see Human Immunodeficiency Viruses 1, 2 and Human T-cell leukemia Viruses I, II)			
Rickettsial diseases			
Fever, rash, vasculitis; arthropod, louse-borne			
Ehrlichiosis, leukopenia	Standard	Yes	Doxycycline, tetracycline
Ehrlichia chaffensis			
Q fever			
Coxiella burnetii			
Pneumonia, hepatosplenomegaly, endocarditis	Standard	Yes	Doxycycline, tetracycline
Rickettsial pox			
Rickettsia akari			
Scab or eschar, rash, regional lymphadenopathy, self-limited	Standard	Yes	Doxycycline, tetracycline, chloramphenicol
Rocky Mountain spotted fever			
Rickettsia rickettsii	Standard	Yes	Doxycycline, chloramphenicol
Typhus (flea-borne)			
Rickettsia typhi	Standard	Yes	Doxycycline (single dose)
Typhus (louse-borne)			
Rickettsia prowazekii	Standard	Yes	Tetracycline, chloramphenicol
Rotavirus			
Diarrhea, vomiting, "winter vomiting disease"	Contact	Yes	
Rubella virus			
Self-limited, mild exanthem with fever; congenital rubella syndrome	Contact	Yes	
Salmonella (see Diarrhea/Gastroenteritis)			
Shigella (see Diarrhea/Gastroenteritis)			
Staphylococcus aureus			
Cellulitis, abscess	Contact	Yes	Oxacillin, dicloxacillin, first-generation cephalosporins, erythromycin, vancomycin
Enterocolitis, diarrhea	Standard	Yes	

Scalded skin syndrome		Contact	Yes (after 24 hrs of effective therapy; discard breast milk for 24 hrs)	Oxacillin, dicloxacillin, vancomycin
Toxic shock syndrome		Standard	Yes*	
Methicillin-resistant *S. aureus* (MRSA)		Contact	Yes*	
Staphylococcus epidermidis	Opportunistic infections	Standard	Yes	Penicillin, erythromycin, cephalosporin
Streptococcus (Group A)	Cellulitis, pharyngitis, pneumonia, myositis/fasciitis, scarlet fever	Standard	Yes (24 hrs after beginning appropriate therapy; discard breast milk for 24 hrs)	
		Contact (for extensive skin infection unable to be covered until after 24 hrs of therapy)	Yes (24 hrs after beginning appropriate therapy; discard breast milk for 24 hrs)	
Streptococcus (Group B)	Urinary tract infection, endometritis, mastitis; infants: sepsis, pneumonia, meningitis, osteomyelitis, arthritis	Standard	Yes* (after 24 hrs of effective therapy); for perinatal exposure, high risk, or suspected illness, infant is given empiric therapy	Penicillin, ampicillin
Streptococcus pneumoniae	Pneumonia, occult bacteremia, otitis media, sinusitis	Standard	Yes	Penicillin, ceftriaxone, vancomycin, cefotaxime, rifampin
Syphilis				
Treponema pallidum	Multisystem, multistage infection with widely varying presentations, congenital infection	Standard	Yes (after 24 hrs of effective therapy; discard breast milk for 24 hrs)	Penicillin
	Open skin lesions of breast or nipples	Contact	No, until 24 hrs of effective therapy in mother if open skin lesions involve the breast	Penicillin

Continued

TABLE E-1   Precautions and breastfeeding recommendations for selected maternal infections[a]—cont'd

Organism, syndrome, or condition[b,c]	Empiric precautions[d]	Breastfeeding acceptable[e]	Compatibility of medications with breastfeeding[f]
Tetanus			
Exotoxin-mediated severe muscular spasms	Standard	Yes (age-appropriate vaccination of the child, no tetanus immune globulin [TIG] necessary for infant)	Penicillin, metronidazole
Clostridium tetani			
Tinea			
Capitis			
Microsporum audouinii	Standard	Yes	Griseofulvin, selenium sulfide shampoo, prednisone
Microsporum canis			
Trichophyton tonsurans			
Corporis, cruris, pedis			
Epidermophyton floccosum	Standard	Yes	Topical agents
Trichophyton canis			
Trichophyton rubrum			
Versicolor			
Malassezia furfur	Standard	Yes	Topical agents, ketoconazole, itraconazole
Toxoplasmosis			
Toxoplasma gondii	Standard	Yes	Pyrimethamine, sulfadiazine
Asymptomatic or mononucleosis-like illness with lymphadenopathy, ocular symptoms; congenital infection			
Toxic shock	See specific agents		
(see *S. aureus*, Streptococcus [Group A])			
Toxin-mediated illness			
Bacillus cereus			
Botulism			
Food poisoning			
Staphylococcal Scalded Skin Syndrome (SSSS)			
Trichinosis			
Trichinella spiralis	Standard	Yes	Mebendazole, thiabendazole, prednisone
Asymptomatic, or may cause myalgia, periorbital edema, myocardial failure, CNS involvement, or pneumonitis			

Infection	Precautions	Breastfeeding	Treatment
Trichomonas vaginalis Vaginitis, urethritis, or asymptomatic infections	Standard	Yes	Metronidazole
Trypanosomiasis			
Trypanosoma brucei "Sleeping sickness"; tsetse fly vector (African)	Standard	No	Suramin, pentamidine, eflornithine, melarsoprol
Trypanosoma cruzi Chagas' disease (American)	Standard	Yes	Nifurtimox, benznidazole
Tuberculosis (see pp. 570-573, Figs. 16-1 and 16-2)	Standard	Yes	
Tularemia			
Francisella tularensis Acute febrile illness with various syndromes; oculoglandular, ulceroglandular, glandular, oropharyngeal, typhoidal, pneumoniae	Standard	Yes	Streptomycin, tetracycline, chloramphenicol
Ureaplasma urealyticum Nongonococcal urethritis (NGU), endometritis, pelvic inflammatory disease	Standard	Yes	Doxycycline, erythromycin, azithromycin
Urinary tract infection			
Group B streptococcus (see Streptococcus [Group B]) Enterobacteriaceal	Standard	Yes	Ampicillin, aminoglycosides, cephalosporin
Staphylococcus saprophyticus	Standard	Yes	Quinolones
Vaginitis			
Bacterial *Candida albicans* (see Candidiasis) *Trichomonas vaginalis*	Standard	Yes	Metronidazole, clindamycin
Varicella-zoster virus (see Herpes viruses)			
Whooping cough *Bordetella parapertussis* and *Bordetella pertussis*; see also Adenovirus, Chlamydia (*Chlamydia pneumoniae*, *Chlamydia trachomatis*), *Mycoplasma pneumoniae*	Droplet (for 5 days of appropriate therapy and chemoprophylaxis for the infant)	Yes, after 5 days of appropriate therapy, BM+, P	Erythromycin, clarithromycin, TMP-SMX
Yersinia enterocolitica Diarrhea, pseudoappendicitis, focal infections, and bacteremia	Contact precautions for incontinent individuals	Yes	Aminoglycosides, cefotoxine, tetracycline, chloramphenicol
Yersinia pseudotuberculosis Fever, rash, abdominal symptoms	Standard	Yes	TMP-SMX

*T*he Lact-Aid Nursing Trainer System

*T*he Lact-Aid nursing trainer system is made up of four parts: (1) the body with permanently attached nursing tube, (2) the clamp ring, (3) the extension tube, and (4) the presterilized Lact-Aid bag with 4-oz capacity.

For convenience in filling and assembling the Lact-Aid system, a bag hanger and funnel have been specially designed. Six T-shaped end tabs provide easy attachment to the nursing bra (Figs. F-1 and F-2).

The filled Lact-Aid is attached to the nursing bra or neck cord between the breasts and is positioned so that the supplement cannot siphon out. The presterilized bag is attached to the body

Fig. F-1.   A, Presterilized, disposable bags have 4-oz capacity. **B,** Lact-Aid system includes detailed instruction booklet plus accessories for filling, cleaning, and use. **C,** Filled Nursing Trainer may be attached directly to the nursing bra as shown or suspended by the neck cord as depicted in Fig. 18-4. (From Avery JL: *Lact-Aid Nursing Trainer instruction book,* rev ed, Athens, Tenn, 1983, Lact-Aid International, Inc., 423-744-9090.)

by the clamp ring. The infant suckles the tip of the nursing tube and the nipple of the breast at the same time. As the infant nurses, supplement is drawn from the bottom of the presterilized bag by the extension tube attached to the bottom of the body. This keeps the infant from swallowing any air that might be trapped in the top of the bag. The body has an orifice designed to provide the best rate of flow, slower than milk flows from the breast, but fast enough to keep from overtiring the infant. The nursing tube carries the supplement to the infant's mouth. It is clear, very

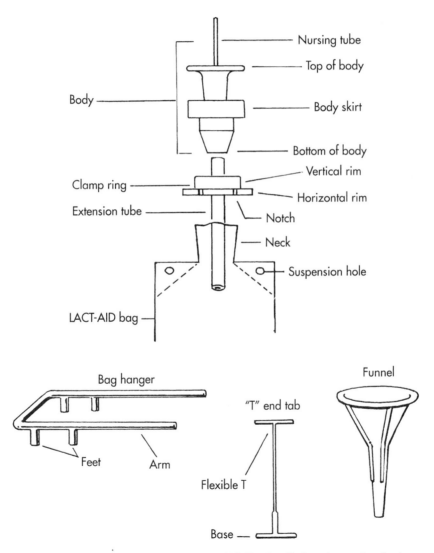

Fig. F-2. Lact-Aid parts. (From Avery JL: *Lact-Aid Nursing Trainer instruction book*, rev ed, Athens, Tenn, 1998, Lact-Aid International, Inc., 423-744-9090.)

soft, and flexible and will not cause the infant's mouth or the nipple any discomfort.

When the infant is put to the breast, the flow of supplement rewards his nursing efforts. This provides a pleasant incentive for the infant to continue nursing, which in turn provides the breasts with suckling stimulation to build up the milk supply. The Lact-Aid is small enough, even when it contains the full 4-oz capacity of supplement, to enable one to nurse discreetly without it showing. It is valuable in adoptive nursing* and in infants diagnosed with failure to thrive (see Chapters 12 and 18).

---

*Avery JL: *A brief discussion of adoptive-nursing: an introduction to the topic,* rev ed, Athens, Tenn, 1998, Lact-Aid International, Inc; and Avery JL: *Induced lactation: a guide for counseling and management,* rev ed, Athens, Tenn, 1998, Lact-Aid International, Inc., P.O. Box 1066, Athens, TN 37371-1066, USA.

$\mathcal{M}$anual expression of breast milk

The health care professional should be familiar with the technique of manual expression and be able to diagnose improper technique.

EXPRESSION OF BREAST MILK

All breastfeeding women should be familiar with the basic technique of manual expression of milk from the breast, and ideally this technique is acquired before discharge from the hospital and with the assistance of the nursery or postpartum nursing staff.

Reasons to express breast milk include the following:

1. Initiating flow to assist the infant to grasp the breast properly
2. Early in lactation when the infant is premature or ill
3. To relieve engorgement
4. To remove milk when it is not possible to nurse the infant at a given feeding
5. To maintain lactation when the infant cannot be fed
6. To pump and save milk for feeding the infant at another time

7. To contribute to a milk bank
8. To pump and discard milk while temporarily on a specific medication

Manual expression is appropriate to initiate the flow before applying a hand pump or an electric pump. Not many women can manually pump large volumes over time without mechanical assistance.

Procedure

Step 1. *Always* wash hands before handling the breast.

Step 2. Breast massage: whether planning to manually express or mechanically pump, preparing the breast for ejecting the milk facilitates the process. The release of oxytocin and the ejection reflex are stimulated by external stimuli: the baby's cry, a picture of the baby, or gentle handling of the breast. Prolactin release and milk production are stimulated by "sucking" stimulation.

After mother finds a comfortable sitting position and is relaxed, the breast is exposed and gently stroked with the fingertips from periphery to areola (Fig. G-1). As this stroking is intensified, one should avoid slipping the hand across skin and irritating tissues. Gently massage. A warm washcloth soak is also helpful in initiating flow through the ducts. Gentle fingertip massage around all quadrants should follow and be repeated several

Modified from Chele Marmet and The Lactation Institute and Breastfeeding Clinic, 16161 Ventura Blvd., Suite 223, Encino, CA 91436.

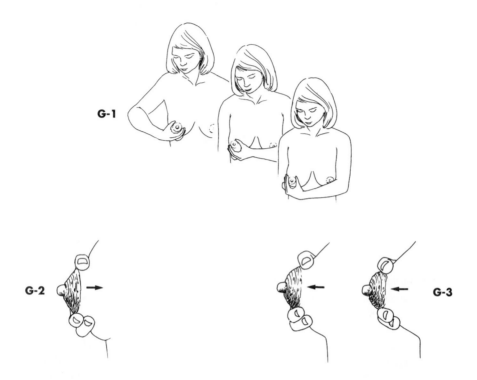

times during extended mechanical pumping. It should not leave red marks or hurt.

Step 3. Position hands on the breast—usually placing the fingers below and thumb on top is natural for most women. One hand placed above and one hand placed below the areola may be easier when the hand is small compared with breast size. The target area is beyond the ampullae, which are the collecting areas of the main ducts that radiate out from the nipple to the areola. The ampullae are about 3 cm from the nipple base, which may not be at the edge of the areola. Press toward the chest wall and then compress the thumb and fingers together (Fig. G-2). Continue to compress the breast while moving the hand away from the chest wall in a "milking" action toward the nipple (Fig. G-3). (Avoid pulling, squeezing, or rubbing motions.) Perform this motion in a repeated rhythmic manner at a comfortable but not abrasive rate. Infant sucking does not involve movement (stroking) of the tongue along the

elongated areola and nipple, but an undulating motion of the tongue itself. Simulating that motion is the goal of manual expression. This action is similar to a peristaltic motion. The hand should be rotated around the breast to massage and stroke all quadrants, including the periphery and the axillae.

Use one or both hands to find the most productive grasp. Preventing trauma is essential, thus avoid squeezing, rubbing, or pulling the breast tissue. Every mother develops her own natural pattern, thus rigid adherence to methods may be counterproductive. Effectiveness is measured by the comfortable release of milk.

Total emptying of the breast will require 20 to 30 minutes of manual stimulation. Warm compresses, hot showers, or suspending the breast in a bowl of warm water may help, especially if there is engorgement or mastitis. Leaning over and gently shaking the breast may help stimulate flow. Manual expression while leaning over may help empty the lower quadrants.

$\mathcal{T}$he storage of human milk*

HUMAN MILK BANKING AND THE HMBANA

The Human Milk Banking Association of North America (HMBANA) was established in 1985, drawing together representatives of donor milk banks and members of the medical community. The goals of HMBANA are to:

1. Provide a forum for networking among experts in the field on issues relating to human milk banking
2. Provide information to the medical community on the benefits and appropriate uses of banked human milk
3. Develop and annually review guidelines for milk banking practices in North America
4. Communicate among member milk banks to ensure adequate supplies for all patients
5. Encourage research into the unique properties of human milk and its uses
6. Act as a liaison between member institutions and governmental regulatory agencies

WHAT IS A HUMAN MILK BANK?

A donor human milk bank is a service established for the purpose of collecting, screening, processing, storing, and distributing donated human milk to meet the specific medical needs of

*From the Human Milk Banking Association of North America, 8 Jan Sebastian Way, Sandwich, MA 02563, (508) 888-4041.

individuals for whom human milk is prescribed by physicians.

A small processing fee is charged by each milk bank on a per-ounce basis.

HOW DOES A HUMAN MILK BANK OPERATE?

Donor human milk banks solicit lactating mothers to donate milk. Donors are carefully screened for health behaviors and tested for communicable diseases before they are accepted as donors.

Donors are taught how to express their milk using sanitary collecting methods.

Donated milk is heat treated to destroy any bacteria or viruses that may be present.

Frozen, heat-treated milk is dispensed to recipients with a medical need for donor milk. A physician's prescription is required.

FREQUENT REASONS FOR PRESCRIBING DONOR MILK

Nutritional uses

Prematurity
Failure to thrive
Malabsorption syndromes
Short-gut syndrome
Renal failure
Feeding intolerance

Inborn errors of metabolism
Postsurgical nutrition
Cardiac problems
Bronchopulmonary dysplasia
Pediatric burn cases

Medicinal/therapeutic uses

Treatment for infectious diseases such as intractable diarrhea, gastroenteritis, infantile botulism, sepsis, pneumonia, and hemorrhagic conjunctivitis
Postsurgical healing (omphalocele, gastroschisis, intestinal obstruction/bowel fistula, colostomy repair)
Immunodeficiency diseases (severe allergies, IgA deficiencies)
Inborn errors of metabolism
Solid-organ transplants (including adults)
Noninfectious intestinal disorders (ulcerative colitis, irritable bowel syndrome)

Preventive uses

Necrotizing enterocolitis
Crohn's disease
Colitis
Allergies to bovine and soy milks/feeding intolerance
During immune suppression therapy

DONOR MILK BANKS IN THE UNITED STATES, CANADA, AND MEXICO

Mothers' Milk Bank
c/o Professional Group
P. O. Box 5730
San Jose, CA 95150
(408) 998-4550

Triangle Mothers' Milk Bank
Wake Medical Center
3000 New Bern Avenue
Raleigh, NC 27610
(919) 250-8599

Wilmington Mothers' Milk Bank
Christiana Hospital
P. O. Box 1665
Wilmington, DE 19579
(302) 733-2340

Mothers' Milk Bank
P/SL Medical Center
1719 East 19th Avenue
Denver, CO 80218
(303) 869-1888

Community Human Milk Bank
Georgetown University Hospital
3800 Reservoir Road
Washington, DC 20007
(202) 784-6455

Regional Milk Bank
UMass/Memorial Medical Center
119 Belmont Street
Worcester, MA 01605
(508) 793-6005

Lactation Support Service
BC Children's Hospital
4480 Oak Street
Vancouver, BC V6H 3V4, Canada
(604) 875-2345, ext. 7607

Banco de Leche Humana
Hospital Amigo del Nino y de la Madre
Centro de Especialidades Medicas Dr. Rafael Lucio
Av Ruiz Cortinez No. 2903
CP 91020, Xalapa, Veracruz, Mexico
52-55-14-45-00

DEFINITIONS

Human milk bank   A human milk bank is a service established for the purpose of collecting, screening, processing, storing, and distributing donated human milk to meet the specific needs of individuals for whom human milk is prescribed by physicians.

Donor milk   Donor milk is voluntarily given by women other than the biologic mother of the recipient.

Preparations

Fresh-raw milk   Milk stored continuously at approximately 4° C for use not longer than 72 hours after expression

Fresh-frozen milk   Fresh-raw milk that has been frozen and held at approximately −20° C for not longer than 12 months

Heat-processed milk   Fresh-raw and/or fresh-frozen milk that has been heated to a minimum of 56° C for 30 minutes

Pooled milk   Milk received from more than one donor

DONOR SELECTION

Definition of a donor

1. Acceptable donors shall be healthy lactating women.
2. The standards of the American Association of Blood Banks for screening donors will be used to determine donor eligibility.
3. Potential donors shall be given educational materials informing them of the characteristics of the high-risk groups or activities that might put them at risk for transmitting blood-borne diseases.

Exclusions

1. Potential donors shall be excluded on the basis of the following:
   a. Receipt of a blood transfusion or blood products within the last 12 months
   b. Regular use of more than 2 oz of hard liquor or its equivalent in 24 hours (Institute of Medicine, 1991)
   c. Regular use of over-the-counter medications or systemic prescriptions, including birth control pills (replacement hormones are acceptable)
   d. Use of megadose vitamins and/or pharmacologically active herbal preparations
   e. Total vegetarians (vegans) who do not supplement their diet with vitamins
   f. Use of illegal drugs
2. A history of hepatitis, systemic disorders of any kind, or chronic infections, (e.g., HIV-I, HTLV-I, tuberculosis, or Epstein-Barr virus), will be sufficient to exclude donation of milk.

Temporary disqualification

Donors shall be instructed to report all infections in the household to the milk bank.

1. Active donors shall be temporarily disqualified from donating milk under the following conditions:
   a. During any acute infection, including clinical mastitis or monilial and fungal infections of the nipple or the breast
   b. During the 4-week period after a case of rubella in the household
   c. During the 4 weeks after the administration of an attenuated virus vaccine to the mother (e.g., polio, measles, mumps, rubella)
   d. During a reactivation of latent infection with herpes simplex virus (HSV) or varicella-zoster
   e. During the 12-hour period after consumption of alcohol (hard liquor, beer, or wine)
2. Any consumption of over-the-counter medication shall be reported to the milk bank

Guidelines for the Establishment and Operation of a Donor Human Milk Bank are available in English from HMBANA for a fee. A Spanish translation is also available on request at no additional cost. The guidelines are reviewed and revised annually. For further information or a copy of the guidelines contact:

HMBANA
Lois D.W. Arnold, MPH, IBCLC
Executive Director
8 Jan Sebastian Way
Sandwich, MA 02563
(508) 888-4041; (888) 232-8809

Recommendations for collection, storage, and handling of a mother's milk for her own infant in the hospital setting can be obtained from the same address.

GUIDELINES FOR STORAGE AND HANDLING MOTHER'S OWN MILK AT HOME

Guidelines for providing the mother's own milk for a hospitalized infant are more stringent than pumping and storing milk for infant feeding in mother's absence at home or at day care.

BOX H-1   Suggestions for milk storage for infant at home

- Wash hands thoroughly.
- Polyethylene bags are acceptable for home use.
- Refrigerate or freeze milk after expressing.
- Use fresh milk whenever possible.
- Freeze milk that will not be used within 2 days.
- Use milk stored in a self-defrosting freezer within 3 months (top of refrigerator).
- Use milk stored in a deep-freeze within 12 months.
- Use the oldest milk first. Date container at time of collection.

When it is not possible for the infant to breastfeed directly, using the mother's fresh or frozen but not heat-treated milk ensures optimal nutritional and immunologic benefits. This milk is handled somewhat differently from donor milk distributed from a bank to an unrelated recipient. Very little special handling of a mother's milk is required. It is important for health professionals not to make storage and handling instructions intimidating or to cause anxiety for the mother by implying that there is great risk of harming the infant if the instructions are not followed.

Handwashing

As with handling any food, clean hands are a key to providing safe milk. Mothers should wash their hands with warm, soapy water before handling their breasts or any equipment or containers.

Containers

Breast milk can be stored in either glass or plastic containers. There are three kinds of plastic containers: clear, hard bottles (polycarbonate); frosted,

---

TABLE H-1   Storage of human milk for home use

Breast milk	Room temperature	Refrigerator	Freezer
Freshly expressed into closed container	6-8 hr (78° F or lower)	3-5 days (39° F or lower)	2 weeks in freezer compartment inside refrigerator 3 months in freezer section of refrigerator with separate door 6-12 months in deep freeze (0° F or lower)
Previously frozen—thawed in refrigerator but not warmed or used	4 hr or less (i.e., next feeding)	Store in refrigerator 24 hr	Do not refreeze
Thawed outside refrigerator in warm water	For completion of feeding	Hold for 4 hr or until next feeding	Do not refreeze
Infant has begun feeding	Only for completion of feeding; then discard	Discard	Discard

Developed from *Recommendations of The Milk Banking Association of North America, Inc.* and current literature. See References, Chapter 20.

flexible bottles (polypropylene); and plastic bags (polyethylene). Any storage causes some loss of protective factors. Although no data are available on the effects of polycarbonate bottles, there are no documented deleterious effects from using them. Glass or polypropylene containers have significant advantages over polyethylene bags in maintaining the stability of the properties in human milk, particularly sIgA, which survives freezing and offers significant protection to the infant (see Chapter 20). The mother expressing milk for a baby at home can chill the milk each time and then add it to a bottle containing already-frozen milk. This is called "layering."

Storage

Untreated expressed breast milk can be bacteriologically safe after sitting at room temperature for up to 8 hours (Table H-1); however, the potential for contamination is greater when any milk is not refrigerated. Therefore where refrigeration is available, it is advisable to store milk in a refrigerator (4° C/39° F). Various studies support storing milk at 4° C from 24 hours to 5 days without increasing bacterial contamination and retaining some cell viability.

Refrigerated milk separates. The skim milk near the bottom of the container may look quite watery, a layer of whole milk will lie in the middle, and the hind milk (cream) will form a dense top layer. Shake the container vigorously to mix the milk before feeding the baby.

Milk can be kept for 3 months in a self-defrosting freezer. It is best to store the milk in the back of the freezer, but not on the bottom, because this area warms during the defrost cycle. Milk can be kept for 12 months in a freezer without a defrost cycle that maintains a temperature of 0° F (−20° C).

STANDARDS FOR COLLECTION AND USE OF MOTHER'S OWN MILK WHEN MOTHER AND INFANT ARE SEPARATED*

In a public institution, hospital, day-care center, or health clinic, universal precautions are mandated whenever handling body fluids, including human milk. Gloves shall be worn. Handwashing after exposure should be carried out as soon as gloves are removed. Strict handwashing is required before and after feeding an infant, whether mother's milk or infant formula is used. Bottles of fresh or frozen mother's milk should be returned to the mother by the caregiver even if the infant has begun to feed from the container. Bottle propping is not permitted.

*Excerpts from *Caring for Our Children, National Health and Safety Performance Standards: Guidelines for Out-of-Home Child Care Programs,* pp 74-78, 117-120, 1992.

Vitamin and mineral supplement needs in normal children in the United States*

GUIDELINES FOR SUPPLEMENTATION

Table I-1 summarizes the following guidelines for the use of supplements in healthy infants and children. The indications for vitamin K and fluoride are discussed in the text only.

Newborn infants

Vitamin K administration to all newborn infants is effective as a prophylaxis against hemorrhagic disease of the newborn. This 1961 recommendation was strongly reaffirmed in 1971 to prevent or minimize the postnatal decline of the vitamin K–dependent coagulation factors (II, VII, IX, and X). Vitamin K_1 is considered the vitamin derivative of choice in a single, intramuscular dose of 0.5 to 1 mg or an oral dose of 1.0 to 2.0 mg. In some instances, the dose may have to be repeated after about 4 to 7 days. The more fat in the milk, the higher the vitamin K level. Enhancing fat level in the milk should be encouraged.

Breastfed infants

The renewed emphasis on human milk as an ideal food has raised the question whether breastfed infants require any vitamin or mineral supplements before the introduction of solid foods. This subject bears further discussion, particularly with respect to the most widely used supplements: vitamins A, C, D, and E, iron, and fluoride.

Rickets is uncommon in the breastfed term infant, despite the fact that human breast milk appears to contain small amounts of vitamin D (i.e., about 22 IU/L). One possible explanation is that the vitamin D in breast milk is in the form of an easily absorbed sulfate analogue, but this needs to be confirmed. The antirachitic properties of breast milk seem to be adequate for the normal term infant of a well-nourished mother. However, if the mother's vitamin D nutrition has been inadequate and if the infant does not benefit from adequate ultraviolet light (because of dark skin color and/or little exposure to light), supplements of 400 IU of vitamin D daily may be indicated.

Vitamin A deficiency rarely occurs in breastfed infants. Historically, vitamin A supplementation was coupled with vitamin D supplementation because both were provided by cod liver oil. Currently, there is little reason to provide vitamin A supplements; thus there would be no harm in

*Modified from American Academy of Pediatrics Committee on Nutrition: *Pediatrics* 66:1015, 1980. Copyright American Academy of Pediatrics, 1980.

TABLE I-1 Guidelines for use of supplements in healthy infants and children*		Vitamins			Minerals
Child	Multivitamin-multimineral	D	E	Folate	Iron
Term infants					
Breastfed	0	±	0	0	±†
Formula fed with iron fortified	0	0	0	0	0
Preterm infants					
Breastfed‡	+‡	+	±§	±‡	+
Formula fed with iron fortified‡	+‡	+	±§	±‡	+†
Older infants (after 6 mo)					
Normal	0	0	0	0	±†
High-risk‖	+	0	0	0	±
Children					
Normal	0	0	0	0	0
High-risk	+	0	0	0	0
Pregnant teenager					
Normal	±	0	0	±	+
High-risk¶	+	0	0	+	+

*Symbols indicate: +, that a supplement is usually indicated; ±, that it is possibly or sometimes indicated; 0, that it is not usually indicated. Vitamin K for newborn infants and fluoride in areas where there is insufficient fluoride in the water supply are not shown.

†Iron-fortified formula and/or infant cereal is a more convenient and reliable source of iron than a supplement.

‡Multivitamin supplement (plus added folate) is needed primarily when calorie intake is below approximately 300 kcal/day or when the infant weighs 2.5 kg; vitamin D should be supplied at least until 6 months of age in breastfed infants. Iron should be started by 2 months of age (see text).

§Vitamin E should be in a form that is well absorbed by small, premature infants. If this form of vitamin E is approved for use in formulas, it need not be given separately to formula-fed infants. Infants fed breast milk are less susceptible to vitamin E deficiency.

‖Multivitamin-multimineral preparation (including iron) is preferred to use of iron alone.

§Multivitamin-multimineral preparation (including iron and folate) is preferred to use of iron alone or iron and folate alone.

omitting vitamin A from supplements designed to provide vitamin D for infants who are breastfed. Similarly, there is no evidence that supplementation with vitamin E is needed for the normal breastfed term infant.

Vitamin B$_{12}$ deficiency has been reported in breastfed infants of strict vegetarian mothers, but this is relatively rare in North America. The report of a 6-month-old infant of a vegan mother with severe megaloblastic anemia and coma is a reminder that the maternal diet strongly influences the concentration of certain water-soluble vitamins in breast milk. Thiamin deficiency can also occur in breastfed infants of thiamin-deficient mothers, but this situation is virtually restricted to infants in developing countries. In the United States, the rare breastfed infants of mothers who are themselves malnourished should receive multivitamin supplements.

Iron deficiency rarely develops before 4 to 6 months of age in breastfed infants because neonatal iron stores can supply the major portion of iron needs during this period. Although breast milk may contain little more than 0.3 mg iron per liter, about half of this iron is absorbed in contrast to the much smaller proportion that is assimilated from other foods. This iron helps to delay the depletion of neonatal iron stores, but other sources of iron are required in midinfancy. In normal, breastfed term infants, the addition to the diet of iron-fortified cereal after 6 months of age probably is desirable to supply adequate amounts of iron.

The supplementation of fluoride in the diet of a healthy breastfed infant is no longer recommended by the Academy of Pediatrics. Evidence supports the contention that there is adequate fluoride in human milk, and fluorosis from excessive amounts is a concern.

The Committee on Nutrition* stated in 1986, "It may not be necessary to give fluoride supplements to breastfed infants who are living in an area where water is adequately fluoridated."

Formula-fed term infants

Infants consuming adequate amounts of commercial cow's-milk formulas that are in keeping with the recommendations of the Committee do not need vitamin and mineral supplementation in the first 6 months of life. They do not require supplements during the latter part of the first year if formula continues to be used in appropriate combination with solid foods. After 4 months of age, iron-fortified formula and/or iron-fortified cereal are convenient sources of iron and are preferable to the use of iron supplements. If powdered or concentrated formula is used, fluoride supplements should be administered only if the community water contains less than 0.3 ppm of fluoride. Ready-to-use formulas are now manufactured with water low in fluoride, and recommendations for fluoride supplementation should be individualized by the pediatrician to provide a total of 0.5 g per day.

Vitamin K deficiency is seen occasionally in infants. It is usually associated with diarrhea and especially with the administration of antibiotics, through a decrease in the synthesis of vitamin K by the intestinal microflora. In the past, the feeding of soy or other non–milk-based formulas was associated with vitamin K deficiency and was related in part to the type of oil used in the formula. In 1976

---

*From the Committee on Nutrition, American Academy of Pediatrics: Fluoride supplementation, *Pediatrics* 77:758, 1986. If the water supply contains less than 0.3 ppm of fluoride, the infant can be supplemented with 0.25 mg fluoride daily.

the Committee recommended that all infant formulas, particularly non–milk-based formulas, be required to contain an appropriate level of vitamin K.

Preterm infants

The needs of preterm infants for certain nutrients are proportionately greater than those of term infants because of the increased demands of a more rapid rate of growth and less complete intestinal absorption.

During the first weeks of life (before consumption of about 300 kcal per day or reaching a body weight of 2.5 kg), a multivitamin supplement that provides the equivalent of the RDAs for term infants should be supplied. The components of this supplement should ideally include vitamin E in a form well absorbed by preterm infants, such as d-α-tocopheryl polyethylene glycol 1000 succinate. Folic acid deficiency has been reported in preterm infants, and folic acid should be included in the regimen. Folic acid is not in liquid multivitamin-multimineral mixes because of its lack of stability. However, because the period of administration will generally be in a hospital, folate can be added to a multivitamin preparation in the hospital pharmacy in a concentration to provide 0.1 mg (the U.S. RDA) per daily dose. The shelf life should be limited to 1 month, and the label should read "shake well" because folate will gradually precipitate. Iron supplementation is best delayed until after the first few weeks of life because extra iron may predispose an infant to anemia when there is insufficient absorption of vitamin E. Neonatal iron stores are still abundant, and iron needs for erythropoiesis are relatively small during the physiologic postnatal decline in hemoglobin concentration.

After several weeks of age, when the infant is consuming more than 300 kcal/day or when the body weight exceeds 2.5 kg, a multivitamin supplement is no longer needed, but it is a convenient method for providing the few specific nutrients that still may be required. These include vitamin D, iron, and possibly folic acid.

There have been sporadic reports of rickets,

particularly in breastfed premature infants. This probably results from the low phosphorus content of breast milk, which has only 150 mg/L in contrast to about 450 mg/L in formulas. The condition is also correctable with phosphate supplementation. However, there is also evidence that vitamin D supplementation is helpful. Iron is required at a level of 2 mg/kg/day beginning at 2 months of age because neonatal iron stores may become depleted earlier than in term infants—before it is appropriate to supply iron in the form of fortified solid foods. Iron-fortified formula also supplies sufficient iron for the prevention of iron deficiency in preterm infants.

$\mathscr{M}$easurements of growth of breastfed infants*

TABLE J-1	**Weight (kg) by age of breastfed boys ages 0 to 12 months**															

Age (mo)	Mean	SD	Z-score												
			−3.0	−2.5	−2.0	−1.5	−1.0	−0.5	0.0	0.5	1.0	1.5	2.0	2.5	3.0
0	3.49	0.40	2.28	2.48	2.68	2.89	3.09	3.29	3.49	3.69	3.89	4.09	4.29	4.49	4.69
1	4.58	0.49	3.11	3.36	3.60	3.84	4.09	4.33	4.58	4.82	5.06	5.31	5.55	5.80	6.04
2	5.50	0.57	3.81	4.09	4.37	4.65	4.94	5.22	5.50	5.78	6.07	6.35	6.63	6.92	7.20
3	6.28	0.63	4.38	4.70	5.01	5.33	5.65	5.97	6.28	6.60	6.92	7.24	7.55	7.87	8.19
4	6.94	0.70	4.85	5.20	5.55	5.89	6.24	6.59	6.94	7.29	7.63	7.98	8.33	8.68	9.02
5	7.48	0.75	5.24	5.61	5.98	6.36	6.73	7.11	7.48	7.85	8.23	8.60	8.98	9.35	9.72
6	7.93	0.79	5.55	5.95	6.35	6.74	7.14	7.53	7.93	8.33	8.72	9.12	9.51	9.91	10.3
7	8.30	0.83	5.82	6.23	6.65	7.06	7.47	7.89	8.30	8.72	9.13	9.54	9.96	10.4	10.8
8	8.62	0.86	6.05	6.48	6.91	7.33	7.76	8.19	8.62	9.04	9.47	9.90	10.3	10.8	11.2
9	8.89	0.87	6.26	6.70	7.14	7.58	8.01	8.45	8.89	9.32	9.76	10.2	10.6	11.1	11.5
10	9.13	0.88	6.48	6.92	7.36	7.81	8.25	8.69	9.13	9.57	10.0	10.5	10.9	11.3	11.8
11	9.37	0.89	6.71	7.15	7.60	8.04	8.48	8.93	9.37	9.81	10.3	10.7	11.1	11.6	12.0
12	9.62	0.88	6.97	7.41	7.85	8.29	8.73	9.17	9.62	10.1	10.5	10.9	11.4	11.8	12.3

*From World Health Organization, 1994.

TABLE J-2	**Weight (kg) by age of breastfed girls ages 0 to 12 months**													

Age (mo)	Mean	SD	Z-score												
			−3.0	−2.5	−2.0	−1.5	−1.0	−0.5	0.0	0.5	1.0	1.5	2.0	2.5	3.0
0	3.44	0.37	2.32	2.51	2.69	2.88	3.06	3.25	3.44	3.62	3.81	3.99	4.18	4.37	4.55
1	4.35	0.45	2.98	3.21	3.44	3.67	3.89	4.12	4.35	4.57	4.80	5.03	5.25	5.48	5.71
2	5.14	0.53	3.55	3.82	4.08	4.34	4.61	4.87	5.14	5.40	5.67	5.93	6.20	6.46	6.73
3	5.82	0.60	4.03	4.33	4.63	4.93	5.23	5.52	5.82	6.12	6.42	6.72	7.02	7.32	7.62
4	6.41	0.66	4.43	4.76	5.09	5.42	5.75	6.08	6.41	6.74	7.07	7.40	7.73	8.06	8.39
5	6.92	0.72	4.77	5.13	5.48	5.84	6.20	6.56	6.92	7.27	7.63	7.99	8.35	8.70	9.06
6	7.35	0.76	5.05	5.44	5.82	6.20	6.58	6.96	7.35	7.73	8.11	8.49	8.87	9.26	9.64
7	7.71	0.81	5.29	5.70	6.10	6.50	6.91	7.31	7.71	8.12	8.52	8.92	9.33	9.73	10.1
8	8.03	0.84	5.50	5.93	6.35	6.77	7.19	7.61	8.03	8.45	8.87	9.29	9.71	10.1	10.6
9	8.31	0.87	5.69	6.13	6.56	7.00	7.44	7.87	8.31	8.74	9.18	9.61	10.0	10.5	10.9
10	8.55	0.89	5.87	6.32	6.77	7.21	7.66	8.11	8.55	9.00	9.45	9.89	10.3	10.8	11.2
11	8.78	0.91	6.06	6.51	6.97	7.42	7.87	8.33	8.78	9.24	9.69	10.1	10.6	11.1	11.5
12	9.00	0.92	6.25	6.71	7.17	7.63	8.09	8.55	9.00	9.46	9.92	10.4	10.8	11.3	11.8

| TABLE J-3 | | Length (cm) by age of breastfed boys ages 1 to 12 months | | | | | | | | | | | | | |

| Age (mo) | Mean | SD | Z-score | | | | | | | | | | | | |
			−3.0	−2.5	−2.0	−1.5	−1.0	−0.5	0.0	0.5	1.0	1.5	2.0	2.5	3.0
1	55.0	1.9	49.2	50.1	51.1	52.1	53.1	54.0	55.0	56.0	56.9	57.9	58.9	59.8	60.8
2	58.5	1.9	52.7	53.7	54.6	55.6	56.5	57.5	58.5	59.4	60.4	61.3	62.3	63.3	64.2
3	61.4	1.9	55.6	56.6	57.6	58.5	59.5	60.4	61.4	62.3	63.3	64.2	65.2	66.1	67.1
4	63.8	1.9	58.1	59.0	60.0	60.9	61.9	62.8	63.8	64.7	65.7	66.6	67.6	68.6	69.5
5	65.8	1.9	60.0	61.0	62.0	62.9	63.9	64.8	65.8	66.7	67.7	68.7	69.6	70.6	71.5
6	67.5	1.9	61.7	62.6	63.6	64.6	65.5	66.5	67.5	68.4	69.4	70.4	71.3	72.3	73.3
7	68.9	2.0	63.0	64.0	65.0	66.0	67.0	67.9	68.9	69.9	70.9	71.8	72.8	73.8	74.8
8	70.2	2.0	64.2	65.2	66.2	67.2	68.2	69.2	70.2	71.2	72.2	73.2	74.2	75.2	76.2
9	71.4	2.0	65.3	66.3	67.3	68.3	69.3	70.4	71.4	72.4	73.4	74.4	75.4	76.5	77.5
10	72.6	2.1	66.3	67.3	68.4	69.4	70.5	71.5	72.6	73.6	74.6	75.7	76.7	77.8	78.8
11	73.8	2.1	67.4	68.5	69.5	70.6	71.7	72.8	73.8	74.9	76.0	77.1	78.1	79.2	80.3
12	75.3	2.2	68.6	69.7	70.8	71.9	73.0	74.2	75.3	76.4	77.5	78.6	79.7	80.8	81.9

| TABLE J-4 | | Length (cm) by age of breastfed girls ages 1 to 12 months | | | | | | | | | | | | | |

| Age (mo) | Mean | SD | Z-score | | | | | | | | | | | | |
			−3.0	−2.5	−2.0	−1.5	−1.0	−0.5	0.0	0.5	1.0	1.5	2.0	2.5	3.0
1	54.1	1.8	48.7	49.6	50.5	51.4	52.3	53.2	54.1	55.0	55.9	56.8	57.7	58.6	59.5
2	57.3	1.8	51.9	52.8	53.7	54.6	55.5	56.4	57.3	58.2	59.1	60.0	60.9	61.9	62.8
3	60.0	1.8	54.5	55.4	56.3	57.3	58.2	59.1	60.0	60.9	61.8	62.8	63.7	64.6	65.5
4	62.3	1.9	56.7	57.6	58.5	59.5	60.4	61.3	62.3	63.2	64.1	65.0	66.0	66.9	67.8
5	64.1	1.9	58.4	59.4	60.3	61.3	62.2	63.2	64.1	65.1	66.0	67.0	67.9	68.9	69.8
6	65.7	1.9	59.9	60.9	61.9	62.8	63.8	64.8	65.7	66.7	67.7	68.7	69.6	70.6	71.6
7	67.1	2.0	61.2	62.2	63.2	64.2	65.2	66.1	67.1	68.1	69.1	70.1	71.1	72.1	73.1
8	68.4	2.0	62.3	63.3	64.3	65.3	66.4	67.4	68.4	69.4	70.5	71.5	72.5	73.5	74.6
9	69.6	2.1	63.3	64.3	65.4	66.4	67.5	68.6	69.6	70.7	71.7	72.8	73.8	74.9	76.0
10	70.8	2.2	64.3	65.4	66.5	67.6	68.7	69.7	70.8	71.9	73.0	74.1	75.2	76.3	77.4
11	72.2	2.3	65.4	66.5	67.6	68.8	69.9	71.0	72.2	73.3	74.4	75.6	76.7	77.8	79.0
12	73.7	2.4	66.6	67.8	69.0	70.1	71.3	72.5	73.7	74.8	76.0	77.2	78.4	79.5	80.7

TABLE J-5   **Weight (kg) by length of breastfed boys ages 1 to 12 months**

Length (cm)	Z-score												
	−3.0	−2.5	−2.0	−1.5	−1.0	−0.5	0.0	0.5	1.0	1.5	2.0	2.5	3.0
50.0	2.70	2.80	2.90	3.01	3.12	3.23	3.35	3.47	3.59	3.72	3.86	4.00	4.14
50.5	2.79	2.89	3.00	3.11	3.22	3.34	3.46	3.59	3.72	3.86	4.00	4.15	4.30
51.0	2.87	2.98	3.09	3.21	3.33	3.45	3.58	3.72	3.85	4.00	4.15	4.30	4.46
51.5	2.96	3.07	3.19	3.31	3.44	3.57	3.70	3.84	3.99	4.14	4.30	4.46	4.63
52.0	3.05	3.16	3.29	3.41	3.54	3.68	3.82	3.97	4.12	4.28	4.45	4.62	4.79
52.5	3.14	3.26	3.39	3.52	3.65	3.80	3.95	4.10	4.26	4.42	4.60	4.78	4.96
53.0	3.23	3.35	3.49	3.62	3.77	3.91	4.07	4.23	4.40	4.57	4.75	4.94	5.13
53.5	3.32	3.45	3.59	3.73	3.88	4.03	4.19	4.36	4.54	4.72	4.91	5.10	5.31
54.0	3.41	3.55	3.69	3.84	3.99	4.15	4.32	4.50	4.68	4.87	5.06	5.27	5.48
54.5	3.50	3.64	3.79	3.95	4.11	4.28	4.45	4.63	4.82	5.02	5.22	5.43	5.65
55.0	3.59	3.74	3.90	4.06	4.22	4.40	4.58	4.77	4.96	5.17	5.38	5.60	5.83
55.5	3.69	3.84	4.00	4.17	4.34	4.52	4.71	4.90	5.11	5.32	5.54	5.77	6.01
56.0	3.78	3.94	4.11	4.28	4.46	4.64	4.84	5.04	5.25	5.47	5.70	5.94	6.19
56.5	3.88	4.04	4.21	4.39	4.58	4.77	4.97	5.18	5.40	5.63	5.86	6.11	6.37
57.0	3.98	4.14	4.32	4.50	4.70	4.89	5.10	5.32	5.54	5.78	6.03	6.28	6.55
57.5	4.07	4.25	4.43	4.62	4.81	5.02	5.24	5.46	5.69	5.94	6.19	6.45	6.73
58.0	4.17	4.35	4.54	4.73	4.93	5.15	5.37	5.60	5.84	6.09	6.35	6.63	6.91
58.5	4.27	4.45	4.65	4.85	5.06	5.27	5.50	5.74	5.99	6.25	6.52	6.80	7.09
59.0	4.37	4.56	4.76	4.96	5.18	5.40	5.64	5.88	6.14	6.40	6.68	6.97	7.27
59.5	4.47	4.66	4.86	5.08	5.30	5.53	5.77	6.02	6.28	6.56	6.84	7.14	7.45
60.0	4.57	4.77	4.98	5.19	5.42	5.66	5.90	6.16	6.43	6.71	7.01	7.31	7.63
60.5	4.67	4.87	5.09	5.31	5.54	5.78	6.04	6.30	6.58	6.87	7.17	7.48	7.81
61.0	4.77	4.98	5.20	5.43	5.66	5.91	6.17	6.44	6.73	7.02	7.33	7.65	7.99
61.5	4.87	5.08	5.31	5.54	5.79	6.04	6.31	6.58	6.87	7.18	7.49	7.82	8.17
62.0	4.97	5.19	5.42	5.66	5.91	6.17	6.44	6.73	7.02	7.33	7.65	7.99	8.34
62.5	5.07	5.30	5.53	5.78	6.03	6.30	6.57	6.86	7.17	7.48	7.81	8.16	8.52
63.0	5.18	5.41	5.64	5.89	6.15	6.42	6.71	7.00	7.31	7.64	7.97	8.33	8.69
63.5	5.28	5.51	5.76	6.01	6.27	6.55	6.84	7.14	7.46	7.79	8.13	8.49	8.86
64.0	5.38	5.62	5.87	6.13	6.40	6.68	6.97	7.28	7.60	7.94	8.29	8.65	9.03

Continued

TABLE J-5	Weight (kg) by length of breastfed boys ages 1 to 12 months—cont'd												

Length (cm)	Z-score												
	−3.0	−2.5	−2.0	−1.5	−1.0	−0.5	0.0	0.5	1.0	1.5	2.0	2.5	3.0
64.5	5.49	5.73	5.98	6.24	6.52	6.81	7.10	7.42	7.74	8.09	8.44	8.81	9.20
65.0	5.59	5.84	6.09	6.36	6.64	6.93	7.24	7.55	7.89	8.23	8.59	8.97	9.37
65.5	5.69	5.94	6.20	6.48	6.76	7.06	7.37	7.69	8.03	8.38	8.75	9.13	9.53
66.0	5.80	6.05	6.32	6.59	6.88	7.18	7.50	7.82	8.17	8.52	8.89	9.28	9.69
66.5	5.90	6.16	6.43	6.71	7.00	7.31	7.62	7.96	8.30	8.66	9.04	9.44	9.85
67.0	6.01	6.27	6.54	6.82	7.12	7.43	7.75	8.09	8.44	8.80	9.19	9.59	10.0
67.5	6.11	6.38	6.65	6.94	7.24	7.55	7.88	8.22	8.57	8.94	9.33	9.73	10.2
68.0	6.22	6.49	6.77	7.06	7.36	7.67	8.00	8.35	8.71	9.08	9.47	9.88	10.3
68.5	6.33	6.60	6.88	7.17	7.48	7.80	8.13	8.48	8.84	9.21	9.61	10.0	10.4
69.0	6.43	6.70	6.99	7.29	7.59	7.92	8.25	8.60	8.97	9.35	9.74	10.2	10.6
69.5	6.54	6.81	7.10	7.40	7.71	8.04	8.37	8.73	9.09	9.48	9.88	10.3	10.7
70.0	6.64	6.92	7.21	7.51	7.83	8.15	8.50	8.85	9.22	9.61	10.0	10.4	10.9
70.5	6.75	7.03	7.32	7.63	7.94	8.27	8.62	8.97	9.34	9.73	10.1	10.6	11.0
71.0	6.86	7.14	7.43	7.74	8.06	8.39	8.73	9.09	9.47	9.85	10.3	10.7	11.1
71.5	6.97	7.25	7.55	7.85	8.17	8.50	8.85	9.21	9.59	9.98	10.4	10.8	11.2
72.0	7.07	7.36	7.66	7.96	8.29	8.62	8.97	9.33	9.70	10.1	10.5	10.9	11.4
72.5	7.18	7.47	7.77	8.08	8.40	8.73	9.08	9.44	9.82	10.2	10.6	11.0	11.5
73.0	7.29	7.58	7.88	8.19	8.51	8.85	9.19	9.56	9.93	10.3	10.7	11.2	11.6
73.5	7.40	7.69	7.99	8.30	8.62	8.96	9.31	9.67	10.0	10.4	10.8	11.3	11.7
74.0	7.51	7.80	8.10	8.41	8.73	9.07	9.42	9.78	10.2	10.5	10.9	11.4	11.8
74.5	7.62	7.91	8.21	8.52	8.84	9.18	9.53	9.89	10.3	10.6	11.1	11.5	11.9
75.0	7.73	8.02	8.32	8.63	8.95	9.29.	9.63	9.99	10.4	10.8	11.2	11.6	12.0
75.5	7.84	8.13	8.43	8.74	9.06	9.39	9.74	10.1	10.5	10.9	11.3	11.7	12.1
76.0	7.96	8.24	8.54	8.85	9.17	9.50	9.84	10.2	10.6	11.0	11.3	11.8	12.2
76.5	8.07	8.35	8.65	8.96	9.28	9.61	9.95	10.3	10.7	11.0	11.4	11.8	12.3
77.0	8.18	8.47	8.76	9.07	9.38	9.71	10.0	10.4	10.8	11.1	11.5	11.9	12.3
77.5	8.30	8.58	8.87	9.18	9.49	9.81	10.2	10.5	10.9	11.2	11.6	12.0	12.4
78.0	8.41	8.69	8.98	9.28	9.60	9.92	10.2	10.6	10.9	11.3	11.7	12.1	12.5
78.5	8.53	8.81	9.09	9.39	9.70	10.0	10.3	10.7	11.0	11.4	11.8	12.2	12.6

TABLE J-6   Weight (kg) by length of breastfed girls ages 1 to 12 months

Length (cm)	−3.0	−2.5	−2.0	−1.5	−1.0	−0.5	0.0	0.5	1.0	1.5	2.0	2.5	3.0
50.0	2.77	2.88	2.98	3.09	3.20	3.32	3.44	3.56	3.69	3.82	3.96	4.11	4.25
50.5	2.85	2.96	3.07	3.18	3.30	3.42	3.55	3.68	3.81	3.95	4.10	4.25	4.40
51.0	2.93	3.04	3.16	3.27	3.40	3.52	3.66	3.79	3.93	4.08	4.23	4.39	4.56
51.5	3.01	3.13	3.25	3.37	3.50	3.63	3.77	3.91	4.06	4.21	4.37	4.54	4.71
52.0	3.09	3.21	3.34	3.47	3.60	3.74	3.88	4.03	4.19	4.35	4.52	4.69	4.87
52.5	3.18	3.30	3.43	3.56	3.70	3.85	4.00	4.15	4.31	4.48	4.66	4.84	5.03
53.0	3.26	3.39	3.52	3.66	3.81	3.96	4.11	4.27	4.44	4.62	4.80	4.99	5.19
53.5	3.34	3.48	3.62	3.76	3.91	4.07	4.23	4.40	4.57	4.76	4.95	5.14	5.35
54.0	3.43	3.57	3.71	3.86	4.02	4.18	4.35	4.52	4.71	4.90	5.09	5.30	5.51
54.5	3.51	3.66	3.81	3.96	4.12	4.29	4.47	4.65	4.84	5.04	5.24	5.45	5.68
55.0	3.60	3.75	3.90	4.06	4.23	4.41	4.59	4.78	4.97	5.18	5.39	5.61	5.84
55.5	3.69	3.84	4.00	4.17	4.34	4.52	4.71	4.90	5.11	5.32	5.54	5.77	6.01
56.0	3.78	3.93	4.10	4.27	4.45	4.63	4.83	5.03	5.24	5.46	5.69	5.93	6.18
56.5	3.86	4.03	4.20	4.37	4.56	4.75	4.95	5.16	5.38	5.60	5.84	6.09	6.34
57.0	3.95	4.12	4.30	4.48	4.67	4.87	5.07	5.29	5.51	5.75	5.99	6.25	6.51
57.5	4.04	4.22	4.40	4.58	4.78	4.98	5.20	5.42	5.65	5.89	6.14	6.41	6.68
58.0	4.13	4.31	4.50	4.69	4.89	5.10	5.32	5.55	5.79	6.04	6.30	6.57	6.85
58.5	4.22	4.41	4.60	4.80	5.00	5.22	5.45	5.68	5.93	6.18	6.45	6.73	7.02
59.0	4.32	4.50	4.70	4.90	5.12	5.34	5.57	5.81	6.06	6.33	6.60	6.89	7.19
59.5	4.41	4.60	4.80	5.01	5.23	5.46	5.69	5.94	6.20	6.47	6.75	7.05	7.36
60.0	4.50	4.70	4.90	5.12	5.34	5.58	5.82	6.07	6.34	6.62	6.91	7.21	7.52
60.5	4.60	4.80	5.01	5.23	5.46	5.70	5.95	6.21	6.48	6.76	7.06	7.37	7.69
61.0	4.69	4.90	5.11	5.34	5.57	5.82	6.07	6.34	6.62	6.91	7.21	7.53	7.86
61.5	4.78	5.00	5.22	5.44	5.68	5.94	6.20	6.47	6.75	7.05	7.36	7.69	8.03
62.0	4.88	5.10	5.32	5.55	5.80	6.06	6.32	6.60	6.89	7.20	7.51	7.84	8.19
62.5	4.98	5.20	5.42	5.66	5.91	6.18	6.45	6.73	7.03	7.34	7.66	8.00	8.35
63.0	5.07	5.30	5.53	5.77	6.03	6.30	6.57	6.86	7.17	7.48	7.81	8.16	8.52

Continued

TABLE J-6   Weight (kg) by length of breastfed girls ages 1 to 12 months—cont'd

Length (cm)	−3.0	−2.5	−2.0	−1.5	−1.0	−0.5	0.0	0.5	1.0	1.5	2.0	2.5	3.0
63.5	5.17	5.40	5.64	5.88	6.14	6.42	6.70	6.99	7.30	7.63	7.96	8.31	8.68
64.0	5.27	5.50	5.74	6.00	6.26	6.54	6.82	7.12	7.44	7.77	8.11	8.47	8.84
64.5	5.37	5.60	5.85	6.11	6.37	6.66	6.95	7.25	7.57	7.91	8.26	8.62	9.00
65.0	5.46	5.70	5.96	6.22	6.49	6.78	7.07	7.38	7.71	8.05	8.40	8.77	9.16
65.5	5.56	5.81	6.06	6.33	6.61	6.90	7.20	7.51	7.84	8.19	8.54	8.92	9.31
66.0	5.66	5.91	6.17	6.44	6.72	7.01	7.32	7.64	7.98	8.32	8.69	9.07	9.46
66.5	5.76	6.02	6.28	6.55	6.84	7.13	7.44	7.77	8.11	8.46	8.83	9.21	9.61
67.0	5.87	6.12	6.39	6.66	6.95	7.25	7.57	7.90	8.24	8.60	8.97	9.36	9.76
67.5	5.97	6.23	6.49	6.77	7.07	7.37	7.69	8.02	8.37	8.73	9.11	9.50	9.91
68.0	6.07	6.33	6.60	6.89	7.18	7.49	7.81	8.15	8.50	8.86	9.24	9.64	10.1
68.5	6.17	6.44	6.71	7.00	7.30	7.61	7.93	8.27	8.63	8.99	9.38	9.78	10.2
69.0	6.28	6.54	6.82	7.11	7.41	7.73	8.05	8.40	8.75	9.12	9.51	9.91	10.3
69.5	6.38	6.65	6.93	7.22	7.53	7.84	8.18	8.52	8.88	9.25	9.64	10.0	10.5
70.0	6.49	6.76	7.04	7.34	7.64	7.96	8.30	8.64	9.00	9.38	9.77	10.2	10.6
70.5	6.59	6.87	7.15	7.45	7.76	8.08	8.41	8.76	9.13	9.50	9.90	10.3	10.7
71.0	6.70	6.98	7.26	7.56	7.87	8.20	8.53	8.88	9.25	9.63	10.0	10.4	10.9
71.5	6.81	7.09	7.37	7.68	7.99	8.31	8.65	9.00	9.37	9.75	10.1	10.6	11.0
72.0	6.92	7.20	7.49	7.79	8.10	8.43	8.77	9.12	9.49	9.87	10.3	10.7	11.1
72.5	7.03	7.31	7.60	7.90	8.22	8.54	8.88	9.24	9.61	9.99	10.4	10.8	11.2
73.0	7.14	7.42	7.71	8.02	8.33	8.66	9.00	9.36	9.72	10.1	10.5	10.9	11.3
73.5	7.25	7.53	7.83	8.13	8.45	8.77	9.12	9.47	9.84	10.2	10.6	11.0	11.5
74.0	7.36	7.65	7.94	8.24	8.56	8.89	9.23	9.59	9.95	10.3	10.7	11.1	11.6
74.5	7.48	7.76	8.05	8.36	8.68	9.00	9.34	9.70	10.1	10.4	10.8	11.3	11.7
75.0	7.59	7.88	8.17	8.47	8.79	9.12	9.46	9.81	10.2	10.6	11.0	11.4	11.8
75.5	7.71	7.99	8.28	8.59	8.90	9.23	9.57	9.92	10.3	10.7	11.1	11.5	11.9
76.0	7.83	8.11	8.40	8.71	9.02	9.35	9.68	10.0	10.4	10.8	11.2	11.6	12.0
76.5	7.94	8.23	8.52	8.82	9.13	9.46	9.80	10.1	10.5	10.9	11.3	11.7	12.1

| TABLE J-7 | **Head circumference by age of breastfed boys ages 1 to 12 months** |

			Z-score													
Age (mo)	Mean	SD	−3.0	−2.5	−2.0	−1.5	−1.0	−0.5	0.0	0.5	1.0	1.5	2.0	2.5	3.0
1	38.1	1.0	35.0	35.5	36.0	36.6	37.1	37.6	38.1	38.7	39.2	39.7	40.2	40.8	41.3
2	40.0	1.1	36.8	37.3	37.8	38.4	38.9	39.4	40.0	40.5	41.0	41.5	42.1	42.6	43.1
3	41.4	1.1	38.2	38.7	39.3	39.8	40.3	40.9	41.4	41.9	42.5	43.0	43.6	44.1	44.6
4	42.6	1.1	39.3	39.9	40.4	41.0	41.5	42.1	42.6	43.1	43.7	44.2	44.8	45.3	45.9
5	43.6	1.1	40.3	40.8	41.4	41.9	42.5	43.0	43.6	44.1	44.7	45.2	45.8	46.4	46.9
6	44.4	1.1	41.0	41.6	42.2	42.7	43.3	43.8	44.4	45.0	45.5	46.1	46.6	47.2	47.8
7	45.1	1.1	41.7	42.3	42.8	43.4	44.0	44.5	45.1	45.7	46.2	46.8	47.4	47.9	48.5
8	45.7	1.2	42.2	42.8	43.4	44.0	44.5	45.1	45.7	46.3	46.8	47.4	48.0	48.6	49.2
9	46.2	1.2	42.7	43.3	43.9	44.5	45.1	45.6	46.2	46.8	47.4	48.0	48.6	49.1	49.7
10	46.7	1.2	43.1	43.7	44.3	44.9	45.5	46.1	46.7	47.3	47.9	48.5	49.0	49.6	50.2
11	47.1	1.2	43.5	44.1	44.7	45.3	45.9	46.5	47.1	47.7	48.3	48.9	49.5	50.1	50.7
12	47.5	1.2	43.9	44.5	45.1	45.7	46.3	46.9	47.5	48.1	48.7	49.3	49.9	50.5	51.1

| TABLE J-8 | **Head circumference by age of breastfed girls ages 1 to 12 months** |

			Z-score													
Age (mo)	Mean	SD	−3.0	−2.5	−2.0	−1.5	−1.0	−0.5	0.0	0.5	1.0	1.5	2.0	2.5	3.0
1	37.4	1.0	34.4	34.9	35.4	35.9	36.4	36.9	37.4	37.9	38.4	38.9	39.4	39.9	40.4
2	39.0	1.0	36.0	36.5	37.0	37.5	38.0	38.5	39.0	39.6	40.1	40.6	41.1	41.6	42.1
3	40.4	1.0	37.3	37.8	38.4	38.9	39.4	39.9	40.4	40.9	41.4	41.9	42.5	43.0	43.5
4	41.5	1.0	38.4	38.9	39.4	40.0	40.5	41.0	41.5	42.0	42.6	43.1	43.6	44.1	44.6
5	42.4	1.1	39.3	39.8	40.3	40.9	41.4	41.9	42.4	43.0	43.5	44.0	44.6	45.1	45.6
6	43.2	1.1	40.0	40.6	41.1	41.6	42.2	42.7	43.2	43.8	44.3	44.8	45.4	45.9	46.4
7	43.9	1.1	40.6	41.2	41.7	42.3	42.8	43.3	43.9	44.4	45.0	45.5	46.1	46.6	47.1
8	44.5	1.1	41.2	41.7	42.3	42.8	43.4	43.9	44.5	45.0	45.6	46.1	46.7	47.2	47.8
9	45.0	1.1	41.6	42.2	42.7	43.3	43.9	44.4	45.0	45.5	46.1	46.6	47.2	47.8	48.3
10	45.4	1.1	42.0	42.6	43.2	43.7	44.3	44.9	45.4	46.0	46.6	47.1	47.7	48.2	48.8
11	45.8	1.1	42.4	43.0	43.6	44.1	44.7	45.3	45.8	46.4	47.0	47.5	48.1	48.7	49.3
12	46.2	1.2	42.7	43.3	43.9	44.5	45.1	45.6	46.2	46.8	47.4	47.9	48.5	49.1	49.7

| TABLE J-9 | | 1-month weight increment (kg/mo) by age of breastfed boys ages 1 to 12 months | | | | | | | | | | | | | |

Interval (mo)	Mean	SD	Z-score												
			−3.0	−2.5	−2.0	−1.5	−1.0	−0.5	0.0	0.5	1.0	1.5	2.0	2.5	3.0
1-2	1.07	0.27	0.25	0.39	0.53	0.66	0.80	0.93	1.07	1.21	1.34	1.48	1.61	1.75	1.89
2-3	0.78	0.24	0.07	0.19	0.31	0.43	0.55	0.66	0.78	0.90	1.02	1.14	1.26	1.37	1.49
3-4	0.63	0.21	−0.00	0.10	0.21	0.31	0.42	0.52	0.63	0.73	0.83	0.94	1.04	1.15	1.25
4-5	0.53	0.19	−0.03	0.06	0.16	0.25	0.35	0.44	0.53	0.63	0.72	0.82	0.91	1.00	1.10
5-6	0.45	0.17	−0.07	0.02	0.11	0.19	0.28	0.37	0.45	0.54	0.63	0.71	0.80	0.89	0.97
6-7	0.33	0.16	−0.16	−0.08	0.00	0.09	0.17	0.25	0.33	0.41	0.50	0.58	0.66	0.74	0.82
7-8	0.34	0.16	−0.14	−0.06	0.02	0.10	0.18	0.26	0.34	0.42	0.50	0.58	0.66	0.74	0.82
8-9	0.29	0.16	−0.19	−0.11	−0.03	0.05	0.13	0.21	0.29	0.38	0.46	0.54	0.62	0.70	0.78
9-10	0.26	0.17	−0.25	−0.16	−0.08	0.01	0.09	0.18	0.26	0.35	0.43	0.52	0.60	0.69	0.77
10-11	0.22	0.18	−0.33	−0.24	−0.15	−0.05	0.04	0.13	0.22	0.31	0.40	0.50	0.59	0.68	0.77
11-12	0.25	0.20	−0.36	−0.26	−0.16	−0.05	0.05	0.15	0.25	0.35	0.45	0.56	0.66	0.76	0.86

| TABLE J-10 | | 1-month weight increment (kg/mo) by age of breastfed girls ages 1 to 12 months | | | | | | | | | | | | | |

Interval (mo)	Mean	SD	Z-score												
			−3.0	−2.5	−2.0	−1.5	−1.0	−0.5	0.0	0.5	1.0	1.5	2.0	2.5	3.0
1-2	0.86	0.23	0.18	0.30	0.41	0.52	0.63	0.75	0.86	0.97	1.08	1.20	1.31	1.42	1.53
2-3	0.69	0.20	0.08	0.18	0.28	0.38	0.48	0.58	0.69	0.79	0.89	0.99	1.09	1.19	1.29
3-4	0.60	0.18	0.05	0.14	0.23	0.32	0.41	0.50	0.60	0.69	0.78	0.87	0.96	1.05	1.15
4-5	0.52	0.17	0.01	0.10	0.18	0.27	0.35	0.44	0.52	0.61	0.69	0.78	0.86	0.95	1.03
5-6	0.42	0.16	−0.07	0.01	0.09	0.17	0.25	0.34	0.42	0.50	0.58	0.66	0.74	0.82	0.90
6-7	0.36	0.16	−0.11	−0.03	0.05	0.13	0.21	0.29	0.36	0.44	0.52	0.60	0.68	0.75	0.83
7-8	0.31	0.16	−0.16	−0.08	−0.01	0.07	0.15	0.23	0.31	0.38	0.46	0.54	0.62	0.70	0.77
8-9	0.25	0.16	−0.23	−0.15	−0.07	0.01	0.09	0.17	0.25	0.33	0.41	0.49	0.57	0.65	0.73
9-10	0.26	0.17	−0.24	−0.16	−0.08	0.01	0.09	0.18	0.26	0.34	0.43	0.51	0.60	0.68	0.76
10-11	0.21	0.18	−0.33	−0.24	−0.15	−0.06	0.03	0.12	0.21	0.30	0.39	0.48	0.57	0.66	0.75
11-12	0.19	0.20	−0.40	−0.30	−0.20	−0.11	−0.01	0.09	0.19	0.29	0.39	0.49	0.59	0.68	0.78

TABLE J-11   **1-month length increment (cm/mo) by age of breastfed boys ages 1 to 12 months**

Interval (mo)	Mean	SD	Z-score												
			−3.0	−2.5	−2.0	−1.5	−1.0	−0.5	0.0	0.5	1.0	1.5	2.0	2.5	3.0
1-2	3.40	0.84	0.89	1.31	1.73	2.14	2.56	2.98	3.40	3.82	4.24	4.66	5.08	5.50	5.92
2-3	3.00	0.78	0.66	1.05	1.44	1.83	2.22	2.61	3.00	3.40	3.79	4.18	4.57	4.96	5.35
3-4	2.34	0.74	0.14	0.50	0.87	1.24	1.61	1.97	2.34	2.71	3.08	3.44	3.81	4.18	4.55
4-5	2.16	0.70	0.06	0.41	0.76	1.11	1.46	1.81	2.16	2.51	2.86	3.21	3.56	3.91	4.26
5-6	1.62	0.67	−0.41	−0.07	0.27	0.60	0.94	1.28	1.62	1.95	2.29	2.63	2.96	3.30	3.64
6-7	1.42	0.66	−0.56	−0.23	0.10	0.43	0.76	1.09	1.42	1.75	2.08	2.41	2.74	3.07	3.40
7-8	1.14	0.65	−0.82	−0.49	−0.17	0.16	0.49	0.81	1.14	1.47	1.79	2.12	2.45	2.78	3.10
8-9	1.36	0.66	−0.61	−0.29	0.04	0.37	0.70	1.03	1.36	1.69	2.01	2.34	2.67	3.00	3.33
9-10	1.40	0.67	−0.61	−0.27	0.06	0.40	0.73	1.07	1.40	1.74	2.08	2.41	2.75	3.08	3.42
10-11	1.32	0.69	−0.76	−0.41	−0.06	0.28	0.63	0.98	1.32	1.67	2.02	2.37	2.71	3.06	3.41
11-12	1.30	0.73	−0.89	−0.52	−0.16	0.21	0.57	0.93	1.30	1.66	2.03	2.39	2.75	3.12	3.48

TABLE J-12   **1-month length increment (cm/mo) by age of breastfed girls ages 1 to 12 months**

Interval (mo)	Mean	SD	Z-score												
			−3.0	−2.5	−2.0	−1.5	−1.0	−0.5	0.0	0.5	1.0	1.5	2.0	2.5	3.0
1-2	3.12	0.74	0.90	1.27	1.64	2.01	2.38	2.75	3.12	3.49	3.86	4.23	4.60	4.97	5.34
2-3	2.80	0.71	0.66	1.01	1.37	1.73	2.08	2.44	2.80	3.15	3.51	3.87	4.22	4.58	4.94
3-4	2.31	0.69	0.25	0.59	0.94	1.28	1.62	1.97	2.31	2.66	3.00	3.35	3.69	4.04	4.38
4-5	1.79	0.67	−0.21	0.12	0.46	0.79	1.13	1.46	1.79	2.13	2.46	2.80	3.13	3.47	3.80
5-6	1.53	0.65	−0.43	−0.10	0.22	0.55	0.87	1.20	1.53	1.85	2.18	2.50	2.83	3.16	3.48
6-7	1.39	0.64	−0.52	−0.21	0.11	0.43	0.75	1.07	1.39	1.71	2.03	2.35	2.67	2.99	3.31
7-8	1.34	0.63	−0.55	−0.23	0.08	0.39	0.71	1.02	1.34	1.65	1.97	2.28	2.60	2.91	3.23
8-9	1.22	0.62	−0.65	−0.34	−0.03	0.29	0.60	0.91	1.22	1.53	1.84	2.15	2.47	2.78	3.09
9-10	1.34	0.62	−0.52	−0.21	0.10	0.41	0.72	1.03	1.34	1.65	1.96	2.27	2.58	2.89	3.20
10-11	1.36	0.62	−0.50	−0.19	0.12	0.43	0.74	1.05	1.36	1.67	1.98	2.29	2.60	2.92	3.23
11-12	1.21	0.62	−0.66	−0.35	−0.03	0.28	0.59	0.90	1.21	1.53	1.84	2.15	2.46	2.77	3.09

Organizations interested in supporting and providing materials for breastfeeding

GOVERNMENT AGENCIES

Food and Nutrition Information Center
National Agricultural Library Building
Room 304
Beltsville, MD 20705
(301) 344-3719

The center serves the information needs of people interested in human nutrition, nutrition education, food service management, consumer education, and food technology. It acquires and lends books, journal articles, and audiovisual materials dealing with these areas of concern, including breastfeeding research and education.

International Nutrition Communication Service
Education Development Center
55 Chapel Street
Newton, MA 02160
(617) 969-7100

Funded by the U.S. Agency for International Development, the service provides support and assistance in designing, implementing, and evalu-

ating nutrition training projects in Third World countries. It has also published the *Nutrition Training Manual Catalogue,* which contains reviews of 116 training manuals. The manuals focus on nutrition in developing countries. Breastfeeding training manuals are included.

National Health Information Clearinghouse
PO Box 1133
Washington, DC 20013
(703) 522-2590 (Metro-DC area)
(800) 336-4797 (outside Metro-DC area)

The Clearinghouse helps the public locate health information by identifying health information resources. Health questions are referred to appropriate health agencies that, in turn, respond directly to inquirers.

World Health Organization
Publications Center, USA
49 Sheridan Avenue
Albany, NY 12210
(518) 436-9686

Publications available include a statement on infant and young child feeding, a breastfeeding guide for use by community health workers, and a study on patterns of breastfeeding.

PRIVATE EDUCATIONAL AND SUPPORT ORGANIZATIONS

Best Start, Inc.*
3500 E. Fletcher Ave., Suite 308
Tampa, FL 33613
(813) 971-2119

Best Start, Inc. is a not-for-profit resource for the social marketing of and training in breastfeeding. The following description is provided by Carol Bryant, PhD, executive director.

Policy development

The Best Start approach calls for local and state coalitions to develop strategies for bringing about institutional and legal changes needed to overcome the barriers created by hospitals, employers, child care facilities and retailers. For example, the Florida Healthy Mothers, Healthy Babies Coalition has developed a set of model hospital policies and accompanying training module for use in enabling administrators and staff to improve the support that they offer breastfeeding mothers. Efforts are also underway to develop more supportive maternity benefits, provide training for child care providers, and encourage retailers to provide comfortable places for mothers to nurse in department stores and malls.

Other components

Other components of a comprehensive social marketing approach include community networking, product development, and public informa-

tion. Outreach to family and friends and the community at large is also important. Classes and activities can be used to provide the community with new information on breastfeeding's advantages and create a more supportive environment for nursing mothers. Many clinic-based programs offer special products such as gift certificates, t-shirts, diapers, shopping bags, and other incentives to breastfeeders. The WIC program is also exploring ways to enhance its food package and use other incentives to offset the draw of the free formula. For example, peer counselors can provide valuable support outside the hospital and clinic setting.

Finally, to increase the acceptance of breastfeeding among women, their families, and the public at large, Best Start has developed public service announcements (PSAs) for radio and television. These PSAs attempt to counter the misinformation and lack of confidence many women have, as well as present the many advantages that breastfeeding offers. News releases, newspaper articles, and advocate appearances on talk shows are also used to improve the image of breastfeeding in the wider society.

Birth and Life Bookstore, Inc.
PO Box 70625
Seattle, WA 98107
(206) 789-4444

The bookstore makes available a large selection of books and pamphlets on breastfeeding, childbirth, and parenting for mothers and health professionals. A 24-page newsletter (published quarterly), *Imprint,* is available free to customers. It contains a review of new publications and a catalog of those that are currently available. A sample newsletter can be obtained on request.

Clearinghouse on Infant Feeding and Maternal
   Nutrition
American Public Health Association
1015 Fifteenth Street, NW
Washington, DC 20005
(202) 789-5712

---

*All materials available in English and Spanish from Best Start, Inc.

The clearinghouse serves as a resource primarily for health professionals who work in Third World countries. They also respond to domestic requests as time and staffing permit. They have a large collection of materials of all types on breastfeeding. They make available bibliographies and lists of resources on a variety of topics, and refer inquiries to appropriate sources for information.

Health Education Associates
211 S. Easton Rd.
Glenside, PA 19038
(215) 659-1149

Health Education Associates make available inexpensive pamphlets and other materials as teaching aids on breastfeeding. They sponsor training programs for breastfeeding counseling and promotion techniques.

Healthy Children 2000
Lactation Associates
254 Conant Road
Weston, MA 021093-1756
(617) 893-3553

International Childbirth Education Association
PO Box 20048
Minneapolis, MN 55420
(800) 328-4815 (outside Minnesota)
(800) 752-4249 (Minnesota residents)

The association's *Bookmarks* catalog has a large selection of books and inexpensive pamphlets on breastfeeding, childbirth, and parenting. They publish *ICEA News,* with news about childbirth, prenatal, and parenting issues; and *ICEA Review,* which provides in-depth review of current perinatal issues. They also have a resource committee on breastfeeding.

Lact-Aid International, Inc.
PO Box 1066
Athens, TN 37371-1066
(615) 744-9090
www.lact-aid.com

Lact-Aid International, Inc. formerly published a quarterly journal, *Keeping Abreast, Journal of Human Nurturing.* They make available back issues of the journal and reprints of selected articles. They also produce and market the Lact-Aid Nursing Trainer and specialize in giving information and consultation on specific breastfeeding situations, including prematurity, relactation, adoptive nursing, and failure to thrive.

Also available is a special counseling service: LAMBS (Lact-Aid Mom's Buddies) are peer counselors ready to assist a mother with the same special problem. Resource LAMBS who have personal experience nursing infants with a variety of problems (e.g., cleft palate, Down syndrome) can be reached by calling the Lact-Aid hotline.

Lactation Institute and Breastfeeding Clinic
16161 Ventura Blvd., Suite 223
Encino, CA 91436
(818) 995-1913

La Leche League International, Inc.
1440 North Meacham Road
Schaumburg, IL 60173
(847) 519-7730; 1-800-LaLeche
La Leche League International Canadian Supply
    Depot
Box 39
Williamsburg, Ontario, Canada KOC 2HO

La Leche's publications catalog includes a large variety and broad scope of materials for mothers and health professionals to use in promoting and supporting breastfeeding. There is also a directory of League area coordinators by state and foreign country. The coordinators can give information about local support groups.

Nursing Mothers Counsel, Inc.
PO Box 50063
Palo Alto, CA 94303
(408) 272-1448

The counsel makes available a variety of publications on breastfeeding for mothers and health professionals.

Wellstart International
Corporate Headquarters
4062 First Avenue
San Diego, CA 92103
(619) 295-5192
FAX: (619) 294-7787

Wellstart International is a private, nonprofit organization dedicated to the global promotion of healthy families through breastfeeding. Its purpose is to promote breastfeeding for future generations, to expand and share knowledge and understanding of breastfeeding and its benefits to families throughout the world, and to provide leadership for global change.

Wellstart International uses the following methodologies to build on existing resources and ensure quality and sustainability:
• Knowledge and skill transfer
• Development of health professional faculty as core resources of in-country expertise
• Short- and long-term technical assistance, follow-up, and field support
• Assessment of infant feeding practices
• Program evaluation, impact appraisal, and trends monitoring
• Network development and utilization
• Policy and economic analyses
• Information dissemination, including publications and meetings
• Funding support for national program activities
These methodologies are used to spread knowledge, skills, and information in the following subject areas:
• Clinical lactation management
• Scientific fundamentals of lactation and breastfeeding
• Communication and social marketing
• Community outreach and mother-to-mother support
• Evaluation and research methodologies
• Education and training methodologies
Wellstart International manages the U.S. Agency for International Development (USAID) funded program, the Lactation Management Education (LME) Program, which is implemented from corporate headquarters in San Diego, California with funding from USAID's Office of Nutrition.

A variety of other activities are also carried out by the organization, including a federally funded education, evaluation, and curriculum development project. Clinical and educational services for local families are also provided at the San Diego facility.

Wellstart International has been designated as a WHO Collaborating Center on Breastfeeding Promotion and Protection, with particular emphasis on lactation management education. The organization has also been involved in a variety of global breastfeeding initiatives, including preparation for the Innocenti Declaration, the World Summit for Children, and the Baby-Friendly Hospital Initiative.

OTHER NATIONAL AND INTERNATIONAL BREASTFEEDING SUPPORT PROGRAMS

For information about Baby-Friendly Hospital Initiative, contact:
Baby Friendly, USA
Karin Cadwell, PhD
Lois Arnold, MPH
8 Jan Sebastian Way #13
Sandwich, MA 02563
(508) 888-8044
FAX: (508) 888-8050

The World Alliance for Breastfeeding Action (WABA) is a network of organizations and individuals dedicated to protecting, promoting, and supporting breastfeeding as a right of all children and women. For information, contact:
WABA Secretariat
World Alliance for Breastfeeding Action
PO Box 1200
10850 Penang
Malaysia
60-4-884-816
FAX: 60-4-872-655

Other international support organizations are:

Ammehejelpen
Postboks 15
Holmen, Oslo 3, Norway

Arbeitsgruppe and Dritte Welt
Postbach 1007
Bern 300, Switzerland

Association for Improvement of Maternity
   Services
61 Dartmouth Park Road
London NW 5, United Kingdom

Australian Lactation Consultants' Association Inc.
PO Box 192
Mawson Act 2607
(06) 290 1920
email: alcagalaxy@interact.net.au

Baby Foods Action Group
103 Gower Street
London WC1E 6AW, United Kingdom

Center for Science in the Public Interest
1779 Church Street, NW
Washington, DC 20036

National Childbirth Trust
Breast-feeding Promotion Group
9 Queensborough Terrace
London W2 3TB, United Kingdom

Nursing Mothers' Association of Australia
   (NMAA)
99 Burwood Road Box 231
Nanawading, Victoria, Australia 3131

Nursing Mothers Counsel, Inc.
PO Box 50063
Palo Alto, CA 94303

Parents Centres of Australia
148 Hereford Street
Forest Lodge, NSW, Australia 2229

War on Want
467 Caledonian Road
London N.7, United Kingdom

INTERNATIONAL ORGANIZATION FOR PHYSICIANS

Academy of Breastfeeding Medicine
PO Box 15945-284
Lenexa, KS 66285-5945
913-541-9077
FAX: 913-541-0156

The Academy of Breastfeeding Medicine is a worldwide organization of physicians dedicated to the promotion, protection, and support of breastfeeding and human lactation. Its mission is to unite into one association members of the various medical specialties with this common purpose. The academy's goals are:
- Physician education
- Expansion of knowledge in both breastfeeding science and human lactation
- Facilitation of optimal breastfeeding practices
- Encouragement of the exchange of information among organizations

LACTATION STUDY CENTER

Lactation Study Center—Encouraging and Promoting Breastfeeding*
   (716) 275-0088, 8 AM to 5 PM EST
   The Lactation Study Center at the University of Rochester Medical Center is a federally funded program that encourages and promotes human lactation and breastfeeding through physician education and support. The goal is to provide the information that will help the practitioner encourage and support breastfeeding for all patients.

*The Lactation Study Center was supported by Grant number MCJ 9104 from the Maternal and Child Health program (Title V, Social Security ACT), Health Resources and Service Administration, Department of Health and Human Services.

Ruth A. Lawrence, MD, Professor of Pediatrics and of Obstetrics/Gynecology, is responsible for the program's development and operation. Linda Friedman, PhD, is responsible for the database.

The computer data bank

The core of the Lactation Study Center program is a networked computer system offering physicians information on issues critical to the success of lactation and breastfeeding.

The bibliography data bank, which is constantly updated, provides immediate access to the latest published references on the subject by searching for an article's primary author, for any author, or for a word in the title, or by using the keyword code (the keyword categorizes papers by subject areas).

The Center can, for example, look up all papers in the collection discussing "anticonvulsant drugs," using a single keyword that will generate a comprehensive list.

The subject data bank has been divided into major category areas, each of which is summarized from thousands of articles from the medical literature.

The drug data bank is updated monthly and includes all the available information about the drug in question, including, if known, its oral availability, whether it appears in the milk, the half-life in maternal plasma and milk, peak time in the maternal plasma and milk, percent protein bound in plasma, percent of adult dose in milk, the maximum amount in a liter of milk, and the ratio of the concentration in milk to the concentration in the maternal plasma.

The biochemistry information can be accessed by the compound name and gives the amount of the compound in various milk fractions; its molecular weight; its solubility properties, including a discussion of the function of the compound in milk; variations related to diet and other factors; the source of the compound; and pertinent references in the literature.

The information on conditions of mother or infant can be identified by name. The information focuses on the effect the condition has on nursing and lactation and what compensatory actions are needed to facilitate the process.

The other categories are organized in outline form and the information is readily retrievable.

Each entry relating to the subject is regularly updated and includes clinically applicable comments and literature references. The presentation is geared for the professional.

How the data bank can help

When a call is made to the Lactation Study Center, the staff searches the data bank and quickly retrieves the information needed. Many inquiries can be answered immediately over the telephone. When that is not possible, a reply will be sent by return mail or by telecopier, if the need is urgent.

The services of the University of Rochester Medical Center's Lactation Study Center are available for a fee to cover costs.

INFORMATION ABOUT EXAMINATION AND CERTIFICATION OF LACTATION CONSULTANTS

Information regarding eligibility to sit the examination for lactation consultants may be obtained by contacting:

International Board of Lactation Consultant
    Examiners (IBLCE)
PO Box 2348
Falls Church, VA 22042-0348
(703) 560-7330
FAX: (703) 560-7332

ORGANIZATION OF LACTATION CONSULTANTS

International Lactation Consultant Association
4101 Lake Boone Trail
Raleigh, NC 26707-3201
(919) 787-5181

$\mathcal{L}$egislation regarding human milk

AVAILABILITY OF HUMAN MILK

State of New York*

An ACT to amend the public health law, in relation to the availability of human breast milk for infant consumption.

The People of the State of New York, represented in Senate and Assembly, do enact as follows:

Section 1. Legislative findings. The legislature hereby finds and declares that human breast milk, the preferred food for all infants, provides a superior, well tolerated nutritional source because of its unique components. It contains substances, lacking in other forms of infant nutrition, which help control infection and aid in preventing infant disease. For premature infants or those with a low birth weight or infants who are allergic to cow's milk and infant formulas, human breast milk is essential.

It shall be the declared policy of the state of

New York that any and all infants requiring human breast milk be assured access to sufficient quantities of wholesome human breast milk, donated by concerned lactating mothers on a continual and systematic basis. The availability of such a supply of human breast milk should be made known to the public so that health providers and families of infants with particular need for human breast milk will be aware of its accessibility.

§2. The public health law is amended by adding a new section twenty-five hundred five to read as follows:

§2505. Human breast milk; collection, storage, and distribution; general powers of the commissioner. The commissioner is hereby empowered to:

(a) adopt regulations and guidelines including, but not limited to donor standards, methods of collection, and standards for storage, and distribution of human breast milk;

(b) conduct educational activities to inform the public and health care providers of the availability of human breast milk for infants determined to require such milk and to inform potential donors of the opportunities for proper donation;

(c) establish rules and regulations to effectuate the provisions of this section.

§3. This act shall take effect immediately.

*From Office of Health Systems Management, Bureau of Standards Development, New York, State Department of Health, Empire State Plaza, Albany NY, 1984.

NEW YORK STATE CODE IN SUPPORT OF BREASTFEEDING (ADDED 1984)

Chapter V
Subchapter A
Article 2
Part 405
Hospitals—minimum standards
(Statutory authority: Public health law § 2803)
405.8 Maternal, child health and newborn services

(10)(i) The hospital, with the advice of the maternity staff, shall formulate a program of instruction and provide assistance for each maternity patient(s) in the fundamentals of (normal) infant care including infant feeding choice and techniques, post-pregnancy care and family planning.

(ii) The hospital shall provide instruction and assistance to each maternity patient who has chosen to breast-feed and shall provide information on the advantages and disadvantages of breast-feeding to women who are undecided as to the feeding method for their infants. As a minimum:

(a) the hospital shall designate at least one person who is thoroughly trained in breast-feeding physiology and management to be responsible for ensuring the implementation of an effective breast-feeding program; and

(b) policies and procedures shall be developed to assist the mother to breast-feed which shall include but not be limited to:

(1) prohibition of the application of standing orders for antilactation drugs;

(2) placement of the infant for breast-feeding immediately following delivery, unless contraindicated;

(3) restriction of the infant's supplemental feedings to those indicated by the medical condition of the infant or of the mother;

(4) provision for the infant to be fed on demand; and

(c) assurance that an educational program has been given as soon after admission as possible which shall include but not be limited to:

(1) the nutritional and physiological aspects of human milk;

(2) the normal process for establishing lactation, including care of breasts, common problems associated with breast-feeding and frequency of feeding;

(3) dietary requirements for breast-feeding;

(4) diseases and medication or other substances which may have an effect on breast-feeding;

(5) sanitary procedures to follow in collecting and storing human milk; and

(6) sources for advice and information available to the mother following discharge.

FLORIDA LEGISLATION— FEBRUARY 1993

House bill no. HB 231
Senate bill no. SB 472

SUBJECT: Encouraging breastfeeding and authorizing breastfeeding in public

1. EFFECT OF PROPOSED CHANGES/ COMMENTS:

This bill would be an endorsement of the importance of Florida infants being breastfed and protect a mother's right to breastfeed whenever and wherever she needs to.

Increasing breastfeeding rates is an international, national and state health priority. Florida has among the lowest breastfeeding rates in the nation. A perceived major barrier for many women to breastfeeding is a fear of embarrassment and harassment when breastfeeding in public. This bill would diminish those fears and make women more secure in their right to breastfeed. More Floridian mothers breastfeeding would lead to decreased infant mortality and morbidity rates. Increased rates of breastfeeding among WIC infants would lead to significant financial savings, due to reduction in illness and associated physician visits, outpatient treatment and hospitalization.

2. ECONOMIC IMPACT AND FISCAL NOTE: None

Florida House of Representatives—1993 CS/HB 231

A bill to be entitled

An act relating to breast feeding; encouraging breast feeding and authorizing breast feeding in public; amending ss. 800.02 and 800.03, F.S.; clarifying language and providing that breast feeding a baby does not violate prohibitions against unnatural and lascivious acts or exposure of sexual organs, and reenacting s. 933.18(7)(b) and (c), F.S., relating to search warrants, to incorporate said amendments in references thereto; amending s. 800.04, F.S.; clarifying language and providing that breast feeding a baby does not violate prohibitions against lewd, lascivious, or indecent conduct in the presence of a child; amending s. 847.001, F.S.; providing that breast feeding a baby does not violate prohibitions against obscenity, is not harmful to minors, and does not constitute unlawful nudity or sexual conduct, and reenacting s. 847.0133(1), F.S., relating to protection of minors, to incorporate said amendment in a reference thereto; providing an effective date.

WHEREAS, the Surgeon General of the United States recommends that babies from birth to 1 year of age be breast fed, unless medically contraindicated, in order to attain an optimal healthy start, and

WHEREAS, despite the Surgeon General's recommendation, statistics reveal a declining percentage of mothers who are choosing to breast feed their babies, and

WHEREAS, nearly half of all new mothers are now choosing formula over breast feeding before they even leave the hospital, only 20 percent are still breast feeding when their babies are 6 months old, and only 6 percent are still breast feeding when their babies are 1 year old, and

WHEREAS, breast milk offers better nutrition, immunity, and digestion, and may raise a baby's IQ, in addition to such other benefits as improved mother-baby bonding, and its encouragement has been established as a major goal of this decade by the World Health Organization and UNICEF, and

WHEREAS, the social constraints of modern society militate against the choice of breast feeding and lead new mothers with demanding time schedules to opt for formula feeding for reasons such as embarrassment and the fear of social ostracism or criminal prosecution, and

WHEREAS, the promotion of family values and infant health demand putting an end to the vicious cycle of embarrassment and ignorance that constricts women and men alike on the subject of breast feeding and represents hostility to mothers and babies in our culture based on archaic and outdated moral taboos, and

WHEREAS, any genuine promotion of family values should encourage public acceptance of this most basic act of nurture between mother and baby, and no mother should be made to feel incriminated or socially ostracized for breast feeding her baby, NOW, THEREFORE,

Be It Enacted by the Legislature of the State of Florida:

Section 1. The breast feeding of a baby is an important and basic act of nurture which must be encourages in the interests of maternal and child health and family values. A mother may breast feed her baby in any location, public or private, where the mother is otherwise authorized to be, irrespective of whether or not the nipple of the mother's breast is covered during or incidental to the breast feeding.

CODING: Additions are underlined.

Section 2. Section 800.02, Florida Statutes, is amended to read:

800.02 Unnatural and lascivious act.—A person who commits any unnatural and lascivious act with another person commits a misdemeanor of the second degree, punishable as provided in s. 775.082 or s. 775.083. A mother's breast-feeding of her baby does not under any circumstance violate this section.

Section 3. Section 800.03, Florida Statutes, is amended to read:

800.03 Exposure of sexual organs.—It is unlawful to expose or exhibit one's sexual organs in public or on the private premises of another, or so near thereto as to be seen from such private premises, in a vulgar or indecent manner, or to be naked in public except in any place provided or set apart for that purpose. Violation of this section is a misdemeanor of the first degree, punishable as provided in s. 775.082 or s. 775.083. A mother's breast feeding of her baby does not under any circumstance violate this section.

Section 4. For the purpose of incorporating the amendments to sections 800.02 and 800.03, Florida Statutes, in references thereto, section 933.18(7)(b) and (c), Florida Statues, are reenacted to read:

933.18 When warrant may be issued for search of private dwelling.—No search warrant shall issue under this chapter or under any other law of this state to search any private dwelling occupied as such unless:

(7) One or more of the following misdemeanor child abuse offenses is being committed there:

(b) Commission of an unnatural and lascivious act with a child, in violation of s. 800.02.

(c) Exposure of sexual organs to a child, in violation of s. 800.03.

If, during a search pursuant to a warrant issued under this section, a child is discovered and appears to be in imminent danger, the law enforcement officer conducting such search may remove the child from the private dwelling and take the child into protective custody pursuant to s. 415.506. The term "private dwelling" shall be construed to include the room or rooms used and occupied, not transiently but solely as a residence, in an apartment house, hotel, boardinghouse, or lodging house. No warrant shall be issued for the search of any private dwelling under any of the conditions hereinabove mentioned except on sworn proof by affidavit of some creditable witness that he has reason to believe that one of said conditions exists, which affidavit shall set forth the facts on which such reason for belief is based.

Section 5. Section 800.04, Florida Statutes, is amended to read:

800.04 Lewd, lascivious, or indecent assault or act upon or in presence of child.—A person who:

(1) Handles, fondles, or assaults any child under the age of 16 years in a lewd, lascivious, or indecent manner;

(2) Commits actual or simulated sexual intercourse, deviate sexual intercourse, sexual bestiality, masturbation, sadomasochistic abuse, actual lewd exhibition of the genitals, or any act or conduct which stimulates that sexual battery is being or will be committed upon any child under the age of 16 years or forces or entices the child to commit any such act;

(3) Commits an act defined as sexual battery under s. 794.011(1)(b) upon any child under the age of 16 years; or

(4) Knowingly commits any lewd or lascivious act in the presence of any child under the age of 16 years, without committing the crime of sexual battery, commits a felony of the second degree, punishable as provided in s. 775.082, s. 775.083, or s. 775.084. Neither the victim's lack of chastity nor the victim's consent is a defense to the crime proscribed by this section. A mother's breast feeding of her baby does not under any circumstance violate this section.

Section 6. Subsections (3), (5), (7), (11), and (13) of section 847.001, Florida Statutes, are amended to read:

847.001 Definitions.—When used in this chapter:

(3) "Harmful to minors" means that quality of any description, exhibition, presentation, or repre-

sentation, in whatever form, of nudity, sexual conduct, or sexual excitement when it:

(a) Predominantly appeals to the prurient, shameful, or morbid interest of minors;

(b) Is patently offensive to prevailing standards in the adult community as a whole with respect to what is suitable material for minors; and

(c) Taken as a whole, is without serious literary, artistic, political, or scientific value for minors.

A mother's breast feeding of her baby is not under any circumstance "harmful to minors."

(5) "Nudity" means the showing of the human male or female genitals, pubic area, or buttocks with less than a fully opaque covering; or the showing of the female breast with less than a fully opaque covering of any portion thereof below the top of the nipple; or the depiction of covered male genitals in a discernibly turgid state. A mother's breast feeding of her baby does not under any circumstance constitute "nudity," irrespective of whether or not the nipple is covered during or incidental to feeding.

(7) "Obscene" means the status of material which:

(a) The average person, applying contemporary community standards, would find, taken as a whole, appeals to the prurient interest;

(b) Depicts or describes, in a patently offensive way, sexual conduct as specifically defined herein; and

(c) Taken as a whole, lacks serious literary, artistic, political, or scientific value.

A mother's breast feeding of her baby is not under any circumstance "obscene."

(11) "Sexual conduct" means actual or simulated sexual intercourse, deviate sexual intercourse, sexual bestiality, masturbation, or sadomasochistic abuse; actual lewd exhibition of the genitals; actual physical contact with a person's clothed or unclothed genitals, pubic area, buttocks, or, if such person is a female, breast; or any act or conduct which constitutes sexual battery or simulates that sexual battery is being or will be committed. A mother's breast feeding of her baby does not under any circumstance constitute "sexual conduct."

$\mathscr{R}$esources for education and training

Breastfeeding: A Special Relationship
Eagle Video Productions
2201 Woodnell Drive
Raleigh, NC 27603

Breastfeeding: The Art of Mothering
Alive Productions, Ltd.
PO Box 72
Port Washington, NY 11050

Best Start: For All the Right Reasons
Other materials listed in the Best Start
Breastfeeding Promotion Catalog
Best Start, Inc.
Suite 308, 3500 E. Fletcher Avenue
Tampa, FL 33613

Breastfeeding Your Preterm Baby
Health Sciences Center for Educational Resources
Distribution Center, SB-56
University of Washington
Seattle, WA 98195
(206) 545-1186

Breastfeeding: Catalog of Products from
Projects Supported by the Bureau of
Maternal and Child Health and Resources
Development 1989
National Center for Education in Maternal and
    Child Health
Rosslyn, VA 22209
(703) 524-7802

Childbirth Graphics,
a division of WRS Group, Inc.
PO Box 21207
Waco, TX 76702-1207
(800) 299-3366

The Learning Curve
Weingart Design
4614 Prospect Ave. #421
Cleveland, OH 44103-4314
(800) 795-9295

Birth and Life Bookstores,
a division of Cascade Healthcare Products, Inc.
141 Commercial Street NE
Salem, OR 97301
(800) 443-9942

Vida Health Communications, Inc.
6 Bigelow Street, Cambridge, MA 02139
(617) 864-4334

Wellstart, Inc.
4062 First Avenue
San Diego, CA 92103
(619) 295-5192

$\mathcal{G}$lossary

acinus   The tube leading to the smallest lobule of a compound gland; it is characterized by a narrow lumen.

adipose tissue   *See* panniculus adiposus.

afferent   Conducting inward to, or toward, the center of an organ, gland, or other structure or area. Applies to sensory nerves, arteries, and lymph vessels.

alactogenesis   Familial puerperal alactogenesis is genetically transmitted isolated prolactin deficiency.

alveolus   A glandular acinus or terminal portion of the alveolar gland where milk is secreted and stored, 0.12 mm in diameter. From 10 to 100 alveoli, or tubulosaccular secretory units, make up a lobulus.

ampulla   Dilated portion of duct. *See* lactiferous sinus.

apocrine   A term descriptive of a gland cell that loses part of its protoplasmic substance.

Apt test   A test, named after its developer, performed on fresh blood to distinguish between adult and fetal hemoglobin. The blood is suspended in saline, and an equal amount of 10% NaOH is added and mixed; adult hemoglobin turns brown, and fetal hemoglobin remains red. A control of known adult blood should also be done.

arborization   Development of a branched appearance.

areola mammae   Areola. The pigmented area surrounding the papilla mammae, or nipple.

autophagic vacuole   Autophagosome. A membrane-bound body within a cell containing degenerating cell organelles.

BALT   Bronchus-associated immunocompetent lymphoid tissue, to which the mammary gland may act as an extension. *See* GALT and MALT.

basal lamina   The layer of material, 50- to 80-mm thick, that lies adjacent to the plasma membrane of the basal surfaces of epithelial cells. It contains collagen and certain carbohydrates. It is often called the *basement membrane.*

casein   A derivative of caseinogen. The fraction of milk protein that forms the tough curd.

colostrum   The first milk. It is a yellow, sticky fluid secreted during the first few days postpartum, which provides nutrition and protection against infectious disease. It contains more protein, less sugar, and much less fat than mature breast milk.

columnar secretory cell   A type of secretory cell in the shape of a hexagonal prism, which appears rectangular when sectioned across the long axis, the length being considerably greater than the width.

Coopers' ligaments   Triangularly shaped ligaments stretching between the mammary gland, the skin, the retinacula cutis, the pectineal ligament, and the chorda obliqua. These underlie the breasts.

corpus mammae   The mammary gland; breast mass after freeing breast from deep attachments and removal of skin, subcutaneous connective tissue, and fat.

creamatocrit   Measurement for estimating the fat content and therefore the caloric content of a milk sample. A microhematocrit tube is filled with milk (usually a mix of foremilk and hind milk) and spun in a microcentrifuge for 15 minutes. The layer of fat is measured as one measures a blood hematocrit.

cross-nursing   The breastfeeding by a lactating woman of a baby who is not her own, usually temporarily, in the role of a child care arrangement.

cuboidal secretory cell   A secretory cell whose height and breadth are of similar size.

cytokines   A generic term for nonantibody proteins that are part of the immune system, including interferon-γ, and interleukin-6.

cytosol   Cell fluid.

doula   An individual who surrounds, interacts with, and aids the mother at any time within the period that includes pregnancy, birth, and lactation; may be a relative, friend, or neighbor and is usually but not necessarily female. One who gives psychologic encouragement and physical assistance to a new mother.

efferent   Carrying impulses away from a nerve center.

ejection reflex   A reflex initiated by the suckling of the infant at the breast, which triggers the pituitary gland to release oxytocin into the bloodstream. The oxytocin causes the myoepithelial cells to contract and eject the milk from the collecting ductules. (Also called *let-down reflex* or *draught*).

engorgement   The swelling and distention of the breasts, usually in the early days of initiation of lactation, caused by vascular dilatation as well as the arrival of the early milk.

eosinophil   A granular leukocyte possessing large conspicuous granules in the cytoplasm and containing a bilobed nucleus.

foremilk   The first milk obtained at the onset of suckling or expression. Contains less fat than later milk of that feeding (i.e., the hind milk).

galactocele   A cystic tumor in the ducts of the breast that contains a milky fluid.

galactagogue   A material or action that stimulates the production of milk.

galactopoiesis   The development of milk in the mammary gland. The maintenance of established lactation.

galactorrhea   Abnormal or inappropriate lactation.

galactose   ($C_6H_{12}O_6$). A simple sugar that is a component of the disaccharide lactose, or milk sugar.

galactosemia   A congenital metabolic disorder in which there is an inability to metabolize galactose because of a deficiency of the enzyme galactose-I-phosphate uridyltransferase. It causes failure to thrive, hepatomegaly, and splenomegaly.

GALT   Gut-associated lymphoid tissue to which the mammary gland may act as an extension. *See* BALT and MALT.

gigantomastia   The excessive enlargement of the breast beyond physiologic needs during pregnancy and lactation.

Golgi apparatus   A specialized region of the cytoplasm, often close to the nucleus, that is composed of flattened cisternae, numerous vesicles, and some larger vacuoles. In secretory cells it is concerned with packaging the secretory product. It is also probably concerned with the secretion of polysaccharides in some cells, but its full range of functions has not yet been elucidated.

heterophagic vacuole   Heterophagosome. A membrane-bound body within a cell, containing ingested material.

hind milk   Milk obtained later during the nursing period, that is, the end of the feeding. This milk is usually high in fat and probably controls appetite.

homocystinuria   A rare inborn error of amino acid metabolism characterized by mental deficiency, epilepsy, dislocation of the lens, growth disturbance, thromboses, and defective hair growth.

hyperadenia   The existence of mammary tissue without nipples.

hypergalactia   The excessive, uncontrolled production of milk over and above the needs of a suckling infant.

hypermastia   The existence of accessory mammary glands.

hyperthelia   The existence of abundant, more or less developed, nipples without accompanying mammary tissue.

immunoglobulin   Protein fraction of globulin, which has been demonstrated to have immunologic properties. Immunoglobulins include IgA, IgG, and IgM—factors in breast milk that protect against infection.

induced lactation   Process by which a nonpuerperal female (or male) is stimulated to lactate.

lactiferous ducts   The main ducts of the mammary gland, which number from 15 to 30 and open onto the nipple. They carry milk to the nipple.

lactiferous sinuses   Dilatations on the lactiferous ducts at the base of the nipple.

Lactobacillus bifidus   Organism of the intestinal tract of breastfed infants.

lactocele   Cystic tumor of the breast caused by the dilatation and obstruction of a milk duct usually filled with milk.

lacto-engineering   The process of enhancing the nutrient value of human milk by adding nutrients obtained by drying and separating out specific nutrients such as protein from pooled human milk.

lactoferrin   An iron-binding protein of external secretions, including human milk. It inhibits the growth of iron-dependent microorganisms in the gut.

lactogenesis   Initiation of milk secretion.

let-down reflex   *See* ejection reflex.

ligand   A low-molecular-weight substance that binds trace elements loosely for ready availability (e.g., zinc ligands in human milk).

lobulus   A subunit of the parenchymal structure of the breast made up of 10 to 100 alveoli, or tubulosaccular secretory units. From 20 to 40 lobuli make up a lobus.

lobus   A subunit of the parenchymal structure of the breast made up of 20 to 40 lobuli. From 15 to 25 lobi are arranged like the spokes of a wheel with the nipple as the central point.

lymphocyte   A mature leukocyte derived through the intermediate stage of lymphoblast from the reticuloendothelium found in lymphatic tissue.

lyophilization   The process of rapidly freeze drying a fluid in a vacuum, which results in a solid.

MALT   Mucosal-associated lymphoid tissue, which includes gut, lung, mammary gland, salivary and lacrimal glands, and genital tract. There is traffic of cells between secretory sites. Immunization at one site may be an effective means of producing immunity at distant sites. *See* GALT and BALT.

mamilla   The nipple; any teatlike structure.

mammogenesis   Growth of the mammary gland.

mastalgia   Painful breasts.

mastitis   Inflammation of the breast, including cellulitis, and occasionally abscess formation.

matrescence   The state of becoming a mother or motherhood as a new event in an individual's life.

megaloblastic anemia   Defective red blood cell formation caused by megaloblastic hyperplasia of the marrow; there are often megaloblasts, or primitive nucleated red cells, in the peripheral blood.

merocrine   Pertaining to the type of secretion in which the active cell remains intact while forming and discharging the secretory product.

mesencephalon   The midbrain.

methylmalonic aciduria   The condition of the urine being acidic from an accumulation of methylmalonic acid caused by an inborn error of metabolism.

milk fever   A syndrome of fever and general malaise associated with early engorgement of the breasts or with sudden weaning from the breast.

mitogen   A substance capable of stimulating cells to enter mitosis.

Montgomery glands   Small prominences, sebaceous glands in the areola of the breast, which become more marked in pregnancy. They number 20 to 24 and secrete a fluid that lubricates the nipple area.

Morgagni's tubercle   Small sinuses into which the miniature ducts of the Montgomery glands open in the epidermis of the areola.

myoepithelial cell   An epithelial cell, usually lying around a glandular acinus, in which part of the cytoplasm has contractile properties, serving to empty the sinus of its secretion.

nonnutritive sucking   The act of suckling the breast with little or no secretion of milk. Infant may suckle when distressed or to be calmed or quieted.

nonpuerperal lactation   The production of milk in a woman who has not given birth.

nucleotides   Compounds derived from nucleic acid by hydrolysis and consisting of phosphoric acid combined with a sugar and a purine or pyrimidine derivative. The milk nucleotides are secreted from glandular epithelial cells.

opsonic   Belonging to or characterized by opsonin, a substance in mammalian blood having the power to render microorganisms and blood cells more easily absorbed by phagocytes.

oxytocin   An octapeptide synthesized in the cell bodies of neurons located mainly in the paraventricular nucleus and in smaller amounts in the supraoptic nucleus of the hypothalamus. Oxytocin stimulates the ejection reflex by stimulation of the myoepithelial cells in the mammary gland.

panniculus adiposus   Adipose tissue. The superficial fascia, which contains fatty pellicles.

papilla mammae   Mamilla. The nipple of the breast.

perinatal   Around birth. The time from conception through birth, delivery, lactation, and at least 28 days postpartum.

plasma cell   Cell derived from the B cell series, which manufactures and secretes antibodies.

prolactin   A hormone present in both male and female and at all ages. During pregnancy it stimulates and prepares the mammary alveolar epithelium for secretory activity. During lactation it stimulates synthesis and secretion of milk. At other ages and in the male it interacts with other steroids.

rachitic   Relating to, characterized by, or affected with rickets.

relactation   Process by which a woman who has given birth but did not initially breastfeed is stimulated to lactate (also applies to reinstituting lactation after it has been discontinued).

squamous epithelium   A sheet of flattened, scalelike epithelium adhering edge to edge.

stroma   The connective tissue basis or framework of an organ.

switch nursing   Putting the infant to one breast for a short time, usually 5 minutes, moving the infant to the other breast for 5 minutes, and then moving the infant back to the first side in an effort to improve milk production.

tail of Spence   The axillary tail of the breast.

transitional milk   The milk produced early in the postpartum period as the colostrum diminishes and the mature milk develops.

tubuloalveolar   Having both tubular and alveolar qualities.

tubulosaccular   Having both tubular and saccular character.

turgescence   The swelling up of a part. The unusual turgid feeling resulting from swelling with fluid.

whey protein   Protein remaining when the curds of casein have been removed. The mixture of proteins present is complex and includes β-lactoglobulin and α-lactalbumin and enzymes.

witch's milk   Product of neonatal galactorrhea caused by absorption of placental prolactin.

$\mathscr{I}$ndex

Page numbers in italics indicate illustrations, *t* indicates tables.